BIOMEDICAL & PHARMACEUTICAL SCIENCES with Patient Care Correlations

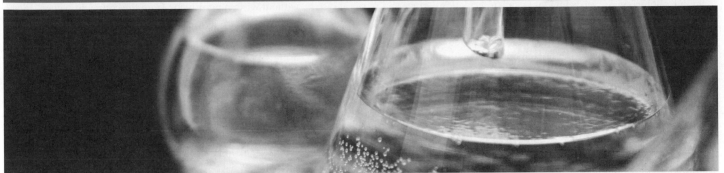

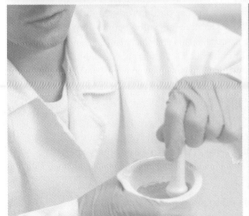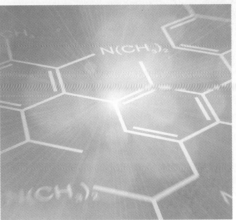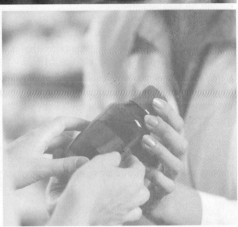

EDITED BY

REZA KARIMI, RPh, PhD

Professor
Associate Dean for Academic Affairs and Assessment
School of Pharmacy
Pacific University
Hillsboro, Oregon

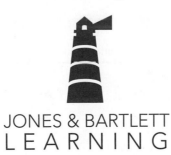

JONES & BARTLETT
LEARNING

World Headquarters
Jones & Bartlett Learning
5 Wall Street
Burlington, MA 01803
978-443-5000
info@jblearning.com
www.jblearning.com

Jones & Bartlett Learning books and products are available through most bookstores and online booksellers. To contact Jones & Bartlett Learning directly, call 800-832-0034, fax 978-443-8000, or visit our website, www.jblearning.com.

Substantial discounts on bulk quantities of Jones & Bartlett Learning publications are available to corporations, professional associations, and other qualified organizations. For details and specific discount information, contact the special sales department at Jones & Bartlett Learning via the above contact information or send an email to specialsales@jblearning.com.

Production Credits

Executive Publisher: William Brottmiller
Executive Editor: Rhonda Dearborn
Editorial Assistant: Sean Fabery
Production Editor: Jill Morton
Marketing Manager: Grace Richards
Composition: Laserwords Private Limited, Chennai, India
Cover Design: Kristin Parker

Photo Research and Permissions Coordinator: Amy Rathburn
Cover and Title Page Images: Several glass beakers, © 26kot/ShutterStock, Inc;
 A pharmacist handing medicine, © Kzenon/ShutterStock, Inc.;
 An abstract chemical formula, © Viktoriya/ShutterStock, Inc.;
 A scientist uses a mortar, © l i g h t p o e t/ShutterStock, Inc.
Printing and Binding: Edwards Brothers Malloy
Cover Printing: Edwards Brothers Malloy

Library of Congress Cataloging-in-Publication Data
Karimi, Reza, author.
 Biomedical and pharmaceutical sciences with patient care correlations / edited by Reza Karimi.
  p. ; cm.
 Includes bibliographical references and index.
 ISBN 978-1-4496-2108-7 – ISBN 1-4496-2108-2
 I. Title.
 [DNLM: 1. Biochemical Phenomena–drug effects. 2. Biopharmaceutics–methods. 3. Physicochemical Processes–drug effects. QU 34]
 RM301.5
 615.7–dc23
                                                                        2013027712
6048

Printed in the United States of America
18 17 16 15 14   10 9 8 7 6 5 4 3 2 1

CONTENTS

I dedicate this book to my son, Kayhan, and his generation for keeping curiosity, motivation, and learning alive.

☒ ch: 2,3,4, 6,7,8,9, 11,12,14

total = 10 ch
5 week

2ch/week

Chapter 2   Introduction to Cell Biology 73

Reza Karimi

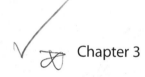

Chapter 4   Introduction to Immunology 205

Reza Karimi and Ian C. Doyle

ACKNOWLEDGEMENTS

First and foremost, I would like to express my heartfelt appreciation to my wife, Fariba, who patiently and compassionately supported me in writing this book. Her tireless discussions about the content and her intelligent advice based on her own pharmacy practice experiences significantly contributed to the quality of this text. Simply put, without her wisdom, patience, intuition, and love, writing this would have been impossible.

I would like to also express my deepest appreciation to my son, Kayhan, who patiently understood the time it took to write this. Kayhan is the motivation and reason for writing this book. His curiosity about the sciences and his desire to learn served as the inspiration and a compass for me to complete this.

I am indebted to my colleagues, Drs. Ian Doyle, Fawzy Elbarbry, Jeffery Fortner, Seher Khan, Pauline Low, Sigrid Roberts, Jennifer Rosselli, Fariba Safaiyan, Susan Stein, Miranda Wilhelm, and Professor Kris Marcus, who contributed to this text. Their experience, knowledge, and commitment to student learning have turned this into a genuine learning resource for pharmacy students.

I would also like to express my deepest gratitude to my school's administration and my faculty and staff colleagues who supported me during the last three and a half years in which I was writing this. I also gratefully acknowledge our pharmacy students at Pacific University for their thirst for exploration and interest in learning, which assisted me in keeping student learning and different learning styles in mind during the writing of this text.

Finally, I would like to express my sincere appreciation for the professional staff at Jones & Bartlett Learning who assisted me in improving the quality of this book. Particularly, I thank Jill Morton for her excellent professional editing assistance and Teresa Reilly for patiently providing guidance and direction for the organization of this book.

INTRODUCTION

As of November 2013, there were 130 colleges and schools of pharmacy with accreditation status in the United States. The Accreditation Council for Pharmacy Education (ACPE) is the only national accreditation agency that oversees pharmacy education in the United States. The curriculum of the doctor of pharmacy degree (PharmD) is offered in different paths, with two employed most frequently. The first path has a three-year curriculum with almost no summer break between two consecutive academic years. In this path the first two years' curricula are mostly didactic and the third year's curriculum is mostly experiential. The second path has a four-year curriculum where students have a break in summer between any two consecutive academic years. Regardless of the paths and curriculum, the ACPE requires that colleges and schools of pharmacy prepare graduates with a comprehensive foundation in four curricular subjects: biomedical; pharmaceutical; clinical; and social, behavioral, and administrative sciences. In addition, at least 5% of the curricular length must be assigned to deliver introductory pharmacy practice experiences (IPPE) and at least 25% of the curricular length must be assigned to deliver advanced pharmacy practice experiences (APPE). Furthermore, the ACPE requires colleges and schools of pharmacy to include in their prerequisite courses at least two years of academic study that include basic sciences, behavioral sciences, social sciences, and communication skills.

In my many years of teaching pharmacy students, I have experienced that students enter the study of pharmacy with a vast variety of prerequisite educations and competencies. There are two major reasons for such a variation. First, students have completed their prerequisite courses at different times since their graduation from their high schools/colleges and, second, students have completed their prerequisite courses at different universities/colleges with different standards of student learning. In addition, I have observed that many first year pharmacy students struggle in different areas of biomedical and pharmaceutical sciences and there is no consistent knowledge level among them. The lack of a consistent knowledge base among students often frustrates faculty, and sometimes student peers as well, as the pace of lecture delivery slows down to explain some of the material from prerequisite courses that students should have learned in the past. This process may lead to instructors being unable to deliver the intended lecture objectives in a timely manner and may produce gaps in the curriculum.

Student learning is the core mission of all colleges and schools of pharmacy in the United States. The landscape of student learning is evolving. Classroom teaching and learning is no longer the norm. Providing a conductive environment that supports active learning and critical-thinking are areas that many faculty strive to achieve. There is growing evidence that integration of didactic learning with experiential experiences assist students in becoming qualified contemporary pharmacists. In order to introduce pharmacy students to biomedical and pharmaceutical sciences and integrate their didactic learning with patient care, I decided to develop *Biomedical and Pharmaceutical Sciences with Patient Care Correlations* to introduce students to the majority of biomedical and pharmaceutical sciences. In addition, in order to provide clinical applications to enhance student learning, many clinical cases—called Learning Bridge assignments in the text—have been generated and are embedded within each chapter. The learning bridge concept was first described in the *American Journal of Pharmaceutical Education* in 2009 (volume 74, issue 3, 2010), which has subsequently proven to be a productive tool for integrating didactic learning with experiential experiences.

It is imperative to address the audience for this book and explain why it is useful for pharmacy students to study this book. First, the audience for this book is first year pharmacy students who ideally have access to this book a few months prior to their matriculation at a PharmD program. This book is written in such a way that many figures, tables, and topics are explained in a simple way that pharmacy students can study on their own. This process will allow students to enter their PharmD programs with a high level of preparation and strong knowledge base in biomedical and pharmaceutical sciences. Second, this book can be offered to preceptors who precept pharmacy students at their experiential sites (pharmacies, clinics, hospitals, etc.). This book can help preceptors familiarize themselves with the pharmacy curriculum and may assist preceptors in invigorating their knowledge of biomedical and pharmaceutical sciences. Third, the goal for this book was not to replace the core pharmacy books. In other words, this book should be used shoulder-to-shoulder with other core books when students are in their first year of study at a PharmD program. For instance, while a faculty member is teaching a complicated topic, he/she can refer to this book in advance and ask students to study a specific topic so that the delivery of the complicated topic in classroom is facilitated.

This book delivers 16 biomedical and pharmaceutical sciences chapters and, as a result, it can be used by faculty in different disciplines. This will be of particular interest for many courses that occur during the first year (for a 3-year curriculum) and/or second year (for a 4-year curriculum) of study in PharmD programs.

This book begins with building blocks of molecules and biological chemistry that pharmacy students will encounter throughout their course of study. This chapter is followed by cell biology and important concepts in cell functions and structure, and the function of biomolecules. The third chapter discusses the basic elements of microbiology and understanding infectious diseases along with the most common existing bacterial, fungal, parasites, and viral microorganisms. The microbiology chapter is followed by a basic introduction to immunology by introducing students to innate and adaptive immunities and various types of hypersensitivities. The introduction to biochemistry chapter begins with basic thermodynamics and metabolism of carbohydrates, proteins, and fatty acids. The important physiological roles that enzymes play in biochemistry are also emphasized in the introduction to biochemistry chapter.

The introduction to pharmacodynamics chapter covers the dynamics and functions of the major signal transduction systems, and the important roles of dose–response relationships and the factors that affect pharmacologic responses. This chapter is followed by an introduction to medicinal chemistry, which describes major metabolic phases and the roles CYP450 isozymes play in drug-drug or drug-food interactions. In addition, the principles behind the structure and function of drugs are addressed in this chapter. The introduction to pharmaceutics delivers basic physical pharmacy, reaction orders, and different dosage forms. This chapter is followed by an introduction to pharmacokinetics that introduces students to basic concepts in drug absorption, distribution, metabolism, and elimination. In addition, the importance and application of bioavailability, the volume of distribution, clearance, and half-life in pharmacokinetics are addressed in the introduction to pharmacokinetics chapter.

The introduction to pharmacology and pathophysiology chapter introduces students to the sympathetic and parasympathetic nervous systems and therapeutic agents that act through the autonomic nervous system. The pharmacology and pathophysiology associated with neurodegenerative diseases, pain, cardiovascular disease, and the respiratory and endocrine systems are addressed in this chapter as well. This chapter is followed by an introduction to toxicology, where various factors that influence drug toxicity are discussed and which provides a list of medications that are most frequently implicated in organ toxicity. The introduction to pharmacogenomics describes common types of genetic variation and how such variation influences pharmacokinetic and pharmacodynamics properties of medications.

The introduction to pharmacognosy brings to light the important roles plants play in the development and production of medications and discusses natural products that are available for common health conditions. In addition, information about safety concerns related to different natural products is discussed in this chapter. This chapter is followed by the introduction to nutrients that discusses the important roles carbohydrates, proteins, and fats play in generating daily calorie intake and the essential roles macronutrients and micronutrients play in maintaining homeostasis. The introduction to calculation introduces students to fundamental calculation skills and facilitates student learning in effectively performing calculations when preparing, dispensing, or recommending medications. The last chapter of this book discusses the important roles drug information, literature evaluation, and biostatistics play in effectively providing evidence-based pharmacotherapy to produce an optimal therapeutic outcome in a patient-care setting.

The following messages may be useful to students, faculty, and preceptors when considering using this book.

- **A message to students:** Study this book at home prior to beginning your first year and then continuously study this book to support and strengthen what you learn during the first and second years of your PharmD program.

- **A message to faculty:** Ask your students to study a pertinent chapter/topic prior to your course in order to prepare students for more complex topics within your course. In addition, direct students to relevant topics in the book during your course to support and strengthen student learning. This entire process will promote student learning and assist you in focusing your limited teaching time on the delivery of more complicated topics. A Test Bank has been provided for instructor support.

- **A message to preceptors:** Read each chapter to invigorate your knowledge base of biomedical and pharmaceutical sciences. Utilize the learning bridge assignments and ask your students to answer the corresponding questions. There is evidence-based data (please see *American Journal of Pharmaceutical Education,* volume 74, issue 3, 2010 and volume 75, issue 3, 2011) indicating that the learning bridge assignments can promote student learning and generate a productive environment for curricular discussions during IPPEs.

Reza Karimi, RPh, PhD

CONTRIBUTORS

Ian C. Doyle, PharmD, BCPS
Assistant Professor
Pacific University
School of Pharmacy
Hillsboro, OR

Fawzy Elbarbry, PhD, RPh
Associate Professor
Pacific University
School of Pharmacy
Hillsboro, OR

Jeffery Fortner, PharmD, RPh
Assistant Professor
Pacific University
School of Pharmacy
Hillsboro, OR

Seher Khan, PhD
Associate Professor
Lake Erie College of Osteopathic Medicine
School of Pharmacy
Erie, PA

Pauline Ann Low, PharmD
Associate Professor
Pacific University
School of Pharmacy
Hillsboro, OR

Kristine B. Marcus, RPh, BCPS, BS Pharm
Associate Professor
Pacific University
School of Pharmacy
Hillsboro, OR

Sigrid Roberts, PhD
Associate Professor
Pacific University
School of Pharmacy
Hillsboro, OR

Jennifer L. Rosselli, PharmD, BCPS, BCACP
Clinical Assistant Professor
Southern Illinois University, Edwardsville
School of Pharmacy
Edwardsville, IL

Fariba Safaiyan, RPh, PhD
Safeway Pharmacy
Portland, OR

Susan M. Stein, DHEd, MS, BS Pharm, RPh
Professor
Pacific University
School of Pharmacy
Hillsboro, OR

Miranda Wilhelm, PharmD
Clinical Assistant Professor
Southern Illinois University, Edwardsville
Edwardsville School of Pharmacy
Edwardsville, IL

REVIEWERS

Dean L. Arneson, PharmD, PhD
Dean
Concordia University, Wisconsin
Mequon, WI

Duc P. Do, PhD
Assistant Professor of Pharmaceutical
Sciences
Chicago State University
College of Pharmacy
Chicago, IL

Abir El-Alfy, PhD
Assistant Professor
Chicago State University
College of Pharmacy
Chicago, IL

Diana Isaacs, PharmD, BCPS
Clinical Assistant Professor
Chicago State University
Chicago, IL

Marketa Marvanova, PharmD, CGP, PhD
Associate Professor of Pharmacy Practice
Chicago State University
College of Pharmacy
Chicago, IL

Syed A. A. Rizvi, MSc, MS, MBA, PhD (Chemistry), PhD (Pharmaceutics)
Professor
Nova Southeastern University
Fort Lauderdale, FL

Rebecca Miller Spivey, PharmD, MBA
Assistant Professor of Pharmacy Practice
Appalachian College of Pharmacy
Oakwood, VA

Hieu T. Tran, PharmD
Professor
Sullivan University
College of Pharmacy
Louisville, KY

Introduction to Biological Chemistry

Reza Karimi

CHAPTER OUTLINE

1. Learn about the basic chemistry related to atoms and molecules. Understand the roles of orbitals and lone-pair electrons in a few common atoms (e.g., N, F, C, O) and comprehend nucleophilic/electrophilic attacks and their impact on oxidation, reduction, addition, and substitution reactions.

2. List and explain the importance of medicinal functional groups that commonly are found in drug molecules and appreciate the important roles that drug structures play in pharmaceutical sciences.

3. Understand basic concepts in acid–base theory and their roles in the structures of drug molecules.

4. Learn about salt formation, ionization, and water solubility of drug molecules, and explain the role of medicinal functional groups in ionization, salt formation, salt hydrolysis, and water solubility of drug molecules.

5. Implement a series of Learning Bridge assignments at your experiential sites to bridge your didactic learning with your experiential experiences.

OBJECTIVES

1. **Brønsted-Lowry acid–base:** definition used to express the acidic or basic properties of acids and bases.

2. **Buffer:** a mixture of an acid and its conjugate base in a solution that causes the solution to resist a pH change.

3. **Compound:** a combination of two or more substances, ingredients, or elements. While the majority of drugs on the market are compounds, not all compounds are drugs.

4. **Conjugate acid:** a base that has gained a proton.

5. **Conjugate base:** an acid that has lost its proton.

6. **Covalence:** the number of covalent bonds present.

7. **Covalent bonding:** bonding in which atoms in a molecule share electrons to fill their outermost shells.

8. **Electrolyte:** a compound that, when dissolved in a solvent (usually water), conducts electricity because it dissociates into ions (charged species).

9. **Electrophile:** an "electron-loving" species.

10. **Functional group:** a group of atoms attached to a molecule that plays an important role in the structure and function of that molecule.

11. **Henderson-Hasselbalch equation:** an equation that is useful when preparing buffer solutions in biochemistry and pharmaceutics. This equation also can be used to estimate the ionization of weakly acidic or basic drugs.

12. **IUPAC:** International Union of Pure and Applied Chemistry; the organization that oversees the rules and guidelines in regard to chemical nomenclature in chemical sciences and makes recommendations on how the nomenclature should be applied.

(continues)

13. **Lone-pair electrons:** pairs of electrons in the valence shell that are not involved in a bond.

14. **Noncovalent bonds:** weak interactions between ions, atoms, and molecules.

15. **Nucleophile:** a "nucleus-loving" species. Its electrons can be used to form a covalent bond with a positively charged molecule.

16. **Octet rule:** atoms have a tendency to lose, gain, or share electrons to reach the same number of electrons as the noble gases (i.e., they try to have eight electrons in their outermost valence shell).

17. **Orbital:** a region in space around the nucleus in which an electron is most likely to be found at any given time.

18. **Oxidation:** a chemical process in which an atom or a molecule loses one or two electrons.

19. **Physical properties:** characteristics of an atom or a molecule that are observed without any chemical change of the atom or molecule.

20. **Reduction:** a chemical process in which an atom or a molecule gains one or two electrons.

21. **Salt hydrolysis:** the reaction of the ions of a salt with water.

22. **Shell:** the grouping of electrons with similar energy into an energy level.

23. **Titration:** an analytical procedure in which a solution (often a base) with known volume and known concentration is added to another solution (an acid) with known volume but unknown concentration. The goal often is to calculate the unknown concentration.

24. **Valence electrons:** the electrons in the outermost shell that determine the chemical properties of the elements.

Introduction

"Introduction to biological chemistry" is an integrated topic that combines the organic chemistry of atoms and molecules with the biological roles that molecules play in our everyday lives. Understanding the science of chemistry begins with atoms, whereas understanding the science of biology begins with molecules. By definition, the smallest object that has a chemical identity is an atom (an element is an atom that has a known atomic number and specific placement in the periodic table). In the essential paths where atoms become molecules and where molecules display their biological and physiological characteristics, the roles of biological chemistry become perceptible. For this reason, it is important not only to appreciate the nature and characteristics of atoms, but also to understand how molecules are built and how the bonds that maintain the integrity of molecules are formed.

Medicinal functional groups are the cornerstone of biological chemistry. Pharmacy students need to fully understand the scope of medicinal functional groups and the key roles they play in pharmaceutical sciences. An understanding of medicinal functional groups is the first instrumental step in comprehending the pharmaceutical topics that will be discussed in this book. The role of medicinal functional groups in pharmacy education remains critical. Indeed, it is these medicinal functional groups that can assist pharmacy students in appreciating the roles that acids and bases play in ionization, salt formation, salt hydrolysis, and water solubility of drug molecules. Similarly, it is the medicinal functional groups that can assist students in predicting which biological role a compound might play. Therefore, learning medicinal functional groups assists students in building a strong foundation to comprehend absorption, distribution, metabolism, and elimination of drug molecules.

This chapter seeks to apply the science of organic chemistry to biological chemistry by addressing important and relevant points without overwhelming students with chemical reactions or detailed biological pathways.

Backbones of Molecules

Chemistry

Chemistry is a science that describes how atoms and molecules react with each other to produce new molecules with unique properties that are different from those of their parent atoms or molecules. While the atoms may be rearranged and redistributed to form new molecules, the chemical nature of the atoms remains the same. For instance, one molecule of acetic acid can be mixed with one molecule of salicylic acid to form acetylsalicylic acid (aspirin). The nature of the oxygen, carbon, and hydrogen atoms remains the same, but the new molecule (aspirin) has different physical and chemical properties than either acetic acid or salicylic acid (**Figure 1.1**).

Physical and Chemical Properties

Physical properties refer to when an atom or a molecule is observed without any chemical change of the substance. For instance, boiling point, melting point, color, and odor are physical properties. Practical examples are when aspirin melts at 143 °C, acetic acid melts at 16.5 °C, and salicylic acid melts at 158 °C. On the other hand, chemical properties are characteristics of an atom or a molecule that can be observed by chemical change of the atom or molecule. For example, the fact that aspirin undergoes hydrolysis is a chemical property that aspirin has.

Compound and Element

Any pure material that can be broken down into simpler substances by a chemical means (but not by a physical means) is a compound. For example, acetylsalicylic acid is a compound that upon hydrolysis (chemical means) is broken into acetic acid and salicylic acid (see the reverse reaction in Figure 1.1). In contrast, a pure substance that cannot be broken down chemically into simpler substances is an element, like Na, C, N, or O.

An atom is the smallest particle of an element that can exist and still retain the chemical properties of that element. An atom consists of (1) electrons (negative electrical charges), found outside the nucleus, and (2) a nucleus that comprises protons (positive electrical charges) and neutrons (no electrical charge) (**Figure 1.2**).

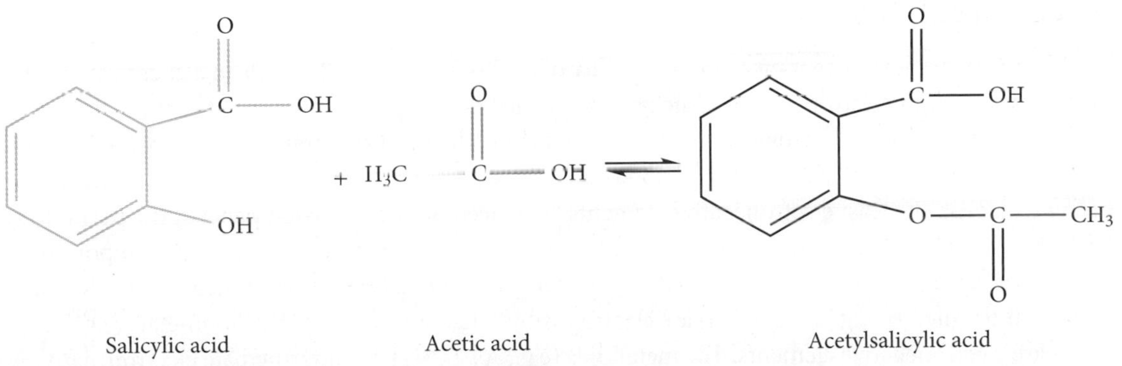

Salicylic acid   Acetic acid   Acetylsalicylic acid

Figure 1.1 Acetic acid (reactant) in a reaction with another reactant, salicylic acid, forms acetylsalicylic acid (product), which has different chemical and physical properties than the two reactants.

The Periodic Table

The order of elements in the periodic table is based on atomic number, which is the same as the number of protons. For instance, while carbon (C) has atomic number 6 (and 6 protons), nitrogen (N) has atomic number 7 (and 7 protons). Given that the numbers of electrons and protons are the same for each element, C has 6 electrons and N has 7 electrons. The periodic table (**Figure 1.3**) can be divided into four sections:

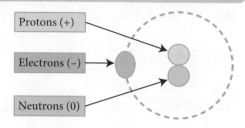

Figure 1.2 An atom with its constituents.

1. Metals: Elements (e.g., Fe, Mg, Ni) are shiny and can conduct electricity.

2. Nonmetals: Nonmetal elements (e.g., C, N, O) have a tendency to gain electrons and become negative ions. They are not shiny and cannot conduct electricity.

3. Metalloids: Metalloids or semimetals (e.g., As, B, Si) have both metallic and nonmetallic properties.

4. Noble gases: Noble gases (e.g., Ne, He, Rn) have a tendency not to combine with any other atoms. As will be discussed later, these elements have a complete set of valence electrons (see octet rule discussed later in this chapter).

Horizontal direction across the periodic table indicates elements with the same valence shells; that is, all of these elements have their valence electrons in the same energy level. For instance, K and Ca have their valence electrons in the same energy level (in this case, in the fourth shell). Vertical direction down the periodic table indicates elements with the same number of electrons in their valence shells. For instance, F and Cl have the same number of electrons in their valence shells.

The atomic number is equal to the number of protons in the nucleus of an atom. Since an atom is electrically neutral, it indicates that the number of protons and electrons must be equal in an atom (so that + and – charges cancel each other and give no net charge). With this definition, one important piece of information comes into view: The atomic number also represents the number of electrons. For instance, the atomic number for carbon is 6 (see the periodic table in Figure 1.3), which means it has 6 protons and 6 electrons. Neutrons have no electrical charges, so their number in an atom is not necessarily the same as the number of protons or electrons. Except for hydrogen atoms, all atoms have protons and neutrons in their nuclei.

The elements in the periodic table are organized into periods and groups. Specifically, there are 7 horizontal rows (periods) and 18 vertical columns (groups). The elements in each group have similar chemical properties. For instance, carbon (C) and silicon (Si) have the same chemical properties.

Electronegativity

The electronegativity concept measures the ability of an atom to attract electrons in a chemical bond. Elements with high electronegativity (such as nonmetals) have a greater ability to attract electrons than elements with low electronegativity (such as metals). The most electronegative elements are found on the upper-right panel of the periodic table (N, O, F, and Cl); they readily accept electrons to become anions. The least electronegative elements are placed on the lower-left panel of the periodic table (Na, K, Rb, Cs, Ba, Fr, and Ra); they readily donate electrons to become cations. A compound such as sodium chloride (NaCl) is formed between electropositive Na and electronegative Cl. Keep in mind that the metals (e.g., Fe, Mg, Ni) are electropositive elements, whereas the nonmetals (e.g., C, N, O) are electronegative elements. The metalloids (e.g., As, B, Si) have intermediate electronegativities. As a rule of thumb, electronegativity increases as you go horizontally from left to right across the periodic table and decreases as you go vertically down the periodic table.

Legend:
- Element — hydrogen
- Atomic Number — 1
- Symbol — H
- *Atomic Mass — 1.01

Metals / Metalloids / Nonmetals

1 IA	2 IIA	3 IIIB	4 IVB	5 VB	6 VIB	7 VIIB	8 VIII	9 VIII	10 VIII	11 IB	12 IIB	13 IIIA	14 IVA	15 VA	16 VIA	17 VIIA	18 VIIIA
hydrogen 1 **H** 1.01																	helium 2 **He** 4.00
lithium 3 **Li** 6.94	beryllium 4 **Be** 9.01											boron 5 **B** 10.81	carbon 6 **C** 12.01	nitrogen 7 **N** 14.01	oxygen 8 **O** 16.00	fluorine 9 **F** 19.00	neon 10 **Ne** 20.18
sodium 11 **Na** 22.99	magnesium 12 **Mg** 24.31											aluminum 13 **Al** 26.98	silicon 14 **Si** 28.09	phosphorus 15 **P** 30.97	sulfur 16 **S** 32.07	chlorine 17 **Cl** 35.45	argon 18 **Ar** 39.95
potassium 19 **K** 39.10	calcium 20 **Ca** 40.08	scandium 21 **Sc** 44.96	titanium 22 **Ti** 47.88	vanadium 23 **V** 50.94	chromium 24 **Cr** 52.00	manganese 25 **Mn** 54.94	iron 26 **Fe** 55.85	cobalt 27 **Co** 58.93	nickel 28 **Ni** 58.69	copper 29 **Cu** 63.55	zinc 30 **Zn** 65.39	gallium 31 **Ga** 69.72	germanium 32 **Ge** 72.61	arsenic 33 **As** 74.92	selenium 34 **Se** 78.96	bromine 35 **Br** 79.90	krypton 36 **Kr** 83.80
rubidium 37 **Rb** 85.47	strontium 38 **Sr** 87.62	yttrium 39 **Y** 88.91	zirconium 40 **Zr** 91.22	niobium 41 **Nb** 92.91	molybdenum 42 **Mo** 95.94	technetium 43 **Tc** (99)	ruthenium 44 **Ru** 101.07	rhodium 45 **Rh** 102.91	palladium 46 **Pd** 106.42	silver 47 **Ag** 107.87	cadmium 48 **Cd** 112.41	indium 49 **In** 114.82	tin 50 **Sn** 118.71	antimony 51 **Sb** 121.75	tellurium 52 **Te** 127.60	iodine 53 **I** 126.90	xenon 54 **Xe** 131.29
cesium 55 **Cs** 132.91	barium 56 **Ba** 137.33	lanthanum 57 **La** 138.91	hafnium 72 **Hf** 178.49	tantalum 73 **Ta** 180.95	tungsten 74 **W** 183.85	rhenium 75 **Re** 186.21	osmium 76 **Os** 190.2	iridium 77 **Ir** 192.22	platinum 78 **Pt** 195.08	gold 79 **Au** 196.97	mercury 80 **Hg** 200.59	thallium 81 **Tl** 204.38	lead 82 **Pb** 207.2	bismuth 83 **Bi** 208.98	polonium 84 **Po** (209)	astatine 85 **At** (210)	radon 86 **Rn** (222)
francium 87 **Fr** (223)	radium 88 **Ra** (226)	actinium 89 **Ac** (227)	rutherfordium 104 **Rf** (261)	dubnium 105 **Db** (262)	seaborgium 106 **Sg** (263)	bohrium 107 **Bh** (262)	hassium 108 **Hs** (265)	meitnerium 109 **Mt** (266)	ununnilium 110 **Uun** (269)	unununium 111 **Uuu** (272)	ununbium 112 **Uub** (277)						

Lanthanide Series

cerium 58 **Ce** 140.12	praseodymium 59 **Pr** 140.91	neodymium 60 **Nd** 144.24	promethium 61 **Pm** (147)	samarium 62 **Sm** 150.36	europium 63 **Eu** 151.97	gadolinium 64 **Gd** 157.25	terbium 65 **Tb** 158.93	dysprosium 66 **Dy** 162.50	holmium 67 **Ho** 164.93	erbium 68 **Er** 167.26	thulium 69 **Tm** 168.93	ytterbium 70 **Yb** 173.04	lutetium 71 **Lu** 174.97

Actinide Series

thorium 90 **Th** 232.04	protactinium 91 **Pa** (231)	uranium 92 **U** 238.03	neptunium 93 **Np** (237)	plutonium 94 **Pu** (244)	americium 95 **Am** (243)	curium 96 **Cm** (247)	berkelium 97 **Bk** (247)	californium 98 **Cf** (251)	einsteinium 99 **Es** (252)	fermium 100 **Fm** (257)	mendelevium 101 **Md** (258)	nobelium 102 **No** (259)	lawrencium 103 **Lr** (260)

*Note: For radioactive elements, the mass number of an important isotope is shown in parenthesis; for thorium and uranium, the atomic mass of the naturally occurring radioisotopes is given.

Figure 1.3　Elements of the periodic table with their symbols and atomic number and weight

What happens if the atoms in a molecule have the same electronegativity? This is the case when two atoms of the same element combine (as in H_2 or Cl_2). Because both Cl atoms have the same electronegativity, both have the same ability to attract the bonding pair of electrons. Electronegativity plays an important role in determining whether a bond is covalent, polar, or ionic (see the discussion of chemical bonds later in this chapter).

The Chemistry of Carbon

The chemistry of carbon compounds is called organic chemistry, and the element carbon is the cornerstone of organic chemistry. The interesting question you might ask is why only carbon, out of the 118 known elements, is the heart of organic chemistry? The answer is simple. If you look at the periodic table, you will find carbon in group 4A (or IVA) (whose members have four valence electrons). In addition, due to its ability to form four hybrid orbitals (see the next section), the carbon atom has the ability to form four strong covalent bonds. Carbon atoms can also react with each other to form long chains of molecules, a phenomenon that is critical in building macromolecules, such as fatty acids, carbohydrates, and nucleic acids (discussed later in this book). Other elements with four valence electrons (e.g., silicon) did not evolve to form macromolecules such as DNA or proteins for the following reasons:

1. Si is larger than the carbon atom and has a lower electronegativity than carbon.

2. When Si reacts with four hydrogen atoms, it forms a silane molecule (SiH_4) that is similar to methane (CH_4). Silane, however, is a very reactive molecule—upon reacting with oxygen (from the air), it explodes immediately. In contrast, methane is a gas that does not explode when it reacts with oxygen.

3. During the oxidation of carbohydrates, the human body produces carbon dioxide (CO_2), a molecule that is readily removed from the lungs by exhalation. When Si is oxidized, it becomes a solid—SiO_2 (silica)—which obviously makes it difficult to exhale from the lungs.

4. Silicon-based molecules are unstable. For example, the largest silicon molecule that has been observed by scientists has only six silicon atoms. This short-length molecule could not contribute to or support the structure of DNA and proteins that have long chains of carbons.

Let's go through some basic concepts in organic chemistry that you will encounter many times throughout this chapter (and even this book):

1. Hybrid orbitals
2. Oxidation–reduction reactions
3. Nucleophiles and electrophiles
4. Chemical bonds
5. Resonance structures

Hybrid Orbitals

Electrons that have similar energy are clustered in an energy level called a shell. The maximum number of electrons in each shell is indicated by the formula $2n^2$, where n is the number of the energy level. For instance, the maximum number of electrons in shell 2 will be 8 and the maximum number in shell 3 will be 18 (**Figure 1.4**).

An orbital is a region in a space around the nucleus where an electron is most likely to be found at any given time. Each orbital can hold a maximum of two electrons with opposite spins. In each shell, there are different types of orbitals (except in shell 1). In shell 1, there is one orbital called *s*; in shell 2, there are one *s* orbital and three *p* orbitals; and so on (**Table 1.1**).

Table 1.1 The Number of Orbitals in an Atom

Shell Number	1	2	3	4
Orbital's name	s	s, p	s, p, d	s, p, d, f
Number of orbitals	1	1, 3	1, 3, 5	1, 3, 5, 7

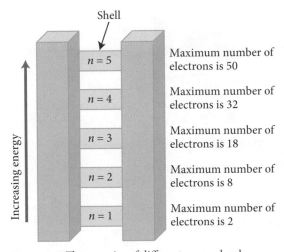

Figure 1.4 The capacity of different energy levels (shells) that can be occupied by electrons.

Adapted from Timberlake KC. Organic and biological chemistry: structures of life. San Francisco: Benjamin Cummings; 2001.

The distribution of electrons among the shells in an orbital diagram (**Figure 1.5**) follows a logic pattern. For example, nitrogen (N) atom has seven electrons (see the arrows in the boxes). The electrons must occupy the lowest-energy orbital available first (in Figure 1.5, s in shell 1) before they move over to the next lowest-energy orbital (s and p in shell 2). Here, electrons fill the p orbital one at a time before any p orbital is completely filled. There is, however, an exception to this rule (see the discussion of hybrid orbitals).

The electrons in the outermost shell determine the chemical properties of the element. These influential electrons, called valence electrons, are located in the valence shell, which is the outermost energy level of an atom. Valence electrons are found in either s or p orbitals, or both. The maximum number of electrons in a valence shell is eight. Nitrogen has five valence electrons, whereas fluorine has seven (**Figure 1.6**).

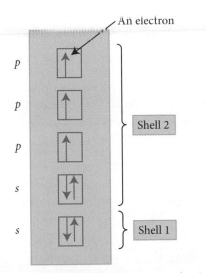

Figure 1.5 Distribution of electrons among the shells in an orbital diagram for a nitrogen atom.

Octet Rule

The octet rule applies when atoms have a tendency to lose, gain, or share electrons to reach the same number of electrons as the noble gases (i.e., they try to have eight electrons in their outermost valence shell). This tendency or rule is applied by an atom as it attempts to become more stable. For instance, an atom with seven electrons (such as fluorine) in its outermost shell would become more stable if it captured another electron.

One of the factors that influences the strength of chemical bonds is the distance of a bond's electrons from each nucleus. **Figure 1.7** demonstrates how the nucleus of chlorine is farther away from the bond pair with a hydrogen atom (compare it with the nucleus of fluorine). The comparison between these two molecules, HF and HCl, indicates that the hydrogen atom is more attracted to the F atom than to the Cl atom.

Hybridized Orbitals and the Lone-Pair Electrons

The topic "hybrid orbitals" is an important concept for understanding many chemical functions and reactions that you will encounter in this chapter. For instance, many enzymes catalyze reactions through nucleophilic or electrophilic attacks. In addition, many drugs are prone to

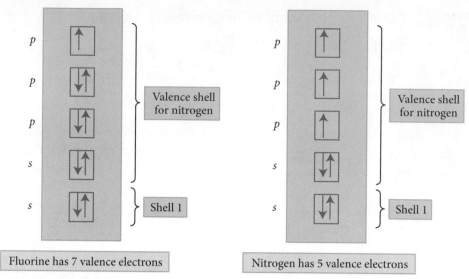

Figure 1.6 Two typical atoms (F and N) and the distribution of their valence electrons.

hydrolysis or metabolism—chemical reactions that are affected by an electrophilic or nucleophilic attack. Furthermore, the way acids and bases accept or donate electrons is related to their existence as electrophiles or nucleophiles. The hybrid orbitals clarify why this behavior occurs: Carbon does not have lone-pair electrons, for example, but

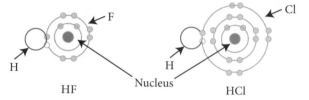

Figure 1.7 The distance between a bond's electrons and the F or Cl nucleus.

nitrogen or oxygen atoms do. The instrumental roles that these lone-pair electrons play in drug action and metabolism are discussed in this chapter.

Hybrid Orbitals

Hybrid orbitals form when atomic orbitals in an atom mix together to enhance its bonding to other atoms. Of particular interest for us here are C, N, and O atoms. Let's return to the carbon atom to explore this concept.

The *s* and *p* orbitals of carbon's second shell (i.e., the valence shell) have very similar energies. As a result, carbon can adapt (hybridize) these orbitals to form the maximum number of chemical bonds. In carbon's hybrid orbitals, a new set of atomic orbitals is constructed so that carbon has four half-filled valence electrons. This makes carbon capable of sharing its electrons with four other atoms. Carbon can enter any of three hybridized atomic states—sp^3, sp^2, and sp—to bind to other elements. **Figure 1.8** illustrates the electron distributions for carbon in its three hybridized atomic states. Of particular interest is the valence electron distribution in the sp^3 hybridized atomic state (the framed boxes represent orbital diagrams for valence electrons).

Single Bond

Analysis of the methane molecule in its sp^3 hybridized state shows how the orbital diagram, which identifies the valence electrons, is filled with four hydrogen electrons (see the light teal arrows in **Figure 1.9**) when carbon atom is bound to four hydrogen atoms to form methane. As Figure 1.9 indicates, the sp^3 orbitals of methane represent a mixture of one $2s$ orbital with three $2p$ orbitals. The bonds between the carbon and hydrogen are called σ (sigma) bonds. All four bonds are equal in regard to strength, bond length, and bond angle.

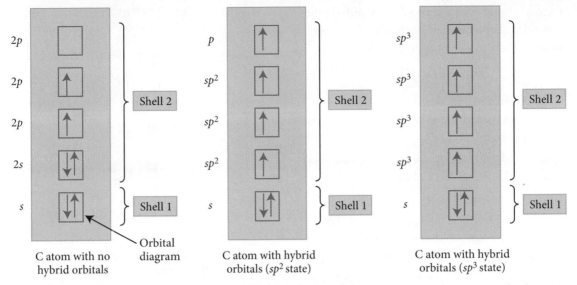

Figure 1.8 Carbon's three hybridized atomic states. Each hybridized state is associated with a unique orbital diagram for the valence electrons.

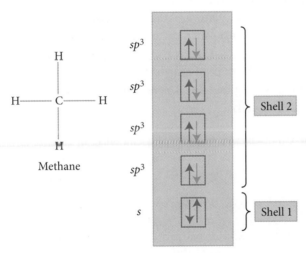

Figure 1.9 The sp^3 orbitals of methane. The orbital diagrams possess valence electrons from both carbon and hydrogen atoms.

Double Bond

In a double bond (for instance, in an ethylene molecule), sp^2 orbitals are present. In carbon, one s orbital is mixed with two p orbitals to form three sp^2 orbitals in the second shell. Two of the sp^2 orbitals, containing one electron each, form a sigma (σ) bond with other carbon atoms (or hydrogen atoms). The third sp^2 also forms a sigma bond with another carbon (for instance, in an ethylene molecule). The last p orbital forms a pi (π) bond with another carbon to form a double bond (**Figure 1.10**).

The electrons in the π bond are not located along an axis between the two carbon atoms, but rather are shared above and below (like a cloud) the sigma bond. Because the electrons in the π bond are above and below the bond, they are more readily donated (**Figure 1.11**).

Ethene (or ethylene) is the simplest alkene molecule. If you place a ripe banana among green tomatoes, you will notice that the green tomatoes undergo the ripening process more rapidly. The reason is that the ripe banana produces ethene, which serves as a plant growth substance. Commercial application of ethene allows many producers to sell fresh fruits. Farmers pick the fruits while they are not mature and ship them to other cities without being worried about the ripening process under the delivery time frame. When the fruits reach their destination, they can be exposed to ethene gas to ripen the fruits.

Triple Bond

In a triple bond (for instance, in an acetylene molecule), the s orbital is mixed with one p orbital to form two sp orbitals in the second shell. The two sp orbitals, which contain one electron each, form a σ bond with a carbon atom and another σ bond with a hydrogen atom. The third and fourth orbitals (*p* orbitals; **Figure 1.12**) form two π bonds with another carbon to create a triple bond. The electrons in the π bonds are not located along an axis between the two carbon atoms, but rather are shared above and below the sigma bond.

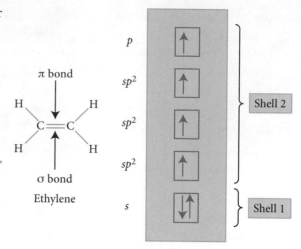

Figure 1.10 Mixing one *s* orbital with two *p* orbitals in the second shell of a carbon atom generates an *sp²* hybridization state.

Use of *s* and *p* Orbitals

When bonds are formed, energy is released and the molecule becomes more stable. For example, two times more energy will be released if carbon binds with four hydrogen atoms than if it binds with two hydrogens (i.e., if it forms CH_4 instead of CH_2). This is one reason carbon atoms try to enter a hybridized state—to form four bonds instead of two bonds, thereby becoming more stable. The new hybrid orbitals are neither *s* nor *p* orbitals, but rather a mixture of the two (hybrid orbitals). The bonds that result from the hybrid orbitals are stronger than the bonds from either *s* or *p* orbitals. Simply put, hybridization provides a means to mix atomic orbitals of slightly different energies to form new orbitals with equal energies. Keep in mind that hybridization occurs within one shell (because of the minimal energy variations among that shell) as opposed to between two shells (because of the large energy variation between shells).

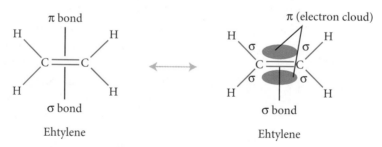

Figure 1.11 Electron cloud in the π bond of an ethylene molecule.

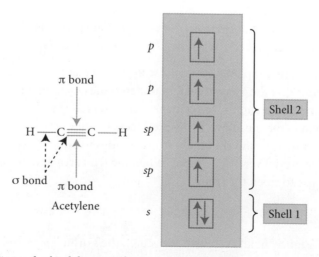

Figure 1.12 Triple bonding and orbital diagrams for an acetylene molecule.

Atoms that bind with just a σ bond (single bond) can rotate about the bond, whereas atoms that bind with a π bond cannot do so unless the π bond is broken. Therefore, a molecule with a double or triple bond is more rigid than a molecule with just a single bond. In addition, multiple bonds result in shorter and shorter bonds; that is, a triple bond is shorter than a double bond, which in turn is shorter than a single bond.

Hybridized States for Nitrogen and Oxygen

The sp^3 hybridized state also applies to nitrogen (N) and oxygen (O). Let's look at nitrogen first. Nitrogen is in group 5A (or VA, see the periodic table in Figure 1.3, which means it has five valence electrons. The electron configuration for nitrogen is shown in **Figure 1.13A**. Nitrogen, like oxygen, tries to adapt to a hybridized state.

Orbital hybridization for nitrogen gives four hybrid orbitals (**Figure 1.13B**). One sp^3 orbital is filled (two electrons) and, therefore, cannot be shared by another element (because it has already the maximum number of electrons that an orbital can have). These two nonbonding electrons are called lone-pair electrons and are not involved in covalent bond formation. (Lone-pair electrons are also called nonbonding electrons and unshared electrons.) The other three sp^3 hybrid orbitals (see the orbital diagrams in Figure 1.13B), each of which has one electron, can be shared with three hydrogen atoms to form ammonia (**Figure 1.14**). Remember, a hybrid orbital can hold only up to two electrons, exactly like a normal orbital. The lone-pair electrons in ammonia are available to be donated to an electron-deficient atom (like H⁺). This is why ammonia has basic properties (we will return to basic properties in another section of this chapter).

Note when the lone-pair electrons are shown as dots around an atom, the model of that atom or molecule is called *Lewis structure*. The ammonia structure shown in Figure 1.14 is a typical Lewis structure.

You might ask why nitrogen's orbitals undergo hybridization when the distribution of electrons in Figure 1.13A is exactly the same as that in Figure 1.13B. Actually, there is a slight energy difference between s and p orbitals, even within the same shell. Nitrogen, by forming hybrid orbitals, will have four hybridized orbitals (sp^3) with exactly the same amount of energy and strength in each of them.

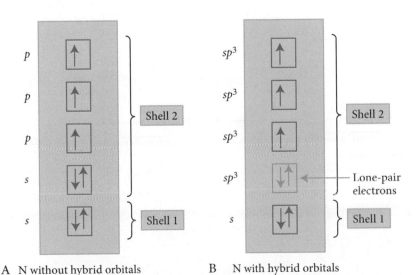

A   N without hybrid orbitals   B   N with hybrid orbitals

Figure 1.13 (A) Nitrogen atom in an isolated form (i.e., without a hybridized state). (B) Nitrogen atom with hybrid orbitals. The lone-pair electrons in the first orbital diagram (sp^3) do not form a covalent bond with other elements, but the electrons in other sp^3 orbitals have the capability to be shared with three other elements.

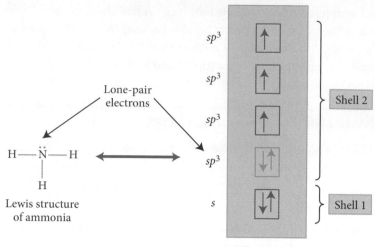

Figure 1.14 The Lewis structure of ammonia with lone-pair electrons and the hybrid atomic orbitals in ammonia.

Oxidation and Reduction Reactions

Oxidation means a loss of electrons; reduction means a gain of electrons. Free electrons are unstable (do not occur), so whenever an electron is released by an oxidation of a molecule, that electron must be accepted in a reduction reaction by another molecule (**Figure 1.15**).

If a carbon atom from an organic compound forms a bond to a more electronegative atom (e.g., to oxygen), the carbon will be oxidized. This occurs because the electrons in the carbon–oxygen bond are drawn ("lost") toward oxygen (recall the electronegativity of oxygen and carbon). Conversely, if the same carbon is bound to hydrogen ("gained"), the carbon atom is reduced.

In the cells of the body, oxidation of organic (carbon) compounds involves the transfer of hydrogen atoms (H), each of which is composed of an electron and a proton. In biochemical reactions, in addition to loss or gain of electrons, a loss of hydrogen may be described as oxidation and a gain of hydrogen as reduction (**Figure 1.16**). More information about biological oxidation–reduction reactions is provided in the *Introduction to Biochemistry* chapter.

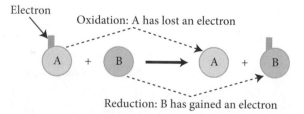

Figure 1.15 In an oxidation reaction, molecule A loses its electron to molecule B, which results in A being oxidized and B being reduced.

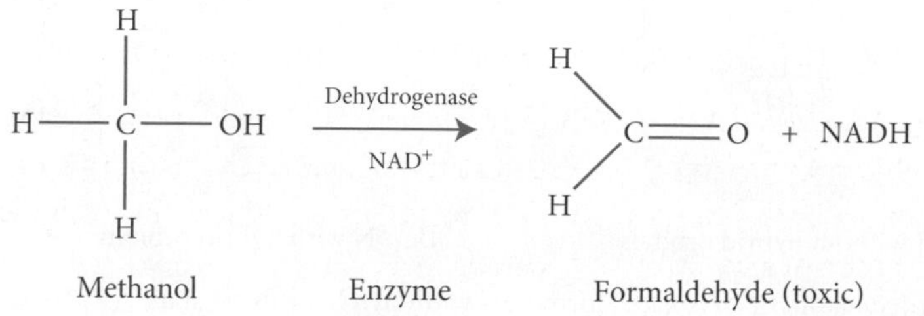

Figure 1.16 The alcohol dehydrogenase enzyme catalyzes the oxidation reaction by transferring two hydrogen atoms from methanol to NAD^+ and the surrounding media.

Important Facts About Alcohols

Alcohols are readily available in many countries and are the most widely encountered poisons in the developed countries. The four alcohols most commonly noted in poisonings are methanol, ethanol, isopropanol, and ethylene glycol. Let's see why these alcohols can be poisonous.

Methanol (CH_3—OH)

Methanol is a clear, colorless liquid that is found in cleaning materials, paints, antifreeze, and windshield washer fluid. It is a toxic solution (causes central nervous system [CNS] depression, blindness, and death) in small amounts of as little as a single mouthful. Methanol forms toxic substances such as formaldehyde and formic acid (see also Figure 1.16). The cause of poisoning is often accidental ingestion due to confusion of this substance with ethanol.

Ethanol (CH_3—CH_2—OH)

Ethanol is a colorless liquid found in many products, ranging from mouthwashes to over-the-counter (OTC) medications to alcoholic beverages. Ethanol is toxic when it is used in high doses. This alcohol is readily absorbed by the stomach and small intestine. Upon digestion, ethanol is oxidized to acetaldehyde by the alcohol dehydrogenase enzyme in hepatocytes, and then further oxidized to acetic acid, which finally is converted to CO_2 and water. This acetaldehyde is believed to give an individual the well-known headache and vomiting symptoms after alcohol consumption. The following reaction shows the metabolism of alcohol by the alcohol dehydrogenase enzyme and aldehyde dehydrogenase enzymes that are found largely in the liver and to some extent in the stomach and brain:

CH_3—CH_2—OH (ethanol) $\rightarrow$ CH_3—CHO (acetaldehyde) $\rightarrow$ CH_3—COOH
(acetic acid) $\rightarrow$ CO_2 and H_2O

While the alcohol dehydrogenase enzyme catalyzes formation of acetaldehyde, the aldehyde dehydrogenase enzyme catalyzes formation of acetate (acetic acid). Due to genetic variations among individuals for expression of the alcohol dehydrogenase enzyme, different individuals may be influenced by different amounts of alcohol consumption. For instance, it has been suggested that women have less of gastric alcohol dehydrogenase than men do. This reduced amount of the alcohol dehydrogenase enzyme results in a longer duration of alcohol in the body, which in turn causes more intoxication among women than among men.

Certain agents can inhibit the alcohol metabolism reaction. For instance, fomepizole (Antizol) is known to inhibit alcohol dehydrogenase, which would otherwise catalyze the metabolism of ethanol, ethylene glycol, and methanol. Consequently, fomepizole is indicated in the treatment of methanol or ethylene glycol poisoning. In contrast, disulfiram (Antabuse), which inhibits the aldehyde dehydrogenase enzyme, is indicated for the treatment of chronic alcoholism. The oral dose is 500 mg/day for 1 to 2 weeks, and this agent should not be taken if ethanol has been consumed within the last 12 hours. Disulfiram prevents oxidation of acetaldehyde to acetic acid, leading to accumulation of acetaldehyde in the blood, which in turn leads to nausea, flushing, headache, palpitation, and vomiting. Because these effects are unpleasant, the patient is less likely to consume alcohol when taking disulfiram.

A few other drugs, when combined with alcohol, also produce a "disulfiram-like" effect. Examples include chloramphenicol (Chloromycetin in Canada), trimethoprim-sulfamethoxazole (Bactrim), cephalosporins, and metronidazole (Flagyl). Given these effects, the drugs should not be taken within 48 hours of alcohol consumption.

Because disulfiram is a hydrophobic agent, it is readily stored in adipose tissue (which makes disulfiram undergo a slow elimination process) and can cross the blood–brain barrier (**Figure 1.17**).

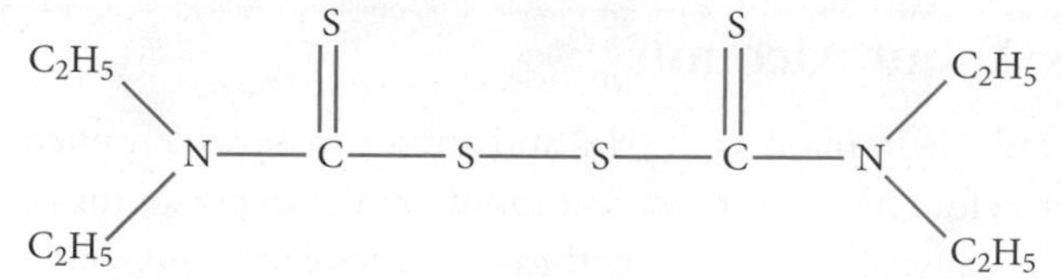

Figure 1.17 Structure of disulfiram, a highly lipid-soluble agent.

The effects of alcohol in lactic acid formation and hypoglycemia are discussed in the *Introduction to Biochemistry* and *Introduction to Pharmacology and Pathophysiology* chapters.

It is interesting to know about the history behind the discovery of disulfiram's healthcare application. In the past, tetraethylthiuram disulfide was used as an antioxidant in some rubber industries. In the early 1900s, workers from rubber industries who were exposed to tetraethylthiuram disulfide developed adverse reactions when they ingested ethanol. Later, tetraethylthiuram disulfide was used as a compound to synthesize the FDA-approved drug disulfiram, which entered the U.S. market in 1951. In addition to inhibiting the aldehyde dehydrogenase enzyme, disulfiram inhibits the dopamine β-hydroxylase enzyme, which is necessary for norepinephrine synthesis from dopamine. As a result, the CNS concentration of dopamine increases and the concentrations of epinephrine and norepinephrine decrease (as you will see in the *Introduction to Pharmacology and Pathophysiology* chapter, dopamine is a precursor to epinephrine and norepinephrine). The latter effect results in a decreased level of norepinephrine and an accumulation of acetaldehyde. Acetaldehyde is an effective vasodilator; the vasodilation, in turn, leads to hypotension.

Isopropanol [CH_3—$CH(OH)$—CH_3]

Isopropanol is found in antifreeze, skin lotions, home cleaning products, and rubbing alcohol (70% isopropyl alcohol). Its effect in causing hypotension and CNS and respiratory depression is two to three times more powerful than that of ethanol. Upon isopropanol ingestion, patients are intoxicated but do not have an odor of ethanol.

Ethylene Glycol (HO—CH_2—CH_2—OH)

Ethylene glycol is found in fire extinguishers, adhesives, air conditioners, and automobile antifreeze. This clear, colorless, sweet-tasting liquid is viscous at room temperature. The enzyme alcohol dehydrogenase converts it to a toxic substance: glycoaldehyde (HO—CH_2—COH). The symptoms of ethylene glycol toxicity include focal or generalized seizures, abdominal pain, nausea, vomiting, and coma.

Learning Bridge 1.1

Joe Smith has been using alcohol for the last 6 months. He has lost his job, and recently his wife filed a divorce petition. However, Joe has been thinking about quitting drinking alcohol and has been seeking help to cope with his alcohol consumption. On a Monday morning, he comes to your pharmacy to fill his disulfiram prescription. While you are asking his date of birth, you notice that he smells of alcohol. The patient denies that he has been drinking alcohol during the last 2 days.

What would you do as an intern pharmacist to help Joe with his medication?

Nucleophiles and Electrophiles

A nucleophile is an electron-rich and a "nucleus-loving" species. It has electrons that can be used to form a covalent bond to an electrophile. Nucleophilic species are either fully negative ions (such

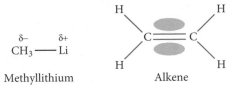

Methyllithium   Alkene

Figure 1.18 The methyl group in methyllithium has higher electron density and is a nucleophile. Similarly, the π bond in the alkene molecule functions as an electron donor, so this molecule is also a nucleophile.

as F^-, I^-, and OH^-); or contain a fairly negative region somewhere in a molecule because of a polar bond (e.g., methyllithium in **Figure 1.18**); or, in the alkene π bond, function as an electron donor (because the electrons in π bonds are above and below the bond, they are more available to be donated, Figure 1.18).

In contrast to a nucleophilic species, an electrophilic species is an electron-deficient and an "electron-loving" species. **Figure 1.19** demonstrates how the positively charged carbon is an electron seeker. A carbocation is an example of an electrophile and carries a positive charge. A neutral carbon atom has four valence electrons, while a charged carbon (C^+) has three valence electrons. C^+ tries to have maximum bonding, so it undergoes rearrangement to form sp^2 hybrid orbitals (Figure 1.19A). The valence electrons for C^+ (three electrons) are distributed among sp^2 orbitals, which can share electrons with other species (Figure 1.19B). Such an interaction leaves the last unhybridized p orbital empty (Figure 1.19C). As shown in Figure 1.19C, the vacant p orbital has a high tendency to accept two electrons so as to follow the octet rule and have a total of eight electrons in the valence shell.

The carbocation is among the most powerful electrophiles; halide anions are among the most powerful nucleophiles. When these two powerful species see each other, they rapidly react with each other (because a nucleus-loving species satisfies an electron-loving species, and vice versa) (**Figure 1.20**). The binding of the Cl anion to the carbocation is called nucleophilic attack, whereas the binding of the carbocation to the Cl anion is called electrophilic attack.

The chemistry of carbonyl compounds is dominated by the polarity of the carbonyl bond. The carbonyl carbon carries a partial positive charge, which makes it highly susceptible to attack by nucleophiles (**Figure 1.21**). Hydroxide ion (a nucleophile) attacks at the electrophilic carbon of the ester C=O, breaks the π bond, and creates a tetrahedral intermediate. This reaction leads to formation of carboxylic acid and an alcohol. This nucleophilic attack explains why esters are prone to hydrolysis (**Figure 1.22**). As you will learn in this chapter, ester is a common functional group for many drugs and a target for hydrolysis and metabolism.

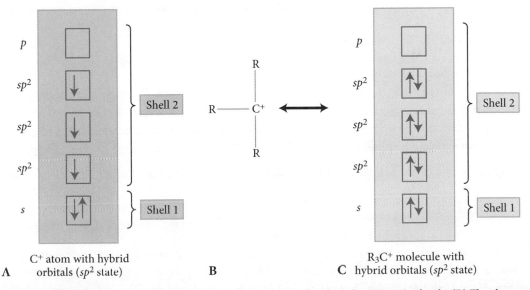

Figure 1.19 (A) The valence electrons for C^+ (three electrons) are distributed among sp^2 orbitals. (B) The electron-deficient C^+ has interacted with three other carbon atoms. (C) The last unhybridized p orbital is empty and has a high tendency to accept two electrons.

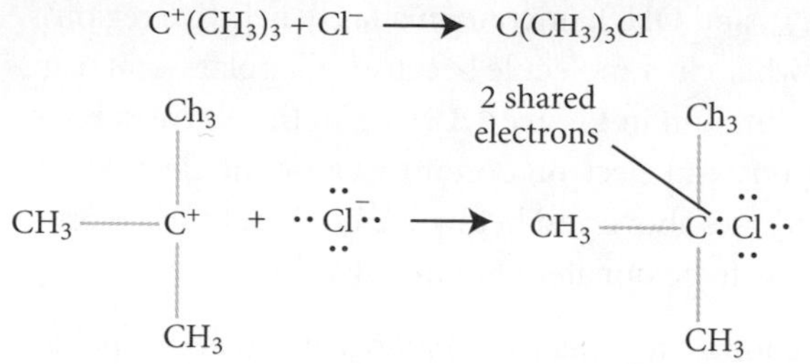

$$C^+(CH_3)_3 + Cl^- \longrightarrow C(CH_3)_3Cl$$

Figure 1.20 When a powerful electrophile (carbocation) meets a powerful nucleophile (halide anion), they rapidly react with each other.

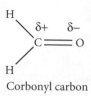

Figure 1.21 Structure of and polarity of the carbonyl carbon.

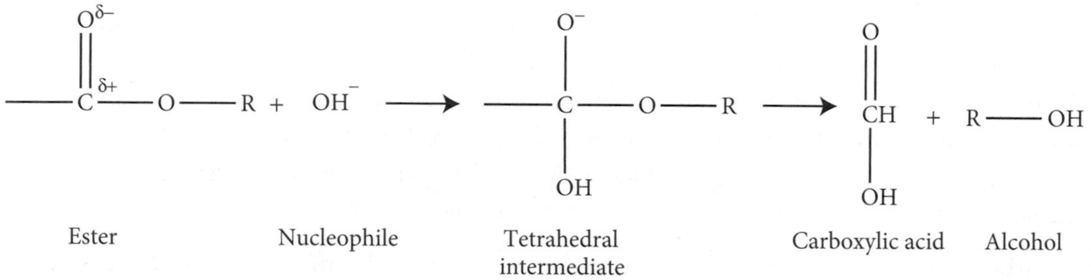

Figure 1.22 Ester molecules are prone to nucleophilic attack and, as a result, are susceptible to hydrolysis.

Learning Bridge 1.2

While you are completing your last day at your introductory pharmacy practice experience (IPPE), a patient is brought to the hospital with signs and symptoms of methanol poisoning—headache, lethargy, blurred vision, vomiting, abdominal pain, and confusion. The patient admits that he drank one mouthful of methanol that he mistakenly believed was ethanol. At the hospital, the attending physician prescribes fomepizole (Antizol).

A. Explain how fomepizole helps to detoxify the methanol poisoning.
B. Why didn't the physician prescribe disulfiram?

Chemical Bonds

The strength of bonds is expressed in units of kilojoules per mole (kJ/mol). The bond energy is the amount of energy that is required to break one mole of the bond. Similarly, it is the amount of energy that is gained when one mole of a bond is formed. For example, 400 kJ/mol of energy is required to break one mole of C—C covalent bonds. To give a simpler example, you need energy to break your pencil into two parts.

Chemical bonds can be divided into two major classes: covalent bonds and noncovalent bonds.

Covalent Bonds

In a covalent bond, atoms in a molecule share electrons to fill their outermost shell. Covalent bonds are responsible for holding atoms together as molecules (**Figure 1.23**). A typical example of a covalent bond is the hydrogen atom that is attached to an oxygen atom to form O—H. The most important covalent bonds in biology (C—C and C—H) have bond energies in the range of 300–400 kJ/mol; they are very strong. Some atoms can form more than one covalent bond. For example, the carbon atom can form four covalent bonds. It is the electron configuration of the atom that

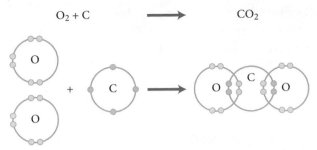

$$O_2 + C \longrightarrow CO_2$$

Figure 1.23 A carbon atom and oxygen atoms share their electrons to fill their outermost shells and, as a result, build a covalent bond.

ultimately determines the number of covalent bonds that are possible. The number of covalent bonds is referred to as covalence.

The covalent bond explains the strong bonding that occurs between hydrogen atoms and oxygen in a water molecule. Covalent bonding also explains why two identical atoms (e.g., Cl_2, H_2) or two atoms with similar electronegativity (C—H) form a molecule. In such a case, because the electronegativity of the atoms is identical or similar, there is no electron that transfers between atoms; instead, electrons are shared between these atoms—a unique characteristic of the covalent bond. When a covalent bond has an unequal sharing of a pair of electrons, it forms a dipole. For instance, hydrogen atoms have much less electronegativity than the oxygen atom in a water molecule. Because of this large electronegativity difference, the oxygen atom draws electrons from the hydrogen atoms, which in turn makes the hydrogen atoms partially positively charged and the oxygen atom partially negatively charged (**Figure 1.24**). This process makes water a dipole molecule. As the name indicates, the dipole molecule has two poles, one positive and one negative. Not all covalent bonds, however, produce dipole molecules.

Polar Bonds

Two identical atoms (such as two carbons) share an electron pair equally, something two unlike atoms cannot do. In a covalent bond between identical atoms, the bound electrons are symmetrically distributed. This bond is also known as a nonpolar covalent bond. By comparison, shared electrons between unlike atoms are found closer to the atom with the higher attraction for the electrons—that is the atom with higher electronegativity. When two atoms share their electrons unequally, they form a polar bond. This bond is also known as a polar covalent bond. Consider HCl. Chlorine is more electronegative (see the periodic table) than hydrogen. Chlorine's electronegativity is not sufficient for Cl to take an electron from hydrogen (otherwise, it would be ionized—see the discussion of ionic bonding later in this section). The bound electrons are shared between H and Cl, but because Cl is more electronegative than H, the shared electrons are pulled toward Cl. The imbalanced electronegativity among Cl and H atoms results in the Cl atom attaining a fractional negative charge (δ^-); for the same reason, the H atom attains a fractional positive charge (δ^+). The structure of this polar bond is shown in **Figure 1.25**.

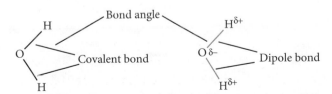

Figure 1.24 A dipole bond is formed when two atoms with different electronegativities share electrons with each other. When an atom is shared between two other atoms, it builds a bond angle. The bond distance is the distance between the nuclei of the bound atoms. Both bond angles and distances characterize the geometry of a molecule.

As you can see, HCl has two electrically distinguishable ends (much like two ends of a magnet). HCl is a dipole (it has two poles). Polar and dipole bonds, however, are different: A polar bond is a type of covalent bond, whereas a dipole is a moment when there are two poles on a molecule. The covalent bond within the HCl molecule is a polar bond but the HCl is a dipole molecule as well. The greater the difference between the electronegativities of the bound atoms, the more polar the bond formed. Keep in mind that the H and carbon atoms have similar electronegativities, so they cannot form a polar bond.

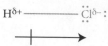

Figure 1.25 The structure of a polar bond. The arrow represents a dipole molecule and the direction of a dipole (direction from the positive pole to the negative pole).

Noncovalent Bonds

Noncovalent interactions (also known as noncovalent bonds) are weak interactions that occur between ions, atoms, and molecules. Such bonds assist some molecules and ions in maintaining their shape and structural integrity. For instance, DNA is composed of two intertwined chains of polynucleotides. While covalent bonds are responsible for holding together the atoms of the nucleotides in each DNA strand, the forces that hold the two strands together are noncovalent hydrogen bonds. The weak hydrogen bond forces are strong enough to keep the two DNA strands attached to each other, yet weak enough to allow the cell to separate the DNA strands from each other to carry out DNA replication and transcription. As another example, consider how amino acids embedded within a protein interact to maintain the structure and function of a protein. In contrast to the covalent bond, no electron sharing occurs between atoms in a noncovalent bond. Instead, in a noncovalent bond, electrons are transferred. As a consequence, a noncovalent bond is not as strong as a covalent bond. Four types of noncovalent bonds exist: ionic bonds, ion–dipole bonds, hydrogen bonds, and van der Waals forces.

Ionic Bonds

Ionic bonds form when one or more electrons are transferred from one atom to another. The ionic bond is the strongest noncovalent bond; it occurs between fully charged positive and negative ions, and it is very common in salt-formed molecules. Molecules that ionize entirely in solutions are electrolytes (a typical example is NaCl). In contrast, molecules that do not ionize in solutions but are very water soluble are nonelectrolytes (polar organic molecules like glucose).

Figure 1.26 depicts a typical ionic bond between Na and Cl ions. In the figure, Na has released one valence electron from its third shell so as to have eight electrons in its second shell and become more stable. Therefore, Na is a good electron donor. In contrast, Cl has seven electrons in its third shell; by gaining one electron, it will complete its valence shell with eight electrons (recall the octet rule) and become more stable. Therefore, Cl is a good electron acceptor. If you mix these two ions, the opposite ions will attract each other—a phenomenon called electrostatic force—leading to the formation of the NaCl salt. This reaction also indicates that an interaction between metals and nonmetals tends to form an ionic bond. However, if a salt with an ionic bond comes in contact

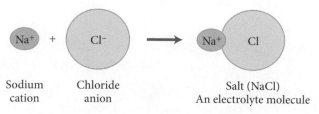

Figure 1.26 Na⁺ and Cl⁻ ions interact with each other to form an ionic bond.

with water, and the attraction between the ions and water subsequently overcomes the attraction between the two ions in an ionic bond, the salt will dissolve into water.

Ion–Dipole Bonds

When an ion (cation or anion) binds to a dipole, it forms an ion–dipole bond (**Figure 1.27**). The ion–dipole bond plays an important role in the water solubility of drugs. Drugs that have free acidic or basic groups have poor aqueous solubility. Salt formation by these groups often improves their solubility, albeit only if the salt is able to dissociate in water (salt formation is explained in another section of this chapter). The topic of solubility is described in detail in the *Introduction to Pharmaceutics* chapter. For now, recognize that the definition of solubility is the amount (gram) of a compound that dissolves in 100 mL of a given solvent (usually in water) and at a specific temperature. For instance, the solubility of sucrose is defined as when 204 grams of sucrose dissolves in 100 mL of water at 20°C.

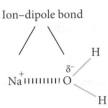

Ion–dipole bond

Figure 1.27 A dipole molecule such as water can form an ion–dipole bond with an ion.

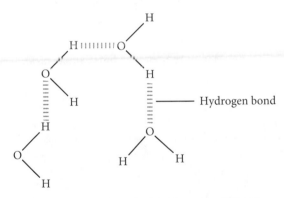

Hydrogen bond

Figure 1.28 Water has a high boiling point (100°C) because of the large number of hydrogen bonds that exist in water.

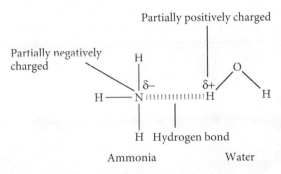

Partially positively charged

Partially negatively charged

Ammonia   Water

Hydrogen bond

Figure 1.29 The partially negatively charged nitrogen of an ammonia molecule interacts with the partially positively charged hydrogen of a water molecule to form a hydrogen bond.

Hydrogen Bonds

Hydrogen bonds are strong chemical bonds. Indeed, it is the hydrogen bonds that explain how water molecules interact with each other to produce a high boiling point (**Figure 1.28**). As explained previously, when a covalent bond forms (like the one between the two hydrogen atoms and one oxygen atom in a water molecule), a dipole bond forms (because of the large electronegativity difference between hydrogen and oxygen). The partially positively charged hydrogen atoms in a dipole molecule (such as in water) can interact with a partially negatively charged atom from another molecule (such as oxygen from another water molecule).

Another example of a hydrogen bond is the interaction that occurs between a water molecule and ammonia—another molecule that contains hydrogen. **Figure 1.29** illustrates how the partially negatively charged nitrogen (of an ammonia molecule) interacts with the partially positively charged hydrogen (of a water molecule). Because both molecules (ammonia and water) are dipoles, the resulting bond is called a dipole–dipole bond as well. However, in a hydrogen bond one of the dipole molecules must contain an electropositive hydrogen—in other words, a hydrogen atom that is bound to an electronegative atom. In the hydrogen bond example shown in Figure 1.28, the hydrogen atom is partially electropositive because it is bound to an electronegative oxygen atom. As mentioned earlier, hydrogen bonds play important roles in stabilizing many macromolecules (e.g., RNA, DNA, proteins).

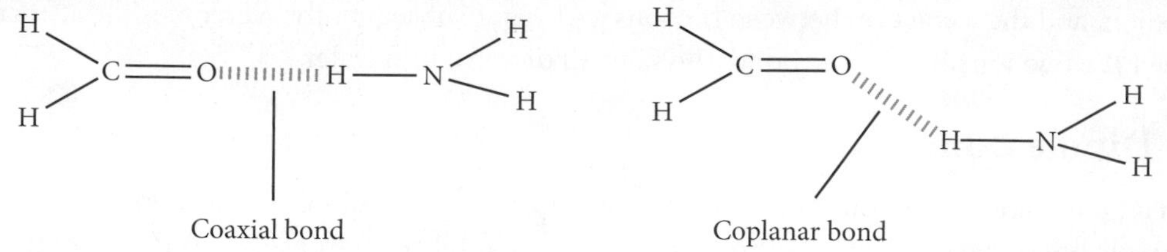

Figure 1.30 Structures of coaxial and coplanar hydrogen bonds.

There are two forms of hydrogen bonds: coaxial and coplanar (**Figure 1.30**). Coaxial hydrogen bonds are stronger than coplanar hydrogen bonds.

Van der Waals Forces

van der Waals forces are the weakest type of interaction between molecules. On average, at any given time the electrons in a nonpolar molecule or atom are distributed around the nucleus. Electrons may, in one instant, be slightly accumulated on one side of the molecule, which results in a small temporary dipole. A temporary dipole may influence the electron distribution of a nearby molecule or atom so that the nearby atom or molecule becomes a dipole—a process called induced dipole. The momentary polarization that causes (forces) attraction between a temporary dipole and an induced dipole is called a London force (**Figure 1.31**). In turn, all molecules in close vicinity, and regardless of their structure, experience London forces.

Although London forces may occur between any two molecules in close vicinity to each other, dipole–dipole forces occur only between polar molecules. However, London forces and dipole–dipole forces make up van der Waals forces. The London forces are temperature dependent (their role becomes more important at low temperatures). This last observation makes sense because, at high temperatures, molecules are not close enough to each other to produce an induced dipole moment. In addition, a steric hindrance negatively affects London forces (i.e., London forces require tight packing of molecules).

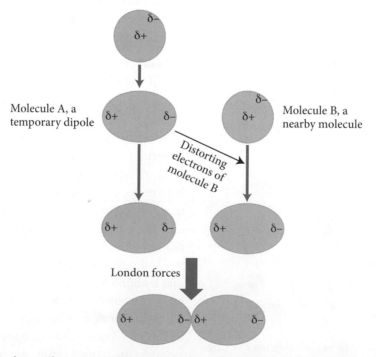

Figure 1.31 London forces. The constant motion and distribution of electrons within the molecule produce momentary polarizations in two nearby molecules (molecules A and B). These polarization processes force molecules A and B to interact with each other.

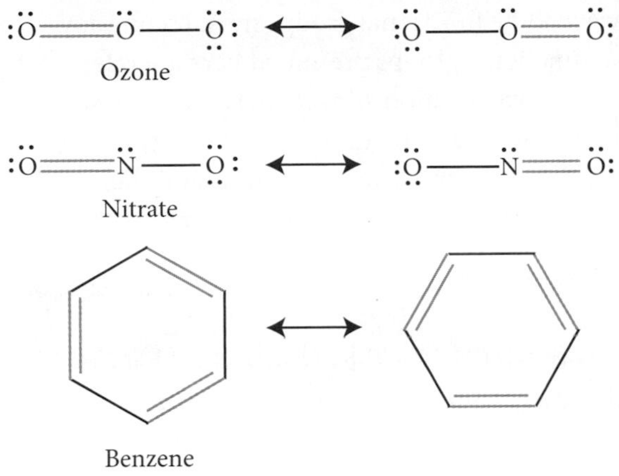

Ozone

Nitrate

Benzene

Figure 1.32 A few examples of molecules that have resonance structures.

Resonance Structures

A resonance structure describes a molecule for which two or more structures with identical arrangements of atoms but different arrangements of electrons can be drawn. **Figure 1.32** demonstrates electron rearrangements in a few examples of molecules with resonance structures.

As an example, let's look at the structure of ozone (O_3). In the ozone molecule shown in Figure 1.32, the electrons in the π bond are not always located between the two atoms of the original bond, but instead are delocalized. This delocalization process enhances the stability of the molecule.

Another example of a molecule with resonance structures is nitrite (NO_2). The electrons in nitrite have been delocalized over the oxygen atoms (as in the ozone molecule). Electrons can be delocalized over many atoms.

Another example of a molecule with resonance structures is a benzene ring. Like the ozone and nitrite molecules, the benzene ring is represented by two resonance structures. In this case, the double-bond electrons are not kept between any two carbons of the ring, but rather are free to move over the entire ring.

Learning Bridge 1.3

Today is your first day of your introductory pharmacy practice experience (IPPE) in a community pharmacy. A grandmother comes to your pharmacy and asks you where she can find aspirin for her 5-year-old granddaughter, Emily. She mentions that Emily has had a low fever since early this morning.

Originally, the customer wanted to give her granddaughter the aspirin tablets that she kept in her medicine cabinet in her bathroom. When she opened the aspirin bottle, however, she noticed a sharp odor of vinegar. The woman noticed immediately that the aspirin tablets' expiration date was 6 months ago. She didn't want to give Emily an old aspirin, so that is why she is at your store today.

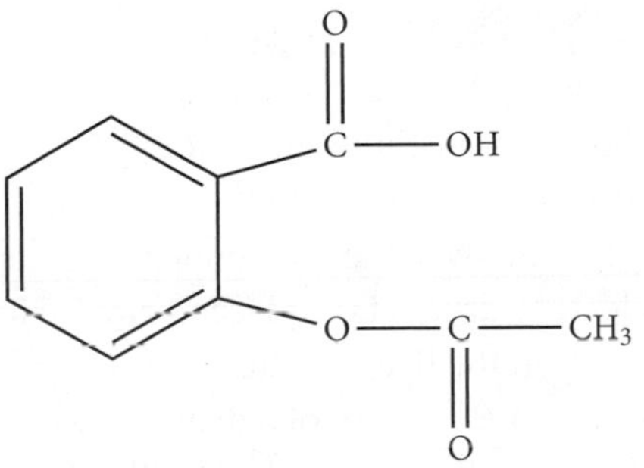

The structure of acetylsalicylic acid is shown in **Exhibit 1.1**.

Exhibit 1.1 Acetylsalicylic acid.

A. How would you explain the vinegar odor of the expired aspirin?
B. What is your reaction when the woman asks you to help her find aspirin for Emily?

Medicinal Functional Groups

Functional groups play important roles in reading structures, categorizing drugs into various classes, and to some extent predicting the pharmacological mechanisms of drugs. This introduction to the organic functional groups provides an overview of the functional groups most commonly encountered in medicinal chemistry. The medicinal functional groups presented here are referred to in many chapters of this book to explain structure–activity relationships (SAR) and to assist students in understanding the principal roles of functional groups. In addition, the functional groups' physicochemical properties in the biochemical and pharmacological realms and their applications in the medical fields, particularly the pharmacy profession, are emphasized.

Nomenclature

The International Union of Pure and Applied Chemistry (IUPAC) is the organization that oversees the rules and guidelines in regard to chemical nomenclature in chemical sciences and makes recommendations on how that nomenclature should be applied. Although this section does not attempt to introduce students to the field of nomenclature for chemical structures, the IUPAC terminology is used to identify and indicate functional groups.

Many molecules are referred to by their common names rather than their IUPAC names. These molecules were identified as pure compounds before their structures were known, so their common names do not provide any information about their structures. Examples of compounds with such names include methane, ethane, benzene, furan, chloroform, and acetic acid. Likewise, many natural compounds are still used under their common names rather than their UIPAC names, such as morphine and limonene.

The following six functional groups are discussed in this chapter:

1.   Alkanes, alkenes, halogenated hydrocarbons, and aromatic hydrocarbons
2.   Alcohols, phenols, and ethers
3.   Aldehydes and ketones
4.   Amines, carboxylic acid, and functional derivatives of carboxylic acids
5.   Sulfonic acids, sulfonamide, and thioethers
6.   The nitro group

Before we go through each functional group, a brief introduction to metabolism will facilitate the discussion of the functional groups' metabolic pathways. A more detailed discussion of metabolism is presented in the *Introduction to Medicinal Chemistry* chapter.

Drug Metabolism

Drug metabolism describes the process in which a drug, through a biological reaction, is transformed into other metabolites. The formation of these metabolites can occur before or after the drugs have reached their sites of action. The metabolism of drugs occurs by more than one pathway. Each pathway consists of a series of metabolic enzymes that catalyze the metabolic reactions. Metabolic reactions of drugs and xenobiotics (foreign chemicals or drugs) take place in two major pathways: Phase I and Phase II. Drug metabolism occurs mainly in the liver, but also to some extent in the blood, kidney, intestine, brain, and lungs. Generally, metabolism of a drug reduces or completely eliminates the drug's pharmacological effect. However, exceptions exist with prodrugs—drugs that become active after they are administered to the body and undergo a metabolic reaction. You will see many examples of prodrugs throughout this book.

Undesirable metabolites are one of the major reasons why a drug may fail to reach the U.S. market—the Food and Drug Administration (FDA) will not approve a drug that produces a toxic metabolite. Therefore, obtaining information about metabolic stability, metabolite formation, and interaction with metabolic enzymes is crucial during the development of a drug. Many pharmaceutical companies have incorporated data analysis regarding metabolites into the discovery phase while developing new drugs.

A major goal of drug metabolism is to make drugs more hydrophilic (water soluble) so that they can be readily excreted by the kidneys. Cytochrome P450 (CYP450) refers to a family of isozymes (also called microsomal enzymes) that are mainly located on the smooth endoplasmic reticulum of the liver. Isozymes are two or more enzymes that catalyze the same reaction but are expressed by different genes.

At least 15 CYP450 isozymes are involved in the metabolism of drugs. Therefore, they are of particular importance when studying drug metabolism and drug interaction. While CYP450 isozymes are mostly seen in the liver, they exist in the intestinal walls as well (albeit in concentrations 20 times less than those found in the liver). The largest amount of these intestinal isozymes is found in the villi of the small intestine.

The hydroxylation reactions of aliphatic compounds, aromatic compounds, and phenols, along with the dealkylation of amines, are catalyzed by CYP450 isozymes. Within the CYP450 system, CYP1A2, CYP2C9, and CYP3A4 are the most abundant isozymes in the liver and account for the metabolism of many drugs. Each CYP450 isozyme is unique and has a distinct role. Drug interactions involving the CYP450 system are common and generally result from either isozyme inhibition or induction. For example, if a drug is a potent CYP450 inhibitor, it may inhibit the metabolism of a co-administered drug, producing a severe adverse effect. Certain foods can enhance or inhibit CYP450 isozyme activity as well.

One of the major roles of the CYP450 system is to facilitate metabolism and detoxification of xenobiotics. As noted earlier, xenobiotic metabolism is divided into two phases: Phase I and Phase II.

Phase I

Phase I introduces new functional groups into the xenobiotics through oxidation, reduction, and hydrolysis by microsomal isozymes. One or more of the CYP450 isozymes may be involved in this pathway. One of the most significant roles played by these isozymes is hydroxylation. Such isozymes (or enzymes) are referred to as mixed-function oxidases or monooxygenases, in recognition of the fact that they catalyze incorporation of one atom of molecular oxygen into the substrate and one atom into water. More detailed information is provided in the *Introduction to Medicinal Chemistry* chapter.

Phase II

Conjugation reactions occur when the xenobiotics react with glucuronic acid, sulfate, or a few amino acids. This pathway usually follows the Phase I reactions. Enzymes involved in Phase II reactions are largely located in the cytosol.

Alkanes

The "-ane" suffix indicates that a molecule is an alkane. Two typical examples are methane (CH_4) and ethane (CH_3—CH_3). In naming an alkane molecule, the name of the longest alkane chain is the parent (base) name for the molecule. In the example shown in **Figure 1.33**, the longest chain is an octane (it has eight carbons), so "octane" will be the parent name for the shown molecule. The lowest number in a chemical structure is given to the substituent (i.e., the methyl group in Figure 1.33).

Alkanes are unable to form hydrogen bonds, ionic bonds, or ion–dipole bonds (recall that there is a very small electronegativity difference between carbon and hydrogen in an alkane molecule). The van der Waals forces are the only forces that drive alkane molecules to interact with each other.

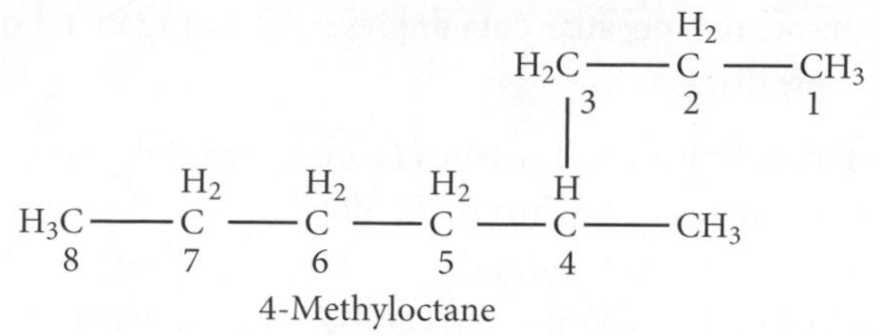

$$H_2C \overset{H_2}{\underset{3}{—}} \overset{}{\underset{2}{C}} — \underset{1}{CH_3}$$

$$H_3C \overset{}{\underset{8}{—}} \overset{H_2}{\underset{7}{C}} \overset{H_2}{\underset{6}{—C}} \overset{H_2}{\underset{5}{—C}} \overset{H}{\underset{4}{—C}} — CH_3$$

4-Methyloctane

Figure 1.33 Structure and the IUPAC name of an alkane molecule. The branched carbon (carbon 4) receives the lowest number. The longest continuous chain is used as the parent name.

Obviously, van der Waals forces exist only for molecules with more than four carbons, as an alkane with four or fewer carbons always takes a gaseous form (e.g., propane). Because alkanes cannot form hydrogen bonds with water molecules, they are water-insoluble molecules (i.e., they are lipid soluble or hydrophobic). Alkanes are colorless, and their melting and boiling points are relatively low. However, as the carbon chain length increases, the melting and boiling points increase due to the involvement of van der Waals forces. In contrast, as the amount of branching increases, the boiling point decreases due to lower van der Waals forces (recall that a steric hindrance reduces van der Waals forces).

Alkanes are mostly excreted as unchanged molecules because they are nonreactive. However, there is an exception: Oxidation of an alkane may occur at the end of the hydrocarbon chain.

Alkenes

The "-ene" suffix indicates that the molecule has a double bond. A typical example is propylene: $CH2=CH—CH_3$. As explained earlier, the name of the longest chain is the parent name for the molecule. The chain is numbered so that the double bond receives the lowest number. Some alkene compounds have more than one double bond (polyenes). A typical example is arachidonic acid, whose structure includes four double bonds inside the arachidonic molecule. Because each double bond decreases the number of hydrogen atoms in the molecule by 2, the general formula for an alkene molecule is C_nH_{2n} (**Figure 1.34**).

Two terms are used to identify the isomers of an alkene molecule:

* *cis* alkene (has the larger substituent on the same side)
* *trans* alkene (has the larger substituent across the double bond)

Despite the fact both maleic acid and fumaric acid have the same number of carbons and double bonds, they have different cellular functions in the citric acid cycle owing to their *cis* and *trans* configurations, respectively (**Figure 1.35**; see also the *Introduction to Biochemistry* chapter).

Alkenes are prone to oxidation (**Figure 1.36**), leading to peroxide formation—a serious pharmaceutical problem. However, the peroxide formation does not affect the *cis* or *trans* configuration of the compound.

Unlike in alkanes, the double bonds in alkenes do not have free bond rotation because of the rigidity of the double bond. As mentioned earlier, double bonds have shorter bond lengths

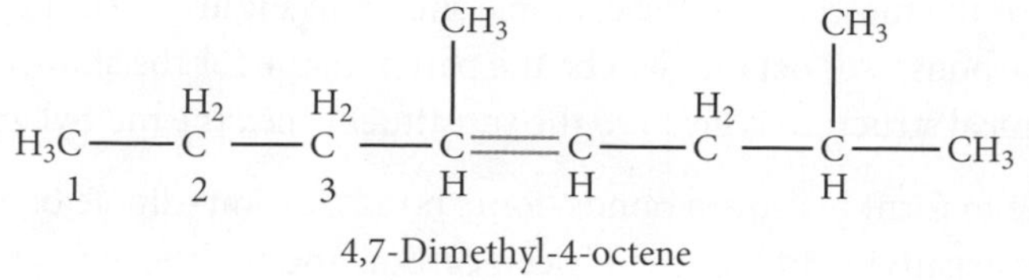

$$H_3C \overset{}{\underset{1}{—}} \overset{H_2}{\underset{2}{C}} \overset{H_2}{\underset{3}{—C}} \overset{CH_3}{\underset{}{—C}} \overset{}{\underset{H}{=}} \overset{}{\underset{H}{C}} \overset{H_2}{—C} \overset{CH_3}{\underset{H}{—C}} — CH_3$$

4,7-Dimethyl-4-octene

Figure 1.34 Structure and IUPAC name of an alkene molecule.

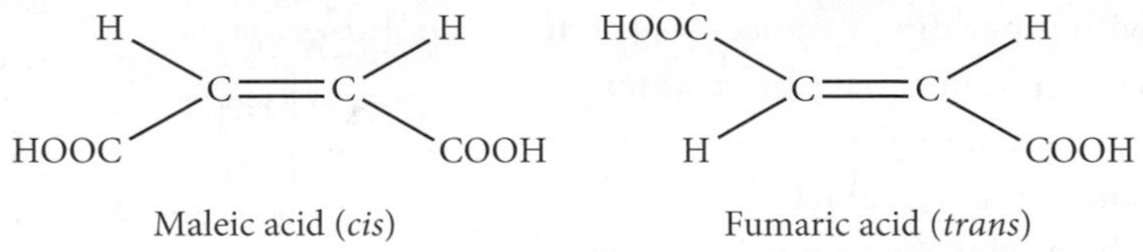

Maleic acid (*cis*)   Fumaric acid (*trans*)

Figure 1.35 Both maleic acid and fumaric acid have the exact same number of carbon, hydrogen, and oxygen atoms. However, due to their *cis* and *trans* configurations, they have totally different cellular functions.

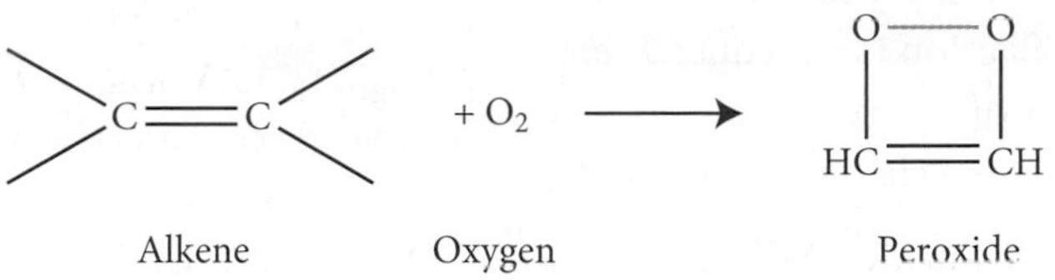

Alkene   Oxygen   Peroxide

Figure 1.36 Incorporation of oxygen into the alkene molecule during an oxidation reaction.

compared with single bonds. Due to alkenes' lack of water solubility, they dissolve in nonpolar solvents (e.g., fat, oil) and are flammable in the presence of oxygen and sparks. Endogenous alkenes (fatty acids from the human body) are reactive (i.e., they undergo hydration, reduction, and epoxidation), with the "addition reaction" being an especially common chemical reaction for these molecules. One example of an addition reaction involving alkenes is hydration of fatty acids (i.e., formation of an alcohol in the presence of water). As mentioned earlier, this reaction occurs because the π bond serves as a nucleophile and, as a result, is vulnerable to electrophilic attack. Just mixing an alkene with water will not cause hydration to occur and produce an alcohol; instead, an enzyme in the body or a strong acid such as H_2SO_4 in an experiment must be present to convert an alkene to an alcohol (**Figure 1.37**). Indeed, the latter experiment is how ethyl alcohol (or ethanol) is produced from ethylene.

Halogenated Hydrocarbons

Halogenated hydrocarbons are molecules in which a halogen atom such as fluorine (F), chlorine (Cl), bromine (Br), or iodine (I) has replaced a hydrogen atom. An example is ethyl bromide (CH_3CH_2Br). Halogenated hydrocarbons are polar molecules because halogen atoms are much more electronegative than carbon. To name a halogenated hydrocarbon, first find the longest chain (parent) and then locate the position of halogen. If halogen is the only substituent, give the halogen group the lowest possible number when naming the molecule (**Figure 1.38**).

Alkyl halides have an important place in the development of a pharmaceutical agent because they can be used as starting compounds for the preparation of other functionally substituted compounds. Monohaloalkanes have a permanent dipole character because of the strongly electronegative halide. However, because alkyl halides are electron-rich molecules, they do not

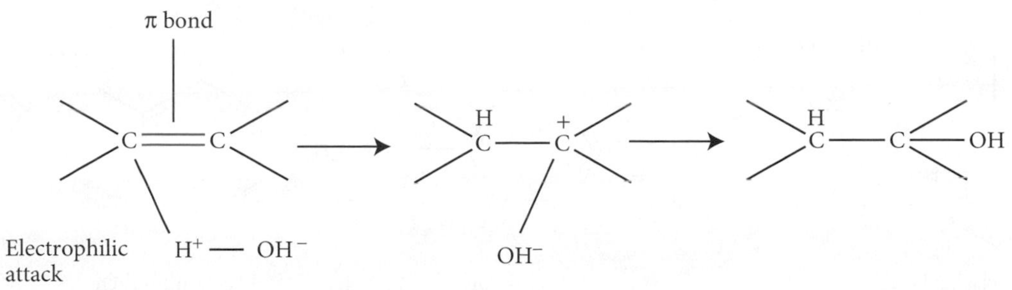

Figure 1.37 The π bond of an alkene molecule serves as a nucleophile and is prone to electrophilic attack.

readily interact with other dipole molecules (such as water) and, as a result, they have poor water solubility (in other words, they are lipid soluble). However, these compounds interact with other molecules through van der Waals forces. In addition, the high lipid solubility of halogens causes halogenated drugs to be reabsorbed from kidney tubules. This physiological process may explain their long duration of action (i.e., reduced renal elimination) and their drug toxicity due to their accumulation in the body. Halogen atoms also can be attached to an alkene to form a vinylic or allylic molecule (**Figure 1.39**).

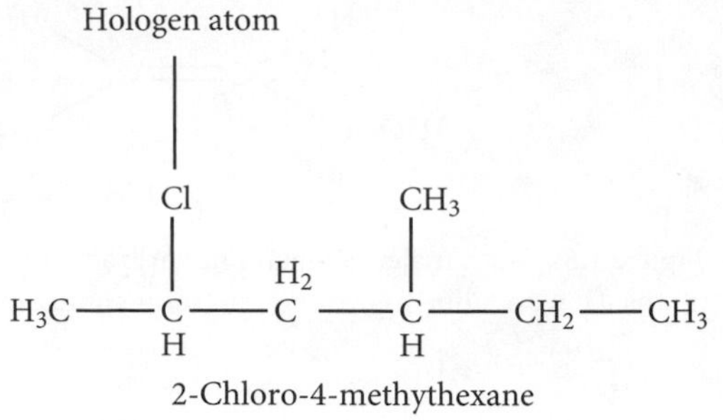

Figure 1.38 Structure and IUPAC name of a halogenated hydrocarbon.

2-Chloro-4-methythexane

Ethyl chloride (Gebauer's Ethyl Chloride) is an anesthetic spray that is used for relief of the skin pain associated with an intravenous (IV) injection or minor sport injury. Because ethyl chloride evaporates rapidly, it cools the skin to reduce pain (which explains why the duration of action is 1 minute or less).

Aromatic Hydrocarbons

Aromatic hydrocarbons have chemistry similar to that of the benzene molecule. These compounds are classified into two categories: benzenoid (or arenes) or nonbenzenoid. Whereas benzenoid aromatic hydrocarbons contain benzene ring(s), nonbenzenoid aromatic hydrocarbons have rings that are either smaller or larger than the benzene ring. The term "aromatic" was used to describe these hydrocarbons because many compounds that have a benzene ring produce an aroma. Not all aromatic hydrocarbons have an aroma, however. For instance, acetylsalicylic acid, ibuprofen, and acetaminophen all have a benzene ring but no aroma (**Figure 1.40**).

Benzene is the most common aromatic parent structure; it has the molecular formula C_6H_6 and is highly unsaturated due to its three double bonds. Substituents on a benzene ring are identified by a unique numbering process that gives the substituents the lowest possible numbers. A prefix is used when only two substituents are attached to a benzene ring: *ortho-* (*o-*): (1–2 placement), *meta-* (*m-*): (1–3 placement), and *para-* (*p-*): (1–4 placement). **Figure 1.41** indicates ortho, meta, and para positions on a benzene ring.

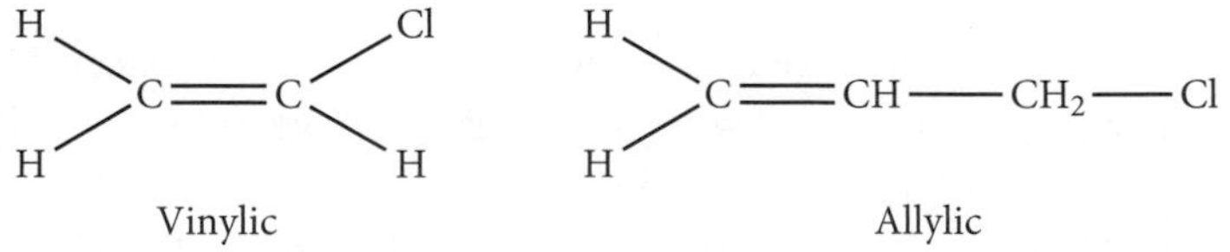

Figure 1.39 Structures of vinylic and allylic molecules.

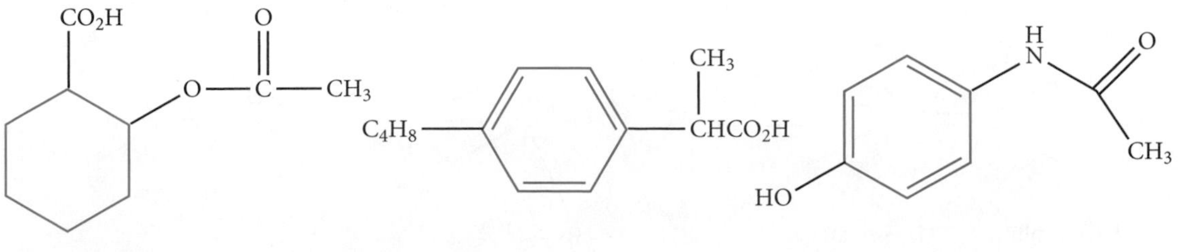

Figure 1.40 A few commonly used analgesic drugs that contain aromatic hydrocarbons.

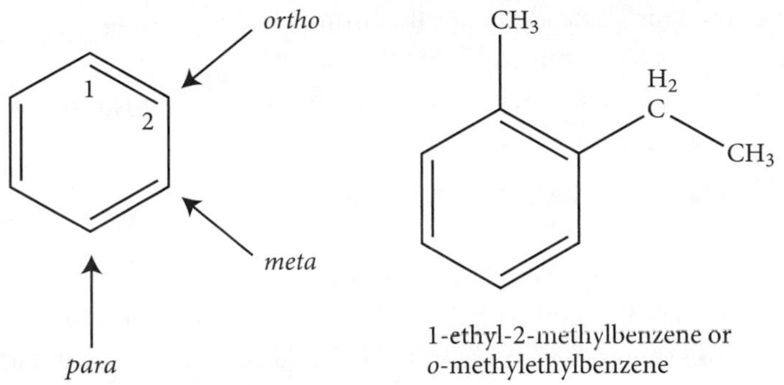

Figure 1.41 Benzene rings are prone to substitution reactions involving the *ortho*, *meta*, or *para* carbon of the benzene ring. The numbering and IUPAC name are shown here.

Because aromatic rings have double bonds, they have a cloud of π electrons above and below the ring (recall the π bonds). Electrophiles, in turn, attack the electron-dense cloud of the benzene ring. **Figure 1.42** shows how the NO_2^- ion, as an electrophile molecule, attacks the double bond and substitutes the hydrogen atom, a mechanism called electrophilic substitution.

Hydroxylation

Hydroxylation of aromatic rings (aromatic hydroxylation) occurs commonly in the liver's microsomal enzymes (i.e., in vivo) during Phase I metabolism. A typical example of a hydroxylation reaction is shown in **Figure 1.43**.

Alcohols

When a hydroxyl group (OH) is the major functional group, the "e" from alkane is dropped and is replaced by "ol." A typical example is methanol (from methane, CH_4, to methanol, CH_3—OH). In

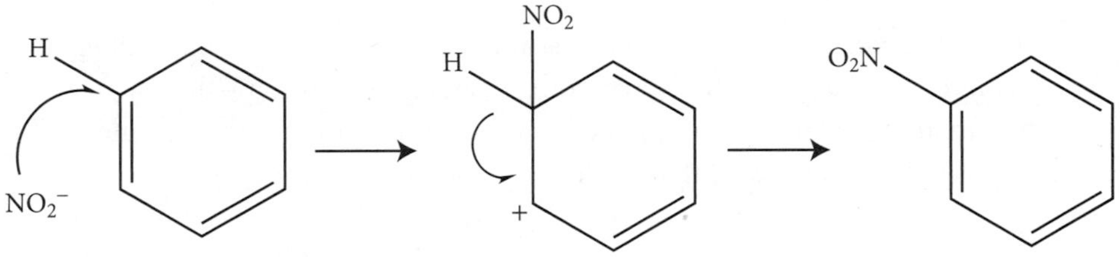

Figure 1.42 Electrophilic substitution reaction on a benzene ring by a nitrite ion.

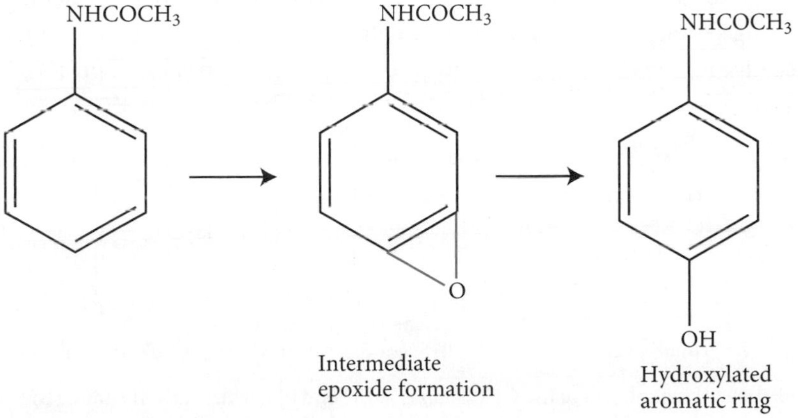

Intermediate
epoxide formation

Hydroxylated
aromatic ring

Figure 1.43 Hydroxylation of an aromatic ring includes formation of an intermediate epoxide.

giving a name to an alcohol molecule, designate the hydroxyl group to have the lowest possible number. When OH is the only functional group, the carbon number that has this group is placed in the front of the chain name (see **Figure 1.44**).

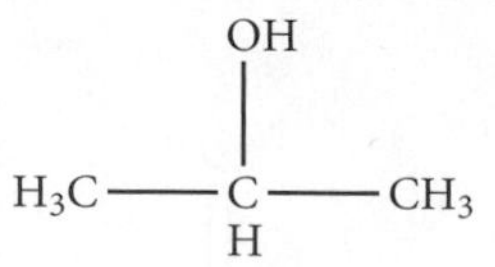

The hydrogen atom attached to the oxygen atom causes alcohols to be dipole molecules. Alcohols are weak acids, are less volatile than the corresponding hydrocarbon, and are water soluble. The water solubility, however, depends on the length of the hydrocarbon attached to the OH group. **Figure 1.45** shows three types of alcohol chains: primary, secondary, and tertiary.

Figure 1.44 Structure of a primary alcohol.

An OH group centered in the molecule has higher water solubility than an OH at the end of the molecule. If a second OH group is added, the water solubility of the alcohol increases. Conversely, the more hydrocarbons are added to the OH functional group, the less water soluble the alcohol is. The C—O bonds of alcohols are polarized because of the electronegative oxygen. This polarization makes the O slightly negative and, therefore, a nucleophile.

Alcohols are readily metabolized in the body. Both primary and secondary alcohols are prone to oxidation (by oxidase enzymes) to form carboxylic acids and ketones. However, tertiary alcohols are stable to oxidation.

Phenol

Phenol is a benzene ring with an attached OH group (**Figure 1.46**). Mono-substituted phenols are named using the prefix *ortho-* (*o-*), *meta-* (*m-*), or *para-* (*p-*) due to the position of the substituent from the phenol's hydroxyl group.

The polar nature of the OH bond, due to the electronegativity difference of the atoms, promotes the formation of hydrogen bonds with other phenol molecules—which also explains why phenol has a high boiling point. Because of the same OH group, and therefore the hydrogen bonds, phenol is highly water soluble as well.

Because of the resonance phenomenon, phenols are more acidic than alcohols: Phenols are at least 100 times more acidic than alcohols. According to an acid definition—that is, the Brønsted-Lowry definition (addressed later in this chapter)—an acid is a substance that donates a hydrogen ion to another molecule or ion. Recall that the hydrogen atom is made of one electron and one proton, so a hydrogen ion (H^+) is a proton. Consequently, an acid is a proton donor. Simply put, both alcohol and phenol, because of the H atoms on their OH groups, can donate protons and thereby act as weak acids, albeit to different extents.

The most important factor that contributes to the fact that phenols are more acidic than alcohols is the aromatic ring system (**Figure 1.47**). Both alcohol and phenol can dissociate protons (being acidic). The negative ion on oxygen in ethoxide (i.e., when ethanol has lost a proton) is localized

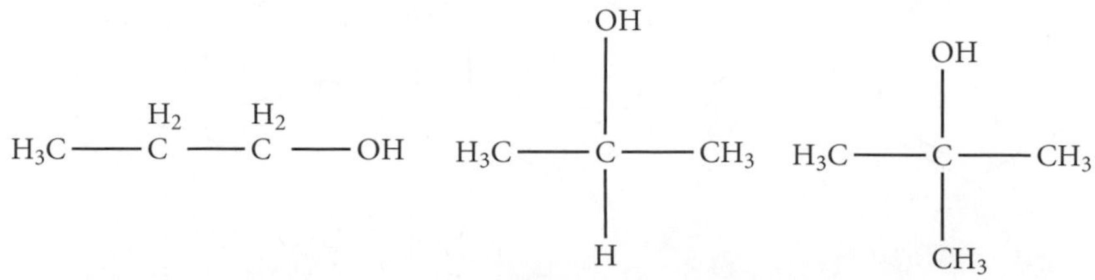

A. Primary alcohol   B. Secondary alcohol   C. Tertiary alcohol

Figure 1.45 (A) Primary alcohol, where the OH group is at the end of a hydrocarbon chain. (B) Secondary alcohol, where the OH group is in the middle of the chain. (C) Tertiary alcohol, where the OH group is attached to a carbon atom that carries no H atoms.

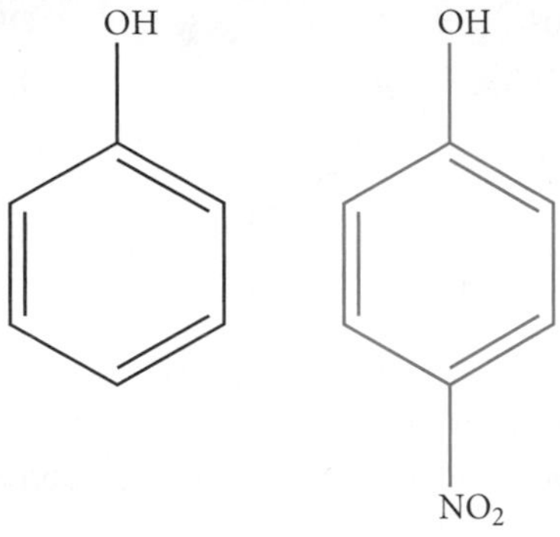

OH

OH

NO$_2$

Phenol   4-Nitrophenol
                 (*p*-nitrophenol)

Figure 1.46 Structures of phenols.

only on the oxygen, and nowhere else. In contrast, the negative ion on a phenoxide ion is delocalized and overlaps with the π electrons (the clouds above and below the aromatic ring). Because of this delocalization, the negative ion is not readily available to attract a proton. This functional property of phenols makes them more acidic than alcohols.

Any electron-withdrawing group such as NO$_2$ or an aromatic ring (aryl group) will draw electrons from an oxygen atom and make the electrons above the oxygen atom less available to attract a proton. This results in a higher acidity. In contrast, an electron-releasing group (alkyl) makes the electrons on oxygen more available to attract a proton, which results in a lower acidity (**Figure 1.48**).

Keep in mind that the addition of a methyl or a halogen (e.g., Cl, F) reduces the water solubility of phenol. The addition of a second OH group (anywhere other than the *ortho* position), however, increases the water solubility of phenol. Salt formation (with Na$^+$ or K$^+$) is an important pharmaceutical reaction because the phenolate ion (phenoxide ion) will interact with water (recall the process of ion–dipole bonding). The liver is the primary site for metabolism of phenol-containing drugs. The metabolism of these drugs is very much like that of alcohols—that is, upon hydroxylation they produce diphenolic substances. Conjugation to glucuronic acid (forming glucuronide) and sulfonation (to produce sulfate conjugate) are the two most common metabolic pathways that occur for phenols during Phase II metabolism (**Figure 1.49**).

Ether

Ether is characterized by having an oxygen atom that links two hydrocarbon groups. Ether has an important place in pharmaceutical industries as a solvent in the preparation of many synthetic drugs. The widely used form of ether is ethyl ether.

The various types of ether are named by naming the two alkyl groups in alphabetic order as separate words and then adding the word "ether" at the end. Most ethers, however, are called by their common names; the IUPAC names are used only when their name is complicated. When both alkyl groups are the same, the prefix "di-" is used in the front of the alkyl name. An example is diethyl ether, which is also simply called ether (**Figure 1.50**).

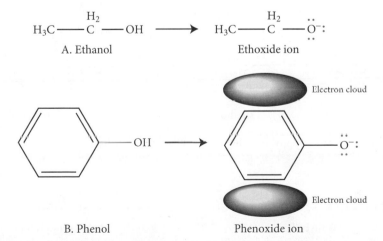

A. Ethanol   Ethoxide ion

                                          Electron cloud

B. Phenol   Phenoxide ion

                                          Electron cloud

Figure 1.47 Alcohols (A) are less acidic than phenols (B) because the negative ion on a phenoxide ion is delocalized and overlaps with the π electrons.

The majority of drugs that contain ether are in the form of aromatic ether (**Figure 1.51**). Examples are codeine (Codeine, Contin, in Canada) and verapamil (Calan).

Ethers have a low boiling point (owing to van der Waals attractions) and poor water solubility (they lack an OH group). Moreover, as the length of the carbon chain increases, the solubility of ethers decreases. Compared with alcohols, ethers are less soluble in water, although they mix well with many organic solvents. Ethers with short carbon chains can form hydrogen bonds to water because the oxygen on ether has lone-pair electrons that bind the hydrogen atom of a water molecule. Ether in contact with O_2 (air) forms peroxides (if peroxide is concentrated, it may explode).

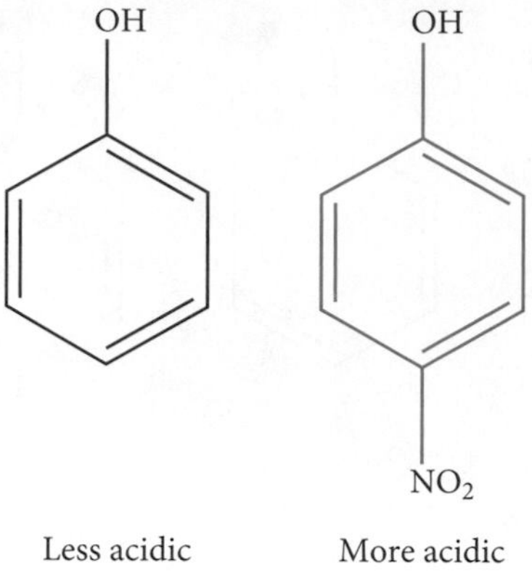

Less acidic   More acidic

Figure 1.48 Two phenol groups with different acidity strengths.

Ether is a colorless liquid, stable, but is light and air sensitive. It is extremely volatile and flammable and, as a result, must be stored carefully. In the 1940s and 1950s, ether was a popular anesthesia agent, but now its use is strongly discouraged. This compound is toxic if ingested, inhaled, or absorbed through skin contact. The anesthetic effect occurs because ether accumulates in the lipids of the neurons and reduces nerve impulse transmission. In general, ethers are excreted unchanged, with one exception: dealkylation, when a short alkyl such as a methyl or ethyl group is lost by enzymatic oxidation in Phase I metabolism (**Figure 1.52**).

Aldehydes and Ketones

Aldehydes and ketones are closely related to each other, in that both contain a carbonyl group. Aldehydes have a high chemical reactivity and, as a result, are important intermediates in the pharmaceutical industry. The longest chain containing the aldehyde group provides the base name for the compound, with the aldehyde group as the first carbon. The suffix "-e" in alkane is replaced by "-al." Aldehydes are produced by oxidation of primary alcohols. As a result, they are easily oxidized to carboxylic acids (**Figure 1.53**). Therefore, aldehydes are sensitive to air oxidation and should not be stored for long periods.

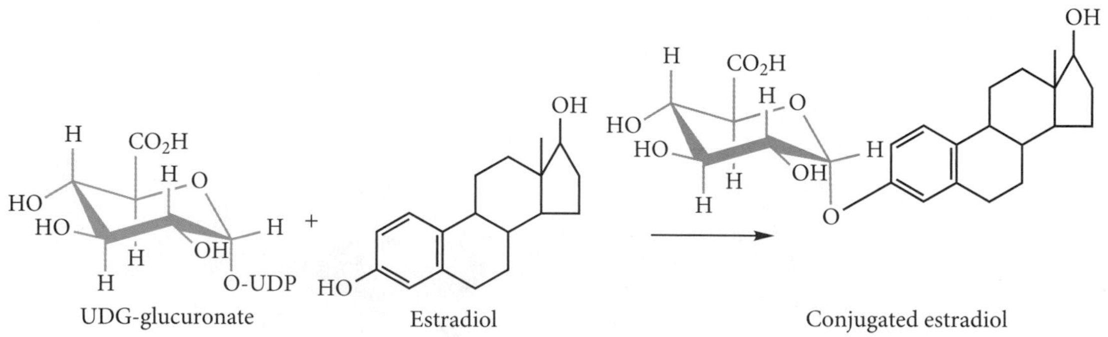

UDG-glucuronate   Estradiol   Conjugated estradiol

Figure 1.49 Glucuronidation of ibuprofen during hepatic Phase II metabolism.

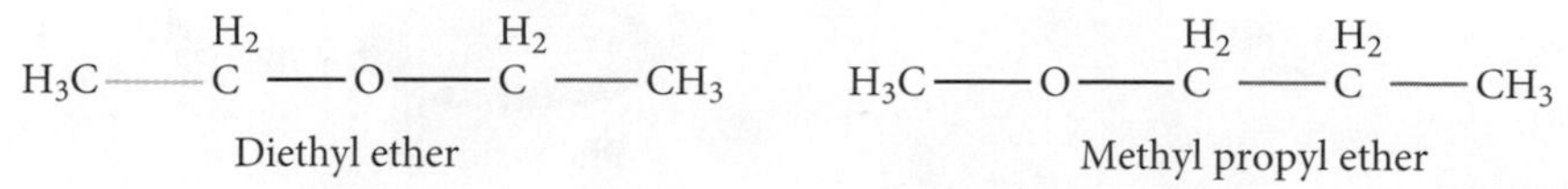

Diethyl ether   Methyl propyl ether

Figure 1.50 Ether names are often designated by common names instead of IUPAC names. They have the chemical structure R—O—R, in which the R can be identical or different aromatic or aliphatic hydrocarbons.

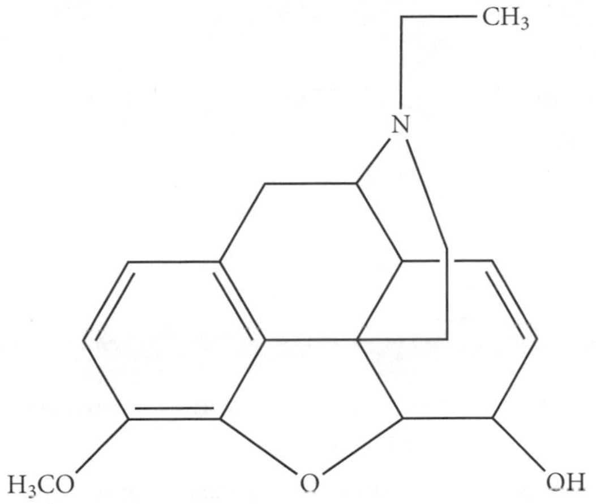

Figure 1.51 Structure of an aromatic ether (codeine).

In naming ketones, you find the longest chain and give the lowest number to the carbonyl group (C=O). The suffix "-e" in alkane is replaced by "-one" (**Figure 1.54**).

The carbonyl group present in aldehydes and ketones is a polar functional group. Ketones have a higher boiling point than other molecules with equal molecular weight. The reason is the dipole–dipole interaction between the carbonyl groups that occurs between the ketone molecules (**Figure 1.55**).

Ketones can form hydrogen bonds to the hydrogen atoms in water, making them water soluble to some extent. As usual, as the length of the chain increases (hydrophobic moiety increases), the water solubility decreases. While aldehydes are reactive to air oxidation (which leads to carboxylic acid formation), ketones are relatively nonreactive. The simplest aldehyde is formaldehyde, a colorless gas with a strong odor. Formaldehyde is toxic; if it comes in contact with the skin, it can cause severe skin irritation, or an ingestion of formaldehyde can lead to coma or death. An aqueous solution of formaldehyde is formalin (containing 37% formaldehyde), which has germicide effects (i.e., kills viruses, bacteria, and fungi) and is used to preserve biological specimens. The germicide effect arises because the aldehyde group of formalin interacts with the amino group of amino acids and thereby changes the structure and function of many essential proteins in viruses, bacteria, and fungi.

The simplest ketone is acetone, a colorless liquid that is used as a solvent in cleaning fluids. In humans, severe starvation or untreated type 1 and 2 diabetes leads to overproduction of a series of

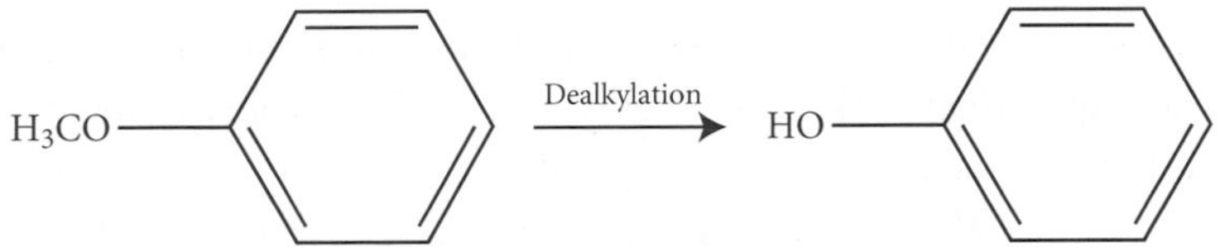

Figure 1.52 Enzymatic oxidation (dealkylation) of an ether during Phase I hepatic metabolism.

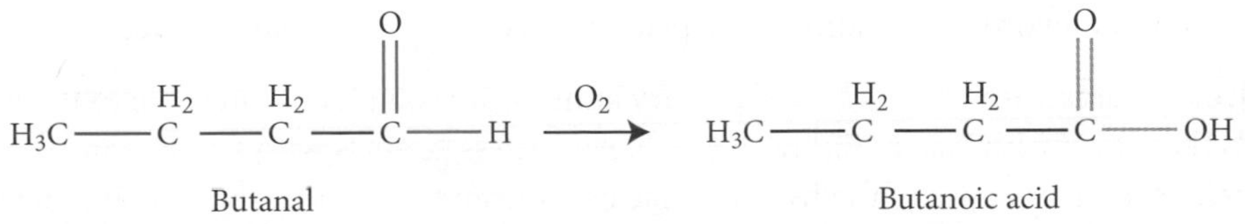

Butanal   Butanoic acid

Figure 1.53 Oxidation of an aldehyde molecule (butanal) to a carboxylic acid (butanoic acid).

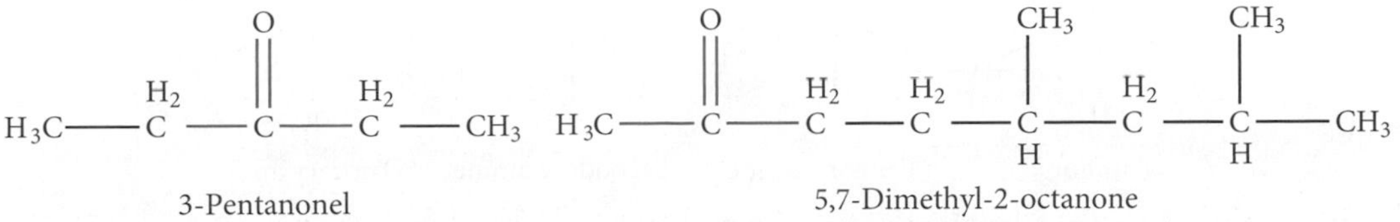

3-Pentanonel   5,7-Dimethyl-2-octanone

Figure 1.54 In the IUPAC system for naming ketones, the suffix "-e" in alkane is replaced by "-one."

acidic molecules called ketone bodies, which can cause a life-threatening condition called diabetic ketoacidosis (see also the *Introduction to Biochemistry* and *Introduction to Pharmacology and Pathophysiology* chapters). Acetone is a ketone body that gives a characteristic odor to the breath, which is sometimes useful in diagnosing untreated diabetes.

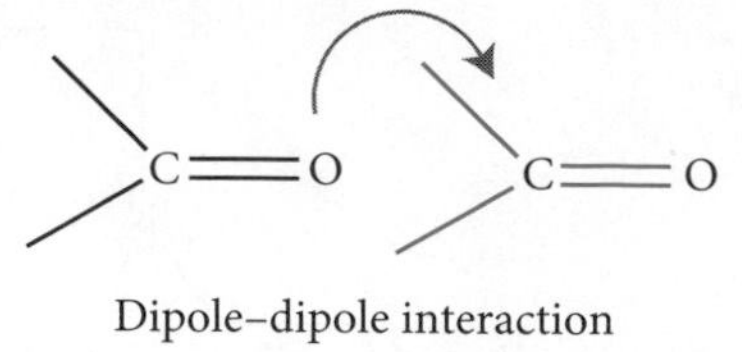

Dipole–dipole interaction

Figure 1.55 Dipole–dipole interaction between two carbonyl groups.

Amines

Most amines are bases (albeit with different strengths) because they can accept a proton. However, while amines usually do not donate a proton, one can find acidic amines such as phenobarbital. Amines are widely used in the structural design of drugs to not only produce a pharmacological effect, but also, due to their basicity, make salts from water-insoluble compounds. The lone pair of electrons on the amine nitrogen plays an important role in the basicity of amines.

Many plants' leaves, roots, and fruits are rich in nitrogen-containing compounds; because their water-based solutions increase the pH of the solutions, they are referred to as alkaloids. Many of these alkaloids are toxic and have a bitter taste—in essence, a warning signal from nature. Some alkaloids are used as analgesics and for the creation of euphoria. You will encounter many examples in this book. The names of amines are similar to the names of alcohols, except that the "e" in the parent alkane name is replaced by "amine." Amines are classified as primary, secondary, and tertiary (similar to alcohols) based on how many alkyl groups are bound to the nitrogen atom (**Figure 1.56**).

In naming amines, you number the carbon chain so as to give the lowest number to the amine group. In secondary and tertiary amines, the largest alkyl group attached to the nitrogen is named as the parent amine. The smaller alkyl groups are named with the prefix "*N*-" followed by the alkyl name, and are listed alphabetically. Common names are used for many aromatic and heterocyclic amines—as is the case for aniline, for instance (**Figure 1.57**).

The most important characteristic of amines is their lone-pair electrons. The melting and boiling points of amines are higher than those of alkanes of similar size because of their hydrogen bonds. The effect of the carbon chain's length on the physical properties is the same as for alkanes— namely, the longer the chain, the higher the boiling point. However, despite the fact that amines are polar molecules, they do not have boiling points as high as those of alcohols. In primary and secondary amines, the hydrogen is bound to nitrogen, which is not as electronegative as oxygen. This characteristic leads to a weak dipole moment. The lowest boiling point is found with tertiary amines, because no hydrogen bonding takes place between the two tertiary amines.

Like alcohols, small amines, including tertiary amines, are soluble in water due to the hydrogen bonds they form with water (**Figure 1.58**). Nevertheless, amines with fewer than six carbons are less water soluble because of the hydrophobic effect from the hydrocarbon chain. The water solubility rank for amines is as follows: primary > secondary > tertiary. This order reflects the fact

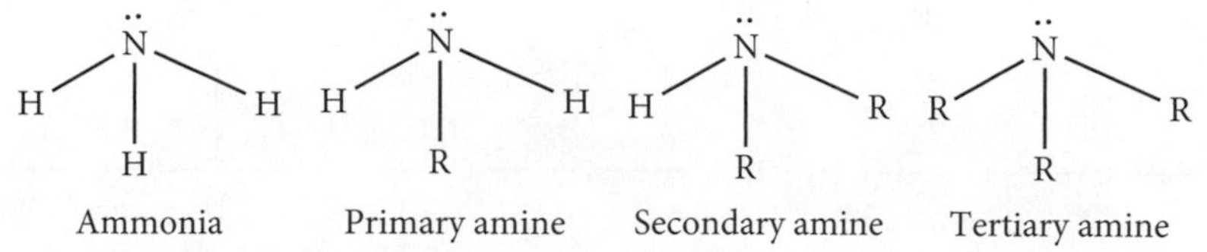

Ammonia   Primary amine   Secondary amine   Tertiary amine

Figure 1.56 Amines are designated as primary, secondary, and tertiary based on the replacement of one, two, or three hydrogen atoms, respectively, on an ammonia molecule.

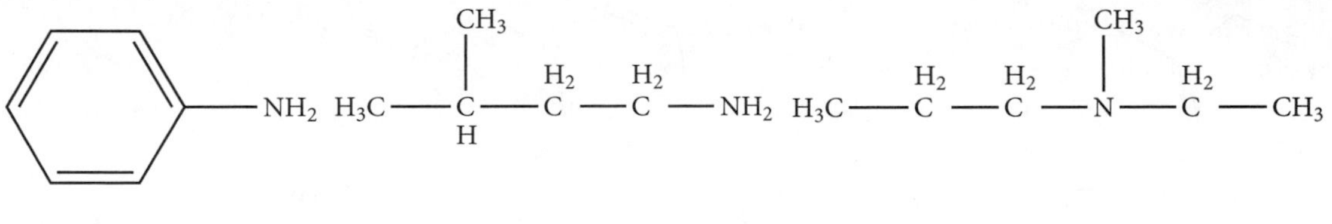

Aniline   3-Methyl-l-butanamine   *N*-Ethyl-*N*-Methyl-l propanamine

Figure 1.57 The parent name of molecules containing an amine is the largest alkyl group attached to the nitrogen atom. Common names are also used to name aromatic and heterocyclic amines (e.g., aniline).

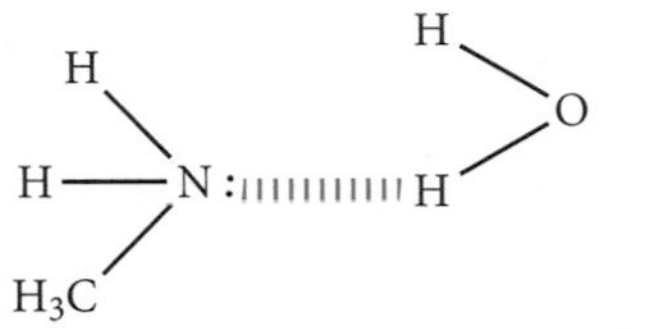

Figure 1.58 Hydrogen bonding between a primary amine and water.

that the nitrogen atom loses its hydrogen atom as it goes from a primary structure to a secondary or tertiary structure.

According to the Brønsted-Lowry definition, a base is a substance that accepts a proton (H$^+$). Because of amine's lone-pair electrons, amines have the ability to accept a proton. Indeed, this property assists amines in the formation of salts (i.e., amines will react with strong acids to form alkyl ammonium salts). Salt formation is a very important process for many drugs if they are to be water soluble, albeit subject to one important condition: The salt should be able to dissociate in water. Among the common acids used for salt formation by drugs containing amines are hydrochloric acid (HCl), sulfuric acid (H$_2$SO$_4$), and phosphoric acid (H$_3$PO$_4$).

The basicity of amines depends on the electron-releasing effect of the functional group that binds to the amines. For instance, electron-releasing groups (alkyl) increase the basicity of amines, whereas electron-withdrawing groups (aryl) reduce the basicity of amines (**Figure 1.59**).

When the aryl groups are attached to the amino group, the electron-withdrawing property of the aryl molecule pulls at the lone-pair electrons of the amine and makes them less available for accepting protons (recall the properties of a weak base). In contrast, the more readily available the lone-pair electrons are, the stronger the base is. In general, basicity declines in the following order:

(CH$_3$)$_3$N > (CH$_3$)$_2$NH > CH$_3$—NH$_2$ > NH$_3$ → Reduced basicity

Dealkylation is one of the major metabolic pathways for secondary and tertiary amines; it results in the formation of aldehyde or ketone groups (**Figure 1.60**). The dealkylation reaction increases the water solubility of an amine-based drug. Recall that a similar mechanism operates with ethers. In contrast, deamination (**Figure 1.61**) often occurs with primary amines, frequently catalyzed by an enzyme called monoamine oxidase (MAO; see the *Introduction to Pharmacology and Pathophysiology* chapter).

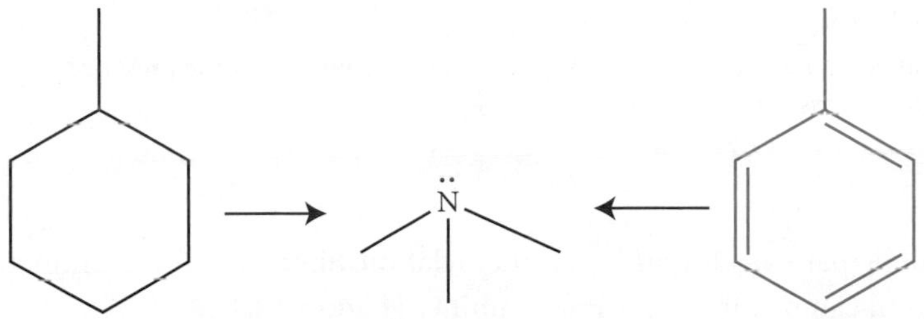

Alkyl group   Aryl group

Figure 1.59 Alkyls are electron-releasing groups and aryls are electron-withdrawing groups. While the former increase the basicity of amines, the latter make amines less basic.

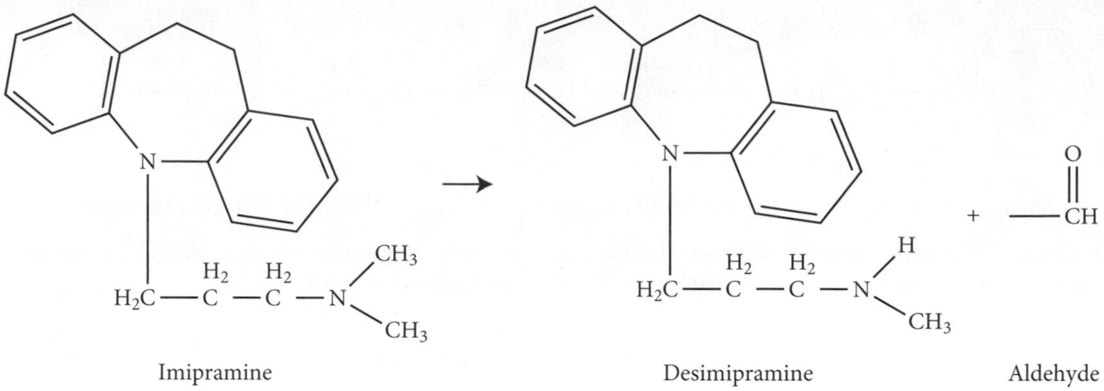

Figure 1.60 Dealkylation of amino groups is a common pathway in the metabolism of secondary and tertiary amines.

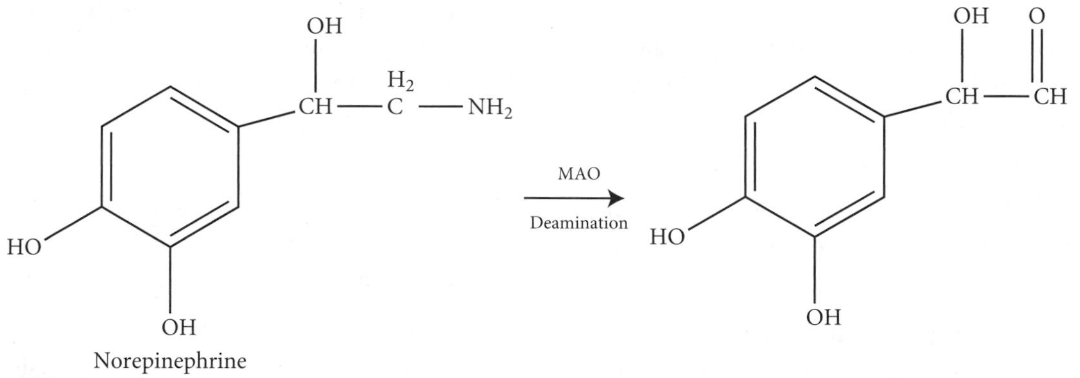

Figure 1.61 Deamination of a primary amine (norepinephrine) by monoamine oxidase (MAO) enzyme.

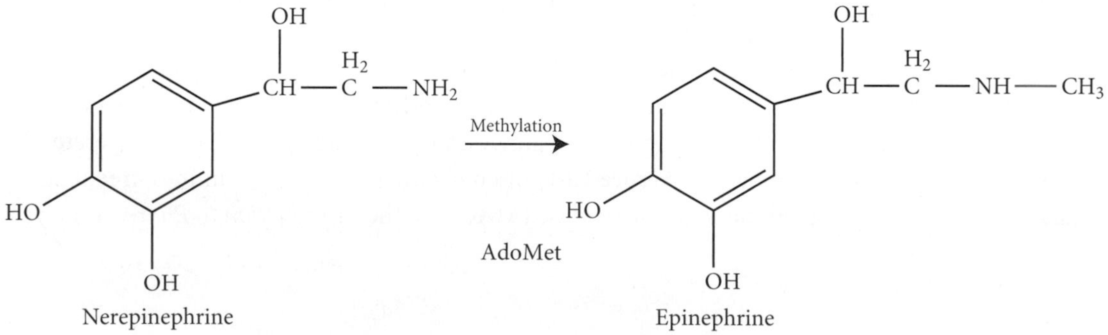

Figure 1.62 Enzymatic methylation of a primary amine (norepinephrine) in the presence of *S*-adenosylmethionine (AdoMet), which functions as a methyl donor.

A minor metabolic pathway for amines is methylation. Similar to the deamination reaction, the methylation reaction can occur with primary amines (**Figure 1.62**).

Glucuronic acid reacts (conjugates) with primary and secondary amines during Phase II hepatic metabolism, which in turn increases the water solubility of amines (**Figure 1.63**).

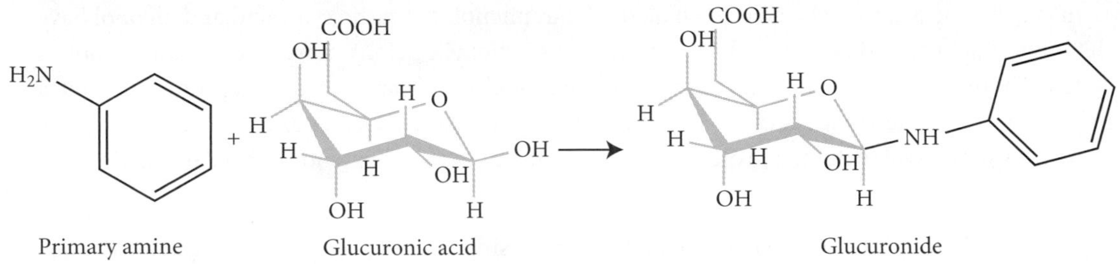

Figure 1.63 Both primary and secondary amines undergo conjugation reaction during Phase II hepatic metabolism, which increases their water solubility.

Learning Bridge 1.4

Amy likes to eat poppy seed bread for breakfast occasionally. Amy's employer implemented a random drug screening test for company employees yesterday. The drug screening test indicated that Amy had morphine in her blood sample. She has never used morphine in her entire life and claimed that the lab result was not accurate. A second lab analysis, however, confirmed the first finding. Amy knows that you are a pharmacy student and hopes that you can assist her in understanding why the drug screening showed traces of morphine. What would be your answer?

Carboxylic Acids

When naming carboxylic acids, the longest chain that contains the carboxyl group is used as the parent name for the molecule; numbering begins from the carbonyl carbon. Carboxylic acids are named by replacing the "e" of the alkane root name with "oic" and adding the word "acid" thereafter (**Figure 1.64**).

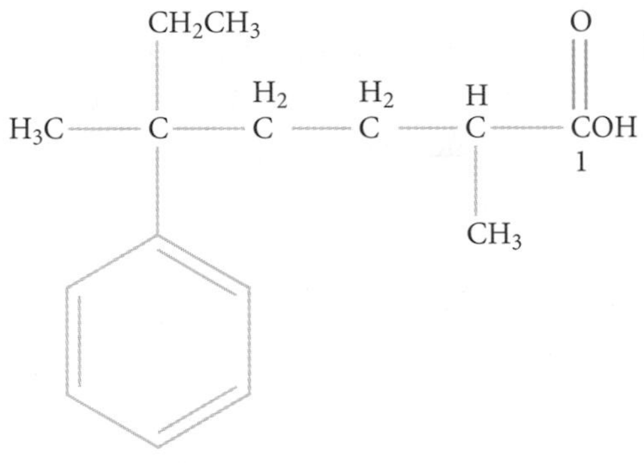

2,5-dimethyl-5-phenylheptanoic aci d

Figure 1.64 IUPAC name of a carboxylic acid molecule.

A carboxylic acid has a relatively high boiling point and high water solubility because of its polar carboxyl group, which enables it to form a hydrogen bond with another carboxyl group. However, as the length of the hydrocarbon chain increases, the water solubility of the carboxylic acid decreases.

Carboxylic acids are acidic due to the resonance stabilization of the carboxylate ion. The available electrons (or the negative charge) are shared equally between the two oxygen atoms. The arrow in **Figure 1.65** indicates the delocalization of electrons; neither of the two oxygen atoms is able to significantly attract a proton.

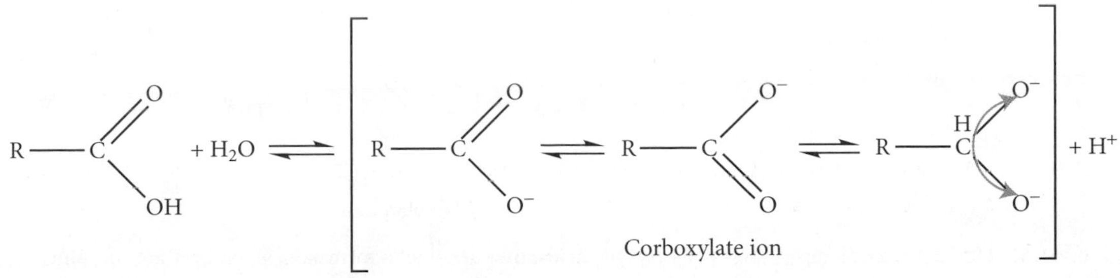

Figure 1.65 Resonance stabilization of the carboxylate ion in a carboxylic acid molecule.

In comparing a carboxylic acid to an alcohol and phenol, the carboxylic acid and alcohol have the highest acidity and lowest acidity, respectively. Carboxylic acid is more acidic than phenol because none of the oxygen atoms in the carboxylic acid significantly attracts a proton. In contrast, in phenol, the oxygen atom is the single most negatively charged species and, therefore, is able to attract, to some weak extent, a proton. Therefore, phenol is a weaker acid than a carboxylic acid.

Similar to amines, the acidity of carboxylic acid depends on the electronic effect of the groups that are attached to the carboxyl group. Electron-releasing groups (alkyls) decrease acidity, whereas electron-withdrawing groups (aryls) increase acidity (**Figure 1.66**); compare this effect with that noted for amino groups.

Because carboxylic acids are acidic molecules, a reaction with a strong base (NaOH) produces a carboxylate salt (**Figure 1.67**). The salt formation increases the water solubility of carboxylic acids. Keep in mind that the salt should be able to dissociate in water to increase the water solubility of the molecule.

It is common for carboxylic acids to undergo Phase II metabolism to conjugate with glycine or glucuronic acid and thereby increase their *in vivo* water solubility.

Functional Derivatives of Carboxylic Acids

Esters

Esters are much less polar than alcohols or carboxylic acids (a polar alcohol is combined with a polar acid to produce a much less polar molecule, so that the two hydroxyl groups disappear), leading to decreased water solubility. The boiling point for esters is low compared with the boiling points for alcohols or carboxylic acids with the same molecular weight. Esters are, however, more soluble in alcohols than in water.

When naming esters, the suffix "-ic" of the carboxylic acid is replaced by "-ate." Esters have two carbon chains separated by an "ether" oxygen; as a result, one has to name both chains separately in the full ester name (**Figure 1.68**). It is the position of the carbonyl group in an ester molecule that dictates which part is the alkyl group and which part is the alkanoate group.

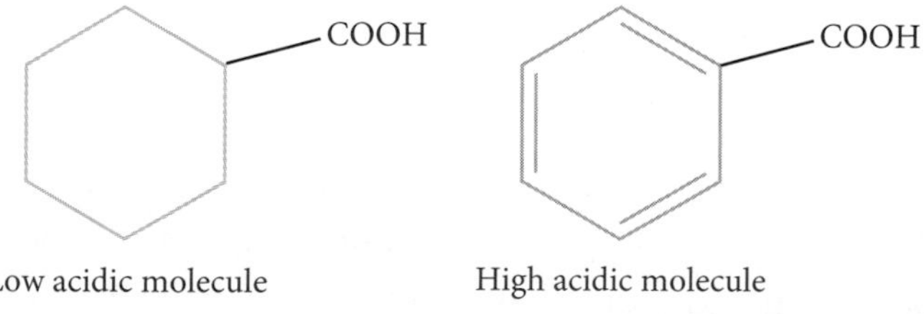

Low acidic molecule   High acidic molecule

Figure 1.66 Alkyl and aryl groups act as electron-releasing and electron-withdrawing groups to carboxylic acids, respectively.

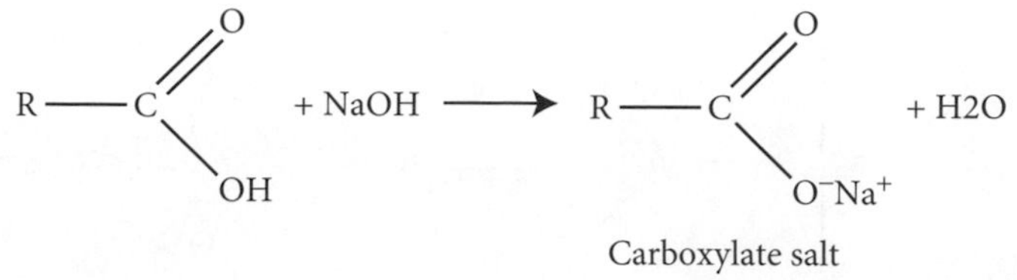

Carboxylate salt

Figure 1.67 Due to the acidic properties of carboxylic acids, they are able to form salts when they are combined with bases.

In a reaction called esterification, a carboxylic acid reacts with an alcohol in the presence of an acid (usually H_2SO_4), which also causes a water molecule to be eliminated from the reaction. Keep in mind that esters are also produced by other pairs of compounds such as an acid anhydride and an alcohol, or an acid chloride and an alcohol, or simply by two different esters. When esters are split apart, in a reaction called hydrolysis, carboxylic acid and an alcohol are formed. Hydrolysis of esters occurs in the presence of water and strong acids such as H_2SO_4 and HCl or esterase enzymes. As a result, esters are prone to hydrolysis, which presents a stability problem that shortens the shelf-life of ester-based drugs.

Many plants and flowers owe their pleasant smells to esters. For instance, methyl butanoate gives the odor to an apple, and pentyl ethanoate gives the odor to a banana (**Figure 1.68**).

In the presence of a strong base (NaOH), ester is converted into a carboxylate salt. This reaction is a typical soap formation (from fats that contain ester groups). The hydrolyzing enzyme, esterase, catalyzes the hydrolysis of the ester to carboxylic acid and alcohol (**Figure 1.69**).

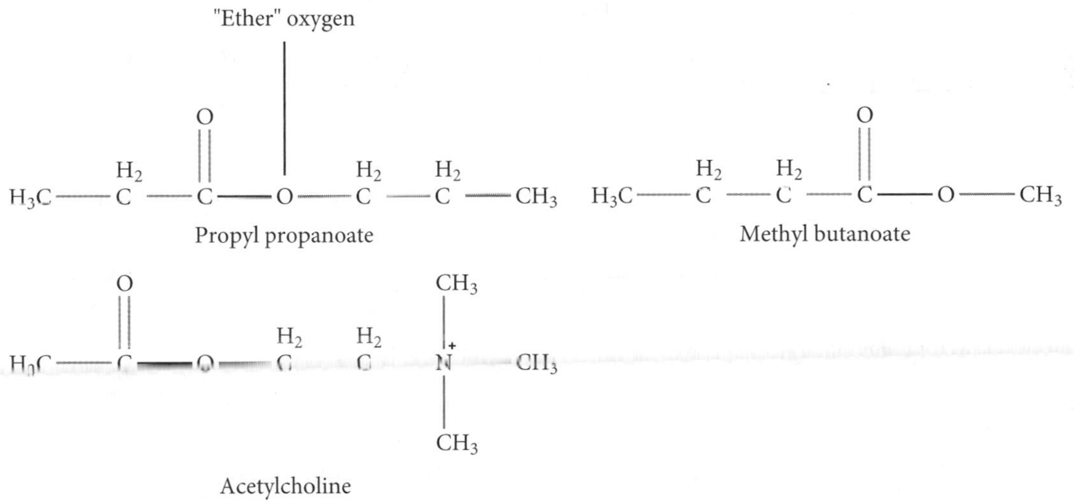

Figure 1.68 Structures of two esters produced by propanol and propanoic acid (propyl propanoate) and by methanol and butyric acid (methyl butanoate). In addition, the structure of the neurotransmitter ester, acetylcholine, is shown.

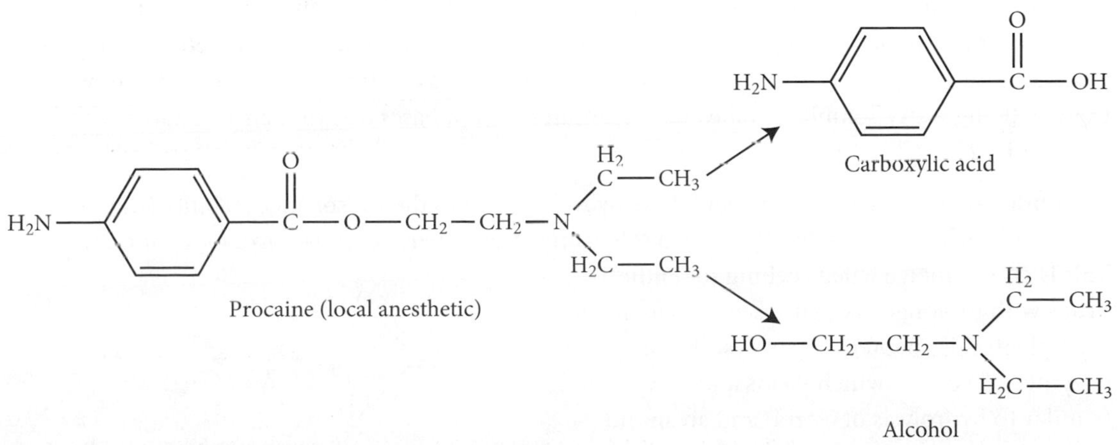

Figure 1.69 Hydrolysis of procaine by esterase enzymes results in the production of alcohol and carboxylic groups.

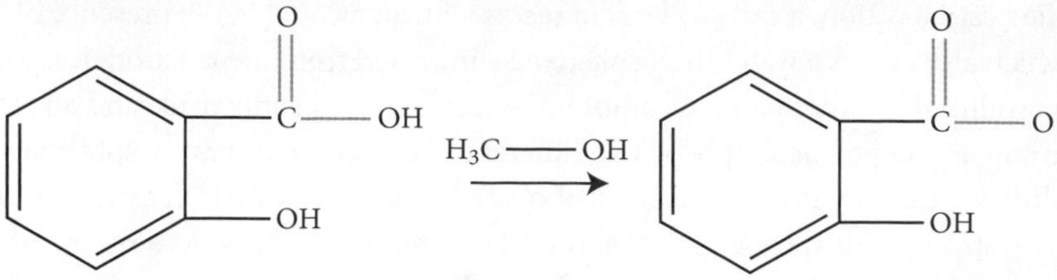

Figure 1.70 Interaction between an acid (salicylic acid) and methanol that produces methyl salicylate.

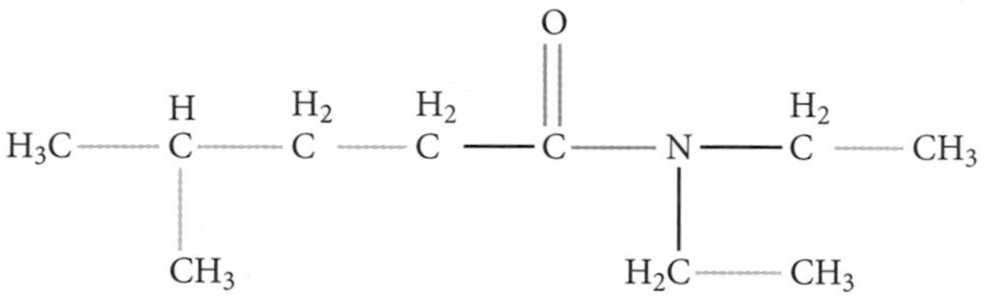

N, N-Diethyl^{-3}-methylbutanamide

Figure 1.71 The IUPAC name of an amide. An amide-containing compound has a characteristic chemical structure that is indicated by the attachment of a nitrogen atom to a carbonyl group.

As shown in **Figure 1.70**, when an acid (salicylic acid) and an alcohol (methanol) interact with each other, an ester (methyl salicylate) is produced. Methyl salicylate (BenGay) is used as a topical drug to temporarily relieve minor muscle pain. Even though it is a topical formulation, if applied extensively to children, this product can result in salicylate poisoning. Heat, young age, and inflammation are all factors that can increase topical salicylate absorption, thereby increasing the risk of salicylate poisoning.

Amides

Amides are derivatives of carboxylic acids in which the hydroxyl group is replaced by a nitrogen group. In naming amides, you find the longest carbon chain and give the lowest number to the carbonyl group. Change the name of the acid by dropping the "oic" or "ic" ending and adding the suffix "-amide" (**Figure 1.71**).

Most amides are solids at room temperature. They have high boiling points, but as more hydrogen atoms are replaced on the nitrogen atom, the boiling point decreases. Regardless of any hydrogen substitution on nitrogen, the carbonyl group is still present—which leads to a dipole–dipole interaction (recall that this property applies to the aldehyde and ketone groups as well). As a result, both substituted and unsubstituted amides can form hydrogen bonds to water, thereby being water soluble. Unlike amines, amides are not bases due to their resonance stability (**Figure 1.72**).

Amides are relatively stable to acid–base hydrolysis due to their resonance stability (the unshared electrons are no longer located solely on N but rather are spread over O, C, and N). This is an advantage when seeking to synthesize drugs with prolonged activity (see the sulfanilamide example in this chapter). Hydrolysis by amidase enzymes can occur, which yields a carboxylic acid (similar to hydrolysis of esters) and an amino group. A typical example is the hydrolysis of lidocaine (Lidoderm) (**Figure 1.73**).

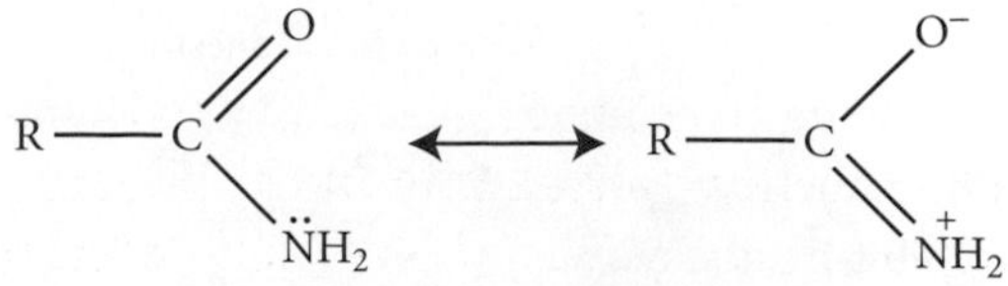

Resonance stability

Figure 1.72 Resonance stability of amides.

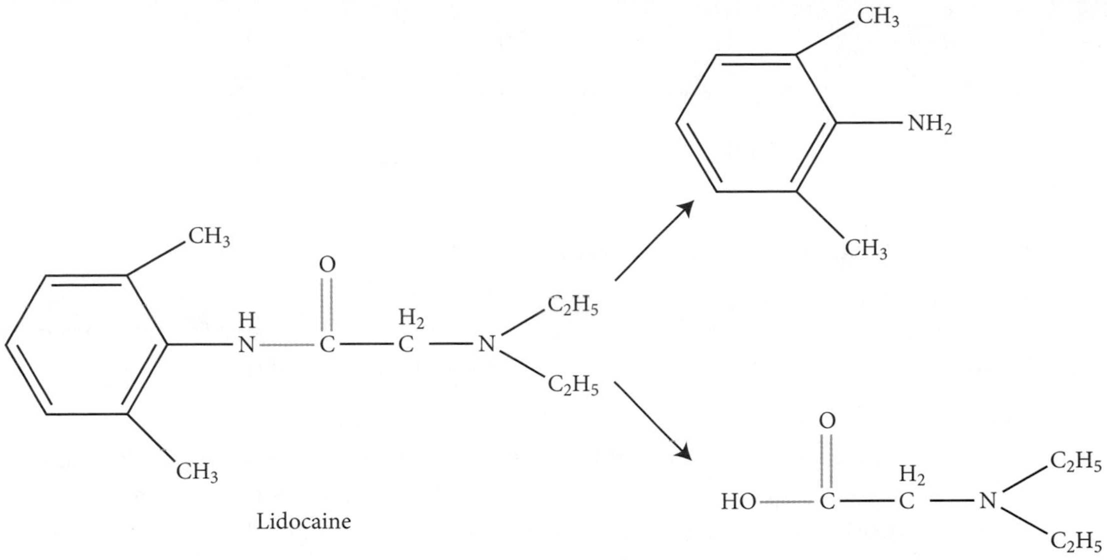

Figure 1.73 Hydrolysis of amides occurs by amidase enzymes during Phase I reactions.

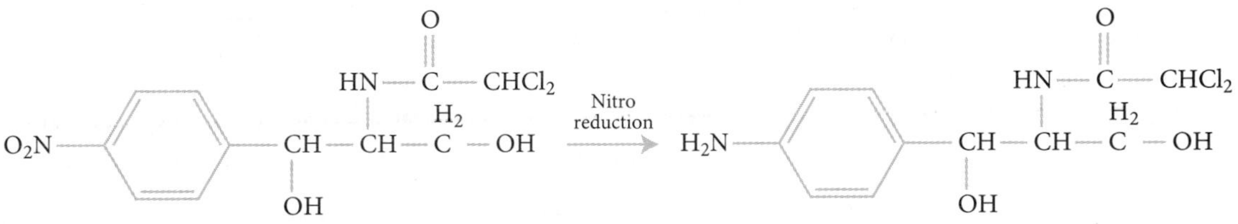

Figure 1.74 Reduction of a nitro group to an amino group is the usual metabolic pathway for nitro groups.

Nitro Groups

Nitro groups consist of a nitrogen atom joined to two oxygen atoms; that is, NO_2. The nitrogen atom is positively charged and the oxygen atoms are partially negatively charged. Nitro groups have a powerful attraction for electrons, meaning that they are strong electron-withdrawing groups. Such groups are commonly found in aromatic chemistry but much less commonly encountered in aliphatic chemistry. Reduction of the nitro group to the corresponding amine is the usual metabolic pathway for drugs that possess a nitro group (**Figure 1.74**). A typical example is the chloramphenicol antibiotic (Chloromycetin, from Canada).

Sulfonic Acids and Sulfonamides

Sulfonic acids are named by first naming the hydrocarbon group as a separate word and then following it with the words "sulfonic acid." Because of the electron-withdrawing property of the SO_2 group, sulfonic acid has a higher acidity than either phenol or carboxylic acid (**Figure 1.75**) Similar to sulfonic acid, a sulfonamide can be named by first naming the carbon group as a separate word and then following it with the word "sulfonamide."

A wide range of drugs contain sulfonamide; these so-called sulfa drugs include diuretics, oral antidiabetic agents, antibiotics, and carbonic anhydrase inhibitors. Sulfa drug antibiotics work by inhibiting nucleic acid (DNA and RNA) synthesis. Such drugs are used to treat a variety of infections—for example, urinary tract infections, infections of the mucous membranes, gut infections, and pneumonia. Today, the antibiotic sulfonamides have largely been replaced by newer antibiotics

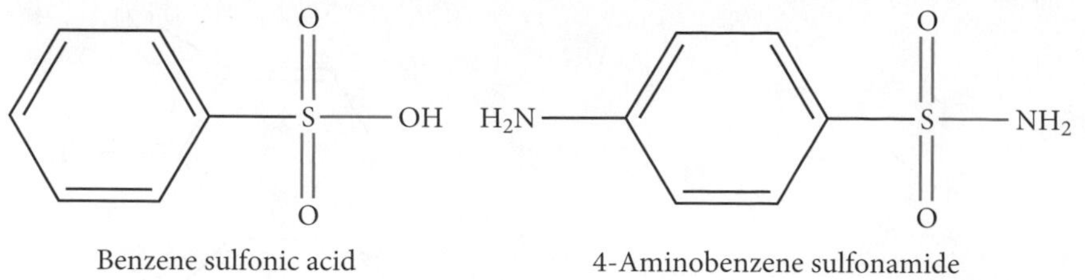

Benzene sulfonic acid   4-Aminobenzene sulfonamide

Figure 1.75 Structures of sulfonic acids and sulfonamides.

owing to the development of bacterial resistance to the older agents. However, a few sulfonamides, including mafenide acetate (Sulfamylon), are still used to treat second- and third-degree burns.

Sulfanilamide (Prontosil) was introduced in the 1930s by the pharmaceutical company Bayer as an antibiotic agent to treat bacterial infections. Prontosil had been shown to inhibit the growth of streptococci. The discovery of Prontosil led to Gerhard Domagk receiving the Nobel Prize in medicine in 1939. When Domagk checked Prontosil on a bacterial culture, the drug did not show any antibacterial effect. However, the research indicated that the drug should have an effective antibacterial effect in humans. Domagk showed that Prontosil was metabolized to sulfanilamide, which explained why Prontosil did not exert any antibacterial effect on a bacterial culture. Prontosil is no longer marketed.

Sulfonamides have low water solubility and weak acidity because the hydrogen attached to the nitrogen is made acidic by the strongly electron-withdrawing SO_2 group. This property ensures that sulfonamides readily form salts with bases. One of the major problems with sulfa drugs, which often justifies their discontinuation in human patients, is that they cause allergic reactions.

Learning Bridge 1.5

Lidocaine (Lidoderm) is a local topical anesthetic. Your job in a pharmaceutical company is to see if you can form a salt of a lidocaine powder. Pick up the lidocaine package insert from your pharmacy site and look at the structure of this compound. As you can see, there are two nitrogen atoms in lidocaine.

A. How would you form a salt of this drug?
B. Which amino group would you use to form the salt? Why?
C. Why do you want to form a salt of the lidocaine powder?

Thioethers

The names of thioethers (or thiols) are formed by using the prefix names for the groups R and R′ in alphabetical order as separate words, then adding the class name "sulfoxide" or "sulfone" (**Figure 1.76**). Thioethers are commonly oxidized to sulfoxide or sulfone (**Figure 1.77**).

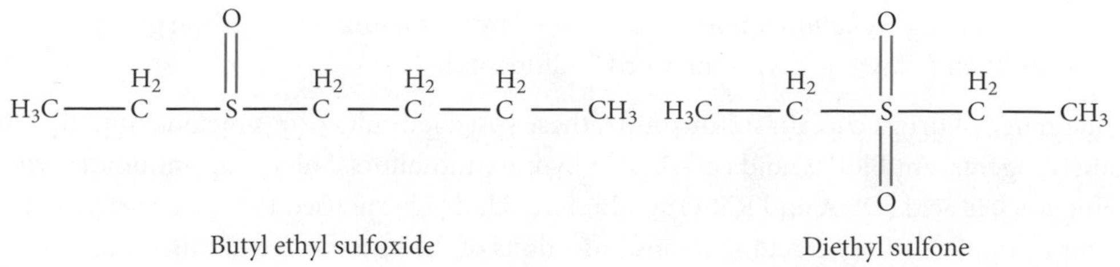

Butyl ethyl sulfoxide   Diethyl sulfone

Figure 1.76 Structures of thioethers.

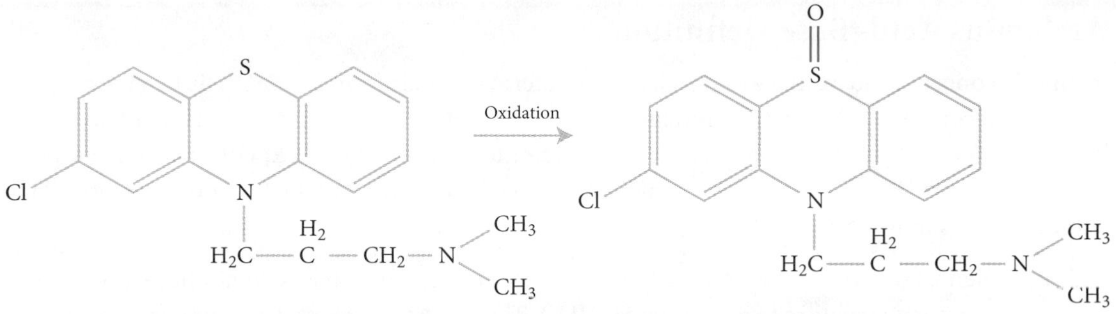

Figure 1.77 Thioethers are commonly oxidized to sulfoxide or sulfone. One example is chlorpromazine, which is used as an antipsychotic and antiemetic drug in the United States and Canada.

Disulfides play an important role in the stability of protein structures (their important biological role is discussed in the *Introduction to Biochemistry* chapter). The formula for disulfides is R—S—S—R. Disulfides are often prone to reduction, where the disulfide bridge is reduced by addition of hydrogen atoms:

$$R-S-S-R \rightarrow R-SH + R-SH$$

Drug Molecules as Acids and Bases

Most drugs are small organic molecules that act in solution as either weak acids or weak bases. To understand drugs and their actions, you must have a good command of acid–base theory. Let's start with the following concepts:

- Electrolytes
- Acid–base definitions
- Acid–base parameters (pH, K_a, and pK_a)

Electrolytes

An electrolyte is a compound that, when dissolved in a solvent (usually water), conducts electricity because it dissociates into ions (charged species). Negative ions move toward a positive terminal (or anode), while positive ions move toward a negative terminal (or cathode). This kind of ion movement allows the passage of electrical current through the solution.

There are two kinds of electrolytes:

- *Strong electrolytes*: These compounds dissociate almost completely into ions in solution, like HCl (a strong acid) or NaOH (a strong base).

- *Weak electrolytes*: These compounds dissociate only to small extent into ions in a solution, like acetic acid (a weak acid). Because many drugs are weak acids, you will find many of them function as weak electrolytes.

Three concepts are used to define acids and bases: (1) Arrhenius acid–base theory, (2) Brønsted-Lowry acid–base theory (often referred to as the Brønsted definition), and (3) Lewis acid–base theory.

Arrhenius Acid–Base Definition

With this concept, acids and bases are classified in terms of their formula and their behavior in water. According to the Arrhenius definition, an acid is a chemical substance that contains a hydrogen atom in its formula and dissociates in water to produce H_3O^+ (i.e., $H_2O + H^+$). Examples include HCl and HNO_3. A base is a chemical substance that contains an OH group in its formula and dissociates in water to yield OH^- (i.e., hydroxide). Examples include KOH and NaOH.

The Arrhenius definition does not include all bases, because some bases do not have any OH groups in their structure (e.g., ammonia, NH_3). The Brønsted-Lowry definition, in contrast, addresses this possibility.

Brønsted-Lowry Acid–Base Definition

With this concept, acids and bases are classified according to their ability to perform a proton (H^+) transfer. An acid is any species that donates a proton; it must have a hydrogen atom in its formula. Thus all Arrhenius acids are also Brønsted-Lowry acids. Examples include HCl and HNO_3. A base is any species that accepts a proton; the base must have lone-pair electrons to accept that proton. Thus all Arrhenius bases are also Brønsted-Lowry bases.

Lewis Acid–Base Definition

The Lewis acid–base definition highlights the role of electron pairs. An acid is any species that accepts an electron pair; an example is the electron-deficient hydrogen ion (H^+). A base is any species that donates an electron pair; an example is the electron-rich ammonia, NH_3:

$$NH_3 + H^+ \rightarrow NH_4^+$$

In this example, H^+ acts as a Lewis acid and accepts a pair of electrons from ammonia. Ammonia is a Lewis base because it donates a pair of electrons to H^+.

The Lewis acid–base definition is much broader than the Brønsted definition. In other words, it includes acids and bases that neither the Arrhenius nor Brønsted definition covers. For example, when an electron-poor molecule, such as BF_3, reacts with ammonia, the BF_3 acts as an acid—a condition that cannot be explained by the Arrhenius and Brønsted definitions (**Figure 1.78**).

In the Lewis model, electron pairs in an acid–base reaction are not given away from base to acid, but rather are shared. Two important conclusions emerge from this model:

1. An electrophile is also an electron-pair acceptor; that is, it is also a Lewis acid.

2. A nucleophile is also an electron-pair donor; that is, it is also a Lewis base.

In this textbook, we will use only the Brønsted-Lowry definition to define an acid or a base.

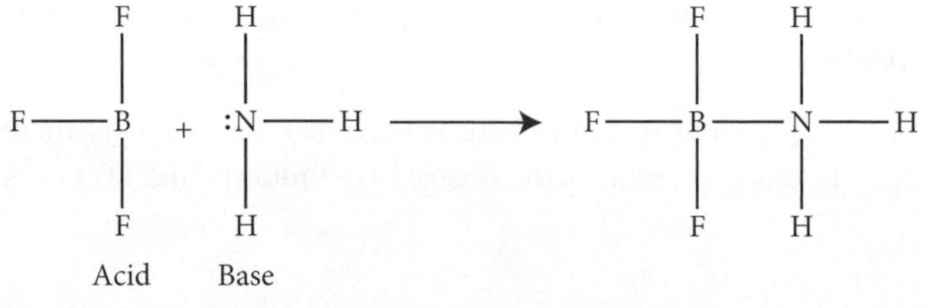

Figure 1.78 BF_3 is a Lewis acid because it is an electron-poor molecule and, as a result, accepts a pair of electrons from ammonia. Ammonia is a Lewis base because it donates a pair of its electrons to BF_3.

Acid–Base Parameters (pH, K_a, and pK_a)

It is important to emphasize a few parameters and concepts in acid–base theory to understand how drugs behave as acids or bases in a solution. Pure water, like any weak acid, slightly dissociates into ions (i.e., OH^- and H_3O^+):

$$H_2O \rightleftharpoons OH^- + H_3O^+ \tag{1.1}$$

Because the dissociation process gives one H_3O^+ ion and one OH^- ion, the concentrations of these two ions are identical. From now on, for simplicity, we will use H^+ instead of H_3O^+. The equilibrium constant for Equation 1.1 is given by the following expression:

$$K_{eq} = \frac{[H^+][OH^-]}{[H_2O]} \tag{1.2}$$

which can be rearranged to give:

$$K_{eq}[H_2O] = [H^+] \times [OH^-] \tag{1.3}$$

The K_{eq} value for water is known (1.8×10^{-16} M). In pure water, the concentration of water is very high: $[H_2O] = 55.5$ M. If we plug these numbers into Equation 1.3, we obtain the ion product of water, K_w:

$$K_{eq}[H_2O] = K_w = [H^+] \times [OH^-] \tag{1.4}$$

$$K_w = 1.8 \times 10^{-16} \text{ M} \times 55.5 \text{ M} = 1 \times 10^{-14} \text{ M}^2 = [H^+] \times [OH^-]$$

As mentioned earlier, in pure water, $[H^+] = [OH^-]$. The last calculation indicates

$$1 \times 10^{-14} \text{ M}^2 = [H^+] \times [OH^-] = [1 \times 10^{-7} \text{ M}] \times [1 \times 10^{-7} \text{ M}]$$

The importance of Equation 1.4 is that it applies to all aqueous solutions that include water. Because K_w is constant for any solution, we can determine the concentration of one species if we know the concentration of the other species. For instance, if an acid is present in water, the concentration of H^+ must be large and the concentration of OH^- must be small.

Example 1.1: The concentration of H^+ in milk is 4.5×10^{-7} M. What is the concentration of OH^- in milk?

Answer: According to Equation 1.4:

$$1 \times 10^{-14} \text{ M}^2 = 4.5 \times 10^{-7} \text{ M} \times [OH^-]$$

$$[OH^-] = 1 \times 10^{-14} \text{ M}^2 / 4.5 \times 10^{-7} \text{ M} = 2.2 \times 10^{-8} \text{ M}$$

It is easier to work with the logarithm (log) of $[H^+]$ to avoid the negative power of 10 (e.g., 1×10^{-x}). Therefore pH = $-\log [H^+]$. The pH for milk in the previous example is

$$pH = -\log [H^+] = -\log (4.5 \times 10^{-7}) = 6.3$$

As you can see, it is easier to say 6.3 than to say the concentration of H^+ is 4.5×10^{-7} M.

If you know the concentration of H^+, you can easily calculate the pH; conversely, if you know the pH, you can easily calculate the concentration of H^+.

$$pH = -\log [H^+]$$

$$[H^+] = \text{antilog of } (-pH)$$

Example 1.2: The large intestine is the most alkaline part of the gastrointestinal tract (its pH is 8.5). What is the concentration of H^+ in the large intestine?

Answer:

$[H^+]$ = antilog of $(-8.5) = 3.16 \times 10^{-9}$ M

The reaction of a weak acid (like acetic acid, hereafter, artificially, called HAc) with water, like any chemical equilibrium, can be expressed by an equation similar to the one that we wrote for water:

$$H_2O + HAc \rightleftharpoons AC^- + H_3O^+ \tag{1.5}$$

Again, for simplicity, we will use H^+ instead of H_3O^+.

In the same way we expressed the equilibrium constant for water, we can express the equilibrium constant for the reaction of an acid with water. In other words, if we multiply the equilibrium constant K_{eq} with the concentration of water, $[H_2O]$, we make a new parameter called K_a.

$$K_{eq} = \frac{[H^+][Ac^-]}{[H_2O][HAc]} \tag{1.6}$$

$$K_{eq}[H_2O] = \frac{[H^+][Ac^-]}{[HAc]} = K_a \tag{1.7}$$

K_a is the dissociation or ionization constant for dissociation of a weak acid—for instance, the dissociation of HAc, acetic acid. Therefore the new reaction at equilibrium will be $HAc \rightleftharpoons AC^- + H_3O^+$ and the ionization constant for this reaction can be expressed as follows:

$$K_a = \frac{[H^+][Ac^-]}{[HAc]} \tag{1.8}$$

As Equation 1.8 indicates, K_a is given by the concentration of the products (H^+ and Ac) divided by the concentration of the reactant (HAc). For the same reason that we mentioned in conjunction with the pH, it is easier to work with the log of K_a to avoid the negative power of 10:

$$pK_a = -\log K_a$$

Strong acids are the acids that completely ionize in a solution. When a strong acid such as HCl dissociates in a solution, the concentrations of the H^+ and conjugate base (Cl^-) are equal to the concentration of the acid:

$$HCl \rightleftharpoons Cl^- + H^+$$

For instance, if you start with 0.7 M HCl, the concentrations of H^+ and Cl^- will be 0.7 M as well. Thus, to measure the pH of a solution containing a strong acid (or base), you need to know only the concentration of that acid (or base).

Example 1.3: What is the pH of a solution when you add 0.3 M nitric acid (a strong acid, HNO_3) into water?

$$HNO_3 \rightleftharpoons NO_3^- + H^+$$

Answer: If you start with 0.3 M HNO_3, the concentrations of H^+ and NO_3^- will be 0.3 M, too.

$$pH = -\log [H^+]$$

$$-\log 0.3 = 0.52$$

Another way to calculate the pH with higher accuracy is to consider the activity of H^+:

$$pH = -\log(\gamma^+ \times [H^+]) \qquad (1.9)$$

where γ^+ is the activity coefficient—that is, the fraction of the actual concentration of the proton that is active. Generally, when you are dealing with nonideal solutions (i.e., solutions with a high concentration of acid or solutions containing many salts), the effective concentration of H^+ is lower than the actual concentration.

Example 1.4: Calculate the pH of 0.1 M HCl with the activity coefficient of 0.83.

Answer: According to Equation 1.9:

$$pH = -\log (\gamma^+ \times [H^+])$$

$$pH = -\log (0.83 \times 0.1 \text{ M}) = 1.08$$

Now that you have learned how to express the dissociation constant, K_a, for weak acids, let's use this constant to calculate the pH of a weak acidic solution. K_a is a constant for a given compound, at a given temperature, and for a weak acid is much less than 1.

Example 1.5: What is the pH of a solution when you add 0.2 M acetic acid (a weak acid, HAc) to water? K_a for acetic acid is 1.74×10^{-5}.

Answer: HAc is a weak acid and will *partially dissociate* in water; that is, HAc (undissociated) will continue to be a significant species in the solution. Thus the solution will contain HAc, Ac^-, and H^+ (**Figure 1.79**).

First write the reaction for the system:

$$HAc \rightleftharpoons AC^- + H_3O^+$$

Next, write the dissociation constant (K_a) for the system:

$$K_a = \frac{[H^+][Ac^-]}{[HAc]}$$

Also write the total concentration of both species in the solution (C_a):

$$C_a = [HAc] + [Ac^-]$$

which we can rewrite as

$$[HAc] = C_a - [Ac^-]$$

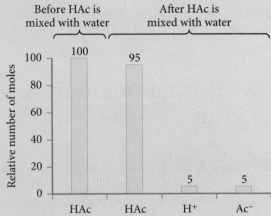

Figure 1.79 When a weak acid is added to water, it will dissociate to only some extent ($\leq 5\%$). The remaining acid ($\geq 95\%$) will remain intact.

Here you are dealing with a weak acid that does not dissociate completely. This means you have to take into account the concentration of HAc because there is a lot of undissociated HAc in the solution (in other words, if all of the HAc was dissociated into Ac^-, no HAc would be left).

Let's rewrite the dissociation constant according to Equation 1.8:

$$K_a = \frac{[H^+][Ac^-]}{C_a - [AC^-]} \qquad (1.10)$$

The concentration of $[Ac^-]$ will be the same as the concentration of $[H^+]$ in the solution, so we can express it as follows:

$$K_a = \frac{[H^+][H^+]}{C_a - [H^+]} \qquad (1.11)$$

which gives

$$[H^+]^2 = K_a (C_a - [H^+]) \qquad (1.12)$$

The square root of Equation 1.12 gives Equation 1.13:

$$[H^+] = \sqrt{K_a(C_a - [H^+])} \qquad (1.13)$$

If the extent of dissociation is small—that is, when you have a weak acid, only 5% of C_a will dissociate ($[H^+] \ll C_a$)—then we have

$$[H^+] = \sqrt{K_a \times C_a} \qquad (1.14)$$

Now let's go back to the original question: What is the pH of a solution when you add 0.2 M acetic acid (a weak acid, HAc) to water? K_a for acetic acid is 1.74×10^{-5}. According to Equation 1.14:

$$H^+ = \sqrt{1.74 \times 10^{-5} \times 0.2 \text{ M}} = 1.86 \times 10^{-3}$$

$$pH = -\log [H^+]; pH = -\log 1.86 \times 10^{-3} = 2.73$$

Check the assumption you made earlier, which was $[H^+] \ll C_a$: $1.8 \times 10^{-3} \ll 0.2$.

In Example 1.5, we did not consider the concentration of H^+ that was contributed by water. Water, as a weak acid, also dissociates; thus the H^+ from water will add to the H^+ that comes from the acid. However, you do not need to account for the concentration of H^+ from water unless you are dealing with a very dilute solution.

Salt Formation, Ionization, and Water Solubility of Drug Molecules

Salt Formation

A salt is formed when an acid is mixed with a base. In such a reaction, the hydrogen atom of the acid is replaced by the cation of the base. Because there are many acids and bases, so there are also many salts. The following reaction is a typical acid–base interaction to form a salt:

$HCl + NaOH \rightarrow NaCl + H_2O$

Acid + Base → Salt + Water

Figure 1.80 shows a salt formation reaction in which a weakly acidic drug is mixed with a strong base (NaOH). Keep in mind that the majority of drugs behave as either weak acids or weak bases.

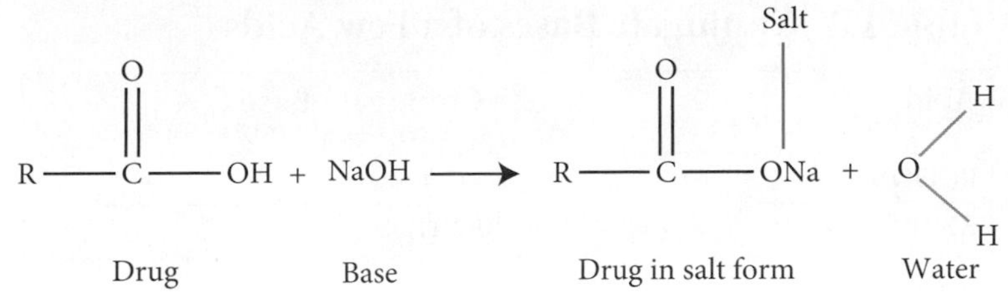

Figure 1.80 Formation of a salt when a weakly acidic drug is mixed with a strong base (NaOH).

Salt Hydrolysis

Most salts are strong electrolytes that completely dissociate into ions in water. When the ions of the salt react with water, the process is called salt hydrolysis. When you think about a salt, realize that the salt, upon dissociation in a solution, changes the pH of the solution. The stronger partner from which the salt is made dominates in the resulting solution. For example, when a salt is formed from a strong acid and a weak base, the salt produces an acidic solution (lower pH of the solution). In other words, the strong acid in this example decrees the final fate of the solution—a low pH.

A few examples of how salts can change the pH of a solution are described here.

Acidic Salt

NH_4Cl (ammonium chloride) is made by mixing a strong acid (HCl) with a weak base (NH_3). If you dissolve NH_4Cl in water, the solution becomes acidic. NH_4Cl, upon dissociation into water, produces NH_4^+, which acts as an acid (because it donates H^+ to the solution) and thereby increases the amount of H^+ in the solution (lowering the pH). In this example, the NH_4Cl is an acidic salt.

NH_4Cl (solid) $\rightarrow NH_4^+$ (aqueous) + Cl^- (aqueous)

$NH_4^+ + H_2O \leftrightarrow NH_3 + H^+$

Basic Salt

If a salt is formed by mixing a strong base with a weak acid, the salt in the solution produces a basic solution (increases the pH of the solution). An example is NaAc (sodium acetate), which is made from a strong base (sodium hydroxide, NaOH) and a weak acid (acetic acid, HAc). The basic (high pH) solution results because Ac^- accepts H^+ from water, which increases the amount of OH^- in the solution. In this case, the NaAc salt is a basic salt.

NaAc (solid) $\rightarrow Ac^-$ (aqueous) + Na^+ (aqueous)

$Ac^- + H_2O \leftrightarrow HAc + OH^-$

If the salt results from the reaction of a strong acid and a strong base, the salt will not change the pH of the solution. An example is table salt, NaCl, which is made from NaOH and HCl. If the salt results from the reaction of a weak acid and a weak base, it will be difficult to predict if the salt will be acidic or basic. Later in this chapter, we show how to calculate the ratio between an acid and its conjugate base by using the Henderson-Hasselbalch equation.

It is important to recognize the conjugate base of an acid. **Table 1.2** identifies a few acids and their conjugate bases.

Table 1.2 Conjugate Bases of a Few Acids

Acid	Conjugate Base
RCOOH	RCOO$^-$
RNH$_3^+$	RNH$_2$
H$_3$PO$_4$	H$_2$PO$_4^-$
H$_2$CO$_3$	HCO$_3^-$

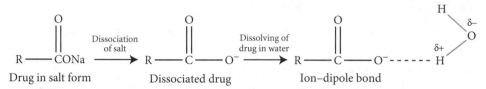

Figure 1.81 Formation of an ion–dipole molecule in a salt hydrolysis process.

Many drugs are provided in the form of salts to increase their water solubility. To confirm this fact, the next time you go to a pharmacy, look at some of the OTC products and see how many of them have "hydrochloride" or "sodium" in their names. When a drug is mixed with NaOH, the drug's name includes "sodium" (e.g., levothyroxine sodium). When a drug is mixed with HCl, the drug's name includes "hydrochloride" (e.g., minocycline hydrochloride).

Figure 1.81 shows how a drug in salt form dissociates first before it interacts with water to form an ion–dipole bond. As seen in the figure, the anion (oxygen) of the drug binds to the electron-deficient region (hydrogen atom) of water.

Example 1.6: Calculate the pH of an 0.3 M solution of NH$_4$Cl (salt). K_b for NH$_3$ is 1.8×10^{-5}.

Answer: NH$_4$Cl is a salt of a weak base (NH3) and a strong acid (HCl). We first write the reaction:

NH4Cl (solid) → NH$_4^+$ (aqueous) + Cl$^-$ (aqueous)

$$NH_4^+ + H_2O \rightleftharpoons NH_3 + H^+$$

The first thing you should think about is whether the salt will act as an acid or a base. In this case, it will work as an acid (see the preceding reaction). Thus what you need to know is K_a, not K_b. The dissociation constant for the acid is

$$K_a = \frac{[NH_3][H^+]}{[NH_4^+]}$$

We utilize the ion product of water to calculate K_a:

$$K_w = K_a \times K_b$$

$$K_a = K_w/K_b$$

We know that $K_w = 1 \times 10^{-14}$ (from the previous section), which in turns means

$$K_a = (1 \times 10^{-14}) / (1.8 \times 10^{-5}) = 5.56 \times 10^{-10}$$

Similar to how we solved the problem for a weak acid (recall the previous section), we can now solve the problem at hand:

$$[H^+] = \sqrt{K_a \times C_a}$$

$$pH = -\log[H^+] = 4.89$$

Example 1.7: What is the pH of an 0.20 M solution of sodium acetate (NaAc)? $K_b = 5.75 \times 10^{-10}$.

Answer: Think about whether the salt will act as an acid or a base. Here, it acts as a base:

NaAc (solid) $\rightarrow$ Ac$^-$ (aqueous) + Na$^+$ (aqueous)

$$AC^- + H_2O \rightleftharpoons HAC + HO^-$$

$$K_b = \frac{[HAc][OH^-]}{[AC^-]}$$

$$[OH^-] = \sqrt{K_b \times C_b}$$

Recall that you have the concentration of OH$^-$, but not H$^+$.

$$[OH^-] = 1.07 \times 10^{-5}$$

To know the pH, you should have the concentration of H$^+$:

$$K_w = [H^+] \times [OH^-]$$

$$[H^+] = K_w/[OH^-]$$

Now one can easily calculate the concentration of H$^+$ and thereby the pH:

$$[H^+] = 1 \times 10^{-14}/[OH^-]$$

$$pH = -\log[H^+] = 9.03$$

So far, you have learned how you can calculate the pH of a solution containing a weak acid. You also have learned that if the extent of dissociation of H$^+$ is low, you can assume that the total concentration of acid in the solution is much higher than the concentration of the dissociated H$^+$ (i.e., Ca >> H$^+$).

But what if you have to deal with an acid for which you have no idea of the extent of H$^+$ dissociation? Could you use the same assumption as we did in the past examples? The short answer is no: If you make the same assumption, you may end up with an incorrect calculation of the pH. If the initial concentration of the weak acid (i.e., when the acid has not yet been in contact with your solution) is at least 100 times higher than its K_a, you can assume that the concentration of H$^+$ that dissociates is negligible compared to the initial concentration of the acid. For instance, in Example 1.6, the initial concentration of the acid (0.3 M) was more than 100 times higher than its K_a (5.56×10^{-10}).

Table 1.3 indicates the strengths of commonly used acidic and basic functional groups. The pK_a values are indicated for the acidic functional groups and for the conjugate acids of the basic functional groups.

Table 1.3 Acid/base Strengths, Based on pK_a Numbers, of Commonly Used Functional Groups in Drug Molecules

Acidic Functional Group	pK_a	Basic Functional Groups	pK_a of Conjugate Acid
R——SO$_3$H	1	R——NH$_2$	10–11
$\overset{\text{O}}{\overset{\|}{\text{R——C——OH}}}$	4–5	$\overset{\text{NH}}{\overset{\|}{\text{R——C——NH}_2}}$	9–10
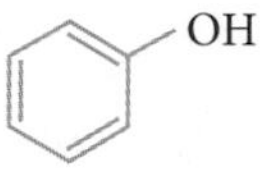 ⬡——OH	8–11	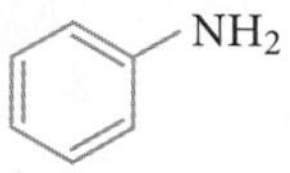 ⬡——NH$_2$	1–5

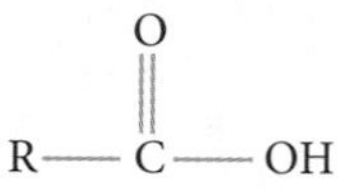

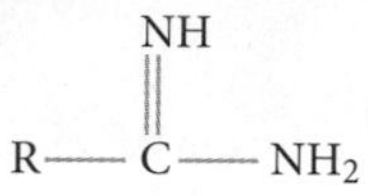

Adapted from Lemke T, Roche V, and Zito W. *Review of Organic Functional Groups: Introduction to Medicinal Organic Chemistry.* Lippincott Williams & Wilkins; 5th edition (2011).

Ionization

Generally, the drugs that are hydrophobic (un-ionized) cross cell membranes more readily than those that are hydrophilic (ionized). Important concepts regarding the acid–base properties of these drugs include the following:

1. Henderson-Hasselbalch equation

2. Titration curve

3. Buffer capacity

Henderson-Hasselbalch Equation

The Henderson-Hasselbalch equation is used to express and calculate the pH of a solution, and thereby to calculate the ionization of a weak acid or base. It fits very well to an acid–base titration curve.

To understand this expression, let's go back to the acetic acid (HAc) ionization and its dissociation constant:

$$HAc \rightleftharpoons AC^- + H^+$$

Because we are interested in knowing the concentration of H$^+$, we can express the dissociation constant as follows:

$$K_a = \frac{[H^+][Ac^-]}{[HAc]} \tag{1.15}$$

which can be rearranged to this expression:

$$[H^+] = K_a \frac{[HAc]}{[Ac^-]} \tag{1.16}$$

We can solve for [H$^+$] by using the negative logarithm of all terms in Equation 1.16:

$$-\log[H^+] = -\log K_a - \log([HAc]/[Ac^-]) \tag{1.17}$$

To cancel the negative sign, we rewrite the last equation to get the Henderson-Hasselbalch equation:

$$pH = pK_a + \log([Ac^-])/[HAc]) \tag{1.18}$$

Equation 1.18 is the same as Equation 1.19, which is also referred to as the Henderson-Hasselbalch equation:

$$pH = pK_a + \log \frac{[\text{Conjugate base}]}{[\text{Acid}]} \qquad (1.19)$$

The Henderson-Hasselbalch equation is a very practical tool when preparing and calculating buffer solutions in a biochemical or compounding laboratory. This equation can be used to estimate the ionization of weakly acidic or basic drugs as well. When a weakly acidic or basic drug is administered and dissolves in the body, the drug ionizes to some extent depending on its pK_a and the pH of the body fluid in which the drug is dissolved in.

We can use the Henderson-Hasselbalch equation to estimate the percentage of ionization of HAc as follows:

For acidic drugs:

$$\% \text{ ionized} = \frac{1 \times 100}{\text{Antilog}\,(pK_a - pH) + 1} \qquad (1.20)$$

For basic drugs:

$$\% \text{ ionized} = \frac{1 \times 100}{\text{Antilog}\,(pH - pK_a) + 1} \qquad (1.21)$$

A few examples will serve to demonstrate how useful Equation 1.20 and Equation 1.21 are.

Example 1.8: What is the percentage ionization of indomethacin (Indocin) ($pK_a = 4.5$; i.e., an acidic drug) in the large intestinal tract (pH = 8.0)?

Answer: We are dealing with an acidic drug, so we use Equation 1.20:

$$\% \text{ ionized} = \frac{1 \times 100}{\text{Antilog}\,(4.5 - 8) + 1} = 99.97\%$$

Example 1.9: What is the percentage ionization of ephedrine ($pK_a = 9.5$; i.e., a basic drug) in the large intestinal tract (pH = 8.0)?

Answer: We are dealing with a basic drug, so we use Equation 1.21:

$$\% \text{ ionized} = \frac{1 \times 100}{\text{Antilog}\,(8 - 9.5) + 1} = 97\%$$

It is very important to know the percentage ionization for a drug. Oral administration of a drug (e.g., tablet, capsule, solution) results in a rapid passage of the drug through the esophagus and into the stomach; upon dissolving there, the drug finds its way quickly into the epithelial cells lining the intestines. The absorption of the drug occurs through the epithelial cells into the blood capillaries of the lamina propria. The blood containing the drug then travels via capillaries to reach the drug's sites of action (see the *Introduction to Pharmacodynamics* and *Introduction to Pharmacokinetics* chapters for more details of drug absorption).

An acidic drug will be un-ionized in an acidic milieu but will become ionized in an alkaline environment. Therefore, an acid in a basic milieu will carry a charge and be unable to directly penetrate cell membranes; by the same token, a base will become ionized in an acidic milieu. Assuming an oral administration of a drug, the drug must go from the lumen of the gastrointestinal (GI) tract to the circulation on the other side of the GI tract. Membranes of the epithelial cells lining the lumen of the GI tract are lipophilic. Un-ionized drugs cross these lipophilic membranes, but ionized drugs do not (**Figure 1.82**). Keep in mind that ionized drugs are hydrophilic, whereas a cell membrane is made of many hydrophobic molecules (see also the *Introduction to Cell Biology* chapter).

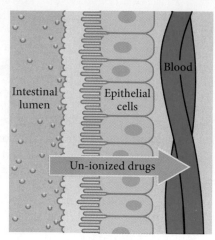

Figure 1.82 An un-ionized drug can readily cross the cell membranes of epithelial cells in the GI tract.

Titration and Buffer Capacity

Titration is an analytical procedure where a solution (often a base) with known volume and known concentration is added to another solution (an acid) with known volume but unknown concentration. This procedure is continued until the acid with unknown concentration has completely reacted with the base. At this point, an equivalence point is reached, where the number of moles of OH^- ions added to the solution equals the number of moles of H^+ ions originally present in the solution. In other words, when you do a titration of a weak acid, the acid dissociates in the solution to yield a small amount of H^+ ions. If you add a base (OH^-) to this solution, the OH^- ions react with the H^+ ions to form water (H_2O). Consequently, more H^+ ions dissociate and more OH^- ions react with H^+ to form more water, until you reach the equivalence point where there is no further H^+ left from the acid to be dissociated.

Learning Bridge 1.6

On the last day of your introductory pharmacy practice experience (IPPE), your preceptor gives you two assignments to see how you would apply your basic sciences knowledge to solve a water solubility problem.

A. Acetylcholi ne has an amino group and is a neurotransmitter that is involved in muscle contraction. Your preceptor asks you this question: If you were in charge of increasing the water solubility of acetylcholine, what could you do to make a salt of this neurotransmitter compound? She asks you to justify your answer. The structure of acetylcholine is shown in **Exhibit 1.2**.

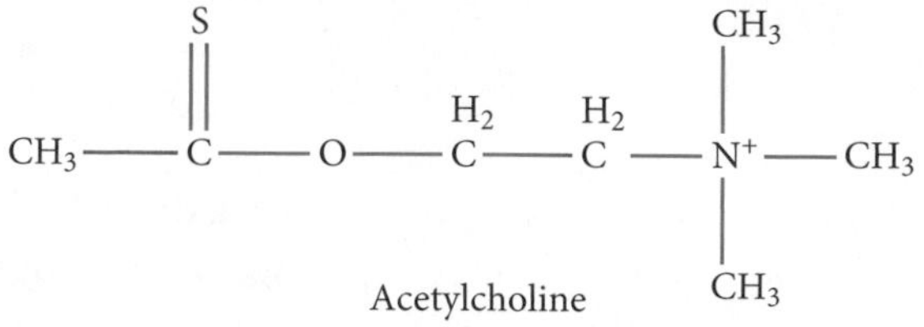

$$CH_3-\overset{\overset{\displaystyle S}{\|}}{C}-O-\overset{H_2}{C}-\overset{H_2}{C}-\overset{\overset{\displaystyle CH_3}{|}}{\underset{\underset{\displaystyle CH_3}{|}}{N^+}}-CH_3$$

Acetylcholine

Exhibit 1.2 Acetylcholine.

B. Levothyroxine is a thyroid hormone that is used to treat hypothyroidism. A solution contains levothyroxine and its salt, levothyroxine sodium. Explain what would happen if an acetic acid solution was added to this solution. The structures of free levothyroxine and its salt form (levothyroxine sodium) are shown in **Exhibit 1.3**.

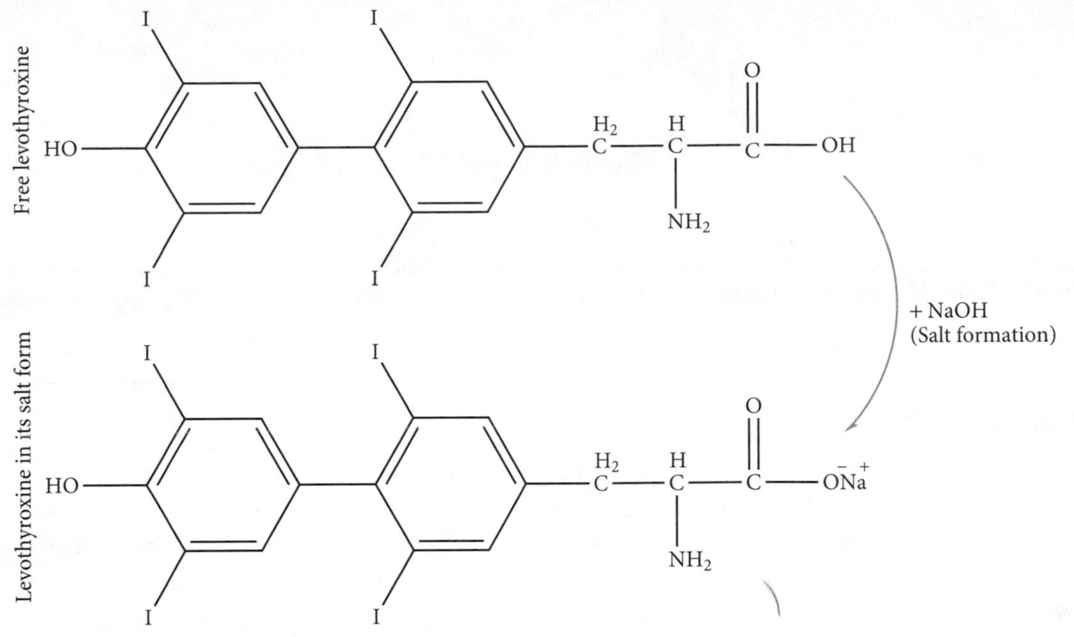

Exhibit 1.3 Free levothyroxine and its salt form (levothyroxine sodium).

Figure 1.83 demonstrates how a titration curve behaves during an acid–base titration experiment. As indicated, when 0.5 NaOH mole equivalent is added, half of the acetic acid has been dissociated so that the concentration of the proton acceptor (the conjugate base, Ac^-) is equal to the concentration of the proton donor (HAc). Based on the titration curve and the Henderson-Hasselbalch equation, if the concentration of the conjugate base is equal to the concentration of the acid, the pH of a solution is exactly the same as the pK_a of the acid (as shown in Figure 1.19 and **Figure 1.84**).

A titration curve shows the buffering range of a solution—that is, the points where the pH changes are minimal upon addition of an acid or a base to the solution. Such a curve allows you to calculate the concentration of an acid or base in a solution and assists you in calculating the pK_a value.

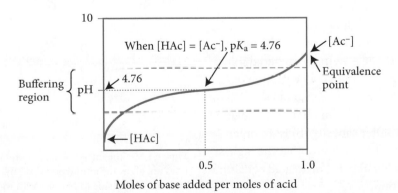

Figure 1.83 A titration curve is produced when a known concentration of strong base (NaOH) is titrated with an unknown concentration of a weak acid (HAc).

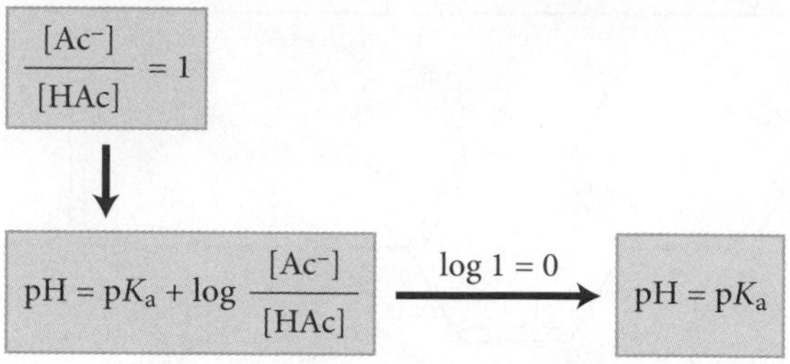

$$\boxed{\dfrac{[Ac^-]}{[HAc]} = 1}$$

$$\boxed{pH = pK_a + \log \dfrac{[Ac^-]}{[HAc]}} \xrightarrow{\log 1 = 0} \boxed{pH = pK_a}$$

Figure 1.84 In a buffer solution, when the concentration of an acid equals the concentration of its conjugate base, the pK_a of the acid equals the pH of the solution.

Learning Bridge 1.7

Suppose you have been asked to calculate the concentration of 10 mL vinegar in one of the compounding labs at your pharmacy program. One technique to measure the concentration of an acid (or a base) is to do a titration experiment. Suppose you add NaOH to the vinegar solution until you reach the equivalence point (you notice the equivalence point by using a pH paper that shows you a pH of 7.0—that is, it identifies when the vinegar is neutralized). To reach the equivalence point, you add 60 mL of 0.1 M NaOH. How would you calculate the concentration of the unknown acid (vinegar)?

Let's go back to Figure 1.83 and see how this titration curve can help us to identify two important pieces of data. First, the region in which the pH changes very little (i.e., −1 and +1 of the pK_a), which in our case is between 3.76 and 5.76, is called the buffering region. Second, the buffering capacity is highest when pH is equal to pK_a—that is, when HAc = Ac$^-$. Thus, when a drug's pK_a is equal to the pH of its milieu (the milieu could be a solution in a beaker, in your blood, in your stomach, or something else), the drug exists as 50% ionized and 50% un-ionized. In other words, the pK_a indicates the form (ionized or un-ionized) that a drug has at a given pH value.

The buffer capacity (β) describes how effectively a buffer can resist changes in the pH of a solution. It can be calculated for a solution by using Equation 1.22, where C is the molar concentration of the acid in the buffered solution. Assuming a constant concentration of C, the closer the dissociation constant (K_a) is to the concentration of the proton (H$^+$) in the solution, the higher the buffer capacity (β) is. In other words, Equation 1.22 indicates that the highest β is achieved when the pK_a of an acid equals the pH of the solution.

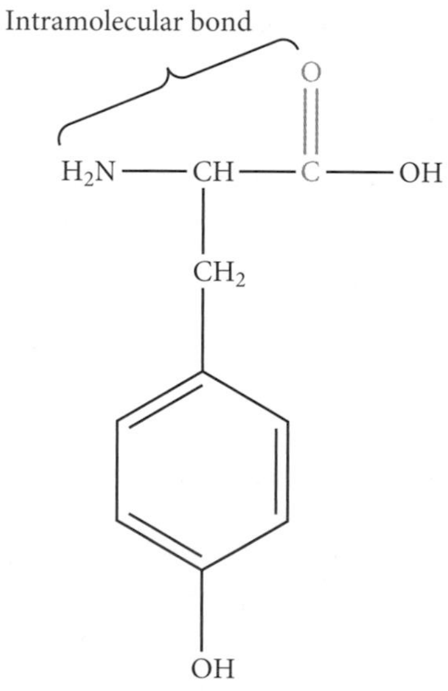

Figure 1.85 The intramolecular bond highlighted here does not allow the amino and carbonyl groups of the amino acid tyrosine to interact with water molecules.

$$\beta = \frac{2.3\,C\,K_a[H^+]}{(K_a + [H^+])^2} \qquad\qquad (1.22)$$

Example 1.10: Assume 0.20 M of an acetic acid solution is added to a solution that has a pH of 3.0. Calculate the buffer capacity for (1) the new solution, (2) a solution that has a pH of 4.76, and (3) a solution that has a pH of 5.76. The pK_a for acetic acid is 4.76.

Answer: First, take the –antilog of pK_a and pH to calculate K_a and $[H^+]$, respectively. Second, use Equation 1.22 to calculate the buffer capacity.

1. 0.008

2. 0.11

3. 0.04

As the results indicate, the highest buffer capacity is achieved when the pK_a is equal to the pH of the solution (i.e., answer 2).

Maintenance of the correct pH in the body is vital because pH alters the ionization of amino acids, the building blocks of proteins. As discussed in the *Introduction to Biochemistry* chapter, a change in the amino acid structure of a protein may change the ionization of the protein and, as a result, lead to inactivation of the protein. The body can tolerate a very small change in the blood's pH (pH 7.4 ± 0.3). A pH outside this range is life threatening because vital proteins lose the integrity of their structures and functions. In addition, distortion of the pH of blood leads to acidosis or alkalosis. The pH of body fluids is maintained by three major buffer systems: (1) HCO_3^-/H_2CO_3, (2) organic phosphates, and (3) proteins. All three buffers are present in the intracellular and extracellular fluids. The concepts of acidosis and alkalosis and the importance of maintaining a buffer system in the human body are discussed in the *Introduction to Nutrients* chapter.

Learning Bridge 1.8

Buffering dosage forms are used as antacids to neutralize "heartburn." While antacids neutralize the excess acid, they do not eliminate the "heartburn" condition. As a result, they should not be used for more than 2 weeks. During one of your intern hours at your introductory pharmacy practice experience (IPPE) site, one of the pharmacy technicians asks you to help her understand how some of the antacids work. She asks you two questions:

A. How does the antacid milk of magnesia work?

B. Alka-Seltzer (Alamag) is an analgesic OTC drug that contains a mixture of sodium bicarbonate ($NaHCO_3$), aspirin, and citric acid. Which of these three components acts as an antacid, and why?

Help the pharmacy technician to understand how the above antacids work.

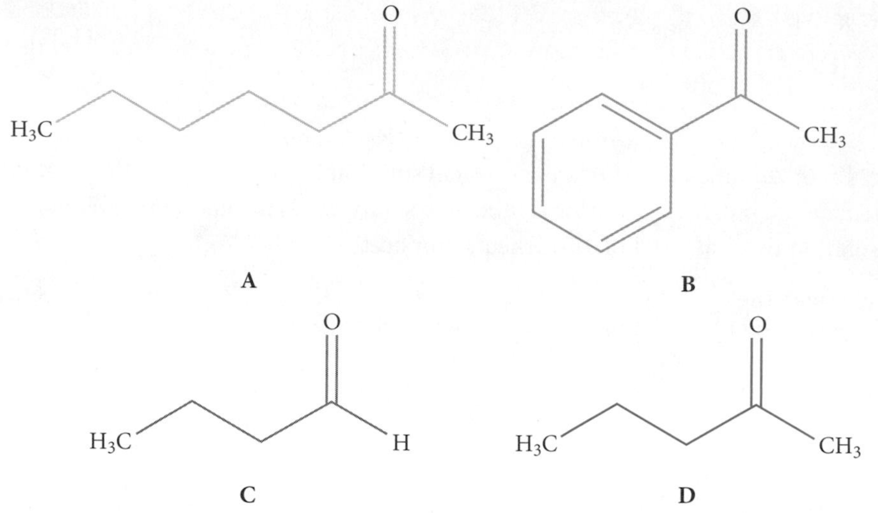

Figure 1.86 Four different molecules with different solubilities in water.

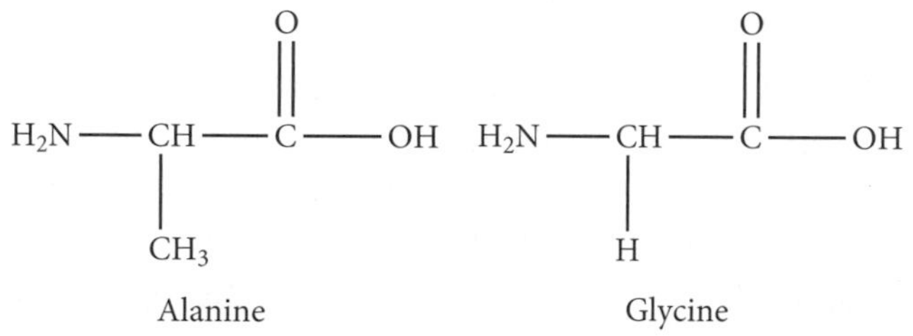

Figure 1.87 The side chains (CH_3 and H) are bound to a similar electronegative atom (C) in both amino acids. No electron attraction occurs between these atoms (between C and H); as a result, their side chain is nonpolar.

Water Solubility of Drug Molecules

For a molecule (drug) to be able to dissolve in water, the intramolecular and intermolecular bonds must first be broken so that water molecules can bind to the functional groups of the drug. Water is an ideal solvent because it is inexpensive, it is inert (i.e., has no pharmacological activity of its own), it is widely available, and its physical and chemical characteristics are well known.

Let's look at the structure of the amino acid tyrosine (**Figure 1.85**). The carboxyl group and amino group of tyrosine have opposite charges and, therefore, can interact with each other (i.e., intramolecular bonding). This means a water molecule cannot undertake an ion–dipole interaction to dissolve tyrosine. The phenol group by itself cannot dissolve tyrosine in water. As a result, tyrosine has a poor solubility in water. To break down the intramolecular bond, one can add NaOH or HCl (salt formation). This reaction enhances the water solubility of the salt.

Let's look at the structure of the four molecules in **Figure 1.86** to see which one has the highest water solubility and which one has the lowest water solubility. Molecule A has the longest carbon groups and, therefore, is hydrophobic (water insoluble). Molecule B has a benzene ring, so it is also hydrophobic. Molecules C and D are both less hydrophobic than A and B. In general, small ketones are more water soluble than small aldehydes. Molecule A is the least water-soluble molecule, and molecule D is the most water-soluble molecule. Generally speaking, functional groups such as amino, hydroxyl, ester, nitro, and amide groups increase the water solubility of a drug, whereas aliphatic carbons, benzene rings, and halogens decrease the water solubility of a drug.

Greater water solubility, to some degree, will usually improve a drug's distribution within the circulatory system and increase its action. Drugs that are administered orally as solids or in the suspension form must be dissolved in the body's gastric fluid (an aqueous milieu) before they can be absorbed and transported to their site of action. The process in which the drug is dissolved in gastric fluid is called dissolution. The rate of dissolution depends on a few chemical and physical factors (these factors are discussed in the *Introduction to Pharmaceutics* chapter). However, the extent of dissolution depends only on the solubility of the drug, which in turn depends on the structure of the drug. Keep in mind that sometimes it is essential for drugs to have poor water solubility to achieve the best effect; for instance, if a drug has to pass through a membrane, it must be significantly hydrophobic.

Let's look at the structure of amino acids alanine and glycine. The R chain plays an important role in the solubility of an amino acid. The R chains of both alanine and glycine are nonpolar, which explains why these two amino acids are not water soluble (**Figure 1.87**).

Learning Bridge 1.9

Amy comes to your pharmacy to ask you about her concern regarding an OTC product that she has been using during the last two days. Amy has been using Anbesol (benzocaine with 0.5% phenol) to relieve the temporary pain of her orthodontic irritation. She just read the label for Anbesol and noticed that it contains phenol. Because Amy knows that phenol is a toxic molecule, she is worried that the phenol may have caused some damage to her mouth.

In addition, Amy mentions that last weekend while she was hiking, she came in contact with poison ivy. She has some skin irritation as a result of this contact and asks you if there is any OTC product to treat the poison ivy exposure.

A. How would you answer Amy's question about Anbesol?
B. How would you answer her question about relief from the poison ivy skin irritation?

Golden Keys for Pharmacy Students

1. Pharmacy education requires a solid foundation in chemistry. The more familiar you are with organic and inorganic chemistry, the better and faster you will understand many pharmaceutical topics, such as medicinal chemistry, biochemistry, pharmacology, and pharmaceutics.

2. Oxidation and reduction are very common reactions in biochemistry and metabolism of drugs. You must learn the basic concepts and mechanisms behind these two types of reactions.

3. Alcohols are readily available in many Western countries, are components of a few medications, and are the most widely available poison in the world.

4. Chemical bonds are divided into two major classes: covalent and noncovalent bonds. Pay special attention to ion–dipole and hydrogen bonds, which play important roles in salt hydrolysis of drugs and the structure and function of proteins, respectively.

5. It is important to recognize the different medicinal functional groups. These functional groups often maintain the integrity, stability, and pharmacological functionality of drugs.

6. Amines and carboxyl groups are the two most commonly encountered functional groups in drug structures. Both of these functional groups are important for salt formation, salt hydrolysis, and water solubility of drugs.

7. It is important to recognize the differences and similarities between amine and amide functional groups.

8. Alkyls are electron-releasing groups; aryls are electron-withdrawing groups. Attachment of these two functional groups to amines and carboxylic acids alters their basicity and acidic strength, respectively.

9. Esters are prone to hydrolysis. Hydrolysis of esters occurs in the presence of water, strong acids such as HCl, and esterase enzymes. Upon hydrolysis of an ester, an alcohol and a carboxylic acid are formed.

10. The Brønsted-Lowry acid–base definition is commonly used to express the acidic or basic properties of acids and bases. One simple reason why this definition is employed is because the proton transfer is readily visible in reaction schemes and equations when basic and acidic drugs participate in salt formation and salt hydrolysis, and for the indication of water solubility.

11. K_a is the dissociation or ionization constant for dissociation of a weak acid. The negative logarithm of K_a and the concentration of protons (H^+) are used in the form of pK_a and pH, respectively.

12. The equation $H^+ = \sqrt{K_a \times C_a}$ is very useful to calculate the pH of a weak acidic solution.

13. The equation $[OH^-] = \sqrt{K_b \times C_b}$ is very useful to calculate the pH of a weak basic solution.

14. A salt is formed when an acid is mixed with a base. Formation of a salt is often used to increase the water solubility of drugs in the pharmaceutical industry. However, if the salt cannot be hydrolyzed in water (i.e., if salt hydrolysis does not occur), the drug will not dissolve in water.

15. If a salt is formed by mixing a strong acid and a weak base, the salt, upon hydrolysis in a solution, reduces the pH of the solution. Conversely, if a salt is formed by mixing a weak acid and a strong base, the salt, upon hydrolysis in a solution, increases the pH of the solution.

16. If the initial concentration of the weak acid (i.e., when the acid has not been in contact with the new solution yet) is at least 100 times higher than its K_a, you can assume that the concentration of dissociated H^+ is negligible.

17. Hydrophobic (un-ionized) drugs cross cell membranes better than hydrophilic (ionized) drugs.

18. The Henderson-Hasselbalch equation is used to calculate the pH of a solution and to calculate the ionization of a weak acid or weak base. It fits very well to an acid–base titration curve. $pH = pK_a + \log \dfrac{[\text{Conjugate base}]}{[\text{Acid}]}$.

19. The percentage of ionization of acidic and basic drugs can be estimated by using two equations: for acidic drugs, $\%\text{ ionized} = \dfrac{1 \times 100}{\text{Antilog}(pK_a - pH) + 1}$, and for basic drugs, $\%\text{ ionized} = \dfrac{1 \times 100}{\text{Antilog}(pH - pK_a) + 1}$.

20. Titration is an analytical procedure where a solution (often a base) with known volume and known concentration is added to another solution (an acid) with known volume but unknown concentration. This procedure is continued until the number of moles of OH⁻ ions added to the solution is equal to the number of moles of H⁺—that is, until an equivalence point is reached.

21. An acidic drug will be un-ionized in an acidic milieu but will ionize in an alkaline environment. Therefore, an acid in a basic milieu will carry a charge and be unable to directly penetrate cell membranes; by the same token, a base will ionize in an acidic milieu.

22. Attachment of functional groups such as amino, hydroxyl, ester, nitro, and amide groups to the structure of drugs increases the water solubility of the drugs. Conversely, attachment of functional groups such as aliphatic carbons, benzene rings, and halogens decreases the water solubility of drugs.

23. If you know the concentration of OH⁻ but not H⁺, use the ion product of water to calculate the concentration of the H⁺: $[K_w] = H^+ \times OH^- = 1 \times 10^{-14}$.

24. A solution containing a strong acid is not a buffer, and its pH can be calculated directly from the acid concentration alone. All of the strong acid dissociates into H⁺. The following equation can be used directly: $pH = -\log[H^+]$.

25. A solution containing a strong base is not a buffer, and the [OH⁻] can be calculated directly from the base concentration alone. If you know [OH⁻], use K_w to calculate [H⁺].

Learning Bridge Answers

1.1 You should refuse to fill this individual's medication, as there is a potential risk for severe nausea, tachycardia and orthostatic hypotension, palpitations, chest pain, and dyspnea. The most alarming side effect is the orthostatic hypotension, which can be fatal. Ask the patient to come back after 24 hours and be observant to ensure that he does not smell of alcohol before you fill his medication. It is very important to be familiar with drugs that produce a "disulfiram-like" effect so that you can counsel patients to avoid using alcohol while taking these medications.

1.2 **A.** In 2001, the FDA approved fomepizole for the treatment of methanol and ethylene glycol poisoning. This drug acts by blocking the alcohol dehydrogenase enzyme, thereby inhibiting oxidization of ethylene glycol and methanol. It has been suggested, based on *in vitro* studies, that fomepizole has approximately 8,000 times higher affinity than ethanol for alcohol dehydrogenase. Sometimes ethanol is given to methanol-intoxicated patients to counteract the effect of methanol, because ethanol has 10–20 times greater affinity for alcohol dehydrogenase than methanol does (a competitive inhibitor of alcohol dehydrogenase enzyme; see the *Introduction to Biochemistry* chapter). This inhibition blocks methanol's access to this enzyme, which in turn impairs the metabolism of methanol (i.e., ethanol or fomepizole keeps the enzyme busy). Recall that it is not the methanol itself that is a killer, but rather its metabolites (formaldehyde and formic acid).

B. Fomepizole (Antizol) is known to inhibit alcohol dehydrogenase, which otherwise catalyzes the metabolism of ethanol, ethylene glycol, and methanol. As a result, fomepizole is indicated in the treatment of methanol or ethylene glycol poisoning. Disulfiram (Antabuse) inhibits the aldehyde dehydrogenase enzyme, so it is not helpful in the case of methanol poisoning.

1.3 **A.** Because acetylsalicylic acid is an ester molecule, it is prone to nucleophilic attack by OH⁻ from the bathroom's moisture (see **Exhibit 1.4**). Aspirin, upon hydrolysis, is broken down into acetic acid (a carboxylic group) and an alcohol group (salicylic acid). Vinegar has 5–10% acetic acid, so the carboxylic acid part (acetic acid) is responsible for the odor of vinegar. Acetic acid is used for formation of acetylsalicylic acid (aspirin) from salicylic acid. When the concentration of acetic acid is greater than 50%, however, the solution can damage the skin, eyes, nose, and mouth.

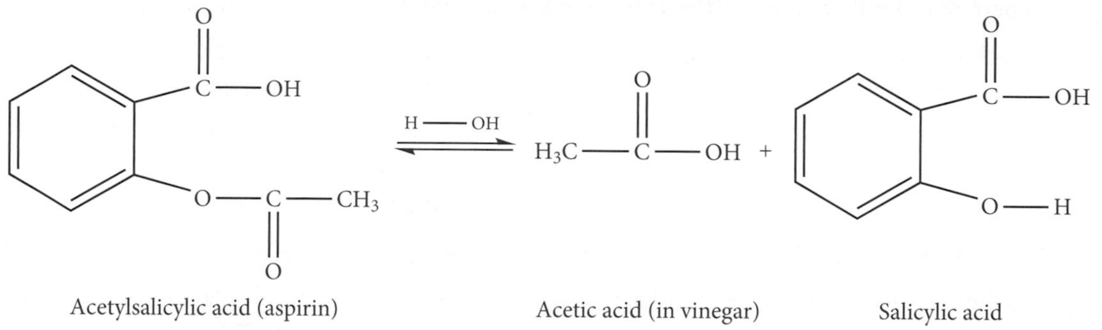

Acetylsalicylic acid (aspirin)   Acetic acid (in vinegar)   Salicylic acid

Exhibit 1.4 Hydrolysis of an ester bond in acetylsalicylic acid (aspirin) produces an acid (a carboxylic group) and an alcohol group (salicylic acid).

Adapted from Timberlake KC. Organic and biological chemistry: structures of life. San Francisco: Benjamin Cummings; 2001.

B. You should advise the woman to not give any aspirin-containing agent to Emily. Aspirin belongs to the category of nonsteroidal anti-inflammatory drugs (NSAIDs). It is most commonly used for its anti-inflammatory effects, but is not recommended for children's fever because it has been associated with Reye syndrome in children. Reye syndrome is a rare, but sometimes fatal condition in children and young adults with viral infection. It may lead to liver damage, cerebral edema, and death. Children with fever should receive acetaminophen or ibuprofen instead of aspirin.

1.4 The opium poppy contains at least 20 alkaloids (e.g., codeine, morphine) (**Exhibit 1.5**). All parts of the poppy, including the seeds, contain morphine. Eating poppy seeds from bread is sufficient to put morphine in Amy's blood sample.

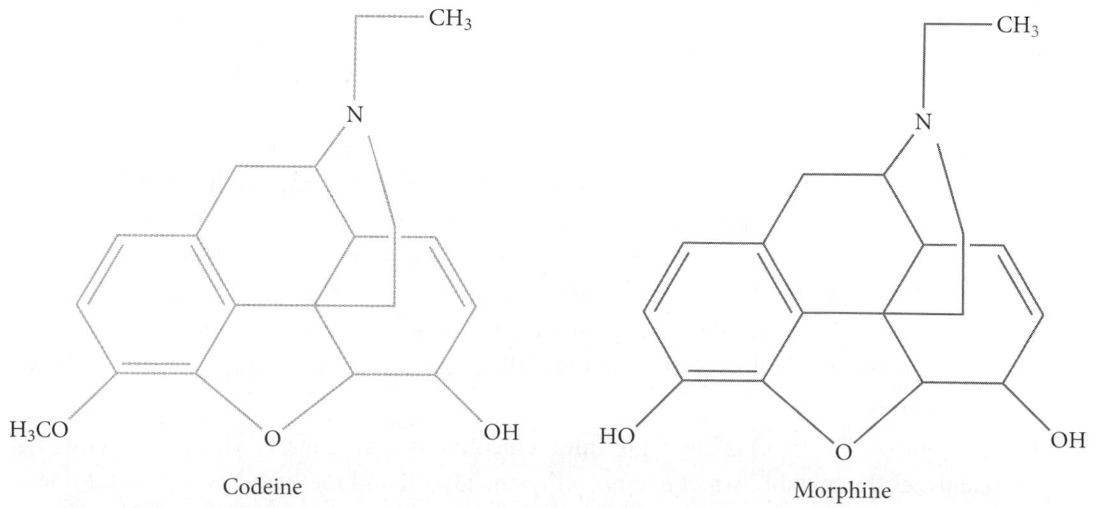

Codeine   Morphine

Exhibit 1.5 Many alkaloids are used as analgesics and for the creation of euphoria.

1.5 The structure of lidocaine is shown in **Exhibit 1.6**.

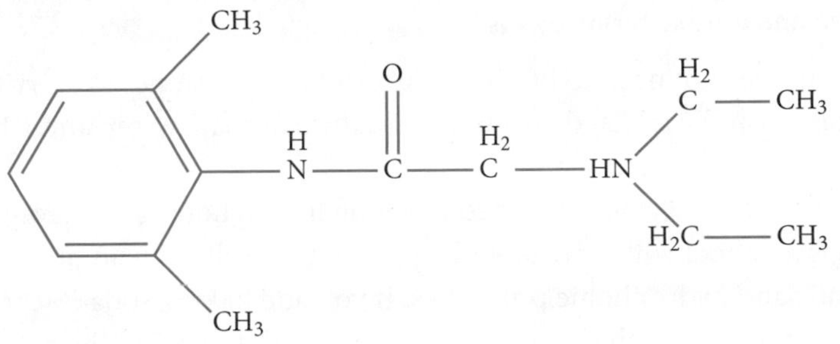

Exhibit 1.6 Lidocaine.

A. Since this drug has a basic amino group, it must work as a basic drug, too. If you mix a base with an acid, you make a salt. Use HCl to make the salt.

B. Unlike amines, amides do not have the basicity property; thus the nitrogen atom in the amide group will not interact with an acid to form a salt.

C. An amine salt is soluble in body fluids (i.e., the salt formation increases the water solubility of the drug).

1.6 **A.** The quaternary nitrogen has no lone-pair electrons that can bind to H^+ from an acid (i.e., it cannot be considered a base). If it is not a base, it cannot make a salt with an acid.

B. This solution has both free levothyroxine and its salt. Acetic acid dissociates to place H^+ into the solution, which will react with levothyroxine sodium to produce more free levothyroxine.

1.7 First write the reaction scheme:

$$HAc + NaOH \rightarrow NaAc + H_2O$$

To determine the molarity (concentration) of the vinegar solution, you need to know the number of moles of acetic acid dissolved in 10 mL of sample; that is, you have the volume but you are looking for the number of moles. First, find out how many moles of NaOH you used to reach the equivalence point. At the equivalence point, the ratio of moles of NaOH added to the moles of acid is 1. Moles of NaOH used: $60 \text{ mL} \times 0.1 \text{ mol/L} = 6 \times 10^{-3}$ mol. This number (6×10^{-3} mol) is exactly the same number of moles of acetic acid used to reach the equivalence point. Now you can calculate the molarity of your sample:

$$6 \times 10^{-3} \text{ mol/10 mL} = 0.60 \text{ mol/L} = 0.60 \text{ M}$$

1.8 **A.** Each molecule of milk of magnesia, $Mg(OH)_2$, is able to collect two protons from the stomach, thereby neutralizing the stomach H^+ by the following reaction:

$$Mg(OH)_2(s) + 2H^+(aq) \rightarrow Mg_2^+(aq) + 2H_2O(l)$$

B. Antacids are bases that neutralize part of the excess stomach acid. Aspirin alone, however, is sufficient to provide the needed analgesic effect. The antacid molecule in Alka-Seltzer is $NaHCO_3$, which is a salt. The $NaHCO_3$ molecule, upon dissolving in water, will produce HCO_3^-, which then serves as a base (accepting protons from the HCl found in the stomach) to form carbonic acid, H_2CO_3. The latter molecule breaks down rapidly to CO_2 and water. Alka-Seltzer in this reaction reduces the H^+, thereby neutralizing the stomach acid.

1.9 **A.** Anbesol contains 0.5% phenol. This relatively small amount of phenol, when the product is used for 1 or 2 days, will not harm either children or adults. The 0.5% phenol has both anesthetic and antibacterial effects.

B. The patient does not need to buy an OTC product to treat her skin irritation; instead, she can simply wash the affected area with a mixture of soap, water, and a basic solution such as baking soda. The molecule in poison ivy that causes skin irritation includes urushiol, a characteristic phenol group attached to a long hydrophobic alkyl group. In other words, urushiol is a phenol with a weak acidic property as well as an amphipathic with both hydrophilic and hydrophobic properties. If you add baking soda (bicarbonate) to a solution of water and soap, the bicarbonate will increase the pH of the solution. Washing the affected area with this solution will ionize the phenol group (through the increased pH) and emulsify the long hydrophobic alkyl group (by the soap through micelle formation). Thus you dissolve the hydrophobic chain with soap, and the phenol ring with water. The overall effect is to wash away the poison ivy from the affected area. Alternatively, you can suggest Ivy Dry, a topical OTC product to apply to the affected area as needed.

Problems and Solutions

Problem 1.1 Oxygen has six valence electrons. Draw the electron configurations in an orbital diagram for oxygen and for a water molecule with hybrid orbitals. In addition, draw the Lewis structure of water and show how many lone-pair electrons can be found on a water molecule.

Solution 1.1 The six valence electrons of oxygen are distributed between four sp^3 hybrid atomic orbitals of the oxygen atom. Oxygen, because of its six electrons, ends up with two lone-pairs and two singly occupied sp^3 hybrid atomic orbitals (figure A). The single occupied orbitals can each overlap with a hydrogen atom to form two O—H bonds (figures B and C).

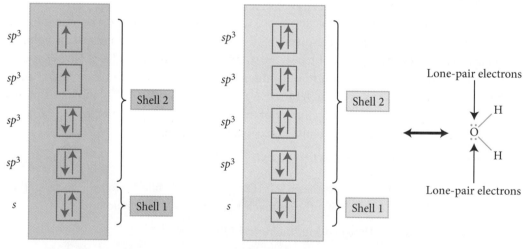

A Oxygen with hybrid orbitals   **B** Water with hybrid orbitals   **C**

Problem 1.2 Draw the Lewis structure and orbital diagram for the formaldehyde molecule (structure shown here). Which kind of hybrid orbitals can you find in the carbon atom of the formaldehyde molecule?

Lewis structure of formaldehyde

Solution 1.2 To predict hybridization in a molecule that has multiple bonds, one can apply the following rules:

1.   If the central atom forms a double bond (like O or C in our example), it has sp^2 hybrid orbitals.

2.   If the central atom forms two double bonds or has a triple bond, it has sp hybrid orbitals.

Because the carbon atom in the formaldehyde molecule has two hydrogen bonds, the carbon forms a double bond with the oxygen atom. As you can see from the carbon's orbital diagrams (figures A and B) and the Lewis structure (figure C), two of the carbon's sp^2 hybrid orbitals form two σ bonds with two hydrogen atoms (figure C). The third sp^2 hybrid orbital forms a σ bond with an sp^2 hybrid orbital of the oxygen atom (figures C and F). Similarly, the p orbital of the carbon atom (figure B) overlaps with the p orbital of the oxygen atom (figure E) and forms a π bond (figure F).

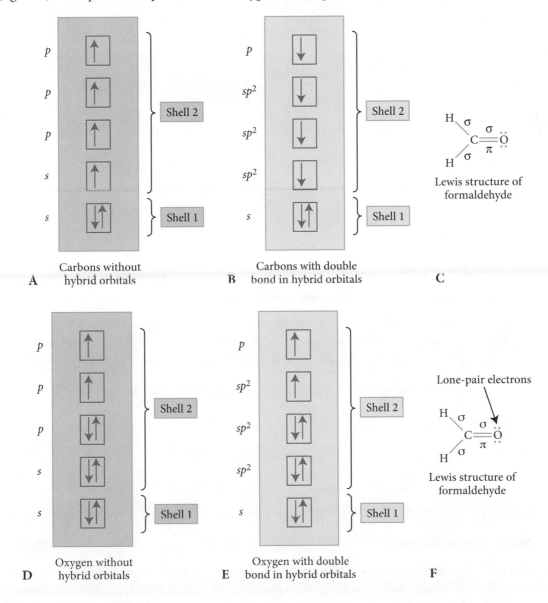

Problem 1.3 Use an orbital diagram to depict how the electrons in each orbital of a phosphorus (P) atom are filled.

Solution 1.3

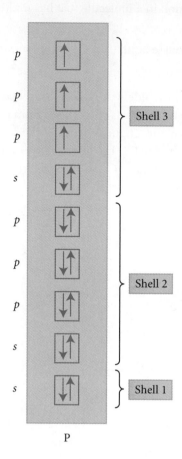

Problem 1.4 How many electrons are present in an atom that has its first and second shells filled and has five electrons in its third shell? Name the element.

Solution 1.4 The first shell of an atom holds two electrons in its *s* orbital, and eight electrons in the second shell (i.e., the second shell has two electrons in the *s* orbital and six electrons in three *p* orbitals). Therefore this element has $2 + 8 + 5 = 15$ electrons; it is phosphorus (see also Problem 1.4).

Problem 1.5 How many electrons does the calcium (Ca^{2+}) ion have in its outermost shell?

A. 2

B. 3

C. 4

D. 5

E. 6

Solution 1.5 A is correct.

Problem 1.6 What is an orbital?

Solution 1.6 An orbital is a region in a space around the nucleus where an electron is most likely to be found. Each orbital can hold a maximum of two electrons. Each shell is populated by different types of orbitals.

Problem 1.7 How would you show the shared and unshared electrons for the H_2S molecule?

$$H : \overset{..}{\underset{..}{S}} : H$$

Solution 1.7 Recall that sulfur and oxygen are in the same column (group) in the periodic table. As a result, sulfur, like oxygen, has six valence electrons. Two of the six electrons are involved with bonds to the hydrogen atoms, so two electron pairs are unbound (four unshared electrons).

Problem 1.8 The atomic orbitals for carbon of methane are considered:

A. *sp* hybridized

B. *sp*² hybridized

C. *sp*³ hybridized

D. unhybridized

Solution 1.8 C; carbon has four valence electrons, with two electrons in the *s* orbital (second shell) and two in the *p* orbital (second shell). Hybridization maximizes the overlap of atomic orbitals when forming bonds. The *s* orbital is mixed with the three *p* orbitals to form a total of four *sp*³ orbitals.

Problem 1.9 What is a nucleophile? Give an example.

Solution 1.9 A nucleophile is a molecule or ion that donates an electron pair to form a new covalent bond. Any molecule, ion, or atom that has electrons that can be shared can be a nucleophile. Examples include Br⁻, OH⁻, and NH_3 (see X⁻ in the figure). Pay attention to why the carbon is partially positively charged (think about the electronegativity difference between C and Cl). The reaction in the figure is also called a substitution reaction (because X displaces Cl). Recall that nucleophiles in the substitution reaction attack the sigma bond (single bond). If they attack the pi (π) bond (double bond), instead, the reaction will be considered an addition reaction.

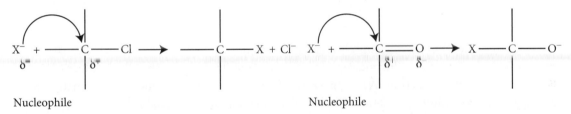

Nucleophile   Nucleophile

Problem 1.10 Why would a water molecule act as both a nucleophile and an electrophile?

Solution 1.10 The oxygen atom of water has two lone pairs and a partial negative charge (δ^-). The oxygen is more electronegative than hydrogen, so water can behave as a nucleophile. A water molecule also can behave as an electrophile because each hydrogen atom bears a δ^+ charge. Only a few molecules can be both nucleophiles and electrophiles.

Problem 1.11 In each of the following instances, indicate whether the substance gains or loses electrons in a redox reaction.

A. A substance undergoing oxidation

B. A substance undergoing reduction

Solution 1.11 A: loses electrons; B: gains electrons.

Problem 1.12 Which of the following molecules has the highest boiling point?

A. Unbranched hexane

B. Branched hexane

C. Unbranched butane

D. Branched ethane

Solution 1.12 A; an unbranched alkane has higher boiling point than a branched alkane because van der Waals attractions are greater for the unbranched alkane than for the branched alkane (the branch acts as a "sticking arm" to increase the intermolecular distances). Remember that as the molecular weight increases, the boiling point increases as well, due to the increased van der Waals attraction between the molecules (however, as mentioned earlier, branching reduces the boiling point).

Problem 1.13 The following formulas are incorrect: N_2H_5, CCl_3. What is wrong with each of these two molecules?

Solution 1.13 Nitrogen forms three bonds and carbon forms four bonds.

Problem 1.14 What is an addition reaction?

Solution 1.14 In an addition reaction, hydrogen (H_2) or a halogen (Cl_2 or Br_2), water (HOH), or a hydrogen halide (HCl or HBr) is added. In an addition reaction, a nucleophile or an electrophile is added to a molecule containing a double bond. In the case of a nucleophile, the double bond is usually between carbon and oxygen (see the figure). In the case of an electrophile, the double bond is between one carbon and another carbon.

Nucleophile

The bottom line: When a nucleophile attacks a sigma bond (single bond), the reaction is a substitution reaction. When the nucleophile (or electrophile) attacks a pi bond (double bond), the reaction is an addition reaction. When an electrophile attacks a double bond in an aromatic ring, the reaction is a substitution reaction. The aromatic ring maintains its double bonds, so it is easier to understand why substitution occurs with an aromatic ring rather than an addition reaction.

Problem 1.15 What is a hydration reaction?

Solution 1.15 A hydration reaction is basically the same as an addition reaction with one exception: Water is added to an alkene (double-bond) molecule. Compare it with the addition reaction.

Water   Alkene   Alcohol

Problem 1.16 Aromatic hydrocarbons have double bonds similar to alkene molecules, however, they are not as prone as alkene to enter into an addition reaction. Why?

Solution 1.16 Aromatic hydrocarbons (aromatic rings) have pi (π) bonds because of the double bonds. The electrons of these double bonds are delocalized, which means they have much more space to move in an aromatic hydrocarbon than if the electrons were in a double bond like that in an alkene molecule. Because electrons repel each other, they are more stable when they have more space to occupy (i.e., the more space electrons have, the less they repel each other). This phenomenon results in more resistance to addition reactions (i.e., makes the aromatic hydrocarbon more stable).

Problem 1.17 One of the common metabolic problems with drugs containing a benzene ring is they can produce a carcinogenic intermediate metabolite during the hydroxylation process. Which of the following reactions is responsible for the carcinogenic intermediate metabolite? Draw the structure of this metabolite.

A. Peroxidation

B. Hydrogenation

C. Epoxidation

D. Reduction

E. Oxidation

Solution 1.17 C is correct.

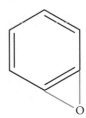

Problem 1.18 What is the IUPAC name for the structure shown?

$$H_3C \longrightarrow \underset{H_2}{C} \longrightarrow \underset{H_2}{C} \longrightarrow \underset{H_2}{C} \longrightarrow N \longrightarrow \underset{H_2}{C} \longrightarrow CH_3$$
$$| \\ CH_3$$

A. *N*-propyl-*N*-ethyl-1-methanamine

D. *N*-ethyl-*N*-methyl-1-butanamine

C. *N*-butyl-*N*-methyl-1-ethananamine

D. *N*,*N*-ethylmethylpropylamine

E. *N*-methyl-*N*-ethyl-1-propanamine

F. Tetra-*N*-ethylmethylpropylamine

Solution 1.18 B is correct.

Problem 1.19 Rank the following amines in order of increasing base strength.

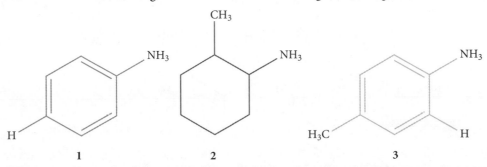

Adapted from Bresnick S. Columbia review: high-yield organic chemistry. Baltimore, MD: Williams and Wilkins; 1996.

A. 1, 2, 3

B. 2, 1, 3

C. 3, 1, 2

D. 2, 3, 1

E. 1, 3, 2

Solution 1.19 E is correct. The lone-pair electrons of the nitrogen atom of compound 1 are delocalized over the aromatic ring, so they are not readily available for accepting protons (decreased basicity). Compound 3 is a stronger base than compound 1 because it has an electron-releasing group (alkyl) on the ring. The strongest base is 2 because it has a longer electron-releasing group (alkyl) in addition to a methyl group, which is also an electron-releasing group. The electron-releasing effect makes the lone-pair electrons on the nitrogen readily available for accepting a proton (increasing the basicity of amines).

Problem 1.20 What is the IUPAC name for the structure shown here?

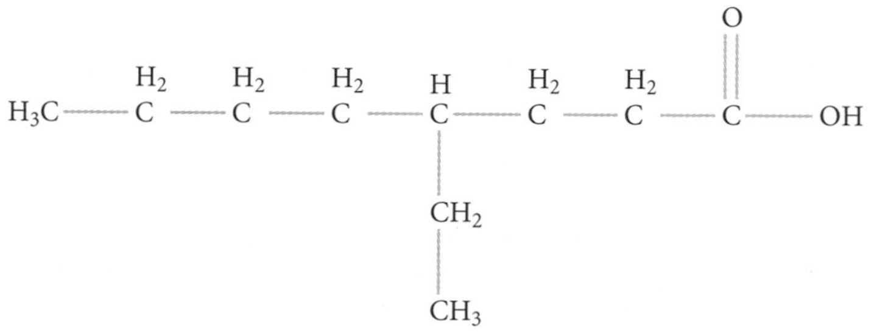

Solution 1.20 4-Ethyloctanoic acid.

Problem 1.21 Which of the following amines is soluble in water?

A. Methylamine

B. Dimethylamine

C. Trimethylamine

D. All of the above

E. None of the above

Solution 1.21 D; small, low-molecular-weight amines are water soluble because they are able to undergo hydrogen binding with water molecules. They do so because the lone-pair electrons on the nitrogen are available to the hydrogen atom from the water molecule.

Problem 1.22 Thymol has a pleasant minty taste. This compound is used by dentists to sterilize a tooth prior to filling it; in addition, it is used in some cough drops. Write the IUPAC name and name the class of compound to which thymol belongs.

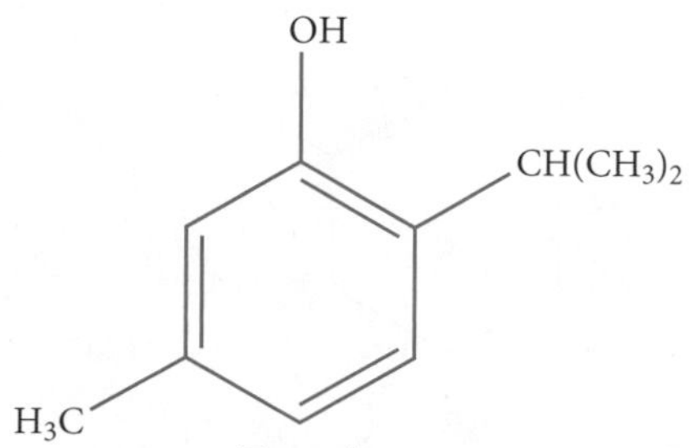

Thymol

Solution 1.22 2-Isopropyl-5-methylphenol; it belongs to the phenol group.

Problem 1.23 Aldehydes undergo oxidation, whereas ketones do not. Why?

Solution 1.23 The carbon–carbon bonds in ketones must be broken for oxidation to occur—a process that requires a lot of energy.

Problem 1.24 Dimethyl ether and ethanol both have a molecular weight of 46 g/mol. Ethanol has a higher melting point than dimethyl ether. Why?

Solution 1.24 Ethanol molecules can form hydrogen bonds with each other, whereas dimethyl ether cannot. Therefore, a higher temperature is required to break down the hydrogen bonds between ethanol molecules.

Problem 1.25 Which of the following answers is (are) correct regarding the ketone and aldehyde functional groups?

I. Both can attract nucleophiles.

II. Both can attract electrophiles.

III. Both can undergo addition reactions.

IV. While a ketone undergoes an addition reaction, an aldehyde undergoes a substitution reaction.

   A. I, II

   B. I, II, III

   C. I, IV

   D. II, IV

   E. I, II, III, IV

Solution 1.25 B; nucleophiles attack C=O at the carbonyl carbon, which is positively polarized, and electrophiles (particularly protons, H^+) attack oxygen, which is negatively polarized. The addition reaction can occur because in a nucleophilic attack, the nucleophile will be added to the carbonyl carbon.

Problem 1.26 What is the concentration of HNO_3 (a strong acid) in a solution that has a pH of 4.0?

Solution 1.26 As the question stated, HNO_3 is a strong acid—and a strong acid dissociates all of its H^+. Thus the concentration of the acid will be the same as the concentration of H^+, which is what you need to calculate pH. To determine the concentration of H^+, you can directly use the pH:

$pH = -\log [H+]$

$[H+] = $ antilog of $-pH$

$[H+] = $ antilog of $-4 = 1 \times 10^{-4}$ M

Be careful with the units of your answer. In this question, the answer should be in the concentration unit, molarity (M).

Problem 1.27 Acetylsalicylic acid (aspirin) is a weak acid with a pK_a of 3.5. Calculate the pH of an 0.05 M solution of aspirin.

Solution 1.27 As the question states, aspirin is a weak acid; as the presented data indicate, you are dealing with a weak acid that weakly (i.e., 5% or less) dissociates H^+. Whenever you deal with a "weak acid" and low dissociation rate for H^+, immediately use the following equation:

$[H^+] = \sqrt{K_a C_a}$

Be careful here: You don't have K_a but rather pK_a, so you must convert pK_a to K_a first:

$pK_a = -\log K_a$

$K_a = $ antilog of $-pK_a$

$K_a = $ antilog of $-3.5 = 3.16 \times 10^{-4}$

$pH = -\log [H+] = 2.40$

Problem 1.28 Erythromycin is an antibiotic that kills the bacteria that cause Legionnaires' disease. Erythromycin is a weak base with a dissociation constant (K_b) of 6.3×10^{-6}. Calculate the pH of an 0.2 M solution of erythromycin.

Solution 1.28 Here you are dealing with a base, so the value of K_b will help you to calculate the pH. When you think about a base, think about the artificial conjugate acid, Ac^-, which reacts with water.

$$Ac^- + H_2O \leftrightarrow HAc + OH^-$$

$$K_b = \frac{[HAc] \times [OH^-]}{[AC^-]}$$

In the same way you solved Problem 1.5, you can solve Problem 1.6, but this time using the following equation:

$$[OH^-] = \sqrt{K_b \, C_b} = 1.12 \times 10^{-3} \text{ M}$$

Remember this number is $[OH^-]$, and not $[H^+]$. Thus, to know pH, you must know $[H^+]$:

$$K_w = [H^+] \times [OH^-] = 1 \times 10^{-14} \text{ M}^2$$

$$[H^+] = 1 \times 10^{-14} \text{ M}^2/[OH^-] = 8.91 \times 10^{-12} \text{ M}$$

$$pH = -\log [H^+] = 11$$

Problem 1.29 How is K_a defined? Write the equation for K_a for the generic weak acid, HAc.

Solution 1.29 K_a is the dissociation constant or ionization constant for an acid and is expressed as follows:

$$K_a = \frac{[H^+] \times [AC^-]}{[HAc]}$$

Problem 1.30 Calculate the pH of a solution of acetic acid, HAc ($pK_a = 4.76$), that contains 0.50 M HAc and 0.05 M Ac^-.

Solution 1.30 Here we can use the Henderson-Hasselbalch equation to calculate the pH:

$$HAc = 0.50 \text{ M and } Ac^- = 0.05 \text{ M}$$

$$pH = pK_a + \log \{[Ac^-]/[HAc]\} = 4.76 + \log \{[0.05]/[0.50]\} = 3.76$$

Problem 1.31 Acetylsalicylic acid (aspirin) is a weak acidic drug with pK_a of 3.5. The pH of the small intestine is 5.5 and the pH of the stomach is 1.5.

Aspirin

A. What is the percentage ionization in the stomach?

B. What is the percentage ionization in the small intestine?

C. Which of these two sites is the absorption site for aspirin? Why?

Solution 1.31 Aspirin is an acidic drug and you want to know the percentage ionization. Thus you should use the equation that gives % ionization of an acid:

$$\% \text{ ionized} = \frac{1 \times 100}{\text{Antilog } (pK_a - pH) + 1}$$

A. 0.99%

B. 99%

C. In the stomach, because aspirin will be almost 100% un-ionized; as an un-ionized molecule, it will penetrate the cell membrane to reach the blood and go to its site of action.

References

1. Bresnick S. *Columbia review: high-yield organic chemistry.* Baltimore, MD: Williams and Wilkins; 1996.
2. Dewick PM. *Essentials of organic chemistry.* United Kingdom: John Wiley & Sons; 2006.
3. Fanta PE, Gaffney A. "Ether." In: *Access Science.* McGraw-Hill; 2008. Available at: http://www .accessscience.com.
4. Fanta PE. "Aldehyde." In: *Access Science.* McGraw-Hill; 2008. Available at: http://www.accessscience .com.
5. Fanta PE. "Amine." In: *AccessScience.* McGraw-Hill; 2008. Available at: http://www.accessscience.com.
6. Fanta PE. "Ester." In: *AccessScience.* McGraw-Hill; 2008. Available at: http://www.accessscience.com.
7. Flomenbaum NE. "Salicylates." In: Flomenbaum NE, ed. *Goldfrank's toxicologic emergencies.* 9th ed. New York: McGraw-Hill; 2011. Available at: http://www.accesspharmacy.com/content .aspx?aID=6510436.
8. Lemke TL, Williams DA, Roche VF, and Zito SW. Foye`s Principles of Medicinal Chemistry, 7th ed. Baltimore. Wolters Kluwer Lippincott Williams & Wilkins, 2012.
9. Garetz BA. "Bond angle and distance." In: *AccessScience.* McGraw-Hill; 2008. Available at: http://www.accessscience.com.
10. Hanson JR. *Functional group chemistry.* Cambridge: Wiley Interscience; 2002.
11. Hart H. "Aromatic hydrocarbon." In: *AccessScience.* McGraw-Hill; 2008. Available at: http://www.accessscience.com.
12. Interactive Chemistry Multimedia Courseware. *Solutions, solubility and precipitation, reaction rates, states of matter, bonding I and II.* Chico, CA: CyberEd; 2001.
13. Koch PM. "Atom." In: *AccessScience.* McGraw-Hill; 2012. Available at: http://www.accessscience .com.
14. Lemke TL, Williams DA, Roche VF, Zito SW. "Disulfiram and disulfiram-like reactions." In: Kuffner EK, ed. *Goldfrank's toxicologic emergencies.* 9th ed. New York: McGraw-Hill; 2011. Available at: http://www.accesspharmacy.com/content.aspx?aID=6521905.
15. Lemke TL, Roche VF, Zito SW. *Review of organic functional groups: introduction to medicinal organic chemistry.* 5th ed. Baltimore: Wolters Kluwer Lippincott Williams & Wilkins, 2012.
16. Moore JM, Rao VNM. "Halogenated hydrocarbon." In: *AccessScience.* McGraw-Hill; 2008. Available at: http://www.accessscience.com.
17. Moss GP. "Chemical nomenclature." In: *AccessScience.* McGraw-Hill; 2008. Available at: http://www.accessscience.com.

18. Masters SB. "The alcohols." In: Katzung BG, Masters SB, Trevor AJ, eds. *Basic and clinical pharmacology.* 12th ed. New York: McGraw-Hill; 2012. Available at: http://www.accesspharmacy .com/content.aspx?aID=55824193.

19. McMurry JE, Castellion ME. *Fundamentals of general, organic, and biological chemistry.* 4th ed. Upper Saddle River, NJ: Pearson Education; 2003.

20. Nelson DL, Cox MM, Lehninger AL. *Principles of biochemistry.* 5th ed. New York: W. H. Freeman and Company; 2008.

21. Osgood M, Ocorr K. *The absolute, ultimate guide to Lehninger principles of biochemistry.* 4th ed. New York: W. H. Freeman and Company; 2005.

22. Ouellette RJ. *Introduction to general, organic and biological chemistry.* 4th ed. Upper Saddle River, NJ: Prentice-Hall; 1997.

23. Patrick GL. *An introduction to medicinal chemistry.* 2nd ed. New York: Oxford University Press; 2001.

24. Segel I. *Biochemical calculations: how to solve mathematical problems in general biochemistry.* 2nd ed. New York: John Wiley & Sons; 1976.

25. Silberberg MS. *Chemistry: the molecular nature of matter and change.* 3rd ed. New York: McGraw-Hill; 2003.

26. Silberberg MS. *Principles of general chemistry.* New York: McGraw-Hill; 2006.

27. Timberlake KC. *Organic and biological chemistry: structures of life.* San Francisco: Benjamin Cummings; 2001.

28. UpToDate. Waltham, MA; 2012. Available at: http://www.uptodate.com/online with subscription.

29. Williams JM. "Hydrogen bond." In: *AccessScience.* McGraw-Hill; 2008. Available at: http://www .accessscience.com.

Introduction to Cell Biology

Reza Karimi

OBJECTIVES

1. Understand prokaryotic and eukaryotic cells and their organelles.

2. Learn the differences between prokaryotes and eukaryotes, including those related to membrane lipids, membrane proteins, and genetic information.

3. Learn the basic cell functions in regard to membrane transporters and cellular diffusion.

4. Comprehend the structure and function of biomolecules such as amino acids, nucleic acids, carbohydrates, proteins, and fatty acids.

5. Understand cell division and the cell cycle.

6. Comprehend the central dogma in cellular biology by learning about the replication, transcription, and protein synthetic machinery.

7. Implement a series of Learning Bridge assignments at your experiential sites to bridge your didactic learning with your experiential experiences.

KEY TERMS AND DEFINITIONS

1. **Amphipathic molecule:** a molecule that has both polar and nonpolar regions.

2. **Autosomes:** all chromosomes, except the X and Y chromosomes.

3. **Charged tRNA:** a transfer RNA that carries an amino acid (is charged with an amino acid).

4. **Chromatid:** a linear double-helix DNA that is millions of base pairs (bp) long.

5. **Chromatin:** a component of the cell nucleus that is composed of a DNA–protein complex.

6. **Chromosome:** a coiled DNA molecule, packed with proteins, that holds genetic information. A chromosome has two chromatids.

7. **Diploid and Haploid:** they refer to the number of chromosomes in a cell. While a parent cell has a diploid number of chromosomes, a daughter cell has a haploid number of chromosomes (half the number of diploid chromosomes).

8. **Dominant:** a genetically determinant gene. A dominant allele overpowers another allele.

9. **Epimer:** one of two sugar molecules that differ only in configuration around one carbon atom.

10. **Exon:** a DNA sequence that is translated.

11. **Gene:** a segment of genetic material that codes for one polypeptide.

12. **Gene expression:** a complex process by which a polypeptide or a protein is synthesized from a gene.

13. **Genetic code:** a code built through the combination of 64 codons. With the exception of termination codons (3 codons), each codon specifies for one of the 20 common amino acids.

(continues)

14. **Genome:** the entire set of genes in all possible chromosomes.

15. **Glycogen:** a polysaccharide that is the major form of carbohydrate storage unit in animals.

16. **Gram-negative bacteria:** bacteria in which the cell wall is composed of three layers—an inner membrane, a thin layer of peptidoglycan, and an outer membrane surrounding the peptidoglycan.

17. **Gram-positive bacteria:** bacteria that have a thicker peptidoglycan layer (90% of their cell wall consists of peptidoglycan). They do not have the outer membrane found in Gram-negative bacteria.

18. **Initiator tRNA:** the first transfer RNA that binds to the P site of a ribosome.

19. **Intron:** a DNA sequence that is not translated.

20. **Meiosis:** a process in eukaryotic cells in which two nuclear divisions occur (meiosis I and meiosis II). The end result of meiosis is production of four daughter cells. Each of these four cells has a haploid number of chromosomes. In humans, the daughter cells develop into gametes, which are sex cells (i.e., sperm or egg). Meiosis occurs only in reproductive organs to produce gametes.

21. **Mitosis:** a process in which a nucleus divides and the genetic material is distributed equally between two identical daughter cells. The end result of mitosis is production of two daughter cells. Each of these cells has a diploid number of chromosomes. Mitosis occurs in all organs.

22. **Monosaccharide:** a single carbohydrate that cannot be hydrolyzed further into other carbohydrates (such as a glucose molecule).

23. **Mutation:** a modification in a DNA structure that can produce permanent changes in the genetic information.

24. **Nucleoside:** a nucleotide without the phosphate group.

25. **Nucleotide:** a molecule that consists of a base, a deoxyribose sugar, and a phosphate.

26. **Peptidyl transferase:** a ribozyme in the large subunit that catalyzes formation of each peptide bond as the ribosome moves along the mRNA.

27. **Plasmids:** small circular DNA that can replicate and be transferred from one cell to another.

28. **Promoter:** a DNA sequence at which RNA polymerase and its cofactors bind to initiate the transcription of a gene.

29. **Recessive:** a characteristic of genes such that when an individual receives two copies of a mutated gene, one from each parent, she or he will develop a disease.

30. **Replication:** a process in which two daughter DNA molecules are synthesized from one parental DNA.

31. **Somatic cell:** a human cell that has 46 chromosomes arranged in 23 pairs—22 autosome pairs and 1 pair of sex chromosomes. In total, humans have 23 pairs of homologous chromosomes.

32. **Symbiotic relationship:** a mutual interaction process between two or more biological species to help each other survive.

33. **Transcription:** a process in which a sequence of a gene is utilized by an RNA polymerase to synthesize an RNA molecule.

34. **Translation:** a process in which a messenger RNA is used by a ribosome to synthesize a polypeptide or a protein.

35. **Wild-type gene:** a normal gene that does not have any mutation, insertion, or deletion.

36. **Zwitterion:** a molecule that is electrically neutral at biological pH (pH 7).

37. **Zygote:** the union of two gametes, a sperm with an egg, producing the first cell (zygote) of an entity that has the full complement of chromosomes, half from the father and half from the mother.

Introduction

Cell biology is one of the building blocks of microbiology, immunology, and biochemistry. All living organisms begin their life's journey by maintaining the integrity of their cells' structure and functions and by promoting accurate cell proliferation and growth. Cells have a unique and complex architecture. Despite many years of intensive research and studies, our knowledge regarding a simple cell, such as *Escherichia coli*, remains limited. While many "big picture" models have been illustrated eloquently, much remains to be learned about the details of these big pictures.

This chapter focuses on describing basic molecules of cells such as carbohydrates, lipids, proteins, compartments of cells and cell membranes, and genes that pharmacy students will encounter many times during their course of study. Understanding these basic molecules and compartments enables students to see the significant structural differences within prokaryotic organisms such as Gram-positive and Gram-negative bacteria and how a prokaryotic organism differs from a eukaryotic organism in regard to cellular structures and functions. In addition, this chapter explains the central dogma (replication, transcription, and translation) that dictates the core targets of many antibiotics available on the market. Due to the complexity of eukaryotic organisms and the fact that many information and many mechanisms are not known yet, much attention in this chapter is paid to the cellular mechanisms of prokaryotic organisms.

Cell Function and Biomolecules

A cell is the basic and functional unit of all living organisms (except viruses) and is highly organized to maintain the life of a tissue, an organ, or an organism. All cells are divided into two major types:

- Prokaryotic: archaebacteria and eubacteria (including photosynthetic organisms). While the former can survive and grow in harsh environments, the latter are commonly referred to as bacteria and often inhabit soil, water, and animals.

- Eukaryotic: protists, fungi, animals, and plants.

Although cells have many similar organelles, they do not have the same function, structure, or shape. For instance, a sperm cell and a pancreatic cell share identical organizations, yet look completely different. There are two organizations that all cells have—a nuclear region and cytoplasm. Extensive similarities are also observed among the eukaryotes, particularly plants and animals (such as cell membrane, DNA, cytoplasm, and ribosomes).

Prokaryotic Organisms

A prokaryotic cell has unique characteristics such as a small size (1 μm in diameter) and lacks a nuclear membrane. Nevertheless, this cell has a region called a nucleoid that contains the cell's DNA. In addition, it has circular DNA—an organization that differs from a eukaryotic cell's linear DNA. Because the size of a prokaryotic cell is small, the DNA must be folded at least 1,000 times to fit into the cell. Indeed, the small size of the prokaryotic cell and its DNA explains the limited number of genes that exist within the prokaryotic DNA. Interestingly, a growing body of evidence suggests that the DNA is packed in an orderly fashion such that specific DNA regions are close to (or far from) one another.

Vast diversity among the prokaryotic cells is observed with regard to their means of generating metabolic energy. For instance, photosynthetic bacteria are grouped into cyanobacteria, purple bacteria, and green bacteria. The cyanobacteria (also called blue-green bacteria) are the largest group of photosynthetic prokaryotes that utilize the energy of sunlight to drive photosynthesis.

They synthesize organic molecules from inorganic molecules and use water as a reducing agent (i.e., as an electron source) to generate oxygen. Cyanobacteria's photosynthetic membranes form multilayered structures known as thylakoids. In contrast, purple and green bacteria, in the absence of oxygen, convert light energy to metabolic energy. The latter two organisms do not use water as a reducing agent and, as a result, do not generate oxygen during their photosynthetic process. Instead, they use hydrogen gas (H_2), hydrogen sulfide (H_2S), and reduced organic molecules as reducing agents.

Whereas aerobic bacteria are solely dependent on consumption of oxygen to produce energy (adenosine triphosphate [ATP]), anaerobic bacteria use electron acceptors other than oxygen in their respiratory mechanism to generate metabolic energy. Another important characteristic of prokaryotes is their ability to carry small circular DNA molecules, known as plasmids. Plasmids can replicate and may be transferred from one cell to another, thereby spreading genetic information throughout a population. A plasmid is neither an organelle nor an organism. Nevertheless, due to its unique structure, it can play a major role in a prokaryotic organism's development of antibiotic resistance.

Some prokaryotic cells interact with other organisms for their survival. While some of these interactions are beneficial, others are detrimental. For instance, the symbiotic relationship that exists within the human gastrointestinal (GI) tract leads to an exchange of mutual nutrition between the bacteria found in this locale and the human host and, as a result, benefits both organisms. For instance, GI-resident bacteria, often referred to as probiotic bacteria, produce vitamins K and B_{12}, short fatty acids that are important for epithelial cell membrane in the large intestine, digestive enzymes, and other substances. Similarly, the human upper GI system is a friendly and nutrition-rich environment for many bacteria, particularly anaerobic bacteria. Conversely, for a parasite (particularly a pathogenic parasite), the symbiotic relationship can be detrimental to the host; it is only the parasite that benefits from such a relationship. Other prokaryotic cells such as mycoplasmas do not have cell walls, but rather use cholesterol from their hosts to build their cell membranes. Keep in mind that prokaryotes are not capable of synthesizing cholesterol.

As mentioned earlier, prokaryotic organisms include eubacteria (also known as simple bacteria) and the archaebacteria. While both of these organisms look similar under a microscope, they differ in their architectures. For instance, one of the major structural differences between them is that bacteria have a peptidoglycan cell wall and a cytoplasmic membrane; both of these protective structures are missing in archaebacteria. In addition, one can find archaebacteria in harsh environments where bacteria cannot survive (such as hot springs).

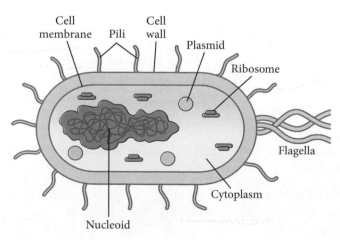

Figure 2.1 A simple form of a prokaryotic cell.

Prokaryotes are single-celled organisms that consist of DNA, cytoplasm, and a surface structure that includes the plasma membrane (**Figure 2.1**). In addition, the following organelles can be found in prokaryotes: nucleoid, cytoskeletal proteins, cytoplasmic membrane, cell wall, flagella, pili, and ribosomes. It is important to appreciate the roles of these organelles in understanding how a prokaryotic cell survives and thrives.

Prokaryote Organelles

Nucleoid

Prokaryotic cells do not have a nucleus; rather, their DNA is contained in a structure known as the nucleoid. When a nucleoid is stained, one can see it under a light microscope. Prokaryotic cells' negatively charged DNA is neutralized by the presence of small polyamines, magnesium ions, and histone-like proteins that assist each prokaryotic cell's DNA in folding and packing inside of the cell. The bacterial DNA has all the necessary information to help a bacterium grow and divide. Because bacterial cells lack nuclei, however, transcription and translation (i.e., synthesis of messenger RNA [mRNA] and protein synthesis, respectively) occur simultaneously; in contrast, in eukaryotes, the mRNA must leave the nucleus to be translated into a protein.

Bacterial DNA can assume topological bonds that are links between DNA molecules and are not joined by any specific chemical bond. Thus these DNA molecules cannot be physically separated because they cross over each other like links in a chain. Some enzymes (topoisomerases) can prevent the formation of these topological bonds, thereby facilitating the replication machinery of prokaryotes. The function of topoisomerases is to relieve the topological stress caused not just by the unwinding of double-stranded DNA during transcription, but also at the replication fork during replication. A series of antibiotics, however, can block the function of topoisomerases. For instance, the function of prokaryotic topoisomerase II (also called DNA-gyrase) is to overwind or underwind a DNA molecule ahead of the replication fork to facilitate DNA replication. Ciprofloxacin (Cipro), which belongs to the family of fluoroquinolone antibiotics, inhibits topoisomerase II function and thereby inhibits bacterial replication (see also the *Introduction to Microbiology* chapter).

The bacterial genes have been named by lowercase italic letter (capital italic letters in eukaryotes—for instance, the *RAS* gene for the RAS protein); for example, *pol* codes for a polymerase enzyme, and *rec* codes for a recombination protein. If more than one gene affects the same process, a fourth capital italic letter is used to identify the bacterial gene, such as in *polA* (for DNA polymerase I) or *recA* (for recombinant protein A). The alphabetical order in which these letters are assigned does not necessarily have to do with the order of the function of proteins (the product of the genes), but rather reflects the order of their discovery. For instance, *polA*, *polB*, and *polC* code for DNA polymerase I, II, and III, respectively, but do not follow this order in exerting their actions during the replication process. When referring to the product of the gene (protein), no italic letters are used and the first letter is a capital. For example, the product of the *recA* gene is the RecA protein.

Cytoskeletal Proteins

Prokaryotic cells have both actin-like and non-actin-like cytoskeletal proteins. While the actin-like proteins assist in giving the cell a shape or localizing intracellular proteins within the cell (i.e., facilitating the movement of vesicles and organelles in the cytoplasm), the non-actin-like proteins assist in determining the cell's shape and regulating DNA segregation and cell division.

Cytoplasmic Membrane (Cell Membrane)

The bacterial cell membrane is made of phospholipids and many proteins. Phospholipids in archaebacteria are ether linked, which means their fatty acids are attached to a glycerol backbone; in contrast, phospholipids are ester linked in bacteria. Many different proteins constitute a large portion of the cell membrane. Approximately, 70% of a prokaryotic cell membrane is built of proteins—a significantly larger proportion than in a eukaryotic cell membrane. A prokaryotic cell membrane does not have any cholesterol, with one notable exception: The *Mycoplasma* bacteria's cell membranes include cholesterol molecules that they obtained from their hosts (similar to other bacteria, *Mycoplasma* does not synthesize cholesterol).

The important roles of the cell membrane are to be selectively permeable to solutes by using membrane proteins to facilitate diffusion of sugars, amino acids, and inorganic ions such as Na^+, K^+, Cl^-, and Ca^{2+}; to facilitate electron transport; to carry out oxidative phosphorylation (only in aerobic bacteria); to release hydrolytic enzymes, including enzymes that are involved in DNA replication, cell-wall polymers, and membrane lipids.

Cell Wall

The bacterial cell wall contains a distinctive structure called peptidoglycan. Archaebacteria, in contrast, do not possess any peptidoglycan. Because of their different cell wall structures, archaebacteria are resistant to many antibiotics that attack the cell wall.

Peptidoglycan plays an important role in the cell wall structure and shape and is important in the classification of bacteria. As its name indicates, peptidoglycan is made of polypeptides and carbohydrates. It has a backbone made up of alternating units of *N*-acetylglucosamine and *N*-acetylmuramic acid. While the backbone is the same in all bacteria, the polypeptide chain varies from species to species. For instance, in Gram-negative bacteria, there are only one or two layers of peptidoglycan. In contrast, in Gram-positive bacteria, there are 40 layers of peptidoglycan, which account for 50% of the cell wall material. The microorganism *Escherichia coli* (E. Coli), which is discussed in many chapters of this book, is a typical Gram-negative bacterium. Gram-positive and Gram-negative bacteria are discussed later in this chapter.

The role of the cell wall is to protect the cell integrity from osmotic pressure; because many solutes enter the cell, the osmotic pressure could burst the cell (see also the *Introduction to Pharmaceutics* chapter). In addition, the cell wall plays an important role in the cell division. The cell wall, in contrast to the cell membrane, does not have a selectively permeable architecture. There are three major layers in the envelope of Gram-negative bacteria: the outer membrane, the peptidoglycan cell wall, and the cytoplasmic or inner membrane. Gram-positive bacteria lack the outer membrane (**Figure 2.2**).

Flagella

Bacterial flagella are thread-like protein fibers (12–30 nm in diameter). A bacterial flagellum consists of a few thousand protein subunits called flagellin. They rotate and drive the cell through its surroundings (Figure 2.1). Flagella are highly antigenic; as a result, upon infection, some of the immune responses are directed against these proteins. A typical example of how the flagella can help bacteria to move is when the *Helicobacter pylori* bacterium (which causes ulcer) uses its flagella to move through the mucus lining of the host to reach the stomach epithelial cells.

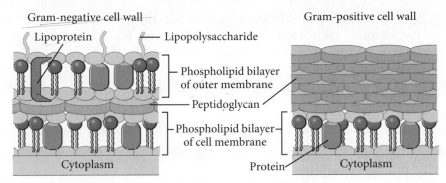

Figure 2.2 The architectures of Gram-negative and Gram-positive cell walls.
Adapted from: Morse SA, Brooks GF, Carroll KC, et al. Cell structure. In: Morse SA, Brooks GF, Carroll KC, et al., eds. *Jawetz, Melnick, and Adelberg's medical microbiology.* 25th ed. New York, NY: McGraw-Hill; 2010:10. Available at: http://www.accesspharmacy.com/content.aspx?aID=6426066.

Pili

Many Gram-negative bacteria have structural protein subunits called pili that assist cells in adhering to the surfaces of other cells. Two classes of pili are distinguished: (1) ordinary pili, which play an important role in the attachment of symbiotic and bacteria to host cells, and (2) sex pili, which play an important role in facilitating the attachment of donor and recipient cells in bacterial conjugation.

Different bacteria produce different pili, which are antigenically useful as they promote the production of antibodies by the host. However, antibodies against the pili of one bacterial species cannot fight the pili of other species. Another problem is that some bacteria can produce pili of different antigenic types. For instance, *Neisseria gonorrhoeae* bacteria are capable of making pili of different antigenic types, yet are able to adhere to cells in the presence of antibodies to their original type of pili. Clinically, another disadvantage for the host cells is that pili can inhibit the phagocytic function of leukocytes (more information about leukocytes is presented in the *Introduction to Immunology* chapter), which results in a longer duration of infection.

Ribosomes

Ribosomes are complex molecules that are made of ribonucleic acid (RNA) and proteins; their role is to translate mRNA into proteins. Structurally, there are significant differences in the ribosomes of prokaryotes and eukaryotes. Indeed, thanks to those differences, many antibiotics can attack only bacteria and are not able to recognize eukaryotic ribosomes. Ribosomes exist in large amounts in all live cells. For instance, it has been estimated that one *E. coli* cell has 20,000 ribosomes, whereas a yeast cell (a simple eukaryotic cell) has 200,000 ribosomes.

Two ribosomal subunits exist: 50S and 30S. The whole ribosomes found in prokaryotes are referred to as 70S ribosomes. The numbers of subunits are not additive (i.e., 50S + 30S will not be called 80S). The S numbers, including the numbers for ribosomal RNA (rRNA) molecules such as 16S and 23S rRNA, refer to centrifugation sedimentation coefficients, which reflect the size of each subunit or RNA molecule.

The smaller subunit (30S) is made of 16S rRNA and 21 proteins. The 16S rRNA contains many regions of self-complement sequences, which are able to form double-helical regions. These double-stranded regions are highly conserved among a wide variety of organisms. The 16S rRNA folds into a three-dimensional structure and is bound by multiple ribosomal proteins (as mentioned earlier, 21 proteins). The larger ribosomal subunit (50S) has two rRNAs: 23S and 5S rRNA.

This subunit also has many ribosomal proteins (36 proteins). The sequences of prokaryotic RNA molecules are known today. While 16S rRNA and 23S rRNA have 1,540 and 2,900 nucleotides, respectively, the length of 5S rRNA is only 120 nucleotides long.

Gram Stain

It is critical to distinguish different classes of bacteria when the goal is to effectively and promptly diagnose an infection caused by a specific class of a species. Obviously, bacterial features that are common (such as DNA, ribosomes, and RNA) to many species cannot be used in this type of diagnostic process.

Bacteria can be divided into two groups on the basis of their cell wall structures and their response to a biochemical test called Gram stain. While Gram-positive bacteria retain a purple dye, Gram-negative bacteria do not retain this dye and, as a result, become translucent. Consequently, Gram-positive bacteria appear to be stained purple under the microscope. Why the purple dye can stain one cell but not another reflects the fundamental differences that exist in the cell envelopes (Figure 2.2).

Gram-Negative Bacteria

The cell wall of a Gram-negative bacterium is composed of three layers: an inner membrane, a thin layer of peptidoglycan, and the outer membrane surrounding the peptidoglycan. The *E. coli* bacterium is an example of a Gram-negative bacterium. Another component of the Gram-negative bacterial cell wall is lipopolysaccharide (LPS), which consists of a complex glycolipid (lipid A) that is attached to a polysaccharide. The role of lipid A is to anchor the LPS molecule to the outer membrane. LPS is important for the function of many Gram-negative bacteria's outer membrane proteins. LPS is, however, very toxic for animal cells (it is also referred to as an endotoxin) because it binds tightly to the host cell surface and is detached only when the cell membrane is lysed. The toxicity is believed to be caused by lipid A rather than the polysaccharide component. Another component of the cell wall is lipoprotein, which is cross-linked to the outer membrane and peptidoglycan layers (Figure 2.2). Lipoprotein is the most abundant protein within Gram-negative cells, with approximately half a million of these molecules being found in each cell. Its role is to anchor the outer membrane to the peptidoglycan layer(s).

The space that separates the inner and outer cell membranes is referred to as the periplasmic space. It contains the peptidoglycan layer and many other proteins and accounts for approximately 30% of the total cell volume. The periplasmic space also contains a high concentration of D-glucose polymer.

Gram-Positive Bacteria

Gram-positive bacteria do not possess an outer membrane, but they do have a much thicker peptidoglycan layer than Gram-negative bacteria; specifically, 90% of their cell wall is composed of peptidoglycan. As a result, they are sensitive to lysozyme enzymes and the penicillin class of antibiotics. *Streptococcus pneumoniae* is an example of a Gram-positive bacterium. Polysaccharides are other carbohydrate molecules that one can find in Gram-positive bacteria.

Animals are capable of synthesizing the hydrolytic enzyme lysozyme. This enzyme, which is found in tears, saliva, and nasal secretions, is an excellent defense mechanism that ruptures the Gram-positive cell wall's peptidoglycan backbone. However, because Gram-negative bacteria have an outer membrane, a lysozyme is not able to reach the tiny peptidoglycan backbone of Gram-negative bacteria. The latter resistance to lysozymes has been confirmed in experimental studies. For instance, in laboratory experiments, one can add ethylene-diaminetetraacetic acid (EDTA) to chelate divalent cations and weaken the outer membrane of the cell wall. This process facilitates the entry of lysozymes and enables them to reach the peptidoglycan backbone.

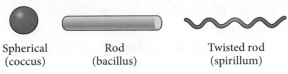

Spherical
(coccus)

Rod
(bacillus)

Twisted rod
(spirillum)

Figure 2.3 The three morphological shapes of bacteria.

Bacteria may take any of the following morphological shapes: spherical (coccus), rod (bacillus), or twisted rod (spirillum) (**Figure 2.3**). For instance, *Staphylococcus aureus* is a spherical Gram-positive bacterium that often is the inhabitant of the skin, nasal passages, and the gastrointestinal tract. The Gram-positive *Bacillus anthracis*, which causes anthrax (skin pustules, fever, and malaise), has the rod morphological shape. The Gram-negative bacterium *Spermillum* morphologically forms a twisted rod and often causes rash, muscle aches, chills, fever, and headache.

Spores

Some bacteria, during their replication process and in a harsh environment, build a very tough coating; the resulting structure is called a spore. Spores assist bacteria in resisting extreme and harsh environments such as heat, cold, radiation, or absence of nutrition, water, or air. The spore-forming bacteria can cause serious infections. For instance, botulism is a type of food poisoning caused by *Clostridium botulinum*.

Eukaryotic Organisms

The eukaryotes include a rich variety of organisms—for example, protists, fungi, plants, and animals (including humans). A eukaryotic cell is distinguished from a prokaryotic cell by the presence of a nucleus. This nucleus contains genetic information that is organized into discrete chromosomes; it is enclosed by a double membrane called the nuclear envelope. Eukaryotes have developed several advanced and complex structures that distinguish them from prokaryotes. For example, a eukaryotic cell contains a variety of organelles that are membrane-bound compartments, such as the nucleus, mitochondria, chloroplasts, endoplasmic reticulum (ER), Golgi apparatus, lysosomes, vacuoles, and peroxisomes. Many of these eukaryotic organelles are discussed in the following section.

Cell Membrane

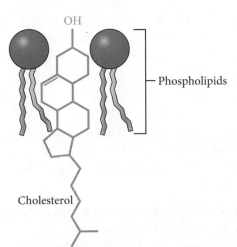

OH

Phospholipids

Cholesterol

Figure 2.4 Cholesterol is inserted between the phospholipids of the membrane bilayer, with its hydroxyl group (gray) close to the hydrophilic head group (teal) of the phospholipids.

The cell membrane is a biological membrane that separates the cytosol from the extracellular environment. The cells of some organisms, such as plants, have an additional layer called the cell wall; animal cells lack such a cell wall. Similar to the roles it plays in prokaryotes, the cell membrane in eukaryotes selectively allows molecules and ions in and out of the cell, regulates the environment of the cell to support reactions within the cytosol, and includes protein receptors to receive external signals. The composition of the cell membrane, which comprises a mixture of phospholipids, proteins, and carbohydrates, provides a barrier against the outside environment and maintains effective transport and signaling systems. A number of proteins serve as selective transporters for protons (H^+), ions (Cl^-, Na^+), and molecules (glucose and amino acids) across the cell membrane.

Cholesterol is another important molecule of cell membranes that, due to its amphipathic nature, is located in the hydrophobic areas of the inner region (**Figure 2.4**).

As mentioned earlier, prokaryotes do not contain any type of cholesterol. Cholesterol is able to modulate membrane fluidity. It is inserted between the phospholipids of the membrane bilayer, such that the hydroxyl group of cholesterol is close to the hydrophilic head group of the phospholipids. This interaction decreases the mobility of the first few CH_2 groups of the phospholipids' hydrocarbon chains and makes the lipid bilayer less fluid. A high concentration of embedded cholesterol molecules, however, blocks the hydrocarbon chains from interacting with each other, which in turn increases the fluidity of the membrane.

Cytoplasm

The cytoplasm is the space that exists between the cell membrane and the nuclear envelope. It is mostly made of water (80%), but also contains proteins, ions, nucleic acids, amino acids, sugars, carbohydrates, and fatty acids. The cytoplasm provides a supportive environment for cell expansion, growth, and reproduction. Keep in mind that cytosol is different from the cytoplasm. The cytoplasm comprises cytosol plus organelles; in other words, cytosol is the liquid component of the cell that is not within organelles.

Nucleus

The organelle in which the cell's genome is located is the nucleus. Found only in eukaryotes, the nucleus has surface receptors and is the largest organelle in the cell. It contains two major components: chromatin, which is composed of a DNA–protein complex, and nucleoplasmic fibrils. Because of the DNA found inside the nucleus, this organelle is considered the storage unit of genetic information for a cell. The DNA is arranged in a very compacted and folded form (approximately 200,000 folds). The entire nucleus is surrounded by a membrane (nuclear envelope). The envelope has holes, called nuclear pores, that allow specific materials—for example, RNA, proteins, and small substances—to pass in and out of the nucleus.

The nucleus has two major functions:

- Synthesize different forms of RNA in a cellular process called transcription. The various RNAs are used to facilitate protein synthesis (translation) in the cytoplasm.

- Prepare a cell for division by allowing the DNA to be duplicated.

The DNA molecules are packed into the nucleus with the help of basic proteins called histones. The DNA of higher eukaryotes must code for all of the specialized proteins found in different tissues and organs; thus these cells contain much more DNA than one would find in a typical prokaryote such as *E. coli*. The genome within a human cell has 3 billion base pairs of nucleotide sequences and an estimated 25,000 genes. The full length of the genome is much larger than this number, however, and the cellular roles of the noncoding genes are not fully understood. A recent multinational research effort indicated that these noncoding DNA molecules, referred to as "junk DNA," may actually be important for regulation of other genes. Keep in mind that there is no simple correlation between the amount of DNA and the complexity of the organism. For instance, an amphibian genome is 50 times larger than the human genome.

Genes are segments of chromosome that contain the information for a functional polypeptide or RNA molecule. A chromosomal DNA segment (or gene) contains three specific nucleotide sequences that are required for replication: (1) the DNA replication origin, (2) a centromere to hold sister chromatids to each other, and (3) telomeres located at each end of the linear chromosome, which are known to protect the end parts of the DNA from losing base-pair sequences. Telomeres are also important because they prevent chromosomes from fusing with each other (**Figure 2.5**).

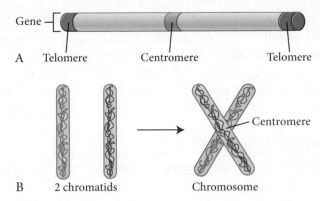

Figure 2.5 (**A**) A linear DNA segment. Both the telomeres and centromere play important roles in the protection and attachment of the sister chromatids, respectively. (**B**) A chromosome made of two chromatids.

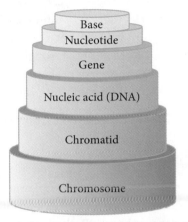

Figure 2.6 A chromosomal pyramid in which the chromosome is the largest molecule and a base (purine or pyrimidine) is the smallest molecule.

The DNA molecule is highly condensed. The human DNA helix occupies too much space to fit easily in a cell. To overcome this problem, small proteins (histones) are responsible for packing the DNA into units called nucleosomes. Histones are proteins rich in amino acid residues with basic side chains (lysine and arginine); as a result, they are positively charged. In turn, there is a tight attraction between histones and the negatively charged phosphates in DNA. **Figure 2.6** illustrates the relationship of a chromosome to its various subcomponents.

Chromosomes

Chromosomes are very long DNA molecules that are associated with packing proteins, or histones. A chromosome carries the organism's hereditary information. Before a cell gets ready to divide by the process called mitosis (discussed later in this chapter), each chromosome is duplicated. A human somatic cell has 46 chromosomes, organized as 23 pairs of chromosomes (while 22 pairs are autosomes, one pair is sex chromosomes). In other words, a somatic cell receives 23 chromosomes from the mother and 23 chromosomes from the father. While females have two X sex chromosomes (XX), males have one X and one Y chromosome (XY). The number of eukaryotic chromosomes ranges from 1 (in an Australian ant) to 190 (in a butterfly species).

In humans, the sex of an individual is determined by the sex chromosomes. Males receive a Y chromosome from their father and an X chromosome from their mother. Similarly, females receive an X chromosome from their father and an X chromosome from their mother. However, there are some exceptions to this rule, such as in Turner's syndrome, which is generally characterized by multiple congenital anomalies. A female who has Turner's syndrome receives only one single X chromosome from one of her parents but does not receive a second X chromosome during meiosis.

Each chromosome is built of two chromatids that are connected with each other by a centromere. Each chromatid possesses a linear DNA double helix that is millions of base pairs long. Each strand of this double helix consists of alternating phosphate and sugar molecules, along with their associated bases. The possible four bases in a DNA molecule are adenine (A), which forms hydrogen bonds with another base, thymine (T), in an opposite DNA strand, and guanine (G), which forms hydrogen bonds with another base, cytosine (C), in an opposite DNA strand.

Endoplasmic Reticulum

The endoplasmic reticulum (ER) is a membrane-bound channel that is attached to the nuclear membrane. It serves as a site for protein synthesis and transport. There are two types of ER: rough and smooth. While rough ER produces glycoproteins and new membrane material that is transported throughout the cell, smooth ER is involved with lipid synthesis and to some extent with carbohydrate metabolism. Like the plasma membrane, the ER is composed of lipid bilayer embedded with proteins.

The membrane of smooth ER has many enzymes that catalyze synthesis of carbohydrates and lipids. One can find a large number of smooth ER sites in cells that carry out extensive lipid synthesis (e.g., in the testes, intestine, and brain). Smooth ER is also where cells detoxify their poisons; thus hepatocytes (liver cells) are rich in smooth ER. In contrast, rough ER surface regions are composed of many ribosomes that produce a "sandpaper" shape. Because of the large number of ribosomes it contains, rough ER is the site of protein synthesis and transport. In other words, the proteins that are synthesized in rough ER are subsequently exported from the cell.

Ribosomes

As described earlier in the discussion of prokaryotic organisms, ribosomes are complex molecules that serve as the sites for protein synthesis. The eukaryotic ribosomes are called 80S ribosomes. They contain two subunits: 40S (a small subunit) and 60S (a large subunit). Both of these subunits are larger than their prokaryotic counterparts. The small subunit has one RNA, 18S rRNA (1,900 nucleotides), which is associated with 33 ribosomal proteins. The large subunit has three RNAs—5S, 5.8S, and 28S (4,700 nucleotides)—which are associated with 49 ribosomal proteins. An easy way to remember the names of the eukaryotic and prokaryotic rRNA molecules is to recognize that the number 8 is found in eukaryotes' ribosomal subunits: The ribosome is 80S, the large subunit has 28S rRNA and 5.8S rRNA, and the small subunit has 18S rRNA.

Golgi Complex

The Golgi complex is a specialized organelle that plays a role in packing and shipping molecules and controls trafficking of different types of proteins. Some of these proteins are destined for secretion, whereas others are bound for incorporation in the extracellular matrix. Basically, the Golgi complex distributes molecules that are synthesized at one location within the cell but used at another location. Of particular importance in this regard are lysosomes, because some of the lysosomal enzymes must be separated from the remaining constituents owing to their potential destructive hydrolytic effects. The important function of the Golgi complex is to ensure that the plasma membrane proteins are able to reach their destinations.

Lysosomes

Lysosomes are relatively large vesicles formed by the Golgi apparatus. They contain hydrolytic enzymes (digestive enzymes) that could destroy the key cellular macromolecules. Because these hydrolytic enzymes are held inside of lysosomes, however, they do not threaten the cellular macromolecules. Lysosomes play an important role in the extracellular breakdown of materials within the cells. They take up foreign invaders such as bacteria, food, and old organelles and digest them into small pieces, which eventually pass from the lysosome into the cytoplasm, where they serve as nutrients.

Peroxisomes

The organelles known as peroxisomes play an important role in protecting the cell from its own production of toxic hydrogen peroxide (H_2O_2). Oxygen accepts electrons and is easily reduced to hydrogen peroxide. Hydrogen peroxide is a toxic molecule because it acts as an oxidizing agent that rapidly destroys cellular components. Peroxisomes are rich in an enzyme called catalase, which catalyzes the breakdown of the hydrogen peroxide into harmless water and oxygen, thereby mitigating its effects:

$$2H_2O_2 \rightarrow 2H_2O + O_2$$

Peroxisomes oxidize long-chain fatty acids that contain more than 20 carbons, making them shorter so that the shorter fatty acids can then be oxidized completely in the mitochondria. Indeed, the toxic hydrogen peroxide is made in peroxisomes because of the oxidation process mentioned previously.

Zellweger syndrome is a devastating disease that arises in individuals (in particular, infants) who do not have functional peroxisomes in the cells of their liver, kidneys, and brain. These patients accumulate very-long-chain fatty acids (VLCFA), particularly in the brain. The physiological abnormalities commonly associated with Zellweger syndrome include an enlarged liver, high levels of cations such as iron and copper in the blood, and vision disturbances. Ingestion of oleic acid and erucic acid (Lorenzo's oil) helps to normalize the level of VLCFA through the competitive inhibitory effect exerted by an enzyme that synthesizes VLCFA.

Mitochondria

Mitochondria are the cells' energy sources. These organelles have two membranes. The outer membrane is permeable, containing many channels that allow passage of ions and small molecules. The outer membrane surrounds inner folded membranes called cristae; due to their folded shape, the cristae increase the surface area of the inner membrane. The cristae play a major role in the synthesis of ATP because they contain enzymes that are involved in oxidative phosphorylation (part of the respiratory chain; see the *Introduction to Biochemistry* chapter). In addition, the cristae contain specific transporters (proteins) that regulate transport of metabolites in and out of the mitochondrial matrix.

Many of the important enzymes that are involved in the citric acid cycle are located in the mitochondrial matrix. Each mitochondrion has its own DNA, RNA, and ribosomes. Compelling evidence indicates that mitochondria and chloroplasts originated from ancient prokaryotic organisms, through engulfment of a prokaryotic cell by a larger cell—a mechanism called endosymbiosis. This origin is also evident from the mitochondrion's size, which is equal to the size of a prokaryotic cell with no sterols in its membrane (i.e., similar to a prokaryotic cell membrane). Because it lacks cholesterol, the mitochondrial membrane is less rigid than the cytoplasmic membrane.

Cytoskeleton

The cytoplasm of all eukaryotic cells is made of a network of protein fibers that supports the form of the cell and attaches organelles to their fixed locations. The three types of protein fibers are distinguished by their size: actin filaments (the thinnest), intermediate filaments, and microtubules (the thickest). Each fiber forms by polymerization of identical subunits into long chains.

The actin filaments are twisted double strands with a function of conferring cell shape and rigidity on the cell surface. The intermediate filaments consist of eight subunits in an overlapping arrangement that provides internal mechanical support for the cell and determines the position of the cell's organelles. Interestingly, once they are synthesized, the intermediate filaments do not break down. The microtubules are tubes made of spiraling two-protein subunits (α, β). Most of the microtubules undergo continual polymerization and depolymerization. Two cytoplasmic proteins, dynein and kinesin, can bind to and move along microtubules using energy from ATP hydrolysis, thereby pulling organelles over a long distance.

Flagella and Cilia

Flagella and cilia are very long organelles (proteins). For instance, the length of flagella is approximately 50 μm and the length of cilia is approximately 10 μm. Both of these proteins, which have the same basic structure and biochemical composition (i.e., they are made of a series of microtubules), move with a wave-like motion to drive the cell through water (as when a sperm cell moves forward) or assist water in moving over the surface of tissue cells.

Learning Bridge 2.1

Amy Johnson comes to your pharmacy to pick up a few vitamins that the family physician has prescribed for Amy's son, who is suffering from a genetic disease called Zellweger syndrome. These lipid-soluble vitamins include vitamins A, D, E, and K.

Amy does not understand why her son needs so many vitamins. She asks you to explain the reason for giving him these lipid-soluble vitamins.

Membranes

Membranes are the boundaries of cells or of the cells' organelles. A variety of molecules, such as phospholipids, proteins, cholesterol, and carbohydrates, are attached to different compartments of a cell membrane (**Figure 2.7**). Each of these molecules plays an important role not only in maintaining the structure of the cell membrane but also in producing its biological functions.

Membrane Lipids

Biological membranes contain specific proteins and lipid components that enable the membranes to perform their unique roles for their cells. Because these membranes are selectively permeable, they retain certain molecules and ions within the cell while excluding others. Membranes have fluidity, meaning the lipid and protein components of the membrane are in constant motion. The fatty acyl chains of the membrane's phospholipids rotate about the C—C bonds along their lengths and move either forward or backward. As a result, lipid molecules, as well as most membrane proteins, diffuse laterally within the membrane bilayer (Figure 2.7).

The fluidity of the lipid side chains inside a biological bilayer increases with the number of double bonds in the fatty acid molecules embedded inside the bilayer. Likewise, the fluidity of a lipid bilayer increases with increasing temperature. For instance, it is known that the bacterium *E. coli* can grow at 20°C as well as at 40°C. At 40°C, the membranes of *E. coli* will contain more saturated fatty acids (fewer double bonds) than are present at 20°C. This variation indicates that a cell can regulate its fatty acid composition to maintain membrane fluidity at different temperatures. Saturated fatty acids

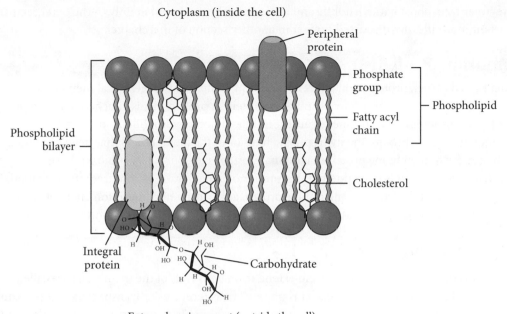

Cytoplasm (inside the cell)

Peripheral
protein

Phosphate
group

Phospholipid

Fatty acyl
chain

Phospholipid
bilayer

Cholesterol

Integral
protein

Carbohydrate

External environment (outside the cell)

Figure 2.7 The structure of a phospholipid bilayer.
Adapted from: Nelson DL, Cox MM. *Principles of biochemistry*, 5th ed. New York, NY: W. H. Freeman and Company; 2008: Chapter 11.

counterbalance the fluidizing effect of high temperature. Because humans maintain a constant body temperature, the fatty acid composition of our membrane lipids is uniform and constant as well.

Lipids move within a membrane bilayer by either of two mechanisms:

- Flip-flop diffusion. This type of diffusion is less likely to occur because the polar head of a phospholipid must span through the hydrophobic environment of the membrane. One family of proteins, known as flippases, facilitates flip-flop diffusion and makes the phospholipid move more rapidly from one side to another side.

- Lateral diffusion. This type of diffusion is more likely to occur because individual lipid molecules freely diffuse laterally within the bilayer. Sometimes the phospholipids move together as a complex unit. For instance, glycerophospholipids cluster together with cholesterol and laterally diffuse as a unit across the cell membrane.

The plasma membrane of an animal cell consists of 45% (by weight) phospholipids and 55% proteins. Phospholipids and sterols are found in both faces of the lipid bilayer (i.e., the sides that face intracellular or extracellular compartments). Integral membrane proteins penetrate or span the lipid bilayer, but peripheral membrane proteins associate at the membrane surface with lipid head groups or integral membrane proteins (Figure 2.7). The carbohydrate moieties of glycolipids and glycoproteins invariably face the extracellular compartment.

The head group of the phospholipids (e.g., serine, ethanolamine, choline) may also be charged and is a polar group. As a result, each phospholipid is an amphipathic molecule, having both polar and nonpolar regions, and forms lipid bilayers spontaneously in water. Such a lipid bilayer serves as the boundary between the cytoplasm and the environment surrounding a cell. One layer of the lipid bilayer faces the external environment, while the other layer faces the cytoplasm. Because the two layers of the membrane face different surroundings, it makes sense that they are quite differ-ent in terms of their composition and structures. Membrane lipids are asymmetrically distributed within the membrane. While phosphatidylethanolamine and phosphatidylserine are found mainly in the inner face, phosphatidylcholine and sphingomyelin are found mainly in the outer face; these important molecules are discussed further in another section of this chapter.

Membrane Proteins

As mentioned earlier, proteins constitute a significant component of biological membranes. In contrast to phospholipids, proteins and glycoprotein (a protein that is attached to a carbohydrate) cannot flip-flop across a membrane because it is difficult for a hydrophilic amino acid or a polar sugar moiety to pass through the hydrophobic interior of the membrane. It has been suggested that the asymmetry of membrane proteins is originally established during their biosynthesis. Keep in mind that a protein that is embedded in the interior of a membrane cannot freely float around. For instance, in the erythrocytes, the membrane protein ankyrin anchors the anion channel proteins to the cytoskeletal protein spectrin, thereby limiting any free diffusion of the anion channel proteins.

Integral Membrane Proteins

The proteins that span the membrane and extend from both ends of the membrane are called integral membrane proteins. These proteins often serve as receptors or transporters that transmit electrical or chemical signals across the membrane; more simply, they may act as channels or pumps that enable small molecules and ions to pass through a membrane.

The shortest α-helix (see the *Introduction to Biochemistry* chapter) segment in a protein that spans a membrane bilayer contains 20 amino acid residues. Because the hydrophobic interior of the membrane is not a friendly environment for the hydrophilic amino acids of an integral protein, the integral proteins fold so that the hydrophilic moieties are mostly in the interior of the proteins, thereby shielding them from the hydrophobic environment of the membrane.

Peripheral Membrane Proteins

Peripheral membrane proteins are attached on the surface of the membrane, often in association with other proteins. For instance, peripheral membrane proteins are attached to membranes through hydrogen bonds or ionic interactions with either integral proteins or the hydrophilic phosphate head groups of membrane phospholipids. Keep in mind that a peripheral protein can be found only on one surface of the membrane—either inside or outside of the cell membrane. Because these proteins are tightly attached to the lipids found in the membrane, to remove integral membrane proteins, it is generally necessary to use detergents.

An example of a peripheral membrane protein is the mitochondrial cytochrome *c*. This protein is associated with the outer surface of the inner mitochondrial membrane. At pH of 7.4 (physiological pH), cytochrome *c* is positively charged. As a consequence, it interacts with the negatively charged phospholipids (such as phosphatidylserine) in the inner mitochondrial membrane.

Integrins

Integrins are a large family of integral membrane proteins that comprise transmembrane glycoproteins; such proteins attach cells to extracellular matrix proteins or to ligands available on other cells. Integrins contain both α and β subunits. Some integrins mediate direct cell-to-cell recognition and interactions. The divalent cation Mg^{2+} and Ca^{2+} binding sites on integrins are essential for their adhesive function. In contrast to the cell-surface receptors for hormones and other signal molecules, integrins have low affinity but high capacity; that is, they weakly bind to their ligands, but are present in high concentrations on the cell surface. This low affinity is necessary because if they were tightly bound to the proteins of the extracellular matrix, integrins would not allow the cell to move freely, causing a very deleterious effect on the cell.

Fibronectin is a major glycoprotein of the extracellular matrix (soluble fibronectin is found in the plasma as well). Fibronectin has two identical subunits that are linked together by two disulfide bridges. Because its gene is very large and includes 50 exons, the RNA transcript undergoes an extensive splicing process to produce as many as 20 different mRNAs in different tissues. Fibronectin plays an important role by binding to integrin in attaching cells to the extracellular matrix. In addition, it assists cells in migrating through the extracellular matrix.

Cadherins and selectins are two other protein families that function similarly to integrins. All three families of integral membrane proteins are involved in cell adhesion. Integrins mediate cell adhesion to proteins of the extracellular matrix (such as collagen and fibronectin), whereas cadherins and selectins mediate cell–cell adhesion. For instance, while cadherins interact with cadherins on the surface of other cells, selectins interact with polysaccharides on the surface of other cells.

Lectins

Lectins are proteins capable of binding specific cell-surface oligosaccharide moieties of glycoproteins so as to mediate cell–cell recognition and adhesion. Indeed, a few microbial toxins and viral capsid proteins, which interact with the cell surface of oligosaccharides, are lectins. For example, lectins of *Helicobacter pylori*, the bacterium that causes gastric ulcer, interact with specific oligosaccharides of the glycoproteins found in gastric epithelial cells.

Membrane Fusion

Fusion of membranes is an important process to facilitate endocytosis, budding of vesicles from Golgi complex, and attachment of a sperm cell to an egg cell. However, some membrane fusion processes can be detrimental. For instance, many viruses utilize a fusion process to enter their host cells. A series of requirements must be met before two membranes can fuse with each other: (1) membranes should recognize each other, (2) their surfaces should be in the vicinity of each other, and (3) their bilayer should be disrupted to form a single bilayer.

Several types of membrane fusion are possible. **Table 2.1** indicates the types and functions of membrane fusion.

Table 2.1 Types of Membrane Fusion That Play Important Cellular and Physiological Roles in Prokaryotic and Eukaryotic Organisms

Type	Function	Organism
Exocytosis	To facilitate exit of molecules from a membrane-bound compartment	Prokaryotes and eukaryotes
Endocytosis	To facilitate entry of molecules into a membrane-bound compartment	Prokaryotes and eukaryotes
Fusion of lysosomes	To facilitate degradation of foreign invaders such as bacteria and old organelles	Eukaryotes
Viral infection	To facilitate entry of a virus into a host cell	None
Sperm and egg	To facilitate development of an embryo	Higher eukaryotes
Budding of vesicles from Golgi apparatus	To facilitate transport of vesicles containing proteins and other molecules to other compartments of a cell	Eukaryotes
Binary fission	To facilitate binary fission of two daughter cells from a single parent cell	Prokaryotes and eukaryotes

Membrane Transporters

The cell membrane functions to isolate the inside of the cell from its environment. It contains a concentrated hydrophobic region that is highly impermeable to most hydrophilic molecules. However, several transport systems exist that assist in transporting nutrients into and waste products out of the cell. A large number of molecules and ions must constantly travel between the inside and outside of the cell to maintain cellular functions. The plasma membrane functions as a selectively permeable membrane that allows only certain molecules and ions to cross into and out of the cell. It also serves to maintain the concentration and composition of ions inside the cell; for many ions, these concentrations and compositions are very different from those found outside the cell. Cells need to communicate with other cells and to be responsive to a series of stimuli and signals; the cell membrane, in turn, plays an instrumental role in cell communications.

Membrane transporters are proteins that are present in both prokaryotic and eukaryotic organisms. These proteins regulate the influx of essential nutrients and ions and the efflux of cellular waste, ions, and xenobiotics. Approximately 2,000 genes in the human genome (i.e., approximately 8% of the total number of human functional genes) code for transporters or transporter-related proteins.

Two general transport mechanisms are involved in membrane transport: diffusion (passive transport and facilitated diffusion) and active transport systems (ion-coupled transport and ATP-driven transport). Both facilitated and active transporters exhibit a few common features:

- There is a specific binding site for the solute.
- The transporter can be saturated with the amount of the solute, so it has a maximum rate of transport.
- There is a binding constant for the solute.
- The transporter can be competitively inhibited by other solutes.

Diffusion

Polar molecules such as amino acids and glucose cannot pass freely through the hydrophobic lipid environment of the bilayer or through the small ion channels that exist on the cell membrane. Instead, the passage of these molecules is facilitated through many integral membrane proteins (transporters). Many of these transporters are specific and bind only a particular substance or class of substances. Molecules and ions that are dissolved in the aqueous part of the cytoplasm or the exterior part of the cell are in constant, random motion. As a result of such motions, they tend to move from sites where they are in high concentration to sites where they are in low concentration. This kind of movement, called diffusion, continues until the concentrations of the molecules in all regions are the same. If the diffusion requires a protein channel, it is called facilitated diffusion; if it does not require a protein channel, it is referred to as a passive diffusion.

Passive Diffusion

Passive diffusion relies on a molecule (or a solute) that diffuses, with no energy requirement, toward a site where the solute is at a lower concentration. Because no protein transporter is involved in this mechanism, no speed or selectivity is involved in the transport of solutes. In the passive diffusion process, few nutrients—including dissolved oxygen, carbon dioxide, and water—diffuse into and out of the cell.

Facilitated Diffusion

Facilitated diffusion is similar to passive diffusion (i.e., no energy is required), but a protein transporter is involved; the latter condition explains why facilitated diffusion is selective in nature.

Proteins, as channels or transporters, facilitate the passage of specific molecules. While the facilitated diffusion is common in simple eukaryotic organisms (yeast), it is rare in prokaryotes. For instance, glycerol is one of the few molecules that enters prokaryotic cells by facilitated diffusion. An example of facilitated diffusion in eukaryotic cells is transport of glucose molecules across the cell membrane. Four transport proteins are known to bind glucose via hydrogen bonds to facilitate the transport of glucose, a hydrophilic molecule, through the hydrophobic membrane.

Active Transport

In an active transport system, energy is employed and a significant solute accumulation occurs in the cytoplasm, with the inside-the-cytoplasm concentration being higher than the external concentration. The energy needed for transport is provided by either electron movement (often an ion) or hydrolysis of an ATP molecule. Depending on the source of energy, two types of active transport mechanisms are possible: ion-coupled transport and ATP-driven transport.

Ion-Coupled Transport

In an ion-coupled transport system, a molecule is moved across the cell membrane at the expense of a previously established ion gradient (e.g., involving protons or sodium ions). Three types of ion-coupled transport systems have been identified: uniport, symport, and antiport (**Figure 2.8**).

The uniporters catalyze the transport of a substrate independent of any coupled ion; that is, they carry only one substrate at a time. In contrast, the symport and antiport types are cotransport systems in which two solutes move through the membrane simultaneously (Figure 2.8). The entry of glucose into erythrocytes is facilitated by the glucose transporter 1 (GluT1) protein. The GluT1 protein is made of 12 transmembrane helical segments whose side-by-side association provides a channel where the hydrophilic parts face the central cavity of the channel. This channel provides hydrogen bonds to the glucose molecule (solute) to facilitate the transport of glucose across the membrane. GluT1 is an example of a uniport system.

Symporters catalyze the concurrent transport of two substrates in the same direction by a single carrier; for example, an Na^+ gradient can permit symport of a glucose molecule.

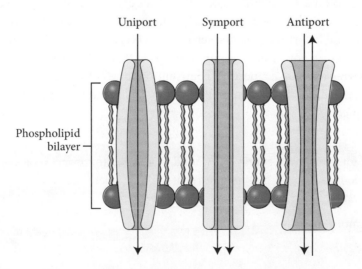

Figure 2.8 Three types of ion-coupled transport systems.

Adapted from: Pandit NK, Soltis RP. *Introduction to pharmaceutical sciences: an integrated approach*, 2nd ed. Baltimore, MD: Walters Kluwer/Lippincott Williams and Wilkins; 2012: Chapter 5.

An example of a symporter is the sodium-glucose transporter (SGL), which actively reabsorbs glucose in the proximal tubule of the kidney. At least two SGL variants exist: SGL-1 and SGL-2. SGL-2 has attracted attention due to its role in reabsorbing glucose in the kidney and as a potential site to inhibit during treatment of type 2 diabetes (see the *Introduction to Pharmacology and Pathophysiology* chapter).

Antiporters catalyze the simultaneous transport of one solute in one direction and the other solute in the opposite direction. For example, the transport of HCO_3^-/Cl^- in and out (exchange) of erythrocytes is facilitated by a chloride–bicarbonate exchanger that is an antiport protein (see also the *Introduction to Nutrients* chapter). Another example of an antiport protein is the Na^+K^+ ATPase enzyme, which pumps two K^+ ions in and three Na^+ ions out of each cell. Both ions must be present to make this transport system an effective mechanism.

With ions and charged molecules, the concentration of the ion and the electrical potential across the membrane are critically important. These two phenomena together constitute the electrochemical gradient that determines the direction of the net movement of ions and charged species in and out of a membrane-bound compartment. An unequal distribution of molecules between the outside and the inside of a membrane is an energy-rich condition. If the molecule also contains a charged species, it gives an electrical potential to the membrane as well. This electrical potential must be taken into consideration when you want to know how much energy is necessary to move that molecule from outside to inside (or vice versa) of a membrane-bound compartment. The Gibbs free energy change (ΔG) for moving ions or molecules can be measured (**Equation 2.1**) when an ion or a molecule goes from a region in which its concentration is C_1 to a region where its concentration is C_2:

$$\Delta G_t = RT \ln (C_2/C_1) + Z F \Delta\psi \tag{2.1}$$

where Z is the charge on the ion, F is the Faraday constant (in J/V-mol), and Ψ is the transmembrane electrical potential (in volts).

If the $\Delta\Psi$ is negative (which is the normal case where the inside of the cell is negative relative to outside) and if Z is a cation and wants to go from outside (C_1) to inside (C_2), the second term of Equation 2.1 ($Z F \Delta\Psi$) makes a negative contribution to ΔG. In addition, if the number of the cations outside the compartment is higher than the number inside, due to the function of the natural logarithm, the first term [$RT \ln (C_2/C_1)$] also makes a negative contribution to the free energy. In contrast, if the ion is an anion that is in low concentration outside of the cell, both terms will make a positive contribution to ΔG. A positive ΔG means input of energy is necessary to drive the action (a nonspontaneous process; see also the *Introduction to Biochemistry* chapter).

Example 2.1: How much free energy is required or released to move 3 moles of Na^+ from inside of a cell (where you have 12 mM Na^+) to outside of the cell (where you have 140 mM Na^+) at 37°C? The following parameters are known for these ion movements:

$R = 8.314$ J/K mol

$T = 310$ K (273 + 37°C)

$F = 96.5$ kJ/V

$\Delta\Psi = 0.07$ V

Here you have to know what the concentrations are:

$C_2 = 140$ mM

$C_1 = 12$ mM

$Z = 1$ because Na^+ has only one charge

Answer: The free energy change (ΔG) for moving ions or molecules can be measured when an ion or a molecule goes from a region in which its concentration is C_1 to a region where its concentration is C_2. Putting these data into Equation 2.1 gives

$\Delta G = 6{,}332 + 6{,}755$ J/mol $= 13{,}087$ J/mol, as we have 3 Na^+ 3
$\times 13{,}098 = 39{,}260$ J/mol $= 39.26$ kJ/mol

The sign is positive, so this amount of energy is required to pump three Na^+ ions from inside to outside of the cell. This makes sense because the system must pump Na^+ against its concentration gradient.

ATP-Driven Transport

Four major classes of ATP-driven active transporters exist: P, F, V, and ABC transporters. All four classes have one or more binding sites for ATP on the cytosolic face of the membrane. Despite the fact these proteins are ATPases (i.e., they hydrolyze ATP molecules), the system is tightly coupled so that the energy is not dissipated.

- *P class*. In this class, ATP is hydrolyzed to pump out three Na^+ ions and pump in two K^+ ions. The P-class ATPase has two subunits, α and β, where the α subunit has a binding site for the ATP molecule. The hydrolysis of ATP occurs only when the Na^+ and K^+ ions are bound to the pump. A significant amount of ATP is hydrolyzed by this mechanism (more than one-third of the body's total ATP is consumed here). The Na^+/K^+ ATPase makes a significant contribution to the electrochemical excitability of neurons. Digoxin (Lanoxin) is a cardiac glycoside that inhibits the Na^+/K^+ ATPase in myocardial cells, which increases the concentration of intracellular sodium. The elevated sodium level increases calcium influx, resulting in enhanced cardiac contractility.

- *F type*. The mitochondrial ATP synthase enzyme belongs to this type; it utilizes a proton gradient across the mitochondrial membrane to synthesize ATP. The F-type ATPase consists of two parts: a peripheral domain, F_1 (which is made of nine different polypetides), and an integral domain, F_0. The whole molecule is called F_0F_1 ATP synthase or simply ATP synthase. ATP synthase can be found in large amounts in the inner mitochondrial membrane, chloroplast, and bacterial membrane (see also the discussion of oxidative phosphorylation in the *Introduction to Biochemistry* chapter).

- *V type*. The V-type transporter has two domains: a peripheral domain, V_1, which is made of multiple subunits, and an integral domain, V_0. The V type actively and selectively transports H^+ across the membranes of the cytoplasmic organelles and vacuoles of plants; a vacuole is an organelle that is filled with water, which produces a hydrostatic pressure, gives rigidity to the plant cell, and has hydrolytic enzymes to digest complex molecules (V stands for vacuole). V-type transporters are found in lysosomes, secretory granules, and vacuole membranes. For instance, the V-type pump creates low pH (high H^+) inside lysosomes to activate proteases and other hydrolytic enzymes because lysosomal hydrolytic enzymes are most active at pH 5.

- *ABC transporters.* The 49 identified genes for ABC transporters can be divided into seven families (ABCA to ABCG). Among the best-known transporters in the ABC superfamily are P-glycoprotein (P-gp, also called multidrug resistance-1 protein [MDR1]) and the cystic fibrosis transmembrane regulator (CFTR).

The CFTR protein is a chloride channel that plays a role in cystic fibrosis (CF). CF is an autosomal recessive disease that is caused by a mutation on chromosome 7 and results in an abnormal mucus production. A functional CFTR acts as a Cl$^-$ channel in epithelial cells and regulates ion transport in the sweat glands. Chloride ion is reabsorbed from the lumen by the CFTR. In individuals with CF, the dysfunctional CFTR fails to reabsorb Cl$^-$, which also affects sodium ion reabsorption. Collectively, these effects result in production of a salty sweat. In addition, an increase of Cl$^-$ concentration within the surface fluid of the lungs provides a suitable milieu for the growth of pathogenic bacteria.

Researchers have shown that growing cancer cells become resistant to anticancer drugs. The reason for such resistance is the expression of the integral protein called P-glycoprotein on the cancer cells. This protein pumps anticancer drugs, via an ATP hydrolysis-dependent mechanism, out of cells before the drugs have any chance to exert their effect (multidrug transporter ATPase). Consequently, multidrug resistance (MDR) is a major problem in chemotherapy treatment. One goal in cancer research is to understand the role of MDR and to find drugs that prevent development of drug resistance in cancer cells.

Learning Bridge 2.2

Amy Johnson comes to your pharmacy with her 7-year-old daughter, Kristin, to receive Kristin's antibiotic tobramycin. The prescription reads as follows:

TOBI 300 mg/5 mL

Solution for nebulization

To be inhaled using a handheld nebulizer every 12 hours for 28 days. Do not mix any other drug with TOBI in the nebulizer.

Refill: 4

You are an intern pharmacist in the pharmacy and have never heard before that antibiotics can be used in an inhaler. You are also wondering why Kristin has been prescribed an antibiotic for such a long time (28 days) with four refills. However, the type of dosage form and the length of the therapy remind you of a specific genetic disease that Kristin may be suffering from. While you are filling the prescription and making ready to counsel the patient, Amy makes a very specific statement that confirms your thinking about the genetic disease: "Each time I kiss Kristin, I feel how salty her skin is."

A. What was the genetic disease that you initially thought about?
B. Why did Amy's statement confirm your thinking about Kristin's disease?
C. How will you counsel Amy about the use of tobramycin?

Ion Channels

Ions are charged species that are repelled by the hydrophobic interior of the membrane bilayer. Because of this resistance, without any help, ions cannot move between the cytoplasm of the cell and the extracellular space. Ion channels, however, can facilitate transport of ions across the cell membrane. These channels open and close in response to external stimuli or events such as binding of a ligand to a receptor or changes in electrical potential across the membrane. The permeability of an ion channel depends on the size and charge density of the ion. For instance, specific channels are available for Na^+, K^+, Ca^{2+}, and Cl^-. The K^+ channel consists of four identical subunits. The specificity of the potassium channel for K^+ over Na^+ is mainly due to the negative carboxyl ends from each of the four subunits that extend into the lumen of the channel and interact with K^+ ions. Consequently, the Na^+ ion, which is smaller than the K^+ ion, is not large enough to interact with the negatively charged subunits.

An ion channel can be either ligand-gated or voltage-gated (see also the *Introduction to Pharmacodynamics* chapter). In a ligand-gated ion channel, the channel can be controlled by opening or closing the gate. For instance, a specific ligand (such as acetylcholine) binds to its receptor (acetylcholine receptor that serves as an ion channel) and opens the channel. In a voltage-gated channel, the gate opens or closes in response to changes in membrane potential. The voltage-gated Na^+ channel is a typical example of an ion channel that is made of a variety of subunits. For instance, the voltage-gated Na^+ channels close when the voltage of the membrane is $-60m$ volt (i.e., when the membrane is at rest) and open when the membrane is depolarized i.e., when inside the cell is positive). In addition to the transporters mentioned previously, certain proteins (channels) facilitate movement of water molecules across erythrocytes and cells of the collecting ducts of the kidneys. These proteins, called aquaporins, are integral membrane proteins. There are 14 different mammalian aquaporins, and even more members of this family are suspected to exist. Crystallographic studies have shown that while these channels permit the passage of water, they prevent the passage of other molecules, particularly ions. Of particular interest is the role of aquaporin-2 (AQP-2) in nephrogenic diabetes insipidus (**Figure 2.9**). Diabetes insipidus is a disease associated with inadequate release or action of antidiuretic hormone (ADH; also known as vasopressin). Without ADH, aquaporin cannot reabsorb water from the collecting ducts, leading to

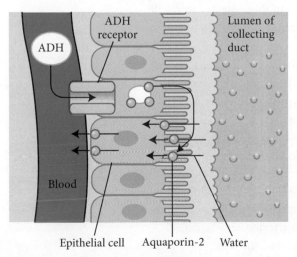

Figure 2.9 ADH binds to its receptor and causes the collecting ducts to activate AQP-2, thereby enhancing transport of water across the epithelial cells.

reduction in water reabsorption and retention. As a result, a large volume of urine (5–10 L) is produced. Vasopressin (Pitressin)—an analog to ADH—is therefore used in the treatment of patients with nephrogenic diabetes insipidus. When exposed to vasopressin, vesicles carrying AQP-2 are positioned into the luminal membrane of epithelial cells, which increases water permeability at the renal tubules of the kidneys.

The interplay between AQP-2 and ADH is important in avoiding dehydration. When a person becomes dehydrated, the blood osmotic pressure rises. Consequently, the hypothalamus secretes large amounts of ADH. The ADH causes the kidney collecting ducts to mobilize AQP-2. This action promotes the reabsorbtion of water through the epithelial cells (the cells that line the collecting ducts in the kidney) into the blood (Figure 2.9). In turn, water is conserved, preventing further dehydration. In addition, dehydration makes the affected person thirsty, and subsequent drinking restores the water volume. In the presence of enough water, ADH will not be released and as a result, the water will not reabsorbed but rather excreted as urine.

Cell Junctions

Cell–cell adhesion is a very common cellular process in animal tissues. Two major forms of cell junctions have been identified: tight junctions and gap junctions (**Figure 2.10**).

In tight junctions, cells are tied to each other with strength and stability. These kinds of junctions can be found in epithelial cells in the intestinal mucosa, in renal tubules, and in certain parts of the ventricular system of the brain (choroid plexus). A series of transmembrane proteins assists in adhering cells together to build the tight junction.

A gap junction permits passage of ions and small molecules (sugars, amino acids, and other molecules with a molecular weight of less than 1,000 Da) from one cell to another by building a channel between cells. Ions and molecules can enter adjacent cells without entering the extracellular matrix, which therefore couples cells together electrically and metabolically. Each channel, which is referred to as a connexon, is built when six protein subunits (each called connexins) bind to each other (Figure 2.10B). Keep in mind that building these channels is not a random process. At least 20 different genes code for connexons in humans, and a mutation in these genes can result in defective communication between cells and have devastating consequences. In animal studies, it has been shown that connexin deletions in mice may result in electrophysiological defects in the heart, female sterility, abnormal bone development, and abnormal growth in the liver. In humans, deficiencies in connexin proteins have been linked to a series of skin disorders such as Clouston syndrome and erythrokeratoderma variabilis, as well as other physiological consequences such as deafness, predisposition to myoclonic epilepsy and arteriosclerosis, cataracts, and idiopathic atrial fibrillation.

Table 2.2 summarizes cellular activities associated with membrane mechanisms in both prokaryotic and eukaryotic organisms.

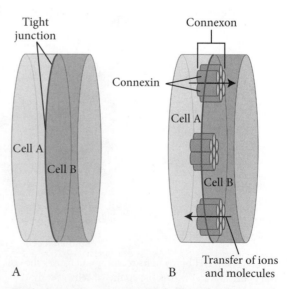

Figure 2.10 Two major types of cell junctions: (A) tight junctions and (B) gap junctions.

Table 2.2 Cellular Activity and Membrane Mechanisms for Prokaryotic and Eukaryotic Organisms

Cellular Activity	Membrane Mechanism	Prokaryotic Cell	Eukaryotic Cell
Cross-membrane movement of small molecules	Diffusion (passive and facilitated)	Yes	Yes
	Active transport	Yes	Yes
Cross-membrane movement of large molecules	Endocytosis (phagocytosis and pinocytosis)	No	Yes
	Exocytosis	No	Yes
Group translocation	Uptake of glucose and mannose (the sugars become phosphorylated during the transport process)	Yes	No
Signal transmission across membranes	Signal transduction	Yes	Yes
	Signal internalization (coupled with endocytosis, such as the low-density lipoprotein [LDL] receptor)	No	Yes
	Movement to intracellular receptors (steroid hormones; a form of diffusion)	No	Yes
Intercellular contact and communication	Passive (simple) diffusion: flow of solute from an area of higher concentration to an area of lower concentration due to random thermal movement.	Yes	Yes
	Facilitated diffusion: passive transport of a solute from an area of higher concentration to an area of lower concentration, mediated by a specific protein transporter	Yes	Yes
	Active transport: transport of a solute across a membrane in the direction of increasing concentration, which requires energy (frequently derived from the hydrolysis of ATP); a specific transporter (pump) is involved	Yes	Yes

---

Learning Bridge 2.3

A 50-year-old woman who is suffering from breast cancer comes to your pharmacy and asks a few questions related to her health condition. She explains how good she felt after taking methotrexate (Rheumatrex) for 1 year. She is very confused now and does not understand why this drug and even other drugs (she tried vincristine—a totally different drug from methotrexate) no longer do any good for her. What would be your comments to this patient?

Structure and Function of Biomolecules

Amino Acids

Amino acids are not only important for the synthesis of proteins, but are also essential for the synthesis of neurotransmitters, hormones, porphyrins, purines, pyrimidines, and urea. Although more than 300 naturally occurring amino acids exist, only 20—the so-called common amino acids (**Table 2.3**)—constitute the building blocks of all proteins. All proteins are made of various compositions of these 20 specific amino acids. As mentioned earlier, several of the amino acids serve as precursors to other molecules. An example is the tyrosine amino acid, which is involved in the formation of thyroid hormones, norepinephrine, and epinephrine hormones. Similarly, the tryptophan amino acid is important for the synthesis of niacin (vitamin B_3) and the neurotransmitter serotonin.

Table 2.3 Common Amino Acids That Are Used by the Protein Synthetic Machinery

Amino Acid	Three-Letter Abbreviation	Symbol
Alanine	Ala	A
*Arginine	Arg	R
Asparagine	Asn	N
Aspartic acid	Asp	D
Cysteine	Cys	C
Glutamic acid	Glu	E
Glutamine	Gln	Q
Glycine	Gly	G
*Histidine	His	H
*Isoleucine	Ile	I
*Leucine	Leu	L
*Lysine	Lys	K
*Methionine	Met	M
*Phenylalanine	Phe	F
Proline	Pro	P
Serine	Ser	S
*Threonine	Thr	T
*Tryptophan	Trp	W
Tyrosine	Tyr	Y
*Valine	Val	V

*Essential amino acids

The α-carbon of all amino acids (except glycine) is bound to four different atoms or groups of atoms, which explains why the α-carbon is a chiral center, or asymmetric. This arrangement indicates that all of the amino acids (except glycine) are enantiomers and optically active. Only the L-enantiomer amino acids are produced in the animal and plant cells and participate in protein synthesis (a more detailed description of chiral molecules and their importance in medicinal chemistry is provided in the *Introduction to Medicinal Chemistry* chapter).

All of the 20 common amino acids share the absolute configuration of L-glyceraldehyde and, as a result, are classified as L-amino acids. While human proteins contain only L-amino acids, there has been an indication that D-serine and D-aspartate may exist in the brain tissue. In contrast, D-alanine and D-glutamate can be found in the cell walls of Gram-positive bacteria. However, some bacterial peptides with D-amino acids are toxic. For instance, the cyanobacterial peptides microcystin and nodularin are very toxic and can cause hepatic cancer. A few peptides with D-amino acids have therapeutic effects, including the antibiotics bacitracin (Baciguent) and Gramicidin A and the antitumor glycopeptide agent bleomycin (Blenoxane, from Canada).

Organisms differ, to a great extent, in their ability to synthesize amino acids. Humans and other higher animals are not able to synthesize 10 of the 20 common L-amino acids (the so-called essential amino acids). As a result, our diet must include adequate amounts of the essential amino acids.

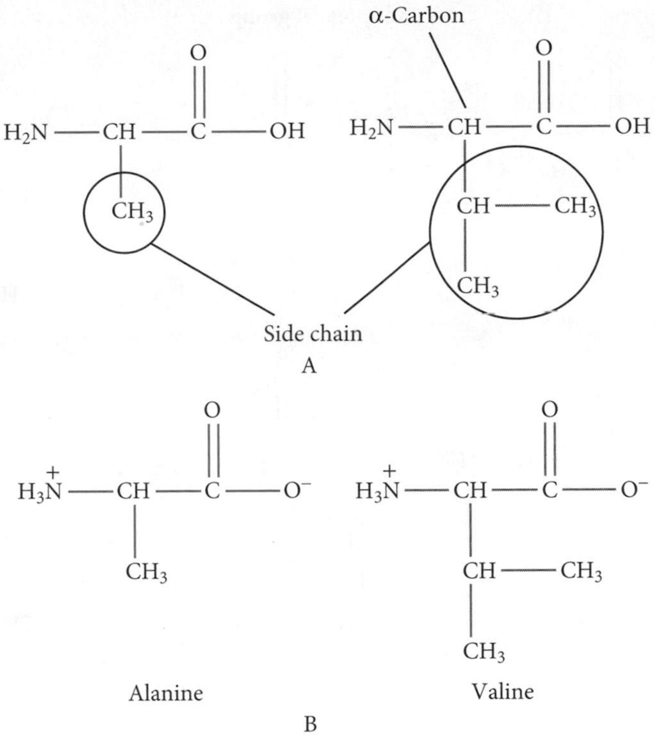

Figure 2.11 The structures of the amino acids alanine and valine and their side chains (R groups). Structure (A) cannot exist in any body fluids. Structure (B) depicts the charged amino acids found in the blood and tissues.

Each amino acid is designated by both a three-letter abbreviation and a one-letter symbol (Table 2.3). For instance, alanine is designated as Ala (abbreviation) and A (symbol). All 20 common amino acids have a carboxyl group and an amino group bound to the same carbon atom, known as the α-carbon. However, amino acids differ from one another in their side chain (R) groups. Because of the presence of amino groups and carboxyl groups in all 20 amino acids, amino acids are charged molecules in the blood and tissues (**Figure 2.11**).

The nonessential amino acids can be synthesized from other amino acids or by using the carbon skeletons from the citric acid cycle intermediates and NH_3 from glutamate. For instance, cysteine and tyrosine can both be synthesized in the body from the essential amino acids methionine and phenylalanine, respectively. The essential amino acids are phenylalanine, threonine, histidine, valine, isoleucine, arginine, tryptophan, methionine, leucine, and lysine.

Keep in mind that arginine is an essential amino acid in the diet of juveniles but not adults.

Characteristics of R (Side Chain) Groups

Five classes of amino acids are defined based on the character of their R (side chain) groups:

1. Nonpolar R group
2. Polar R group
3. Aromatic R group
4. Positively charged R group (basic)
5. Negatively charged R group (acidic)

Nonpolar R group

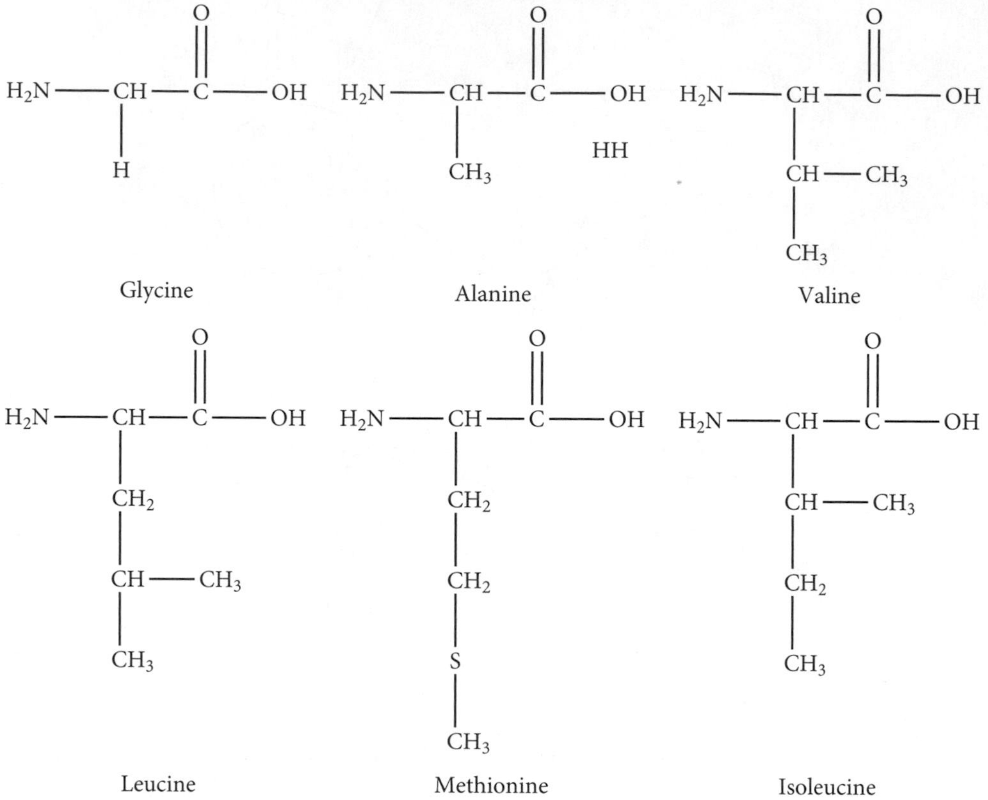

Figure 2.12 The structures of amino acids with nonpolar R groups.

Nonpolar R Group

The R group is hydrophobic and stabilizes the structure of protein by hydrophobic interaction. The hydrophobic character is important for purification of proteins in research laboratories (i.e., by a column chromatography, in which a hydrophobic protein attaches to a hydrophobic column to separate that protein from other less hydrophobic proteins). Nonpolar amino acid residues cluster within the protein, where they engage in hydrophobic interactions with similar nonpolar amino acids. This process creates a hydrophobic environment within an enzyme where chemical reactions can be catalyzed (**Figure 2.12**).

Polar R Group

The R group in this class is hydrophilic, so it readily interacts with water (**Figure 2.13A**). Polar R groups often present on the surface of a protein, where they can interact with the hydrophilic intracellular or extracellular environment of the cells. Cysteine is a unique amino acid that with another cysteine, upon oxidation, builds a disulfide (S—S) bridge to form cystine. The disulfide bridge is an important reaction for the formation of active structural domains in a large number of proteins (**Figure 2.13B**). The primary alcohol group of serine amino acid residue and the primary thioalcohol (—SH) group of cysteine amino acid residue are effective nucleophiles that donate electrons during enzymatic catalysis. The secondary alcohol group of threonine, although a nucleophile, cannot perform the same function in a catalytic reaction.

Aromatic R Group

These amino acids are hydrophobic amino acids (**Figure 2.14**). All of them absorb, to different extents, ultraviolet (UV) light—a very powerful tool for quantitative measurement of proteins

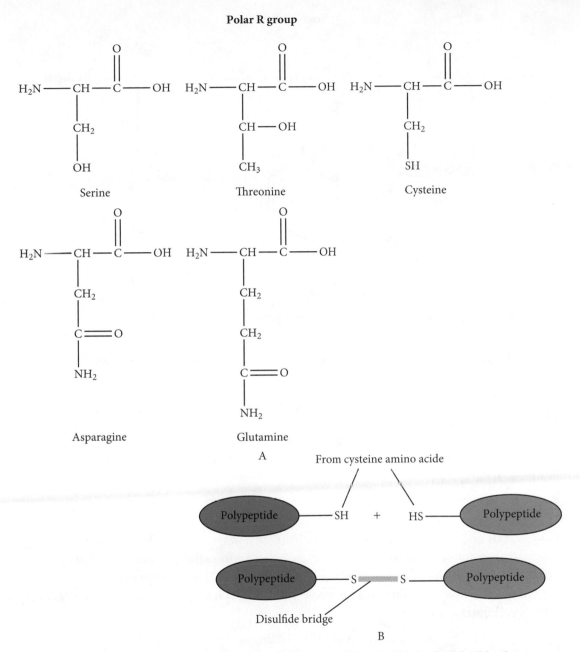

Figure 2.13 (A) The structures of amino acids with polar R groups. (B) A disulfide bridge is built by the interaction of two cysteine amino acids.

(at 280-nm wavelength). Tryptophan, however, absorbs UV light approximately 10 times more efficiently than the other two aromatic amino acids. As a result, tryptophan, in a protein, makes the major contribution to absorb light. All three aromatic amino acids are involved in the synthesis of neurotransmitters (see also the *Introduction to Pharmacology and Pathophysiology* chapter). The primary OH group of tyrosine participates in reactions with regulatory enzymes whose catalytic activity depends on the phosphorylation of the OH group (see the *Introduction to Pharmacodynamics* chapter).

Positively Charged R Group (Basic)

These hydrophilic amino acids have basic side chains at neutral pH. Their side chains contain nitrogen. Because of nitrogen's basicity, it tends to bind protons, thereby becoming positively

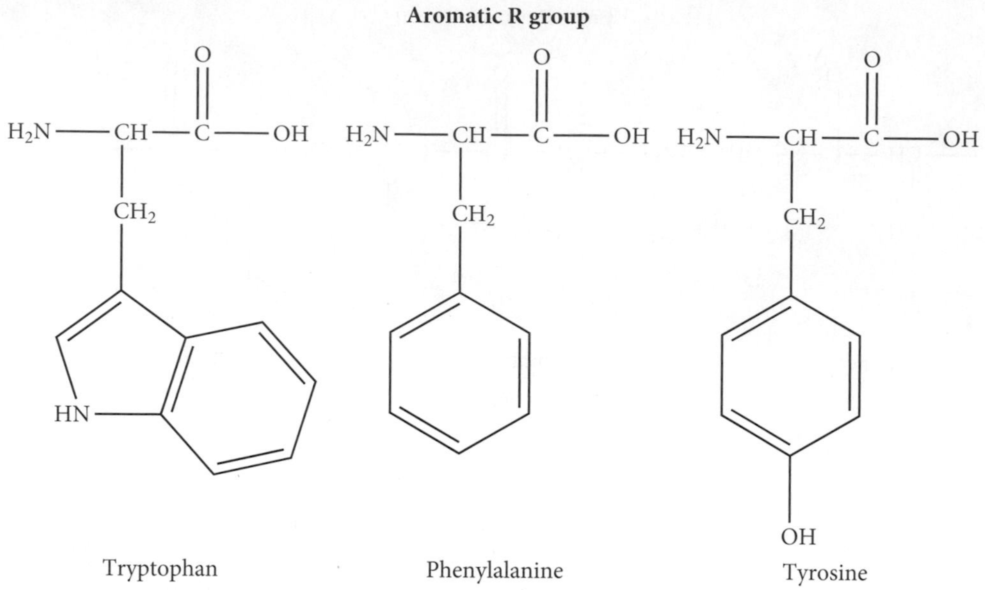

Aromatic R group

Figure 2.14 The structures of amino acids with aromatic R groups.

charged (**Figure 2.15A**). The charged R groups tend to stabilize specific protein conformations via ionic interactions or salt bridges.

Negatively Charged R Group (Acidic)

These amino acids have acidic side chains at neutral pH (**Figure 2.15B**). Their side chains have carboxyl groups whose pK_a values are low enough that they lose protons and thereby become negatively charged molecules.

Zwitterions

The —COOH and —NH$_2$ groups attached to the α-carbon in amino acids are capable of being ionized, similar to the acidic and basic R groups of the amino acids. An amino acid with no ionizable R group is electrically neutral at biological pH (pH 7); such an entity is referred to as a zwitterion. For instance, glycine in an aqueous solution (such as in the blood) is in the form of a zwitterion (**Figure 2.16**).

Amino acids in the blood and tissues exist as zwitterions. The uncharged glycine (Figure 2.16) cannot exist in an aqueous solution because any pH low enough to protonate the carboxyl group will also protonate the amino group, thereby making the amino group a positively charged species.

As mentioned in the *Introduction to Biological Chemistry* chapter, the acid strengths of weak acids are expressed by their pK_a values. For amino acids that have multiple dissociable protons, the pK_a for each acidic group (or conjugate acid) is indicated by replacing the subscript "a" with a number (**Table 2.4**). The net charge of any amino acid will depend on the pH of the aqueous environment in which the amino acid is dissolved. The pH that makes the net charge of an amino acid be zero is equivalent to the isoelectric point (pI). Glycine is positively charged in a pH lower than its pI; it is negatively charged in a pH higher than its pI.

The pI is the mean of a molecule's two pK_a values: pI = $(pK_1 + pK_2)/2$. For instance, for the amino acid phenylalanine that has two dissociating groups, pK_1 (R—COOH) is 2.2 and pK_2 (R—NH$_3^+$) is 9.2. The pI of phenylalanine is the mean of these two dissociation constants, which is 5.7. The pI plays an important role in a clinical laboratory (or a research laboratory where

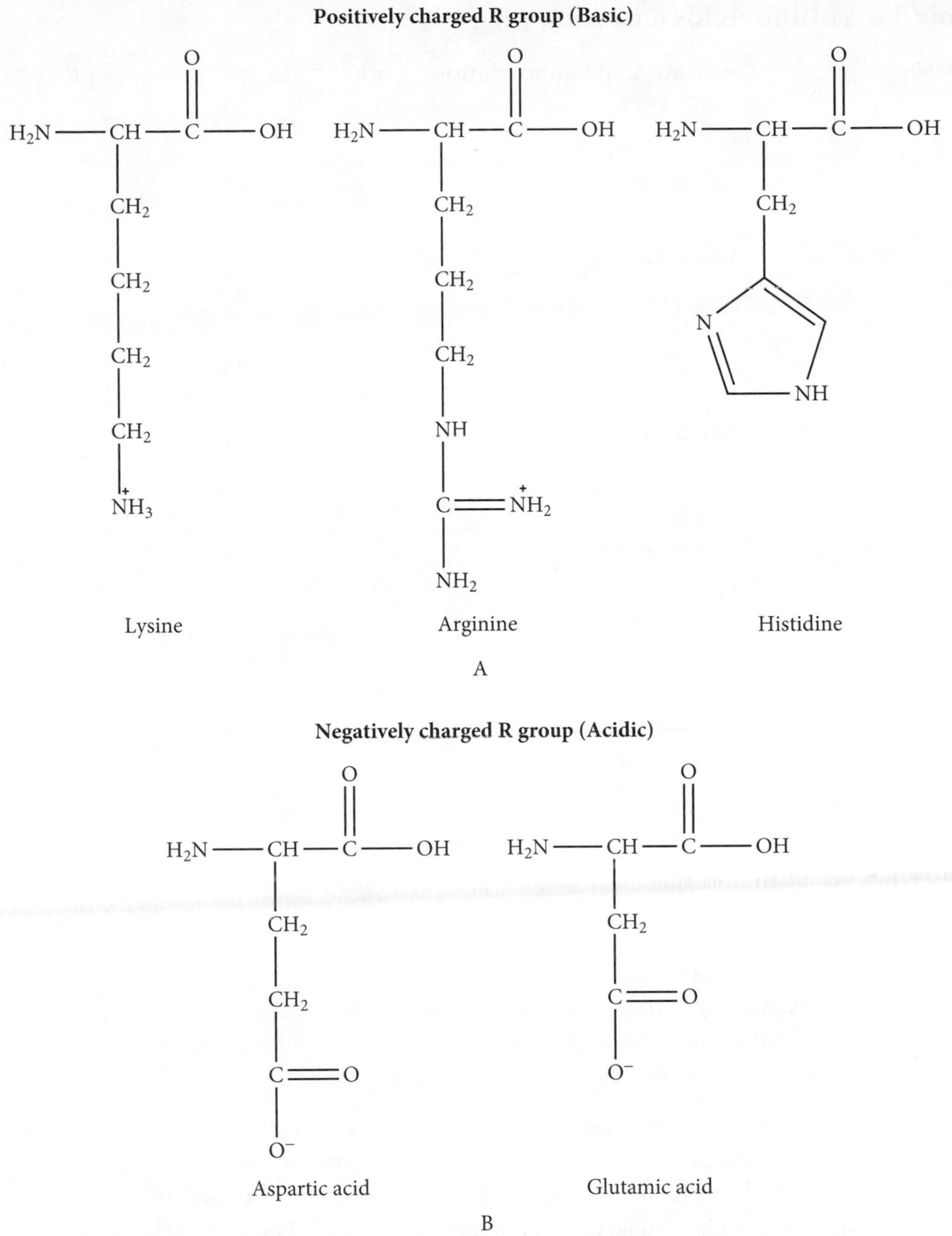

Positively charged R group (Basic)

Lysine

Arginine

Histidine

A

Negatively charged R group (Acidic)

Aspartic acid

Glutamic acid

B

Figure 2.15 The structures of amino acids with positively charged (A) and negatively charged (B) R groups.

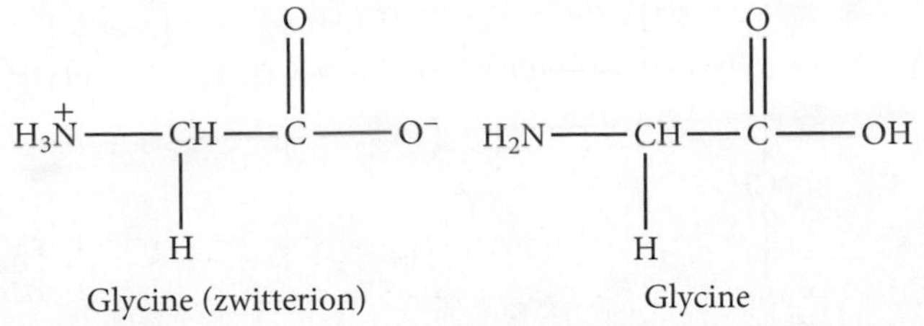

Glycine (zwitterion)

Glycine

Figure 2.16 Glycine is both positively and negatively charged at a neutral pH and, as a result, is a zwitterion.

Table 2.4 Amino Acids and Their pK_a Values

R Group	Amino Acid (Abbreviation)	pK_1 α-COOH	pK_2 α-NH$_2$	pK_3 (R Group)
Nonpolar	Glycine (Gly)	2.4	9.8	
	Alanine (Ala)	2.4	9.9	
	Valine (Val)	2.2	9.7	
	Leucine (Leu)	2.3	9.7	
	Methionine (Met)	2.1	9.3	
	Isoleucine (Ile)	2.3	9.8	
Polar	Serine (Ser)	2.2	9.2	
	Threonine (Thr)	2.1	9.1	
	Cysteine (Sys)	1.9	10.8	8.3
	Asparagine (Asn)	2.1	8.8	
	Glutamine (Gln)	2.2	9.1	
Aromatic	Tryptophan (Trp)	2.4	9.4	
	Phenylalanine (Phe)	2.2	9.2	
	Tyrosine (Tyr)	2.2	9.1	10.1
Positively charged	Lysine (Lys)	2.2	9.2	10.8
	Arginine (Arg)	1.8	9.0	12.5
	Histidine (His)	1.8	9.3	6.0
Negatively charged	Aspartic acid (Asp)	2.0	9.9	3.9
	Glutamic acid (Glu)	2.1	9.5	4.1

Adapted from: Nelson DL, Cox MM. *Principles of biochemistry*, 5th ed. New York: W. H. Freeman and Company; 2008: Chapter 3.

purification of proteins takes place), because it assists in selecting the appropriate conditions for electrophoretic separations of proteins. For instance, at pH 7.0, one can separate two proteins with pI values of 6.0 and 9.0 because the first protein with a pI of 6.0 will have a net positive charge and the second protein with a pI of 9.0 will have a net negative charge.

A growing body of evidence indicates that the amino acid selenocysteine can be considered the "21st amino acid." Similar to the other 20 amino acids, selenocysteine is an L-amino acid that is found in a few proteins, including a few peroxidases and reductase enzymes. The selenium atom replaces the sulfur of its analog, cysteine (**Figure 2.17**). It is believed that selenocysteine is inserted into polypeptides during translation. However, there is no codon in the genetic code (see the *Introduction to Biochemistry* chapter) that is specific for selenocysteine. Metabolism of

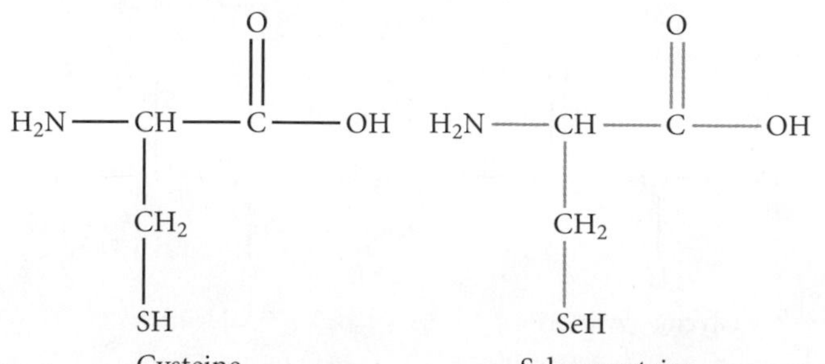

Figure 2.17 Selenocysteine mimics the amino acid cysteine.

selenocysteine can produce selenium—a mineral that humans need to consume daily in an amount of approximately 100 µg (although as much as 400 µg is tolerable). Selenium is believed to improve feelings of well-being and mood. It has been suggested that selenium deficiency reduces synthesis of triiodothyronine (T_3) from thyroxine (T_4) and that taking a selenium supplement might increase conversion of T_4 to T_3 in elderly patients (see also the *Introduction to Pharmacology and Pathophysiology* chapter). However, patients who are iodine and selenium deficient should not receive selenium supplements alone because this treatment might exacerbate the thyroid hormone deficiency (hypothyroidism). Liver, fish, broccoli, garlic, and onions are rich in selenium.

Proteins

Proteins are functional macromolecules that perform essential and specific functions. They are found both intracellularly and extracellularly, and can be embedded in or extended from a membrane. In the cytoskeleton, proteins (tubules and microtubules) participate in maintaining cellular shape and physical integrity; in muscles, proteins (actin and myosin) participate in muscle contraction and relaxation; in the blood, proteins (hemoglobin, albumin, and antibodies) bind and transfer oxygen or fatty acids or defend against foreign agents; and as enzymes, proteins (kinases and proteases) are involved in essential catalytic activities. In addition, proteins are found as membrane-bound or intracellular receptors that respond to external hormones and other ligands.

The life span of proteins begins with gene expression and translation, matures through post-translational modifications, and metabolizes through oxidation and deamination back to the original building blocks (amino acids) to either provide energy (through amino acid oxidation) or to recycle the amino acids to produce other proteins (protein synthesis). Reflecting proteins' unique multifunctional properties, many diseases are caused by nonfunctional proteins.

Proteins fold into their native (active) conformation by twisting and turning so that their backbone forms a series of stable structures. Between two amino acids in a protein chain is a peptide bond (covalent bond) involving carbonyl carbon and a nitrogen atom (**Figure 2.18**). Due to the delocalization of electrons over the peptide bond, only two bonds per amino acid are able to rotate. It is the primary structure of a protein that indicates the exact order of the amino acid residues that exist in the protein. In addition, the primary structure dictates the final form they will take as they twist and turn after post-translational modifications (see also the *Introduction to Biochemistry* chapter).

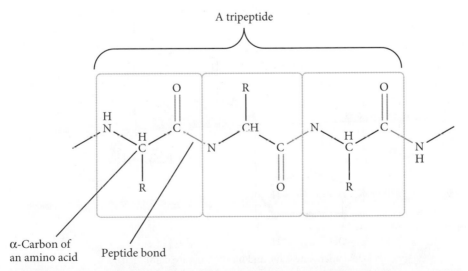

Figure 2.18 Structure of a tripeptide in which a peptide bond is formed between two amino acid residues. The peptide bond is not able to rotate due to the delocalization of electrons over the peptide bond.

Proteins may have any of four different structures: primary, secondary, tertiary, or quaternary. While the primary structure is built by a linear polymer of amino acids linked together by peptide bonds (Figure 2.18), the secondary structure assumes two folding models: the α-helix and the β-sheet. Both α-helices and β-sheets project their side chains outward. In the secondary structure, the amino acid residues are generally near each other. In contrast to the secondary structure, the tertiary structure is strongly influenced by amino acid residues that are very far apart in sequence, and interactions between the R groups play an important role in maintaining the structural integrity of the tertiary structure. A quaternary structure is formed when two or more polypeptide chains (or subunits, as they are often called) attach to one another. More detailed information about these structures is provided in the *Introduction to Biochemistry* chapter.

Nucleic Acids

DNA

Nucleotides are the building blocks of nucleic acids, which serve as storage units for our genetic information. Two cellular types of nucleic acid exist: ribonucleic acid (RNA) and deoxyribonucleic acid (DNA). Nucleotides are also the primary carriers of chemical energy in cells (ATP, GTP), structural components of electron carrier coenzymes (NAD^+, $NADP^+$, FAD, and FMN), and cellular second messengers (cAMP, cGMP). DNA is a polymer synthesized by attachment of nucleotide units. The nucleotide unit includes a base, a deoxyribose sugar, and a phosphate group. It is the nitrogenous base that determines the identity of the nucleotide. A nucleotide without the phosphate group is called a nucleoside. In **Figure 2.19**, the nucleotide is deoxyadenylate and the nucleoside (the black color without the teal phosphate group) is deoxyadenosine.

There are two major purine bases, adenine (A) and guanine (G), and three pyrimidine bases, cytosine (C), thymine (T), and uracil (U) (**Figure 2.20**). DNA includes all of these bases except uracil. In RNA, uracil replaces thymine. Each of the bases is linked to a sugar via a β-glycosyl linkage (Figure 2.19). In addition to these bases, traces of 5-methylcytosine, 5-hydroxymethylcytosine, pseudouridine, and *N*-methylated heterocycles are found in DNA and RNA molecules.

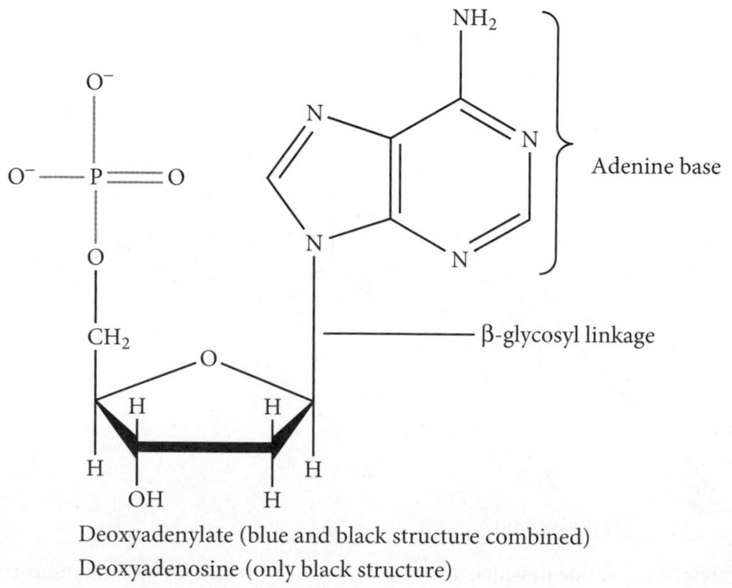

Deoxyadenylate (blue and black structure combined)
Deoxyadenosine (only black structure)

Figure 2.19 The structure of deoxyadenylate.

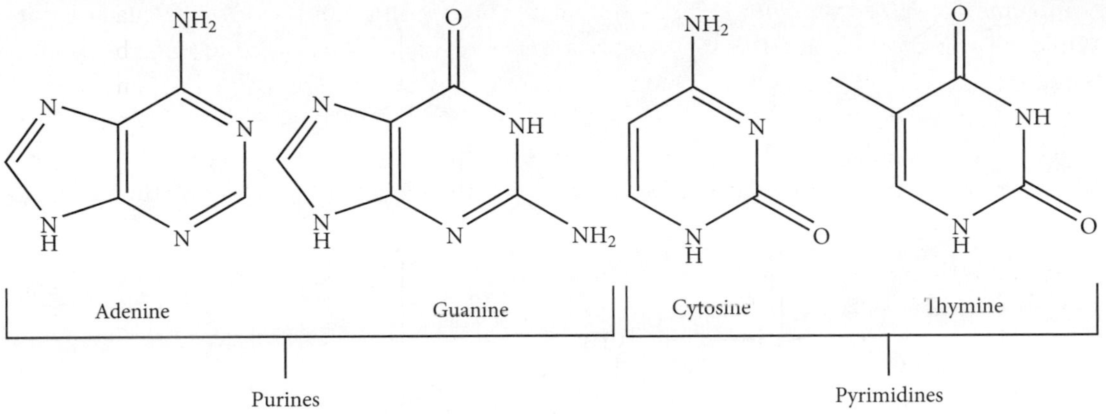

Figure 2.20 The structures of purine and pyrimidine bases found in DNA.

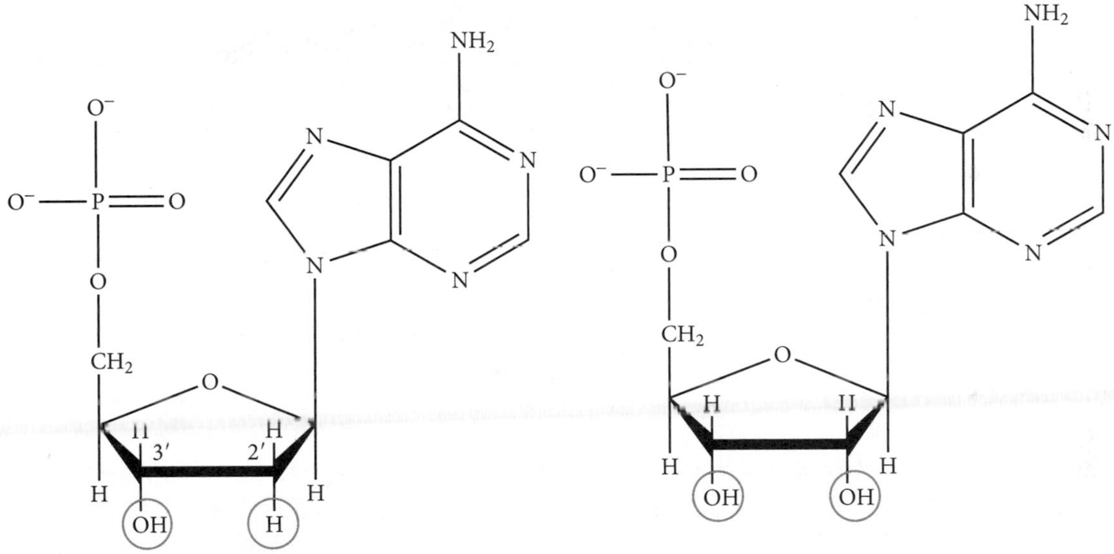

Figure 2.21 The structures of deoxyribonucleic acid and ribonucleic acid.

As mentioned earlier, nucleotides consist of a sugar, a nitrogenous base, and at least a phosphoryl group. Because nucleotides are complex molecules, a method is needed to distinguish the carbons in the base from the carbons in the sugar moiety. For this reason, the carbons of the sugar part are designated with a prime sign. The nitrogenous base, however, determines the identity of the nucleotide. As the DNA name indicates, *deoxy*ribonucleic acid lacks an —OH group at the 2′ position of the ribose, whereas ribonucleic acid contains —OH groups at both the 2′ and 3′ positions of the ribose ring (**Figure 2.21**). Approximately, 90% of a cell's nucleic acids is RNA; the remaining 10% is DNA.

In any given molecule of DNA, the concentration of adenine (A) is equal to the concentration of thymine (T), and the concentration of cytosine (C) is equal to the concentration of guanine (G). This indicates that A base-pairs with T, while G base-pairs with C. In other words, the base pairs build two complementary chains. A duplex of DNA is formed by these two complementary chains in an antiparallel manner. In both DNA and RNA synthesis, the 5′-phosphate of one nucleotide attaches to the 3′-OH of another nucleotide (**Figure 2.22**). Each nucleotide residue is added to the 3′-OH of the nucleic acid, which indicates the chain's growth is always in the 5′ to 3′ direction.

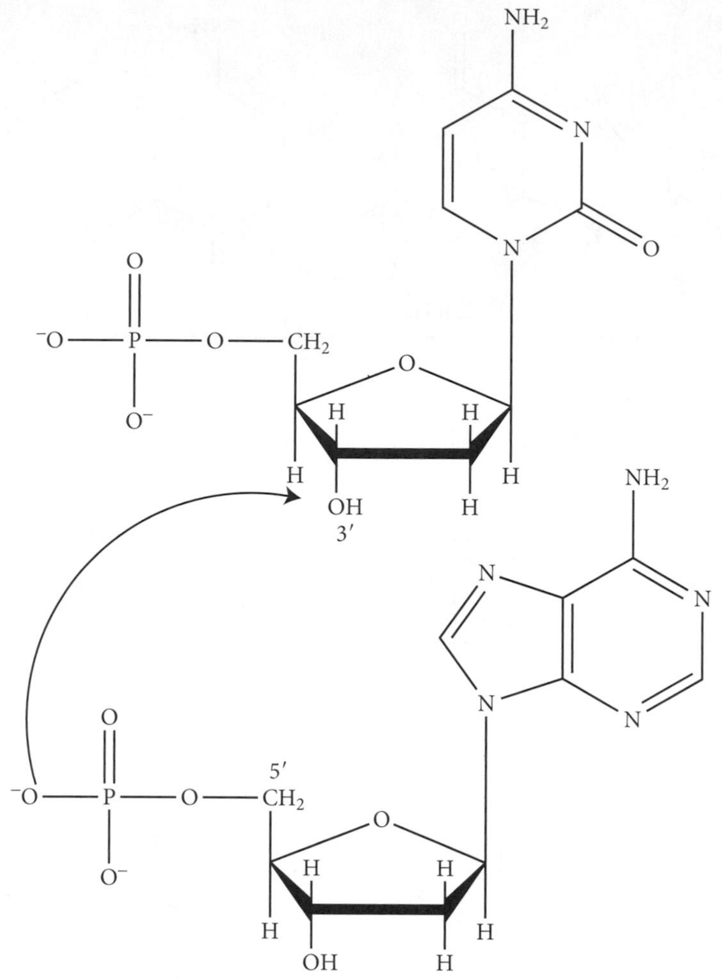

Figure 2.22 In a growing nucleic acid chain, the 5′-phosphate group of one nucleotide attaches to the 3′-OH of another nucleotide.

Because DNA replication occurs much faster in cancer cells than in normal cells, synthetic analogs of both purine and pyrimidine bases can serve as anticancer drugs. In other words, these anticancer drugs either inhibit an enzyme of nucleotide biosynthesis or are incorporated into DNA or RNA molecules to slow or inhibit cell growth (see also the *Introduction to Medicinal Chemistry* chapter).

A gene is an essential unit of DNA nucleotides that contains the information for the synthesis of a single polypeptide chain. The basic structure of a typical eukaryotic gene has both coding and noncoding regions. In eukaryotes, but not in prokaryotes, the DNA sequences of the genes that code for the formation of proteins are broken into several segments called exons. Theses sequences are separated from other DNA sequences (introns) that are not translated. At the beginning of the gene is an important sequence called a promoter; it is the site at which RNA polymerase and its cofactors bind to initiate transcription (synthesis of RNA). This promoter region often includes a thymidine–adenine–thymidine–adenine (TATA) sequence (also called a TATA box), which ensures that the transcription process is initiated at the right location. After the coding region (at the 5′ end), there are other sequences that are involved in the regulation of the transcription; they include enhancer and silencer sequences.

Both DNA and RNA are water soluble because the backbone (i.e., the phosphate and the sugar residue) of both DNA and RNA are hydrophilic. The pK_a of the phosphate group is near zero, so

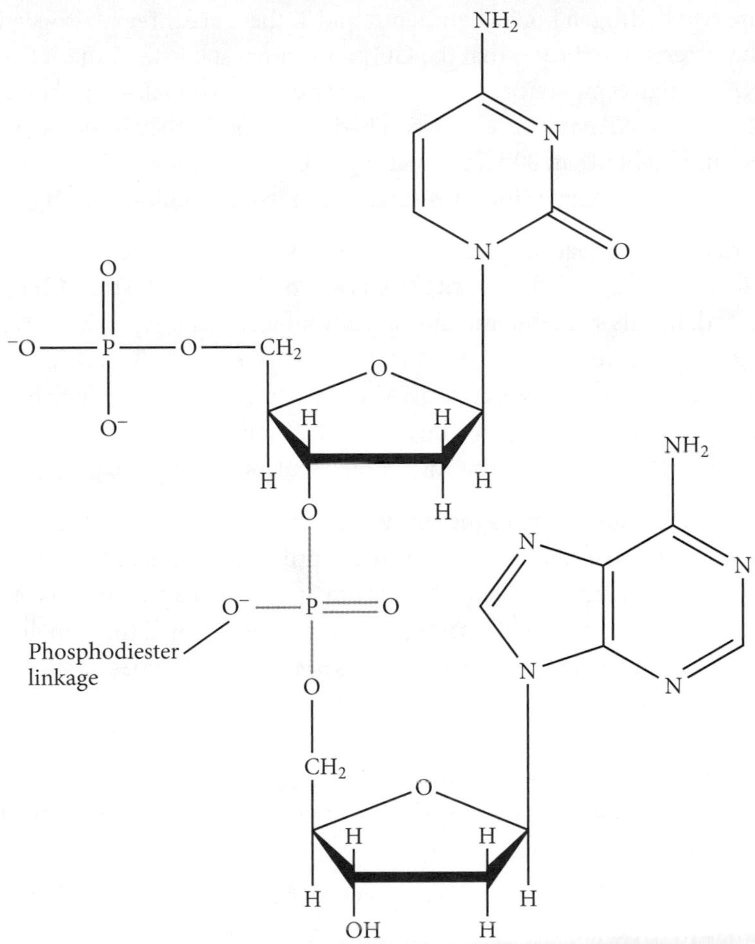

Figure 2.23 Phosphodiester linkage of adjacent nucleotides is found in both RNA and DNA.

this molecule is fully negatively charged at pH 7. It is the phosphodiester linkage that links adjacent nucleotides in both RNA and DNA. The nitrogenous bases are the side groups that are joined by a backbone at a regular interval.

As is indicated in **Figure 2.23**, the 5′-phosphoryl group of a mononucleotide esterifies to a hydroxyl group (the 3′-OH of the pentose) of another nucleotide by forming a phosphodiester linkage. The 3′,5′-phosphodiester linkage builds the "backbone" of DNA (or RNA). Interestingly, the hydrolysis of the phosphodiester linkage is thermodynamically favored. That is to say, the hydrolysis has a negative Gibbs free energy ($-\Delta G$; see also the *Introduction to Biochemistry* chapter). Having a favorable ΔG, however, does not dictate the speed of a reaction. As a result, in the absence of phosphodiesterase enzymes, hydrolysis of the phosphodiester bonds occurs very slowly over a long period of time. This explains why the structure of DNA is so stable that one can find a conserved intact DNA sequence in old fossils. By comparison, RNA molecules are much less stable than DNA because the 2′-hydroxyl group of RNA (recall that DNA lacks this hydroxyl group) functions as a nucleophile (see the *Introduction to Biological Chemistry* chapter) during hydrolysis of the phosphodiester bond.

In solution, the two strands of DNA find each other and form a double helix by hydrogen bonds. This kind of base pair is called a Watson–Crick base pair, in honor of the scientists James Watson and Francis Crick, who discovered the structure of DNA in 1953. Together with another scientist, Maurice Wilkins, Watson and Crick were awarded the Nobel Prize in medicine in 1962.

While there are two hydrogen bonds between A and T, there are three hydrogen bonds between G and C. This characteristic indicates that the GC pair is more stable than the AT pair. If you heat a solution of DNA, at high temperatures the hydrogen bonds will break—a phenomenon called melting of DNA. Because AT pairs have only two hydrogen bonds, they undergo a melting process first. At a temperature higher than 80°C, the melting of GC pairs follows the AT melting, such that the double-stranded DNA separates into two single-stranded molecules.

Watson and Crick showed that each strand of the DNA was a template for the other strand. During cell division, the two strands separate from each other; for each strand, a new daughter strand is synthesized. In this synthetic manner, a DNA molecule can reproduce (replicate) itself without changing its structure. Three different forms of DNA exist: A, B, and Z. The B-form DNA predominates in aqueous solution, whereas DNA in dehydration form (i.e., when the humidity of DNA is less than 75%) favors the A form. The Z-form DNA, in contrast to A and B forms, has a left-handed helical structure; it may play a role in the regulation of gene expression.

In 1944, Oswald Avery and his colleagues provided compelling evidence that the DNA is indeed the genetic material found in a cell. Their experiments produced data showing that DNA, when isolated from the virulent (disease-causing) bacterium *Streptococcus pneumoniae* and mixed with a living cell of a nonvirulent strain of the same bacterium, transformed the nonvirulent strain to a virulent strain. In 1950, Erwin Chargaff outlined a series of unique rules about DNA molecules known as Chargaff's rules:

1. Different species have different base compositions of DNA.

2. DNA molecules from different tissues within the same species have the same base composition.

3. The base composition of DNA in a given species remains constant regardless of the organism's age, nutritional state, or changing environment.

4. In all species' DNA molecules, the number of A nucleotides equals the number of T nucleotides, and the number of C nucleotides equals the number of G nucleotides, which indicates that the number of A + G is equal to the number of T + C.

A modification in DNA structure that produces permanent changes in the genetic information is called a mutation. In addition, when organisms copy their DNA, mistakes may occur occasionally. These mistakes may be random errors that arise during copying or they may be a result of DNA damage from radiation or chemical mutagens (i.e., substances that produce mutations). For instance, UV radiation causes two adjacent thymine bases on the same DNA to form a dimer. The resulting kink in the double helix at that site may interfere with DNA replication and transcription. (UV radiation is used to sterilize the surface area of hoods and laboratory places where bacterial contamination is a problem.)

Two frequently encountered DNA sequences are the palindrome and the mirror repeat (**Figure 2.24**).

*   A *palindrome sequence* is a strand of DNA where one strand reads the same as the opposite strand in the reverse direction (much like the phrase "Lonely Tylenol," which reads the same from both directions). The palindrome structure can promote development of unusual forms of DNA and RNA called hairpin and cruciform forms, depending on whether they occur in single-strand or double-strand DNA, respectively. The palindromes are sites where restriction enzymes (enzymes from microorganisms that restrict or cut up DNA) act and cut nucleic acids. In nature, the role of these enzymes is to destroy foreign DNA that

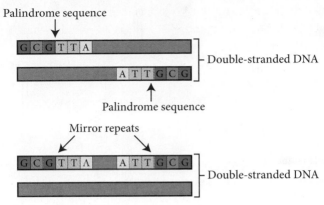

Figure 2.24 Palindrome and mirror repeat DNA sequences.

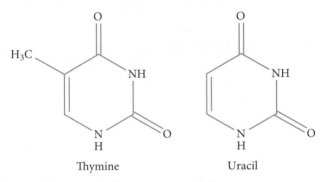

Figure 2.25 Uracil and thymine have very similar structures.

invades the bacterial cell. In the research laboratory, they are used extensively for genetic engineering (i.e., to cut two different strands of DNA and then join them to produce a specific DNA sequence).

- A *mirror repeat* is formed when the inverted repeat occurs in one of the DNA strands. The mirror repeats do not have complementary sequences within the same strand and, as a result, no hairpin structure is possible.

RNA

RNA contains an OH group at both the 2′ and 3′ positions of the ribose ring (Figure 2.21). The same bases that attach to the ribose group in DNA occur in RNA as well, with the exception that in RNA, thymine is replaced by uracil. Uracil does not have a methyl group, but rather a hydrogen atom at the C-5 position of the pyrimidine (**Figure 2.25**). Cytosine spontaneously deaminates to uracil in DNA (**Figure 2.26**), in a common mutation that occurs almost 100 times per day in the human genome. The newly formed uracil, however, is removed from DNA by an effective and accurate DNA repair system.

Although DNA and RNA structurally are similar, there are a few distinct differences between them.

1. In RNA, the sugar is a ribose with two hydroxyl groups (at the 2′ and 3′ carbons).

2. An RNA molecule contains adenine, guanine, and cytosine, but no thymine; instead, it has another base, uracil.

3. RNA exists as a single strand, whereas DNA exists as a double-stranded helical molecule. The single strand of RNA, because of complementary sequences along the RNA, is capable

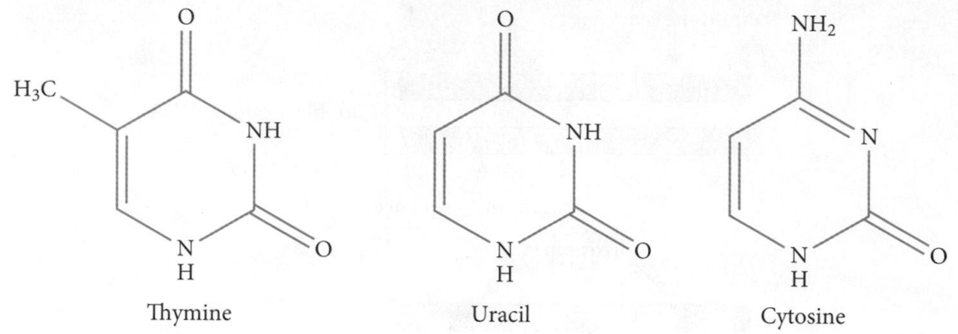

Figure 2.26 Cytosine spontaneously deaminates to uracil in DNA, causing a mutation.

of folding back on itself to form a double-stranded molecule. This secondary structure of RNA often results in a hairpin, a loop, or a bulge that significantly affects the function of the RNA.

4. Because the RNA molecule is complementary to only one of the two strands of a DNA molecule, its guanine number does not necessarily equal its cytosine number (the same is true for the number of adenine and uracil subunits).

Learning Bridge 2.4

A representative from a pharmaceutical company, CancerCut, comes to your pharmacy to give you and your preceptor a few pamphlets that the company has produced about a new FDA-approved anticancer drug. The representative talks to you and your preceptor about how effectively the new anticancer drug works to stop the growth of cancer cells. While he is talking about how effectively the thymine of cancer cells is targeted by the anticancer drug, he mentions that the drug does not affect RNA because RNA does not have thymine, but rather uracil.

Your preceptor asks the representative why DNA contains thymine rather than uracil. The representative tries to find an answer first in his pamphlet and later on in his iPad, but without any success. The representative turns to you and says, "Well, you are an intern and have just completed basic sciences. Why don't you answer this question?"

Try to answer the question by using your knowledge from cell biology.

There are four RNA molecules with distinct functions: messenger RNA (mRNA), ribosomal RNA (rRNA), transfer RNA (tRNA), and small nuclear RNA (snRNA).

Messenger RNA

Messenger RNA serves as a template for protein synthesis and is directly synthesized during the transcription of a gene. It works as an intermediate between DNA and protein. Transcription begins at a specific site on the DNA known as the promoter and ends at a terminator sequence. Each gene has its own promoter(s). In mammalian cells, the mRNA molecule is first synthesized in the nucleus before it appears in the cytoplasm. In the nucleus, the unprocessed mRNA is processed (i.e., undergoes maturation) before entering the cytoplasm. Therefore, the length of an mRNA in the nucleus could be 10- to 50-fold longer than the mature mRNA molecules found in the cytoplasm.

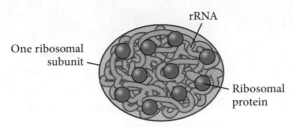

Figure 2.27 A ribosomal subunit is built by a few ribosomal RNA molecules and many ribosomal proteins.

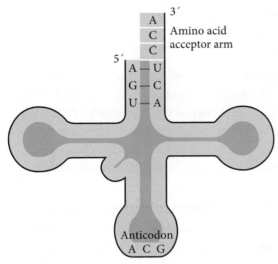

Figure 2.28 An artificial tRNA molecule with an anticodon loop and an amino acid acceptor arm (or stem).

There are two types of mRNAs:

- Monocistronic: when an mRNA molecule codes for one polypeptide (or protein). Most mRNAs in eukaryotes are monocistronic.

- Polycistronic: when an mRNA molecule codes for more than one polypeptide (or protein). Prokaryotes have both mRNA types.

Ribosomal RNA

Ribosomal RNA is an abundant cytoplasmic RNA molecule that, together with proteins, builds the body of the ribosome. There are four different rRNAs in eukaryotic cells and three different rRNAs in prokaryotic cells, each with a different size (**Figure 2.27**).

Transfer RNA

Transfer RNAs serve as adapter molecules for transferring amino acids to ribosomes for the translation of mRNA sequences into polymerized amino acids. For each kind of amino acid, there is a specific tRNA. Two important parts of a tRNA molecule are the aminoacyl attachment site (also called the acceptor stem) and the anticodon (**Figure 2.28**). The anticodon, which includes three bases, base pairs with the appropriate codon in the mRNA. This interaction allows the amino acid, carried by the tRNA, to be incorporated into the polypeptide or protein chain during the translation process. During periods of protein synthesis (translation), many ribosomes attach to and read an mRNA molecule to form a complex called a polysome. More than 20 tRNA molecules are present in every cell, at least one (but often several) corresponding to each of the 20 amino acids that are used in the protein synthetic machinery. Although each specific tRNA differs structurally from the others, they have many features in common.

Small Nuclear RNA

Small nuclear RNA sequences exist only in eukaryotic organisms. They are not directly involved in protein synthesis but play important roles in RNA processing.

Carbohydrates

Carbohydrates are important components of human nutrients (see also the *Introduction to Nutrients* chapter) and are largely found in plants. Although the human body can make carbohydrates from proteins, the majority of carbohydrates in the body are derived from plants. Carbohydrates are mainly consumed in the diet in the form of polysaccharides and disaccharides.

Carbohydrates are organic molecules. The simple sugars are monosaccharides that include pentoses (five carbons, or ribose) and hexoses (six carbons, or glucose); they perform both structural roles (e.g., ribose and deoxyribose in nucleic acids) and functional roles (e.g., inositol 1,4,5-trisphosphate acts as a cellular signaling molecule, as discussed in the *Introduction to Pharmacodynamics* chapter) in the body. Plants synthesize glucose from carbon dioxide and water via photosynthesis, storing the glucose as a polysaccharide (starch). In addition, plants use glucose to synthesize the cellulose of plants' cell walls.

More complex carbohydrates (disaccharides and polysaccharides) must be broken down to their building blocks (monosaccharides) before they are fully absorbed. The human intestinal tract contains many harmless microorganisms, whose glycoside hydrolases break down complex polysaccharides. In addition, humans use our own enzymes—namely, the alpha-amylases in salivary and pancreatic secretions—to cleave the interior 1,4-glucose linkages in large polymers of starch, thereby turning these large molecules into smaller fragments (disaccharides, trisaccharides, and oligosaccharides).

Oligosaccharidases and disaccharidases in the brush border of enterocytes are digested into monosaccharides, glucose, galactose, and fructose (**Figure 2.29**). While glucose and galactose, together with two Na^+ ions, are absorbed across the apical membrane of enterocytes by the SGLT-1 transporter, fructose is absorbed into the cell by facilitated diffusion through the apical membrane by another transporter, GLUT-5. All three hexoses (glucose, galactose, and fructose) depart the cell by facilitated diffusion through the GLUT-2 transporter, which is located in the basolateral membrane.

A deficiency of the SGLT-1 transporter, caused by mutation in its gene, impairs glucose and galactose absorption. Affected patients develop diarrhea when they consume sugars that contain glucose and galactose because they cannot absorb Na^+, monosaccharides, and water. However, because fructose is not transported by SGLT-1, its digestion does not cause diarrhea. Other serious diseases associated with carbohydrate metabolism include diabetes mellitus (DM), galactosemia, glycogen storage diseases, and lactose intolerance. Some of these diseases will be discussed in this book.

There are three classes of carbohydrates: monosaccharides, disaccharides, and polysaccharides.

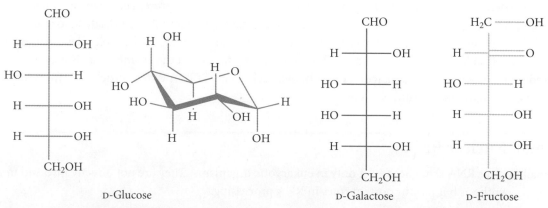

Figure 2.29 Monosaccharide hexoses—glucose, galactose, and fructose—are absorbed into our cells through monosaccharide transporter proteins.

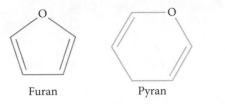

Figure 2.30 Monosaccharides contain either five (furan) or six carbons (pyran).

Monosaccharides

Monosaccharides are the simplest sugars; they cannot be hydrolyzed further into other carbohydrates. Depending on the number of carbon atoms, monosaccharides are classified as trioses, tetroses, pentoses, hexoses, or heptoses. Monosaccharides can have two forms: straight chain or cyclic structure. The monosaccharides with either five (furan) or six carbons (pyran) (**Figure 2.30**) assume the form of a five-membered ring (furanose) or a six-membered ring (pyranose). When glucose is in a solution, more than 99% is in the pyranose form. Monosaccharides are colorless, are water soluble, and have a sweet taste.

If the carbonyl group (C=O) is in the end of the molecule (i.e., when building an aldehyde functional group), the monosaccharide is an aldose; an example is glucose or galactose (see Figure 2.29). If the carbonyl group (C=O) is in any other position of the molecule (i.e., ketone), then the monosaccharide is a ketose; an example is fructose (see Figure 2.29).

Monosaccharide rings can exist in two forms: chair form and boat form. Because of the eclipsed conformation for the boat form, this form is less stable than the chair form (**Figure 2.31**).

Glucose

As shown in **Figure 2.32A**, the structure of glucose can be either linear (Fischer projection) or cyclic (chair and Haworth projection). The Haworth projection is the most common form that represents the cyclic structure of glucose. The cyclic structure is built when a hemiacetal forms by a reaction between the aldehyde group and a hydroxyl group (**Figure 2.33**). When both the carbonyl group and the alcohol are part of the same molecule (as in monosaccharides), they form a stable cyclic molecule. The cyclic structure is thermodynamically favored. You will encounter the essential role of glucose in the *Introduction to Biochemistry* chapter; for now, simply recognize that glucose is an essential molecule for life and one of the main sources that produces the high-energy-yielding molecule, ATP. Glucose molecules that are not used immediately or stored in the liver can be converted to fat for future use. Although we can synthesize fatty acids from glucose, however, we cannot synthesize glucose from fatty acids.

Similar to amino acids, monosaccharides exist in D and L isomers, which are determined by their spatial relationships to D or L glyceraldehyde isomers. The orientation of the H and OH groups on carbon 5 dictates whether the sugar qualifies as a D or L isomer. When the OH group is on the right, the isomer is D; when the OH group is on the left, the isomer is L. Most naturally occurring monosaccharides take the form of the D isomer (Figure 2.32B). The majority of

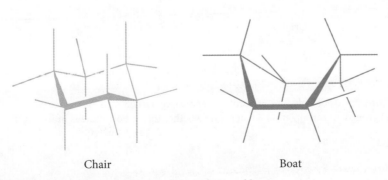

Figure 2.31 Monosaccharide rings can exist in two forms: chair and boat.

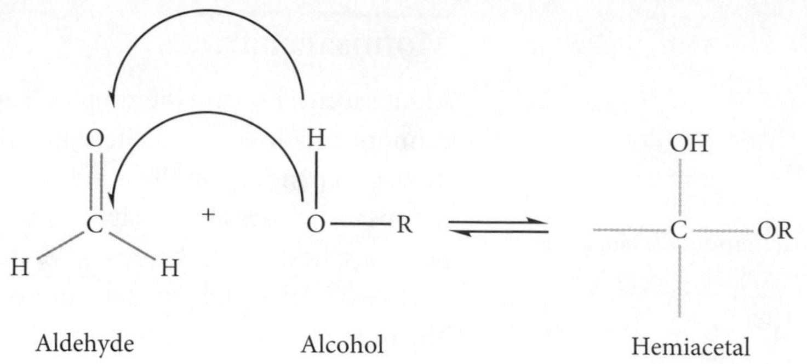

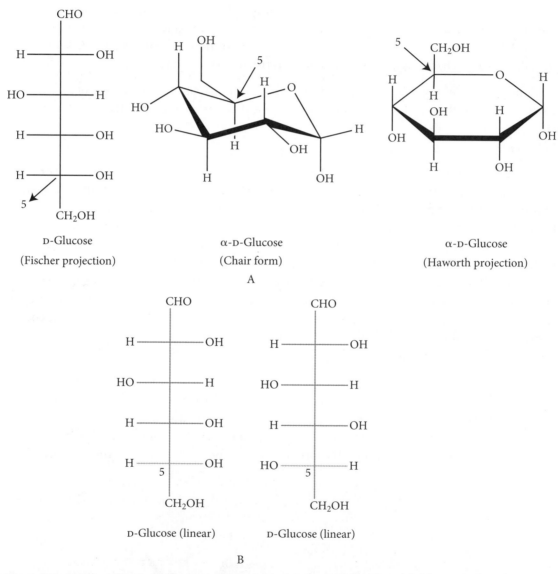

Figure 2.32 Hemiacetal is formed by a reaction between an aldehyde group and a hydroxyl group.

D-Glucose
(Fischer projection)

α-D-Glucose
(Chair form)

α-D-Glucose
(Haworth projection)

A

D-Glucose (linear)

D-Glucose (linear)

B

Figure 2.33 (A) Three forms of a glucose molecule: linear (Fischer), chair, and Haworth projections. (B) The H and OH groups on carbon atom 5 determine whether the carbohydrate is in its D or L form.

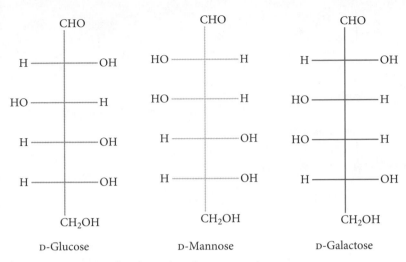

Figure 2.34 D-Glucose/D-mannose and D-glucose/D-galactose are epimers.

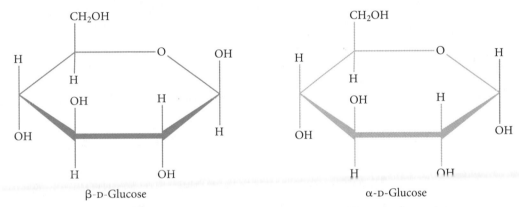

Figure 2.35 Mutarotation of a glucose molecule that can be in both α and β configurations. If the OH group on C_1 exists in the α form, the hydroxyl group is pointing down; if it is in the β form, the hydroxyl group is pointing up.

the monosaccharides that occur in mammals are found as D isomers, and the enzymes that can metabolize them are specific for the D isomer.

Two sugar molecules that differ only in configuration around one carbon atom are called epimers. Examples include D-glucose and D-mannose as well as D-glucose and D-galactose (**Figure 2.34**). The two most biologically important epimers of glucose are mannose (epimerized at carbon 2) and galactose (epimerized at carbon 4). Simple sugars such as glucose and fructose are absorbed directly and readily through the gastrointestinal tract. However, more complex sugars, such as lactose (D-glucose + D-galactose) and sucrose (D-glucose + D-fructose), are first broken down in the gastrointestinal tract so that they can be absorbed. Absorbed glucose is either stored in the liver, as glycogen, or used in glycolysis to produce ATP as an energy source (both mechanisms are discussed in the *Introduction to Biochemistry* chapter).

Glucose exists largely as cyclic hemiacetal. The C_1 carbon becomes chiral and is called the anomeric carbon. In other words, the anomeric carbon is the carbonyl carbon of a sugar, which is involved in ring formation. The new OH group (on C_1) can exist in an α form (the hydroxyl group on carbon 1 is pointing down) or a β form (the hydroxyl group on carbon 1 is pointing up). Carbohydrates can undergo mutarotation; that is, they can change spontaneously between the α and β configurations. In a solution, 38% of the total glucose will be in the form of α-glucose and 62% will appear as β-glucose (**Figure 2.35**).

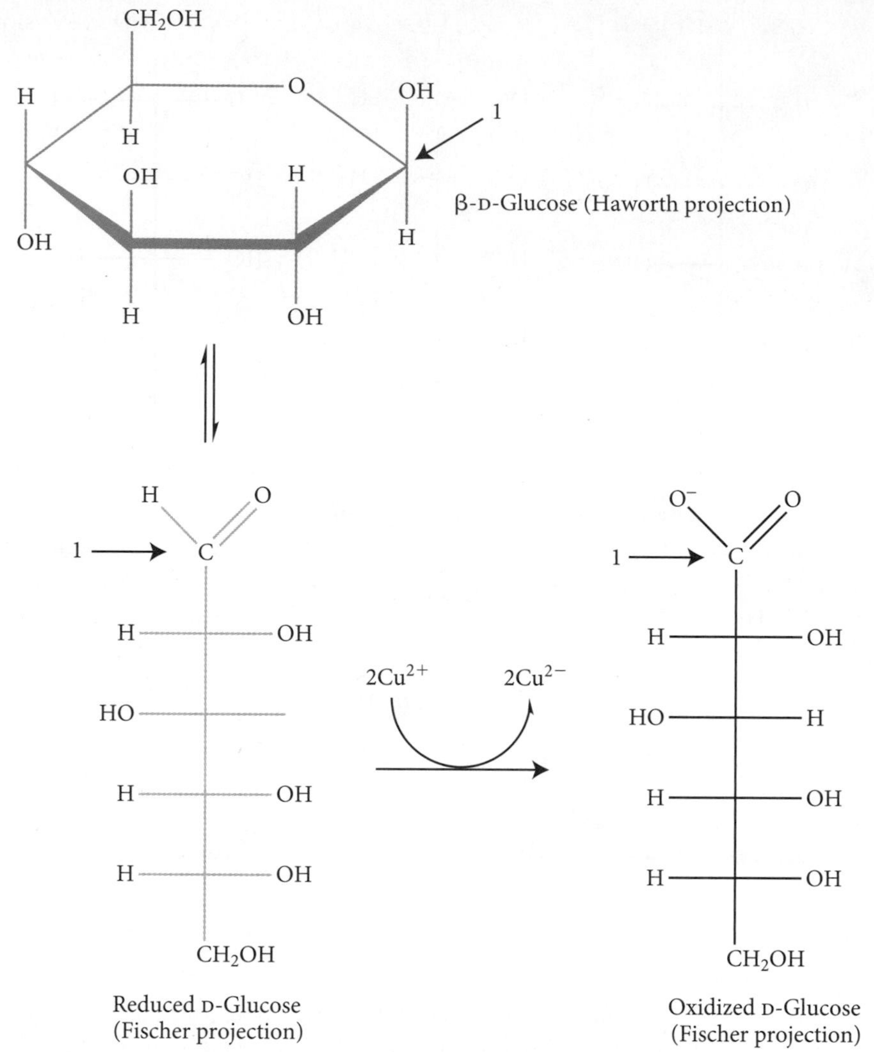

Figure 2.36 Monosaccharides (including glucose) act as mild reducing agents because the carbonyl carbon in the linear chain can be oxidized to form a carboxylate group.

Adapted from: Nelson DL, Cox MM. *Principles of biochemistry*, 5th ed. New York, NY: W. H. Freeman and Company; 2008: Chapter 7.

Some monosaccharides (including glucose) act as mild reducing agents because the carbonyl carbon in the straight chain can be oxidized to form a carboxylate group (recall that aldehyde is prone to oxidation). Monosaccharides that are cyclic are not reducing sugars because they do not have a carbonyl carbon group that can be oxidized (**Figure 2.36**). The reducing agent, of course, donates electrons. In the reducing reaction, the linear glucose donates an electron (i.e., the electron that comes from H) to the cupric ion (Cu^{2+}).

Some monosaccharides have nitrogen atom in their rings—for instance, D-glucosamine (**Figure 2.37**), which is a constituent of hyaluronic acid, and D-galactosamine, which is a constituent of chondroitin. A few antibiotics (erythromycin, neomycin) contain amino sugars, which are important for their antibacterial activity.

Disaccharides

A disaccharide is built when two monosaccharides are linked together (condensed). A glycosidic bond forms when covalent bonds are created between the anomeric hydroxyl of a cyclic sugar

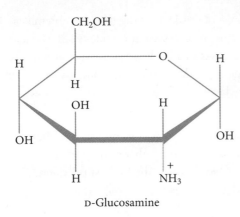

D-Glucosamine

Figure 2.37 Structure of a nitrogen-containing sugar molecule, glucosamine.

and the hydroxyl of a second sugar. Physiologically important disaccharides include sucrose (the sugar crystals used in the kitchen, which consist of bonded glucose–fructose), lactose (mammalian milk and formula, which consist of bonded glucose–galactose), and maltose (a starch that consists of bonded glucose–glucose; **Figure 2.38**). Maltose is produced from oligosaccharide starch—that is, when the disaccharide is obtained by partial hydrolysis of starch. In contrast, cellobiose is a disaccharide that is obtained by partial hydrolysis of cellulose.

Maltose and cellobiose are biologically different. While cellobiose cannot be digested by humans, maltose is digested without difficulty. Any glucose in our food is absorbed without the need for digestion. Ruminant animals have in their rumens microorganisms that produce the enzyme cellulase, which is able to split the ($\beta1 \rightarrow 4$) linkages in cellulose to release glucose. Humans, in contrast, do not have the cellulase enzyme; as a result, they cannot digest cellulose.

One of the most common problems with the digestion of carbohydrates relates to lactose. Lactose is a disaccharide (D-glucose–D-galactose) whose ingestion causes medical problems if a

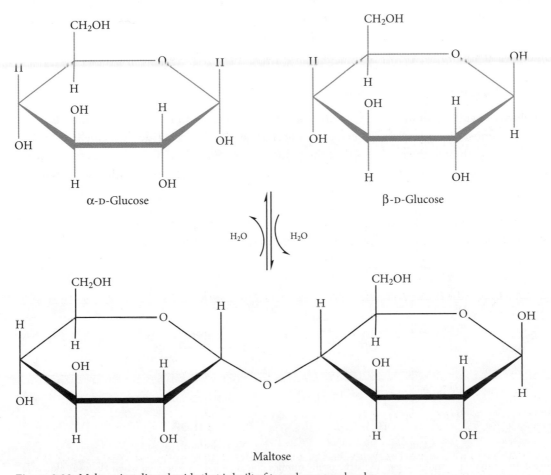

Maltose

Figure 2.38 Maltose is a disaccharide that is built of two glucose molecules.

person develops lactose intolerance. The underlying cause of this lactose digestion problem is a reduction of lactase enzyme activity in adults. This enzyme is expressed at high levels in the jejunum of neonatal and infant humans, but its activity decreases in adulthood in many parts of the world. Two types of lactase deficiency exist: primary and secondary. In primary lactase deficiency, a mutation or absence of lactase is the cause. Secondary lactase deficiency is caused by mucosal disease or mucosal injury in the small intestine.

In a number of non-Caucasian groups, primary lactase deficiency is common in adulthood. Indeed, Northern European and North American Caucasians are the only populations that maintain small intestinal lactase activity throughout their adulthood. The highest prevalence of lactase deficiency is found among Hispanic (50%), Mediterranean (60–85%), African (85–100%), and Asian (90–100%) adults. If lactase is deficient or its activity is reduced, this sugar is not absorbed. The unabsorbed lactose draws in and retains water in the small intestine, which causes abdominal pain (cramps), nausea, and diarrhea. Symptoms are often experienced after consumption of lactose-rich food, particularly milk (as little as 200 mL). Sadly, the lactase enzyme activity is decreased significantly in many areas where milk products are an important part of the adult diet. Lactaid is an over-the-counter product that temporarily relieves the symptoms of lactose intolerance by providing the body with sufficient lactase to digest lactose.

Some individuals develop diarrhea when they consume large amounts of sorbitol. This effect explains why sorbitol is used as a laxative compound (it has also been indicated as a diuretic). Sorbitol is included in diabetic candy and is listed as an inactive ingredient in some other products. In addition, this disaccharide can be found in fruits such as apples, pears, and peaches. Sorbitol is minimally absorbed in humans because of lack of an intestinal absorptive transport mechanism. Sorbitol is produced by animals when glucose is reduced—that is, when glucose's aldehyde group at carbon 1 is reduced to an alcohol group (**Figure 2.39**). This molecule causes cataracts in diabetic patients (see the *Introduction to Pharmacology and Pathophysiology* chapter).

Polysaccharides

The majority of carbohydrates found in nature are polysaccharides, most of which contain the D-glucose monosaccharide unit. The end of a disaccharide or polysaccharide molecule that has a free anomeric carbon in the chain is called the reducing end (**Figure 2.40**). Polysaccharides with a single monosaccharide building block are called homopolysaccharides (e.g., cellulose, starch,

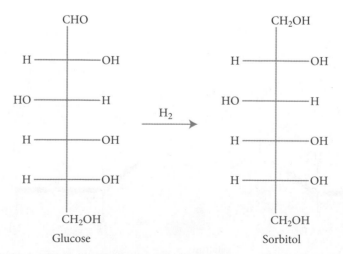

Figure 2.39 Sorbitol is another sugar that structurally mimics glucose and is synthesized when glucose's aldehyde group at carbon 1 is reduced to an alcohol group.

Cells

	Prokaryotic - Single celled – No cholesterol	Eukaryotic

Types	- archaebacteria
	- Eubacteria
	
	- Eubacteria - peptidoglycan
	  cell wall
	    - cytoplasmic membrane
		- protists
		  - fungi
		    - animals
		      - plants

	- Nucleoid
	- circular DNA
	- Plasmids.
	   - replicate & transfer
	     - Antibiotic resistance
	-
		- Nuclear membrane
		- linear DNA

energy	- Photosynthesis - use
	  light & thylakoids
	  - inorganic → organic med
	  - reducing agent = H_2O,
	     H_2, or H_2S
	
	   - aerobic - O_2 to get ATP
	   - anaerobic - NAD to get ATP	

gram ⊕ = $\dfrac{\text{Phospholipid}}{\text{Peptidoglycan}}$
$\dfrac{\text{Phospholipid}}{\text{Cytoplasm}}$ ↓

gram ⊖ = $\dfrac{\text{Peptidoglycan}}{\text{Phospholipid}}$ ↓
Cytoplasm

<u>Pili</u> = on gram ⊖
- sex & ordinary Pili
  ↓   ↳ attach
  conjugation   to host

Prokaryotic cells
- Nucleoid
- small
- circular DNA
- Plasmids
- Photosynthetic Bacteria = use light to inorganic → organic molecule
    - aerobic vs anaerobic   use H_2O or H_2 or
                                                                        H_2S
                                                                    as reducing agent
                                                    thylakoids
              use electron acceptors to
                    generate metabolism
                 - in GI-tract
    cyanobacteria (blue-green bacteria) - Photosynthetic aerobe w/H_2O
    purple -   → H_2 or H_2S Photosynthetic
    green -
    myco bacteria

Nucleoid
- histone-like proteins + magnesium ions + small polyamines
            = rap up DNA into Nucleoid
    - Topoisomerase- prevent topological bands
            - unwind DNA in transcription & replication Fork

Cytoskeletal Protein
- actin-like & non-actin-like proteins
    ↳ maintain shape   ↳ regulate DNA segregation
    facilitate movement   & cell Division
                                            · Determine shape

Ribosomes - RNA + proteins - translate mRNA→A protein
    - 50S & 30S = subunits = 70S Ribosome
            ↳ sedimentation coefficient
    - rRNA = 16S & 23S   ↳ two 23S & 5S rRNA
            ↳+   36 proteins
            21 proteins

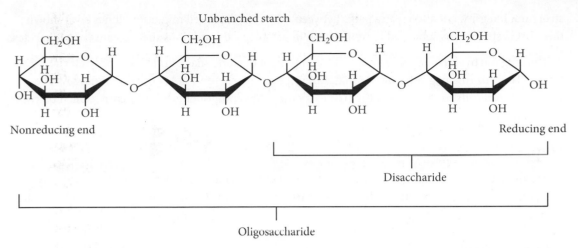

Figure 2.40 Polysaccharides with a single monosaccharide building block (in this example, glucose) are called homopolysaccharides.

and glycogen; Figure 2.40). Polysaccharides with more than one type of monosaccharide are called heteropolysaccharides (e.g., peptidoglycan).

The two most important polysaccharides are starch (in plants) and glycogen (in animals). Starch is the main storage source of carbohydrate in plant cells. The structure of starch is similar to that of glycogen, except that it has a much lower degree of branching. Unbranched starch is known as amylose, whereas branched starch is called amylopectin. Alpha-amylase is an enzyme that is found in saliva and in pancreatic secretions in the small intestine. This enzyme cleaves the α-1,4 linkage in starch to produce oligosaccharide (two to nine monosaccharide molecules) and disaccharide (two monosaccharide molecules). Oligosaccharides are condensed products of three to 10 monosaccharides.

Let's go through a few important polysaccharides that play important roles in physiology and biology.

Glycogen

The glycogen polysaccharide is the major carbohydrate storage unit in animals. It has a very compact structure, which allows large amounts of carbohydrates to be stored in a small volume with an insignificant effect on cellular osmolarity. Glycogen is largely found in the liver and muscle. In fact, the liver has a higher concentration of glycogen than any other body tissue. Because the total mass of muscle is higher than the mass of liver, however, muscle stores twice as much glycogen as the liver.

The human body stores glucose as a highly branched molecule (glycogen) rather than as linear polymers. This preference occurs because the enzymes that catalyze degradation of glycogen to release glucose for metabolism act only on the nonreducing ends of glycogen (Figure 2.40). Having extensive branching produces more nonreducing ends for enzymatic attack than one would find in a linear polymer. As a result, branched polymers increase the substrate concentration of these enzymes, which in turn increases the catalytic rate. Consequently, the body is able to quickly adjust to low blood glucose levels. The role of the substrate concentration in increasing an enzyme's catalytic rate is discussed in the *Introduction to Biochemistry* chapter.

Glycosaminoglycans

Glycosaminoglycan (GAG) is another polysaccharide that is highly negatively charged and is located on the surface of cells or in the extracellular matrix (ECM). The rigidity of GAG not only provides structural integrity, but also creates paths between cells to facilitate cell migration. It has been shown that GAG's structure is subjected to modulation in pathological conditions such as cancer and diabetes.

The enzyme hyaluronidase is found as a component of some snake and insect or bacterial toxins. This enzyme degrades hyaluronate, an important structural GAG in animal tissues. The degradation results in invasion of the tissues by the other components of the toxins, which disrupts the cell membranes of the target cells.

Heparin

Through its unique and highly negatively charged pentasaccharide, heparin binds to positively charged amino acids in antithrombin III (in particular, lysine). This action activates antithrombin III and enables it to work as an effective inhibitor of the blood clotting cascade (**Figure 2.41**).

Glycoconjugates

The interaction of proteoglycan with other extracellular matrix components (i.e., collagen and fibronectin) and the membrane proteins known as integrins not only anchors cells to the extracellular matrix, but also provides paths that facilitate the migration of cells in developing tissue. There are three types of glycoconjugates:

1. Proteoglycans: proteins covalently attached to GAGs (such as chondroitin sulfate and keratin sulfate), where the carbohydrate (polysaccharide) fraction is larger than the protein fraction. The polysaccharides normally attach to the hydroxyl group of a serine residue in the protein fraction.

2. Glycoproteins: proteins covalently attached to carbohydrate, where the protein part is bigger than the carbohydrate part. More than 50% of all eukaryotic proteins carry covalently attached oligosaccharide or polysaccharide chains. Glycoproteins are classified into two groups:

    a. *N*-linked glycoproteins: glycans are linked to the side chain amide group in an asparagine amino acid residue.
    b. *O*-linked glycoproteins: glycans are linked to the hydroxyl group of a threonine or serine amino acid residue.

3. Glycolipids: carbohydrates attached to lipids. These glycoconjugates play important roles in specific biological processes. The lipid fraction forms a complex with a polysaccharide through a glycosidic linkage.

There are two important glycolipids:

1. Gangliosides are membrane lipids of eukaryotic cells that are found on the outer face of the plasma membrane. The most complex gangliosides are sphingolipids, which represent

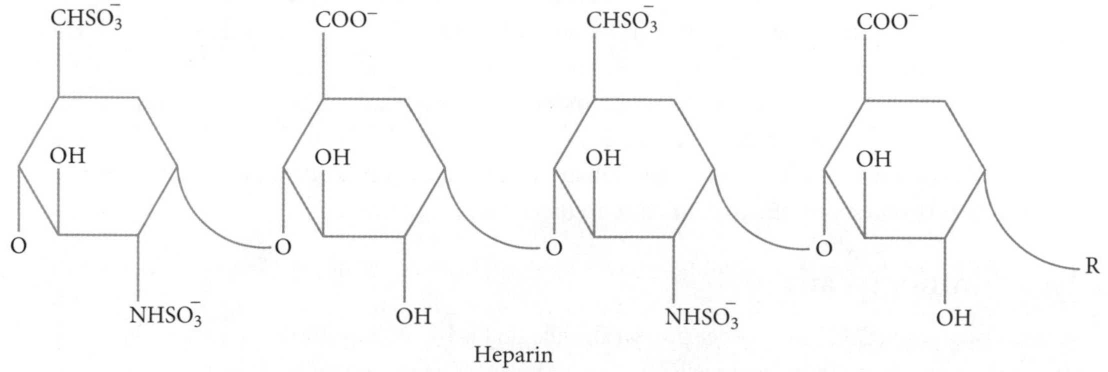

Heparin

Figure 2.41 Heparin is a highly negatively charged polysaccharide that inhibits the blood clotting cascade.

Table 2.5 Three Major Differences Between Proteoglycans and Glycoproteins

Proteoglycan	Glycoprotein
Protein part smaller than GAG	Protein part larger than GAG
Long unbranched GAG chains	Short branched GAG chains
Repeating disaccharides	Nonrepeating disaccharides
All mammalian cells produce proteoglycans, which are mainly found in connective tissue (cartilage)	Found in both the extracellular matrix and the Golgi complex and lysosomes
Examples: heparin and chondroitin	Examples: mucins and immunoglobulins

GAG: Glycosaminoglycan.

approximately 5% to 8% of the total lipids in the brain. The carbohydrate moiety extends beyond the surface of the membrane and, therefore, is involved in cell–cell recognition, binding sites for hormones, and bacterial toxins. It is the carbohydrate moieties of certain sphingolipids that determine the different types of human blood groups.

2. Lipopolysaccharides (LPSs) are membrane lipids; that is, they are found on the outer face of the plasma membrane of Gram-negative bacteria. The LPSs are potential targets for vertebrate antibodies that seek to fight an infection caused by the bacteria. As mentioned earlier, LPSs are the major toxins of Gram-negative bacteria, and are also called endotoxins in this context. The main pathological effects associated with LPSs are shock, fever, hypotension, and thrombosis—collectively referred to as septic shock. Endotoxins may be released by growing bacterial cells or by invading cells that have been lysed by lysozymes or certain antibiotics (penicillins).

Table 2.5 summarizes a few important differences between proteoglycans and glycoproteins.

As explained elsewhere in this chapter, peptidoglycans are the rigid components of the bacterial cell walls and form when a peptide is cross-linked to a polysaccharide chain. This cross-link is important for protection against cell lysis. The cell wall is the site of action of many important antibiotics. The relatively small number of penicillin-binding proteins (PBPs), such as carboxypeptidases, endopeptidases, and transpeptidases, reside in the bacterial inner membrane; their role is to perform construction of, repair, and maintain the integrity of the bacterial cell wall. One of the major mechanisms by which penicillin kills invasive bacteria is the inhibition of the bacterial transpeptidases.

Learning Bridge 2.5

A 38-year-old car mechanic comes to your pharmacy to pick up his omeprazole refill. At the counter, he asks to speak with you, the intern pharmacist. The patient explains that since yesterday afternoon, he has experienced abdominal cramps, diarrhea, and bloating. You notice additional signs of dehydration (such as anxiety and rapid breathing). The customer denies taking any medication except omeprazole. He explains that the diarrhea and bloating symptoms occurred 30 minutes after he ate ice cream and drank a glass of milk yesterday afternoon.

The patient asks you why he has these symptoms. He is also wondering if any OTC products are available that can help him with his symptoms.

A. Identify the cause of the patient's problems and explain why he is experiencing the symptoms.
B. Suggest an OTC product to assist in reducing his symptoms.
C. Is there any food that this patient can eat to reduce his symptoms?

Lipids

Fats or lipids are a source of energy needed in human nutrition. Fats are an important component of our daily diet, and at least a minimum ingestion is essential (see also the *Introduction to Nutrients* chapter). All lipids are hydrophobic and, therefore, water insoluble. Because lipids are hydrophobic, however, they are soluble in nonpolar solvents such as ether and chloroform. Lipids perform many essential cellular functions: They are basic components of cell membranes (bilayer); they produce energy (β oxidation of fats); they produce steroid hormones (e.g., progesterone, testosterone, vitamin D); and they serve as carriers for fat-soluble vitamins (vitamins A, D, E, and K). These roles are discussed further in the *Introduction to Nutrients* chapter.

Similar to proteins and carbohydrates, lipids need to be broken down prior to their absorption. Fatty acids that have a length of less than 10 carbon atoms can pass through cells and enter the blood directly. Uptake and transport of long-chain fatty acids (and some phospholipids), however, requires a specialized fatty acid transporter protein—the so-called microvillous membrane fatty acid binding protein.

Lipids are divided into two major classes: storage lipids and membrane lipids.

Storage Lipids

Storage lipids, which include triacylglycerols, are made from two types of molecules:

- Glycerol, with a hydroxyl group on each of its three carbons (**Figure 2.42**)
- Fatty acids, which include a long-chain aliphatic carboxylic acid (Figure 2.42)

When a glycerol molecule esterifies to three fatty acid molecules, a triacylglycerol molecule is synthesized (Figure 2.42).

Glycerol

Glycerol is a sweet-tasting molecule that in liquid form is syrupy. It has three carbons, each bonded to a hydroxyl group (Figure 2.42). As a result, glycerol is hydrophilic and water soluble. The stereochemistry of the three carbons of glycerol is not identical. While our naked eyes do not differentiate between these three carbons, enzymes that act on glycerol clearly distinguish between them. For instance, glycerol kinase phosphorylates only carbon 3 to produce glycerol 3-phosphate (see also the *Introduction to Biochemistry* chapter).

Glycerol is the backbone of many glycerophospholipids that play important roles in the structure and function of cell membranes. Because it is also the backbone of triacylglycerol, glycerol is an important part of both storage and membrane lipids.

Fatty Acids

Fatty acids are carboxylic acids with long hydrocarbon chains, ranging in length from 4 to 36 carbons. Each fatty acid includes a hydrophobic "tail" (long hydrocarbon chain) and a hydrophilic "head" (carboxyl group) (**Figure 2.43**). However, when the "head" is attached (esterified) to a glycerol molecule, the whole molecule is hydrophobic. Fatty acids differ from one another in two respects: the number of carbon atoms that are bound together and the kind of bonds between the carbon atoms (i.e., single bonds versus double bonds).

Fatty acids occur in the body both as esters (the main form) and as unesterified molecules (free fatty acids). Fatty acids that occur in natural fats usually have an even number of carbon atoms. Three types of fatty acids are distinguished: saturated, monounsaturated, and

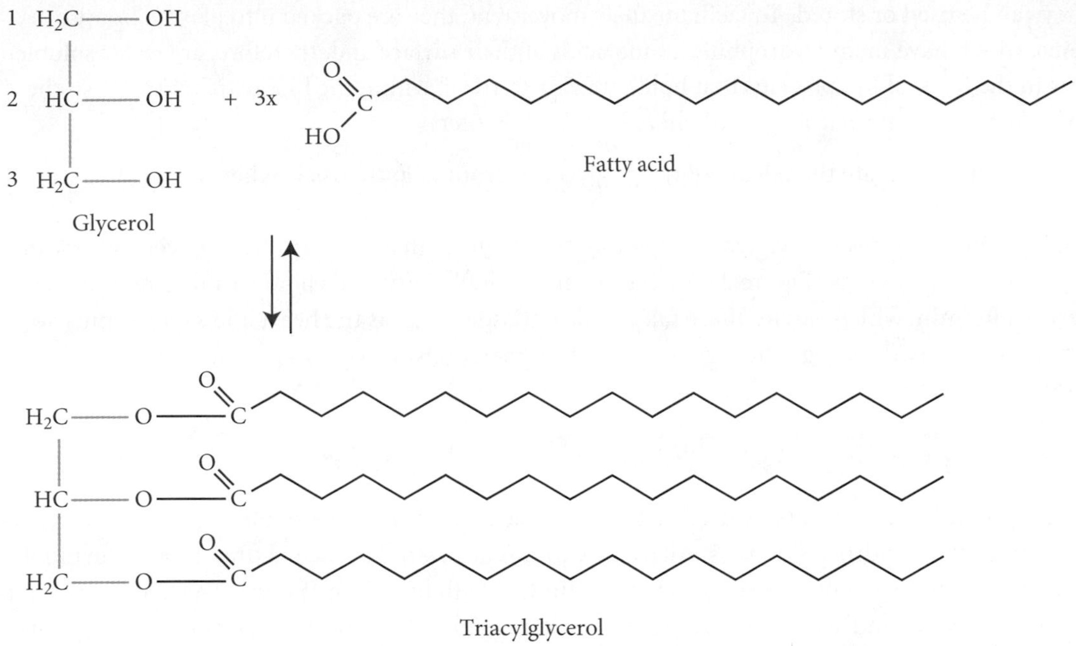

Figure 2.42 Structures of glycerol and fatty acid molecules that interact with each other to produce a triacylglycerol molecule.

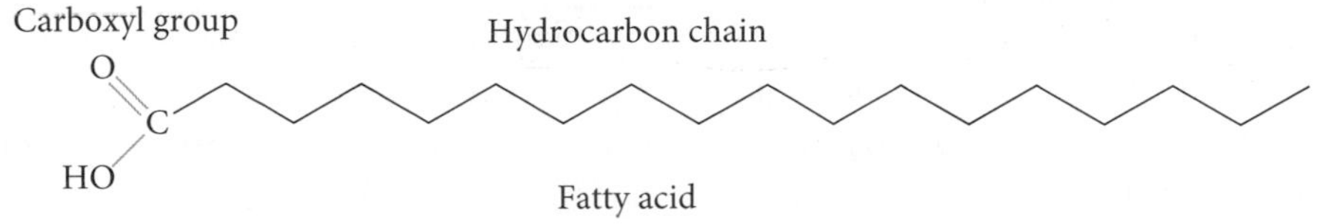

Figure 2.43 Structure of a fatty acid molecule. While the carboxyl group is hydrophilic, the hydrocarbon chain is hydrophobic.

polyunsaturated. The nomenclature for fatty acids is dictated by how long the hydrocarbon is and whether it is saturated or unsaturated. For instance, the name of a saturated fatty acid with 18 carbons ends in -*anoic* (octadecanoic acid), while the name of an unsaturated fatty acid of the same length but with double bonds ends in -*enoic* (octadecenoic acid).

In a fatty acid, the carboxyl carbon is counted as carbon number 1, and the carbon atoms next to the carboxyl carbon (i.e., carbons 2, 3, and 4) are known as α-, β-, and γ-carbons, respectively. The terminal methyl carbon is known as the ω-carbon. A variety of symbols are used to indicate the number and position of the double bonds. For instance, Δ^{11} indicates a double bond on the eleventh carbon (between carbons 11 and 12) of the fatty acid; ω^7 indicates a double bond on the seventh carbon counting from the ω-carbon (numbered from the opposite terminal carbon).

Triacylglycerols

Most people consume between 60 and 150 g of lipids every day. These dietary lipids are not digested in the mouth or stomach, but rather in the small intestine. The majority of these lipids (approximately 90%) are in the form of triacylglycerol. The remaining 10% are in the form of cholesterol, cholesteryl esters, phospholipids, and free fatty acids. Triacylglycerols (sometimes called by their older name, triglycerides) are storage lipids. In fact, triacylglycerol is the largest energy-storing molecule because both its backbone (glycerol) and its three fatty acids can be oxidized to produce many ATP molecules.

Both endogenous (from the body) and exogenous (from food) triacylglycerols are hydrophobic. As a consequence, they have a hard time traveling from their tissue of origin to the tissues in which they can be used or stored. To facilitate their movement, they are packed into plasma lipoproteins, which have many hydrophilic amino acids at their surface and, therefore, are water soluble. It is in the form of lipoproteins that lipids are able to travel within the bloodstream (see also the *Introduction to Pharmacology and Pathophysiology* chapter).

Hormones regulate the release of triacylglycerols from adipose tissue when we need energy between meals. For instance, when not much glucose is available for energy, the hormone epinephrine activates triacylglycerol lipases—the enzymes that convert triacylglycerols back to glycerol and fatty acids (Figure 2.42). The water-insoluble fatty acids bind to a plasma protein, serum albumin, which carries these fatty acids to tissues such as the heart and skeletal muscles, where they provide energy through a β-oxidation metabolism (see also the *Introduction to Biochemistry* chapter).

Saturated Fatty Acids

Saturated fatty acids are mostly derived from animal sources and have single bonds between the carbons in their hydrocarbon tails. All of the carbons are bound to the maximum possible number of hydrogen atoms; in other words, they are saturated with hydrogen (**Figure 2.44**). Saturated fatty acids are straight and, as a result, can readily pack together—a factor that explains why they have a solid form at room temperature (25°C).

Monounsaturated Fatty Acids

Monounsaturated fatty acids are mostly derived from plants, have one double bond between some of the carbons, and have a curve in their shape. Because of this curve, unsaturated fatty acids cannot pack as closely together as do saturated fatty acids (Figure 2.44). In turn, they remain in a liquid form at room temperature. However, they start to solidify at lower temperatures.

Polyunsaturated Fatty Acids

Polyunsaturated fatty acids have two or more double bonds across their long hydrocarbon chain. These fats are liquid at room temperature. Fish oils, for example, are 20 to 24 carbons long. Although these are very long chains, fish oils remain liquid because they are highly unsaturated (polyunsaturated) fats. Their polyunsaturated nature means that consumption of these oils helps lessen the possibility that a person might develop heart disease (see also the *Introduction to Pharmacology and Pathophysiology* chapter).

Membrane Lipids

Membrane lipids constitute approximately 50% of the mass of the plasma membrane in the cells of most animals. They are amphipathic molecules (i.e., they have both hydrophilic and hydrophobic properties). Membrane lipids have many functions, including determining what enters or exits a cell. Membrane lipids are divided into four groups: phospholipids, glycolipids, sterols, and ether lipids.

Phospholipids

Phospholipids are made from either glycerol or sphingosine. In both forms, the third fatty acid is replaced by a polar phosphate group. Based on their backbone, two subclasses of phospholipids are distinguished: glycerophospholipids and sphingolipids (**Figure 2.45**). The most abundant phospholipids are glycerophospholipids, which contain two fatty acids and one phosphate group. Many important molecules such as arachidonic acid in animals and the essential fatty acids in plants are made from glycerophospholipids.

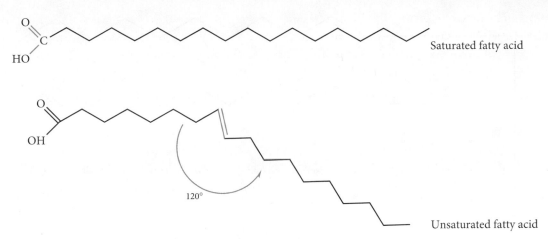

Figure 2.44 A mixture of saturated and unsaturated fatty acids.

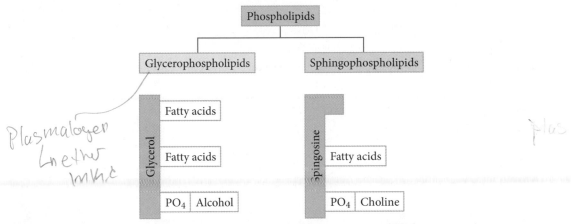

Figure 2.45 There are two subclasses of phospholipids: glycerophospholipids and sphingolipids. The most abundant phospholipids are glycerophospholipids.

Adapted from: Nelson DL, Cox MM. *Principles of biochemistry,* 5th ed. New York, NY: W. H. Freeman and Company; 2008; Chapter 10.

Phospholipids may also take the form of ether lipids, of which plasmalogen is one example. Plasmalogen is structurally different from glycerophospholipids because the long-chain acyl group attached to carbon 1 of glycerol is ether linked; in glycerophospholipids, this group is ester linked. In addition, there is a double bond between carbons 1 and 2 of the fatty acyl chain in plasmalogen (**Figure 2.46**).

Approximately 50% of the phospholipids found in the heart tissue of vertebrates consists of plasmalogens. It is not clear why humans have plasmalogens in our membranes but obviously, because they contain ether instead of ester, these membrane lipids are not prone to hydrolysis by phospholipase enzymes. Platelet-activating factor is another ether-based lipid that is produced by basophils to aggregate platelets. Platelet-activating factor is also involved in releasing the neurotransmitter serotonin from platelets.

Sphingolipids contain, instead of glycerol, a long-chain base as their backbone; this structure is called sphingosine. When a fatty acid is attached to the sphingosine amino group, a molecule called ceramide is formed; ceramide is the parent of all sphingolipids (**Figure 2.47**). The terminal OH group of ceramide usually has other groups attached to it to give different sphingolipids.

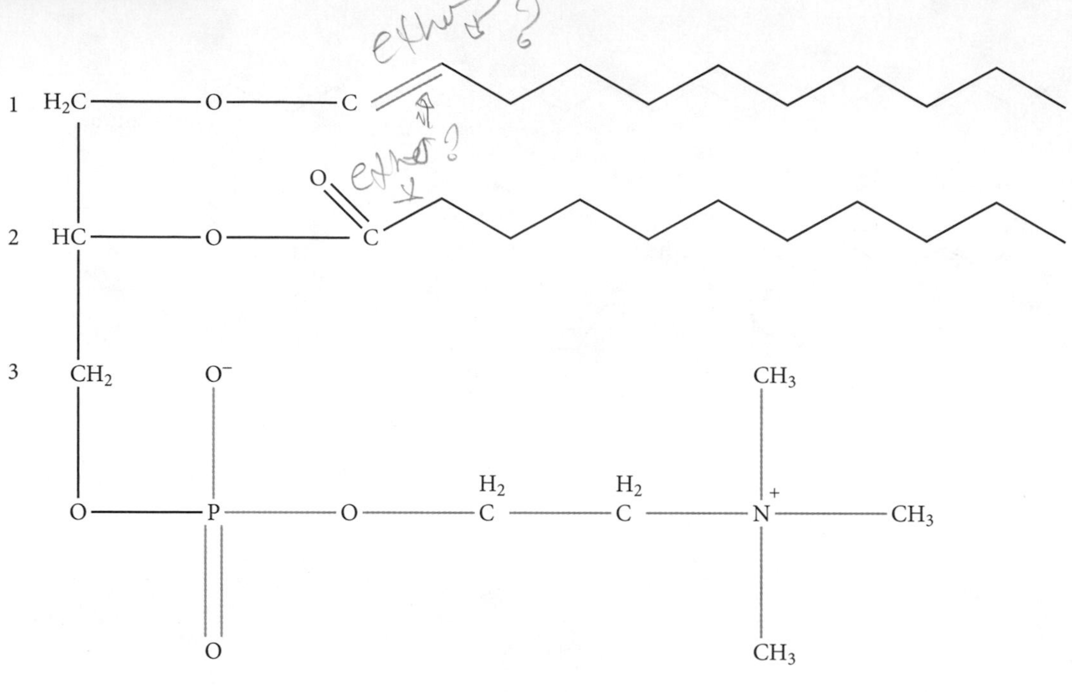

Figure 2.46 Plasmalogen is an ether lipid that has a different function and structure compared with a glycerophospholipid.

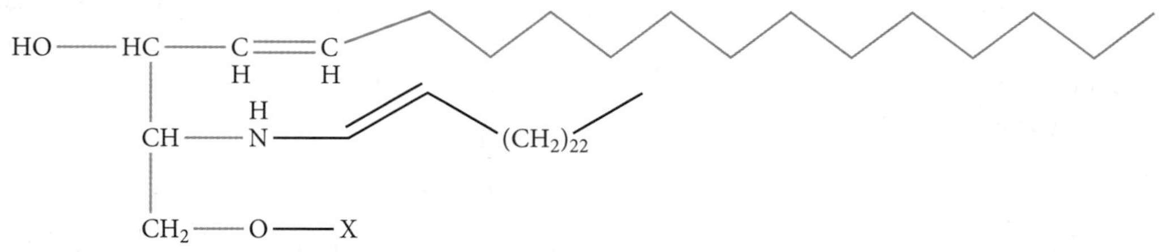

Figure 2.47 The generic structure of a sphingolipid. The structure indicates a sphingosine.

Because the polar head (X) group of sphingomyelins is either phosphocholine or phosphoethanolamine (i.e., has phosphate), these fatty acids are classified as phospholipids. Sphingolipids are prominent in the myelin sheath that structurally surrounds the axons of some neurons.

Sterols

Sterols are common in mammalian cell membranes. They cannot, however, be found in bacterial membranes. Eukaryotic cells synthesize their own sterols. The characteristic structure of sterols is a four-member fused ring (three 6-carbon rings and one 5-carbon ring). One of the major sterols in the cell membrane is cholesterol (**Figure 2.48**). Sterols also serve as precursors for steroid hormones and bile acids.

Cholesterol is unique among membrane lipids in that it contains a hydrocarbon fused-ring structure and lacks a fatty acyl chain. Cholesterol molecules make the membrane bilayer stronger and more flexible; indeed, if the plasma membrane did not contain cholesterol, cells would be very stiff. Cholesterol occurs in all animal cells. Plants, fungi, and protists make other sterols instead of cholesterol—for example, ergosterol.

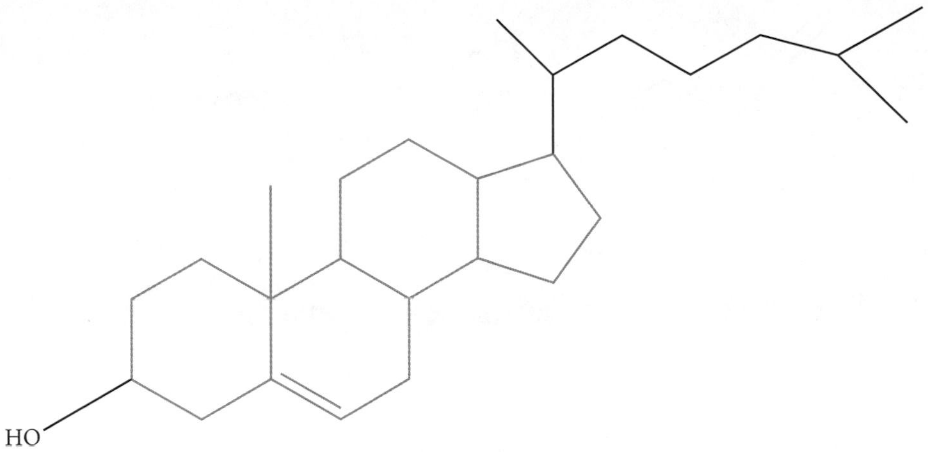

Cholesterol

Figure 2.48 Cholesterol is a sterol that has four fused rings and a hydrophilic group (hydroxyl group).

Cholesteryl ester is the major form of cholesterol in the plasma; it is produced when a fatty acid is esterified to cholesterol. This esterification process occurs in the liver. Because of the esterification reaction, cholesteryl ester is hydrophobic and, therefore, needs a lipoprotein to transport it to other tissues.

The membrane lipids are continually degraded and replaced by new synthesized lipids. A series of enzymes acts on the constituents of the membrane. One typical example is the phospholipases that serve to catalyze cleavage of acyl or phosphoacyl moieties from glycerophospholipids. Degradation of lipids occurs mainly in the lysosomes. It is important to have metabolic turnover of these lipids because a deficiency in phospholipases leads to accumulation of phospholipids.

Phospholipase A_2, which exists in most mammalian cells, is known to attack phospholipids containing arachidonic acid in a manner that releases this arachidonic acid (which is characterized by 20 carbons) at the middle carbon of membrane phospholipids (**Figure 2.49**). The arachidonic acid is then oxygenated by separate mechanisms to produce prostaglandins or thromboxane (by the action of cyclooxygenases) or leukotrienes (by the action of the lipoxygenase enzyme). Prostaglandins, thromboxanes, and leukotrienes are physiologically important molecules that are collectively called eicosanoids. Eicosanoids have potent physiological effects at low concentrations and are synthesized in all mammalian cells except erythrocytes (see also the *Introduction to Biochemistry* chapter).

Two essential fatty acids—linoleic acid and linolenic acid—are precursors to arachidonyl-coenzyme A (CoA). Humans cannot synthesize linoleic acid and linolenic acid; instead, we must include them in our diet to be able to synthesize arachidonic acid (see also the *Introduction to Biochemistry* and *Introduction to Nutrients* chapters).

Prostaglandins contain a five-carbon ring and in many tissues regulate the synthesis of the intracellular messenger cAMP, which in turn mediates the action of many hormones. (The role of the cAMP is discussed in the *Introduction to Pharmacodynamics* chapter.) In addition, prostaglandins regulate the secretion of gastric mucin to protect the gastric mucosa from the gastric acid and proteolytic enzymes found in the stomach. Nonsteroidal anti-inflammatory drugs (NSAIDs) such as ibuprofen, aspirin, and naproxen are known to inhibit the synthesis of prostaglandins from arachidonic acids. By comparison, thromboxane is known to induce constriction of blood vessels and platelet aggregation, both of which are early steps in the blood clotting cascade. As a result, aspirin, in low doses, acts as a prophylactic agent to prevent heart attack by reducing the synthesis of thromboxanes.

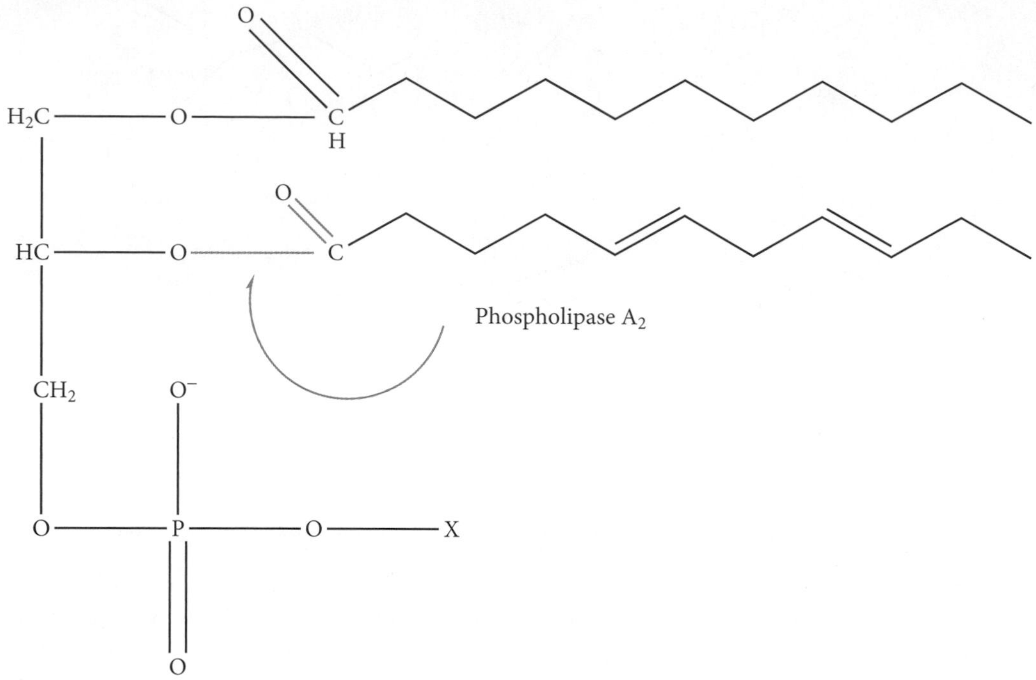

Phospholipids containing arachidonic acid

Figure 2.49 Phospholipase A$_2$ attacks phospholipids containing arachidonic acid to release arachidonic acid.

Leukotrienes are potent inflammatory mediators. Both immunological and nonimmunological stimuli can activate the phospholipase A$_2$ enzyme to release arachidonic acid, which in turn is metabolized to produce leukotrienes. Several types of leukotrienes exist. For instance, leukotriene D$_4$ induces contraction of the muscles lining the airways to the lung. Therefore, overproduction of leukotrienes causes asthmatic attacks. Inhibition of leukotriene synthesis is a good approach in the treatment of patients with asthma (see also the *Introduction to Pharmacology and Pathophysiology* chapter).

A few serious diseases are associated with a lack of phospholipid metabolism. For instance, Niemann-Pick and Tay-Sachs diseases are caused by mutations in the genes that code for enzymes that catalyze metabolism of phospholipids. In Niemann-Pick disease, the sphingomyelinase enzyme is defective and cannot catalyze reactions involving sphingomyelin, which results in the accumulation of sphingomyelin in the brain, spleen, and liver. The buildup of these molecules leads to mental retardation. In Tay-Sachs disease, because of a deficiency in the enzyme hexosaminidase A, gangliosides accumulate in the brain and spleen. Currently, there is no cure for these devastating diseases; instead, medical attention has focused on detecting these diseases in fetuses via amniocentesis. **Table 2.6** summarizes a series of enzyme deficiencies that cause abnormalities in the metabolism of lipids (which collectively is referred to as lipidosis).

Another important molecule found in the inner face of cell membrane is phosphatidylinositol. Phosphatidylinositol undergoes two phosphorylation reactions to produce phosphatidylinositol 4,5-bisphosphate, which is rich in arachidonic acid. Phosphatidylinositols play important roles in the regulation of many enzymes by enhancing either intracellular Ca^{2+} release or the stimulation of protein phosphorylation (see also the *Introduction to Pharmacodynamics* chapter).

While relatively few drugs target lipids, the mechanism of action for the majority of the available drugs is to disrupt the lipid structure of the cell membranes. One example is amphotericin B, a treatment for severe systemic and central nervous system infections caused by detrimental fungal species, particularly *Candida* and *Aspergillus* species. *Candida* infections are most commonly seen in patients with granulocytopenia (i.e., patients who have low amounts of granular leukocytes in

Table 2.6 Enzyme Deficiencies That Cause Lipid-Related Diseases

Disease	Lipid Accumulation	Enzyme Deficiency	Primary Organs Involved
Gaucher	Glucocerebroside	Glucosylceramide β-glucosidase	Liver, spleen, brain
Niemann-Pick	Sphingomyelin	Sphingomyelinase	Brain, liver, spleen
Krabbe	Galactocerebroside	Galactosylceramide β-glucosidase	Brain
Fabry	Ceramide trihexoside	α-Galactosidase	Kidney
Tay-Sachs	Ganglioside GM$_2$	β-Hexosaminidase A	Brain
Wolman	Cholesterol esters and glycerides	Not well characterized	Liver, kidney
Cholesterol ester storage disease	Cholesterol esters and triglycerides	Cholesteryl ester hydrolase	Liver, spleen, lymph nodes, elsewhere
Cerebro-tendino-sus xanthomatosis	Dihydrocholesterol (cholestanol)	Sterol hydroxylase in bile acid synthetic pathway	Central nervous system, eyes, tendons
β-Sitosterolemia and xanthomatosis	Plant sterols	Not well characterized	Tendons, skin, circulatory system
Refsum	Phytanic acid	Phytanic acid hydroxylase	Central nervous system, skin, bone

Reproduced from: Woodbury CP. *Biochemistry for the pharmaceutical sciences*. Jones & Bartlett Learning; 2012.

their blood). Amphotericin B (Fungizone, from Canada) is an amphipathic substance. This drug binds the fungal cell membrane sterol (i.e., ergosterol), thereby disrupting the osmotic integrity of the fungal membrane and leading to cellular death (**Figure 2.50**). Despite the fact that amphotericin B is a very toxic drug, it is the treatment of choice for many detrimental fungal infections. Due to its hydrophilic groups, this drug cannot cross the blood–brain barrier. Consequently, to reach the central nervous system, it must be administrated intrathecally—that is, by injection into the spinal cord.

Allylamines are another type of drugs that target the cell membranes of fungi. Terbinafine (Lamisil) belongs to this group. Terbinafine acts by inhibiting squalene epoxidase. This enzyme is important to synthesize ergosterol, an essential component of fungal cell membranes. Therefore, inhibition of squalene epoxidase blocks the biosynthesis of ergosterol, which finally leads to the loss of the cell membrane's integrity.

Learning Bridge 2.6

Joe Smith is a 28-years-old car salesman who comes to your pharmacy to buy a "painkiller" for his headaches, which seem to occur once every other week. He has been using Bufferin tablets, but each time he takes the recommended dose of one or two tablets, he experiences excruciating pain in his stomach. To alleviate his stomach pain, Joe has used Advil. Unfortunately, not only has this medication not helped him with his stomach pain, but it has actually worsened his stomach pain.

A. Explain to Joe why he experiences stomach pain when he takes Bufferin.
B. Explain to Joe why Advil will not help him with his stomach pain and why this medication is increasing, rather than decreasing, his pain.
C. Suggest an OTC product that will help alleviate Joe's stomach and headache pain.

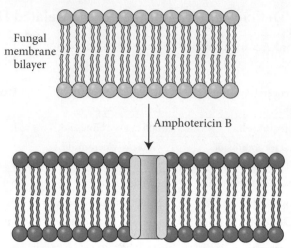

Fungal membrane bilayer

Amphotericin B

Figure 2.50 Amphotericin B has a mixed hydrophobic and hydrophilic structure that forms a tunnel through the fungal cell membrane, thereby disrupting the osmotic integrity of the cell.

Bacterial Cell Division and the Cell Cycle

All cells undergo cell division during their life span. DNA replication is an essential aspect of cellular and viral reproduction. Both accuracy and efficiency are essential considerations in the replication process. DNA replication, however, is far more accurate than any other enzyme-catalyzed process.

Replication is a semiconservative DNA duplication, which means each DNA strand serves as a template for a new strand, with the result being two new DNA molecules (**Figure 2.51**). Each new DNA molecule has one old strand and one new strand. In other words, each DNA molecule contains one parental strand and one newly synthesized strand.

Cell growth in bacteria is accomplished by binary fission—that is, production of two daughter cells from a single parent cell. Due to the simplicity of the rod-shaped *E. coli* bacterium, researchers were able to extensively study binary fission in this organism.

As mentioned earlier, replication of the cell's DNA (genome) is essential to support cell growth. Prokaryotic DNA comprises a single supercoiled circular DNA. During cell growth, the parent cell elongates first to form a partition, which is also referred to as a septum. Bacteria lack a mitotic spindle, so the septum is formed to separate the two DNA molecules produced by the replication machinery (**Figure 2.52**).

During the formation of the septum, and prior to the actual cell division, the replication begins at a specific location on the DNA molecule called "ori." The DNA molecule begins to unwind at the ori to synthesize two new strands, forming a replication fork as it does so. A number of proteins are associated with the replication fork that facilitate the DNA replication. The synthesis of the new DNA always proceeds in the $5' \rightarrow 3'$ direction. As a consequence, one daughter strand would be expected to undergo $3' \rightarrow 5'$ synthesis—an impossible process. The solution to this dilemma is that one strand of the newly synthesized DNA is first produced in small fragments (Okazaki fragments) in the $5' \rightarrow 3'$ direction. As the replication fork moves, the Okazaki fragments join each other covalently by DNA ligase to form one of the daughter strands (**Figure 2.53**).

As the entire double-stranded DNA is replicated, each copy of the DNA molecule is attached to the plasma membrane. An active membrane synthesis occurs between the sites of attachment of the two daughter DNAs to form two daughter cells. Interestingly, both chloroplasts and mitochondria contain a single, circular chromosome. In addition, these two organelles replicate

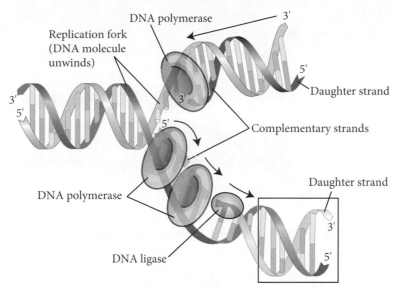

Figure 2.51 The mechanism of replication is semiconservative, which means each DNA strand serves as a template for a new strand, resulting in the synthesis of two new DNA molecules. DNA polymerase and ligase enzymes and the replication fork are also shown in this figure.

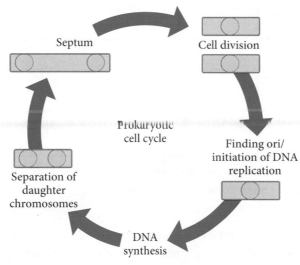

Figure 2.52 Prokaryotic cell growth is accomplished by binary fission—that is, production of two daughter cells from a single parent cell.

their chromosomes and undergo binary fission, similar to prokaryotic cells, within the cytoplasm of eukaryotic cells.

Cell Growth

Cell growth has three distinct features: biomass production, cell production, and cell survival. Each of these features is dependent upon a series of factors. For instance, biomass production depends on the environment (water, pH, temperature, nutrients such as carbons and nitrogen, energy) and the enzymatic machinery required to synthesize the necessary products (DNA, RNA, proteins). Cell production, in addition to biomass production, depends on DNA replication and subsequent cell division. Cell survival depends on the stress to which the cells are exposed. Many bacteria are able to survive by differentiating into resistant resting forms (such as spores); others may adjust their metabolic rate when nutrition is scarce. Bacteria grow well when all three features are provided in a medium.

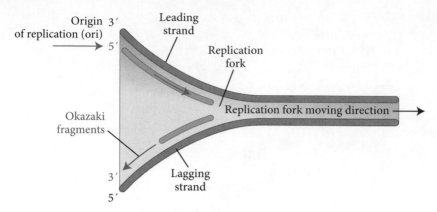

Figure 2.53 DNA replication is initiated at the origin of replication (ori). The leading strand directs continuous synthesis of the new strand, whereas the lagging strand directs the synthesis of Okazaki fragments.
Adapted from: Nelson DL, Cox MM. *Principles of biochemistry*, 5th ed. New York, NY: W. H. Freeman and Company; 2008; Chapter 25.

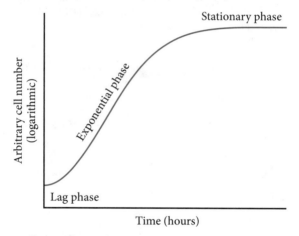

Figure 2.54 A general pattern of bacterial growth in a cultural medium.

Because bacteria grow rapidly, after an extended culturing period, cells exhaust their external and internal resources and enter a stationary phase. To avoid the stationary phase, it is necessary to keep diluting the culture in a fresh nutrient-rich medium. During the diluting process, cells adjust to the new medium and the cell growth enters a lag phase, in which the number of cells does not increase but the cells are actively making preparations for growth. During the lag phase, cells synthesize ribosomes and other necessary factors for protein synthesis. After the lag phase, DNA replication is initiated, which is the beginning of the exponential phase. During the exponential phase, cells divide regularly by binary fission at a constant rate. The growth continues until some nutrient becomes scarce or some toxic product accumulates, which results in a stationary phase where cell growth ceases (**Figure 2.54**).

Most of our understanding about bacterial cell growth has come from studying isolated cell lines that grow under optimal conditions. In a natural environment, however, many bacteria compete with each other while they are under nutritional stress, which may result in a physiologic condition that is quite different from what has been observed in the experimental test tube.

Even a simple organism such as *E. coli* has not provided all answers to our questions about cell growth and cell division. For instance, it is known that *E. coli*, under normal growth condition, uses only 10% of the coding capacity of its genome. Two explanations have been proposed for why many genes are not used during normal cell growth. First, these genes may have been needed in the past but then became silenced. Second, these genes may be functional but are part of systems that work only when under stress (e.g., in the face of genetic damage, starvation, or oxidation). For instance, approximately 46 genes are involved in protecting *E. coli* against temperature shocks. Similarly, approximately 50 genes are active in this organism during starvation.

Bacteria and yeasts can grow in a liquid medium or on a solid medium, usually in a 2% agar. All of these culture media provide water, minerals, nitrogen, carbon, and energy, and sometimes vitamins or other growth factors. Different organisms, however, may require different media to support their cell growth. For instance, while prototrophic bacteria (organisms that are able to synthesize their required growth factors) can meet all of their needs from a single organic carbon source in the presence of a few ions (K^+, Mg^{2+}, Fe^{3+}, PO_4^{3-}, and SO_4^{2-}), the auxotrophic bacteria (organisms that are not able to synthesize their required growth factors) lack various biosynthetic pathways and, as a result, require amino acids, nucleic acid bases, and vitamins. In contrast, facultative anaerobes grow only in the absence of oxygen.

Because cultures isolated from nature often contain a mixture of different organisms, the best way to produce a pure culture (i.e., a culture that has cells of one kind and for which all progeny are of a single cell) is by subculturing a single colony. Test cultures in the laboratory are grown in small flasks, whereas large cultures grown in fermentors that have room for hundreds of liters are used to produce antibiotics or other microbial products. The cells are often separated from the culture fluid by centrifugation or filtration.

Eukaryotic Cell Growth and the Cell Cycle

In contrast to prokaryotic cells, the daughter cells in eukaryotic cells may differ from their parent cell in terms of size, shape, and differentiation phase. In addition, the growth time depends on the specific eukaryotic cell. For instance, while it takes 8 minutes for an embryonic cell to initiate and complete a cell cycle, it takes more than 10 hours for most other rapidly dividing somatic cells to finish their cell cycle. Conversely, many somatic cells do not divide frequently. For example, hepatocytes divide only once per year, and mature neurons never divide.

The eukaryotic cell cycle comprises two periods: (1) a long interphase representing the time in which the cell is actively involved in reproducing its components and (2) a short period of mitosis in which the actual process of cell division into two daughter cells occurs. Five phases, each of a different duration, take place during the complete eukaryotic cell cycle (**Figure 2.55**).

After each cell division, there is a time gap (G_1 phase) before the synthesis of DNA begins.

1. G_1 phase: The cell is metabolically active, and synthesis of RNA and proteins occur. While DNA precursors are made, no actual DNA synthesis occurs during this phase. In addition, at the end of this phase, there is a restriction point such that once a cell passes this point, it is committed to enter the S phase. It takes 6–12 hours to complete the entire G_1 phase.

2. S phase: DNA replication occurs, and the number of chromosomes doubles, which results in the formation of two sister chromatids. In addition, the cell continues to synthesize proteins and RNA. It takes 6–8 hours to complete the entire S phase.

3. G_2 phase: While no DNA synthesis occurs in this phase, the cell continues RNA and protein synthesis. It takes 3–4 hours to complete the entire G_2 phase.

4. M phase: Mitosis (nuclear division) and cytokinesis (cell division) occur, which results in two daughter cells. It takes only 1–2 hours to complete the entire M phase.

5. G_0 phase: Terminally differentiated cells indefinitely withdraw from the cell cycle.

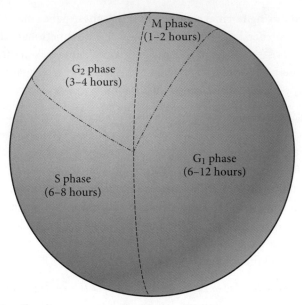

Figure 2.55 The eukaryotic cell cycle.

Adapted from: Nelson DL, Cox MM. *Principles of biochemistry*, 5th ed. New York, NY: W. H. Freeman and Company; 2008; Chapter 12.

Interphase in a cell cycle refers to the time that elapses between one M phase and the next cell cycle; it usually accounts for 90% or more of the total cell cycle time. The cells that are produced by a series of mitotic divisions (in the phases described previously) and generate the entire organism are called somatic cells. While during embryonic development most of the somatic cells proceed through the cell cycle, during adult time many cells enter the G_0 phase and are terminally differentiated or no longer divide.

As was mentioned earlier, during the M phase of the cell cycle, the separation of replicated nuclei takes place and results in two identical daughter nuclei. During mitosis, six different phases occur: prophase, prometaphase (or late prophase), metaphase, anaphase, telophase, and cytokinesis. In rapidly proliferating eukaryotic cells, an M phase occurs once every 16–24 hours. A brief discussion of each phase is important to understand the mitotic process.

Prophase

During the S phase, two sister chromatids are produced. At the beginning of prophase, these sister chromatids are condensed but remain attached at a specific sequence of DNA necessary for chromosome separation called the centromere. During interphase, the centrosome, which is a large cytoplasmic organelle that serves to organize microtubules, divides to produce two sets of centrioles. The centrioles are made of microtubules and are also able to duplicate during interphase; they begin to move to opposite ends of the nucleus to form separate poles. While these centrioles move away from each other, the microtubules disassemble. The role of centrioles is to produce the microtubules, which in turn are the components of the cytoskeleton that provide both shape and structure to a cell. The new microtubules begin to extend from the centriole pairs in all directions to form the mitotic spindle. There is a variation among organisms in regard to the number of microtubules that make up the mitotic spindle. The microtubules that connect at the center of the chromatid pairs are called kinetochore microtubules; others that extend to the opposite pole are called polar microtubules (**Figure 2.56**).

Prometaphase

Prometaphase, also called late prophase, begins with the breakdown of the nuclear membrane. During this phase of the cell cycle, the kinetochore microtubules interact with the chromosomes

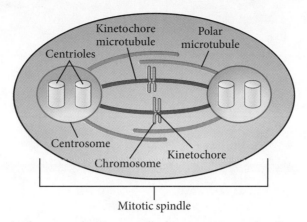

Figure 2.56 A centrosome is a large cytoplasmic organelle that serves to organize microtubules and is duplicated during the S phase of the cell cycle. Each centrosome has two centrioles. While the kinetochore microtubule connects the kinetochore to the poles, the polar microtubules begin to overlap halfway through the mitotic spindle. Adapted from: Keyormarsi K, O'Leary N, Pardee AB. Cell division. In: *AccessScience*. New York, NY: McGraw-Hill; 2012. Available at: http://www.accessscience.com.

to form protein complexes at their centromeres, and the polar microtubules are stabilized through cross-linking of microtubule binding proteins (Figure 2.56). These microtubules are protected from disassembly by the constant formation of new microtubules from tubulin molecules in the cytosol. The stabilization of these microtubules is critical for effective mitosis to occur.

Drugs that inhibit assembly of microtubules do not allow the cells to complete their mitosis. One example is colchicine (Colcrys). Colchicine is used for the treatment of acute gout attack and for prophylactic treatment of gout. It is known to disrupt cytoskeletal functions by inhibiting microtubule formation, which in turn prevents cellular movement of the neutrophils that are associated with causing some gout symptoms. Colchicine is often given together with probenecid (Benuryl, from Canada), an analgesic drug, to improve chronic gouty arthritis because probenecid, at a therapeutic dose, blocks reabsorption of uric acid in the kidney's proximal tubules (i.e., increases excretion of uric acid into urine). Patients who are taking colchicine experience alopecia (hair loss) because in addition to exerting its tubulin effect, this drug binds to the mitotic spindle and thereby blocks cell division.

Metaphase

During metaphase, the kinetochore microtubules from both poles evenly align their chromosomes in one plane, called the metaphase plate, which is halfway between the spindle poles. This even-alignment process is a result of a counterbalance generated by the opposing kinetochores. Each sister chromatid is now at right angles to the opposite poles. During the mitotic process, metaphase lasts about 30 minutes in mammalian cells (the longest span of time during mitosis).

Anaphase

During anaphase, which comprises two stages, the sister chromatids are separated and move to opposite spindle poles to assemble and form the nucleus of the new cell. During the first stage, a sister chromatid pair separates at the kinetochore and is directed to the opposite pole as the kinetochore microtubules begin to shorten at a rate of 1 micrometer per minute. As the sister chromatids reach the opposite poles, the microtubules disassemble. During the second stage, the disassembling polar microtubules begin to elongate so that the two poles of the spindle move apart (**Figure 2.57**).

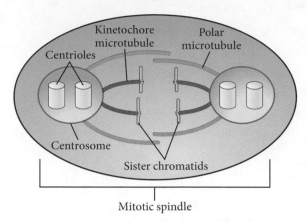

Figure 2.57 During anaphase, the microtubules of the mitotic spindle play critical roles in separating the sister chromatids. The sister chromatids, once separated, move to opposite spindle poles to assemble and form the nucleus of a new cell. This process is facilitated by shortening of the kinetochore microtubule and elongation of the polar microtubules.

Adapted from: Keyormarsi K, O'Leary N, Pardee AB. Cell division. In: *AccessScience*. New York, NY: McGraw-Hill; 2012. Available at: http://www.accessscience.com.

Telophase

Telophase is the final phase of mitosis. During this phase, the sister chromatids arrive at each separate pole, the kinetochore microtubules disappear, and the polar microtubules continue to elongate. A nuclear envelope begins to form around each group of sister chromatids.

Cytokinesis

Cytokinesis, which stands for cell division, begins during anaphase and ends the mitotic process. During this phase, the cytoplasm is cleaved and produces two daughter cells. The forces to cleave the cytoplasm are generated through actin–myosin interactions. The cleavage is an accurate process so that the two daughter cells are of approximately equal size and have similar properties.

Replication, Transcription, and Translation

During the process of cell division, the cell's DNA must be replicated to allow formation of the two daughter cells. When a gene is expressed, a single-strand RNA (mRNA) is synthesized, in a process referred to as transcription. The mRNA is then used by ribosomes and many other molecules and proteins to polymerize amino acids into proteins, in a process referred to as translation. A closer look at all these three processes is important to understand cell survival and growth.

Replication

DNA replication is an essential aspect of cellular and viral reproduction. Accurate, efficient, and rapid duplication of DNA have a significant impact on the replication process. As mentioned earlier, DNA replication is a semiconservative mechanism that utilizes each DNA strand as a template for a new strand, resulting in a new DNA molecule. The final products are two daughter DNA molecules.

DNA replication is the most accurate enzyme-catalyzed process. It has been estimated that the error rate per base pair for each round of replication is approximately 10^{-9}; that is, only one wrong base pair is incorporated per 1 billion correct base pairs. Compared to protein synthesis (translation) or transcription, DNA replication is 100,000 times more accurate. One of the main reasons for this high accuracy is that all DNA polymerases have a proofreading capability.

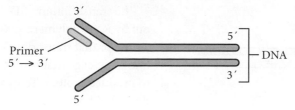

Figure 2.58 All DNA polymerases catalyze DNA synthesis only in the 5′ → 3′ direction.

Figure 2.53 demonstrated the movement of the replication fork during the replication process. The strand of DNA that is synthesized continuously in the same direction as the replication fork moves is termed the leading strand. The strand of DNA that is synthesized in fragments (Okazaki fragments) in the opposite direction to the movement of the replication fork is called the lagging strand. DNA ligase seals the DNA at the boundaries between the synthesized Okazaki fragments. This replication process, though it appears simple in description, requires accurate and efficient replication machinery that includes many proteins and molecules. DNA polymerases play essential roles in the replication machinery.

The synthesis of a DNA molecule is quite similar in prokaryotes and eukaryotes. Because the replication process is much less complex in prokaryotic cells, a great deal is known about this process, at least as it is experienced by the *E. coli* bacterium. Replication can be divided into three stages: initiation; elongation, and termination. To save cellular energy, initiation is the major target for the regulation of replication; in other words, if something goes wrong, it is better to stop replication at the beginning of the process when the energy cost is tolerable.

All DNA polymerases catalyze DNA synthesis only in the 5′ → 3′ direction. DNA polymerases require a primer, which is a short, single-strand nucleic acid attached at the site where replication is to begin (**Figure 2.58**). Primers of DNA can then be elongated by a DNA polymerase. The primer is synthesized by an enzyme called primase, and the primer is removed after the Okazaki fragment is synthesized. The ability of a polymerase to remain associated with the template strand during replication is known as processivity. The higher the processivity of the enzyme, the higher the probability of completely and successfully synthesizing a DNA molecule. For DNA polymerases to synthesize DNA, the DNA must encounter a free 3′-OH deoxyribose at the end of a DNA chain, which then serves as the substrate for attachment of the 5′-phosphate of a deoxyribonucleoside triphosphate of the incoming nucleotide.

During the elongation process, the parental DNA is unwound by DNA helicases, which causes topological stress. This topological stress, however, is relieved by topoisomerases. Each separated strand is then stabilized by a single-stranded DNA-binding protein (SSB). From here on, both leading and lagging strands will be synthesized by different mechanisms.

Transcription

Transcription is the mechanism by which a sequence of DNA is utilized by specific proteins, RNA polymerases, to generate an RNA molecule that is complementary to one of the DNA strands. There are three main types of RNA—mRNA, tRNA, and rRNA—which are directly used by the protein synthetic machinery during the translation process. In the prokaryotic cell, protein synthesis starts using the mRNA even as it is still being synthesized. In contrast, both tRNA and rRNA are first completely transcribed and then undergo post-transcriptional processing and modification before they are used in the protein synthesis process.

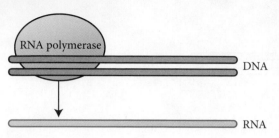

Figure 2.59 RNA polymerase is an enzyme that synthesizes a single-stranded RNA molecule.

The transcription of DNA to RNA is carried out by RNA polymerase(s). RNA polymerase is a protein that transcribes genetic information into a message that can be read by the ribosome to produce protein. To express a gene, the gene must first be recognized by an RNA polymerase (**Figure 2.59**). Unlike DNA polymerase, RNA polymerase does not require a primer to initiate transcription because certain sequences (promoters) are automatically recognized by RNA polymerases. Prokaryotes have one RNA polymerase and eukaryotes have three distinct RNA polymerases that catalyze the synthesis of all three RNA classes (mRNA, tRNA, and rRNA).

Because the *E. coli* transcription process is quite well understood, we focus on prokaryotic transcription to describe the mechanism of RNA synthesis. The *E. coli* RNA polymerase is composed of a core enzyme that has two α subunits; one subunit each for β, β′, and ω; and a sixth subunit called σ factor. The σ factor plays an essential role in recognizing the transcriptional initiation site and unwinding the DNA double helix. Once the elongation starts, the σ factor dissociates from the core enzyme. It is the core enzyme that carries out the actual polymerization of RNA (i.e., transcription).

To begin the transcription process, the DNA is temporarily unwound at some point over a short distance (approximately 17 base pairs) to make a transcriptional bubble that moves with RNA synthesis. The DNA is unwound ahead and rewound behind as RNA is transcribed—a process that would create a topological problem on the DNA, except that topoisomerases are available to reduce any DNA tension. **Table 2.7** demonstrates differences and similarities between DNA polymerases and RNA polymerases.

Similar to the replication process, the transcription process includes three steps: initiation, elongation, and termination. In the initiation step, the σ factor of RNA polymerase binds to a specific DNA sequence called a promoter. The DNA base pairs that correspond to the beginning of an RNA molecule are numbered with positive numbers, whereas those located prior to the RNA start site are numbered with negative numbers (**Figure 2.60**). While the promoter's length varies (in the range of 20 to 200 base pairs) in different DNA molecules, two short sequences (–10 and –35) are similar in different bacterial species. The –35 and –10 regions play important roles in the initiation of transcription. Mutation in these regions will significantly decrease the rate of

Table 2.7 Similarities and Differences Between DNA Polymerases and RNA Polymerases

Similarity	Differences
Use nucleoside triphosphates as substrates.	RNA polymerase does not require a primer; a DNA polymerase does. An RNA polymerase requires a promoter to initiate transcription; a DNA polymerase does not.
Require Mg^{2+} and Zn^{2+}.	RNA polymerase lacks the $3' \rightarrow 5'$ proofreading exonuclease activity that is present in DNA polymerases. As a result, accuracy is much higher in DNA replication than in RNA transcription.
Produce an antiparallel complement to the DNA template and synthesize nucleic acids in the $5' \rightarrow 3'$ direction.	Prokaryotes have one RNA polymerase; there are five DNA polymerases.

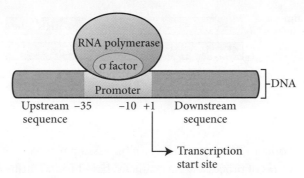

Figure 2.60 The σ factor of the RNA polymerase recognizes the promoter region of the DNA to initiate the transcription process.

transcription. Many promoters for RNA polymerase II contain a sequence called a TATA box that occurs approximately 20 to 25 base pairs upstream from the start site.

The RNA polymerase binds to the promoter region by first forming a closed complex (i.e., when the DNA double helix is not unwound). The closed complex converts to an open complex by unwinding of a short region of the promoter (from −10 to +2). The RNA polymerase travels along the DNA away from the promoter region and, after synthesis of a short sequence of the new RNA (approximately 10 nucleotides), the σ subunit dissociates. Here, the rest of the polymerase (i.e., the core enzyme) leaves the promoter and becomes committed to productively elongating the RNA.

The specific sequences to which *E. coli* RNA polymerase binds generally contain more A/T base pairs than G/C base pairs because the A/T base pairs are stabilized by two hydrogen bonds rather than the three hydrogen bonds for G/C pairs. Regulation can occur at any stage of transcription (i.e., at initiation, elongation, or termination), although it most commonly occurs at initiation. Ultimately, the DNA sequence at the promoter (or a nearby DNA sequence) determines how the DNA is transcribed and regulated, although proteins carry out the instructions.

Upon completion of the initiation stage, an α subunit leaves the RNA polymerase, which decreases the affinity of RNA polymerase for the promoter. From this point forward, the core enzyme of RNA polymerase is converted to an active transcription complex. RNA polymerase continues to elongate the RNA by successively adding one nucleotide after another to the growing RNA chain in the 5′ → 3′ direction. Here, the β subunit has a major role by being involved in phosphodiester bond formation. The antibiotic rifampicin (Rifadin) binds to the β subunits, for example, thereby inhibiting prokaryotic transcription. In the termination step, some structural changes cause the RNA polymerase to slow or to stop its action, which in turn disrupts the RNA–DNA hybrid; as a result, the RNA polymerase is removed from the DNA and the transcription process terminates.

Strong evidence indicates that several types of RNAs can serve as catalysts. These RNA molecules are referred to as ribozymes. One typical example is peptidyltransferase, which is a component of the large ribosomal subunit. This ribozyme is able to catalyze peptide formation during the translation process (see the discussion of translation elsewhere in this chapter).

RNA Processing

Many RNA transcripts are modified before they begin to function in protein synthesis. In particular, the goal of RNA processing is to produce a mature mRNA or a functional tRNA or rRNA from a primary transcript. The eukaryotic mRNA is produced in the nucleus and must be exported into the cytosol for translation. However, before it is ready to participate in protein synthesis in the cytoplasm, it undergoes extensive processing in the nucleus. As a result, the primary transcript may include introns that must be removed before translation can occur.

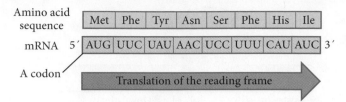

Figure 2.61 Codons that specify an amino acid sequence in a reading frame of mRNA.

For this reason, eukaryotic mRNA must undergo a processing mechanism before it can be used as a protein template. A series of processing mechanisms have been identified. The largest class of RNA processing mechanism comprises the spliceosomal introns. Five snRNAs (U1, U2, U4, U5, and U6) and their associated proteins (small nuclear ribonucleoproteins [snRNPs]) are involved in this splicing mechanism. The ribonucleoproteins, in the presence of ATP molecules, form a large complex (50 proteins) called a spliceosome. The spliceosome removes an intron and joins two neighboring exons together. Unlike eukaryotes, prokaryotes do not have spliceosomes.

tRNA also undergoes RNA processing. Surprisingly, tRNAs have several bases in addition to the four bases normally found in RNA. The unusual bases in tRNA are made by first incorporating the usual four bases into a tRNA precursor, which is then modified by specific enzymes. In addition, short sequences at the 5′ and 3′ ends of the primary tRNA transcript are removed by RNase P and D, respectively. A specific enzyme then adds CCA at the 3′ end, which is a necessary step in the tRNA processing. This 3′-CCA end is the same for all functional tRNA molecules and plays a critical role in translation because it is the site for amino acid attachment (see Figure 2.28 or Figure 2.62).

Translation

Protein synthesis entails translation of the genetic information into proteins. The translation process requires a mechanism to bring the mRNA together with other molecules so as to catalyze polymerization of amino acids into a protein. The coding genes are organized into nucleotide units called codons, identified by three-letter designations such as UUU, ACC, and AUG; the codons correspond to the nucleotides found in the gene. Altogether, 64 codons make up the entire genetic code. Each codon can specify an amino acid, but more than one codon can also be used to specify a given amino acid. For instance, the UUU and UUC codons can both specify the same amino acid, phenylalanine. Each single mRNA has an initiation codon (AUG), a stop codon (UAA, UAG, or UGA), and a binding site for a ribosome that is always upstream of the AUG codon. A set of continuous triplet codons in an mRNA read by a ribosome is called a reading frame (**Figure 2.61**).

The major components of the protein synthetic machinery are amino acids, mRNA, ribosomes, tRNA, and aminoacyl-tRNA synthetase. Keep in mind that while there are 64 codons in the genetic code, only 20 amino acids are found in the human genetic code. This mystery arises because in the anticodon–codon interaction, the first base in a tRNA's anticodon experiences a flexibility or "wobble." This "wobble" allows one specific tRNA to read more than one codon. The "wobble hypothesis" explains why, for instance, both the UUC and UUU codons (which code for the amino acid phenylalanine) can be read by the same tRNA (phenylalanine).

Two important selection steps occur during the translation process (1) to select a correct amino acid for a correct tRNA and (2) to select a correct charged tRNA for a correct codon. The first selection process is accomplished by an enzyme called aminoacyl-tRNA synthetase. To charge a tRNA with an amino acid, the amino acid must be activated by reacting with an ATP molecule to form aminoacyl-AMP. In a subsequent reaction, this activated molecule (aminoacyl-AMP) interacts with a tRNA to form a charged tRNA. Both reactions are catalyzed by the same enzyme, aminoacyl-tRNA synthetase. The aminoacyl-tRNA synthetase attaches an amino acid covalently to the CCA end (3′ end) of a tRNA (**Figure 2.62**).

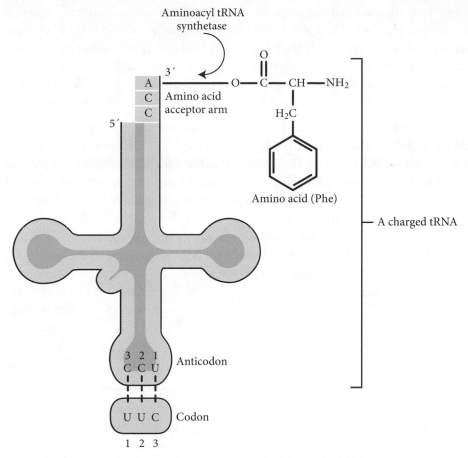

Figure 2.62 The first base in a tRNA's anticodon experiences a flexibility or "wobble."

Aminoacyl-tRNA synthetases have proofreading activity that can check whether an amino acid is linked with its correct tRNA, which ultimately will reduce the error rate for the translation process. Each amino acid has its own specific aminoacyl-tRNA synthetase; because humans have 20 amino acids, then, we must have 20 aminoacyl tRNA synthetases as well.

Learning Bridge 2.7

While you are working in the pharmacy as an intern during one of your introductory pharmacy practice experiences, a physician calls you to prescribe mupirocin (Bactroban Cream) for his patient, Joe, who is a 23 year-old first-year medical student. The prescription reads:

Mupirocin cream, 2%, 15 g

Apply to affected area t.i.d. for 5 days

Refill: 0

Joe comes to your pharmacy to pick up his medication. He has a few questions about this antibiotic:

A. How does this antibiotic clear the bacterial infection?
B. How should he apply this medication on his face?
C. Are there any side effects associated with this medication?

Similar to the replication and transcription processes, the protein synthetic machinery moves through initiation, elongation, and termination steps. Because translation is better understood in prokaryotes than in eukaryotes, only the prokaryotic translation is discussed here. Prokaryotic mRNA includes a so-called Shine-Dalgarno sequence that is found upstream of the initiation codon. This sequence base pairs with a complementary sequence in the 16S rRNA of the ribosome, thereby facilitating the attachment of the 30S ribosomal subunit to mRNA (**Figure 2.63**).

After attachment of the 30S ribosomal subunit to the mRNA, the initiator tRNA, fMet-tRNAf^Met, is brought to the AUG codon by initiation factor 2 (IF2) and GTP. The ternary complex (IF2-GTP-initiator tRNA) places the fMet-tRNAf^Met in the P site (fMet-tRNAf^Met is the only tRNA that can bind to the P site during the initiation process) to form a 30S initiation complex. The role of initiation factor 3 (IF3) is to prevent a premature association of the 50S subunit with the 30S subunit. It has been suggested that initiation factor 1 (IF1) occupies the A site to make sure that no charged tRNA binds to the A site during the initiation step. After the formation of the 30S initiation complex, the 50S subunit joins the 30S subunit to form a 70S initiation complex in which GTP is hydrolyzed to GDP and all three initiation factors, including GDP, depart the 70S ribosome. This 70S initiation complex has three tRNA binding sites: A site (acceptor), P site (peptidyl), and E site (exit of deacylated tRNA). At the A site is the codon corresponding to the upcoming aminoacyl-tRNA (**Figure 2.64**).

During the elongation phase of translation, a charged tRNA is brought to the A site by the elongation factor EF-Tu and a GTP molecule. The charged tRNA is placed into the A site, the GTP is hydrolyzed, and the EF-Tu/GDP leaves the ribosome. The last GTP hydrolysis is a crucial step in maintaining the accuracy in translation, because it allows a correctly charged tRNA to be selected for the A site and an incorrectly charged tRNA to be rejected from the ribosome. The Tu/GDP is exchanged for Tu/GTP by another elongation factor (EF-Ts), thereby ensuring that the recycled EF-Tu/GTP is ready to bring another charged tRNA.

After both the P and A sites have been occupied by the initiator tRNA and elongator charged tRNA, respectively, the amino acid of the initiator tRNA is transferred to the amino acid of the charged tRNA in the A site. This step is catalyzed by peptidyl transferase (ribozyme), which is an integral part of the 50S subunit (**Figure 2.65**).

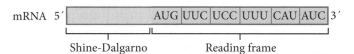

Figure 2.63 The Shine-Dalgarno sequence is found only in prokaryotes and facilitates binding of the 30S ribosomal subunit to mRNA.

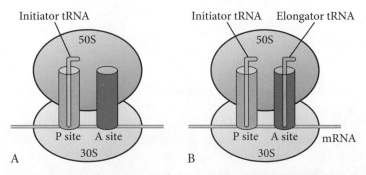

Figure 2.64 **(A)** The 70S initiation complex is ready to accept the first elongator tRNA at the A site. **(B)** The elongator tRNA is placed on the A site and the ribosome is ready to build the first dipeptide.

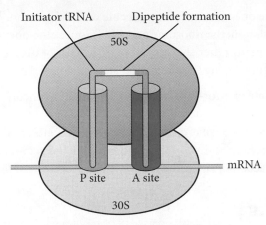

Figure 2.65 Peptidyl transferase from the 50S subunit catalyzes the binding of the two amino acids from the tRNA that are attached to the P and A sites of the ribosome.

After forming the first dipeptidyl-tRNA at the A site, the ribosome is ready to move along the mRNA by one codon. This movement is catalyzed by another elongation factor, EF-G, in a step referred to as translocation (**Figure 2.66**). After the translocation process (ribosome movement), the uncharged tRNA (deacylated tRNA) leaves the E site and the dipeptidyl-tRNA remains at the P site. The empty A site is ready to accept the next elongator aminoacyl-tRNA.

The net result of one turn of each elongation cycle is that the polypeptide grows by one amino acid residue and the ribosome moves along the mRNA by one codon. The elongation process is repeated until the full length of a polypeptide is synthesized and a termination signal (a stop codon) is reached. Any of a series of antibiotics (e.g., tetracyclines, aminoglycosides, macrolides) may inhibit the elongation step of the protein synthetic machinery; these medications are discussed in the *Introduction to Microbiology* chapter.

Termination begins when one of the stop codons (UAA, UAG, or UGA) moves into the A site of the ribosome. No functional tRNA corresponds to these codons. One of the release factors (RF1 or RF2) recognizes the stop codon and enters the A site to remove the synthesized polypeptide from the last tRNA at the P site. A ribosomal recycling factor (RRF), working together with EF-G and a GTP molecule, facilitates the dissociation of 70S into the 50S and 30S subunits. In addition, IF3 dissociates the last deacylated tRNA from the 30S subunit to recycle the 30S subunit for another round of 70S formation.

The accuracy of translation is an important aspect of fidelity for the entire process that has been fairly well investigated and established. As mentioned earlier, two mechanisms facilitate accuracy in translation: (1) selection of the correct amino acid and correct tRNA, which is carried out by aminoacyl-tRNA synthetase, and (2) selection of the correct charged tRNA for the A site of the ribosome, which is carried out by elongation factor Tu (EF-Tu) and the ribosome. In charging a tRNA with an amino acid, one aminoacyl-tRNA synthetase selects not only the one correct amino

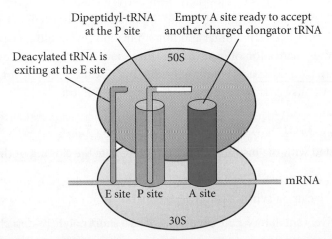

Figure 2.66 Elongation factor G (EF-G) translocates the ribosome by one codon along the mRNA after each peptide bond is formed.

acid out of the 20 possible amino acids, but also the one correct tRNA molecule out of the many possible tRNAs. In the elongating pathway of translation, the ribosome and EF-Tu select the one correct aminoacyl-tRNA (charged tRNA) over the many other charged tRNAs. The cost of the latter selection process is the GTP hydrolysis that occurs during the elongation step.

The process of translation is quite accurate. The rate of error—that is, incorporation of an incorrect amino acid into a protein—is less than 1×10^{-4}. Thus one incorrect amino acid, for every correct 10,000 amino acids, is incorporated into a protein. This level of error in translation is tolerated by the cell, even though the accuracy of the translation process is at least 10 times poorer than the accuracy of transcription and 100,000 times poorer than the accuracy of the DNA replication process.

Cell Biology in Biotechnology

For many years scientists have used microorganisms such as bacteria and fungi as living factories to produce useful drugs. A typical example of the use of microbes in biotechnology is the production of antibiotics such as penicillin, which is synthesized by a fungus called *Penicillium*, and streptomycin, which is produced by the bacterium *Streptomyces griseus*. Many proteins of therapeutic value are synthesized by animals, albeit often only in small amounts. In addition, purification of these proteins is difficult and expensive. Gene cloning together with the large-scale growth of recombinant DNA in bacterial cultures offers an inexpensive and more reliable way of producing therapeutic proteins. These techniques have allowed the cloning of human genes (see also the *Introduction to Pharmacogenomics* chapter) and the expression of encoding proteins with therapeutic action in specialized host systems. A remarkable property of a cloned gene is that it is expressed in an organism entirely different from the organism that originally expressed it.

Bacterial cells offer simplicity, short generation times, and large yields with low costs. The expression in bacteria, however, is not without problems. Some of the proteins that are expressed in bacteria can fill 10% or more of the mass of the bacterium, which can be detrimental to the host organism, or they may fail to be folded properly. The unfolded—and insoluble—proteins are called inclusion bodies. The inability of prokaryotes to glycosylate or phosphorylate proteins is another problems. To solve these problems, yeast has been often used to express a mammalian gene. Yeast is a simple eukaryote that mimics mammalian cells in many ways, but can grow as quickly and inexpensively as bacteria.

Several successes have already been achieved in the realms of biotechnology and biopharmaceuticals as a result of gene cloning, by producing nonbacterial proteins that are of therapeutic value in *E. coli*. Insulin, for example, has traditionally been derived from the pancreases of pigs and cows. Treating diabetic patients with this kind of insulin is associated with problems, however. Notably, there are slight differences between animal and human insulin that could give rise to adverse effects. In addition, the purification of insulin from these sources is a difficult process. A more satisfactory procedure would be to use human insulin, but obviously that is not ethical. So what is the solution? The short answer is cloning of the insulin gene in *E. coli*.

Recombinant Insulin

Two features associated with the insulin polypeptides facilitate the cloning of the insulin gene:

- Insulin is not modified after translation (i.e., it is not glycosylated or phosphorylated), so it could be active upon synthesis in the bacteria.

- Insulin is a relatively small molecule consisting of two short polypeptides: chain A and chain B.

To make recombinant insulin, a few steps must be taken carefully. First, the gene must be synthesized; that is, trinucleotides should be synthesized representing all possible codons in the

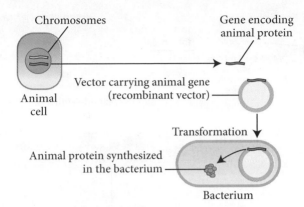

Figure 2.67 Cloning of an animal gene into a vector that can be expressed following transformation of the vector within a host organism (bacterial).

Adapted from Nelson DL, Cox MM. *Principles of biochemistry*, 5th ed. New York, NY: W. H. Freeman and Company; 2008; Chapter 9.

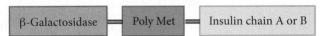

Figure 2.68 Three polypeptides that are synthesized by inserting the insulin gene downstream of the β-galactosidase and poly Met genes.

order that is dictated by the amino acid sequences of the A and B chains. The artificial insulin gene should not necessarily have the exact same gene sequence as long as alternative codons correspond to correct amino acids in the polypeptide sequence. That is, due to the "wobble hypothesis," the UUC codon (which specifies the amino acid phenylalanine) can also be used instead of the UUU codon (which also corresponds to phenylalanine).

Second, an expression vector is needed to carry these artificial genes (i.e., the genes for chain A and B) into *E. coli* (a mechanism called transformation; see **Figure 2.67**). Third, an expression system is needed to control the gene expression. This task is carried out by inserting the gene for A and B next to a *lac* promoter. The *lac* promoter makes it possible to express the insulin more effectively and in large amounts. With this approach, the gene for the A chain or the B chain is inserted downstream of a polymethionine sequence and a *lacZ* gene (this gene produces β-galactosidase). When the *lacZ* gene is transcribed, the insulin gene is transcribed as well. Translation of this polycistronic mRNA yields the polypeptides shown in **Figure 2.68**.

The poly Met plays a role in the cleaving of the product (insulin) chain from the β-galactosidase by cyanogen bromide: CNBr cleaves the peptide bond on the carboxyl side of Met. Because the insulin chains do not have any methionine amino acid, they are not affected by CNBr. The amplified A and B chains are mixed together to form the active recombinant insulin (**Figure 2.69**).

Recombinant Human Growth Hormone

Human growth hormone (hGH) is a protein that contains 191 amino acid residues. The hGH protein is produced in the pituitary gland and regulates growth and development. Children born with hGH deficiency will never achieve normal growth. Regular injections of growth hormone can, however, stimulate the growth of children with such a deficiency and assist them in reaching near-normal heights. In the past, only the human protein has worked in this application. For many years, this hGH protein has been purified from human cadavers. Unfortunately, a number of children were infected with a fatal virus from some of these cadavers.

Gene cloning has emerged as a powerful tool to produce a pure hGH that could eliminate any contamination problem from the human cadavers. Similar to the insulin gene, the hGH gene

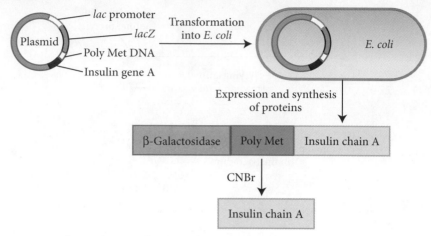

Figure 2.69 Expression of recombinant insulin chains in *E. coli* bacteria.
Adapted from: Brown TA. *Gene cloning: an introduction.* London: VNR International; 1986: Chapter 12.

can be expressed in bacteria. However, a potential problem was the need to purify hGH from hundreds of other bacterial proteins. As a solution, a DNA fragment encoding a bacterial signal sequence that specifies secretion of a bacterial protein was inserted in the front of the hGH coding sequence.

After transformation of a vector that includes the gene for hGH into bacteria, hGH is synthesized. The bacterial signal sequence targets the protein for secretion into the periplasmic space between the inner and outer bacterial membranes (**Figure 2.70**). The hGH protein that is bound to the signal sequence accumulates in the periplasmic space, and the bond is cleaved by bacterial proteases. Next, the hGH protein is released by disrupting the cell membranes of *E. coli* cells. The hGH produced in this way will avoid contamination with hundreds of other cytosolic proteins, which in turn facilitates hGH purification (Figure 2.70).

Production of Recombinant Vaccines

The importance of vaccines in immunology and protection against invading bacteria and viruses is discussed in the *Introduction to Immunology* chapter. Briefly, injection of a vaccine into the bloodstream stimulates the host's immune system to synthesize antibodies that will protect the body against subsequent infections.

Recombinant DNA technology allows for the production of a subunit vaccine. A subunit vaccine makes use of just a small portion of a pathogen. The first successful subunit vaccine was produced for hepatitis B virus (HBV). This virus is known to infect the liver; it causes liver damage and, in some cases, hepatic cancer. HBV consists of two proteins: a core protein that is associated with the virus genome and a surface protein referred to as a coat protein (subunit). While the core protein does not have any antigenic property, it plays a valuable role in the diagnosis of infection caused by HBV. In contrast, the coat protein, HBsAg, forms large aggregates in the blood of infected patients and is a potential vaccine to fight HBV.

Initially, efforts to clone the HBV genome in *E. coli* failed. Next, researchers sought to use yeast as the host organism for the production of a vaccine against HBV. One sequence of the HBV DNA is responsible for the production of the virus's protein coat. After the identified DNA sequence is added to a yeast expression vector and this vector is transformed into a yeast cell, the yeast cell incorporates the viral DNA into its own DNA and produces the protein coat of hepatitis B. The isolated hepatitis B protein produced by the yeast cells does not contain the viral genome and, as a result, can safely be administered as a vaccine (**Figure 2.71**).

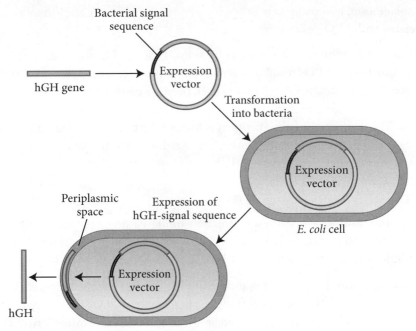

Figure 2.70 Use of the recombinant DNA technology in expressing recombinant hGH protein in *E. coli* bacteria.
Adapted from: Watson JD, Gilman M, Witkowski J, Zoller M. *Recombinant DNA*, 2nd ed. New York, NY: Scientific American Books; 1992: Chapter 23.

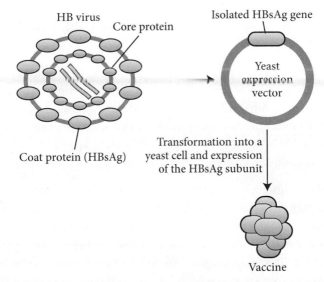

Figure 2.71 Use of recombinant DNA technology in expressing recombinant HBsAg vaccine in eukaryotic (yeast) cells.
Adapted from: Watson JD, Gilman M, Witkowski J, Zoller M. *Recombinant DNA*, 2nd ed. New York, NY: Scientific American Books; 1992: Chapter 23.

Recombinant Erythropoietin

Erythropoietin (EPO) is a glycoprotein hormone that consists of 165 amino acids and 4 carbohydrate chains. This hormone is produced in the kidneys and plays an important role in the production of erythrocytes. When the oxygen level in the blood is low (hypoxia), the kidney cells produce EPO, which travels to the bone marrow and binds to specific receptors to stimulate proliferation and differentiation of erythroid cells (a more detailed mechanism is presented in the *Introduction to Pharmacodynamics* chapter). More erythrocytes will then be produced and, in turn, more oxygen will be sent to the tissues. Patients with chronic kidney disease, patients who undergo bone marrow transplantation, and patients with cancer who receive chemotherapy may all suffer from anemia associated with EPO deficiency.

In contrast to the situation with recombinant insulin, a bacterial host is not a feasible mechanism for the production of EPO (recall that glycosylation does not occur in bacteria). The cloned human EPO gene (recombinant EPO) has, however, been successfully implanted into Chinese hamster ovary cells. These tissue culture cells secrete EPO into the culture fluid, from which EPO is then purified. The drug epoetin alfa (Epogen) is used in the treatment of anemia in patients with chronic kidney disease or anemia caused by the use of zidovudine (Retrovir) in patients infected with the human immunodeficiency virus (HIV).

Production of Monoclonal Antibodies

Antibodies are proteins that selectively and precisely bind to a single target among millions of others (see also the *Introduction to Immunology* chapter). It has been a goal for many scientists to produce antibodies that can be administered as drugs to fight infections or to destroy tumor cells.

The conventional method of producing such drugs has been to inject a rabbit with a specific antigen, thereby stimulating the rabbit's defense mechanism to produce the desired antibody. Collected blood from the rabbit has the desired antibodies. There are, however, two problems with this method:

- The antibody is not pure; that is, the desired antibody is mixed together with many other proteins and antibodies.

- Only a small quantity of usable antibody can be produced in this manner.

Monoclonal antibody (MAb) technology allows researchers to produce large amounts of pure antibodies that come from only one type of cell. Simply put, the strategy is to (1) obtain one type of cell that can produce the desired antibodies naturally and (2) obtain another cell that can grow continually (endlessly) in a cell culture. A hybrid that combines these two cells can then serve as a factory that produces a large quantity of pure antibodies. In MAb technology, tumor cells that grow extensively are fused with mammalian cells that produce the desired antibody to yield a hybridoma. Because these antibodies are produced by only one cell type, they are referred to as monoclonal antibodies.

When using the MAb technology, an antigen that can produce the desired antibody is injected into a mouse. Subsequently, the cells that produce the antibody are isolated from the mouse's spleen. Spleen cells die after a few days in culture, because they have a short life span. Thus, to produce a continuous source of the desired antibody, the spleen cells are fused with myeloma cells to produce a hybrid cell line (hybridoma). It is important to select myeloma cells that do not produce any antibody by themselves and that are also sensitive to a medium called hypoxanthine aminopterin-thymidine (HAT) (**Figure 2.72**).

Myeloma cells lack the enzyme hypoxanthine guanosine phosphoribosyl transferase (HGPRT). The HGPRT enzyme enables cells to synthesize purines from hypoxanthine. When cells are exposed to HAT, they are fully dependent on HGPRT for survival. The HGPRT enzyme is in the B cells, so only the fused cells survive in the HAT medium; in other words, the unfused myeloma die due to the lack of HGPRT enzyme and the unfused spleen cells die due to their short life span.

The fused cells grow continuously in culture. Given the chance that the original culture might include more than one hybridoma cell, ideally one should isolate a single cell that produced the desired antibody and then subculture it. This subculture produces a monoclonal antibody. By scaling up the size of the cell culture of the successful clones, it becomes possible to produce a large quantity of the desired monoclonal antibody.

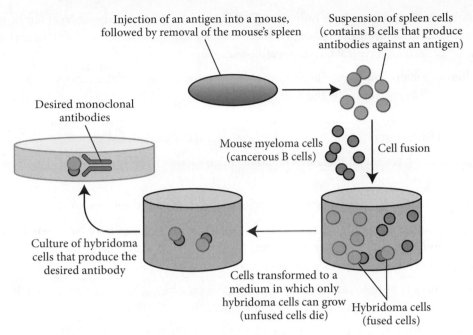

Figure 2.72 Use of monoclonal antibody (MAb) technology.
Adapted from: Shargel L, Wu-Pong S, Yu AB. Targeted drug delivery systems and biotechnological products.
In *Applied biopharmaceutics and pharmacokinetics*, 6th ed. New York, NY: McGraw-Hill; 2012: Chapter 18.

Today, monoclonal antibodies have many applications. One example is the home pregnancy test in which a woman places a drop of her urine onto a paper that is coated with MAb against the pregnancy hormone human chorionic gonadotropin (hCG). Approximately 2 weeks postconception, the placenta produces hCG. The OTC pregnancy kit (many examples are available in the market) contains an antibody that is specific for the β subunit of hCG. A color will be developed if the MAb binds the hormone.

Another example of a monoclonal antibody is trastuzumab (Herceptin). This drug blocks human epidermal growth factor receptor 2 (HER2), which is expressed on breast cancer cells, thereby preventing these cells from receiving signals to grow and divide.

Golden Keys for Pharmacy Students

1. All cells can be classified into one of two types: (1) prokaryotic: archaebacteria and eubacteria; or (2) eukaryotic: protists, fungi, animals, and plants.

2. A prokaryotic cell lacks a nuclear membrane but has a region called a nucleoid that contains DNA.

3. The bacterial cell wall contains a unique structure called peptidoglycan, which, as the name indicates, is made of polypeptides and carbohydrates.

4. Aerobic bacteria are solely dependent on consumption of oxygen to produce energy (ATP); anaerobic bacteria use electron acceptors other than oxygen in their respiratory chain mechanism to generate ATP.

5. Plasmids are able to carry genetic information from one bacterium to another—a process that may protect a bacterium from an antibacterial agent.

6. Approximately 70% of a prokaryotic cell membrane is built of proteins—a significantly higher percentage than in a eukaryotic cell membrane.

7. Gram-negative bacteria have only one or two layers of peptidoglycan, whereas Gram-positive bacteria have 40 layers of peptidoglycan that account for 50% of their cell wall material. *Escherichia coli* is a typical Gram-negative bacterium.

8. Different bacteria produce different pili that are antigenically useful, as they promote the production of antibodies by the host.

9. Bacterial lipopolysaccharide (endotoxin) is toxic to animal cells because it binds tightly to the host cell surface and detaches only when the cell membrane is lysed.

10. Bacteria can have any of three morphological shapes: spherical (coccus), rod (bacillus), or twisted rod (spirillum).

11. The genome within a human cell has 3 billion base pairs of nucleotide sequence.

12. Histones are proteins that are rich in amino acid residues and that have basic side chains (lysine and arginine). Consequently, there is a tight attraction between histones and the negatively charged phosphates in DNA.

13. The fluidity of the lipid side chains within a membrane bilayer is usually increased by an increasing number of double bonds in fatty acids.

14. The pI is the mean of a molecule's two pK_a values: $pI = (pK_1 + pK_2)/2$.

15. In a DNA molecule, the number of adenine nucleotides (A) is equal to the number of thymine nucleotides (T), and the number of cytosine (C) nucleotides is equal to the number of guanine (G) nucleotides.

16. While humans can synthesize fatty acids from carbohydrates, we cannot synthesize carbohydrates from fatty acids.

17. Fibronectin plays an important role in the attachment of cells to the extracellular matrix. In addition, it assists a cell in migrating through the extracellular matrix.

18. Two general mechanisms are involved in membrane transport: diffusion (passive and facilitated) and active transport systems. While passive transport does not require energy, active transport does.

19. There are four major classes of ATP-driven active transporters: P, F, V, and ABC. All four classes have one or more binding sites for ATP on the cytosolic face of the membrane. The well-known mitochondrial ATP synthase enzyme belongs to the F type.

20. Expression of an integral protein called P-glycoprotein on cancer cells pumps anticancer drugs, in an ATP hydrolysis-dependent mechanism, out of these cells.

21. Ions are charged species that are repelled by the hydrophobic environment of a membrane bilayer. As a result, the presence of ion channels facilitates transport of ions across the cell membrane.

22. In a tight cell–cell junction, cells are tied to each other with strength and stability. In a gap cell–cell junction, movement of ions and small molecules (sugars, amino acids, and other molecules with a molecular weight of less than 1,000 Da) from one cell to another is feasible by going through a channel that is built between cells.

23. Amino acids are important not only for the synthesis of proteins, but also for the synthesis of other amino acids, neurotransmitters, hormones, porphyrins, purines, pyrimidines, and urea.

24. There are more than 300 naturally occurring amino acids, but only 20 (the so-called common amino acids) constitute the building blocks of all proteins.

25. Humans and other higher animals are not able to synthesize 10 (the so-called essential amino acids) of the 20 common L-amino acids. For this reason, the human diet must contain adequate amounts of these essential amino acids.

26. Four different structures are possible for proteins: primary, secondary, tertiary, and quaternary.

27. Nucleotides are the building blocks of nucleic acids, including ribonucleic acid (RNA) and deoxyribonucleic acid (DNA).

28. During cell division, a DNA molecule can reproduce (replicate) itself without changing its structure.

29. There are four RNA molecules, each with a distinct function: mRNA, tRNA, rRNA, and snRNA.

30. Starch (in plants) and glycogen (in animals) are the two most important polysaccharides.

31. Lipids are a vital component of nutrition and perform necessary functions, such as being a basic component of cell membranes (bilayer), production of energy in the form of ATP molecules (β-oxidation of fatty acids), synthesis of steroid hormones (progesterone, testosterone, vitamin D), and acting as a carrier for fat-soluble vitamins (vitamins A, D, E, and K).

32. Triacylglycerols are the chemical form of lipids found in food as well as in the body.

33. Sterols are common in mammalian cell membranes, but are not found in bacterial membranes. The characteristic structure of sterols is four fused rings (three 6-carbon rings and one 5-carbon ring).

34. Prostaglandins contain a five-carbon ring. They act in many tissues by regulating the synthesis of the intracellular messenger cAMP, which in turn mediates the action of many hormones.

35. Many RNA transcripts are modified and matured before they function in protein synthesis—a mechanism referred to as RNA processing.

36. Two important selection steps in translation are (1) to select the correct amino acid for the correct tRNA and (2) to select the correctly charged tRNA for the correct codon at the A site of a ribosome.

37. Gene cloning, together with the large-scale growth of recombinant DNA in bacterial or yeast cultures, offers an inexpensive and more reliable method of producing therapeutic proteins.

38. Monoclonal antibody (MAb) technology is used to produce a large amount of antibodies that are generated from only one type of cell.

Learning Bridge Answers

2.1 These vitamins are lipid soluble. Because Amy's son has Zellweger syndrome, he has difficulty absorbing lipids (fats), which results in his body having inadequate storage of the lipid-soluble vitamins. Amy's son lacks functional peroxisomes. This peroxisomal deficiency results in a few abnormal biochemical reactions, particularly in the oxidation of very-long-chain fatty acids. Lipid-soluble vitamins are critical in many biochemical reactions and pathways, such as cell differentiation (vitamin A), Ca^{2+} and phosphate metabolism (vitamin D), prevention of oxidative damage and protection of neurons (vitamin E), and inhibition of a blood clotting process (vitamin K).

2.2 **A.** Tobramycin (TOBI) is a typical antibiotic that is used in an inhaler to treat cystic fibrosis (CF); it clears *Pseudomonas aeruginosa,* the bacterium commonly found in patients with

CF. Tobramycin inhibits the bacterial protein synthetic machinery. The FDA approved the use of TOBI in patients with CF in 1998. CF is an autosomal recessive disease caused by a mutation on chromosome 7 that results in abnormal mucus production. Kristin needs to be on prophylactic treatment to avoid lung infection for the rest of her life.

B. The salty skin can be explained by the dysfunctional CFTR, which is typically the cause of CF. CFTR is responsible for reabsorbing chloride ion; its failure to do so can impact sodium ion reabsorption as well. Together, these effects produce a salty sweat.

C. As the physician has pointed out, Amy should not mix any other medications in the TOBI inhaler. Because TOBI can cause bronchospasm, if Kristin is also using a bronchodilator, it is important that she use the bronchodilator first before inhaling TOBI.

2.3 The development of resistance to cytotoxic drugs is a concerning problem with cancer chemotherapy. P-glycoprotein (P-gp; also termed multidrug resistance-1 protein [MDR1]) pumps the drug, through an ATP hydrolysis-dependent mechanism, out of the cell before giving the drug any chance to exert its effect. Once this pump develops on the cancer cells, other anticancer drugs that are not functionally or structurally related to the first drug used can also be pumped out of the cancer cells.

2.4 Cytosine spontaneously deaminates to uracil in DNA—a relatively common mutation that occurs every day in the human genome. The newly formed mutated uracil (let's call it "bad uracil") is removed from DNA by a DNA repair system. If DNA contained uracil (let's call it "good uracil") instead of thymine, the repair system would not be able to distinguish between "good uracil" and "bad uracil" (because both would look exactly the same) and removal of the "bad uracil" would be very difficult, leading to a permanent mutation during the DNA replication process (i.e., DNA synthesis). To resolve this dilemma, evolution has increased the fidelity of DNA synthesis by incorporating thymine rather than uracil into the DNA sequences (see Figure 2.26).

2.5 **A.** The patient is likely to have a lactase deficiency (lactose intolerance) because both milk and milk-derived products (butter, ice cream, cheese) are rich in lactose. He should reduce the amount of lactose products he consumes. The lactase enzyme is known to metabolize lactose into glucose and galactose in the digestive system. To metabolize lactose, a person needs to have a functional or adequate amount of lactase. A lack of or reduction in lactase activity results in the accumulation of lactose, which will then be passed to the colon. As the lactose accumulates, an osmotic imbalance will result. When concentration of something is higher on one side of an osmotic compartment, the water will move to that side to reduce the concentration of those materials. In this case, an excess of fluid will enter the intestinal tract from the tissues, resulting in diarrhea. The bacteria that are in the colon will use lactose as substrates for fermentation, resulting in production of gas (CO_2). It is this gas that causes abdominal cramping and bloating.

B. Suggest enzymatic lactase supplements such as Lac-Dose or Lactaid Fast Act, one to two capsules to be taken with milk or a meal. If these OTC products do not help him with his symptoms, the patient needs to consult with his physician. If he is limiting his consumption of milk or milk-derived products, he will benefit from using Ca^{2+} supplements as well.

C. Yogurt is made from milk; the companies that make the yogurt add microorganisms to convert milk to yogurt. The same microorganisms that are present in the yogurt will metabolize lactose. Be sure the yogurt has live bacterial cultures. Yogurt with killed bacteria will not work in this context.

2.6 **A.** Joe's stomach pain likely has to do with his taking Bufferin, which contains acetyl salicylic acid (ASA), the same ingredient found in aspirin. He should immediately stop taking Bufferin and Advil, because he is at risk to develop ulcer. ASA inhibits synthesis of prostaglandin. Prostaglandin regulates the secretion of gastric mucin so as to protect gastric mucosa from the low pH in the gastric acid. In other words, less prostaglandin causes more exposure of gastric mucosa to the gastric acid, which explains Joe's excruciating pain.

B. Both Bufferin and Advil (ibuprofen) belong to the class known as nonsteroidal anti-inflammatory drugs (NSAIDs). These two medications add to, rather than reduce, his stomach pain.

C. Suggest a non-NSAID such as acetaminophen (Tylenol), 500 mg, 1–2 tablets as needed per pain but not to exceed 6–7 tablets/day. In addition, advise Joe that Tylenol will cause drowsiness so he should not operate machinery after taking his tablets. Because acetaminophen is included in many OTC and prescription drugs, it is imperative to ask Joe about his other current medications to avoid any hepatic toxicity caused by an overdose of acetaminophen.

2.7 **A.** Mupirocin inhibits the enzymatic activity of the bacterial isoleucyl-tRNA synthetase, which attaches the amino acid Ile to tRNA^{Ile}. This inhibition does not allow the tRNA^{Ile} to be charged with the amino acid Ile. As a result, an incorporation of amino acid Ile into bacterial proteins does not occur, which ultimately leads to the presence of many non-functional proteins that kill the bacteria.

B. He should avoid contact with his eyes. If skin irritation occurs, he should discontinue this medication and contact his physician.

C. Because this antibiotic is a topical medication and not a systemic agent, the side effects are minimal. However, he may experience minor stinging on his face.

Problems and Solutions

Problem 2.1 Which of the following bacterial organelles assists bacteria in adhering to the surfaces of other cells?

A. Cytoskeletal proteins
B. Cytoplasmic membrane
C. Pili
D. Nucleus
E. Flagella

Solution 2.1 **C** is correct.

Problem 2.2 What is the function of an animal's lysozyme?

Solution 2.2 Animals are capable of synthesizing the hydrolytic enzyme lysozyme. This enzyme is found in tears, saliva, and nasal secretions and is an excellent defense mechanism to rupture Gram-positive cell walls' peptidoglycan backbone. However, due to Gram-negative bacteria's outer membrane, a lysozyme cannot reach the tiny peptidoglycan backbone of such bacteria.

Problem 2.3 Which of the following antibiotics might be useful in clearing a bacterial infection?

A. An antibiotic that attacks 16S rRNA
B. An antibiotic that attacks 18S rRNA
C. An antibiotic that attacks 23S rRNA

    D. An antibiotic that attacks 80S ribosomes

    E. An antibiotic that attacks 60S ribosomal subunits

Solution 2.3 A and C are correct; 18S rRNA, 80S ribosomes, and 60S ribosomal subunits are all found in eukaryotic cells.

Problem 2.4 Name two major functions of the cell nucleus.

Solution 2.4 (1) Prepare a cell for division by allowing the DNA to be duplicated; (2) synthesize different forms of rRNAs during the transcription process to facilitate protein synthesis (translation).

Problem 2.5 An *E. coli* bacterium can grow at a temperature of 40°C. This indicates that the membranes of the *E. coli* bacterium contain:

    A. more saturated fatty acids at 40°C than at a lower temperature.

    B. fewer saturated fatty acids at 40°C than at a lower temperature.

    C. more proteins that diffuse laterally through the membrane.

    D. fewer proteins that diffuse laterally through the membrane.

Solution 2.5 A is correct; the more saturated a fatty acid is, the fewer double bonds it has—a fact that allows it to regulate its fatty acid composition to maintain the membrane fluidity at a higher temperature. In other words, saturated fatty acids counterbalance the fluidizing effect of high temperature.

Problem 2.6 Why does the polypeptide backbone of an integral protein that is a polar group pass along the hydrophobic interior of the membrane?

Solution 2.6 The integral proteins fold so that the hydrophilic moieties are mostly in the interior of the proteins so as to exclude them from the hydrophobic environment of the membrane.

Problem 2.7 Which transport system is the best match for Na^+K^+ ATPase? Why?

Solution 2.7 An antiport system that pumps two K^+ ions in and three Na^+ ions out. Both ions need to be present to make this transport system functional.

Problem 2.8 Which kinds of forces hold an integral membrane protein and a peripheral membrane protein to a biological membrane?

Solution 2.8 Hydrophobic interactions between hydrophobic amino acid residues and the fatty acyl chains of the membrane bilayer play an important role in attaching integral membrane proteins to the membrane. Hydrogen bonds between the charged and polar side chains of amino acids and the polar head groups of membrane lipids are mainly responsible for attaching the peripheral membrane proteins.

Problem 2.9 Which of the following statements is correct?

    A. A ribonucleotide is attached to a base through a phosphodiester linkage, whereas a deoxyribonucleotide is attached to a base through a glycosyl linkage.

    B. A deoxyribonucleotide has hydrogen instead of a hydroxyl group at the 2′ position.

    C. A ribonucleotide has an extra –OH group at carbon 4.

    D. A ribonucleotide can attach to adenine, and a deoxyribonucleotide can attach to guanine.

Solution 2.9 B is correct.

Problem 2.10 What is an amphipathic molecule?

Solution 2.10 An amphipathic molecule has both hydrophilic and hydrophobic regions. An example of an amphipathic compound is the phospholipid molecule, which plays an important role in the formation of the lipid bilayer of membranes.

Problem 2.11 Why does an ion need a channel to pass through a cell membrane?

Solution 2.11 Ions are charged species that can easily interact with water and other polar molecules. Because they cannot interact with the hydrophobic molecules of a cell membrane, however, they are repelled by the nonpolar nature of the membrane. As a result, ions need the assistance of a channel to pass through the hydrophobic interior of the membrane bilayer.

Problem 2.12 Indicate whether the following statements are true or false.

- **A.** mRNA is chemically a stable molecule.
- **B.** The genetic code consists only of bases that code for amino acids.
- **C.** There are millions of genetic codes in humans.
- **D.** Three types of RNAs—rRNA, mRNA, and tRNA—are produced during transcription.

Solution 2.12 A. False. B. False. C. False. D. True.

Problem 2.13 Name one significant structural difference between glycogen and starch.

Solution 2.13 Glycogen is found only as a highly branched carbohydrate polymer in animals. In contrast, starch can take the form of both branched and linear carbohydrate polymers and is found in plants. The branched form of starch has a much lower degree of branching than glycogen.

Problem 2.14 Which of the following steps in translation is catalyzed by peptidyltransferase?

- **A.** Binding of charged tRNA to the A site of ribosomes
- **B.** Binding of deacylated tRNA to the P site of ribosomes
- **C.** Translocation of the ribosome along the mRNA
- **D.** Peptide formation
- **E.** Association of the 30S subunit to the 50S subunit

Solution 2.14 D is correct.

Problem 2.15 True or false: Glycogen is the main storage for carbohydrates in both plants and animals.

Solution 2.15 False; glycogen is the storage unit for carbohydrates (glucose) in animals.

Problem 2.16 Bill, an 18-year-old student, comes to your pharmacy and complains about having intestinal problems. He explains that shortly after drinking milk he has experienced abdominal cramps, bloating, gas, and diarrhea.

- **A.** Identify the problem.
- **B.** What would you suggest if Bill is a friend and is coming over your house?

Solution 2.16 A. Bill most likely has a lactase deficiency problem. Milk contains a large amount of lactose (disaccharide). The lactose must be cleaved into glucose and galactose by the lactase enzyme in the intestinal microvilli before it can be absorbed through the intestinal tract.

B. You can suggest that Bill drink yogurt. Yogurt is made from milk, and the company that makes the yogurt has added microorganisms to it to convert the milk to yogurt. The same microorganisms, which are still in the yogurt, will also metabolize lactose.

Problem 2.17 Regarding the Watson-Crick structure of DNA, which of the following statements is (are) correct?

- **A.** The two strands are antiparallel to each other.
- **B.** The base content must be the same in both strands.
- **C.** The nucleotides do not carry phosphate groups.
- **D.** The 2′-hydroxyl groups in ribose are prone to oxidation.
- **E.** The two strands have complementary sequences.

Solution 2.17 A and E are correct.

Problem 2.18 Which of the following organelles is responsible for the degradation of lipids?

- **A.** Nucleus
- **B.** Lysosome
- **C.** Cytoplasm
- **D.** Mitochondria
- **E.** ER

Solution 2.18 B is correct.

References

1. Arthur LK. Bacterial growth. In: *AccessScience.* New York, NY: McGraw-Hill; 2008. Available at: http://www.accessscience.com.

2. Barrett KE, Barman SM, Boitano S, Brooks HL. Overview of cellular physiology in medical physiology. In: Barrett KE, Barman SM, Boitano S, Brooks HL, eds. *Ganong's review of medical physiology*, 24th ed. New York, NY: McGraw-Hill; 2012. Available at: http://www.accesspharmacy.com/content.aspx?aID=56260315.

3. Bender DA, Mayes PA. Carbohydrates of physiologic significance. In: Murray RK, Bender DA, Botham KM, et al. *Harper's illustrated biochemistry*, 28th ed. New York, NY: McGraw-Hill; 2009. Available at: http://www.accessmedicine.com/content.aspx?aID=5226612.

4. Binder HJ. Disorders of absorption. In: Fauci AS, Kasper DL, Jameson JL, et al., eds. *Harrison's principles of internal medicine*, 18th ed. New York, NY: McGraw-Hill; 2012. Available at: http://www.accesspharmacy.com/content.aspx?aID=9132182.

5. Borst P, Elferink RO. Mammalian ABC transporters in health and disease. *Annu Rev Biochem.* 2002;71:537–592.

6. Botham KM, Mayes PA. Lipids of physiologic significance. In: Murray RK, Kennelly PJ, Rodwell VW, et al., eds. *Harper's illustrated biochemistry*, 29th ed. New York, NY: McGraw-Hill; 2011. Available at: http://www.accesspharmacy.com/content.aspx?aID=55882446.

7. Brimacombe R, Wittmann HG, Joseph S. Ribosomes. In: *AccessScience.* New York, NY: McGraw-Hill; 2012. Available at: http://www.accessscience.com.

8. Brown TA. *Gene cloning: an introduction.* London: VNR International; 1986.

9. Damian RT. Parasitology. In: *AccessScience.* New York, NY: McGraw-Hill; 2008. Available at: http://www.accessscience.com.

10. Spector DL. Cell nucleus. In: *AccessScience.* New York, NY: McGraw-Hill; 2008. Available at: http://www.accessscience.com.

11. Davis BD, Foster JW, Kallio RE. Culture. In: *AccessScience.* New York, NY: McGraw-Hill; 2008. Available at: http://www.accessscience.com.

12. Dzieczkowski JS, Anderson KC. Transfusion biology and therapy. In: Fauci AS, Braunwald E, Kasper DL, et al. *Harrison's principles of internal medicine*, 17th ed. New York, NY: 2008. Available at: http://www.accesspharmacy.com/content.aspx?aID=2866013.

13. Goodman SR. Cell (biology). In: *AccessScience.* New York, NY: McGraw-Hill; 2012. Available at: http://www.accessscience.com.

14. Johansson M, Zhang J, Ehrenberg M. Genetic code translation displays a linear trade-off between efficiency and accuracy of tRNA selection. *PNAS.* 2012;109(1):131–136.

15. Karimi R, Pavlov MY, Buckingham RH, Ehrenberg M. Novel roles for classical factors at the interface between translation termination and initiation. *Mol Cell.* 1999;3:601–609.

16. Karimi R, Brumfield T, Brumfield F, et al. Zellweger syndrome: a genetic disorder that alters lipid biosynthesis and metabolism. *Internet J Pharmacol.* 2007;5:1.

17. Kennelly PJ, Rodwell VW. Amino acids and peptides. In: Murray RK, Kennelly PJ, Rodwell VW, et al., eds. *Harper's illustrated biochemistry*, 29th ed. New York, NY: McGraw-Hill; 2011. Available at: http://www.accesspharmacy.com/content.aspx?aID=55881220.

18. Keyormarsi K, O'Leary N, Pardee AB. Cell division. In: *AccessScience*. New York, NY: McGraw-Hill; 2008. Available at: http://www.accessscience.com.

19. Mills JC, Stappenbeck TS, Bunnett NW. Gastrointestinal disease. In: McPhee SJ, Hammer GD. *Pathophysiology of disease: an introduction to clinical medicine*, 6th ed. New York, NY: McGraw-Hill; 2010. Available at: http://www.accesspharmacy.com/content.aspx?aID=5369402.

20. Morse SA, Brooks GF, Carroll KC, et al. Cell structure. In: Morse SA, Brooks GF, Carroll KC, et al., eds. *Jawetz, Melnick, and Adelberg's medical microbiology*, 25th ed. New York, NY: McGraw-Hill; 2010:10. Available at: http://www.accesspharmacy.com/content.aspx?aID=6426066.

21. Mount DB. Fluid and electrolyte disturbances. In: Fauci AS, Kasper DL, Jameson JL, et al., eds. *Harrison's principles of internal medicine*, 18th ed. New York, NY: McGraw-Hill. Available at: http://www.accesspharmacy.com/content.aspx?aID=9097635. Accessed November 21, 2012.

22. Murray RK, Keeley FW. The extracellular matrix. In: Murray RK, Kennelly PJ, Rodwell VW, et al., eds. *Harper's illustrated biochemistry*, 29th ed. New York, NY: McGraw-Hill; 2011. Available at: http://www.accesspharmacy.com/content.aspx?aID=55886054.

23. Murray RK, Granner DK. Membranes: structure and function. In: Murray RK, Kennelly PJ, Rodwell VW, et al., eds. *Harper's illustrated biochemistry*, 29th ed. New York, NY: McGraw-Hill; 2011. Available at: http://www.accesspharmacy.com/content.aspx?aID=55884978.

24. Murray RK. Glycoproteins. In: Murray RK, Kennelly PJ, Rodwell VW, et al., eds. *Harper's illustrated biochemistry*, 29th ed. New York, NY: McGraw-Hill; 2011. Available at: http://www.accesspharmacy.com/content.aspx?aID=55885875.

25. Nelson DL, Cox MM. *Principles of biochemistry*, 5th ed. New York, NY: W. H. Freeman and Company; 2008.

26. Pandit NK, Soltis RP. *Introduction to pharmaceutical sciences, an integrated approach*, 2nd ed. Baltimore, MD: Walters Kluwer, Lippincott Williams and Wilkins; 2012.

27. Pierce M. Prokaryotae. In: *AccessScience*. New York, NY: McGraw-Hill; 2008. Available at: http://www.accessscience.com.

28. Rodwell VW. Nucleotides. In: Murray RK, Bender DA, Botham KM, et al., eds. *Harper's illustrated biochemistry*, 28th ed. New York, NY: McGraw-Hill; 2009. Available at: http://www.accesspharmacy.com/content.aspx?aID=5228081.

29. Satir P. Cilia and flagella. In: *AccessScience*. New York, NY: McGraw-Hill; 2012. Available at: http://www.accessscience.com.

30. Shargel L, Wu-Pong S, Yu AB. Targeted drug delivery systems and biotechnological products. In: Shargel L, Wu-Pong S, Yu AB, eds. *Applied biopharmaceutics and pharmacokinetics*, 6th ed. New York, NY: McGraw-Hill; 2012. Available at: http://www.accesspharmacy.com/content.aspx?aID=56606300.

31. UpToDate. Waltham, MA: 2012. Available at: http://www.uptodate.com/online with subscription.

32. Watson JD, Gilman M, Witkowski J, Zoller M. *Recombinant DNA*, 2nd ed. New York: Scientific American Books; 1992: Chapter 23.

33. Wright CC, Vera YY. Cystic fibrosis. In: Talbert RL, DiPiro JT, Matzke GR, et al., eds. *Pharmacotherapy: a pathophysiologic approach*, 8th ed. New York, NY: McGraw-Hill; 2011. Available at: http://www.accesspharmacy.com/content.aspx?aID=7977119.

CHAPTER 3

Introduction to Microbiology

Reza Karimi

OBJECTIVES

1. Understand the epidemiology and social issues behind infectious diseases.

2. Know and list transmission pathways of pathogenic microorganisms.

3. Recognize the normal and pathogenic microorganisms and the various sciences that study infectious agents.

4. Appreciate the most common existing bacterial, fungal, parasitic, and viral microorganisms.

5. Recognize which factors cause a compromised immune system.

6. Understand infectious diseases and know which agents are used to treat infectious diseases.

7. Appreciate the importance of anti-HIV agents on the market in treating patients with HIV.

8. Know the different classes of antibiotics and their mechanisms of action.

9. Learn about different mechanisms that cause a resistance to antibiotics.

10. Implement a series of Learning Bridge assignments at your experiential sites to bridge your didactic learning with your experiential experiences.

KEY TERMS AND DEFINITIONS

1. **Antibiotics:** molecules (synthetic, semisynthetic, or natural) that are effective when they inhibit the growth of or kill a microorganism.

2. **Bactericidal agent:** an antibacterial agent that can eliminate an infection caused by bacteria.

3. **Bacteriology:** the science that exclusively studies bacteria and their living habits.

4. **Bacteriostatic agent:** an antibacterial agent that does not kill bacteria, but rather inhibits the growth of a bacterial organism.

5. **β-lactam antibiotics:** agents that have a unique four-membered ring that plays an important role in the inhibition of bacterial cell wall synthesis.

6. **Beta-lactamase:** an enzyme that is produced by many bacteria and that plays a major role in the development of antibiotic resistance.

7. **Community-acquired pneumonia (CAP):** an acute pulmonary infection that is acquired in the community; it is different from hospital-acquired (nosocomial) pneumonia.

8. **Endemic:** when a disease is not eradicated and occurs frequently in a specific area or population.

9. **Epidemic:** an occurrence of a contagious disease that spreads rapidly. When an epidemic occurs widely over a very large area, it is called a pandemic.

(continues)

10. **Epidemiology:** the study of microorganism-related patterns, causes, and prevention of human diseases.

11. **Granulocytopenia:** a condition characterized by a reduced number of white blood cells.

12. **Microbiology:** a dynamic science that identifies, classifies, and studies the structure and function of a wide range of microorganisms, including bacteria, protozoa, algae, fungi, viruses, and rickettsia.

13. **Minimal inhibitory concentration (MIC):** the lowest concentration of an antimicrobial agent that can inhibit the growth of an organism in a defined growth medium after 18–24 hours of incubation in that medium.

14. **Mycology:** the study of fungal infection.

15. **Parasitology:** the study of parasitic diseases.

16. **Pathogenicity:** the ability of microorganisms, including bacteria, fungi, protozoa, viruses, and parasites, to cause infectious diseases.

17. **Penicillin-binding proteins (PBPs):** bacterial membrane proteins that act as receptors for β-lactam antibiotics.

18. **Peptidoglycans:** molecules that consist of polysaccharides and a highly cross-linked polypeptide.

19. **Plasmids:** circular DNA molecules that are separated from a host DNA. Plasmids can replicate independently of the host DNA and usually occur in bacteria.

20. **Subclinical infection:** a viral infection that does not produce any symptom in the host; also called inapparent infection.

21. **Transmission:** the process in which pathogenic microorganisms spread from one host to another.

22. **Transpeptidases:** bacterial enzymes that catalyze the cross-linking of peptidoglycans during cell wall synthesis.

23. **Vertical transmission:** mother-to-child transmission of an infectious agent during pregnancy.

24. **Virology:** the science that studies viruses, including their structure, classification, and reproduction.

Introduction

The field of microbiology comprises a dynamic and complex science that is associated with infectious diseases. The science of microbiology identifies, classifies, and studies the structure and function of microorganisms such as bacteria, protozoa, algae, fungi, viruses, and rickettsia. As a result, microbiology interacts with many other sciences, such as cell and molecular biology, immunology, biochemistry, biotechnology, parasitology, virology, and medicine. Both basic and applied microbiological research are areas of interest within the pharmaceutical and biotechnology, academic, and government sectors. Thanks to endless efforts from the academic sector to examine the structure and function of macro-molecules such as proteins, polysaccharides, nucleic acids, and lipids, combined with a mutual interest in collaboration with the pharmaceutical and biotechnology sector, many milestone outcomes have been achieved. A typical example is the development of the recombinant gene cloning technique that utilizes restriction enzymes to cleave specific sites within genes and chromosomes. Such techniques have been employed in various types of microorganisms to develop many hormones (such as insulin, glucagon, growth factors, and proteins) and drugs (such as antibiotics, vaccines, and antifungal agents) that are the cornerstone therapies in fighting many diseases and disorders. In addition, the Human Genome Project of the 1990s and early 2000s was a milestone effort that mapped and determined the DNA sequences of all 23 human chromosomes, which ultimately will allow for better diagnosis of and improved therapeutic outcomes for many genetic diseases.

A knowledge of microbiology is vital to understand infectious diseases and their effects on patient care. In this chapter, the basic elements of microbiology and a few medically important microorganisms and their specific harmful effects to humans are described. The biochemical and pharmacological roles of antimicrobial classes are described, and mechanisms developed to exert resistance to antibiotics are illustrated.

Normal and Pathogenic Microorganisms

Microorganisms (bacteria, viruses, parasites, and fungi) can be harmless, harmful, or beneficial. If they are harmful (i.e., they cause diseases), they are called pathogenic microorganisms. If they are beneficial (i.e., both the microorganism and the infected host derive advantages from their relationship), they are called commensal microorganisms, or simply commensals. A typical example of commensals is the bacteria that live in the gastrointestinal (GI) tract, particularly in the large intestine (colon), in a coexisting manner that does not cause any disease. These bacteria, which are called "intestinal microflora," assist in preventing the invasion of the host by disease-causing bacteria such as *Salmonella*, *Shigella*, and *Campylobacter* species. In exchange for this benefit, the host provides nutrients to support the intestinal microflora's metabolic needs and growth.

The GI tract of an adult human contains an estimated 100 trillion bacteria (approximately 1 kilogram of bacteria), with the smallest number found in the stomach and the highest number occurring in the colon. These intestinal microflora create a tight junction between epithelial cells, resulting in a barrier against the passage of drugs between these cells. Administration of antibiotics, particularly macrolides (e.g., erythromycin, azithromycin), often causes a reduction in the intestinal microflora population. This reduction, in turn, results in inactivation of a few drugs that are largely dependent on the microflora's metabolism to exert their effects.

A typical example of the role of intestinal microflora on drugs can be seen with oral contraceptives (OCs). While there is no compelling evidence that antibiotics alter the effects of OCs, you might advise your patients of the potential risk that antibiotics (particularly penicillin derivatives) might reduce the effectiveness of OCs. Upon entering the liver, estrogen (the basis of many OCs) forms conjugated estrogen, which in turn travels to the gallbladder; the contents of the gallbladder are then emptied into the duodenum of the small intestine (**Figure 3.1**). The intestinal microflora produce enzymes that hydrolyze conjugated estrogens to free estrogen,

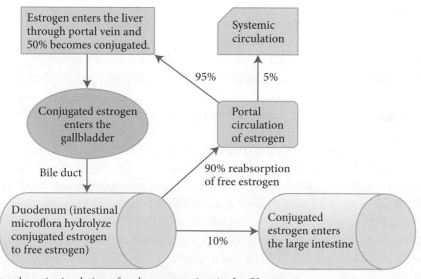

Figure 3.1 Enterohepatic circulation of oral contraceptives in the GI system.

Adapted from Barrett KE, Gastrointestinal Physiology, Section IV. Transport and Metabolic Functions of the Liver. *AccessMedicine*. New York: McGraw-Hill; 2006, Chapter 10.

thereby permitting enterohepatic circulation of OCs. The overall effect of the enterohepatic circulation is to provide more OC and, ultimately, a greater effect. Reducing the microflora population, however, reduces the effect of the enterohepatic circulation on OCs. Indeed, a significant amount (98%) of bile acids, which also have steroid structures, returns to the liver through the enterohepatic circulation.

Because pathogenic microorganisms cause diseases, and sometimes life-threatening ones, they have been given much more attention than harmless or beneficial microorganisms. Essentially, microorganisms that cannot be fought by the host's immune system are classified as pathogenic microorganisms. A few important examples are identified here:

- Gram-positive bacteria such as *Staphylococcus aureus* and *S. epidermidis*, which have a tendency to invade the skin as well as catheters and other implanted devices
- Gram-negative bacteria such as *E. coli* and the deadly *Pseudomonas aeruginosa*, both of which causes granulocytopenia
- Acid-fast bacteria such as *Mycobacterium tuberculosis* (TB) and the related *Actinomycetes*, to which mostly elderly patients and AIDS patients are vulnerable (the acid-fast stain technique can identify pathogenic microorganisms that retain carbol fuchsin red dye)
- Protozoa such as *Toxoplasma gondii* and *Cryptosporidium*, which can be deadly in severely immunocompromised AIDS patients
- Fungi such as *Cryptococcus neoformans*, which causes meningitis, especially in patients with AIDS, cancer, and diabetes

The host's site of infection plays an important role in the designation of these pathogenic microorganisms. For instance, while *Bacteroides*, *Prevotella*, and *Haemophilus* species are associated with respiratory tract infections, poxviruses and *Trichophyton* species commonly infect the skin. *Staphylococcus* species cause a series of infections affecting the respiratory, gastrointestinal, and genitourinary tracts and skin, eyes, and ears. Before pathogenic organisms are further discussed, it is worth reviewing the most commonly used terms in microbiology.

Epidemiology

The study of microorganism patterns, causes, and prevention of human diseases is called *epidemiology*. In contrast, *epidemic* refers to an occurrence of a contagious disease that spreads rapidly. When an epidemic occurs widely over a very large area, it is called a pandemic. Typical examples of epidemics are food poisoning and influenza outbreaks within a community. The influenza pandemic that killed many young individuals in 1918–1919 and the most recent flu pandemic in 2009 (influenza virus H1N1), which caused a serious concern in the United States, are examples of pandemic cases. The job of epidemiologists is to review and determine what causes such outbreaks across a population. For instance, epidemiologists worked together to determine what caused the *Salmonella* outbreaks during 2008–2009 in the United States.

If a disease is not eradicated and occurs frequently in a specific area or population, it is referred to as *endemic*. For instance, malaria is endemic in many countries.

Behavioral Science/Health Education

The term *behavioral science/health education* refers to information-based campaigns such as those aimed at stopping the spread of sexually transmitted diseases, such as herpes and HIV/AIDS; helping youth recognize the dangers of binge drinking; and promoting seatbelt use. The major focus of behavioral science/health education is to educate and persuade people to make healthy choices in their daily lives. Key areas within behavioral science/health education are mental health, aging and prevention of disease, and public health practice.

Biostatistics

Biostatistics is used to identify trends in a disease outbreak, to determine whether a disease has become prevalent in a specific area, and to illuminate trends in disease and prevention measure outcomes. Two terms are often used to describe the number of people who have a specific disease: (1) *point prevalence*, which indicates the number of individuals who have the disease at any one time, and (2) *period prevalence*, which indicates the number of individuals who have the disease during a given period. A more detailed description of biostatistics is provided in the *Introduction to Drug Information, Literature Evaluation, and Biostatistics* chapter.

Virulence and Pathogenicity

The terms *virulence* and *pathogenicity* mean the same thing and are used interchangeably in medical literature. Pathogenic microorganisms include bacteria, fungi, protozoa, viruses, and parasites that cause infectious diseases; the ability to cause a disease is referred to as pathogenicity. However, factors related to the host's medical and physical condition (e.g., age, gender, immune system, genetic factors) also play an important role in the pathogenicity of the microorganisms. For instance, transplant recipients and cancer patients are often susceptible to microorganisms that would not be virulent to healthy hosts.

A microorganism that causes an infectious disease because of the host's inability to fight back is called an opportunistic pathogen. A typical example is the *Mycobacterium tuberculosis* bacterium, which upon infecting its host may cause pulmonary tuberculosis. If the patient has a healthy immune system that can fight this bacterium, he or she is unlikely to become clinically ill upon encountering it. In contrast, if an individual has a deficient immune system (as is the case for patients with AIDS, for example), the progress of *M. tuberculosis* infection is much different and the patient may die from the disease. Another example is the protozoan *Pneumocystis jiroveci*. It infects nearly everyone, but causes a problem only when the immune system is compromised (such as in AIDS patients) or when the host's body is weakened by hematologic cancers or malnutrition. Today, this microorganism represents a life-threatening opportunistic infection only in AIDS patients.

Transmission

Pathogenic microorganisms have the ability to spread themselves from one host to another, a process that is called *transmission*. Transmission can occur by four major pathways: (1) contact with the microorganism; (2) airborne inhalation; (3) being carried by a vehicle; and (4) vector-borne spread. These pathways are discussed further in another section of this chapter.

Sampling the Infected Body

It is imperative to sample the infected body (or fluid) before an antimicrobial therapy is administered. While various body fluids—such as blood, sputum, urine, stool, and wound or sinus drainage—may all be used for this purpose, blood cultures are the most common way to sample an infected body. Nevertheless, other, more challenging-to-obtain samples such as spinal fluid (when meningitis is suspected) and joint fluid (when arthritis is suspected) are sometimes used because they provide for better identification of specific pathogens.

There are two rationales for sampling the infected body. First, a Gram stain test or an acid-fast test can rapidly identify a class of pathogen. Second, if an antimicrobial therapy is employed first and then one attempts to identify the pathogen, the result may be a false-negative culture simply because the therapy affected the cellular and chemical composition of the infected body. The latter problem may be seen when a patient develops a urinary tract infection, meningitis, or septic arthritis.

Biomarkers

Biomarkers are biologic markers that are routinely used to distinguish between bacterial and nonbacterial causes of pneumonia, for example. The two most frequently used biomarkers for infections are procalcitonin (PCT) and C-reactive protein (CRP).

PCT is a precursor of the calcitonin protein that is released by parenchymal cells as a response to bacterial toxins. As a result, it is a good indicator of pneumonia, particularly when the serum concentration of PCT is more than 0.25 µg/L (generally, when the serum concentration of PCT is more than 2 µg/L, a bacterial infection is present). While the serum concentration of PCT is high in patients with bacterial infections, it is low in patients with viral infections.

CRP is released in response to acute and chronic inflammatory conditions caused by bacterial, viral, or fungal infections; rheumatic fever; malignancy; inflammatory bowel disease; vascular inflammation and cardiovascular disease; and tissue injury. The cause of the elevated concentration of CRP is the release of interleukin-6 and other cytokines (see also the *Introduction to Immunology* chapter) that are known to trigger the synthesis of CRP by the liver.

In addition, the erythrocyte sedimentation rate (ESR) measures the sedimentation rate of the red blood cells over a period of 1 hour. If inflammation is present, the large amount of fibrinogen in the blood causes erythrocytes to become attached to each other and, as a result, increases their sedimentation rate. The ESR lacks specificity and sensitivity as a means to measure inflammation because the serum level of red blood cells can be increased with advanced age and any number of diseases.

Transmission of Pathogenic Microorganisms

As mentioned earlier, pathogenic microorganisms can be transmitted to animals in several different ways. Let's go through these common routes, as they play an important role in diagnosis and identification of the infectious pathogenic microorganism.

Contact with the Microorganism

A typical example of contact transmission is the spread of a pathogenic microorganism by direct sexual contact. In indirect contact, a contaminated device (e.g., a needle) is the cause of the spread. Droplets that are coughed or sneezed into the air are another means by which pathogens are transmitted to nearby individuals; streptococcal pharyngitis (strep throat) and measles are spread in this way, for example.

Airborne Inhalation

In airborne transmission, pathogenic microorganisms are attached to dust particles or aerosols are contaminated with specific pathogenic microorganisms. These microorganisms can persist in the air for hours and days. Two microorganisms whose transmission via the airborne route causes major concerns are *Mycobacterium tuberculosis* (TB) and varicella-zoster virus (chickenpox), both of which can threaten air travelers and the community at large. For this reason, patients with infectious TB should postpone air travel until they become noninfectious. If an air traveler with one of these diseases comes to the attention of public health authorities, they have the obligation to inform the concerned airline of the infectious passenger and request that boarding of the patient be denied.

Transmission Through a Vehicle

Transmission of microorganisms can occur through a variety of vehicles: contaminated food (e.g., *E. coli*, mycotoxins, *Salmonella*), water (cholera), or blood (e.g., blood transfusion with human immunodeficiency virus [HIV]– infected or hepatitis B–infected blood).

Vector-Borne Spread

In this means of transmission, an intermediate organism such as an insect or tick is responsible for spreading the pathogenic microorganism. For example, *Plasmodium falciparum* (which causes malaria) is spread by mosquitoes, *Rickettsia rickettsii* (which causes spotted fever) is spread by ticks, and *Borrelia burgdorferi* (which causes Lyme disease) is transmitted by the bite of an infected tick.

Infection of the Host

No matter which route of pathogenic transmission is followed, pathogenic microorganisms follow a common pattern to infect a host. They first enter the host through the respiratory, gastrointestinal, or genitourinary tract or through a skin cut or other damage. At that point, they interact with specific tissues or cells within the host. For instance, HIV interacts with the membranes of specific T cells—that is, CD4 cells—to infect its host (see also the *Introduction to Immunology* chapter). The influenza A virus targets epithelial cells of the respiratory tract to cause the flu symptoms (e.g., fever, headache, tiredness, cough, sore throat, muscle aches).

In addition to directly interacting with the tissues and cells in their areas of first contact, pathogenic microorganisms can travel through the blood or lymphatic system to reach a variety of secondary tissues and organs. For example, *Neisseria meningitidis* enters the respiratory tract of humans and spreads through the bloodstream into the brain and spinal cord to cause meningitis, a life-threatening disease. Meningitis is identified by the high number of white blood cells (WBCs) in the cerebrospinal fluid, along with symptoms such as fever, headache, photophobia, neck rigidity, diarrhea, vomiting, and altered mental status. It is treated with at least two different antibiotics (such as ampicillin and an aminoglycoside type, both of which are discussed later in this chapter).

A wide range of pathogenic microorganisms are able to produce harmful toxins that either cause tissue and cell damage at the site of infection or interfere with a metabolic pathway of the host. For example, the toxins produced by *Staphylococcus aureus* and *Clostridium botulinum* are responsible for food poisoning. Some of these toxins resist environmental or immunological measures intended to protect the host from infection. For instance, *S. aureus* produces heat-stable toxins that are not eliminated by cooking the food. The signs and symptoms caused by the *S. aureus* toxins include nausea, diarrhea, muscle tenderness, fever, abnormally low blood pressure, and formation of blisters.

Toxic shock syndrome (TSS), which first came to public notice in 1980, is a deadly illness that is caused by the toxin TSST-1. TSST-1 is produced by some strains of *Staphylococcus.* It was discovered that this toxin can become attached to tampons, thereby allowing the staphylococci to multiply in the vagina. Hundreds of young women became infected in this way before the infective route was recognized. Symptoms of TSS include high fever, low blood pressure, malaise, and confusion, which can rapidly progress to stupor, coma, and multiple organ failure. Patients with symptoms of TSS should receive immediate treatment to reduce their risk of death from this condition.

The *Clostridium tetani* toxin blocks the normal relaxation impulses of the nerves and causes severe muscle spasms characteristic of tetanus. The toxins produced by *Bordetella pertussis* (which causes whooping cough) and by *Vibrio cholerae* (which causes cholera) both interfere with signal transduction mechanisms in mammalian cells. These toxins are enzymes that catalyze structural changes in host proteins that act in various signal transductions. For instance, an attachment of ADP-ribose prevents the host's G proteins from cycling between their GDP-bound (inactive) and GTP-bound (active) forms. This inhibition interferes with normal signal transduction and the metabolic events that are dependent on the signaling systems (see also the *Introduction to Pharmacodynamics* chapter). Infection with *V. cholerae* causes severe diarrhea, which, if not treated, causes patients to enter shock and finally die. While it is critical to use antibiotics to treat *V. cholerae*, diarrhea caused by *Salmonella* or *E. coli* should not be treated with drugs unless the infection is severe.

Compromised Immune System

While anyone can develop a compromised immune system, a few factors play key roles in the evolution of this condition—namely, age, disease, medications, and medical devices. In addition, malnutrition, stress, lack of rest, and cigarette smoking can lead to a compromised immune system. Because the existence of a compromised immune system is a major concern in infectious diseases, a more detailed description and causes of this condition are provided here.

Age and Immune System Compromise

Elderly individuals have less effective immune systems than younger individuals because the ability of the immune system to fight pathogenic microorganisms declines with age. This is true for both the innate and acquired immune systems (see also the *Introduction to Immunology* chapter). For example, the response that produces fever upon an encounter with infectious bacteria does not usually occur in elderly patients; approximately 20% of individuals older than age 65 with serious bacterial infections do not develop such fevers. The reason is the older adult's central nervous system (CNS) is less responsive to immune signals.

In addition, newborn infants (0–1 month of age) have immature immune systems. Both of these generations—the elderly and infants—are prone to opportunistic infections.

Medical Conditions and Immune System Compromise

A series of well-known diseases renders patients especially vulnerable to infection with opportunistic microorganisms. For example, AIDS, cancer, diabetes, cystic fibrosis, sickle cell anemia, asthma, severe burns, and cirrhosis all diminish the effectiveness of the immune system. In rare cases of cancer, the tumor itself may obstruct or physically invade vital organs, resulting in other forms of immune system compromise.

Drugs and Immune System Compromise

Certain drugs work as immunosuppressive agents or cause side effects that reduce the effectiveness of the immune system of patients. For instance, steroid drugs (corticosteroids), prolonged use of antibiotics, alcohol, and anticancer drugs all diminish the effectiveness of the immune system. Granulocytopenia is a phenomenon in which the number of white blood cells decreases as a result of an underlying hematologic cancer, cancer chemotherapy, or infection with aerobic bacteria and fungi. For instance, individuals with granulocytopenia are prone to colonization by *Candida albicans*, a fungus that causes blood and organ infections.

Medical Devices and Immune System Compromise

Patients with mechanical devices such as prosthetic heart valves, intravenous catheters, or intravascular needles are at risk for infection by organisms that can enter their organs through these devices. The microorganism that most commonly enters organs or tissues by a device is *Staphylococcus aureus*. Indeed, it is through this route that many hospital-acquired infections occur.

Microbiology and Infectious Diseases

The terms *bacteriology* and *microbiology* are often perceived by students as the same science and terminology. While these two fields have many similar features, they do not study the same science. For instance, both bacteriology and microbiology deal with organisms that are invisible to the naked eye and require a microscope to visualize the organisms. Indeed, bacteriology is a precursor science to microbiology. Bacteriology refers to the science that studies exclusively bacteria and their living habits. By comparison, microbiology refers to a dynamic science that identifies, classifies, and studies the structure and function of a wide range of microorganisms, including bacteria, protozoa, algae, fungi, viruses, and rickettsia.

Nineteenth-century pioneers in the field of biology, including Louis Pasteur (discovery of the first vaccine for rabies and anthrax), Robert Koch (discovery of the cause of tuberculosis), Theobald Smith (discovery of *Salmonella*), and other scientists of the early twentieth century, laid the groundwork for bacteriology, and their bacteriological discoveries led to better understanding of many of today's infectious diseases. The landmark discovery of the fungus *Penicillium* by Alexander Fleming in the 1920s led to the development of the penicillin antibiotic to treat bacterial infections. This discovery was soon followed by other important antibiotic findings—for example, streptomycin and tetracycline—in the 1940s. Scientists in the fields of biochemistry, molecular biology, and immunology often use microbes to study basic living processes such as metabolism, photosynthesis, enzymatic catalysis, gene action and expression, population dynamics, and immune responsiveness.

The diagnosis of an infection often is made in a laboratory to which samples of body fluids, such as sputum, urine, blood, and respiratory or genital secretions, are sent for analysis. These samples are incubated on agar plates and examined by microbiologists to determine the types of microorganisms present and their pattern of antibiotic susceptibility. The results are shared with healthcare providers, who then select an appropriate antibiotic to kill the infectious microorganisms. In addition, microscopes are used to count the number of white blood cells observed in specimens, which often is an indication of infectious diseases.

As was discussed in the *Introduction to Cell Biology* chapter, organisms are classified into three distinct groups: prokaryotes, eukaryotes, and archaebacteria. While eukaryotes are the most complicated organisms, having advanced structures and functions, prokaryotes are simple organisms that, due to their simplicity, have been studied extensively in an effort to understand eukaryotic organisms. Archaebacteria live in harsh environments such as those characterized by extreme temperature, pressure, or salty conditions.

The contribution from the government sector is of paramount importance in regard to epidemiology: the detection and elimination of a wide range of diseases having microbial causes. Many federal agencies are responsible for monitoring potential epidemics and the development of drugs or vaccines to fight pathogenic microorganisms. The U.S. Food and Drug Administration (FDA), which is a subdivision within the U.S. Department of Health and Human Services, is responsible for protecting public health through monitoring and regulation of food safety, tobacco products, dietary supplements, prescription and over-the-counter (OTC) medications, medical devices, veterinary products, and cosmetics.

The Science of Infectious Agents

A few words about the sciences that study infectious agents such as fungi (mycology), parasites (*parasitology*), and viruses (virology) are in order before these agents are described in depth in this chapter.

Mycology

Mycology is the study of fungal infection, including fungi's genetic and biochemical properties. Fungi are eukaryotic organisms. As a result, they have many eukaryotic organelles, such as mitochondria; a Golgi apparatus; an endoplasmic reticulum (ER); ribosomes; a nucleus; a cytoplasmic membrane containing lipids, glycoproteins, and sterols; and a cytoskeleton. In addition and in contrast to higher eukaryotes (animals), the cells of fungi possess a rigid cell wall.

Fungi can be classified into two major groups: molds and yeasts. Dimorphic fungi constitute a third minor group; they consist of a mixture of molds and yeasts. Typical examples of yeasts are *Candida* and *Cryptococcus*; typical examples of molds are *Aspergillus* and *Rhizopus*. A major difference between yeasts and molds is that while yeasts can invade animals, molds are found in the environment as a free-living organism. It has been suggested that molds cause fewer infections compared with yeasts. However, the *Aspergillus* species of molds cause severe clinical infections characterized by high mortality.

Most fungal infections are not as severe as bacterial or viral infections, but rather are simply bothersome for patients. For instance, while ringworm and athlete's foot are annoying, they do not cause any severe clinical consequences. Additionally, some fungi, including *Saccharomyces*, are harmless—in fact, they are used to produce ethanol and carbon dioxide in the processes of brewing and baking. A few severe fungi cause severe illness, however, including blastomycosis, coccidioidomycosis, and histoplasmosis. The severity of fungal disease also depends on whether the patient's immune system is compromised. Thus an understanding of patients' production of antibodies and other immunological mediators is important in selecting the right medications to counteract fungal infections. Keep in mind that fungi grow more slowly than bacteria.

The diagnostic tool most commonly used in a laboratory to identify fungi in fluid specimens is calcofluor white stain. This stain binds to fungi, which can then be examined via fluorescent microscopy.

Parasitology

The science that studies parasitic diseases such as malaria and Chagas disease is called parasitology. In a microbiology lab, a clinical microbiologist examines specimens in blood and intestinal parasites in feces to isolate and identify parasitic agents. These examinations are performed by microscopic investigation and the parasitic agents are identified on the basis of their characteristic structure.

Virology

Virology is the science that studies viruses, including their structure, classification, and reproduction. Due to the complexity involved in growing viruses outside of the living host, fertilized chicken eggs have often been used for this purpose. This approach has allowed many large hospitals and state departments of health to grow and identify viruses rather than sending samples to microbiology laboratories. Use of antibodies to identify viruses has proved a valuable means to diagnose viral infection. Despite the fact there are relatively few drugs that can fight different classes of viruses, early identification of a particular virus assists clinicians in ruling out the use of antibiotics that fight only bacterial infections. Common viruses that cause diseases include influenza, herpes, chickenpox, the common cold, and many nonspecific respiratory infections.

Fungi

Fungi have a nucleus, are usually filamentous, and are spore-bearing organisms that reproduce both sexually and asexually. Their survival depends solely on absorption of nutrients from either living or dead organisms; as a result, they work as decomposers and recycle carbon and minerals. Fungi are among the oldest organisms on the earth. Indeed, the oldest terrestrial fungi are hyphae, which are approximately 430 million years old. Approximately 80,000 species of fungi have been identified, but fewer than 50 species cause fungal infections of animals. Fungi live in plants, animals, or other fungi. Examples of fungi are yeasts, mildews, rusts, mushrooms, and truffles. Interestingly, there is a similarity between the ribosomes of animals and fungi.

The fungi that engage in asexual reproduction are extremely diverse. Asexual reproduction most commonly occurs when various types of fungal offspring swim or are forcibly discharged from the parent. In contrast to asexual reproduction, sexual reproduction occurs in a majority of species of all classes.

Many pharmaceutical companies are utilizing fungi to produce medicines. For instance, some statin drugs—such as pravastatin (Pravachol), simvastatin (Zocor), and lovastatin (Mevacor)—are effective cholesterol-reducing agents that are derived from mevinolin, which is produced by *Aspergillus terreus*. Other examples include the antibiotics amoxicillin (Moxatag) and ceftriaxone (Rocephin), as well as cyclosporine (Gengraf), which is an immunosuppressive agent. Because some fungi cause life-threatening infections, a variety of antifungal agents have been developed to treat patients who are infected with these pathogens.

Three echinocandins are effective in treating fungal infections. The pharmacological mechanism of echinocandins is inhibition of glucan synthase in susceptible fungi, thereby blocking the formation of $1,3$-β-D-glucan, which is an important component of the fungal cell wall. This mechanism of action has almost no side effects in human host cells. A typical example of an echinocandin is caspofungin (Cancidas). Caspofungin's minimal drug–drug interactions have made this drug one of the agents of choice to treat fungal infections caused by *Candida* and *Aspergillus*. Newer antifungal agents include members of the azole class (all of which possess a five-membered heterocyclic ring that includes two double bonds; **Figure 3.2**), such as fluconazole (Diflucan), itraconazole (Sporanox), voriconazole (VFEND), and posaconazole (Noxafil).

Because fungi are eukaryotes, there are many cellular similarities between fungi and animals. As a result, there are only a few pathways by which to inhibit the growth of fungi without

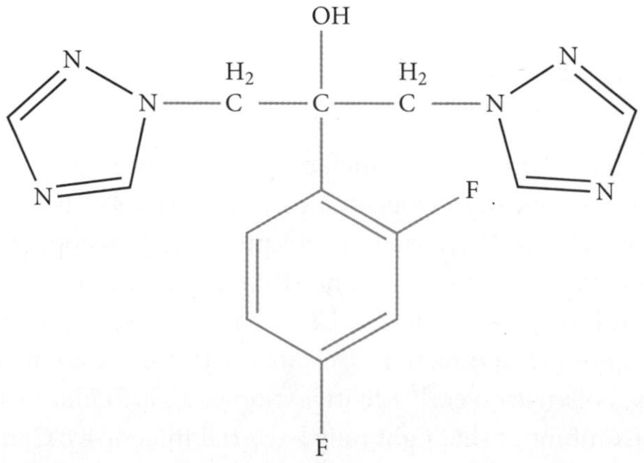

Fluconazole

Figure 3.2 Structure of fluconazole, which belongs to the azole class. An azole contains a five-membered heterocyclic ring with two double bonds.

harming the host. The pharmacological mechanism employed by the azoles is the inhibition of 14-α-lanosterol demethylase, which in turn inhibits the formation of the fungi's sterol, ergosterol. In this way, the integrity of the cell membrane is destroyed.

Some animals are especially prone to fungal infections. For example, the fungal disease caused by *Actinomycetes* affects cattle, swine, and horses. In cattle, this infection is called lumpy jaw and may be treated with iodine or by local injection of streptomycin (Streptomycin for Injection, from Canada) in severe cases. Most fungal infections (so-called mycoses) develop gradually and follow a prolonged course.

Patients who undergo transplantation are prone to fungal infections, particularly those individuals who are on broad-spectrum antibiotics. *Candida* infections are most commonly seen in this setting, especially in patients with granulocytopenia. After the prophylactic use of fluconazole became common practice, infections with resistant fungi (particularly *Aspergillus*, *Fusarium*, *Scedosporium*, and *Penicillium*) emerged as a problem. The development of resistance has led to calls to replace fluconazole with other agents such as caspofungin, voriconazole, and posaconazole.

It is critical to differentiate clinical resistance from microbial resistance. The former refers to *in vivo* development of resistance to an antifungal agent that is caused by factors other than microbial resistance. For instance, clinical resistance may emerge when the antifungal agent cannot reach the site of infection or when the immune system cannot eliminate the fungus. In contrast, the microbial resistance refers to *in vitro* development of resistance, when the fungus no longer responds to an antifungal agent.

Four mechanisms have been identified as underlying causes of azole antifungal resistance: (1) mutations in the gene for 14-α-lanosterol demethylase (the enzyme that synthesizes ergosterol); (2) cellular rejection of the drug by multidrug efflux transport pumps; (3) posttranslational modification of 14-α-lanosterol demethylase; and (4) alteration of fungi's cell membrane proteins.

Learning Bridge 3.1

A physician calls you to discuss an antifungal agent, fluconazole, that he has prescribed for his patient to treat esophageal infection caused by *Candida*. He is concerned that the antifungal agent is no longer working. The physician wants to prescribe itraconazole, which he believes is more effective as a treatment for the esophageal infection. When you ask him if his patient is using any other medications, he responds, "Yes, I have also prescribed sucralfate to treat the patient's duodenal ulcers."

A. What is (are) the problem(s)?
B. What is (are) your recommendation(s)?

Parasites

Parasites are divided into two groups: protozoa and helminths. Both types of organisms affect the CNS, but particularly in patients with a suppressed immune system—for example, HIV-infected patients. Protozoa are single-celled eukaryotes that are similar to a yeast cell in terms of their small size (in the range of micrometers) and simplicity, whereas helminths are multicellular worms with complex organ systems with a wide range of sizes (from less than 1 millimeter to 1 meter). Pathological parasites that cause diseases such as malaria, babesiosis, Lyme disease, and Chagas disease are capable of passing from one patient to another through blood transmission. Often, donors' migration and travel are the cause of spreading parasitic infections. As a result, parasitic infections are the most prevalent diseases in underdeveloped nations and are global health problems that have resulted in high morbidity and mortality.

A few major factors related to parasites enable them to spread widely. For instance, there are challenges such as relatively few effective vaccines, development of drug resistance by parasites, and a lack of new antiparasitic agents (many new agents in the United States are approved by the FDA for use only as investigational medications). Today, the most effective way to control a parasitic infection is chemotherapy. In addition, only a few vaccines (which remain in clinical trials) have shown progress against schistosomiasis, hookworm, and leishmaniasis.

The physiologic interactions of parasites with their hosts comprise a complex process in which metabolic dependency is the key to the parasite's survival. For instance, the common intestinal roundworm, *Ascaris*, which uses the host's intestinal contents for nourishment, depends on the host's ATP molecules and other basic molecules for synthesis of proteins and essential cofactors. Similarly, *Diphyllobothrium latum* takes up vitamin B_{12} so effectively that the host may develop pernicious anemia.

The immune system's ability to fight parasites is not as strong as it is for bacteria and viruses. Therefore, many parasites are able to escape the immune response. The best-known evasive technique used by parasites is production of an antigenic variation—an approach employed by African trypanosomes, for example. These parasites produce a glycoprotein that fully covers the entire parasite. However, each variant surface glycoprotein is antigenic, such that its production stimulates the synthesis of host antibodies that bind with high specificity to the surface glycoprotein to eliminate the *Trypanosoma* parasite. These parasites, however, are able to produce a variety of surface glycoproteins through genetic means. Consequently, the trypanosome may not be recognized by the host antibodies and is not cleared from the blood. In some cases, the result is a balance—that is, coexistence—between host and parasite.

Parasitic *Trypanosoma* species cause the devastating disease known as human African trypanosomiasis (HAT) or, more simply, African sleeping sickness. Two forms of this disease occur: one in East Africa and one in West and Central Africa. Both forms are transmitted by the tsetse fly. Approximately 50 million people are afflicted by HAT in tropical areas, and mortality is high with many of these infections. Because parasitic trypanosomes use glycolysis as their only source of energy, the enzymes involved in glycolysis (i.e., multi-enzymatic reactions that oxidize one glucose molecule to two pyruvate molecules; see the *Introduction to Biochemistry* chapter for more details) are good targets for drug development. One especially promising target 3-phosphate dehydrogenase (see also the *Introduction to Biochemistry* chapter), which plays a central role in glycolysis and is an essential pathway for parasitic survival.

Malaria

Malaria is a parasitic infectious disease that is transmitted by the bite of an infected *Anopheles* mosquito. Approximately one-third of the world population lives in areas that are affected by malaria organisms—clearly, malaria is a global health issue. Nearly 400 million new infections are reported annually, and malaria causes approximately 2 million deaths globally due to a lack of prophylaxis (prevention) for this disease, inadequate or inappropriate chemoprophylaxis (use of drugs as a preventive tool), and a lack of medical care. Most cases of malaria in the United States involve travelers from the endemic areas. The symptoms of malaria are similar to those associated with bacterial and viral infections, and include fever, chills, sweats, headache, malaise, fatigue, myalgia, and nausea and vomiting. These symptoms usually appear 1–2 weeks after the infection occurs. There are four main strains of malaria (*Plasmodium falciparum, P. vivax, P. malariae,* and *P. ovale*), of which *P. falciparum* is the most dangerous. This strain is discussed in more detail in the next subsection.

Plasmodium falciparum Malaria

Plasmodium falciparum is a protozoan parasite that causes malaria in humans, is the deadliest malarial organism, and has successfully developed resistance to several antimalarial agents. While *P. falciparum* can be transmitted by blood transfusion, congenitally, and by infected needles, most infections occur by the mosquito bite.

Gametocytes, the sexual stages of the malaria parasite, fuse to produce sporozoites. These sporozoites travel from the mosquito's salivary glands into the host animal's circulation and localize in animals' hepatocytes. There, they multiply and then cause hepatocytes to rupture so that the invaders can enter erythrocytes. This infectious process takes approximately 2 days. Both young children (6 to 36 months) and nonimmune pregnant women are at especially high risk for malaria infections.

To avoid malarial complications such as hypoglycemia, pulmonary edema, and renal failure, it is very important to accurately diagnose malaria and promptly initiate antimalarial therapy within 48 to 72 hours of infection. Similarly, to avoid malaria infections, particularly when travel is planned in areas where the disease is endemic, one can take prophylactic chloroquine phosphate (Aralen), 500 mg/week, 1–2 weeks prior to travel, during the travel period, and continuing for another 4 weeks after leaving the endemic area. If a chloroquine-resistant problem is suspected, one can use mefloquine (Lariam, from Canada), 250 mg weekly beginning 2–3 weeks before travel and continuing until 4 weeks after returning from the endemic area. In addition, the affected individual needs to use the antibiotic doxycycline (Adoxa), 100 mg, 1–2 days before travel and continuing until 4 weeks after returning from the affected area. It is worth mentioning that the FDA issued a boxed warning for Lariam in July 2013 due to its adverse effects such as "ringing in the ears, depression, and hallucinations."

Free Radicals and Malaria Prevention

Hydrogen peroxide (H_2O_2) and hydroxyl free radicals are highly toxic to cells. If they are not destroyed, they will damage lipids in the cell membrane, causing hemolysis of erythrocytes. One mechanism to break down H_2O_2 involves catalase, which is found inside peroxisomes (see also the *Introduction to Cell Biology* chapter). Glutathione, which is an abundant tripeptide molecule in most cells, also helps to degrade H_2O_2. In fact, glutathione not only helps to degrade H_2O_2 but also reduces hydroxyl free radicals. During these reactions, glutathione itself is oxidized (**Figure 3.3**). The enzyme that reduces (regenerates) glutathione uses NADPH as a coenzyme.

Glucose-6-phosphate dehydrogenase (G6PD) enzyme is one of the cytosolic enzymes that is involved in the oxidation of glucose-6-phosphate into nucleotides, a pathway referred to as the pentose phosphate pathway (see also the *Introduction to Biochemistry* chapter). One NADP⁺ molecule is reduced to NADPH by the G6PD enzyme in the course of this pathway. A deficiency in the G6PD enzyme means less NADPH generation and, therefore, a less reduced form of glutathione. In turn, hemolysis occurs more readily in G6PD-deficient individuals (400 million people worldwide). Certain foods that contain divicine

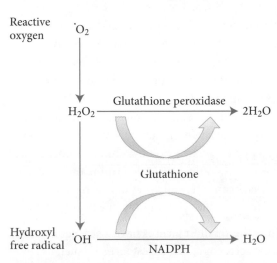

Figure 3.3 Reduced NADPH and glutathione protect erythrocytes' cell membranes from attacks by reactive oxygen and hydrogen peroxide.
Adapted from: Nelson DL, Cox MM. *Principles of biochemistry*, 5th ed. New York: W. H. Freeman and Company; 2008: Chapter 14.

(e.g., fava beans) and some antimalarial agents such as primaquine produce H_2O_2, which can cause a hemolytic anemia (massive destruction of erythrocytes) in G6PD-deficient individuals. Fortunately (and amazingly), several deficiencies in G6PD activity have been observed to be associated with resistance to *P. falciparum*, particularly among individuals of Mediterranean and African descent. This resistance arises because the parasite is very sensitive to a level of oxidative stress that is tolerable to G6PD-deficient individuals.

Learning Bridge 3.2

Joe Smith, a 26-year-old college student, visits the pharmacy where you are completing your introductory pharmacy practice experiences. Joe comes to the counter and wants to talk to you. He has been diagnosed with pernicious anemia, which is a vitamin B_{12} deficiency. Joe has never had any vitamin deficiency before, and his diet is rich in proteins and vitamins. While his vitamin B_{12} medication is being filled, he asks you why he has suddenly developed pernicious anemia and also experienced abdominal discomfort, loss of appetite, and weight loss during the past 6 weeks. You review his medical records and do not see any sign of a gastrointestinal deficiency in the absorption of cobalamin (vitamin B_{12}).

A.   What is your first reaction? How would you explain the vitamin B_{12} deficiency?
B.   Do you have any suggestion for Joe's prescriber?

Viruses

Viruses do not have cells, but rather are acellular active agents whose remarkable genomes can easily adapt to changing environments. However, viruses are not able to survive outside their host cells. In other words, viruses are nucleic acid molecules that can enter cells and redirect the host's enzymatic machinery to replicate the virus's genome and encode proteins capable of forming protective shells around the virus. Some viruses are capable of incorporating their genetic information, as DNA, into the host's chromosomes.

All viruses share two characteristics: (1) They have a nucleic acid genome (as DNA or as RNA) that is surrounded by a protective protein shell called a capsid (which in turn may be enclosed within an envelope made of lipids, proteins, and carbohydrates) and (2) they are not able to reproduce independently of the host's cells because they are obligate intracellular species. Both of these characteristics indicate that viruses can replicate only within host cells because their nucleic acids do not encode enzymes that are necessary for the synthesis of proteins, carbohydrates, or lipids. In addition, viruses are incapable of producing high-energy phosphates. Essentially, viral nucleic acids encode the proteins necessary to replicate, package, and insert their genome within the biochemical environment of host cells. Proteins, most often glycoproteins, in the capsid determine the specificity of interaction of a virus with its host cell. While viruses can infect all types of organisms (plant, animal, fungi, and bacteria), the majority of viruses infect specific types of only one host species.

Viruses range from 10 to 400 nm in diameter. While the smallest viruses have a size equal to that of a ribosome and are not visible under a light microscope, the largest viruses (such as vaccinia) are readily visible via light microscopy.

Despite the similar terminology used to label viroids, virusoids, virions, and prions, they are different agents. For instance, viroids are naked (there is no capsid), cyclical, mostly double-stranded small RNAs that are replicated by the cellular RNA polymerase II and infect only plants. In contrast, virusoids are nucleic acids that need assistance from helper viruses to package their nucleic acids into virus-like particles. A virion is a complete virus particle, with this term indicating both the intactness of the viral structure and the property of infectiousness.

The story for prions is totally different. Prions are infectious abnormal proteins that are able to spread beyond the host. The cellular and normal form of the prion protein (PrP^c) is encoded by the host's chromosomal DNA. It has a molecular weight of 33–35 kDa, and its secondary structure is mainly organized into α-helices and is sensitive to proteases. PrP^c is expressed on the surface of neurons. The abnormal form of this protein (PrP^{res}), however, has the same amino acid sequence as PrP^c but its secondary structure is mainly organized into β-sheets that have exposed hydrophobic regions of PrP^{res}. A newly synthesized PrP^{res} molecule triggers the production of more PrP^{res}. Due to the hydrophobic nature of PrP^{res}, these molecules become attached to each other to form insoluble protease-resistant aggregates. Prions have been shown to cause neurodegenerative problems such as Creutzfeldt-Jakob disease, Gerstmann-Sträussler disease, kuru, fatal familial insomnia, and human bovine spongiform encephalopathy (BSE; widely known as mad cow disease). The study of prions continues, as much remains to be learned about these infectious proteins.

Viral genomes are very diverse. Two major families of viruses are distinguished based on their genomes: one with a DNA genome and one with an RNA genome (but never both). For instance, circovirus has a single-stranded DNA and rotavirus has a double-stranded RNA. However, the shape of their genomes may vary; for example, some genomes are linear, whereas others are circular. Some viral genomes consist of one molecule, whereas other viral genomes contain as many as 12 molecules (fragmented genome). There is also wide variation in the sizes of viral genomes: Some double-stranded genomes range from 3,000 to 280,000 base pairs, while other single-stranded genomes range from 5,000 to 27,000 nucleotides in size.

Viruses cause both serious and minor diseases, including poliomyelitis, hepatitis, influenza, the common cold, measles, mumps, chickenpox, herpes, rubella, hemorrhagic fevers, and encephalitis. Retroviruses have an enzyme called reverse transcriptase that plays an important role in synthesizing a DNA copy of the RNA genome, which is then integrated into the host cell's genome. Retroviruses have caused devastating health problems such as leukemias, lymphomas, sarcomas, and acquired immune deficiency syndrome (AIDS) among animals. Clearly, these viruses deserve a closer look into their structures and functions.

Retroviruses

Retroviruses are organized into seven genera, with letters in the Greek alphabet being used to distinguish those genera. Among retroviruses one can find Alpharetrovirus (avian leukosis virus), Betaretrovirus (mouse mammary tumor virus, which often infects mice, certain species of monkeys, and sheep), Gammaretrovirus (murine leukemia virus), Deltaretrovirus (bovine leukemia virus), Epsilonretrovirus (Walleye dermal sarcoma virus), Lentivirus (human immunodeficiency virus), and Spumavirus (chimpanzee foamy virus).

Retroviruses are characterized by (1) an RNA genome, (2) a reverse transcriptase enzyme, (3) a dense core and an envelope that surrounds the core, and (4) synthesis of a DNA that is a copy of the viral RNA and integration of that DNA into the host cell's genome (a mechanism that is essential for the viral reproductive cycle).

Retroviruses may be sexually transmitted, as is the case with HIV. In addition, HIV can be passed from mother to infant during gestation (vertical transmission), at birth, or through breast-feeding. Effective treatments are available that can prevent transmission from an infected mother to her child. In addition, infection may occur through the respiratory tract (i.e., when a virus enters the mouth or nose) or through the circulatory system (i.e., via blood transfusion or use of contaminated needles). While some of retroviruses are transmitted through insect bites, thankfully

HIV is not. The role of HIV in the development of AIDS and the use of drugs in the treatment of HIV-infected patients are discussed later in this chapter.

Infectious Diseases

Infectious diseases are serious pathological health issues that, if not treated, may lead to life-threatening consequences. The host's susceptibility, the infectious agent, and the external environment play important roles in the development of an infection, particularly in children, the elderly, and patients with compromised immune systems. The infectious agent can be either exogenous (foreign) or endogenous (i.e., one that is cultured in a specific tissue in the body of the host but is not causing any disease in the host). In other words, an infection arrives when a foreign agent invades the host or when an endogenous agent overcomes the host's innate immune system.

The foreign agent can also come from another host that functions as a reservoir or acts as a vector for an infectious agent. For example, the bacteria *Borrelia burgdorferi* is stored in the white-footed mouse and upon infection of the host's bloodstream causes Lyme disease. The *Ixodes* tick is a vector, and the bacteria can be injected into animals by the bite of infected ticks and causes paralysis of the animal.

The study and elimination of an infectious disease requires understanding of the hierarchical process that starts with pathogenesis at the level of the population, then addresses infected individuals, followed by identification of the cells (that are infected or produced as a result of the infection), and finally considers the genes involved in the infection. For instance, the spread of *Mycobacterium tuberculosis* in homeless shelters, prisons, and the community at large occurs at the level of a population. At the individual level, this bacterium can be transmitted through inhalation of respiratory droplets. At the cellular level, the bacteria activate T cells, which seek to fight the infection. Clearly, then, patients with compromised T-cell levels (e.g., individuals with AIDS) are at greater risk of infection with *M. tuberculosis*. Because the *M. tuberculosis* bacteria multiply inside macrophages of their host, at the genetic level individuals with polymorphisms in their macrophage genes that are unregulated upon infection are at higher risk for tuberculosis. In contrast to most other pathogenic microorganisms, which are killed within these macrophages, *M. tuberculosis* thrives and grows inside the macrophages.

Depending on the microorganism, the kind of infection experienced may also be related to the specific bacterium involved. For instance, *Streptococcus pneumoniae* causes pneumonia and meningitis, whereas *E. coli* causes gastrointestinal and urinary tract infections.

Viruses Causing Infectious Diseases

The viral replication cycle is the most important factor in viral infections. While some of these infections may lead to cell death, hyperplasia, or cancer, others may not produce any disease. In fact, most viral infections do not produce a disease. A viral infection that does not produce any symptom in the host is referred to as an inapparent or subclinical infection. If a virus can cause signs of disease in its host, it is referred to as a pathogenic virus.

Viral pathogenesis proceeds through a series of steps: attachment and entry of the virus into the host's cell, replication of the viral genome, multiplication of the virus, cellular attack and injury, host immune response, elimination of the virus by the immune system, and viral shedding. In the past, the number of copies of virus per milliliter of blood was called the viral load (this term is still used by many laboratories). More recently, the number of international units per liter (IU/L) has been adopted as a means to quantify infection. **Figure 3.4** indicates the paths taken by and infections caused by pathogenic viruses.

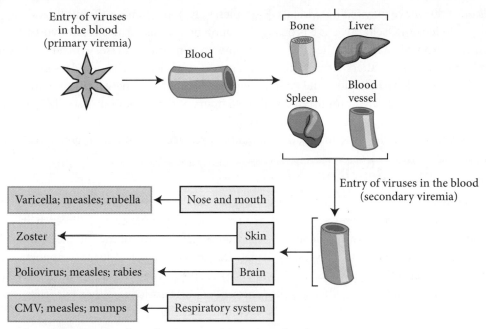

Figure 3.4 Spreading of viruses through primary and secondary viremia.
Adapted from: Brooks GF, Carroll KC, Butel JS, Morse SA, Mietzner TA. *Jawetz, Melnick, & Adelberg's medical microbiology*, 25th ed. New York: McGraw-Hill.

Influenza

Influenza is a viral infection that causes illness on a global scale. Worldwide, 500,00 people die from influenza each year. Influenza infection is most common during winter season, but it can occur at any time during the year.

Three types of influenza are distinguished: A, B, and C. While types A and B are very common, type C is rarely seen in humans. Both influenza A and B cause acute respiratory illness mainly because the viral replication occurs only in the respiratory tract. While clinical diagnosis of influenza is a challenge, signs and symptoms are known to include fever, headache, myalgia, sore throat, rhinitis, nonproductive cough, and weakness. Often, patients with uncomplicated influenza gradually improve in 2–7 days. Other patients may experience persistent symptoms of weakness, so-called post-influenza asthenia, for several weeks.

The route of transmission and infection by the influenza virus is often through sneezing and coughing—that is, from the respiratory secretions of infected persons. In addition, contact with objects that are contaminated with respiratory droplets is a source of transmission.

Although the treatment of influenza is manageable, and to some extent the disease is preventable, this infection has increased morbidity and mortality in certain high-risk populations. Pneumonia is the major complication of influenza and occurs most frequently in children younger than 2 years; adults aged 65 or older; patients with asthma, heart disease, diabetes mellitus, epilepsy, stroke, or immunosuppression; and pregnant women (even within 2 weeks after delivery).

The Centers for Disease Control and Prevention (CDC), in collaboration with the World Health Organization, globally and actively tracks influenza virus isolates to facilitate preparation of the annual influenza vaccine. The two most common influenza vaccines that are available for seasonal vaccination are the trivalent influenza vaccine (TIV) and the live-attenuated influenza vaccine (LAIV). These two vaccines protect against influenza A subtypes H3N2 and H1N1 and influenza B virus. A few other anti-influenza agents are also used to fight the influenza A and influenza B viruses once they have infected individuals. Examples include oseltamivir (Tamiflu) and zanamivir (Relenza). Oseltamivir is a prodrug that upon hydrolysis forms oseltamivir carboxylate. Oseltamivir carboxylate inhibits the viral enzyme known as neuraminidase, which is important for viral reproduction (it alters virus particle aggregation and release). Zanamivir is not a prodrug but, similar to oseltamivir, inhibits the viral neuraminidase enzyme. These anti-influenza agents are most effective if they are administered within 48 hours of the onset of illness. The use of anti-influenza agents for prophylaxis is most effective when these medications are given as adjuncts to the annual vaccination; in other words, they should not replace the annual influenza vaccination.

Human Immunodeficiency Virus

HIV, a member of the retrovirus family, causes severe viral disease in which the host's immune system becomes severely compromised. Patients who have acquired HIV eventually reach an endpoint that is known as acquired immunodeficiency syndrome (AIDS). One of the unique characteristics of HIV is the virus's capacity to irreversibly deplete the host's T-helper-inducer lymphocytes (CD4$^+$ lymphocytes; see also the *Introduction to Immunology* chapter). The destruction of these lymphocytes compromises the body's ability to fight recurrent opportunistic infections by viruses, fungi, bacteria, protozoa, and tumors (e.g., Kaposi's sarcoma and lymphomas).

HIV infection may be transmitted by various pathways, including sexual intercourse (heterosexual and homosexual), blood transfusion and blood products, intravenous needles, vertical transmission, and breast milk. Detection of HIV infection is achieved by a few different methods, such as detecting antibodies to the virus, detecting the viral p24 antigen, and detecting viral RNA. In 2012, the FDA approved an over-the-counter (OTC) home test, OraQuick, that is able to detect the presence of HIV in saliva by using a mouth swab. This home test may assist HIV-infected patients in beginning a treatment course more quickly. Currently, the most commonly used HIV test relies on the detection of antibody to HIV. Thanks to careful screening methods of donors' blood, the risk of HIV-1 infection via blood transfusion is now low (1 infection per 2 million transfusions). No cases of HIV-2 infection have occurred in the United States since 1992, as this type has relatively poor ability to infect humans. HIV-2 infection is largely confined to West Africa.

One of the major problems with HIV is the virus's ability to integrate its genetic material into the host's DNA, which makes it very challenging to eliminate the virus. As a result of this challenge, the medications available today aim to slow the progress of the viral growth and to prevent the spread of the virus. The best methods for preventing transmission of HIV infection are to avoid unprotected sexual intercourse and to not share infected needles or medical devices (e.g., insulin pens). In January 2013, it was reported that a hospital in the state of New York used HIV-contaminated insulin pens to inject insulin into other diabetes patients, which exposed more than 700 patients to HIV, hepatitis B, and hepatitis C infections.

Because HIV-infected patients are immunocompromised patients, they are prone to secondary opportunistic infections, particularly if their CD4 levels are low (fewer than 200 CD4$^+$ lymphocytes/μL). Two common opportunistic organisms in this population are *Pneumocystis jiroveci* and cytomegalovirus, neither of which causes severe health problems in healthy individuals. In addition, *Streptococcus pneumoniae* causes secondary infection in HIV-infected individuals. Indeed, it is the secondary infections that cause morbidity and mortality in HIV-infected patients. For this reason, these patients are vaccinated against pneumococci (pneumococcal vaccine) and receive prophylactic treatment for infections with pathogenic organisms such as *P. jiroveci*, *Mycobacterium tuberculosis*, and *M. avium*.

The goals for HIV treatment are to increase patients' longevity, improve the quality of their lives, improve their immune function, and prevent further transmission of the infection. The most effective treatment is to reduce HIV replication and achieve a plasma HIV RNA concentration of less than 50 RNA/mL. Keep in mind that while the amount of RNA in the plasma indicates the extent of HIV replication, the CD4 cell counts indicate to what extent the HIV replication has caused CD4 cell destruction. In turn, taking both measurements (CD4 and RNA counts) on a regular basis is important to follow the progression of the HIV infection. The rates of disease progression differ among patients with HIV, so the course of therapy should be individualized based on patients' RNA and CD4 cell counts.

A number of drug therapies are available for the treatment of patients with HIV.

Nucleoside Reverse Transcriptase Inhibitors

Nucleoside reverse transcriptase inhibitors (NRTIs) are known to interfere with viral reverse transcriptase enzyme, resulting in inhibition of the viral replication. The major adverse effects associated with NRTIs include lactic acidosis and severe hepatomegaly (i.e., an enlarged liver). Agents in this class include zidovudine (Retrovir), lamivudine (Epivir), and abacavir (Ziagen). While zidovudine is a thymidine analog, lamivudine is a cytosine analog and abacavir is a guanosine analog. All of these agents are prodrugs and require phosphorylation to become active agents. Healthcare providers must be careful not to use zidovudine with stavudin, as both need thymidine for their activity and, as a result, can antagonize each other.

Non-nucleoside Reverse Transcriptase Inhibitors

Non-nucleoside reverse transcriptase inhibitors (NNRTIs) bind to another site on the viral reverse transcriptase enzyme to inhibit this enzyme. The major adverse effects associated with NNRTIs are rash and hepatoxicity. In HIV treatment, usually one NNRTI is used with two NRTIs. A few examples of NNRTI are efavirenz (Sustiva), nevirapine (Viramune), and delavirdine (Rescriptor). Unlike NRTIs, NNRTI agents do not require intracellular phosphorylation to exert their antiviral activity; thus they are not prodrugs.

Protease Inhibitors

Protease inhibitors (PIs) bind to the viral protease and competitively inhibit cleavage of the HIV viral gag-Pol polyprotein. The viral cleavage of gag-Pol polyprotein is crucial to produce the functional proteins that are required for the viral maturation process. Many of the anti-HIV agents that have "vir" at the ends of their names belong to this class: indinavir (Crixivan), atazanavir (Reyataz), ritonavir (Norvir), and fosamprenavir (Lexiva). Indinavir can cause kidney stones, and pharmacists should advise patients to drink at least 48 ounces (1.5 L) of water each day to reduce this risk. Both atazanavir and indinavir require the acidic environment of the stomach for their absorption; for this reason, any antacids should be taken at least a few hours after administration of these agents. The major adverse effects with PIs are gastrointestinal intolerance and rash. All PIs are CYP3A4 inhibitors, so potential drug–drug interactions are a concern. Patients on PIs should be monitored 3–4 weeks after beginning therapy for glucose, liver function test (LFT), lipids, and total cholesterol levels. (Atazanavir is the only PI that does not cause hyperlipidemia.) To ensure an effective therapeutic outcome, a PI is used with two other NRTIs.

Atazanavir is frequently used as an antiviral agent in treatment-naive HIV-infected patients. In addition, it is used in the treatment of HIV-infected patients who are intolerant of other antiretroviral drugs. Because a Pgp-mediated efflux mechanism plays an important role in reducing the antiviral absorption of atazanavir, it has been suggested that co-administration of ritonavir might inhibit Pgp-mediated efflux of atazanavir and, as a result, increase the absorption of atazanavir. Ritonavir is also used as an atazanavir "enhancer" due to its ability to inhibit CYP3A4-mediated metabolism of atazanavir in the intestinal mucosa.

A notably effective treatment regimen for HIV-infected patients combines two NRTIs with one NNRTI or one PI. For instance, zidovudine and lamivudine (two NRTIs) may be combined with efavirenz (an NNRTI). For postexposure therapy (e.g., when a nurse has an HIV-infected needlestick), treatment should begin within 2 hours of the accident and consist of combination therapy with zidovudine/lamivudine/nelfinavir for 4 weeks.

When several anti-HIV agents (three to four drugs) are taken in combination, the regimen is called highly active antiretroviral therapy (HAART). HAART is employed, for example, for the treatment of pregnant women who are HIV positive. Because efavirenz crosses the placenta, it has teratogenic effects; as a result, it should be avoided during pregnancy. In pregnant women, then, HAART should begin after the first trimester. Zidovudine is a good choice for pregnant women, as it has shown to reduce the risk of transmission of HIV to the fetus. In addition, zidovudine should be given both during labor and to the infant during the first 6 weeks of life.

A breakthrough in HIV treatment was reported in March 3, 2013. According to this report, a newborn infant who was infected with HIV, through vertical transmission from her mother, was given a combination of three anti-HIV agents—zidovudine, lamivudine, and nevirapine 30 hours after she was born. No treatment was given to the mother during pregnancy. The baby girl continued with zidovudine, lamivudine, and a co-formulated lopinavir/ritonavir for another 18 months; thereafter, the treatment, for an unknown reason, stopped. Ten months after discontinuation of the combination therapy, the child's blood samples showed very low viral levels and undetectable HIV-specific antibodies in her serum. Although more research needs to be carried out to fully understand this breakthrough, the result suggests that implementation of combination therapy upon the delivery of HIV-infected infants might be both beneficial and critical.

In August 2012, the FDA approved a new combination agent, Stribild (formerly called the Quad), which includes four active ingredients: elvitegravir 150 mg (PI); emtricitabine 200 mg (NRTI); tenofovir disoproxil fumarate 300 mg (NRTI); and cobicistat 150 mg (an inhibitor of CYP3A4 with no anti-HIV effect). Stribild is to be taken once daily. This drug is used for HIV-infected patients who have not yet been treated with other anti-HIV agents (treatment-naive patients).

Entry Inhibitors

Glycoprotein 120 (gp120) is HIV's envelope protein, which has affinity for the host CD4's glycoprotein. The binding between viral gp120 and the host CD4 glycoprotein induces conformational changes in gp120 that allow it to bind to another receptor (CCR5) on CD4 cells. The overall effect is to stabilize the binding of gp120 to the CD4 cell, thereby enabling HIV to fuse its membrane with the CD4 cell. This membrane fusion facilitates the entry of HIV into the CD4 cell.

Only two agents classified as entry inhibitors are available in the United States to treat HIV: enfuvirtide (Fuzeon) and maraviroc (Selzentry). Enfuvirtide blocks the entry of the virus into CD4 cells by inhibiting the conformational changes in the viral gp41 that are essential in the membrane fusion mechanism. Maraviroc selectively and reversibly blocks the host CD4's CCR5 receptor and destabilizes binding of the viral gp120 to the CD4 cell. Vicriviroc, another agent currently under FDA review, has a similar mechanism of action to maraviroc. While enfuvirtide is administered subcutaneously, maraviroc is taken orally.

Hepatitis A Virus

Hepatitis A virus (HAV) is an RNA virus that usually spreads by the oral–fecal route, in overcrowded areas, and in persons with poor hygiene. It has an incubation period of 15–45 days. HAV is not detectable in the blood but can be detected by serologic methods (i.e., in other bodily fluids).

The HAV target is usually children and young adults. This hepatitis virus is not usually transmitted by transfusion. Infection with HAV is largely asymptomatic and does not lead to chronic disease.

Hepatitis B Virus

Infection with hepatitis B virus (HBV) is a serious and major public health problem, as this infection can spread rapidly and horizontally from one patient to another. HBV infection is associated with a significant risk of death caused by liver disease.

HBV is a DNA virus. Upon infection and attachment of the virion to the liver cells' surface receptors, the virus begins to replicate. Interestingly, HBV is not pathogenic to cells, but rather stimulates the release of T cells that are cytotoxic to hepatocytes; this effect is responsible for most of the hepatic damage that causes cirrhosis and hepatocellular carcinoma (HCC).

More than 2 billion people worldwide have been acutely infected with HBV. The most widely affected areas, however, are sub-Saharan Africa, Asia, the Amazon, and southern parts of Eastern and Central Europe. Every year, approximately 1 million people die worldwide as a result of cirrhosis and HCC.

HBV transmission may occur via sexual contact (both homosexual and heterosexual), parenterally (including injection-drug use), and perinatally (5 months before and 1 month after birth). While vertical transmission is most common in areas with high HBV prevalence, horizontal transmission (from child to child) is most common in the intermediate-prevalence areas. As a result, donated blood is screened for HBV, using hepatitis B surface antigen (HbsAg) as a marker for this infection. Vaccination of individuals who are receiving long-term transfusions is necessary to prevent infection caused by transfusion (the transfusion risk of HBV infection is 1 in 63,000). Concentrations of HBV are high in the blood, serum, and wound exudates of infected persons. While HBV is detectable in semen, vaginal fluid, and saliva, its concentration is low in urine, feces, sweat, tears, and breast milk.

Hepatitis C Virus

Hepatitis C virus (HCV) damages the liver by causing chronic active hepatitis, cirrhosis, and liver failure. Although the prevalence of HCV infection worldwide is 3%, the infection rate in North America is in the range of 1% to 2%. The major route of HVC transmission is through blood transfusion, although the overall risk of acquiring HCV through transfusion is small. Unfortunately, a large number of patients who use intravenous drugs for at least one year become infected with HCV. This factor explains why blood donations are always tested for antibodies to HCV and HCV's RNA. Other risk factors for HCV transmission include vaccination practices, tattoos, piercing, cocaine snorting, homosexual relationships, and multiple sexual partners. In addition, vertical transmission from mothers to their infants can occur.

The only method that can definitively confirm a diagnosis of cirrhosis is liver biopsy. For this reason, it is recommended that liver biopsy be performed prior to initiating treatment for this disease. A second principle in the management of patients with HCV infection is to eliminate any factors that might potentially contribute to progression of HCV disease. When they receive their initial therapy, patients will be advised to stop drinking alcohol, watch their body mass, avoid toxic drugs, and, if possible, be vaccinated against hepatitis A and B. No vaccination against HCV is available, however.

The FDA expedited its review of and recently approved telaprevir (Incivek), which has been shown to be effective against existing HCV infection. Telaprevir binds reversibly to the virus's serine protease to block the replication of HCV. However, it is recommended that this drug be used with other antiviral agents such as peg-interferon-α and ribavirin. If the patient's liver enzymes are normal and there is no detectable HCV RNA in the blood 6 months after treatment, one can consider the virus to be eradicated from the patient's body. Other agents used to treat HCV include synthetic interferon and the antiviral agent ribavirin (Virazole).

Most animal viruses are inhibited by interferons. Interferons (IFNs) are potent cytokines that have antiviral, immunomodulating, and antiproliferative activities (see also the *Introduction to Immunology* chapter). There are three major classes of human IFNs—α, β, and γ—which have different levels of antiviral activity. While IFN-α and IFN-β are synthesized by almost all virus-infected cells, the synthesis of IFN-γ is confined to only a few cells, such as T lymphocytes, macrophages, and natural killer (NK) cells, that respond to antigenic stimuli or specific cytokines. In other words, IFN-γ has less antiviral activity but more potent immunoregulatory effects and enhances the expression of class I and II major histocompatibility complex (MHC) molecules (see also the *Introduction to Immunology* chapter). By comparison, IFN-α and IFN-β have antiviral and antiproliferative actions; stimulate the cytotoxic T lymphocytes (CTLs), NK cells, and macrophages; and up-regulate class I MHC molecules. The use of recombinant technology has enabled pharmaceutical companies to produce large quantities of human interferons (a few agents will be introduced in the following sections). Unfortunately, these agents are associated with numerous side effects. For instance, an injection of an IFN dose of 2 million units (MU) or more causes adverse effects such as flu-like symptoms (fever, chills, headache, myalgia, arthralgia, nausea, vomiting, and diarrhea).

When an interferon is used alone, the complete eradication of the HCV virus is seen in fewer than 20% of patients. By comparison, ribavirin has poor antiviral activity but good immunomodulatory activity. Similarly, when ribavirin is used alone, it does not provide any significant antiviral response and, as a result, patients continue to be HCV-RNA positive. A combination of interferon α-2b (Intron A) injection and ribavirin, however, has been shown to increase the rate of HCV eradication, particularly in patients who have relapsed after α-interferon therapy or when the α-interferon therapy has not been effective.

Cytomegalovirus

Cytomegalovirus (CMV) is one of the most common infectious viruses, affecting approximately 50% to 90% of the population in industrialized nations and 90% to 100% of the population in developing countries. The major route of transmission for this virus is sexual contact. CMV infection is asymptomatic in healthy individuals, and the virus is not a major cause of congenital infection. However, because this virus causes a latent infection, patients with compromised immune systems (e.g., patients with AIDS, cancer patients who are treated with chemotherapy, CMV-seronegative transplant recipients) or those with immature immune systems (neonates) are at risk of latent infection.

Food-Borne Pathogens

Food-borne pathogens are toxins that are released by pathogenic microorganisms in contaminated food and cause food poisoning—an acute gastrointestinal or neurologic disorder. Although most cases of food poisoning are caused by bacteria, viruses and chemical food contaminations can result in food poisoning as well. The food-borne pathogens that most often cause food poisoning include *Brucella*, *Campylobacter jejuni*, *E. coli*, *Listeria monocytogenes*, *Salmonella*, *Shigella*, *Vibrio*, and *Yersinia*. These organisms enter the body through ingestion. The two most prevalent food-borne pathogens are *Salmonella* and *C. jejuni*. Indeed, *Salmonella* causes food poisoning in 40,000 individuals, on average, in the United States every year.

Some food-borne pathogens produce heat-stable toxins that will not be eliminated by cooking. For example, the toxin produced by *Staphylococcus aureus* remains active in foods even after cooking; that is, while cooking kills the bacterium, it does not inactivate the toxin. As a result, within 30 minutes to 4 hours after consuming the contaminated food, the infected individual develops severe vomiting and diarrhea. Staphylococcal infections are estimated to cause 20% to 40% of all food-borne outbreaks in the United States.

Salmonella bacteria cause gastroenteritis, which results in symptoms such as fever, diarrhea, and vomiting 1–2 days after ingestion. *Salmonella* bacteria are commonly found in meats and eggs, but they are easily eliminated by cooking. Infected raw meat can transmit the bacteria to ready-to-eat foods, thereby causing food poisoning.

Similar to *Salmonella*, *Shigella* bacteria cause gastroenteritis. However, *Shigella*'s route of infection is not through food, but rather via fecal–oral contact or feces-contaminated water. Keeping food hot (more than 63°C) or cold (less than 7°C) will prevent most of the food-borne pathogens from growing so that they might not subsequently cause food-borne illnesses. However, *L. monocytogenes*—a psychrophylic (cold-loving) pathogen—is an exception; it is not controlled by hot/cold methods. Another technique, and perhaps the least expensive one, is to keep food in an environment containing at least 3% salt (NaCl), as most food-borne pathogens cannot grow in such a medium. The high salt concentration inhibits the protein synthetic machinery of bacteria.

Not all bacteria cause food poisoning. In fact, some of them impede the growth of other bacteria. For instance, *Streptococcus thermophilus*, *Lactobacillus bulgaricus*, *Leuconostoc*, *Pediococcus*, and *Micrococcus* are used to preserve food because they oxidize sugars, which are needed by the contaminated and competing bacteria, to lactic acid, thereby inhibiting the growth of the contaminated bacteria.

Despite the fact glucosteroid drugs are known to reduce the effectiveness of the immune system, in a few infectious diseases they benefit patients. For instance, in patients with AIDS and pneumonia (i.e., when patients with AIDS are also infected with *P. jiroveci*) and with moderate to severe hypoxia (when tissues do not have adequate access to oxygen), administration of hydrocortisone (Cortef), 50 mg three times daily, increases oxygenation and, in turn, reduces respiratory failure. Hydrocortisone may also be used in the most severe complication of sepsis, septic shock, as it has been shown to reduce the effects of the cytokines that are induced by the disease.

Antibiotics

Antibiotics are molecules that are synthesized either *in vitro* or *in vivo*. They are effective when they inhibit the growth of a microorganism (bacteriostatic) or when they kill the entire microorganism (bactericidal). Indeed, the first antibiotic was used more than 2,500 years ago in China, where moldy soybean was applied to infectious sites. However, real evidence of an antimicrobial effect was not seen until 1877 when Louis Pasteur and J. F. Joubert observed that an infectious amount of anthrax bacilli could be killed by concomitant infections with other antibiotic-producing bacteria.

Perhaps the first real antibiotic was Prontosil (sulfamethoxazole), which was discovered by the Nobel Prize winner Gerhard Domagk from Germany; his work showed that Prontosil could interfere with the metabolism of microorganisms. This new finding opened up a whole new era in medicine. Later, Alexander Fleming discovered penicillin (the general name for one group of β-lactam antibiotics) in the early 1940s. Soon after, cephalosporins (another group of β-lactam antibiotics) and streptomycin (a type of aminoglycoside) were discovered in two different research laboratories. Since the 1940s, many antibiotics with therapeutic effects have been isolated, identified, and synthesized.

While some of the antibiotics are produced by fungi (e.g., penicillin is produced by the fungi *Penicillium notatum* and *Penicillium chrysogenum*), others are produced by bacteria (*Actinomycetes*). Many other antibiotics are synthesized by pharmaceutical companies (e.g., clotrimazole). In addition, chemical modifications of existing natural antibiotics have resulted in the production of semisynthetic antibiotics; for example, clarithromycin (Biaxin) is produced from erythromycin. While some of these medications have been marketed as "safe antibiotics," many others have shown drug–drug interactions (mainly through inhibition of metabolic enzymes) or side effects that range from minor problems such as dizziness, stomach upset, and diarrhea, to serious allergy reactions and severe skin rashes. Therefore, when selecting the right antibiotic for patients, it is imperative to consider whether a concomitant drug therapy could pharmacokinetically or pharmacodynamically affect the risk of side effects or alter therapeutic outcomes.

Resistance is a major problem that emerges with the frequent use of antibiotics. Because of this potential, the therapeutic value of many antibiotics is reduced when they are used without precautions and in unnecessary clinical situations. One issue that has both positively and negatively affected the use of antibiotics is the emergence of drug-resistant bacterial strains. It has positively affected the antibiotic market in that the number of antibiotics has increased significantly since the 1940s as scientists have sought to overcome many infectious diseases and to eliminate the resistance problem. It has negatively affected medical practice in that higher doses have been used to kill resistant bacteria, which has often resulted in drug toxicities. An example of the positive impact is the resistance to penicillin that was recognized soon after its introduction, which ultimately resulted in the development of another class of antibiotics, the cephalosporins. An example of negative impact is the use of high doses of chloramphenicol (serum concentrations greater than 100 mg/L) that cause "gray baby syndrome," which is characterized by adverse effects such as abdominal distension, vomiting, metabolic acidosis, cyanosis, hypothermia, and hypotension. These adverse effects can occur with patients of any age, from children to adults.

Antibiotics can be classified according to their mechanism of action. The three major classes of antibiotics identified on this basis are cell wall inhibitors, protein synthesis inhibitors, and nucleic acid synthesis inhibitors.

Cell Wall Synthesis Inhibitors

Because the cell membrane plays an important role in functioning as a selective barrier and as the site of action for enzymes involved in the biosynthesis of components of the cell envelope (see the *Introduction to Cell Biology* chapter), a series of antibiotics has been developed to prevent bacterial cell wall synthesis, integrity, and functioning, with the goal of producing bactericidal or bacteriostatic effects. The bacterial cell wall has a rigid structure that maintains the shape and size of the bacterium. The rigidity of this cell wall is imparted by cross-linking of peptides inside the peptidoglycans, which is a catalytic function of transpeptidase enzymes. Damage to the rigid cell wall by a lysozyme (such as that found in human tears and saliva) or an antibiotic that inhibits cell wall synthesis will result in the destruction of an infectious bacterium.

One frequently prescribed group of antibiotics that act on the bacterial cell wall is the β-lactam antibiotics. These medications have a characteristic structure known as a β-lactam ring (**Figure 3.5**). The major reason why resistance to β-lactam antibiotics develops is the production of the beta-lactamase enzyme. If this enzyme cleaves penicillins, it is called penicillinase; if it cleaves cephalosporins, it is called cephalosporinase; if it cleaves both, it is called beta-lactamase. Beta-lactamase enzymes are expressed by bacterial genes. Drugs that are resistant to the enzymatic activity of penicillinase include the piperacillin/tazobactam combination (Zosyn), the amoxicillin/clavulanate combination (Augmentin), and nafcillin (Nallpen, from Canada).

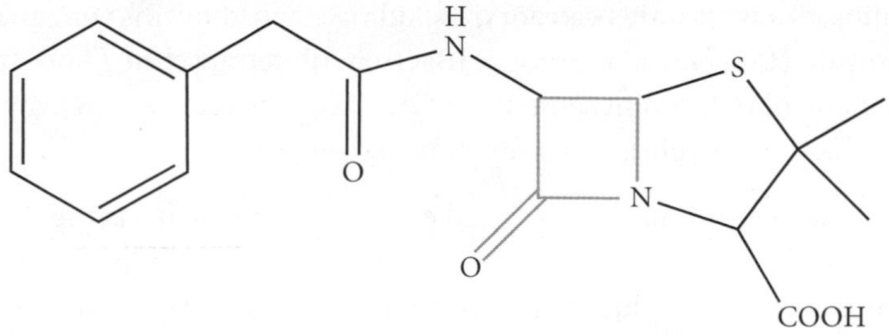

Figure 3.5 The structure of penicillin G (Pfizerpen). The β-lactam ring is shown in teal.

Cephalosporin antibiotics are classified into four generations. First-generation cephalosporins have the highest effectiveness against Gram-positive bacteria but only modest effectiveness against Gram-negative bacteria. Second-generation cephalosporins have moderately better activity against Gram-negative organisms. Third-generation cephalosporins have activity against Gram-positive organisms and are more potent against the Enterobacteriaceae. The last generation in this class (fourth generation) includes the antimicrobial spectrum of all of the third-generation cephalosporins but also has increased stability to beta-lactamases.

As was discussed in the *Introduction to Cell Biology* chapter, Gram-positive bacteria have a much thicker layer of peptidoglycan than Gram-negative bacteria. More than 50 antibiotics, with a wide range of spectra and clinical applications, are available, all of which act as cell wall synthesis inhibitors. The initial step in the destruction process is binding of the antibiotic to cell receptors (so-called penicillin binding proteins [PBPs]). The next step is to inhibit the transpeptidation reaction so as to prevent peptidoglycan synthesis. Three to six PBPs exist, a few of which are transpeptidases.

Four major classes of antibiotics within this category are penicillins, cephalosporins, vancomycin (Vancocin), and cycloserine (Seromycin); these agents all effectively inhibit bacterial cell wall synthesis. While vancomycin, fosfomycin (Monurol), and bacitracin (Baciguent) inhibit cell wall synthesis, they are not as effective as the β-lactam drugs because they need to penetrate the cells to inhibit the early steps in the biosynthesis of the peptidoglycan. Penicillin is often the antibiotic of choice for infections caused by Gram-positive bacteria such as *Streptococcus pyogenes*, which causes strep throat. When treating a penicillin-allergic patient who has inflammation of the inner layer of the heart (endocarditis), however, vancomycin is a better choice.

Beta-lactam contains a characteristic four-membered ring that is common to all of the β-lactam drugs (Figure 3.5). Interestingly, the β-lactam antibiotics do not harm mammalian cells because animals do not have peptidoglycan in their cell walls. Indeed, the difference in Gram-positive and Gram-negative bacteria's sensitivity to penicillins or cephalosporins reflects structural differences that are found in bacterial cell walls (i.e., the amount of peptidoglycan, the presence of receptors and lipids, chemical nature of cross-linking in the peptidoglycan).

Other antibiotics act on the cell membrane rather than the cell wall. For instance, daptomycin (Cubicin), which is a cyclic lipopeptide antibiotic, binds to the cell membrane and causes depolarization of the bacterial membrane and inhibit intracellular synthesis of DNA and RNA. This antibiotic is approved to clear *Staphylococcus aureus* in the treatment of sepsis and skin and soft-tissue infections caused by Gram-positive bacteria and bacteria that are resistant to β-lactam agents and vancomycin.

Protein Synthesis Inhibitors

Because of differences that exist in the protein synthetic machinery of prokaryotic and eukaryotic organisms, many antibiotics have been developed to target bacterial protein synthesis. There are many classes of antibiotics within this category, including erythromycins (one member is Erythrocin), lincomycin (Lincocin), mupirocin (Bactroban), tetracycline (Apo-Tetra, from Canada), chloramphenicol (Chloromycetin, from Canada), linezolid (Zyvox), aminoglycosides (neomycin, gentamicin, kanamycin), and streptomycin.

One major difference between prokaryotic and eukaryotic organisms is the structure of their ribosomes. As was described in the *Introduction to Cell Biology* chapter, prokaryotes have 70S ribosomes, whereas eukaryotes, including mammalian cells, have 80S ribosomes. The ribosomal RNA (rRNA) and ribosomal proteins that assemble ribosomes are sufficiently different that researchers have been able to find antibiotics that act on only prokaryotic ribosomes. Indeed, the efforts by Ramakrishnan, Steitz, and Yonath to identify the structure of ribosomes and to elucidate ribosomes' roles in binding antibiotics were awarded the Nobel Prize in chemistry in 2009. Given the large number of antibiotics in this category, it is helpful to differentiate the various classes of protein synthesis inhibitors so as to take a closer look at their mechanisms of action.

Erythromycins

Erythromycins are classified as macrolide antibiotics. All macrolides have a macrocyclic lactone ring (which is why they are called macrolides) that is attached to carbohydrates. These agents bind to the 23S RNA of the 50S subunit of ribosome and block the translocation step that is catalyzed by the protein known as elongation factor G (EF-G) (**Figure 3.6**). Early resistance to macrolides severely limited their use, but subsequent structural changes to erythromycin resulted in the production of other useful antibiotics such as azithromycin (Zithromax), clarithromycin (Biaxin), and telithromycin (Ketek). Erythromycin is the oldest of the macrolides (was developed in the 1950s), but it has been prescribed less often since other effective macrolides have been developed. Clarithromycin is more effective than erythromycin in the treatment of staphylococcal and streptococcal infections.

Resistance is an emerging issue with macrolides because of at least three problems with these agents:

- Macrolides do not readily enter bacterial cells.
- Some bacterial strains have developed a pump at their cell membrane that rejects antibiotics, pushing them out of the cell (efflux).

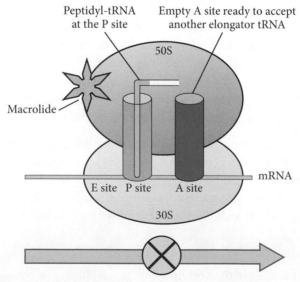

Figure 3.6 Macrolide antibiotics inhibit the role of elongation factor G (EF-G) and, as a result, inhibit translocation of the 70S ribosome along the mRNA.

- Some bacteria are able to methylate their ribosomal 50S subunit so that macrolides are no longer able to bind to the bacterial 50S subunit.

Telithromycin is good choice for treating patients infected with erythromycin-resistant bacteria. Structurally, telithromycin differs from erythromycin in that telithromycin binds to the 50S subunit more tightly, which makes it difficult for the bacteria to pump this antibiotic out.

Among the macrolides, azithromycin is the only agent that does not inhibit cytochrome P-450 isozymes. The toxicity of many macrolides is low, but in March 2013 the FDA issued a warning about a potential adverse effect from azithromycin. It was suggested that azithromycin might cause abnormal changes in the electrical activity of the heart leading to fatal arrhythmias, particularly among patients with existing QT-interval prolongation, hypokalemia, or hypomagnesemia.

Lincosamides

Clindamycin (Cleocin HCl) and lincomycin (Lincocin), similar to erythromycin, bind to the 50S subunit and, as a result, resemble macrolides in their binding site and mechanism of action (Figure 3.6). Chromosomal mutants that block binding of clindamycin to the 50S subunit cause bacterial resistance. Because both lincosamide antibiotics and erythromycin bind to the 50S subunit, concomitant administration of these drugs is not recommended so as to avoid any competition for the same binding site on the 50S subunit.

Mupirocin

Mupirocin is active against a wide range of Gram-positive bacteria. This agent is used in an ointment form for treatment of impetigo (a bacterial skin infection) caused by susceptible strains of *Staphylococcus* and *Streptococcus*. When isoleucyl-tRNA synthetase attaches the amino acid Ile to tRNA^{Ile}, mupirocin inhibits the enzymatic activity of the isoleucyl-tRNA synthetase by blocking the binding site of the intermediate substrate (Ile-AMP) (**Figure 3.7**). A lack of charged tRNA^{Ile} (i.e., Ile-tRNA^{Ile}) results in the inhibition of protein synthesis that requires Ile residue; in other words, many proteins are synthesized that lack the Ile amino acid, which results in truncated and nonfunctional proteins.

Tetracyclines

Tetracycline antibiotics and their derivatives are broad-spectrum antibiotics that bind to the 16S rRNA of the 30S ribosomal subunit and inhibit translation. They block the A site of ribosomes and do not allow charged tRNAs to participate in the protein synthesis (**Figure 3.8**). Because eukaryotes do not have 16S rRNA (recall that humans have 28S rRNA), these antibiotics do not harm humans. Similar to the case with macrolides, the efflux mechanism causes bacterial resistance to tetracyclines. Because tetracyclines chelate cations such as Ca^{2+}, they may cause teeth discoloration and result in abnormal bone growth in a growing child. For this reason, tetracyclines are contraindicated in children younger than 8 years.

Chloramphenicol

Chloramphenicol blocks elongation of protein synthesis by acting as a competitive inhibitor of the peptidyltransferase complex, thereby inhibiting formation of peptide bonds (**Figure 3.9**). Chloramphenicol is bacteriostatic, so the growth of bacteria resumes when administration of this agent is withdrawn or stopped by patients. Chloramphenicol has been shown to be effective in eradicating bacterial infections, but it is rarely used as routine antibacterial therapy because of its toxic side effects.

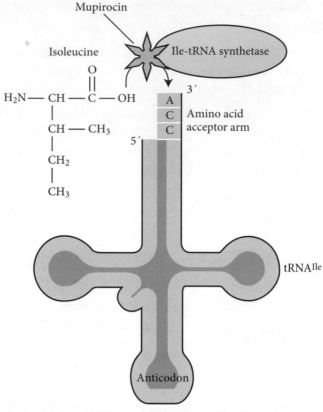

Figure 3.7 Binding of isoleucine amino acid (Ile) to bacterial Ile-tRNA is blocked by mupirocin.

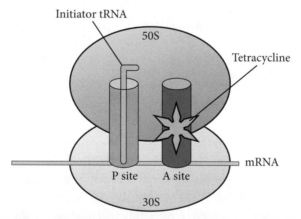

Figure 3.8 Binding of tetracycline antibiotics blocks the A site of the ribosome and inhibits binding of any charged tRNA to the ribosome.

Oxazolidinones

Linezolid is the only member of the oxazolidinone family of antibiotics that is approved by the FDA for the treatment of bacterial infections (a few other oxazolidinones are in clinical development). This antibiotic binds to the bacterial 23S rRNA of the large subunit (50S subunit), thereby inhibiting the formation of the 70S initiation complex (**Figure 3.10**). Linezolid displays both bactericidal (against streptococci) and bacteriostatic (against enterococci and staphylococci) effects. In addition, it is moderately effective against *Mycobacterium tuberculosis*. Because this agent has an

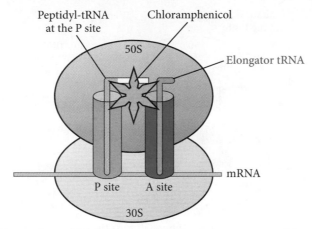

Figure 3.9 Binding of chloramphenicol inhibits peptidyltransferase, a component of the 50S subunit, thereby inhibiting bacterial peptide formation.

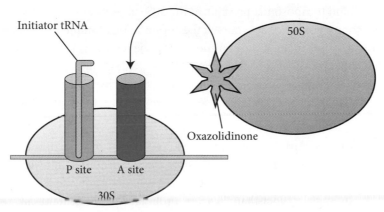

Figure 3.10 Oxazolidinone inhibits binding of the 50S subunit to the 30S subunit, thereby inhibiting the formation of the 70S initiation complex.

inhibitory mechanism that is unique and different from that of other antibiotics, it is used to treat penicillin-resistant strains of *S. pneumoniae*; methicillin-resistant, vancomycin-intermediate, and vancomycin-resistant strains of staphylococci; and vancomycin-resistant strains of enterococci.

Linezolid is a weak, nonspecific inhibitor of the monoamine oxidase enzyme as well. This enzyme metabolizes a few neurotransmitters, including serotonin in the brain (see also the *Introduction to Pharmacology and Pathophysiology* chapter). Consequently, in patients taking serotonergic medications (such as selective serotonin reuptake inhibitors), linezolid increases the level of serotonin, which can lead to the devastating side effect known as serotonin syndrome. This syndrome is characterized by confusion, muscle twitching, excessive sweating, trouble with coordination, and fever. One of the benefits of using linezolid, however, is that it is neither a substrate nor an inhibitor of CYP isozymes.

Aminoglycosides

The major role of aminoglycosides is to create errors in the protein synthetic machinery of bacterial organisms. Many antibiotics are included in this class—for example, streptomycin, neomycin (Neo-Fradin), amikacin, gentamicin (Gentamicin Injection, from Canada), tobramycin (TOBI), and kanamycin. Streptomycin and neomycin have been extensively studied over the past 30 years.

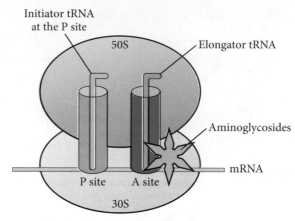

Figure 3.11 Binding of aminoglycosides to the 30S subunit distorts the selection of the correct charged tRNA at the A site of ribosomes.

Aminoglycosides bind to ribosomal proteins in the 30S subunits and 16S rRNA, thereby interfering with the selectivity process that occurs at the codon/anticodon interaction (**Figure 3.11**). The latter mechanism causes many wrong amino acids to be incorporated into bacterial polypeptides or proteins, a lethal process for bacteria. For instance, it is known that neomycin binds to the 16S rRNA of the 30S subunit and increases errors in translation by increasing the binding stability of incorrect charged tRNA at the A site of ribosomes. Neomycin is often used topically to treat minor skin infections.

Aminoglycosides—particularly gentamicin—are known to accumulate in the proximal tubule of the kidney, which results in nephrotoxicity. Plasma levels of gentamicin lower than 2 mg/mL are considered safe. A few factors contribute to the nephrotoxicity adverse effect associated with aminoglycosides, including age older than 70 years, prolonged use of gentamicin, and concurrent therapy with amphotericin B (Fungizone) or cisplatin. Resistance of bacteria to aminoglycosides can be caused by either a nucleotide change in the 16S rRNA or an amino acid change in the 30S ribosomal proteins; production of bacterial adenylating, phosphorylating, or acetylating enzymes that destroy aminoglycosides; or a decrease in the active transport of the aminoglycoside into the cell. The last resistance mechanism, however, is plasmid mediated.

Nucleic Acid Synthesis Inhibitors

Because DNA replication and transcription have direct roles in cell growth and reproduction, both replication and transcription are cellular targets of many available antitumor drugs. The drugs that act on DNA can be classified into five groups: antimetabolites, intercalating drugs, alkylating drugs, anthracyclines, and antisense RNA. These classes are discussed in more depth in the *Introduction to Medicinal Chemistry* chapter.

Fluoroquinolone

Ciprofloxacin (Cipro), gatifloxacin (Zymaxid), gemifloxacin (Factive), levofloxacin (Levaquin), moxifloxacin (Avelox), norfloxacin (Noroxin), and oflaxacin (Apo-Oflox) inhibit DNA gyrase (also called bacterial topoisomerase II). Gemifloxacin, moxifloxacin, and gatifloxacin are the newest fluoroquinolones on the market. The role of DNA gyrase is to overwind or underwind a DNA molecule ahead of the replication fork so as to facilitate the activity of the DNA replication enzymes that are involved in the replication and transcription of the bacterial DNA (**Figure 3.12**). Fluoroquinolones are rarely linked to life-threatening overdose, but they are associated with some notable adverse effects. Of particular concern is their use in children and pregnant women,

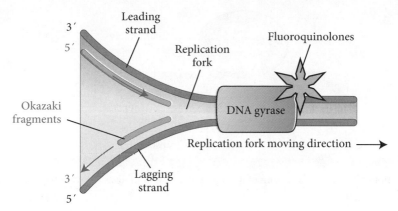

Figure 3.12 Fluoroquinolones inhibit bacterial DNA gyrase, which is known to work ahead of the replication fork. Adapted from: Nelson DL, Cox MM. *Principles of biochemistry*, 5th ed. New York: W. H. Freeman and Company; 2008; Chapter 25.

because it is known that these agents adversely affect developing cartilage and bone. In addition, fluoroquinolones cause tendon rupture, so their use should be discontinued with any signs or symptoms of tendon rupture and in athletes who suffer from painful and swollen tendons.

Gemifloxacin tablets were approved by the FDA in 2003 for the treatment of mild to moderate community-acquired pneumonia (CAP) as well as pneumonia caused by multidrug-resistant strains of *S. pneumoniae* (MDRSP). In addition, gemifloxacin is indicated for acute exacerbations of chronic bronchitis. However, 14% of women older than the age of 40 who used gemifloxacin for longer than 7 days experienced rashes. To prevent this adverse effect, the course of therapy has been changed to 5 days.

The best therapy for prostate infection is ciprofloxacin, 500 mg every 12 hours for 28 days, because ciprofloxacin becomes concentrated in the prostate fluid.

Concurrent use of fluoroquinolones and NSAIDs lowers the seizure threshold. Therefore, one has to use fluoroquinolones with caution in patients with CNS disorders, particularly those with seizure. In addition, ciprofloxacin, a commonly prescribed drug, is a strong inhibitor of the cytochrome P450 enzyme, CYP1A2. As a result, there is a risk of drug interactions if it is used concurrently with drugs that are metabolized by CYP1A2 (e.g., the muscle relaxant tizanidine [Zanaflex]).

Rifampin

Rifampin (Rifadin; also called Rifampicin) and its derivatives rifapentine (Priftin) and rifabutin (Mycobutin) are useful antibiotics in the treatment of *Mycobacterium tuberculosis* infection. Rifampin is effective against most Gram-positive and Gram-negative bacteria and is very active against *Staphylococcus aureus*, coagulase-negative staphylococci, *Neisseria meningitidis*, and *Haemophilus influenzae*. This agent blocks the β subunit of RNA polymerase by binding to an allosteric site of the RNA polymerase enzyme rather than to the active site of the enzyme (**Figure 3.13**). The key problem with this antibiotic is that resistance develops rapidly if it is used as a single agent. For this reason, rifampin is used often with other drugs in therapy for tuberculosis. Rifampin resistance can develop when there is a mutation in the β subunit of RNA polymerase.

Rifampin is a potent inducer of CYP isozymes 1A2, 2C9, 2C19, and 3A4. As a result, drug–drug interactions occur between rifampin and some of the drugs used in the treatment of HIV-infected patients (protease inhibitors and non-nucleoside reverse transcriptase inhibitors), as well as between rifampin and digoxin (Lanoxin), ketoconazole (Apo-Ketoconazole from Canada), propranolol (Inderal), metoprolol (Lopressor), verapamil (Calan), methadone (Dolophine), and corticosteroids, among others.

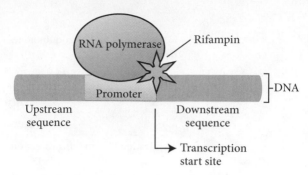

Figure 3.13 Rifampin binds to the β subunit of RNA polymerase and inhibits the transcription process.

In the case of *M. tuberculosis,* isoniazid (Isotamine, from Canada) is prescribed for 9 months together with rifampin for 2 months. In addition, patients must take vitamin B_6 as long as they continue to use isoniazid because isoniazid is known to deplete vitamin B_6 (pyridoxine; see also the *Introduction to Nutrients* chapter). During the past four decades, rifampin has been used as a 10 mg/kg dose in the treatment of *M. tuberculosis.* However, a new ongoing study has indicated that increasing the dose to at least 3 times this level can achieve a far better therapeutic outcome.

Antibiotic Resistance Mechanisms

Antibiotic resistance may arise through several different mechanisms:

- Inactivation of antibiotics by bacterial enzymes. For instance, resistance may be caused by bacterial beta-lactamase. An example is the resistance of *Staphylococcus aureus* to penicillins.

- Alteration of the bacterial membrane that prevents antibiotics from entering the bacterial cell. For instance, mutations of bacterial porin may prevent hydrophilic antibiotics from entering the bacterial cells. Resistance to penicillins can be caused by this mechanism. Alternatively, the bacterial membrane compositions may mutate and change so that an antibiotic cannot enter the bacterial cell. For instance, the attraction of positively charged aminoglycosides to the negatively charged intracellular environment of bacteria can be disrupted by a reduced membrane permeability. The resistance of *Staphylococcus* to aminoglycoside antibiotics is an example.

- Formation of a membrane efflux that pumps out antibiotics from bacterial cells. For instance, tetracyclines may be ejected by an active efflux mechanism that develops in bacterial cells. *Staphylococcus aureus* develops resistance to tetracyclines by employing such an efflux mechanism.

- Alterations of bacterial proteins that change the binding of antibiotics to the bacterial cell wall, ribosomes, or other essential bacterial proteins. Binding of erythromycin to ribosomes is impaired in this way, which explains *S. aureus* and enterococcal resistance to erythromycin.

- Development of alternative pathways to overcome an inhibited enzyme. For instance, enterococcal bacteria are dependent on thymidine. When an antibiotic, such as trimethoprim (Primsol), inhibits the synthesis of the bacterial thymidine, the bacteria are able to utilize exogenous thymidine to support their growth. As a result, the bacteria develop resistance against trimethoprim.

Learning Bridge 3.3

During one of your introductory pharmacy practice experiences, Kristen brings a prescription to your pharmacy for her son Brad. Brad is a 5-year-old boy who has been infected with *Streptococcus pyogenes* and during the past 2 days has been complaining of sore throat and pain in his throat. The prescription reads:

Azithromycin 200 mg/5 mL suspension

Sig: give 10 mL qd × 5 days

A. Kristen is a biology teacher and asks you to explain how azithromycin works as an antibacterial agent. Use what you have learned in this chapter to explain to your preceptor and to Kristen how azithromycin works. In addition, do a literature search at your site and tell your preceptor which specific RNA (it should have an associated digit number) is the binding site for azithromycin.

B. What is (are) the most common side effect(s) associated with the use of azithromycin that Kristen should know?

Learning Bridge 3.4

Eva is a 42-year-old gymnastics trainer who works for a high school in Portland, Oregon. During the past 48 hours, she has been experiencing fever, stabbing chest pains, coughs, and difficulty in breathing. Eva visited her primary care physician for these symptoms and was diagnosed with community-acquired pneumonia (CAP). Her physician prescribed gemifloxacin, 320 mg once daily for 14 days.

One week after she began using the medication, Eva comes to your pharmacy and complains about pain in her swollen ankle, particularly when she is in the gym training her students. In addition, she has rashes over her hands and face. Eva is worried that these problems might have been caused by gemifloxacin and asks you for advice.

A. Is there any link between the use of gemifloxacin and the pain in Eva's ankle? Why?
B. Is there any link between the use of gemifloxacin and her rashes? Why?
C. What would you tell Eva?

Learning Bridge 3.5

David is a 22-year-old student who has been infected with *M. tuberculosis*. He has experienced symptoms such as weight loss, fever, night sweats, and persistent cough and productive sputum. David's physician has prescribed isonizide (200 mg/day) for 9 months and rifampin and pyrazinamide for 2 months. David began his course of therapy 2 weeks ago.

David comes to your pharmacy and complains about malaise. He also mentions that yesterday, when he was driving to school, he became lost and had difficulty seeing street signs. The mental confusion has seriously concerned David, and he is worried that he has developed mild Alzheimer's disease.

(continues)

(*continued*)

A. Is there any link between David's vision and his medications?

B. Is there any link between his malaise and his medications?

C. Is there any link between his mental status and his medications?

D. What suggestions do you have for David?

Learning Bridge 3.6

During the last day of your introductory pharmacy practice experience, one of the pharmacy technicians who is printing the label for a new prescription, ciprofloxacin (Cipro), requests your preceptor to give an override so that she can continue printing the label and filling the prescription. Your preceptor asks you to investigate why there is an override warning for filling ciprofloxacin. Upon reviewing the patient profile, you see that the patient is currently using tizanidine (Zanaflex) 4 mg 1 tid prn, for her muscle spasms.

A. Why is there an override warning regarding filling of ciprofloxacin for this patient?

B. What is your suggestion to your preceptor?

Golden Keys for Pharmacy Students

1. Inflammatory markers such as C-reactive protein, erythrocyte sedimentation rate, and tumor necrosis factor (TNF) may increase during infection and are good signals of infectious diseases.

2. Indinavir can cause kidney stones, so pharmacists should advise patients to drink at least 48 ounces (1.5 L) of water each day to reduce this risk.

3. The bacteria that most commonly cause community-acquired pneumonia (CAP) are *Mycoplasma pneumoniae*, *Streptococcus pneumoniae*, and *Haemophilus influenzae*.

4. The best therapy for prostate infection is ciprofloxacin, because it becomes concentrated in the prostate fluid.

5. Oseltamivir is the widest-spectrum antiviral used against influenza (both types A and B) and is indicated for both prophylaxis and treatment of influenza infections.

6. Clarithromycin is more effective than erythromycin in the treatment of staphylococcal and streptococcal infections.

7. Drugs that are resistant to penicillinase include the piperacillin/tazobactam combination (Zosyn), the amoxicillin/clavulanate combination (Augmentin), and nafcillin (Nallpen, from Canada).

8. To treat *M. tuberculosis* infection, isoniazid is prescribed for 9 months together with a 2-month course of rifampin.

9. Meningitis is identified by an abnormally large number of white blood cells in the cerebrospinal fluid combined with symptoms such as fever, headache, photophobia, neck rigidity, diarrhea, vomiting, and altered mental status. It is treated with at least two different antibiotics (such as ampicillin and an aminoglycoside).

10. Toxins produced by *Staphylococcus aureus* and *Clostridium botulinum* are responsible for food poisoning.

11. *Vibrio cholerae* causes severe diarrhea, which, if not treated, causes patients to develop shock and finally die.

12. AIDS, cancer, diabetes, cystic fibrosis, sickle cell anemia, asthma, severe burns, and cirrhosis all reduce the effectiveness of patients' immune systems.

13. Steroid drugs (corticosteroids), prolonged use of antibiotics, alcohol, and anticancer drugs also reduce the effectiveness of the immune system.

14. Many pharmaceutical companies are utilizing fungi to generate medicines. For example, pravastatin, simvastatin, and lovastatin are derived from mevinolin, which is produced by *Aspergillus terreus*.

15. Because fungi are eukaryotes, there are many cellular similarities between fungi and animals.

16. Patients who undergo transplantation are prone to fungal infections, particularly those who are taking broad-spectrum antibiotics.

17. The immune system's ability to fight parasites is not as effective as its ability to defend against bacteria and viruses. Therefore, many parasites may escape the immune response.

18. Malaria is a parasitic infectious disease that is transmitted by bites of infected *Anopheles* mosquitoes.

19. *Plasmodium falciparum* is the deadliest malarial organism and, unfortunately, has developed resistance to several antimalarial agents.

20. While *P. falciparum* can be transmitted by blood transfusion, congenitally, and by contaminated needles, most infections occur through mosquito bites.

21. Hydrogen peroxide (H_2O_2) and hydroxyl free radicals are highly toxic to the cells. If they are not destroyed, they will damage lipids in the cell membrane, causing hemolysis of erythrocytes.

22. Viruses do not have a cell structure, but rather are acellular active agents with remarkable genomes that easily adapt to changing environments.

23. Viral genomes are very diverse. Two major families of viruses are distinguished based on their genomes: viruses with a DNA genome and viruses with an RNA genome (but never both).

24. Influenza is a viral infection and a global illness. Worldwide, 500,000 people die from influenza each year.

25. There are three types of influenza: A, B, and C. While types A and B are very common, type C is rarely seen in humans.

26. The route of transmission and infection by the influenza virus is often through sneezing and coughing—that is, from the respiratory secretions of infected persons.

27. The influenza vaccines that are most widely available for seasonal vaccination are the trivalent influenza vaccine (TIV) and the live-attenuated influenza vaccine (LAIV).

28. The human immunodeficiency virus (HIV), a member of the retrovirus family, causes a severe viral disease in which the host's immune system is compromised.

29. Because HIV-infected patients are immunocompromised patients, they are prone to secondary opportunistic infections, particularly if their CD4 levels are low (less than 200 CD4$^+$ lymphocytes/µL).

30. Currently, NRTIs, NNRTIs, PIs, and entry inhibitors are available to treat HIV infection.

31. Vertical transmission of HIV may be prevented through either HAART or zidovudine single-agent therapy.

32. Any HIV-infected patient who has a CD4 count of less than 200/μL or an opportunistic infection should start HIV therapy.

33. An effective treatment regimen for HIV-infected patients combines two NRTIs and either one NNRTI or one PI.

34. The goals for patients with HIV treatment are to increase their longevity, improve the quality of their lives, improve their immune function, and prevent further transmission.

35. Infection with hepatitis B virus is a major public health problem, as this virus can spread from one patient to another quite rapidly and is associated with a significant risk of death caused by a liver disease.

36. *Salmonella* bacteria are commonly found in meats and eggs, but are eliminated by cooking.

37. Currently, no vaccine against hepatitis C virus is available.

38. Because differences exist in the protein synthetic machinery of prokaryotic and eukaryotic organisms, many antibiotics have been developed that target bacterial protein synthesis.

39. The major role of aminoglycosides is to create errors in the protein synthetic machinery of bacterial organisms.

40. Fluoroquinolones adversely affect developing cartilage and bone and can cause tendon rupture.

41. The most common form of antibiotic resistance is inactivation of antibiotics by bacterial enzymes. For example, resistance may emerge due to the activity of bacterial beta-lactamase.

Learning Bridge Answers

3.1 **A.** There are two major problems:

1. Drug–drug interaction. The azole antifungal drugs interact with many other drugs. For instance, sucralfate decreases the absorption of fluconazole.

2. Resistance may have played an important role here by making fluconazole less effective. Four mechanisms have been identified as underlying causes for azole antifungal resistance: (i) mutations in the gene for 14-α-lanosterol demethylase (the enzyme that synthesizes ergosterol); (ii) cellular rejection of the drug by the multidrug efflux transport pumps; (iii) post-translational modification of 14-α-lanosterol demethylase; and (iv) alteration of fungi's cell membrane proteins.

B. For the reasons mentioned previously, it seems that another azole agent, itraconazole, will not help the patient. Because the patient also needs to take care of his ulcer, it is important to continue with sucralfate and replace fluconazole with intravenous (IV) caspofungin (Cancidas). An oral dosage form is not available for caspofungin, but the IV route will eliminate any absorption interference from the sucralfate therapy, which will benefit this patient.

3.2 **A.** Because the patient does not seem to have malnutrition or a deficiency in the ability of his GI system to absorb cobalamin, the cause of the pernicious anemia must be something else. One cause of pernicious anemia is infection with *Diphyllobothrium latum*, a parasite that takes up vitamin B_{12}. Indeed, the weight loss confirms this parasite infection.

B. Praziquantel (Biltricide) can readily eliminate the parasite. Call the patient's healthcare provider and share your thoughts about *D. latum* and the effectiveness of praziquantel. A single dose of 5–10 mg/kg is often adequate to eradicate this parasite and treat an infected patient.

If you are interested in learning more about cobalamin deficiency and the role of the GI tract in cobalamin absorption, read the *Introduction to Nutrients* chapter.

3.3 A. Azithromycin is the generic name for Zithromax, which belongs to the class of drugs known as macrolides. Macrolides bind to the prokaryotic 23rRNA of the 50S ribosomal subunit and block the elongation factor G (EF-G) from translocating ribosomes along the mRNA, thereby inhibiting the bacterial protein synthetic machinery.

B. Diarrhea. You might suggest giving Brad yogurt if he has diarrhea because of azithromycin. However, persistent or severe diarrhea should be reported to his pediatrician. Azithromycin may also cause abnormal changes in the electrical activity of the heart leading to fatal arrhythmias, particularly in patients with existing QT-interval prolongation, hypokalemia, or hypomagnesemia.

3.4 A. Fluoroquinolones are known to damage cartilage and bone and can cause tendon rupture. It is likely that the pain in her swollen ankle comes from the tendon rupture.

B. Her rashes are also likely associated with the use of gemifloxacin. Gemifloxacin is known to cause rashes in 14% of women older than the age of 40 who use gemifloxacin for longer than 7 days. To avoid this adverse effect, the course of therapy has been changed to 5 days.

C. Eva should discontinue gemifloxacin and contact her physician. Because she has been using gemifloxacin for 7 days, the course of therapy may have been adequate, which can be confirmed by her physician with a lab test.

3.5 A. Blurred vision is one of the significant adverse effects from isoniazid and may explain the patient's impaired vision.

B. One of the major side effects of pyrazinamide is malaise.

C. Isoniazid can bind pyridoxal phosphate (PLP), which comes from pyridoxine (vitamin B_6), and induce a vitamin B_6 deficiency. Because PLP is important for the synthesis of a few neurotransmitters (e.g., decarboxylase enzymes that convert histidine to histamine, glutamate to GABA, tryptophan to serotonin, and dopa to dopamine), David's altered mental status is likely caused by the vitamin B_6 deficiency. A vitamin B_6 supplement is needed to complement his isoniazid therapy.

D. Suggest to David to continue to take a vitamin B_6 supplement (25 mg/day) as long as he is using isoniazid. If his mental status does not improve after one week, he should contact his physician to identify the cause of his altered mental status. In addition, advise David to take his isoniazid tablets 1 hour before meals on an empty stomach. The malaise adverse effect will stop when pyrazinamide is stopped after 2 months, and David should not worry that he is developing Alzheimer's disease.

3.6 A. Tizanidine is extensively metabolized in the liver by CYP1A2. Ciprofloxacin is a strong inhibitor of CYP1A2. This drug interaction may inhibit tizanidine's metabolism, leading to significantly increased serum levels of this drug. Increased serum levels of tizanidine have been associated with a drop in the blood pressure, somnolence, and impaired psychomotor performance. A decreased heart rate has also been observed. Concurrent use of tizanidine and ciprofloxacin is contraindicated and is marked with the warning "Risk X: avoid combination."

B. Suggest to your preceptor that you call the patient's physician and ask him or her to change the ciprofloxacin to another antibiotic. If the patient took her last tizanidine dose more than 20 hours ago (tizanidine has a short half-life of 2.5 hours), it should have been eliminated from her plasma, so it is safe for her to take ciprofloxacin. Patients should never concurrently use ciprofloxacin and tizanidine.

Problems and Solutions

Problem 3.1 Which of the following best describes the term *epidemiology*?

A. The study of microorganism patterns, causes, and prevention of human diseases
B. An occurrence of a contagious disease that spreads rapidly
C. When a disease occurs widely over a very large area
D. The ability of microorganisms, including bacteria, fungi, protozoa, viruses, and parasites, to cause infectious diseases

Solution 3.1 A is correct. B is epidemic, C is pandemic, and D is pathogenicity.

Problem 3.2 Which of the following statements is incorrect in regard to GI bacteria?

A. The GI tract of an adult human contains approximately 1 kg of bacteria.
B. The largest amounts of bacteria are found in the colon.
C. The GI bacteria create a tight junction between epithelial cells, which results in formation of a barrier to allow drugs to pass between these cells.
D. Steroid drugs reduce the intestinal bacteria.
E. Administration of antibiotics, such as erythromycin and azithromycin, reduces the intestinal bacteria.

Solution 3.2 D is correct.

Problem 3.3 The enterohepatic circulation is an important mechanism that allows _____ to be more available in the GI system.

A. antibiotics
B. antacids
C. antidiabetic agents
D. oral contraceptives
E. antiviral agents

Solution 3.3 D is correct.

Problem 3.4 What does *granulocytopenia* mean? Give an example.

Solution 3.4 Granulocytopenia refers to a reduced number of white blood cells as a result of an underlying hematologic cancer, cancer chemotherapy, or infection with aerobic bacteria and fungi. For instance, individuals with granulocytopenia are prone to infection with *Candida albicans*, a fungus that causes blood and organ infections.

Problem 3.5 Which of the following factors does (do) not lead to a compromised immune system?

A. Age and disease
B. Medications and medical devices
C. Malnutrition and stress
D. Cigarette smoking
E. Extensive aerobic exercise

Solution 3.5 E is correct. Indeed, it has been reported that regular exercise increases the amount of perforin. Perforin is a molecule that is important for natural killer (NK) cells and cytotoxic T cells to effectively fight viruses and tumor cells (see also the *Introduction to Immunology* chapter).

Problem 3.6 What is the study of fungal infection called?

    A. Fungiology
    B. Mycology
    C. Virology
    D. Microbiology

Solution 3.6 While D can be correct, B is the best answer. The word "fungiology" is a made-up term.

Problem 3.7 Which of the following statements is incorrect regarding fungi?

    A. Fungi have a nucleus and reproduce both sexually and asexually.
    B. Fungi's survival depends solely on absorption of nutrients from either living or dead organisms.
    C. There are approximately 80,000 species of fungi but fewer than 50 species cause fungal infections of animals.
    D. Fungi are ~~prokaryotic~~ organisms. *eukaryote*
    E. Fungi live in plants, animals, or other fungi.

Solution 3.7 D is incorrect; fungi are simple eukaryotic organisms.

Problem 3.8 Differentiate between clinical resistance and microbial resistance.

Solution 3.8 Clinical resistance refers to *in vivo* development of resistance to an antifungal agent that is caused by factors other than microbial resistance—for instance, when resistance emerges because the antifungal agent cannot reach the site of infection or when the immune system cannot eliminate the fungus. Microbial resistance refers to *in vitro* development of resistance—that is, when the fungus does not respond to an antifungal agent during *in vitro* susceptibility testing.

Problem 3.9 Which of the following mechanisms is not an underlying cause of azole antifungal resistance?

    A. Mutations in the gene for 14-α-lanosterol demethylase (the enzyme that synthesizes ergosterol)
    B. Modification of the fungi's ribosomes
    C. Cellular rejection of the drug by the multidrug efflux transport pumps
    D. Post-translational modification of 14-α-lanosterol demethylase
    E. Alteration of fungi's cell membrane proteins

Solution 3.9 B is not an underlying cause for azole antifungal resistance.

Problem 3.10 True or False: The immune system's ability to fight parasites is not as effective as its ability to protect against bacteria and viruses. Therefore, many parasites have the ability to escape the immune response.

Solution 3.10 True.

Problem 3.11 Which parasite causes human African trypanosomiasis (African sleeping sickness)?

    A. *Ascaris*
    B. *Diphyllobothrium latum*
    C. *Trypanosoma*
    D. *Plasmodium falciparum*

Solution 3.11 C is correct. A is a common intestinal roundworm, B causes vitamin B$_{12}$ deficiency, and D causes malaria.

Problem 3.12 Which of the following statements about malaria is incorrect?

A. Malaria is a parasitic infectious disease that is transmitted by the bites of infected *Anopheles* mosquitoes.

B. Approximately one-third of the world's population lives in areas that are affected by malaria organisms, which indicates that malaria is a global health issue.

C. Approximately 2 million deaths occur globally due to a lack of prophylactic approach, inadequate or inappropriate chemoprophylaxis, and a lack of medical care for malaria.

D. Most cases of malaria in the United States involve travelers from the endemic areas.

E. Malaria symptoms are different from symptoms associated with bacterial and viral infections.

Solution 3.12 E is correct; malaria symptoms are similar to symptoms of bacterial and viral infections and include fever, chills, sweats, headache, malaise, fatigue, myalgia, and nausea and vomiting.

Problem 3.13 Define the following virology-related terms: viroids, virusoids, virions.

Solution 3.13 Viroids are naked (there is no capsid), cyclical, mostly double-stranded small RNAs that are replicated by the cellular RNA polymerase II and infect only plants. Virusoids are nucleic acids that need assistance from helper viruses to package their nucleic acids into virus-like particles. A virion is a complete virus particle, with this term indicating both the intactness of the viral structure and the property of infectiousness.

Problem 3.14 Which of the following statements is (are) correct in regard to retroviruses? Choose all that apply.

A. Retroviruses have an RNA genome.

B. Retroviruses have a reverse transcriptase enzyme.

C. Retroviruses have a dense core and an envelope that surrounds the core.

D. Retroviruses can synthesize a DNA copy of the viral RNA and integrate that DNA into the host cell's genome.

E. Retroviruses have DNA as their genome.

Solution 3.14 All are correct except E.

Problem 3.15 Which of the following statements is correct regarding treatment of patients with HIV infection?

A. An effective treatment for HIV-infected patients is to use two NRTIs and one NNRTI or one PI.

B. An effective treatment for HIV-infected patients is to use two PIs and two NRTIs.

C. An effective treatment for HIV-infected patients is to use one NRTI and one NNRTI.

D. An effective treatment for HIV-infected patients is to use one NRTI and two PIs.

Solution 3.15 A is correct.

Problem 3.16 Which of the following proteins facilitate(s) binding of HIV to the host's CD4 cells? Choose all that apply.

A. Glycoprotein 120 (gp120)

B. Chemokine CCR5

C. TNF

D. HIV proteases

Solution 3.16 Both A and B are correct; A is from HIV, B is from the host's CD4 cell.

Problem 3.17 Which of the following antibiotics blocks the translocation step in the protein synthetic machinery?

   A.   Streptomycin
   B.   Neomycin
   C.   Erythromycin
   D.   Chloramphenicol
   E.   Tetracycline

Solution 3.17 C is correct; erythromycin blocks the elongation factor G (EF-G), which in turn blocks ribosomes from translocating on an mRNA during bacterial protein synthesis.

Problem 3.18 Which of the following statements is correct regarding antibacterial agents that act on bacterial cell wall synthesis?

   A.   The major cause for developing resistance to β-lactam antibiotics is the production of beta-lactamase enzyme.
   B.   The major cause for developing resistance to β-lactam antibiotics is the production of an enzyme that alters ribosomes.
   C.   Both ribosomal RNA (rRNA) and ribosomal proteins play important roles in development of resistance.
   D.   The lactam ring plays a major role in antibacterial agents that act on bacterial cell wall synthesis.

Solution 3.18 A is correct. While the lactam ring is important, it is not capable of inhibiting bacterial cell wall synthesis by itself.

Problem 3.19 Describe how mupirocin inhibits the bacterial protein synthetic machinery.

Solution 3.19 Mupirocin inhibits the enzymatic activity of the isoleucyl-tRNA synthetase by blocking the binding site of the intermediate substrate (Ile–AMP). This results in lack of a charged-tRNA^{Ile} during the bacterial protein synthesis.

Problem 3.20 Which of the following antibiotics blocks the A site of ribosomes and does not allow a charged tRNA to participate in protein synthesis?

   A.   Neomycin
   B.   Erythromycin
   C.   Mupirocin
   D.   Tetracycline
   E.   Gentamicin

Solution 3.20 D is correct.

References

1.   Anandan V. Parasitic diseases. In: Talbert RL, DiPiro JT, Matzke GR, et al., eds. *Pharmacotherapy: A pathophysiologic approach.* 8th ed. New York, NY: McGraw-Hill; 2011. Available at: http://www .accesspharmacy.com/content.aspx?aID–8003911.

2.   Annane D. Resurrection of steroids for sepsis resuscitation. *Minerva Anesthesiol.* 2002;68(4):127–131.

3.   Annane D, Cavaillon JM. Corticosteroids in sepsis: from bench to bedside? *Shock.* 2003;20(3):197–207.

4.   Arya N, Girgraph N, Levy G. Hepatitis C. In: *AccessScience.* New York, NY: McGraw-Hill; 2003. Available at: http://www.accessscience.com. Association of Schools of Public Health. Available at: http://www.whatispublichealth.org/about/index.html.

5. Bloch KC. Infectious diseases. In: McPhee SJ, Hammer GD. *Pathophysiology of disease: an intro- duction to clinical medicine.* 6th ed. 2000. Available at: http://www.accesspharmacy.com/content .aspx?aID=5366994.

6. Brimacombe R, Wittmann HG, Joseph S. Ribosomes. In: *AccessScience.* New York, NY: McGraw-Hill; 2008. Available at: http://www.accessscience.com.

7. Brooks GF, Carroll KC, Butel JS, et al. The science of microbiology. In: Brooks GF, Carroll KC, Butel JS, et al., eds. *Jawetz, Melnick, & Adelberg's medical microbiology.* 25th ed. 2010. Available at: http://www.accesspharmacy.com/content.aspx?aID=6426001.

8. Brooks GF, Carroll KC, Butel JS, et al. The growth, survival, and death of microorganisms. In: Brooks GF, Carroll KC, Butel JS, et al., eds. *Jawetz, Melnick, & Adelberg's medical microbiology.* 25th ed. New York, NY: McGraw-Hill; 2010. Available at: http://www.accesspharmacy.com /content.aspx?aID=6426424.

9. Brooks GF, Carroll KC, Butel JS, et al. Antimicrobial chemotherapy. In: Brooks GF, Carroll KC, Butel JS, et al., eds. *Jawetz, Melnick, & Adelberg's medical microbiology.* 25th ed. New York, NY: McGraw-Hill; 2010. Available at: http://www.accesspharmacy.com/content.aspx?aID=6429657.

10. Carver PL. Invasive fungal infections. In: Talbert RL, DiPiro JT, Matzke GR, et al., eds. *Pharmacotherapy: a pathophysiologic approach.* 8th ed. New York, NY: McGraw-Hill; 2011. Available at: http://www.accesspharmacy.com/content.aspx?aID=8005562.

11. Cohen JO. Toxic shock syndrome. In: *AccessScience.* New York, NY: McGraw-Hill; 2008. Available at: http://www.accessscience.com.

12. Dabbs DJ. Herpes. In: *AccessScience.* New York, NY: McGraw-Hill; 2008. Available at: http://www.accessscience.com.

13. Deming P, Mercier RC, Pai MP. Viral hepatitis. In: DiPiro JT, Talbert RL, Yee GC, et al., eds. *Pharmacotherapy: a pathophysiologic approach.* 7th ed. American College of Clinical Pharmacy; 2008. Available at: http://www.accesspharmacy.com/content.aspx?aID=3201001.

14. Doyle M. Food poisoning. In: *AccessScience.* New York, NY: McGraw-Hill; 2008. Available at: http://www.accessscience.com.

15. Ebadi M. *Desk reference of clinical pharmacology.* 2nd ed. CRC Press; 2007.

16. Hammar SP. Hepatitis. In: *AccessScience.* New York, NY: McGraw-Hill; 2008. Available at: http://www.accessscience.com.

17. Handsfield HH. Sexually transmitted diseases. In: *AccessScience.* New York, NY: McGraw-Hill; 2008. Available at: http://www.accessscience.com.

18. Feldman SF, Ruth NE. Public health. In: Nemire RE, Kier KL. *Pharmacy student survival guide.* 2nd ed. New York, NY: McGraw-Hill; 2009; 521–535.

19. Finberg R, Fingeroth J. Infections in transplant recipients. In: Fauci AS, Braunwald E, Kasper DL, et al. *Harrison's principles of internal medicine.* 17th ed. New York, NY: McGraw-Hill; 2008. Available at: http://www.accesspharmacy.com/content.aspx?aID=2893988, 2008.

20. Fine JS. Pediatric principles. In: Fine JS, ed. *Goldfrank's toxicologic emergencies.* 9th ed. New York, NY: McGraw-Hill; 2011. Available at: http://www.accesspharmacy.com/content.aspx?aID=6509216.

21. Flexner C. Antiretroviral agents and treatment of HIV infection. In: Chabner BA, Brunton LL, Knollmann BC, eds. *Goodman & Gilman's the pharmacological basis of therapeutics.* 12th ed. New York, NY: McGraw-Hill; 2011. Available at: http://www.accesspharmacy.com/content. aspx?aID=16679561.

22. Fred W, Elliott K. Medical virology. In: Fauci AS, Braunwald E, Kasper DL, et al. *Harrison's prin- ciples of internal medicine.* 17th ed. New York, NY: 2008. Available at: http://www.accesspharmacy .com/content.aspx?aID=2873184.

23. Gladwin M, Trattler B. *Clinical microbiology made ridiculously simple.* Miami, FL: MedMaster; 2004.

24. Gourley DR, Eoff JC, eds. *The APhA complete review for pharmacy*. 9th ed. Washington, DC: APhA; 2012.

25. Hayden FG. Antiviral agents (nonretroviral). In: Brunton LL, Lazo JS, Parker KL. *Goodman & Gilman's the pharmacological basis of therapeutics*. 11th ed. New York, NY: McGraw-Hill; 2005. Available at: http://www.accesspharmacy.com/content.aspx?aID=950476.

26. Johnson RR, Williams WA, Albaugh R. Agricultural science (animal). In: *AccessScience*. New York, NY: McGraw-Hill; 2008. Available at: http://www.accessscience.com.

27. Joklik WK, Pierce MM. Virus. In: *AccessScience*. New York, NY: McGraw-Hill; 2008. Available at: http://www.accessscience.com.

28. Kennelly PJ, Rodwell VW. Proteins: higher orders of structure. In: Murray RK, Kennelly PJ, Rodwell VW, et al., eds. *Harper's illustrated biochemistry*. 29th ed. New York, NY: McGraw-Hill; 2011. Available at: http://www.accesspharmacy.com/content.aspx?aID=55881356.

29. Kis O, Zastre JA, Hoque T, et al. Role of drug efflux and uptake transporters in atazanavir intestinal permeability and drug–drug interactions. *Pharm Res*. 2013;30:1050–1064.

30. Lewis JS. Antifungal agents. In: *AccessScience*. New York, NY: McGraw-Hill; 2007. Available at: http://www.accessscience.com.

31. MacDougall C. Protein synthesis inhibitors and miscellaneous antibacterial agents. In: Chabner BA, Brunton LL, Knollman BC, eds. *Goodman & Gilman's the pharmacological basis of therapeutics*. 12th ed. New York, NY: McGraw-Hill; 2011. Available at: http://www.accesspharmacy.com/content.aspx?aID=16677888.

32. Macher AM, Goosby EP. Acquired immune deficiency syndrome (AIDS). In: *AccessScience*. New York, NY: McGraw-Hill; 2008. Available at: http://www.accessscience.com.

33. Marx PA. Retrovirus. In: *AccessScience*. New York, NY: McGraw-Hill; 2008. Available at: http://www.accessscience.com.

34. McNamara PJ. Infectious disease. In: *AccessScience*. New City, NY: McGraw-Hill; 2008. Available at: http://www.accessscience.com.

35. Montville TJ. Food microbiology. In: *AccessScience*. New York, NY: McGraw-Hill; 2008. Available at: http://www.accessscience.com.

36. Moore TA. Agents used to treat parasitic infections. In: Fauci AS, Kasper DL, Jameson JL, et al., eds. *Harrison's principles of internal medicine*. 18th ed. New York, NY: McGraw-Hill; 2012. Available at: http://www.accesspharmacy.com/content.aspx?aID=9111202.

37. Morse SA, Brooks GF, Carroll KC, et al. Pathogenesis and control of viral diseases. In: Morse SA, Brooks GF, Carroll KC, et al., eds. *Jawetz, Melnick, & Adelberg's medical microbiology*. 25th ed. New York, NY: McGraw-Hill; 2010. Available at: http://www.accesspharmacy.com/content.aspx?aID=6430454.

38. Morse SA, Brooks GF, Carroll KC, et al. Medical mycology. In: Morse SA, Brooks GF, Carroll KC, et al., eds. *Jawetz, Melnick, & Adelberg's medical microbiology*. 25th ed. New York: McGraw-Hill; 2010. Available at: http://www.accesspharmacy.com/content.aspx?aID=6432990.

39. Murphy R. Opportunistic infections. In: *AccessScience*. New York, NY: McGraw-Hill; 2008. Available at: http://www.accessscience.com.

40. Nelson DL, Cox MM. *Principles of biochemistry*. 5th ed. New York, NY: W. H. Freeman and Company; 2008.

41. Neofytos D, Horn D, Anaissie E, et al. Epidemiology and outcome of invasive fungal infection in adult hematopoietic stem cell transplant recipients: analysis of Multicenter Prospective Antifungal Therapy (PATH) Alliance registry. *Clin Infect Dis*. 2009;48:265–273.

42. Njoku JC, Hermsen ED. Influenza. In: Talbert RL, DiPiro JT, Matzke GR, et al., eds. *Pharmacotherapy: a pathophysiologic approach*. 8th ed. New York, NY: McGraw-Hill; 2011. Available at: http://www.accesspharmacy.com/content.aspx?aID=8002170.

43. Pierce MM, Reichmann ME. Virus classification. In: *AccessScience*. New York, NY: McGraw-Hill; 2008. Available at: http://www.accessscience.com.

44. Pringle CR. *The classification of vertebrate viruses*. Hoboken, NJ: John Wiley & Sons; 2010.

45. Sanglard D, Odds FC. Resistance of *Candida* species to antifungal agents: molecular mechanisms and clinical consequences. *Lancet Infect Dis*. 2002;2:73185.

46. Schimmer BP, Parker KL. Adrenocorticotropic hormone; adrenocortical steroids and their synthetic analogs; inhibitors of the synthesis and actions of adrenocortical hormones. In: Brunton LL, Lazo JS, Parker KL. *Goodman & Gilman's the pharmacological basis of therapeutics*. 11th ed. New York, NY: McGraw-Hill; 2006.

47. Slain D. Invasive fungal infections. In: Slain D, ed. *McGraw-Hill's NAPLEX® review guide*. New York, NY: McGraw-Hill; 2011. Available at: http://www.accesspharmacy.com/content. aspx?aID=7252384.

48. Stork CM. Antibacterials, antifungals, and antivirals. In: Nelson LS, Lewin NA, Howland MA, et al. *Goldfrank's toxicologic emergencies*. 9th ed. New York, NY: McGraw-Hill; 2010. Available at: http://www.accesspharmacy.com/content.aspx?aID=6515644.

49. Talbert RL, DiPiro JT, Matzke GR, et al. Antimicrobial regimen selection. In: Talbert RL, DiPiro JT, Matzke GR, et al., eds. *Pharmacotherapy: a pathophysiologic approach*. 8th ed. New York, NY: McGraw-Hill; 2011. Available at: http://www.accesspharmacy.com/content.aspx?aID=8001114.

50. Tilton RC, Spiegel CA. Clinical microbiology. In: *AccessScience*. New York, NY: McGraw-Hill; 2008. Available at: http://www.accessscience.com.

51. Trevor AJ, Katzung BG, Masters SB. Beta-lactam antibiotics and other cell wall synthesis inhibitors. In: Trevor AJ, Katzung BG, Masters SB. *Pharmacology: examination & board review*. 9th ed. New York, NY: McGraw-Hill; 2010. Available at: http://www.accesspharmacy.com/content .aspx?aID=6546134.

52. Tunkel AR, Hartman BJ, Kaplan SL, et al. Practice guidelines for the management of bacterial meningitis. *Clin Infect Dis*. 2004;39:1267–1284.

53. UpToDate. Waltham, MA: 2012. Available at: http://www.uptodate.com/online with subscription.

54. U.S. Department of Health and Human Services, National Institutes of Health, National Institute of Allergy and Infectious Diseases (NIAID). 2013. Available at: http://www.niaid.nih.gov/news /newsreleases/2013/Pages/toddlerfunctionallycured.aspx.

55. Voss EW. Microbiology. In: *AccessScience*. New York, NY: McGraw-Hill; 2008. Available at: http://www.accessscience.com.

56. Weis F, Andres BF, Kaczmarek I, et al.. Daptomycin for eradication of a systemic infection with a methicillin-resistant *Staphylococcus aureus* in a biventricular assist device recipient. *Ann Thorac Surg*. 2007;84:269–270.

57. Wilkinson B. Virulence. In: *AccessScience*. New York, NY: McGraw-Hill; 2008. Available at: http://www.accessscience.com.

58. Wildman HG. Fungi (medicine). In: *AccessScience*. New York, NY: McGraw-Hill; 2001. Available at: http://www.accessscience.com.

Introduction to Immunology

Reza Karimi
Ian C. Doyle

OBJECTIVES

1. Describe the organs and cells that are involved in the human immune system.

2. Identify the roles of the various subtypes of helper T cells and major histocompatibility complexes.

3. Define humoral immunity and identify the structure and function of antibodies; recognize biological drugs that act as antibodies.

4. Summarize the host cellular responses and the roles of antigens in fighting infections.

5. Define cytokines and understand the roles of highlighted cytokines.

6. List and differentiate the various types of hypersensitivities and mediators in the development of hypersensitivity reactions.

7. Explain the clinical features of systemic lupus erythematosus (SLE) and give examples of drugs that cause SLE.

8. Discuss immune deficiencies and opportunistic infections caused by pathogenic organisms.

9. Define the different phases of HIV progression.

10. Discuss vaccines, the vaccination process, and the therapeutic usefulness of vaccines.

11. Implement a series of Learning Bridge assignments at your experiential sites to bridge your didactic learning with your experiential experiences.

KEY TERMS AND DEFINITIONS

1. **Antigen:** a molecule that triggers the production of an antibody by the immune system.

2. **Apoptosis:** a regulated process of programmed cell death.

3. **Chemokines:** low-molecular-weight proteins that attract neutrophils and leukocytes to the areas of inflammation.

4. **Cluster of differentiation (CD):** cell surface proteins that are present on lymphocytes.

5. **Complement:** a group of more than 30 serum proteins that, when activated, initiate an inflammatory response, phagocytosis of antigens, and lysis of cells.

6. **ELISA:** Enzyme-linked immunosorbent assay; an analytical method to detect an antibody against a specific antigen.

7. **Epitope:** a specific part of an antigen that is directly recognized by antibodies and T-cell receptors.

8. **Granulocytopenia:** a medical condition characterized by a reduced number of blood granulocytes (neutrophils, eosinophils, and basophils).

9. **Hapten:** a foreign chemical that, when attached to an endogenous protein, is recognized by the immune system.

(continues)

10. **Immunization:** the induction of immunity by any means, including an active or passive process that may or may not involve a vaccine.

11. **Interleukins:** cytokines that primarily serve as communicators between leukocytes.

12. **Leukocytopenia:** a medical condition characterized by a decreased white blood cell count in blood (fewer than 4,500 cells/mm^3).

13. **Leukocytosis:** a medical condition characterized by an increased white blood cell count in blood (more than 11,000 cells/mm^3).

14. **Lymphadenopathy:** enlarged lymph nodes; common in HIV-infected individuals.

15. **Lymphocytosis:** an increased blood concentration of lymphocytes (more than 4×10^9 cells/mm^3).

16. **Lymphokines:** cytokines that are secreted from lymphocytes.

17. **Major histocompatibility complex (MHC):** a series of genes found on chromosome 6 in humans; also called human leukocyte antigen (HLA) complex.

18. **Monoclonal antibody:** an antibody (immunoglobulin) that is synthesized by a single clone of plasma B cells.

19. **Monokines:** cytokines that are secreted from monocytes or macrophages.

20. **Naive T lymphocytes:** T cells that have not yet been exposed to an antigen.

21. **Neutropenia:** a medical condition characterized by an abnormally low number of neutrophils in the blood.

22. **Opsonization:** the action of coating an infectious agent by antibodies or complement components so that the complex effectively becomes engulfed by phagocytes, initiating phagocytosis.

23. **Phagocytosis:** the process by which a cell is engulfed and destroyed.

24. **Plasma viremia:** the presence of a virus in the bloodstream.

25. **Polyclonal antibodies:** a collection of antibodies (immunoglobulins) that are produced by many different lineages of plasma B cells.

26. **Primary viremia:** the spread of a virus from the initial site of infection to the bloodstream.

27. **Secondary viremia:** the state in which primary viremia reaches additional tissues via the bloodstream.

28. **Vaccine:** a preparation, usually biologic, that evokes an immune response in the body to that substance.

29. **Vaccination:** administration of a vaccine with the intent to provoke immunity.

Introduction

Immunology is the science that studies an organism's immune system and its ability to generate specific and nonspecific defense mechanisms. Since the English physician Edward Jenner initiated the fight against smallpox in 1796, the world of science has witnessed many discoveries concerned with defense mechanisms. Similarly, our understanding of genetic and environmental factors and their influences on various diseases of the immune system have grown dramatically. These enormous advances have contributed significantly to the field of immunology. Today, immunology is concerned with examining how a host is protected from invading infectious agents and with exploring the important roles that the human immune system plays in allergy, autoimmune disease, transplant rejection, and fighting tumors.

This chapter introduces the basic elements of immunology, providing an overview of innate and adaptive immunities, the essential molecules in evolving defense mechanisms of the human immune system, and the varying degrees of immune responses that develop secondary to allergen exposure. In addition, the vital roles that vaccination and manipulation of the immune system play in protecting the human body from invading infectious agents and tumors are addressed.

The Immune System: Overview and Divisions

The immune system plays a crucial role in our everyday survival by fighting viruses, bacteria, parasites, and toxins produced by some pathogenic bacteria during an infection. Animals have both specific and nonspecific defense mechanisms against pathogenic organisms. In addition, several other means of protecting against pathogenic microorganisms are available. For instance, an animal's skin is a nonspecific mechanism (physical barrier) that protects the animal from infection. Other examples of defense mechanisms include the lysozymes found in saliva and tears; the normal flora in the lower gastrointestinal tract; and mucous membranes in which mucous neck cells secrete mucins—large glycoproteins that form a mucus layer that adheres to the surface of epithelial cells of the stomach and protects these cells from gastric acid and potentially invasive bacteria.

The human immune system includes both cells that fight infectious pathogens and cells that produce mediators that assist the body in fighting foreign invaders. During embryonic development, blood cell precursors form and accumulate in the liver and yolk sac. However, in postnatal life, it is the stem cells from bone marrow that differentiate into cells of the myeloid line (monocytes, macrophages, neutrophils, basophils, eosinophils, erythrocytes, platelets, dendritic cells) and lymphoid line (B and T lymphocytes). Lymphocytes account for some 15% to 40% of all white blood cells (WBCs). A complete blood count (CBC) is a routine laboratory test that indicates the hemoglobin (Hgb) content, hematocrit (Hct), and number of white blood cells and red blood cells (RBCs) in the blood. The WBC count often alerts healthcare providers to the presence of an infection. When the number of WBCs is increased, the condition is referred to as leukocytosis; this state may be attributable to factors such as infection, certain cancers, trauma, emotion, stress, thyroid storm, and use of corticosteroids.

There are two types of lymphocytes: T cells and B cells. The ratio of T cells to B cells is approximately 3:1. **Figure 4.1** depicts the formation of various types of cells from bone marrow stem cells.

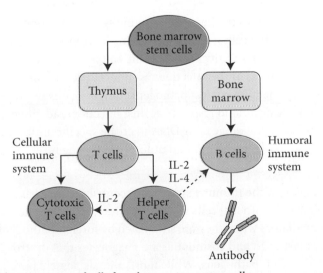

Figure 4.1 Formation of various types of cells from bone marrow stem cells.

Table 4.1 Major Differences Between Innate and Adaptive Immunities

	Innate Immunity	Adaptive Immunity
Molecules and cells	Complement proteins, granulocytes (basophils, eosinophils, and neutrophils), mast cells, macrophages, dendritic cells, and natural killer cells	Immunoglobulin, B cells, CD4$^+$ and CD8$^+$ T cells
Function and efficiency	Rapid response to destroy foreign or infected cells, but with a lower potency	Slow response to destroy infected cells, but with a higher potency
Specificity	While effectively recognizing pathogens, does not embrace specificity	Very specific
Memory	Does not develop memory	Develops memory that protects the host upon reentry of the same pathogens
Antigen-presenting cells	Macrophages and dendritic cells	B cells
Reaction time	Hours	Days

The immune system is organized into two major immune-response types: adaptive immunity and innate immunity. Adaptive immunity includes B cells and the antibodies they produce, as well as CD4$^+$ (helper) and CD8$^+$ (cytotoxic) T lymphocytes that differentiate, grow, adapt, and develop memory predicated on the presentation of specific antigens. Innate immunity consists of complement proteins, granulocytes (basophils, eosinophils, and neutrophils), mast cells, macrophages, dendritic cells, and natural killer (NK) cells. These cells respond to lipids and carbohydrates that are specific to bacterial cell walls, tumors, and transplanted cells. The cells that provide innate immunity do not need antigen stimulation to develop or grow, so they are always ready to provide the first line of defense against infections. **Table 4.1** indicates differences between adaptive and innate immunities.

Adaptive immunity is further divided into two groups: humoral-mediated and cell-mediated immunities. While the humoral immune system is activated to fight bacterial and viral infections that are found in the "humor" (*humor*, a Latin word, means "fluid") or serum (i.e., extracellular invaders prior to their entry into host cells), the cellular immune system fights cells that are already infected by viruses or parasites.

Antibodies are the key players in the humoral immune system. Antibodies are produced by B lymphocytes (or B cells). In the cellular immune system, T lymphocytes (or T cells) are the key players (Figure 4.1). Innate immunity is nonspecific and is always prepared to fight a broad array of organisms (i.e., regardless of the infectious agents). However, innate immunity defense mechanisms offer limited protection against pathogenic microorganisms. While innate immunity includes genes that provide a rapid response against infections, adaptive immunity utilizes B cells, which have the ability to rearrange their DNA to create specific antibodies to bind individual antigens. Innate immunity exists from birth and utilizes preexisting receptors to recognize and eliminate pathogens.

Other cells not belonging to the immune system also contribute to innate immune responses. For example, endothelial and epithelial cells release cytokines upon their activation—that is, they release inflammatory mediators when they are stimulated by foreign pathogens. In contrast, macrophages, neutrophils, mast cells, and eosinophils are phagocytes that destroy invading pathogens upon recognition of the foreign pathogens. While most animals possess both types of immunities, some—such as insects and other invertebrates—rely solely on their innate immunities.

Both humoral- and cell-mediated responses of the adaptive immune system share three important features:

- They are diverse (i.e., they can respond to millions of different antigens).
- They can possess memory (i.e., they are ready to be produced in large amounts should the body be exposed to the same antigen for a second time).
- They are specific (i.e., their actions are directed against the antigen that initiated the immune response).

Lymph Nodes and Lymph

Lymph nodes are bean-shaped tissues that, from a morphologic standpoint, have reticular cells and fibers that are organized into a cortex and a medulla. A lymph node is surrounded by a collagenous capsule and has a groove, called a hilum, where blood vessels enter and leave. The lymph nodes are usually found in the armpits, on both sides of the neck, and in the groin and legs. They are responsible for draining and filtering soluble antigens from interstitial fluid. Antigen-presenting cells (dendritic cells and macrophages) and lymphocytes (B and T cells) may then encounter the trapped antigens in the lymph nodes and initiate an immune response. The lymph that comes to a lymph node from a tumor, an infected tissue, or an inflamed area may also contain cancer cells, bacteria, or cytokines, respectively.

Within the circulatory system, when arterial blood reaches the capillaries, interstitial fluid is formed. While a small volume of this interstitial fluid returns to the venous flow via the capillaries, a larger proportion of it enters the lymphatic vessels to form lymph. Lymph is a clear fluid primarily composed of water containing lymphocytes and proteins. It enters the lymph nodes through afferent lymphatic vessels, flows through a series of channels called sinuses, and departs the nodes through efferent lymphatic vessels at the hilum (**Figure 4.2**). After leaving the node, the lymph flow empties into larger lymphatic channels leading to the thoracic duct, which in turn drains into the left subclavian vein. In this way, the lymph returns to the systemic circulation. As noted earlier, abnormal cells such as neoplastic cells can be trapped and removed from the lymph nodes as part of the lymph flow.

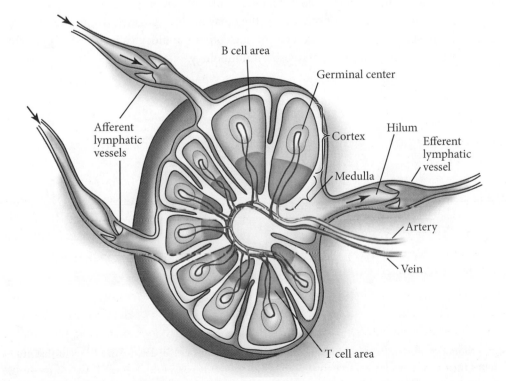

Figure 4.2 The anatomy of a lymph node.

The structure of lymph vessels differs from the structure of blood vessels in several ways. For instance, there is very little, if any, basal lamina under the endothelium, and there are no tight intercellular connections between endothelial cells.

A swollen lymph node is an indication of the presence of additional lymphocytes, which in turn is an indication that the body is fighting an infection. Thus the lymph nodes are the primary sites of immune response to tissue antigens. Indeed, because lymph nodes are found in the underarm, during the regional spread of cancer cells, these cells—particularly breast cancer cells—spread first to the underarm lymph nodes. For this reason, identifying whether the lymph nodes contain cancer cells is an important indicator when diagnosing breast cancer. It is from these lymph nodes that the breast cancer cells can metastasize to bones, liver, lungs, and other parts of the body. Lymphoseek (technetium-99m [Tc-99m] tilmanocept) injection is a new diagnostic imaging agent approved by the FDA in March 2013. It is employed to locate lymph nodes in patients with breast cancer or melanoma, so that surgeons can then remove tumor-draining lymph nodes from patients.

Leukocytes

Leukocytes are white blood cells. There are approximately 4,000–11,000 WBC/µL of human blood. Many agents and drugs inhibit WBC production when they are given to patients in high doses or for prolonged use (e.g., alcohol, penicillins, ganciclovir).

There are two groups of WBCs: agranulocytes, which include monocytes (macrophages) and lymphocytes (B and T cells); and granulocytes, which include neutrophils, basophils, and eosinophils. Lymphocytes account for 15% to 40% of total WBCs (on average, 30%). In addition, lymphocytes include the so-called natural killer cells. Collectively, these cells provide powerful defense mechanisms against tumors, viruses, bacteria, and parasites. **Figure 4.3** depicts different cells within the lymphoid line.

Agranulocytes

Agranulocytes, as the name indicates, do not have cytoplasmic granules. As a consequence, their morphology is different from that of other cells; they may be distinguished from other cells based on size, chromatin structure, and the presence of nucleoli. Agranulocytes include lymphocytes and monocytes—both of which play crucial roles in immunology.

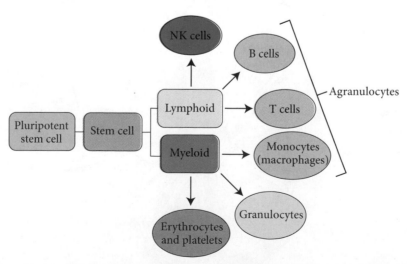

Figure 4.3 Monocytes, granulocytes, and B, T, and NK cells provide powerful defense mechanisms that protect the body against tumors, viruses, bacteria, and parasites.

Adapted from: Shen WC, Stan GL. *Immunology for pharmacy students.* Harwood Academic Publisher; 1999.

Monocytes and Macrophages

Monocytes originate in the bone marrow, circulate briefly in the blood (for 1–2 days), and then migrate into tissues to become macrophages. One way to differentiate between monocytes and macrophages is that macrophages have an increased number of Fc receptors (a protein that binds an antibody; see also Figure 4.8) and complement receptors.

Macrophages are found in the liver, spleen, gastrointestinal tract, lymph nodes, brain, bone, and connective tissue. In addition to their important role in the immune system, macrophages salvage iron from the degraded hemoglobin of old erythrocytes and return iron to the plasma iron transport protein (transferrin), thereby ensuring that iron is delivered to the bone marrow. Hydrocortisone—a steroid that is used as an anti-inflammatory agent, as an immunosuppressant, and for rheumatic disorders—decreases the population of neutrophils at the site of inflammation and inhibits macrophage function.

Macrophages play roles in three important processes: phagocytosis, antigen presentation, and cytokine production.

- In their phagocytic role, macrophages ingest bacteria, viruses, and other pathogens. Their Fc receptors interact with the Fc ligand of immunoglobulin G (IgG) to enhance the uptake of opsonized organisms. Upon ingestion, the microbe-containing phagosome fuses with a lysosome (forming a phagolysosome), killing the microbe by subjecting it to reactive oxygen, reactive nitrogen, and lysosomal enzymes.

- In their antigen-presenting role, following ingestion and degradation of the foreign agent, macrophages break the invader down into polypeptide fragments and present these fragments on the cell surface in conjunction with class II MHC proteins. The MHC II-fragment complex then interacts with the T-cell receptor (TCR) of CD4⁺ cells.

- In their cytokine-producing role, macrophages secrete several cytokines, interleukin-1 (IL-1), IL-8, and TNF (tumor necrosis factor). While IL-1 activates helper T cells, IL-8 attracts neutrophils and T cells to the site of infection. TNF is an important inflammatory mediator that is discussed in more depth later in this chapter.

Lymphocytes

All lymphocyte progenitor cells originate in the bone marrow. There are two main classes of lymphocytes: T lymphocytes (T cells), which kill viruses and tumor cells, and B lymphocytes (B cells), which produce antibodies.

T Cells

The thymus produces two types of T cells: cytotoxic T cells and helper T cells (the letter "T" refers to the thymus). Cytotoxic T cells and helper T cells constitute 35% and 65%, respectively, of the total T cell count. In the thymus, T cells express both antigen receptors and various CD (cluster of differentiation) proteins. The CD proteins can function as receptors or ligands. Initially, T cells express both CD4/CD8 (double-positives). However, through a selection process mediated by proteins collectively known as the major histocompatibility complex (MHC), they proceed to express either CD4 or CD8 before they leave the thymus. A small percentage (less than 5% of the lymphocyte population) of CD4/CD8 double-positive cells enter the periphery prematurely, particularly during viral infections. However, the exact mechanism of this premature release is not known.

While double-positive cells are processed in the cortex of the thymus, single-positive cells (differentiated into either CD4 or CD8) are processed in the medulla. The MHC proteins play two major roles in the immune system: (1) They assist the thymus in selecting T cells (positive selection) and (2) they present antigens to T cells so as to activate those T cells. In addition, the MHC proteins play an important role in the process of graft rejection.

Like T cells, B cells also undergo selection, albeit not in the thymus. The B cells that possess antigen receptors for self-proteins are eliminated to avoid any occurrence of autoimmune diseases. However, the site of this selection is not yet fully known.

All viruses multiply in the cytoplasm of the cells they infect. Because they do not have their own biosynthetic machinery, they can begin to replicate only when situated within the infected cells. Unfortunately, inside the cells, viruses are not detected by circulating antibodies. Therefore, a mechanism for their detection and elimination is needed. With the help of the cytotoxic T lymphocytes (CTLs; known also as CD8 cells) and NK cells, virally infected cells can be recognized and killed. The elimination of infected cells without destruction of other healthy cells requires that these CTL and NK cells be specific, powerful, and accurate.

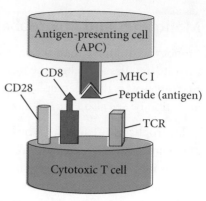

Figure 4.4 T cell receptors (TCR) play an important role in the recognition of a presented antigen.

Adapted from: Janeway CA, Travers P, Walport M. *Immunobiology: the immune system in health and disease.* 4th ed. New York: Elsevier Science /Garland; 1999: Chapter 8.

During T-cell development in the thymus, the double-positive T cell synthesizes a specific antigen receptor called the T-cell receptor (TCR). The unique gene rearrangement that occurs in the T cell results in the receptor being encoded early in the T-cell differentiation process. It accounts for the T cell's distinctive ability to recognize millions of different antigens.

In addition to the TCR, the T cell has two other co-receptors, CD4 and CD8, that enhance the binding interaction of TCR and MHC proteins (**Figure 4.4**). While the CD receptor for helper T cells is called CD4, the CD receptor for cytotoxic T cells is called CD8.

Not all T cells develop in the thymus. Notably, approximately 40% of all T cells develop in the gastrointestinal tract, in gut-associated lymphoid tissue (GALT). These lymphocytes are found in the epithelial layer of mucosal linings in the gastrointestinal tract and are called intraepithelial lymphocytes (IELs). IELs provide protection against intestinal pathogens. However, because these IELs have different antigen receptors than do the thymus-derived lymphocytes, they cannot substitute for thymus-derived lymphocytes. For instance, despite having effective IELs, patients with the immune deficiency disease known as DiGeorge syndrome are not immune to many infections.

Cytotoxic T Lymphocytes

As was discussed in the *Introduction to Microbiology* chapter, viruses infect only nucleated cells so that they can use the cellular replication, transcription, and protein synthetic machinery of the host cells. To kill an intracellular virus, then, the cytotoxic T cell must first lyse (rupture) the infected cell by recognizing and responding to the presented antigenic peptides encoded by the virus on the host cell's surface. Prior to this cell lysis, a series of events must take place. First, the antigen in the cytosol of the host cell is cleaved into small peptides by a complex of proteases known as the proteasome. Second, the peptide fragments are transported from the cytosol into the lumen of the endoplasmic reticulum (ER). Third, in the ER, the fragments become attached to an MHC class I molecule, which then is exported as a complex (peptide–class I) to the Golgi apparatus. In the final step, the peptide–class I complex appears at the cell surface where it can be recognized by a cytotoxic T cell.

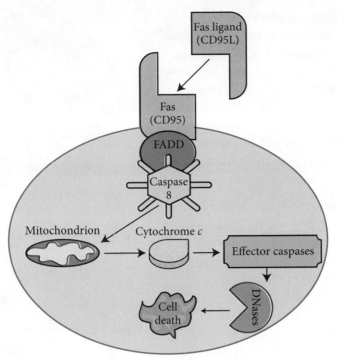

Figure 4.5 The Fas-FasL mechanism induces cell death.
Adapted from: Nelson DL, Cox MM, Lehninger AL. *Principles of biochemistry.* 5th ed. New York: W. H. Freeman and Company; 2008: Chapter 12.

There are two mechanisms by which cytotoxic T cells kill virally infected cells or tumor cells: the Fas-FasL mechanism and the granule-exocytosis mechanism.

Fas-FasL Mechanism. A series of cytoplasmic proteases called caspases is synthesized as inactive proteins (zymogen) in normal cells, but become activated (active proteases) upon receiving apoptotic signals. Caspases play important roles in the apoptotic process; apoptosis is a highly regulated process by which cells are genetically programmed for death. Because active caspases are proteases, they are capable of hydrolyzing their target proteins.

In the Fas-FasL mechanism, the Fas ligand (also referred to as CD95L) binds to its receptor, Fas (also referred to as CD95), on the surface of the target cell, which in turn is bound to a cytosolic protein called FADD (**Figure 4.5**). The Fas ligand is expressed mainly on $CD8^+$ CTL and NK cells. FADD sends a signal to procaspase 8 (zymogen) to undergo self-activation to form active caspase 8. Mitochondria are targets for the activated caspase 8. This protease causes the release of cytochrome *c*. Cytochrome *c*, together with caspase 8, then activates other caspases called effector caspases. The effector caspases, in turn, degrade cellular proteins and activate a nuclease (DNase) to digest the cell's DNA, which results in the cell's death. The dead cells are then recognized by phagocytes and are fully destroyed.

Granule-Exocytosis Mechanism. Tumor cells expressing low levels of Fas could still be eliminated by cytotoxic T lymphocytes and NK cells thanks to the granule-exocytosis mechanism. When CTL (or NK cells) recognizes its target cells (virally infected cells or tumor cells), CTL releases cytoplasmic-effective molecules such as granzymes and granules containing the pore-forming protein, perforin, into the intracellular space. Perforin is an effective protein that, even in extremely low concentration (less than 10^{-9} M), makes a large pore in the target cell. This pore forms when perforin binds to the phospholipids of the target cell's membrane through a calcium-dependent mechanism. The damage to the cell membrane created by making pores allows granzymes to penetrate the target cell and induce cell death (**Figure 4.6**). The granules also contain granulysin, a protein that has an antimicrobial effect against bacteria, fungi, and parasites. Although they possess effective mechanisms to kill virally infected cells or tumor cells, cytotoxic T cells can also harm normal tissue. For example, they recognize the self-antigens of melanocytes and, as a result, contribute to the development of skin patches lacking pigments (i.e., causes pathogenesis vitiligo).

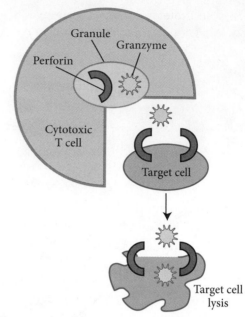

Figure 4.6 Granule-exocytosis–mediated cell death.

Multiple granzymes have been identified from granules of cytotoxic lymphocytes. Specifically, five granzymes are found in the human body: A, B, G, H, and K. Granzymes A and B are major cytotoxic serine proteases of CTL and NK cells. The exact role of granzyme B (also known as granzyme 2 or serine protease B) in CTL and NK cells is not fully understood. A current model of granzyme B's role suggests that it binds to its receptor—the mannose-6-phosphate/insulin-like growth factor II receptor—to enter the cytosol of its target cells. In the target cells, granzyme B activates the caspase cascade, which in turn activates DNase, which finally leads to cell death (similar to the Fas-FasL mechanism). Figure 4.6 demonstrates that the perforin molecules make pores in the membrane of the virally infected cell, rupture the cell membrane, and allow the entry of granzymes, particularly granzyme B, into the cytosol of the target cell.

A few diseases have been linked to high concentrations of granzyme B. For instance, patients with Hodgkin's disease have elevated concentrations of granzyme B in their lymph glands. In addition, patients with rheumatoid arthritis present with high concentrations of granzymes A and B. Granzyme B is also found in monocytes, resting T cells, and B cells, albeit at much lower concentrations. After the cytotoxic cells have killed the tumor or virally infected cells, they must be removed to prevent them from attacking other cells. CTLs induce apoptosis in each other and even in themselves.

Mammalian erythrocytes do not have nuclei and, therefore, cannot support viral replication. In turn, viruses do not infect erythrocytes. Cytotoxic T cells destroy virally infected cells by recognizing MHC class I molecules, which are expressed on all nucleated cells. Erythrocytes do not express MHC class I, so an infection of these cells may go undetected by cytotoxic T cells. For example, the lack of MHC class I molecules in the erythrocytes means that *Plasmodium* species (see also the *Introduction to Microbiology* chapter), which cause malaria, can live in erythrocytes and ultimately modify the membrane permeability of erythrocytes.

Zymogen

The role of protein degradation is to prevent accumulation of abnormal, damaged, or unwanted proteins and to permit the recycling of amino acids in many biochemical reactions, particularly in the synthesis of proteins. Rapidly degraded proteins include defective proteins, damaged proteins, and proteins that are no longer required at a particular stage in the cell cycle. Protein degradation is catalyzed by special enzymes called proteases. Many proteases are synthesized in inactive forms called zymogen, which then can be activated by proteolytic cleavage. Specific cleavage causes conformational changes that expose the active site of the enzyme, thereby converting it to an active enzyme. Proteases play important roles both in the degradation of abnormal proteins and in many physiological processes such as infection, cell growth, apoptosis (granzymes), and blood clotting.

Apoptosis

Many organisms demonstrate a regulated process of programmed cell death called apoptosis. The typical morphologic picture of an apoptotic cell emerges when a cell's DNA is fragmented and the cell is shrunken because the cell's nuclear and cytoplasmic materials are condensed. It is important to emphasize the important benefits that apoptosis offers, including elimination of a cell injury or elimination of a cell with mutagenic DNA damage to provide a mechanism for tissue repair. Conversely, alteration in an apoptotic process can lead to cancer, neurodegeneration, and autoimmune diseases.

During apoptosis, the changes that occur in the cell membrane result in the presentation of phosphatidylserine on the outer surface of the cell. Phosphatidylserine acts as a signal for apoptosis because it is recognized by macrophages, which then phagocytize the dead cell. Interestingly, because the membrane of the apoptotic cell remains unchanged, the contents of the cell are not released. In contrast, in necrotic cell death, the cell contents are released, resulting in an inflammatory response. Consequently, apoptosis does not induce an inflammatory response. Two types of signaling mechanisms can trigger apoptosis: (1) the external apoptosis signaling pathway, which includes ligands such as TNF, FAS, and TNF-related apoptosis-inducing ligand (TRAIL); and (2) the internal apoptosis signaling pathway, which includes DNA and mitochondrial damages.

Helper T Cells

T cells that express the CD4 surface antigen are designated as helper T cells. When CD4 cells are fully developed and matured, they can be divided into two major classes: Th1 and Th2. When activated, both types of helper cells are capable of releasing different cytokines. While extracellular antigens stimulate the generation of Th2 cells, pathogens that accumulate inside a macrophage stimulate the generation of Th1 cells. In addition to these two major cells, there are CD4$^+$ cells called Th17 and T_{reg} cells, although they are not produced to the same extent as Th1 and Th2 cells.

Human immunodeficiency virus (HIV) infects and destroys CD4 cells. CD4 cells play important roles in the activation of macrophages, CTL, NK cells, and B cells, and stimulate the secretion of a series of factors that induce growth and differentiation of lymphoid cells. Consequently, destruction of CD4 cells by HIV predisposes HIV-infected patients to opportunistic infections, tumors, dementia, and finally death. Both monocytes and macrophages play central roles in the dissemination and pathogenesis of HIV infection because they carry the CD4 molecules that act as receptors for HIV. This is of particular concern because monocytes and macrophages are the major cell types infected with HIV in the brain, which might explain the development of neuropsychiatric symptoms associated with HIV infection.

T Helper 1 (Th1). The Th1 cells activate predominantly macrophages and their antigen-presenting capacity to kill intracellular pathogens. They also stimulate B cells to produce immunoglobulin G (IgG) to facilitate the removal of extracellular pathogens by phagocytic cells. The Th1 cells also cause delayed-type hypersensitivity responses. They mainly release cytokines such as interferon-gamma (IFN-γ) and IL-2 and, by "helping" other cell types, indirectly clear intracellular pathogens. The IL-2 stimulates proliferation of cytotoxic T cells and B cells as well (Figure 4.1). Interestingly, the IFN-γ and IL-12 released by Th1 are important for Th1 differentiation and the inhibition of Th2 cells' proliferation. For instance, IFN-γ induces the signal transducer and activator of transcription (STAT) 1 and 4 and other transcription factors in promoting Th1 cell differentiation.

T Helper 2 (Th2). Th2 cells release mainly IL-4, IL-5, IL-13, and IL-25 cytokines and play an important role in the production of immunoglobulin E (IgE) and differentiation of mast cells and eosinophils. The production of IgE and differentiation of mast cells are key factors in the development of allergies. Although allergies are irritating to humans, Th2 cells are beneficial and effective in fighting other types of infectious invaders, including helminths (various types of parasitic worms). Th2 cells are also able to activate B cells with subsequent production of IgM, IgA, IgE, and weakly opsonizing subtypes of IgG. The Th2 cytokine, IL-10, is known to inhibit Th1 cell activation, thereby limiting the production of Th1 cytokines.

It is important to differentiate among the cytokine profiles of the various types of helper T cells. Activated Th1 cells secrete cytokines IL-2, IFN-γ, IL-3, TNF-α, TNF-β, and a stimulating factor called GM-CSF (granulocyte-macrophage colony-stimulating factor) that stimulate proliferation, differentiation, and functional activity of neutrophils, eosinophils, monocytes, and macrophages. Activated Th2 cells secrete IL-3, IL-4, IL-5, IL-6, IL-10, and IL-13. Medications such as sargramostim (Leukine) have been developed that mimic the effects of Th1 activity. Sargramostim is an analog of GM-CSF and is used, for example, to augment the effects of cytotoxic therapy in the treatment of acute myelogenous leukemia in older patients (older than 55 years of age).

Th17 Cells. Th17 cells produce IL-17. These cells play an important role in the immune responses to a few specific extracellular pathogens and fungi; they are also involved with autoimmune inflammatory disorders. Prostaglandin E_2, IL-23, and IL-175 all play vital roles in the differentiation of CD4$^+$ T cells into Th17 cells. Th17 cells are found in large quantities in the intestinal lamina propria. Normal intestinal bacteria are important for their activation. Not surprisingly, then, patients who use long-term broad-spectrum antibiotics have fewer active Th17 cells, which might explain why they are at increased risk of gastrointestinal infections with *Candida albicans* and *Clostridium difficile*. In addition, because of their residence in the intestinal lamina propria, Th17 cells are important for the maintenance of epithelial integrity. Transcription factor STAT3 is important for the differentiation of Th17 cells. Patients who lack Th17 cells are at increased risk for infection with the various species of *Staphylococcus* or *Candida*.

T_{reg} Cells. Regulatory T cells—T_{reg} cells—regulate expression of CD3, which is associated with the T-cell antigen receptor (TCR; **Figure 4.7**); CD4; and CD25, which is a receptor with low affinity for IL-2. However, T_{reg} cells account for only 5% to 10% of all CD4$^+$ cells. The association of CD3 with TCR enhances the signaling processes involved in the activation of T_{reg} cells. Unlike other helper T cell types, T_{reg} cells (which are sometimes referred to as suppressor T cells) suppress immune responses, produce anti-inflammatory cytokines (IL-10, TGF-β, and IL-35), reduce the availability of IL-2, and reverse the activation state of antigen-presenting cells. The expression of a transcription factor, FoxP3, plays an important role in T_{reg} cells' immune suppressive functions. Patients with immune dysregulation and autoimmune diseases (e.g., X-linked diseases characterized by polyendocrinopathy and enteropathy; systemic lupus erythematosus), for example, have inactive genes for FoxP3. As a result, these patients cannot generate T_{reg} cells.

Table 4.2 summarizes the roles of the various helper T cells.

Natural Killer Cells

Natural killer cells do not have any CD4 or CD8 proteins. Nevertheless, they carry out an essential activity by recognizing and killing virus-infected cells, tumor cells, and antibody-coated target cells without the need for recognition of class I or class II MHC proteins. In addition, virus-infected and tumor cells that down-regulate MHC class I expression (the process of recognizing "self" cells) are susceptible to destruction by NK cells. This is an important defense mechanism because many cells, after having been infected by a virus, lose their ability to synthesize and display class I MHC proteins. For example, NK cells are vital for patients with severe combined immunodeficiency disease (SCID), in which CD8–MHC I recognition and interleukin signaling is compromised. NK

Table 4.2 Roles of Helper T Cells in the Immune System

Th1 Cells	Th2 Cells	Th17 Cells	T_reg Cells
• Activate macrophages to kill intracellular pathogens • Stimulate B cells to produce IgG • Release IL-2 to stimulate proliferation of cytotoxic T cells and B cells • Inhibit Th2 cells' proliferation	• Release IL-4, IL-5, IL-13, and IL-25 cytokines and stimulate production of IgE and differentiation of mast cells and eosinophils • Activate B cells, with subsequent production of IgM, IgA, and IgE • Fight various types of parasitic worms • Inhibit the activation of Th1 cells	• Produce the IL-17 cytokine • Provide an immune response to extracellular pathogens and fungi • Play a role in autoimmune inflammatory disorders • Prostaglandin E_2, IL-23, and IL-175 play vital roles in the differentiation of $CD4^+$ T cells into Th17 cells • Intestinal bacteria are important for their activation	• Regulate expression of CD3, which is associated with TCR • Suppress immune responses • Produce anti-inflammatory cytokines (IL-10, TGF-β, and IL-35) • Reduce the availability of IL-2 • Reverse the activation state of antigen-presenting cells

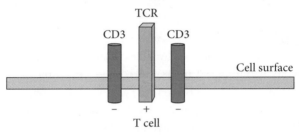

Figure 4.7 The negatively charged amino acids of the CD3 transmembrane domains interact with the positively charged amino acids of the T cell antigen-receptor (TCR) transmembrane domains.

cells participate in two important mechanisms that protect the human body: (1) They kill virus-infected cells and (2) they produce the IFN-γ that activates macrophages to kill bacteria.

While NK cells can kill without antibody mediation, the IgG antibody enhances their effectiveness, in a process called antibody-dependent cellular cytotoxicity. In addition, cytokines such as IL-12 produced by macrophages, CD122 (an IL-2 receptor), and INF-α and INF-β produced by virus-infected cells are all effective activators of NK cells. NK cells are part of the innate immune system and immediately kill virally infected cells (i.e., they are active all the time). Because CTL and NK cells are effective means of killing virally infected and tumor cells, it is important to recognize the differences and similarities between these cells (**Table 4.3**). Certain drugs are known to suppress NK cell effectiveness, including prednisolone (Orapred), theophylline (Theo-24), and salicylates (e.g., aspirin).

Major Histocompatibility Complex

MHC proteins are present on the surface of all nucleated cells, including specialized immune system cells. Antigen fragments derived from external proteins are bound to the MHC proteins and subsequently displayed on cell surfaces to initiate an immune response. An accurate selection process eliminates the cells with MHC complexes that might bind normal cellular proteins, leaving behind only those cells with MHC complexes that bind foreign proteins. As a result, the MHC has a crucial role in the immune system's ability to discriminate between self and non-self. The genes of the MHC are located on human chromosome number 6. The human MHC genes that produce MHC molecules are called human leukocyte antigens (HLA).

Table 4.3 Comparison of Natural Killer Cells and Cytotoxic T Cells

Type	NK Cells	CTL
Property	Have granules; act on the Fas-FasL mechanism to induce apoptosis; have perforin and serine proteases (granzymes); do not express antigen-specific receptors	Have granules; act on the Fas-FasL mechanism to induce apoptosis; have perforin and serine proteases (granzymes)
Function	Cell lytic activity through granule-exocytosis mechanism; lytic activity is enhanced by high levels of alpha and beta interferons	Cell lytic activity through granule-exocytosis mechanism
Activation	Active all the time; able to kill target cells without being restricted by MHC; resting NK cells express CD122 (an IL-2 receptor) and, upon binding to IL-2, exhibit better cytotoxic activity	Require antigen and MHC class I molecules for their activation; produce IL-2 for their own proliferation and are active when they have differentiated from naive T cells into cytotoxic T cells
Memory	Lack immunological memory	Provide memory responses against latent or persistent viral infections

There are two MHC classes: I and II.

- *MHC class I molecule:* A protein encoded by genes of the MHC, which actively participates in antigen presentation to cytotoxic T (CD8) cells. MHC class I molecules are found on all nucleated cells and have the ability to present self or non-self proteins (fragments of a virus that have entered the cell) to scanning immune cells. Every individual can produce up to six MHC class I types, with the end result that any two individuals are unlikely to have the same set.

- *MHC class II molecule:* A protein encoded by genes of the MHC, which actively participates in antigen presentation to helper T cells (CD4 cells). MHC class II molecules are found primarily on antigen-presenting cells such as macrophages. MHC II binds and displays peptides derived from external proteins digested by the cells (rather than peptides derived from cellular proteins). Every individual can produce up to 12 MHC II types; as with MHC class I, this diversity makes it unlikely that two individuals will have the same set of class II molecules.

Antigen-Presenting Cells

Most foreign antigens are not recognized by the immune system unless the foreign antigens are processed by immune cells known as antigen-presenting cells (APCs). APCs include macrophages, B cells, and dendritic cells. These cells engulf the pathogen, enzymatically ingest and degrade it, and then display the pathogen's peptide fragments (peptides that are 11–22 amino acids long) on their cell surfaces with the help of their MHC molecules, particularly their MHC class II molecules. Macrophages and dendritic cells participate in both adaptive and innate immunities; that is, both kill different pathogens and present antigens to helper T cells. Interestingly, neutrophils are also phagocytes, but do not present antigens to helper T cells; thus they function only as innate immune system cells. Indeed, the first step in the activation of the T lymphocyte occurs when the antigen–MHC II complex is recognized by its TCR.

Dendritic cells express class II MHC proteins and present antigens to CD4+ T cells. These cells serve as the main stimulators of the primary antibody response—a key role in immunity. The label "dendritic" is given to them because they resemble neuronal dendrites, a characteristic that makes them very efficient in attaching to foreign materials. Dendritic cells are located primarily under the skin (e.g., Langerhans cells in the skin). They migrate from their peripheral location in the skin to local lymph nodes to present foreign antigens to helper T cells. Because APCs also express MHC class I molecules, they, too, can present antigens: either self-antigens or viral antigens (secondary to having been infected).

Table 4.4 summarizes the functions of APCs in the immune system.

Table 4.4 Roles of Antigen-Presenting Cells in the Immune System

Characteristic	Macrophages	Dendritic Cells	B Cells
MHC I expression	Interact with CD8⁺ (CTL)	Interact with CD8⁺ (CTL)	Interact with CD8⁺ (CTL)
MHC II expression	Interact with CD4⁺ T (helper) cells	Interact with CD4⁺ T (helper) cells; up-regulated by inflammatory cytokines, particularly by TNF-α	Interact with CD4⁺ cells, which leads to secretion of IL-4 and IL-5, which in turn stimulate B cells to differentiate into memory B cells
Effect on microbes	Ingestion and killing of microbes	Ingestion and killing of microbes	Ingestion and killing of microbes
Location	Lymphoid tissue, connective tissue, liver, spleen, gastrointestinal tract, lymph nodes, and brain	Skin and mucosa, lymphoid tissue, and connective tissue	Peripheral blood and lymphoid tissue
Function	Migrate to the site of inflammation, engulf pathogens, and express MHC II	Main inducers of the primary antibody response; activate innate lymphocytes, particularly NK cells; are themselves activated after antigen recognition and particle engulfment, which results in increased expression of their MHC II, B7, CD40, and adhesion molecules	Use their immunoglobulin receptors to present specific antigens to T cells; synthesize and release additional immunoglobulin
Antigen presented	Peptides, viral antigens, and allergens	Intracellular and extracellular antigens	Toxins, viruses, and soluble antigens

---

Learning Bridge 4.1

During your introductory pharmacy practice experience activities at your pharmacy, David, a 31-year-old cab driver, comes to your pharmacy to pick up his refill medications. David's medications are as follows:

> Prednisolone, 20 mg tablet; take 1 pill by mouth daily.
> Theophylline, 300 mg capsule; take 1 capsule by mouth daily.

These medications are prescribed for David's allergy and his occasional respiratory problem (he claims that sometimes he has difficulty breathing during extensive aerobic exercise).

For the last 3 weeks, David has been feeling weak with a persistent headache and has noticed a sore throat and swollen lymph glands—typical symptoms of an infection with Epstein-Barr virus (EBV). Indeed, he was diagnosed with EBV, but his physician has not prescribed any medication to treat his infection (currently there is no effective treatment for EBV). Today, David wants to buy an OTC aspirin to treat his headache; he also asks you to request that his physician switch him from theophylline to Proventil (his wife has suggested strongly that Proventil is very effective for respiratory problems).

(continues)

(*continued*)

All three of these medications—prednisolone, theophylline, and aspirin—suppress a specific immune cell type that might have promoted the EBV infection as well. Identify the cell and explain how these medications suppress that particular cell type. What suggestion do you have for David?

B Cells

B cells belong to the humoral immune system and are directed to fight bacterial infections and extracellular viruses. They are produced and mature in the bone marrow (the source for the letter "B" in their name). Because of the unique human natural genetic rearrangement and recombination mechanism, B cells can produce millions of diverse glycoproteins called immunoglobulin molecules (antibodies), each of which is coded against a specific antigen. The activation of functional B cells requires that two steps be completed: (1) The immunoglobulin attached to the B cell's surface (also called the B-cell receptor) recognizes the antigen and (2) the B cell receives stimulation from growth factors released by activated CD4[+] T cells, such as IL-4, IL-5, and IL-6. Upon activation, the majority of B cells morph into plasma cells, producing and secreting immense amounts of the same immunoglobulin (antibody) that is on the B cell's surface. A fraction of the activated B cells does not differentiate into plasma cells, but rather becomes memory cells, ready for subsequent attacks by that same antigen. In addition, some B cells may become activated without help from CD4[+] T cells. However, their responses are weak, and they do not produce memory B cells.

An immunoglobulin (Ig) molecule is constructed from two identical heavy chains and two identical light chains (each chain being a polypeptide) that are arranged in a symmetric fashion to form a Y-shaped structure. The terms "light" and "heavy" refer to the molecular weight of the chains. In addition, each chain has two distinct regions: a variable region in which the sequence of amino acids varies among immunoglobulin molecules, and a constant region that is conserved within each class of immunoglobulin molecules. The two antigen-binding sites are called Fab fragments. The opposite end of the "Y" is called the Fc fragment and has no antigen-binding activity (**Figure 4.8**). Each immunoglobulin contains an antigen-binding site (paratope) that is specific for a particular portion of an antigen (epitope or an antigenic determinant) (**Figure 4.9**).

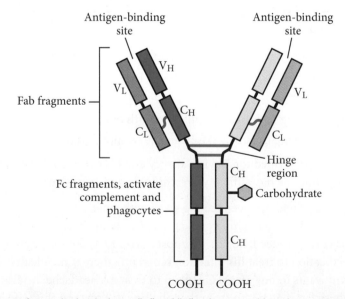

Figure 4.8 The structure of an antibody. The letters "V" and "C" indicate variable and constant polypeptides, respectively. The letters "L" and "H" indicate light and heavy chains, respectively. Four disulfide bridges hold the molecule together.
Adapted from: Nelson DL, Cox MM, Lehninger AL. *Principles of biochemistry.* 5th ed. New York: W. H. Freeman and Company; 2008: Chapter 5.

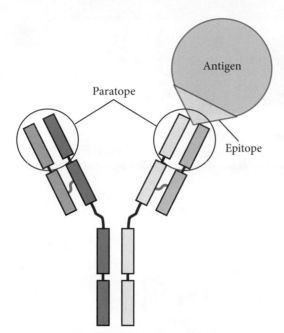

Figure 4.9 The component of an antibody that recognizes a specific component of an antigen (epitope) is referred to as a paratope.

Most chemicals and medications, and their metabolites, are not large enough to be recognized by the immune system. For an immunoglobulin to recognize these chemicals, they must be combined with an endogenous protein (hapten) to form an antigen. Immunogens may also be combined with substances called adjuvants that enhance the immune response. Adjuvants stimulate the immune system's response to the target antigen, but, unlike haptens, they do not confer immunity in themselves. Adjuvants can also act as a local irritant that amplifies its immune response. For instance, the aluminum present in the tetanus, diphtheria, and pertussis vaccine works in this way.

Four internal disulfide bonds in the immunoglobulin bridge the heavy chains to each other and the light chain to the heavy chain (Figure 4.8). The amino acids in the light chain and the heavy chain form the V regions that produce two identical antigen-binding sites. These V regions serve as the amino-terminal sequence of the heavy and light chains and are highly variable (hence the "V" designation) among different immunoglobulin molecules. In contrast, the carboxyl-terminal regions are called constant ("C") regions because their structures do not differ among immunoglobulin molecules of the same class or subclass. The C regions provide stability for the immunoglobulin molecule.

Gene recombination and rearrangement are essential factors for ensuring that humans produce immunoglobulin that is both accurate in terms of the binding antigen and adequate in number. The genes for an immunoglobulin's polypeptide chains are divided into segments, with multiple versions of each segment being available. For instance, the genes for immunoglobulin molecules are located in three unlinked chromosomes: Chromosome 14 has the gene for the heavy-chain classes, including 39 functional heavy-chain variable-region (VH) genes; chromosome 2 has the gene for κ light chains, including 40 functional light-chain variable-region genes (V_κ genes); and chromosome 22 has the gene for λ light chains, including 41 functional light-chain variable-region genes (V_λ genes).

It is through different attachments of these variable genes that humans produce millions of specific antibodies despite the fact that the human genome is made of only 35,000 genes. One B cell makes one antibody in response to a specific antigen. This antibody works as a receptor on the B cell's membrane, capable of binding with high affinity to that specific antigen and becoming activated following the antigen binding. The specific binding between antibody and antigen is a result of the structural and chemical properties (such as size, charge, and hydrophobicity) of the antigen and the antigen-binding site of the antibody. Upon binding of an antigen to its antigen-binding site on the antibody, the conformations of both the antigen and the binding site change. These conformational changes result in tighter binding (induced fit which is described further in the *Introduction to Biochemistry* chapter).

As noted earlier, B cells are a component of the memory of the adaptive immune system. Should the same infectious agent (antigen) invade the body again, the B cells that make the specific antibodies to it will be ready to attack it immediately. Indeed, the B cells are able to make their antibodies more quickly and in greater amounts upon reencountering the antigen than they did the first time the antigen invaded.

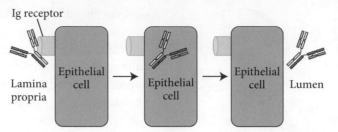

Figure 4.10 The Fc component of IgA interacts with the Ig receptor, which is expressed on the epithelial cell membrane, to facilitate the passage of IgA through the epithelial cells into the lumen, which is in contact with the external environment.

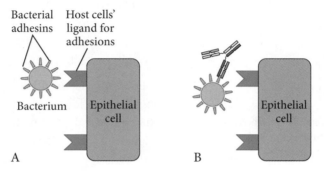

Figure 4.11 Bacterial attack in the absence (A) and presence (B) of IgA. IgA is able to block the interaction of bacterial adhesins with the host epithelial cell's ligands.

There are five classes of human immunoglobulin molecules, each of which plays a different role in the immune defense strategy. Each Ig class is based on the same "Y"-shaped structure discussed previously.

Immunoglobulin A (IgA)

IgA is found largely in body fluids such as tears and saliva, as well as in the nasal, respiratory, urinary, and gastrointestinal tracts; it is present in large quantities at mucosal sites. IgA constitutes approximately 10% of the total plasma immunoglobulin molecules, with a serum concentration of less than 5 mg/mL. It is known, however, that a 70-kg adult can produce as much as 2 g of IgA, making it the most abundant Ig in the body. The major role for IgA is in mucosal immunity: It prevents foreign substances from adhering to mucosal surfaces (epithelial cells) so that foreign substances cannot enter the blood circulation (**Figures 4.10** and **4.11**).

There are two subclasses of IgA, designated as IgA_1 and IgA_2, of which IgA_1 is the most abundant subclass (accounting for approximately 85% of the total IgA in plasma). IgA has a relatively short half-life of approximately 6 days. Because it is secreted in breast milk, its mechanism is important to neonatal immunity. IgA can be found as a monomer, dimer, or trimer through which the interaction of the multitrimer (Y-shaped structures) is facilitated by the so-called J chain. Neutrophils, eosinophils, and monocytes bear specific Fc receptors (FcR) for IgA molecules.

Berger's disease, an autoimmune disease, is caused by defective glycosylation of IgA_1 that results in one of the most common forms of glomerulonephritis, IgA nephropathy. In this disease, the carbohydrate moiety in the hinge region of IgA_1 (see Figure 4.8) is recognized and attacked by anti-glycan IgG or IgA_1 antibodies. This immune complex escapes the normal clearance mechanisms in the circulation and is deposited in the renal mesangium, the inner layer of the glomerulus (see also the *Introduction to Pharmacology and Pathophysiology* chapter), where it causes glomerular injury.

In addition, the glomerular IgA deposits can cause Henoch-Schönlein purpura, a disease that is characterized by skin rash, arthritis, and abdominal pain in children or adolescents.

Immunoglobulin D (IgD)

IgD molecules are found exclusively attached to the membranes of B cells (and hence are membrane-bound Ig molecules); they represent the second antibody class to be expressed during B-cell development. IgD is found only in trace amounts in the human body, accounting for less than 1% of all plasma immunoglobulin molecules (with a serum concentration of less than 0.5 mg/mL). While IgD's role is not fully understood, it can serve as an antigen receptor for naive B cells. IgD does not penetrate extravascular spaces efficiently and cannot cross the placental barrier.

Immunoglobulin E (IgE)

Under normal circumstances, IgE molecules are found only in trace amounts in the circulation; they represent only 0.004% of the total plasma immunoglobulin molecules and have a serum concentration of 17–450 ng/mL. While mast cells, basophils, and eosinophils have high-affinity receptors, B cells and dendritic cells have low-affinity receptors for the Fc portion of IgE. One role of IgE is to activate mast cells, basophils, and eosinophils. Its principal role is to combat parasites and to function in hypersensitivity reactions (allergic responses). In recognition of this activity, IgE molecules are called reaginic antibodies. In patients with parasitic infestation and atopic diseases, the amount of plasma IgE is very high (as much as 20 times higher than normal).

IgE, as a monomeric structure, binds via its Fc region to receptors on basophils and mast cells. The binding of cell-bound IgE antibody to antigens stimulates the release of a series of potent molecules, such as vasoactive amines, lipid-derived inflammatory mediators, proteases, and proteoglycans. In turn, these mediators produce the rapid consequences of immediate hypersensitivity, including vascular leakage, vasodilation, and bronchoconstriction (**Figure 4.12**). In addition to these potent molecules, the binding of antigen stimulates release of cytokines (e.g., TNF, ILs) from mast cells. These cytokines are responsible for the late phase of the immediate hypersensitivity response.

Immunoglobulin G (IgG)

The IgG antibody constitutes approximately 80% of the total immunoglobulin molecules in adult plasma, with a serum concentration of 8–16 mg/mL. The IgG molecules effectively penetrate

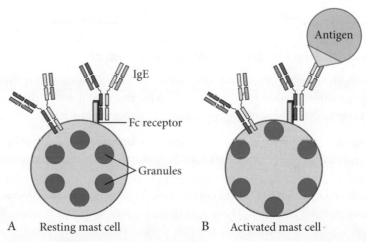

Figure 4.12 In the absence of antigen, mast cells are in a resting state (A). Upon binding of an antigen to IgE (B), the mast cell's granules diffuse to the cell membrane to release their potent inflammatory mediators (e.g., histamine, proteases).

extravascular spaces and the placental barrier to provide passive immunity to the newborn (see the discussion of passive immunity near the end of this chapter). In addition, they work efficiently to coat microorganisms and thereby speed their uptake by phagocytic cells of the immune system. IgG plays an important role in neonatal protection from foreign substances because it is the only immunoglobulin class that can cross the placenta. Similar to IgA, IgG can be secreted into breast milk as well.

Upon secondary exposure to an antigen, the IgG production machinery results in this immuno-globulin being the major antibody found in plasma, with an average half-life of 23 days. It exhibits a high affinity for antigens.

IgG molecules can be divided into four major subclasses: IgG_1, IgG_2, IgG_3, and IgG_4. IgG_1 is present in the largest amount (65% of total IgG in plasma) and IgG_4 in the smallest amount. Each of these subclasses has a specific heavy-chain C region that mediates different effector functions. Consequently, the IgG subclasses have different roles in the immune system. For instance, while IgG_1 and IgG_3 activate complement via the classic pathway, IgG_2 is a poor activator of this system. IgG_4 does not activate the complement system at all. IgG coats (opsonizes) antigens to allow phagocytosis of the antigen by a macrophage.

Immunoglobulin M (IgM)

Five IgM molecules combine to create star-shaped clusters (pentamers) that are joined at their C-terminals and stabilized by the J chain. IgM tends to remain in the circulation, where it is the major effector of the primary antibody response in killing bacteria due to the increased number of Fab regions per molecule. IgM molecules are termed macroglobulins because of their large molecular weight (900 kDa). They constitute only 7% of the total immunoglobulin molecules in adult plasma, with a serum concentration of 0.5–2.0 mg/mL.

The attachment of B cell membrane–bound IgM to antigen activates naive B cells. IgM is the first Ig molecule to be expressed during B-cell development (primary antibody response). Despite the fact that IgM has a low affinity for its antigen, it can activate the complement cascade. It is very effective in responding to multivalent antigens (i.e., polysaccharides with repeating epitopes). However, its pentameric structure allows for multiple low-affinity interactions, which result in an overall stronger attachment to antigens (**Figure 4.13**). IgM activity is also associated with autoimmune diseases. For instance, IgM antibodies against IgG molecules are present in high amounts in rheumatoid arthritis and a few other diseases affecting collagen.

Table 4.5 summarizes the roles of the various immunoglobulin molecules.

Monoclonal Antibodies Versus Polyclonal Antibodies

A monoclonal antibody differs from a polyclonal antibody in that monoclonal antibodies are synthesized by a population of identical, or "cloned," cells. Polyclonal antibodies are produced by many different B lymphocytes responding to different epitopes on one antigen.

Many biologic drugs available for treatment of autoimmune diseases are synthesized as mono-clonal antibodies, including adalimumab (Humira), rituximab (Rituxan), cetuximab (Erbitux), and ibritumomab (Zevalin). The *Introduction to Cell Biology* chapter describes how these monoclonal antibodies are produced by pharmaceutical companies. As you perhaps have guessed, the "-mab" suffix stands for monoclonal antibody. These agents are becoming the treatment of choice in many

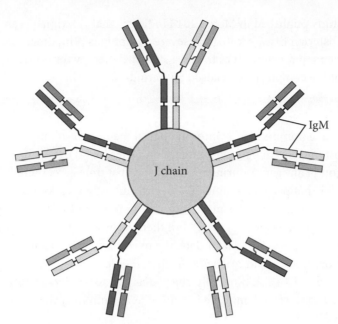

Figure 4.13 The pentameric form of five joined IgM proteins provides an overall high affinity to antigens. The held IgM proteins are connected together by the joining (J) chain.

Adapted from: Nelson DL, Cox MM, Lehninger AL. *Principles of biochemistry.* 5th ed. New York: W. H. Freeman and Company; 2008: Chapter 5.

Table 4.5 Roles of Immunoglobulin Molecules in the Immune System

IgA	IgD	IgE	IgG	IgM
• Found largely in body fluids and in the nasal, respiratory, urinary, and GI tracts • Serum concentration < 5 mg/mL • Prevents foreign substances from adhering to mucosal surfaces (epithelial cells) • Half-life of approximately 6 days • Secreted into breast milk	• Exclusively attached to the membranes of B cells • Serum concentration < 0.5 mg/mL • Serves as an antigen receptor for naive B cells • Cannot cross the placental barrier	• Serum concentration = 17–450 ng/mL • Activates mast cells, basophils, and eosinophils • Combats parasites and functions in hypersensitivity reactions (allergic responses) • Stimulates the release of a series of potent molecules such as vasoactive amines, lipid-derived inflammatory mediators, proteases, and proteoglycans	• Penetrates extravascular spaces and the placental barrier to provide passive immunity to the newborn • Serum concentration = 8–16 mg/mL • The only Ig class that can cross the placenta • Secreted into breast milk • Upon secondary exposure to an antigen, IgG is the major serum antibody • Half-life of 23 days	• Star-shaped pentamer • Remains in the circulation, where it is the major effector of the primary antibody response in killing bacteria • Serum concentration = 0.5–2.0 mg/mL • Associated with autoimmune diseases

diseases. Indeed, a study published in March 2013 indicates that rituximab is an effective treatment for the severe skin blistering disease known as severe pemphigus. Rituximab is currently being evaluated as a replacement for steroids as the new standard therapy for severe pemphigus; its use would avoid many of the complications caused by steroids.

Immunological Memory

A key feature of adaptive immunity is its immunological memory. Both primary and secondary responses play important roles in fighting an infection. After initial exposure to a given antigen (for instance, injection of antigen A during immunization) at time zero, there is no serum antibody concentration for that particular antigen. However, after two weeks, the amount of serum antibody reaches its maximum level (primary response or immunologic priming). This high concentration persists for a few days (plateau), but then declines. If the same antigen enters the body (e.g., booster immunization) at a later date, the maximum level of antibody concentration is produced much more quickly and reaches a much higher level (secondary response or immunologic memory) (**Figure 4.14**). Additionally, the plateau persists for a longer time than during the primary immune response and, in some instances (e.g., immunity to measles), the antibody concentration remains high for life.

Granulocytes

Neutrophils, eosinophils, basophils, and mast cells are all part of and involved in the innate immune system. They are called granulocytes because they contain granules in their cytoplasm, along with inflammatory mediators or digestive enzymes. These cells play key roles in the removal of pathogens.

Neutrophils

Neutrophils make up 55% to 70% of the total number of WBCs. Neutrophils serve as the primary human protection against invasive bacteria. They move rapidly from the bloodstream into infected or inflamed tissue in response to IL-8, C3a, and C5a (C3a and C5a are components of the complement system). The roles of the complement system and interleukins are described in other sections of this chapter.

To reach the affected tissues, the circulating neutrophils pass through the capillaries by adhering to the endothelial (lining) cells of the capillaries. After reaching the site of inflammation, neutrophils recognize and then remove the pathogen by phagocytosis. During the phagocytic process, the pathogen is taken into the neutrophil's cytoplasmic lysosome. Subsequently, the granular contents of a neutrophil are released into the lysosome to destroy the engulfed pathogen.

Neutrophils are key cells involved in an immune response system called acute inflammatory response. The unique characteristics of

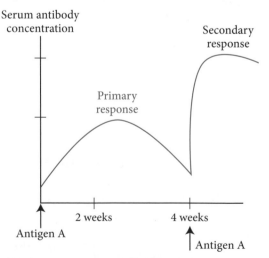

Figure 4.14 Primary and secondary immune responses result from the initial and subsequent antigen attacks, respectively.

an acute inflammatory response are an increase in the vascular permeability, entry of activated neutrophils into the tissues, and activation of platelets.

Eosinophils

Eosinophils are phagocytic cells that account for 3% of the WBC total. Similar to neutrophils, they move from the bloodstream into the infected tissues. While they do not play a crucial role in fighting bacterial infections and have less phagocytic activity than neutrophils, eosinophils are effective in fighting parasites. Eosinophils are activated by their high-affinity receptor (Fc receptor) for IgE to release their granules, which in turn release cationic proteins, leukotriene C4, IL-3, and reactive oxygen species to cause lysis of the parasite. Although these reactions are often beneficial, the same cells and molecules are also involved in other disease states, including the airway inflammatory response in asthma. Consequently, these molecules can actually worsen an allergic response and injure the airway tissue.

Eosinophilia is the state in which there are more than 500 eosinophils/µL blood (in severe cases, one can find more than 1,500 cells/µL blood). Eosinophilia is often caused by an allergic reaction to either iodides or drugs such as aspirin, antibiotics, sulfonamides, nitrofurantoin, penicillins, and cephalosporins, or by medical conditions such as hay fever, asthma, eczema, and rheumatoid arthritis. IL-5 plays a major role in the eosinophil's growth. Mepolizumab and reslizumab (currently not available in the United States) are monoclonal anti-IL-5 antibodies that have been developed to bind IL-5, thereby arresting eosinophil-driven inflammatory reactions.

Basophils

Basophils account for 0.5% to 1% of the total WBC population and, through their high-affinity receptors (FcεRI) for IgE, are involved in immediate allergic responses. These responses range from mild urticaria and rhinitis to severe anaphylactic shock. Similar to mast cells, basophils, upon activation by binding of specific antigens to cell-fixed IgE molecules, release their granule contents; these contents include heparin (an anticoagulant), histamine (a powerful vasodilator), leukotriene B_4, prostaglandins, and platelet-activating factor (PAF) (Figure 4.12).

While a smaller than normal number of basophils is rarely observed, a high concentration of basophils is indicative of several forms of myeloid leukemia. Should many basophils become activated at once, shock may occur as a result of the increased release of histamine and other vasoactive mediators.

Mast Cells

Mast cells are granulocytes that are found in plentiful numbers in tissues that come into contact with the external environment—for example, skin, lungs, nasal mucosa, and connective tissue. Similar to basophils, mast cells release the contents of their granules upon activation by antigens that bind to the IgE molecules that have coated the mast cell surface (Figure 4.12). The granule contents of mast cells include proteoglycans, histamine, heparin, and serotonin.

Basophils and mast cells differ in several ways. Most significantly, basophils are mature cells that circulate in the blood and enter tissues but do not reside in tissues, whereas mast cells complete their maturation in the tissues. Mast cells are involved in inflammatory responses initiated by IgE and IgG, where the inflammation reaction serves as a defense against invading parasites.

Table 4.6 Normal Blood Levels of Leukocytes and Differential in Adults

Cell	Range (cells/mm³)*	Range (10⁹ cells/L)*	Percent Leukocytes
WBC	4,000–11,000	4–11	100
Neutrophils	2,000–7,700	1.8–8.3	57
Immature neutrophils (band neutrophils)	0–10,000	0–10	3
Lymphocytes	1,000–4,800	1–4.8	30
Monocytes	300–800	0.3–0.8	6
Eosinophils	0–700	0–0.7	3
Basophils	0–200	0–0.2	1

*1 mm³ equals 1 μL.

In addition, mast cells release TNF in response to bacterial products. Significant release of the contents of mast cell granules can lead to anaphylaxis.

Table 4.6 indicates the normal ranges for the total WBC and the different percentages of each type of leukocyte (i.e., differential). While the longevity of many of these cells in the blood is unknown, it is known that neutrophils and monocytes have a life span of 7 hours and 3 days, respectively.

Learning Bridge 4.2

While participating in introductory pharmacy practice experience at your pharmacy, you review the medical records of your patient, Amy Johnson. Amy has type 1 diabetes and has come to your pharmacy to obtain the fexofenadine tablets (Allegra) that she is using for her allergy. Upon reviewing her medical records, you notice that when Amy visited a clinic 2 days ago, her CBC indicated the following blood counts, as shown on her medical records:

> WBC: 12,000 cells/mm³
>
> Neutrophils: 9,800 cells/mm³ or 82%
>
> Eosinophils: 200 cells/mm³ or 1.7%
>
> Basophils: 150 cells/mm³ or 1.2%
>
> Lymphocytes: 1,500 cells/mm³ or 13%
>
> Monocytes: 350 cells/mm³ or 3%

There was no indication of infection, and her physician has not prescribed any antibiotic for Amy. Based on the provided information and lab data, answer the following questions that your preceptor has posed to you:

A. Are Amy's blood counts normal? Explain why or why not.

B. What does an abnormal level of each cell tell you about Amy's status?

C. What advice do you have for Amy?

> **Learning Bridge 4.3**
>
> Amy returns to your pharmacy to buy an anti-itch OTC product. She shows you her hands and arms, which are covered with severe rashes. You ask her to have a seat while looking at her medical records. According to her record, Amy has a urinary tract infection (UTI) that began 3 days ago. The infection was caused by a strain of *E. coli* susceptible to nitrofurantoin (Macrobid). Amy's records indicate that she has been using this antibiotic at 100 mg every 12 hours during the last 3 days. Records also indicate that her eosinophils are high (1,200 cells per μL of blood).
>
> Your preceptor asks you to answer the following questions about Amy's medical conditions:
>
> **A.** Why are Amy's eosinophils high?
> **B.** What should Amy do to remedy her severe skin rashes and itching problem?

Cluster of Differentiation

The cluster of differentiation (CD) is a designation for cell surface proteins that are present on lymphocytes. CD molecules can function as ligands and receptors (but not both) on a cell. For instance, CD2 serves as a ligand to the CD58 receptor.

Approximately 350 CD molecules are found in humans. A few important CD molecules are highlighted here:

- CD2: This 50-kDa protein is found on all T lymphocytes. Its role is to facilitate cell–cell adhesion by binding to the CD58 receptor that is expressed on erythrocytes, leukocytes, and endothelial, epithelial, and connective tissue cells. Blocking of CD2 by monoclonal antibodies inhibits T-lymphocyte functions. CD2, in addition to carrying out its adhesion function between T cells and APCs, plays an important role in signal transduction.

- CD4: This protein functions as a co-receptor for MHC class II to facilitate recognition of peptide antigens by T helper cells. It is also a co-receptor for HIV gp120.

- CD8: This protein functions as a co-receptor for MHC class I to facilitate recognition of peptide antigens by cytotoxic T cells.

- CD23: This protein is expressed in mature B cells, activated macrophages, eosinophils, dendritic cells, and platelets. It has a low affinity for IgE but is able to regulate IgE synthesis.

- CD28: This 44-kDa protein is an important receptor for T cells. Approximately 90% and 50% of CD4$^+$ and CD8$^+$ cells, respectively, express this receptor. CD28 has an affinity for CD80 and CD86, and it stabilizes and prolongs the synapses between T cells and antigen-presenting cells. In addition, the binding of CD28 to its ligands (CD80 and CD86) is important for T cell activation and proliferation. CD28 plays an important role in the stabilization of IL-2 mRNA as well.

Cytokines

Cytokines are principal proteins that regulate (capable of up- and down-regulating) immune responses by affecting cellular activation, migration, growth, differentiation, and cell-surface molecule expression. Interestingly, cytokines act like hormones; that is, the same cytokine can be produced by different cells, can act on the same cell that secretes them (similar to autocrine hormones), can act on a nearby cell (similar to paracrine hormones), and can travel through the peripheral circulation or lymphatics to act on a far-reaching cell (similar to endocrine hormones). For example, IL-6 is produced at a distant inflammatory site but can reach the liver to enhance its acute-phase protein production.

Cytokines stimulate humoral and cellular immune responses and activate phagocytic cells. To date, more than 100 cytokines have been identified. In addition to lymphocytes and macrophages, other cells such as endothelial cells and neurons can release cytokines. Cytokines that primarily target leukocytes are referred to as interleukins. Cytokines that are secreted from lymphocytes are referred to as lymphokines, and cytokines that are secreted from monocytes or macrophages are called monokines. The cytokine family includes these other important proteins: various interleukins (IL); tumor necrosis factor-α (TNF-α); lymphotoxin (TNF-β); interferon-α, -β, and -γ (IFN); various chemokines; and CD40 ligands.

Cytokines are expressed rapidly in response to injury, inflammation, and infectious disease to promote a quick immune response. As a consequence, they have significant effects on the regulation of immune responses and the pathogenesis of many infectious diseases. Indeed, the important functions that cytokines carry out in promoting an immune response have encouraged many pharmaceutical and biotechnology companies to produce drugs that mimic the roles of cytokines. As a result, many cytokines are used routinely as therapeutic agents.

So far, 29 ILs have been identified, and more are expected to be recognized. For instance, IL-1 stimulates B-cell growth and antibody production; IL-2 promotes the proliferation and activity of CD4 cells, cytotoxic T lymphocytes, and natural killer (NK) cells; IL-5 stimulates differentiation of eosinophils; and IL-10 inactivates macrophages, which in turn decreases the rate of generation of cytokines from T cells. The intracellular proteins known as interferons induce the expression of antiviral cellular genes that can destroy viral mRNA and/or inhibit the synthesis of viral proteins. Conversely, TNF acts to promote inflammation. In recognition of this role, monoclonal antibodies that block TNF-α (TNF-α blockers) have been developed to treat inflammatory conditions such as rheumatoid arthritis, psoriasis, and Crohn's disease. When used to treat rheumatoid arthritis, TNF-α blockers are referred to as disease-modifying antirheumatic drugs (DMARDs).

A few OTC products are known to affect the role or production of some cytokines. For example, cytokines (IL-1, IL-6, and TNF-α) are known to increase prostaglandin production in and near the hypothalamus. The response to this prostaglandin synthesis is fever. Because NSAIDs inhibit prostaglandin synthesis, the hypothalamus receives no signal to produce fever. In contrast, echinacea is reported to increase the production of interferons, tumor necrosis factor, and IL-1. This natural product may be contraindicated in transplant patients taking immunosuppressants because it might stimulate immunological rejection of the organ. One must be vigilant in reviewing patients' medical records to avoid any unnecessary suppression or potentiation of an immune response.

Chemokines

Chemokines (chemotactic cytokines) are proteins of low molecular weight that attract neutrophils and leukocytes to areas of inflammation. In addition, they act in the regulation of cell growth and angiogenesis. More than 40 chemokine molecules have been identified. Their receptors are classified as G protein–coupled receptors (serpentine receptors; see also the *Introduction to*

Pharmacodynamics chapter). To respond to a chemokine, a cell must have a specific receptor to that particular chemokine. One example of a chemokine is IL-8, which is able to bind to specific surface receptors on neutrophils and induce these cells to migrate into tissues.

Interferons

Interferons are potent cytokines that play essential roles in initiating immune responses. There are three major classes of human interferons: IFN-α, IFN-β, and IFN-γ. Virtually all human cells can synthesize IFN-α and IFN-β in response to viral infections that are caused by double-stranded viral RNA or in response to a stimulation by IL-1, IL-2, and TNF. IFN-α and IFN-β stimulate the cytotoxic activity of lymphocytes, NK cells, and macrophages and up-regulate MHC class I antigen presentation. IFN actions are directed against the infected cell and focus on limiting viral replication (as mentioned earlier, by inducing the host virus-infected cell's expression of proteins that can destroy viral mRNA). At least 20 subtypes of IFN-α and 2 subtypes of IFN-β exist, but they all act on the identical receptor, and their genes are located on chromosome 9.

The third type of IFN, IFN-γ, has been shown to have less antiviral activity. It is produced mainly by NK cells or when T lymphocytes respond to IL-12. However, IFN-γ is more potent than the other forms of IFN in its ability to activate macrophages and to increase the expression of MHC class II antigens. There is only one type of IFN-γ, which acts on its unique receptor; this receptor differs from the IFN-α and IFN-β receptors (i.e., while both IFN-α and IFN-β bind to the IFN-α receptor, IFN-γ binds to a different receptor). The gene for IFN-γ is located on chromosome 12.

Upon binding to their receptors, interferons initiate expression of certain enzymes, inhibit cell proliferation, stimulate immune responses by increasing the phagocytosis of macrophages, and enhance the cytotoxic effect of T lymphocytes. Analogs of IFNs have been developed and are critical elements of the treatment of chronic hepatitis B virus infection. Unfortunately, poor responses are seen in patients with suppressed immune systems, including HIV-infected patients. Currently available IFNs come in injectable dosage forms: intramuscular (IM), subcutaneous (SC), or intravenous (IV). DNA recombinant technology allows for the production of highly purified IFNs that are effective in fighting viral infections.

Following are the most commonly used recombinant interferons:

- IFN-α2b (Intron A) is produced by utilizing *E. coli* bacteria. This recombinant interferon is identical to the natural IFN-α2 that human cells produce and secrete in response to viral infections. The recombinant IFN-α2b is used to fight tumors, including hairy cell leukemia, malignant melanoma, follicular lymphoma, and Kaposi's sarcoma in patients with AIDS. In addition, it is used for chronic HBV infection and, in combination with other antiviral agents, as a treatment for chronic hepatitis C and condylomata acuminate (a sexually transmitted disease).

- IFN-γ1b (Actimmune) stimulates phagocytes' generation of the free-radical metabolites that are toxic to many microorganisms. This agent is useful in treating chronic granulomatous disease because phagocytes in patients with this disease cannot generate free-radical metabolites.

- IFN-β 1a (Avonex) and IFN-β 1b (Betaseron) are used to treat the relapsing form of multiple sclerosis (MS). They reduce the frequency of clinical exacerbations, although their exact mechanism of action is not known.

Learning Bridge 4.4

Joe Smith is a biology teacher who works in a middle school in Oregon. He was diagnosed with rheumatoid arthritis 4 months ago. He comes to your pharmacy to receive his medication, adalimumab. Joe has been using another monoclonal antibody, infliximab. Both of these agents are disease-modifying antirheumatic drugs (DMARDs). Joe was also using methotrexate together with infliximab. However, when his physician switched Joe to adalimumab, he asked Joe to stop using both infliximab and methotrexate.

While you are filling his new prescription, Joe asks you to explain how adalimumab works. He also wonders why he should stop using infliximab and methotrexate. In addition, Joe has noticed that his hair has been receding since he began use of these drugs. He wonders whether there is any drug that can stop his hair loss.

The Complement System

The cell-killing effects of innate and adaptive immunities are mediated in part by a system that includes more than 30 plasma proteins, of which many are proteases (zymogens) that become activated by proteolytic cleavage. The name "complement system" reflects the fact that it "complements" the effects of antibodies. The activation of the complement system is tightly regulated to avoid any damage to host tissues. The regulation mechanism is carried out by regulatory proteins that are concentrated in the blood plasma.

The C3 protein plays a central role in the activation of the complement system. Cleavage of C3 results in the production of C3a and C3b. C3b is able to coat pathogen surfaces to facilitate phagocytosis. C3, C3b, and the terminal components C5–C9 (also referred to as the membrane-attack complex) play significant roles in the complement system by lysing pathogens (**Figure 4.15**).

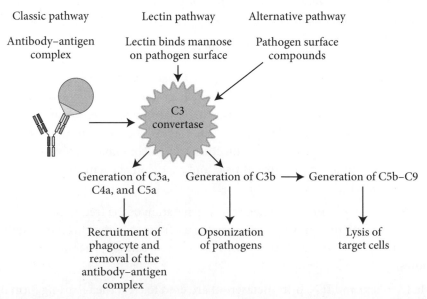

Figure 4.15 A summary of the complement system's pathways. While the classic pathway is activated by an antigen–antibody complex, the lectin and alternative pathways are activated by other mechanisms that are independent of antibodies.

Adapted from: Ray CG, Ryan KJ. Immune response to infection. In: Ray CG, Ryan KJ, eds. *Sherris medical microbiology.* 5th ed. New York, NY: McGraw-Hill; 2010. Available at: http://www.accessmedicine.com/content.aspx?aID=6936356.

Three different pathways, or enzyme cascades, activate the complement system: (1) the classic pathway, which is triggered by immune complexes; (2) the mannose-binding lectin pathway, which is triggered when a lectin molecule (see the *Introduction to Cell Biology* chapter) binds mannose groups on the surface of pathogens; and (3) the alternative pathway, which is triggered by binding to a pathogen's surface components. The proteins involved in the complement system have three distinct functions: (1) They serve in part as a bridge from innate to adaptive immunity by activating B cells and aiding immune memory; (2) they assist in killing invading organisms by opsonization, chemotaxis, and eventually causing cell lysis; and (3) they help dispose of waste products after apoptosis.

The concentration of the complement factors can be reduced due to a high rate of utilization of the complement system during a series of medical conditions such as acute inflammation caused by systemic lupus erythematosus, rheumatoid arthritis, or collagen vascular disorders, among others. In addition, in severe liver failure, the quantity of several components of the complement system—such as C2, C3, C4, and factors B and D—is reduced.

Hypersensitivity

Immune responses are key to the development of hypersensitivity. Hypersensitivity reactions are divided into four types, I–IV. While types I–III are mediated by antibodies, type IV is mediated by cells. There are two phases in which hypersensitivity occurs: the sensitization phase and the effector phase. While the former occurs upon initial exposure to an antigen, the latter involves immunologic memory and occurs upon subsequent exposure to the initial antigen.

Type I Hypersensitivity

Type I hypersensitivity, or immediate hypersensitivity, causes urticaria (skin rash with bumps), anaphylaxis, asthma, or hay fever (rhinitis) following ingestion of antigen-containing food or medications or inhalation of allergens. The immediate allergic reaction reflects the interaction of an antigen to a preexisting IgE that is bound to blood basophils or tissue mast cells (**Figure 4.16**). Immediate therapy is needed to counteract the systemic anaphylaxis caused by insect bites or contact with specific food or drug allergens. A typical type I allergy reaction is hypersensitivity to penicillin, which occurs within one to two minutes after ingestion. To remedy this reaction, the patient must receive competitive H_1 antagonists, an epinephrine injection, cromolyn sodium (a mast cell stabilizer), and injectable (or topical) steroids. The most important remedy, of course, is the withdrawal of the penicillin agent. However, because bacterial infections need to be treated, penicillin must be replaced with another antibacterial agent.

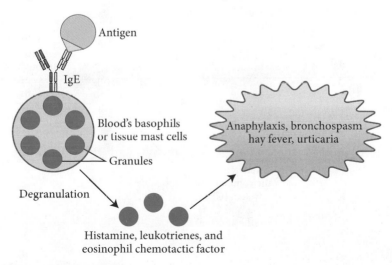

Figure 4.16 Type I hypersensitivity reaction.

Type II Hypersensitivity

A type II hypersensitivity reaction occurs in autoimmune disorders when IgG and IgM that react to self-antigens are produced. A typical example is Graves's disease (hyperthyroidism), in which the body produces antibodies that serve as agonists to the thyroid-stimulating hormone (TSH) receptor; the result is hypersecretion of the thyroid hormone, T_4.

In addition, type II reactions can occur secondary to a blood transfusion reaction when the blood is not cross-matched accurately. As a result of IgG attachment, the complement system becomes activated, leading to lysis of the transfused erythrocytes. Another example of type II hypersensitivity is when anti-Rh IgG antibodies, generated by an Rh-negative mother, cross the placenta and attack the Rh-positive fetus's erythrocytes, resulting in cell destruction.

In addition, a type II reaction can occur when penicillin binds to cell-surface proteins and attracts immunoglobulins, which then leads to hemolytic anemia. This penicillin reaction is not as immediate as the reaction seen in type I hypersensitivity, and it takes a few hours to a few days before the onset of the allergic reaction occurs. The withdrawal of the penicillin medication is important in the course of treatment.

Figure 4.17 depicts a type II hypersensitivity reaction.

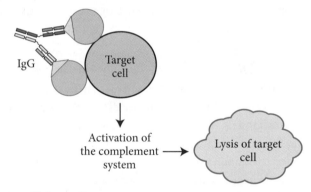

Figure 4.17 Type II hypersensitivity reaction.

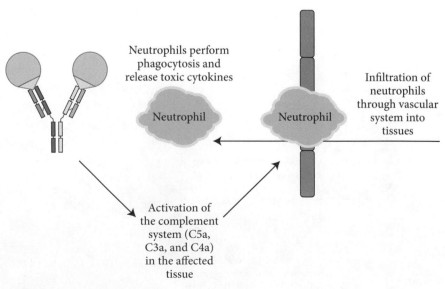

Figure 4.18 Type III hypersensitivity reaction.

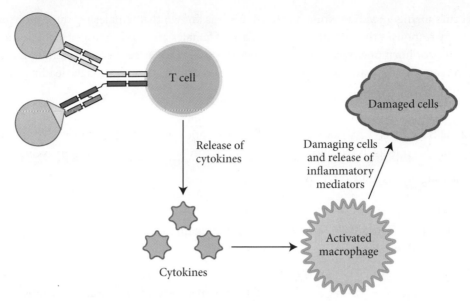

Figure 4.19 Type IV hypersensitivity reaction.

Type III Hypersensitivity

A type III allergic reaction is caused by persistent circulating immune complexes. In contrast to the immediacy of a type I reaction, the clinical symptoms of type III hypersensitivity appear three to four days after exposure to an antigen. In a type III reaction, the complement system is activated by antibody–antigen interaction in which a series of complement proteins (C5a, C3a, C4a) with anaphylatoxic and chemotactic properties are produced (**Figure 4.18**). These proteins enhance vascular permeability and attract neutrophils to the site of complex deposition in tissues. The lytic enzymes released by neutrophils and the complement proteins can cause destruction at the sites of their accumulation in the form of skin rashes, glomerulonephritis, rheumatoid arthritis, and systemic lupus erythematosus. Type III hypersensitivity is caused by many drugs, including penicillin, sulfonamide, and thiouracil. The most useful therapy is to withdraw the drug and administer antihistamine or corticosteroid agents.

Type IV Hypersensitivity

As mentioned earlier, type IV hypersensitivity is mediated through direct contact of antigens with immune cells (i.e., it is not mediated by antibody) and causes extensive tissue damage. In a type IV reaction, cytokines are released from T cells, thus promoting migration and influx of macrophages to the site where antigen is found (**Figure 4.19**). At different ends of the spectrum of diseases mediated by type IV hypersensitivity are contact dermatitis (mild) and attacks by T cells on the beta cells of the pancreas (inducing type 1 diabetes). The type IV hypersensitivity reaction is delayed (for more than 12 hours) because T cells, when activated, need to attract macrophages to the site of antigens. Topical or injectable corticosteroid therapy (depending on the site of reaction) can suppress the T cells' and macrophages' functions.

Systemic Lupus Erythematosus

Systemic lupus erythematosus (SLE) is an inflammatory autoimmune disease characterized by cell damage and mediated by tissue-binding autoantibodies and immune complexes. Discoid lupus is a form of lupus dermatitis that is confined to the skin (i.e., does not affect internal organs). When internal organs are involved, the condition is much more severe and is referred to as SLE. The prevalence of SLE in the United States is 0.05% of the population.

SLE occurs mainly in young women ages 18–35. It is known that females produce more extensive antibody responses than do males, particularly if females are using estrogen-containing oral contraceptives or hormone replacement therapy. This difference arises because estradiol, when binding to receptors on T and B lymphocytes, increases activation of these cells, leading to prolonged immune responses.

In addition, SLE causes anemia, leukopenia, and thrombocytopenia. Furthermore, infection with Epstein-Barr virus (EBV) can trigger SLE in susceptible individuals because EBV not only activates, but also infects, B lymphocytes. It can survive in B lymphocytes for many years.

The following agents are known to trigger SLE:

- Hydralazine (Apo-Hydralazine, from Canada), a vasodilator used for high blood pressure
- Quinidine (Apo-Quinidine, from Canada) and procainamide (Apo-Procainamide, from Canada), used for abnormal heart rhythms
- Phenytoin (Dilantin), used for epilepsy
- Isoniazid (Isotamine, from Canada), used for the treatment of infections caused by *M. tuberculosis*
- D-Penicillamine (Depen), used for rheumatoid arthritis
- Methyldopa (Apo-Methyldopa, from Canada), used for the management of moderate to severe hypertension
- Chlorpromazine (Largactil, from Canada), used for the treatment of schizophrenia and for control of nausea and vomiting

Drug-induced SLE accounts for fewer than 5% of cases and usually resolves when the medication is withdrawn.

Symptoms of patients with SLE include fatigue; low-grade fever; loss of appetite; weight loss (prior to diagnosis) or weight gain (often occurs after diagnosis when treatment has been initiated); muscle pain; arthritis (particularly joints in hands); ulcers of the mouth and nose; "butterfly" rash (a characteristic rash over both cheeks and the nose having the shape of a butterfly); unusual sensitivity to sunlight (photosensitivity); inflammation of the linings that surround the lungs (pleuritis) and heart (pericarditis and myocarditis); leukopenia and thrombocytopenia; glomerulonephritis; and poor circulation in the fingers and toes with sensation of cold (Raynaud's phenomenon). The most commonly experienced symptoms are fatigue, fever, and weight loss, which occur in nearly all patients.

Currently, there is no cure for SLE. Thus the goal of treatment is to control symptoms and minimize damage to internal organs by decreasing inflammation. Mild symptoms are treated with NSAIDs. Severe symptoms are treated with steroids: methylprednisolone (Medrol), hydrocortisone (Cortef), or dexamethasone (Dexamethasone Intensol). Cyclophosphamide (Procytox) and mycophenolate (CellCept) are immunosuppressants that may be useful if steroids are not effective. An immunosuppressant, as its name indicates, suppresses the immune system by inhibiting or destroying those cells that produce antibodies (B cells) or mediate inflammation and cell destruction (T cells). Approximately 30% of all patients with SLE take an immunosuppressant. Other classes of drugs are available that might provide remission of the disease.

Patients with SLE are prone to infections. It is important to assist patients in protecting themselves against *Pneumocystis jiroveci* (formerly *P. carinii*) pneumonia, particularly if they are neutropenic. The recommended prophylactic antibiotic treatment is dapsone 100 mg, three times a week. One must take care not to administer medications that might cause SLE flares. For example, sulfonamide antibiotics should be avoided in SLE patients.

Learning Bridge 4.5

While participating in your last advanced pharmacy practice experience (APPE) just before graduation, you are teamed with a medical group that includes an attending physician, a nurse, and a pharmacist who is also your preceptor. During morning rounds at the clinic and review of the medical record of a patient who has SLE, your preceptor notices that one of the medications might not benefit the patient; a drug change is indicated. The following agents appear on the patient's medical records:

> Methylprednisolone (Medrol), taking a tapering-dose schedule by mouth
>
> Naproxen (Aleve), 500 mg by mouth daily
>
> Azathioprine (Imuran), 150 mg by mouth daily
>
> Trimethoprim-sulfamethoxazole (Bactrim), 160/800 mg, one tablet daily for urinary tract infection

Answer the following inquiries that have been put to you by your preceptor:

A. Identify the dubious drug that should be discontinued.
B. Is it important to replace the dubious drug? Why?
C. What suggestion do you have to replace the dubious drug?

Immune Deficiencies

Immune deficiencies can be genetic diseases or have causation by a viral infection (infection with HIV being the best-known virally caused immune deficiency). In addition, toxins released by bacteria can function as "superantigens." Superantigens are antigens that bind and react nonspecifically with multiple T-cell receptor molecules to activate T cells nonspecifically. Initially, superantigens may cause stimulation of T cells, but ultimately they suppress the immune response, which in turn allows a pathogen to grow. As a result, a patient with an immune deficiency is highly susceptible to infections. No matter what the cause of the immune deficiency, affected patients often have low amounts of serum antibodies, have altered phagocytic cells, or lack B or T cells.

Sometimes, the pathogen avoids the immune response by altering its antigenic structure and function. For instance, the influenza virus changes its antigenic function through mutational mechanisms that promote formation of new antigenic phenotypes, which in turn cause a reoccurrence of infection with the virus. Similarly, trypanosomes and streptococci alter their surface glycoproteins and surface carbohydrate antigens, respectively.

In addition to these factors, some medications cause immune deficiencies that reduce a patient's resistance to infectious diseases. Examples of these medications include prolonged antibiotic therapy, steroids, immunosuppressive agents, and cytotoxic drugs. Furthermore, some specific medical conditions—for example, uncontrolled diabetes, granulocytopenia, leukemias, and hypogammaglobulinemia—render patients susceptible to infection. Some of these medical conditions are caused by drugs rather than by a physiological deficiency. For instance, granulocytopenia (or agranulocytosis) occurs in 0.1% of patients who receive sulfonamide antibiotics; it might take a few weeks for these individuals' levels of neutrophils, eosinophils, and basophils to return to normal after the sulfonamide is withdrawn.

Analytical Methods

Several different analytical methods may be used to test a patient's immune deficiency. It is well known that many immune deficiencies are related to malnutrition, severe trauma, severe burns, or cancer. In addition to the white blood cell count with differential, cell-mediated immunity techniques are commonly employed to diagnose an immune deficiency.

Enzyme-Linked Immunosorbent Assay

The reaction that occurs between an antigen and an antibody is highly specific. This specificity, in turn, can be utilized to identify an immune deficiency. Enzyme-linked immunosorbent assay (ELISA) is a very effective method for identifying whether there is serum antibody against a specific antigen. Antisera (antibodies suspended in serum) often contain complex mixtures of antibodies, which make these samples ineffective as the basis for a specific test. In addition, cross-reactions between related antigens may potentially occur. In contrast, monoclonal antibodies are effective tools for identifying immune deficiencies because they have a single known specificity and are homogeneous.

To measure an antibody, a solid plate is probed (fixed) with a known antigen. The plate is then incubated with an antibody (the primary antibody, which is the serum antibody) against the fixed antigen. This antibody will bind specifically to the fixed antigen. After a few washing procedures to remove unbound (unspecific) antibody from the plate, a secondary antibody carrying an enzyme (the linked enzyme, often horseradish peroxidase) is added to the first antibody. A substrate specific to the linked enzyme is catalyzed to develop a color that allows the technician to detect the antigen as a direct result of the amount of antibody bound.

ELISA is an effective way to detect antibodies to HIV proteins (antigens) in blood samples (**Figure 14.20**).

Immunoblotting

Immunoblotting (also called Western blot) is another analytical method for detection of an antigen in a mixture of other polypeptides or proteins (i.e., other antigens). In this technique, sodium dodecyl sulfate (SDS)–polyacrylamide gel electrophoresis (PAGE) is used to detect the antigen of interest. The principle is similar to ELISA, except that, rather than using a plate to fix the antigen, the antigen is separated from other polypeptides on an SDS gel, which is then transferred by electrophoresis to a nitrocellulose membrane. The nitrocellulose membrane reacts with the patient's antibody (**Figure 4.21**). A secondary antibody carrying an enzyme (the linked enzyme, often horseradish peroxidase) is added to the first antibody. The antigen then becomes visible as a band on the nitrocellulose membrane. Because there is specific binding between the antibody and its antigen, all other antibodies are washed out; that is, none of the other antigens in the mixture is detected. This technique is important as a second test for an ELISA-positive HIV result to confirm the presence of an antibody to specific HIV antigens in a patient's serum.

In 2012, the FDA approved an OTC HIV test, OraQuick. This product can be used at home to detect the presence of HIV in saliva. The sample is collected via a mouth swab; that is, the gums are swabbed using the special cotton pad provided with the test. The test result is seen in less than 1 hour. Blood or plasma samples can also be used with this product. Indeed, in a study from 2009, it was shown that the test was equally effective at detecting HIV in both saliva and blood (blood taken from a fingerstick) samples.

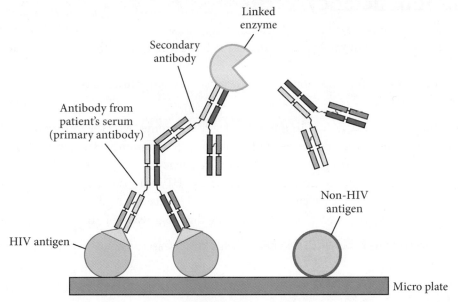

Formation of colored product catalyzed by the linked enzyme indicates the presence of HIV antigen.

Figure 4.20 ELISA is used routinely to detect infection caused by HIV.

Adapted from: Nelson DL, Cox MM, Lehninger AL. *Principles of biochemistry.* 5th ed. New York: W. H. Freeman and Company; 2008: Chapter 5.

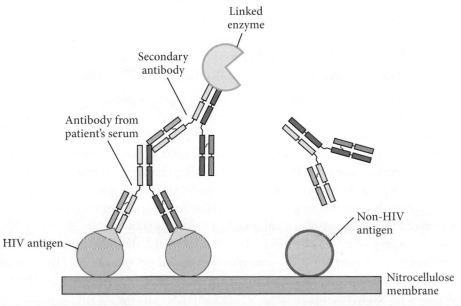

Formation of colored product catalyzed by the linked enzyme indicates the presence of HIV antigen.

Figure 4.21 Immunoblotting assay is used as a second test to confirm a positive HIV result from an ELISA test.

Adapted from: Nelson DL, Cox MM, Lehninger AL. *Principles of biochemistry.* 5th ed. New York: W. H. Freeman and Company; 2008: Chapter 5.

Opportunistic Infections Caused by Human Immunodeficiency Virus

Opportunistic infections are caused by bacteria, fungi, viruses, or parasites that infect compromised immune systems, but rarely cause a disease in hosts with an effective immune system. The characteristics of opportunistic infections are described in the *Introduction to Microbiology* chapter. In this section, HIV infection, one of the most prevalent causes of opportunistic infections, is discussed.

HIV and the associated acquired immunodeficiency syndrome (AIDS) expose patients to a series of infections due to the development of a compromised immune system in HIV-infected patients. HIV replication and a progressive immune deficiency take place throughout the course of HIV infection. As a result, the clinical consequences of HIV infection begin with the primary infection, enter into a prolonged asymptomatic state, and proceed to an advanced state. Adequate and appropriate therapy plays a major role in slowing the progression of HIV.

HIV-infected patients experience two phases with this disease: an acute phase and a chronic phase.

Acute Phase

Approximately half of all patients experience an acute clinical phase approximately one month after their initial infection with HIV. During this acute phase, levels of plasma viremia increase, and typical clinical symptoms such as fever, skin rash, pharyngitis, and myalgia appear. These symptoms occur less frequently in patients who have been infected by contaminated injections, compared with those who have been infected by sexual contact. The acute symptoms usually subside after a few weeks as patients' immune responses to HIV develop and the levels of plasma viremia decrease.

Opportunistic infections may occur during this phase as a result of the reduced numbers of $CD4^+$ and $CD8^+$ cells. Later in the disease course, the number of $CD8^+$ cells increases, which reduces the $CD4^+$:$CD8^+$ ratio. Another possible medical scenario is that a lower ratio is caused by a constant level of $CD8^+$ cells, coincident with a smaller number of $CD4^+$ cells.

Chronic Phase

The acute phase of HIV infection is followed by a prolonged period of clinical latency, referred to as the chronic phase. The length of time from the initial infection to the development of clinical disease varies to a great extent in HIV-infected patients, but the average time for disease progression in untreated patients is 10 years. In these individuals, virus replication is an ongoing and progressive process. The rate of disease progression is directly correlated with the HIV's genome (i.e., RNA levels): Progression of symptoms is faster in patients with high levels of HIV RNA. If patients have a low level of HIV RNA (fewer than 50 copies/mL), they are called "nonprogressors" and show little decline in their $CD4^+$ cell counts over extended periods of time. The average rate of $CD4^+$ cell decrease is $50/\mu L$/year during the asymptomatic period of HIV infection. However, the immunodeficiency becomes severe if the $CD4^+$ population falls below $200/\mu L$, at which time the patient is at high risk for opportunistic infections and neoplasms.

Overall, the symptoms of HIV disease depend on the changes in the $CD4^+$ count and can appear at any time during the course of HIV infection. The peak of severe and life-threatening complications occurs when patients' $CD4^+$ T cell counts are lower than $200/\mu L$. As mentioned earlier, HIV infection places patients at risk for opportunistic infections (while HIV is the primary infection, the opportunistic infections are secondary infections). Most importantly, HIV-infected patients are prone to infections with cytomegalovirus (CMV), *Pneumocystis jiroveci* pneumonia (PCP), and *Mycobacterium avium* complex (MAC). Approximately 50% of all deaths among AIDS patients is related to the fact that patients' CD4+ counts are low. Use of combination antiretroviral therapy has been shown to reduce the incidence of opportunistic infections (see the discussion of treatment options in the *Introduction to Microbiology* chapter). Unfortunately, patients with HIV infection may develop other medical complications as well, including cardiovascular, pulmonary, renal, and hepatic diseases.

Two complications that occur during all stages of HIV infection are acute bronchitis and sinusitis, albeit to a greater extent in patients with low CD4+ counts. Symptoms such as fever, nasal congestion, and headache are commonly observed. The high incidence of sinusitis is caused by an increased frequency of infection with *H. influenzae* and *Streptococcus pneumoniae*. Pulmonary disease is another prevalent complication of HIV infection, as pneumonia is very common in patients, often caused by unicellular fungus *P. jiroveci* infection or mycobacterial infections.

As part of the treatment of patients infected with HIV, it is clearly important to observe for other symptoms and their progress. One way to improve the treatment of HIV complications is to use combination antiretroviral therapy in conjunction with effective primary and secondary prophylaxis for opportunistic infections. Statistical data from 1997 through 2001 showed that rates of Kaposi's sarcoma and opportunistic infections such as CMV, PCP, and MAC declined in HIV-infected patients, even when patients' CD4+ counts were lower than 100/µL, owing to widespread adoption of this therapeutic regimen.

Vaccination and Immunization

One of the successes of modern medicine is the development of vaccines against infectious diseases. Vaccines, after injection into the body, stimulate the immune system to synthesize antibodies that will protect the body against subsequent infection. Vaccination is the most cost-effective health intervention on a broad scale, according to the World Health Organization (WHO), and has had a significant impact on the world's health. Millions of lives are saved each year by vaccines. Immunization with vaccines is central to controlling and improving morbidity and mortality, particularly among infants and children.

Vaccination, simply put, means inoculation of individuals with weakened or destroyed strains of a pathogen (attenuation) that, in a live form, would cause a disease. Vaccines may also consist of recombinant virus particles that have no infective power. Vaccination has a long history, dating back to the late 1700s when Edward Jenner, a physician, discovered vaccinia (cowpox); when administered to humans, vaccinia protected them from the fatal disease smallpox.

In recent years, vaccination has come under intense scrutiny. Claims have been made that some of the nonpathogenic components of vaccination have caused neurological problems, most commonly cited as being autism and attention-deficit/hyperactivity disorder, diabetes, allergic reactions, and autoimmune diseases. As a result, a growing number of individuals and families have opted out of vaccination programs. So far, the claims of harm from vaccines appear to be unfounded. Perhaps the only benefits that such opposition to vaccines can bring to our society are the development of safer vaccination procedures and enhanced education for the general public about the benefits and risks of vaccination. Of particular concern is the need to educate parents about how important and valuable childhood immunization is.

Today, more than 50 biologic products for immunization are licensed in the United States. Many antigens also are available for routine immunization of infants, children, adolescents, and adults. Other vaccines are intended to protect adolescent girls from human papillomavirus (HPV), thereby preventing them from developing cervical cancer, or to protect elderly individuals from herpes zoster, thereby preventing them from developing—or at least mitigating the effects of—zoster (shingles). In 2011, the Centers for Disease Control and Prevention's Advisory Committee on Immunization Practices (ACIP) recommended that, in addition to adolescent females, all 11- to 12-year-old males be vaccinated against HPV. Still other vaccines have been developed in response to outbreaks (polio and H1N1 flu vaccines), and others have been created for prophylaxis in travelers (yellow fever).

Research is ongoing to provide vaccines for different pathogens, with some areas proving more fruitful than others. For instance, researchers successfully created Hib (*Haemophilus influenzae* type B) conjugate vaccines for immunization of infants and children younger than 5 years of age to protect them from Hib infection, whose sequelae include meningitis and pneumonia. In contrast, development efforts directed toward vaccines against eukaryotic pathogens (protozoa and helminths) and HIV have not resulted in any promising outcomes to date.

Allergy is one of the important factors that must be considered carefully to avoid any life-threatening consequence associated with vaccination. Any patient who has experienced an anaphylactic reaction to a vaccine in the past should not receive that vaccine again. Other contraindications to vaccination include pregnancy—for live-virus vaccines (and some selected inactivated-virus vaccines); immunosuppressive disease—for live-virus vaccines (and some selected inactivated-virus vaccines); and untreated tuberculosis—for attenuated-virus vaccines. Caution should also be exercised when patients have acute or severe illness, recent administration of biological antibodies, history of thrombocytopenia with measles–mumps–rubella (MMR) vaccine administration, high fever, shock, or seizure.

Proper storage is necessary to ensure the potency and activity of vaccines. Most vaccines require refrigerated or frozen storage. Precautions should be taken to store vaccines not in refrigerator doors, but rather in the middle of the refrigerator. Temperature monitoring and documentation thereof are required.

As a result of a worldwide inoculation program, the disease known as smallpox was eradicated; subsequently, routine smallpox vaccination was eliminated from healthcare programs. Measles is another example of a disease that affected many children in the past but, due to vaccination, has been virtually eliminated. Outbreaks of the disease, at least in the United States, continue to occur in patients who have elected to not be vaccinated. Other successful immunization campaigns in the United States have targeted rubella and congenital rubella syndrome, neonatal tetanus, and diphtheria. It is important to maintain global vaccination programs, however, as diseases may rebound if the world's guard is let down. For example, poliovirus infection, though it has been eradicated in many countries, has reappeared in a few African and Middle Eastern countries. In addition, while the natural disease has been eradicated, smallpox vaccination is being reconsidered owing to potential concerns about the use of the smallpox virus in bioterrorism.

Immunization and vaccination are not synonymous. Simply put, an immunization process does not require a vaccine (immunization could occur from natural disease course, such as happens with chickenpox), whereas a vaccination process does not guarantee immunity against a pathogen. The latter condition reflects the possibility that an individual's immune response might be different on a genetic level from others', such that all individuals may not respond identically to the same vaccine. During an immunization process, if a vaccine is administered, the vaccine carries antigens from living or killed pathogens that might include protein or carbohydrate molecules from these organisms. These antigens stimulate antibodies or activate T cells to recognize a particular antigen from the pathogen. In most cases, exposure to these antigens will confer immunity, but occasionally and rarely a patient's immune system does not respond appropriately. Sometimes it will be necessary to check antibody titers in these patients to ensure that the vaccine was effective. Only in rare cases have these vaccine antigens harmed recipients. Also of concern are the vaccine formulations' non-antigenic constituents, which enhance the efficacy of certain vaccine types, but are responsible for many of the adverse events associated with vaccines.

The first successful subunit vaccine was produced for hepatitis B virus, which is known to infect the liver, cause liver damage, and, in some cases, cause cancer. This virus consists of two proteins: the core protein associated with the virus genome and the coat protein (subunit). The core protein is not a useful antigenic molecule to serve as a vaccine, but it has a valuable function in diagnosis of the disease. The coat protein or surface antigen, known as HBsAg, forms large aggregates in the blood of infected patients. Development of the vaccine using a "decoy" of this surface protein has proved a very effective means of preventing infection when individuals are later exposed to the "real" HBV (also see the discussion in the *Introduction to Cell Biology* chapter dealing with the development of recombinant vaccines).

Two forms of immunization are possible: active and passive. While the former produces lifelong protection, the latter provides only temporary protection. Sometimes (but not always), the two types of immunization may complement each other and thereby create effective protection against a pathogen. For example, the combination of hepatitis B vaccine (active) and hepatitis B immunoglobulin (passive) is often administered following accidental exposure to HBV-infected blood. The hepatitis B Ig will attach itself to the virus and facilitate its clearance via the complement system and macrophage activity. Hepatitis B Ig has short activity, however, with a half-life of approximately three weeks. Meanwhile, the hepatitis B vaccine can stimulate development of T and B cells that will provide lifelong immunological memory against the HBV.

There are no contraindications to simultaneous administration of two vaccines (even live-attenuated viruses with inactivated viruses). Live-attenuated vaccines must be separated from concurrent administration of biological antibody (such as hepatitis B Ig) because of concerns that the antibody might bind the vaccine, but it is not necessary to separate biological products from inactivated vaccine. The following simple rules are important to consider with regard to vaccination.

1. If two live-attenuated vaccines are to be given at different times, make sure that there is at least a four-week interval between their administration.

2. If two inactivated vaccines are to be given at different times, a specified time interval between vaccine products does not need to be observed.

3. If one live-attenuated vaccine and one inactivated vaccine are to be given at different times, a specified time interval between vaccine products does not need to be observed.

Active Immunization (with Live or Inactive Vaccines)

Active immunization is a process in which the body's own immune system reacts in the expected manner but with a delayed onset, producing a lifelong protection. This phenomenon can happen as a result of encounter with natural disease or by vaccination, both of which result in the production of memory B cells. Active immunity is established by administration of either attenuated or inactivated viruses. An attenuated virus is a live organism that has been altered so that it no longer multiplies in an inoculated organism. However, it retains its immunogenic function and, compared with an inactivated virus, produces longer-lasting immunity. Because the viruses found in such vaccines are not killed but rather are attenuated, live vaccines might cause mild illness. Examples of diseases for which such vaccines are available include measles, mumps, rotavirus, rubella, typhoid, varicella, vaccinia (smallpox), and yellow fever.

An inactivated vaccine is a chemically killed derivative of the actual infectious agent that might include only subunits (subvirions) of that agent—for example, bacterial cell-wall polysaccharides, conjugated bacterial cell-wall polysaccharides, or inactivated toxins. Because these particles cannot replicate, they cannot cause disease. Due to their nature, inactivated vaccines often require patients to receive multiple doses and periodic boosters to maintain immunity. Examples of inactive vaccines include those directed against anthrax, diphtheria, Hib, hepatitis A and B, influenza (injectable), polio (injectable), rabies, and tetanus.

Both types of vaccines have both advantages and disadvantages. Despite the fact that they confer longer immunity, live vaccines are not always the best options. Indeed, the live oral polio vaccine (OPV) no longer is recommended in the United States because there is a slight risk of a virulence reversion. Given that OPV is inexpensive and widely available, WHO still recommends its use in developing countries.

To avoid any negative effect on the production of antibodies, at least a four-week interval must separate administrations of the same vaccine—a factor that is built into vaccination schedules. Vaccine dosing intervals vary greatly between products as well as between the initial vaccination series versus the booster for that vaccine. Some booster intervals are as long as 10 years (e.g., the tetanus toxoid). In other cases, no boosters are required for lifelong immunity. For example, MMR vaccination consisting of the two doses routinely administered in adolescence generally provides lifelong protection against measles, mumps, and rubella. In contrast, influenza vaccination is recommended one time each year, as the viruses in the community change from year to year. Another common theme among vaccine schedules is that the time interval between later doses in a series increases (months to years, not monthly as in the beginning of the series). Except in the case of typhoid vaccine, it is very unusual to restart a series from the beginning if a patient gets off schedule.

Passive Immunization

Passive immunization is, as it sounds, a short-term immunity that wanes over time. Produced in humans, in other animals, or *in vitro,* these immunologic products are designed to transfer the immunity developed in one subject (animal, human) to another (human, the patient). Only immunoglobulins are used to provide passive immunization. Administration of T cells or B cells is infeasible and difficult, and the preparation might be rejected by the host immune response. Recombinant cytokines (interferons) have been used in the treatment of some hematologic and infectious diseases, but they are simply messengers between our own immune cells and do not confer any passive immunity. In contrast to active immunity's slow response, passive immunity has a rapid onset, but lasts for only a brief duration. Passive immunity is the type of immunity that infants receive from their mothers (Ig) through placental transfer and breastfeeding.

Antibodies derived from human sera have a longer half-life (approximately 23 days for IgG antibodies) compared to antibodies from animals (approximately one week). As a result, the administered dose amounts from human antibody sources are much smaller than those from animal sources.

Passive immunization has proven to benefit the following groups:

- Patients who are unable to produce antibodies (congenital agammaglobulinemia)
- Patients who cannot receive active immunization (due to a contraindication)
- Patients in whom treatment is contraindicated because of immunization
- Individuals who do not have access to active immunization

The injection of human immunoglobulins can be moderately painful and may cause transient hypotension and pruritus. Patients with IgA deficiency may develop hypersensitivity reactions to the injected immunoglobulin. In addition, if the antibodies are derived from animals, hypersensitivity reactions may occur. However, antibodies from rodents or lagomorphs rarely cause hypersensitivity reactions in humans. To avoid any anaphylactic reactions, patients should be tested for hypersensitivity reactions.

A few examples of passive immunizations are antivenin (for black widow spider bite and snake bite); botulism antitoxin (for botulism); diphtheria antitoxin (for diphtheria); and hepatitis B immune globulin, known also as HBIG (for hepatitis B, as soon as possible after percutaneous or sexual exposure to HBV).

The following link from the Centers for Disease Control and Prevention provides the recommended immunization schedule for persons aged zero through 6 years and ages 7 through 18 years: http://www.cdc.gov/vaccines/schedules/index.html.

Vaccines as Immunotherapy

The use of vaccines as treatments for diseases, particularly cancer, has been studied for decades. Ideally, such treatments would stimulate our own immune system to engage and destroy cancer cells. In 2010, the FDA approved sipuleucel-T (Provenge) to accomplish just that, using antigen presentation as the mechanism of action to alert cytotoxic T cells. As noted earlier in this chapter, cytotoxic T cells have tumor-cell killing properties.

The production process for sipuleucel-T is unique and specific to each patient. Sipuleucel-T consists of the recombinant antigen protein known as prostatic acid phosphatase (PAP), which must be incubated with the patient's own APCs. The PAP antigen is expressed on the surfaces of most prostate cancer cells. In the sipuleucel-T process, the patient first donates his APCs through a blood donation process called leukapheresis. The blood sample is then sent to a central manufacturing facility, where the APCs are mixed with the recombinant protein, PAP, which is fused to a cytokine, GM-CSF (an immune-cell activator). Presentation of the PAP antigen causes activation of the APC. The APC matures, expressing PAP on its MHC complexes, and is ready for reinfusion into the patient. This entire process takes approximately four days.

The sipuleucel-T dose is, at a minimum, 50 million autologous CD54$^+$ APCs that were activated by the PAP fusion protein. This dose is administered every two weeks for three total doses. Once the activated APCs are reintroduced, they will display the cancer antigen to the patient's cytotoxic T cells, stimulating their activation. These T cells, in turn, will attack and kill those prostate cancer cells that express PAP.

Advances in immunotherapy or therapeutic vaccines are providing new treatment options for many patients with cancer. By programming human immune cells with the target antigen, it might be possible to fight disease without subjecting the patient to the undesirable side effects of traditional chemotherapeutic medicine.

Learning Bridge 4.6

During your health system introductory pharmacy practice experience, your preceptor shows you two medications, basiliximab (Simulect) and cyclosporine (Sandimmune). He asks you to answer the following questions regarding the above agents:

A. Compare the mechanisms of action for these two agents. How are they the same, yet different?

B. What are the routes of administration for these medications? What does the route indicate about the indication and use?

C. Can these two medications be given concomitantly? If so, comment on the risks.

D. What is the origin of basiliximab?

Golden Keys for Pharmacy Students

1. The immune system is organized into two major immunities: innate immunity and adaptive immunity. Adaptive immunity is divided further into two groups: humoral-mediated and cell-mediated immunity.

2. Innate immunity is nonspecific and is always present and prepared to fight a broad array of organisms. Adaptive immunity is specific and utilizes B and T cells.

3. Antibodies that are produced by B lymphocytes (B cells) constitute the humoral immune system. T lymphocytes (T cells) are the key players in the cellular immune system.

4. Lymph nodes are usually found in the axilla, on both sides of the neck, and in the groin, legs, and some other areas of the body. They are responsible for draining and filtering antigens from interstitial fluid. As a result, antigen-presenting cells (dendritic cells and macrophages) and lymphocytes (B and T cells) may encounter trapped antigens in the lymph nodes.

5. Lymph is a clear fluid that contains lymphocytes and proteins.

6. A swollen lymph node is an indication of the buildup of lymphocytes, which in turn indicates that the body is fighting an infection. Lymph nodes are the primary sites of immune response to tissue antigens.

7. Because the lymph nodes are found in the axilla, during a regional spread of cancer cells, such as may occur in breast cancer, cells spread first to these lymph nodes. In turn, identifying whether the lymph nodes contain cancer cells is important when diagnosing breast cancer.

8. Leukocytes, also known as white blood cells (WBCs), are divided into two groups: agranulocytes, which include monocytes (macrophages) and lymphocytes (B and T cells), and granulocytes, which include neutrophils, basophils, and eosinophils.

9. Monocytes originate in the bone marrow, circulate briefly in the blood (one to three days), and then migrate into tissues to become macrophages.

10. Macrophages play important roles in three processes in the human immune system: phagocytosis, antigen presentation, and cytokine production.

11. All lymphocyte progenitor cells originate in the bone marrow. There are two main classes of lymphocytes: T lymphocytes (T cells), which kill viruses/tumor cells, and B lymphocytes (B cells), which produce antibodies.

12. Cytotoxic T cells kill virally infected cells and tumor cells by two means: the Fas-FasL mechanism and the granule-exocytosis mechanism.

13. Multiple granzymes have been identified from granules of cytotoxic lymphocytes. Granzymes A and B are major cytotoxic serine proteases of CTL and NK cells.

14. Mammalian erythrocytes do not have nuclei, so they do not support viral replication. In turn, viruses do not infect erythrocytes.

15. T cells that express only the CD4 surface antigen are designated as helper T cells, also known as CD4 cells.

16. CD4 cells play important roles in the activation of macrophages, CTL, NK cells, and B cells. They also stimulate the secretion of a series of cytokines that induce growth and differentiation of lymphoid cells.

17. The human immunodeficiency virus (HIV) infects and destroys CD4 cells. The destruction of CD4 cells by this virus predisposes HIV-infected patients to opportunistic infections, tumors, dementia, and often death.

18. Th1 cells activate predominantly macrophages and their antigen-presenting capacity to kill intracellular pathogens; they also stimulate B cells to produce immunoglobulin G (IgG) to facilitate the removal of extracellular pathogens by phagocytic cells.

19. Th2 cells release mainly the IL-4, IL-5, IL-13, and IL-25 cytokines and play an important role in the production of immunoglobulin E (IgE) and differentiation of mast cells and eosinophils.

20. NK cells do not have any CD4 or CD8 proteins. However, they play important roles in recognizing and killing virus-infected cells, tumor cells, and antibody-coated target cells without any involvement of class I or class II MHC proteins.

21. The majority of foreign antigens will not be recognized by the immune system unless the antigens are processed by antigen-presenting cells (APCs). APCs include macrophages, B cells, and dendritic cells.

22. Because of humans' unique natural genetic rearrangement and recombination mechanisms, B cells can produce millions of diverse immunoglobulin molecules.

23. The major role for IgA is in mucosal immunity: It prevents foreign substances from adhering to mucosal surfaces (epithelial cells) so that those substances cannot enter the blood circulation.

24. The role of IgD is not fully understood, but it can serve as an antigen receptor on the surface of naive B cells.

25. IgG plays an important role in neonatal protection from foreign substances—it is the only immunoglobulin class that can cross the placenta. Similar to IgA, it can also be secreted in breast milk.

26. After secondary exposure to an antigen, IgG is the major antibody that is found in the plasma. It has an average half-life of 23 days.

27. The role of IgE is to activate mast cells, basophils, and eosinophils; it also stimulates allergic reactions.

28. The attachment of membrane-bound IgM to antigens activates naive B cells. It is the first Ig molecule to be expressed during B-cell development (i.e., during the primary antibody response).

29. Neutrophils, eosinophils, basophils, and mast cells are granulocytes—so named because they have granules.

30. Cytokines are important proteins that regulate (up or down) immune responses by affecting cellular activation, migration, growth, differentiation, and cell-surface molecule expression.

31. Cytokines that primarily target leukocytes are referred to as interleukins, cytokines that are secreted from lymphocytes are referred to as lymphokines, and cytokines that are secreted from monocytes or macrophages are called monokines.

32. Interferons are potent cytokines and polypeptides that play important roles in initiating immune responses. There are three major classes of human interferons: IFN-α, IFN-β, and IFN-γ.

33. Three different pathways, or enzyme cascades, activate the complement system: the classic pathway, which is triggered by immune complexes; the mannose-binding lectin pathway, which is triggered when a lectin molecule binds to mannose groups on the surface of pathogens; and the alternative pathway, which is triggered by binding to a pathogen's surface components.

34. Hypersensitivity has been classified into four types, I–IV. While types I–III are mediated by antibodies, type IV is mediated by cells.

35. Systemic lupus erythematosus (SLE) is an autoimmune disease characterized by cell damage and mediated by tissue-binding autoantibodies and immune complexes.

36. Discoid lupus is a form of lupus dermatitis that is confined to the skin (i.e., not affecting internal organs). When internal organs are involved, the condition is much more severe and is referred to as systemic lupus erythematosus.

37. Prolonged antibiotic therapy, steroids, immunosuppressive agents, and cytotoxic drugs can cause immune deficiencies that reduce a patient's resistance to infectious diseases.

38. Immunoblotting (Western blot) is an analytical method to detect an antigen in a mixture of other antigens. Gel electrophoresis is used to detect the antigen of interest.

39. One treatment approach that has been shown to benefit HIV-infected patients is the use of combination antiretroviral therapy in conjunction with primary and secondary prophylaxis for opportunistic infections.

40. Once vaccines are injected, they stimulate the immune system to synthesize antibodies that will protect the body against subsequent infection.

41 Vaccination means inoculation of individuals with weakened or destroyed strains (attenuation), or components thereof, of a pathogen that in a live form would cause a disease.

42. Two forms of immunizations are distinguished: active and passive. While the former produces lifelong protection, the latter provides only temporary protection.

43. If two live-attenuated vaccines are to be given at different times, at least a four-week interval should separate their administration. If two inactivated vaccines are to be given at different times, no specific interval is required. If one activated vaccine and one inactivated vaccine are to be given at different times, they may be administered without regard to each other.

44. Active immunization is a process in which the body's own immune system reacts with a delayed onset, but produces lifelong protection.

45. Passive immunization immunologic products are produced in humans, in animals, or *in vitro*. These immunologic products are designed to transfer the immunity developed in one subject (animal, human) to another (human, the patient). Immunoglobulins are used in passive immunization therapy. Administration of T cells or B cells is not practical and is difficult, and the products might be rejected by host immune responses.

46. Leukocytopenia is caused by primary/secondary immunodeficiency and infection (HIV/AIDS).

47. Many chemotherapy drugs (including cyclophosphamide) that are designed to kill rapidly dividing cells can cause leukocytopenia. Many agents and drugs inhibit WBC production when they are given in high doses or over prolonged periods. Examples include alcohol, penicillins, and ganciclovir.

48. When the WBC count is stated to be "3.1," it really means 3,100 cells/mm^3.

Learning Bridge Answers

4.1 Drugs that increase the synthesis of cAMP appear to reduce the lytic activity of NK cells. In addition, both glucocorticoids (prednisolone) and salicylates (aspirin) appear to reduce the cytotoxic activity of NK cells. Additionally, glucocorticoids inhibit the production of IL-2, which in turn can decrease communication to and subsequent activation of NK cells.

You might suggest that David's physician consider alternative therapy and discontinue theophylline. Use of these three medications in combination will have additive effects on immunosuppression, and theophylline probably is providing less benefit for David than prednisolone. Unfortunately, switching from theophylline to albuterol (Proventil) will not benefit David because albuterol also enhances the synthesis of cAMP. David can be counseled to modify his exercise routine to avoid triggers that exacerbate his occasional respiratory problem. In addition, suggest to David that he use acetaminophen (Tylenol) instead of aspirin.

4.2 **A.** Except for the unusually large percentage of neutrophils (82%, when the normal level is around 60%), all other values are in the normal range.

B. An elevated WBC count (leukocytosis) is often an indication of infection. This is usually a result of increased production of granulocytes (neutrophils, basophils, and eosinophils). However, a number of other, more detailed cell counts can help further the diagnostic process. Leukocytosis may be the result of a variety of circumstances: infection, leukemic cancers, trauma, thyroid storm, or corticosteroids. Elevated lymphocytes (lymphocytosis) can occur with hepatitis, chickenpox, herpes simplex, or herpes zoster. Recall that lymphocytes are a type of leukocyte. An elevated number of eosinophils may be a sign of allergic disorders, allergic drug reactions, and parasitic infections. An elevated number of monocytes may indicate chronic inflammation, viral and parasitic infections, or tuberculosis. An elevated number of basophils is an indication of hypersensitivity reactions to food or drugs. An elevated number of neutrophils (neutrophilia) is often caused by infection, diabetic ketoacidosis, stress, burns, acute inflammation, or use of corticosteroids. Because Amy has diabetes and could develop signs and symptoms of the life-threatening condition known as ketoacidosis, we would expect that her WBC would indicate neutrophilia.

C. You can counsel her that fexofenadine is an antihistamine. As such, it will inhibit the effects of histamine released from eosinophils owing to her allergies. Given that her eosinophil count is within normal limits, this patient is not at risk for having an exacerbated reaction.

4.3 **A.** One of the side effects of nitrofurantoin is allergic reaction presenting as rash. Eosinophilia (when the number of eosinophils is greater than 500 cells/μL blood) combined with rash is a confirmatory finding that the patient is having an allergic reaction to the agent. Many other agents also cause eosinophilia, including sulfonamides, penicillins, and cephalosporins.

B. Amy should immediately stop using nitrofurantoin. You also should immediately contact her physician and ask him or her to prescribe another antibiotic. There is no OTC product that can resolve this patient's severe rashes. Glucocorticoids such as oral prednisone can help control the inflammatory reaction and reduce the number of eosinophils, thereby alleviating the severity of the allergic reaction. Oral antihistamines such as diphenhydramine will inhibit the inflammatory and itching effects caused by histamine released from the eosinophils. Theoretically, because IL-5 plays a major role in the eosinophil growth, one could administer a monoclonal anti-IL-5 antibody to bind IL-5 and thereby slow the development of more eosinophils. Unfortunately, this type of therapy is better at preventing reactions than treating current episodes (nor is the product currently available).

4.4   Adalimumab is a humanized monoclonal antibody (similar to human IgG) that binds to TNF and inhibits the binding of TNF to its receptors on inflammatory cells. Infliximab is a chimeric fusion of human and mouse IgG. Not only does methotrexate have activity against rheumatoid arthritis, but it was administered together with infliximab because Joe's body might potentially see infliximab as a foreign protein (due to the mouse component) and produce antibody against it, thereby reducing the efficacy of infliximab. To avoid production of antibodies to infliximab, Joe should take an oral formation of methotrexate as long as he continues to use infliximab.

Because adalimumab is a humanized IgG, it has no foreign component; thus it is less antigenic than infliximab. Adalimumab is available as injection pens (40 mg) and is administered subcutaneously every other week. Because this immunoglobulin reduces Joe's immune responses, he must take the same precautions regarding infections.

Joe's alopecia (hair loss) was caused most likely by methotrexate; now that he has stopped using it, his hair growth should return to its previous level.

You should also advise Joe that he should continue to be careful with live-attenuated vaccines. Administration of live-attenuated vaccines must be separated from administration of biological drugs that promote immunosuppression (e.g., adalimumab, infliximab) because the immune response to the vaccination might be blunted. This might result in failed protection against disease. It is not necessary to separate administration of biological products from administration of inactivated vaccines.

4.5   **A.** Trimethoprim-sulfamethoxazole causes SLE to flare and should be avoided in patients with SLE.

   B. Yes, it is, because the patient has a UTI requiring treatment. Patients with SLE are often prone to infections. Additionally, as the patient is taking an immunosuppressant (azathioprine), its action will increase the patient's risk of developing infection. Vigilant long-term monitoring for infection is warranted.

   C. Trimethoprim-sulfamethoxazole should be discontinued and another antibiotic started in its place. Given the lack of a urine culture to guide therapy in this example, an appropriate alternative would be levofloxacin (Levaquin), 500 mg by mouth daily. A closer examination of the patient's history will determine the length of therapy indicated.

4.6   **A.** Basiliximab is a monoclonal antibody that functions as an immunosuppressive agent. It specifically binds to and blocks the interleukin-2 receptor α-chain (IL-2Rα, known also as CD25 antigen) on the surface of activated T-lymphocytes.

Cyclosporine inhibits calcineurin phosphatase, which results in reduced IL-2 gene transcription. The final outcome is a decrease in IL-2 synthesis.

Both agents reduce the effectiveness of IL-2 communication between cells, limiting clonal expansion of T cells. Basiliximab blocks IL-2 on the outside of the T cell, while cyclosporine blocks "secretion" of IL-2 from inside the T cell.

   B. Basiliximab: IV; cyclosporine: PO or IV. Cyclosporine IV is prescribed only for in-hospital use due to its risk and adverse effects, and for finite periods of use. Oral cyclosporine is easily taken at home, and is intended for long-term immunosuppression.

C. Basiliximab and cyclosporine are given together on a short-term basis (a few days). Basiliximab continues to exert its effect, providing practitioners with time to tailor the cyclosporine dose without being overly concerned about low concentration levels that might contribute to rejection. These two agents, when given together, have additive immunosuppression and adverse reactions. The additive T cell suppression is theoretical, in that basiliximab is blocking IL-2 receptors, while the addition or reduction of IL-2 production has a limited effect on the "blocked" T cells.

D. Basiliximab is a chimeric (murine/human) monoclonal antibody, produced by recombinant DNA technology. It is an IgG, but is specific for only one antigen (CD25).

Problems and Solutions

Problem 4.1 Which of the following statements about WBC is correct?

A. It is the WBC number that often tells us about an infection.
B. When the number of WBCs is enhanced, the condition is referred to as leukocytosis.
C. Increases in the number of WBCs can be caused by infection, leukemia, trauma, emotion, stress, thyroid storm, or use of corticosteroids.
D. Only A and B.
E. All of the above.

Solution 4.1 E is correct.

Problem 4.2 The lymph nodes are found in

A. the armpits.
B. on both sides of the neck.
C. in the groin.
D. the legs.
E. All of the above.
F. A, B, and C.

Solution 4.2 E is correct.

Problem 4.3 Which of the following statements about white blood cells is (are) correct?

A. Leukocytes are referred to as white blood cells.
B. The human body contains approximately 400–11,000 WBCs/μL blood.
C. WBCs include both agranulocytes and granulocytes.
D. Lymphocytes account for 60% of the total number of WBCs.
E. Both A and B.
F. Both A and C.
G. All of the above.

Solution 4.3 F is correct. B is not correct because the normal WBC range is 4000–11,000 WBCs/μL blood. Lymphocytes account for 30% of total WBCs.

Problem 4.4 Which of the following cells are synonymous with monocytes?

A. Macrophages
B. Eosinophils
C. Basophils
D. B cells
E. T cells

Solution 4.4 A is correct. Monocytes originate in the bone marrow, circulate briefly in the blood (one to three days), and then migrate into tissues to become macrophages.

Problem 4.5 Name three major functions of macrophages.

Solution 4.5 Phagocytosis, antigen presentation, and cytokine production.

Problem 4.6 Which of the following cells are lymphocytes? Choose all that apply.

    A. T cells
    B. B cells
    C. Macrophages
    D. Monocytes
    E. Eosinophils

Solution 4.6 A and B are correct. All lymphocyte progenitor cells originate in the bone marrow. T lymphocytes (T cells) kill viruses and tumor cells, and B lymphocytes (B cells) produce antibodies.

Problem 4.7 Name two mechanisms by which cytotoxic T cells kill virally infected cells or tumor cells.

Solution 4.7 Fas-FasL mechanism and granule-exocytosis mechanism.

Problem 4.8 Describe the role of perforin in the granule-exocytosis mechanism.

Solution 4.8 Perforin is an effective protein that, even in extremely low concentration (less than 10^{-9} M), makes large pores in the target cell. The pores form when perforin binds to phospholipids of the target cell's membrane through a calcium-dependent mechanism. As a result, the damage to the cell membrane allows granzymes to penetrate into the target cell to induce cell death.

Problem 4.9 Which of the following granule-exocytosis molecules are found in high concentrations in patients with rheumatoid arthritis?

    A. Granzymes A and B
    B. Perforin
    C. Granzymes G and H
    D. Granzymes G, H, and K

Solution 4.9 A is correct.

Problem 4.10 Many proteases are synthesized in inactive forms called

    A. caspases.
    B. zymogens.
    C. complement proteins.
    D. cytokines.
    E. perforin.

Solution 4.10 B is correct.

Problem 4.11 Which of the following immunoglobulin molecules is the first Ig molecule to be expressed during B-cell development (i.e., during the primary antibody response)?

    A. IgA
    B. IgD
    C. IgE
    D. IgG
    E. IgM

Solution 4.11 E is correct. The attachment of membrane-bound IgM to antigen activates naive B cells. IgM is, therefore, the first Ig molecule to be expressed during the B cell's development.

Problem 4.12 Neutrophils, eosinophils, basophils, monocytes, and lymphocytes are effective cells of the human immune system. Describe the consequences that arise as a result of having an unusually large number of these cells. In addition, indicate the normal percentages of these cells in a WBC count.

Solution 4.12 Normal levels: neutrophils, 60%; lymphocytes, 30%; monocytes, 6%; eosinophils, 3%; basophils, 1%. An elevated WBC count (leukocytosis) is often an indication of infection because it signals increased production of granulocytes (neutrophils, basophils, and eosinophils). An elevated number of neutrophils (neutrophilia) may be caused by infection, diabetic ketoacidosis, stress, burns, acute inflammation, or use of corticosteroids. Elevated lymphocytes are observed in hepatitis, chickenpox, herpes simplex, and herpes zoster. An elevated number of eosinophils is a sign of allergic disorders, allergic drug reactions, or parasitic infections. An elevated number of basophils is an indication of hypersensitivity reactions to food or drugs.

Problem 4.13 Upon administering penicillin, patients develop rashes within two to three minutes. This is an example of

- **A.** type I hypersensitivity.
- **B.** type II hypersensitivity.
- **C.** type III hypersensitivity.
- **D.** type IV hypersensitivity.
- **E.** having a high IgG level.

Solution 4.13 A is correct. Type I hypersensitivity, or immediate hypersensitivity, causes urticaria (skin rash with bumps), anaphylaxis, asthma, or hay fever (rhinitis) and occurs after ingestion of food, medication, or airborne allergens. The immediate allergic reaction occurs because of interaction of an antigen with a preexisting IgE that is bound to blood basophils or tissue mast cells.

Problem 4.14 Upon administering penicillin, a patient develops rashes after 24 hours. This is an example of

- **A.** type I hypersensitivity.
- **B.** type II hypersensitivity.
- **C.** type III hypersensitivity.
- **D.** type IV hypersensitivity.
- **E.** having a high IgG level.

Solution 4.14 D is correct. Type IV hypersensitivity reaction is delayed, occurring more than 12 hours after contact with the allergen. The response is delayed because, when T cells become activated, they need to attract macrophages to the sites of antigens, which is a relatively slow process compared to other types of hypersensitivity.

Problem 4.15 Which of the following drugs does not trigger SLE?

- **A.** Hydralazine
- **B.** Quinidine
- **C.** Acetaminophen
- **D.** Phenytoin
- **E.** Isoniazid
- **F.** D-Penicillamine

Solution 4.15 C is correct.

Problem 4.16 A patient who is diagnosed with SLE, but has only mild symptoms, would be treated with

    A. NSAIDs.
    B. methylprednisolone.
    C. hydrocortisone.
    D. cyclophosphamide.
    E. mycophenolate.

Solution 4.16 A is correct. All other of the other choices are used to treat SLE associated with severe symptoms.

Problem 4.17 For which indication would a mast cell stabilizer be best used?

    A. Autoimmune disorders
    B. Immune deficiencies
    C. A disease characterized by excessive histamine release
    D. A disease characterized by excessive serotonin release

Solution 4.17 C is correct.

Problem 4.18 Rejection of transplanted organs is primarily associated with which types of antigens?

    A. Epitopes
    B. Haptens
    C. CD antigens
    D. MHC proteins

Solution 4.18 D is correct.

Problem 4.19 In a kidney transplant patient, which type of T cell would be attracted to the MHC class I protein on the donated kidney, stimulating rejection, and why?

Solution 4.19 Cytotoxic T lymphocytes (CD8 cells). These T cells see the MHC class I protein as "foreign" and would kill the cell.

Problem 4.20 Echinacea is reported to increase the production of

    A. interferon.
    B. tumor necrosis factor.
    C. IL-1.
    D. all of the above.

Solution 4.20 D is correct.

References

1. Anassi E, Ndefo UA. Sipuleucel-T (Provenge) injection. *Pharmacy Therap.* 2011; 36:197–202.
2. Barrett KE, Barman SM, Boitano S, Brooks HL. Blood as a circulatory fluid and the dynamics of blood and lymph flow. In: Barrett KE, Barman SM, Boitano S, Brooks HL, eds. *Ganong's review of medical physiology.* 24th ed. New York, NY: McGraw-Hill; 2012. Available at: http://www.accesspharmacy.com/content.aspx?aID=56264612.
3. Barrett KE, Barman SM, Boitano S, Brooks H. Immunity, infection, and inflammation. In: Barrett KE, Barman SM, Boitano S, Brooks H, eds. *Ganong's review of medical physiology.* 23rd ed. New York, NY: McGraw-Hill Professional; 2009. Available at: http://www.accesspharmacy.com/content.aspx?aID=5242699.
4. Blumenthal DK, Garrison JC. Pharmacodynamics: molecular mechanisms of drug action. In: Chabner BA, Brunton LL, Knollman BC, eds. *Goodman & Gilman's the pharmacological basis of*

therapeutics. 12th ed. New York, NY: McGraw-Hill; 2011. Available at: http://www.accesspharmacy .com/content.aspx?aID=16658452.

5. Borja-Hart N, Whalen KL. Interpretation of clinical laboratory data. In: Kier KL, Nemire RE, eds. *Pharmacy student survival guide.* 2nd ed. New York, NY: McGraw-Hill; 2009. Available at: http://www.accesspharmacy.com/content.aspx?aID=5257616.

6. Brooks GF, Carroll KC, Butel JS, et al. Immunology. In: Brooks GF, Carroll KC, Butel JS, et al., eds. *Jawetz, Melnick, & Adelberg's medical microbiology.* 25th ed. New York, NY: McGraw-Hill; 2010. Available at: http://www.accessmedicine.com/content.aspx?aID=6427017.

7. Brooks GF, Carroll KC, Butel JS, et al. Pathogenesis and control of viral diseases. In: Brooks GF, Carroll KC, Butel JS, et al., eds. *Jawetz, Melnick, & Adelberg's medical microbiology.* 25th ed. New York, NY: McGraw-Hill; 2010. Available at: http://www.accessmedicine.com/content. aspx?aID=6430454.

8. Burns EA. Immune system. In: *AccessScience.* New York, NY: McGraw-Hill; 2000. Available at: http://www.accessscience.com.

9. Colliou N, Picard D, Caillot F., et al. Long-term remissions of severe pemphigus after rituximab therapy are associated with prolonged failure of desmoglein B cell response. *Sci Transl Med.* 2013; 5:175.

10. Delves PJ, Roitt IM. The immune system: first of two parts. *N Engl J Med.* 2000; 343:37–49.

11. Doherty GM. Preoperative care. In: Doherty GM. *Current diagnosis & treatment: surgery.* 13th ed. New York, NY: McGraw-Hill; 2010. Available at: http://www.accessmedicine.com/content .aspx?aID=5211032.

12. Fauci AS, Lane HC. Human immunodeficiency virus disease: AIDS and related disorders. In: Fauci AS, Braunwald E, Kasper DL, et al. *Harrison's principles of internal medicine.* 17th ed. New York, NY: McGraw-Hill; 2008. Available at: http://www.accessmedicine.com/content .aspx?aID=2904810.

13. Fraser SA, Karimi R, Michalak M, Hudig D. Perforin lytic activity is controlled by calreticulin. *J Immunol.* 2000; 164: 4150–5.

14. Gourley DR, Eoff JC, eds. *APhA complete review for pharmacy.* 9th ed. Washington, DC: American Pharmacists Association; 2012.

15. Grosser T, Smyth E. Anti-inflammatory, antipyretic, and analgesic agents: pharmacotherapy of gout. In: Chabner BA, Brunton LL, Knollman BC, eds. *Goodman & Gilman's the pharmacological basis of therapeutics.* 12th ed. New York, NY: McGraw-Hill; 2011. Available at: http://www.accesspharmacy.com/content.aspx?aID=16670422.

16. Hahn BH. Systemic lupus erythematosus. In: Fauci AS, Braunwald E, Kasper DL, et al. *Harrison's principles of internal medicine.* 17th ed. New York, NY: McGraw-Hill; 2008. Available at: http://www.accessmedicine.com/content.aspx?aID=2858970.

17. Hall PD, Pilch NW, Atchley DH. Function and evaluation of the immune system. In: Talbert RL, DiPiro JT, Matzke GR, et al., eds. *Pharmacotherapy: a pathophysiologic approach.* 8th ed. New York, NY: McGraw-Hill; 2011. Available at: http://www.accesspharmacy.com/content .aspx?aID=7995409.

18. Hall PD, Weimert NA. Function and evaluation of the immune system. In: DiPiro JT, Talbert RL, Yee GC, et al. *Pharmacotherapy: a pathophysiologic approach.* 7th ed. New York, NY: McGraw-Hill; 2008. Available at: http://www.accesspharmacy.com/content.aspx?aID=3210102.

19. Hayden FG. Antiviral agents (nonretroviral). In: Brunton LL, Lazo JS, Parker KL. *Goodman & Gilman's the pharmacological basis of therapeutics.* 11th ed. New York, NY: McGraw-Hill; 2006. Available at: http://www.accessmedicine.com/content.aspx?aID=950476. Haynes BF, Soderberg KA, Fauci AS. Introduction to the immune system. In: Fauci AS, Braunwald E, Kasper DL, et al. *Harrison's principles of internal medicine.* 17th ed. New York, NY: McGraw-Hill; 2008. Available at: http://www.accessmedicine.com/content.aspx?aID=2858331. Holland SM, Gallin JI. Disorders of granulocytes and monocytes. In: Fauci AS, Kasper DL, Jameson JL, et al., eds. *Harrison's principles*

of internal medicine. 18th ed. New York, NY: McGraw-Hill; 2012. Available at: http://www.accesspharmacy.com/content.aspx?aID=9113657.

20.   Janeway CA, Travers P, Walport M. *Immunobiology: The immune system in health and disease.* 4th ed. New York: Elsevier Science /Garland; 1999: Chapter 8.

21.   Kantoff PW, Higano CS, Shore ND, et al. Sipuleucel-T immunotherapy for castration-resistant prostate cancer. *N Engl J Med.* 2010; 363:411–422.

22.   Katzung BG. Vaccines, immune globulins, and other complex biologic products. In: Katzung BG. *Basic & clinical pharmacology.* 11th ed. New York, NY: McGraw-Hill; 2009. Available at: http://www.accessmedicine.com/content.aspx?aID=4517462.

23.   Keusch GT, Bart KJ, Miller M. Immunization principles and vaccine use. In: Fauci AS, Braunwald E, Kasper DL, Hauser SL, et al. *Harrison's principles of internal medicine.* 17th ed. New York, NY: McGraw-Hill; 2008. Available at: http://www.accessmedicine.com/content.aspx?aID=2901633.

24.   Kipps TJ. The organization and structure of lymphoid tissues. In: Lichtman MA, Kipps TJ, Seligsohn U, et al. *Williams hematology.* 8th ed. New York, NY: McGraw-Hill; 2010. Available at: http://www.accessmedicine.com/content.aspx?aID=6115884.

25.   Kipps TJ. Functions of B lymphocytes and plasma cells in immunoglobulin production. In: Lichtman MA, Kipps TJ, Seligsohn U, et al. *Williams hematology.* 8th ed. New York, NY: McGraw-Hill; 2010. Available at: http://www.accessmedicine.com/content.aspx?aID=6115884.

26.   Kipps TJ. Functions of T lymphocytes: T-cell receptors for antigen. In: Lichtman MA, Kipps TJ, Seligsohn U, et al. *Williams hematology.* 8th ed. New York, NY: McGraw-Hill; 2010. Available at: http://www.accessmedicine.com/content.aspx?aID=6115884.

27.   Kipps TJ. The cluster of differentiation antigens. In: Lichtman MA, Kipps TJ, Seligsohn U, et al. *Williams hematology.* 8th ed. New York, NY: McGraw-Hill; 2008. Available at: http://www.accessmedicine.com/content.aspx?aID=6121852. Krensky AM, Vincenti F, Bennett WM. Immunosuppressants, tolerogens, and immunostimulants. In: Brunton LL, Lazo JS, Parker K. *Goodman & Gilman's the pharmacological basis of therapeutics.* 11th ed. New York, NY: McGraw-Hill; 2006. Available at: http://www.accessmedicine.com/content.aspx?aID=951722.

28.   Kurschus FC, Jenne DE. Delivery and therapeutic potential of human granzyme B. *Immunol Rev.* 2010; 235(1):159–171.

29.   Lake DF, Briggs AD, Akporiaye ET. Immunopharmacology. In: Katzung BG, Masters SB, Trevor AJ, eds. *Basic & clinical pharmacology.* 12th ed. New York, NY: McGraw-Hill; 2012. Available at: http://www.accesspharmacy.com/content.aspx?aID=55831418.

30.   Lee LA. Humoral immunity and complement. In: Wolff K, Goldsmith LA, Katz SI, et al. *Fitzpatrick's dermatology in general medicine.* 7th ed. New York, NY: McGraw-Hill; 2007. Available at: http://www.accessmedicine.com/content.aspx?aID=2954799.

31.   Levinson W. Immunity. In: Levinson W. *Review of medical microbiology and immunology.* 11th ed. New York, NY: McGraw-Hill; 2010. Available at: http://www.accessmedicine.com/content.aspx?aID=6458813.

32.   Levinson W. Cellular basis of the immune response. In: Levinson W. *Review of medical microbiology and immunology.* 11th ed. New York, NY: McGraw-Hill; 2010. Available at: http://www.accessmedicine.com/content.aspx?aID=6458977.

33.   Madan RA, Gulley JL, Kantoff PW. Demystifying immunotherapy in prostate cancer. *Cancer J.* 2013;19:50–58.

34.   Mescher AL. The immune system and lymphoid organs. In: Mescher AL, ed. *Junqueira's basic histology: text & atlas.* 12th ed. New York, NY: McGraw-Hill; 1010. Available at: http://www.accessmedicine.com/content.aspx?aID=6181867.

35.   Modlin RL, Kim J, Maurer D, et al. Innate and adaptive immunity in the skin. In: Wolff K, Goldsmith LA, Katz SI, et al. *Fitzpatrick's dermatology in general medicine.* 7th ed. New York, NY: McGraw-Hill; 2007. Available at: http://www.accessmedicine.com/content.aspx?aID=29535662007.

36. Murray RK. Red and white blood cells. In: Murray RK, Kennelly PJ, Rodwell VW, et al., eds. *Harper's illustrated biochemistry.* 29th ed. New York, NY: McGraw-Hill; 2011. Available at: http://www.accesspharmacy.com/content.aspx?aID=55886752.

37. Nelson DL, Cox MM. *Principles of biochemistry.* 5th ed. New York: W. H. Freeman and Company; 2008.

38. Ortolani C, Forti E, Radin E, et al. Cytofluorimetric identification of two populations of double positive (CD4$^+$,CD8$^+$) T lymphocytes in human peripheral blood. *Biochem Biophys Res Commun.* 1993;191:601–609.

39. Petri M. Systemic lupus erythematosus. In: Imboden JB, Hellmann DB, Stone JH. *Current rheumatology diagnosis & treatment.* 2nd ed. New York, NY: McGraw-Hill; 2007. Available at: http://www.accessmedicine.com/content.aspx?aID=2725464.

40. Ray CG, Ryan KJ. Immune response to infection. In: Ray CG, Ryan KJ, eds. *Sherris medical microbiology.* 5th ed. New York, NY: McGraw-Hill; 2010. Available at: http://www.accessmedicine.com/content.aspx?aID=6936356.

41. Rybak MJ, Aeschlimann JR, Laplante KL. Laboratory tests to direct antimicrobial pharmacotherapy. In: Talbert RL, DiPiro JT, Matzke GR, et al., eds. *Pharmacotherapy: a pathophysiologic approach.* 8th ed. New York, NY: McGraw-Hill; 2011. Available at: http://www.accesspharmacy.com/content.aspx?aID=8000915.

42. Saavedra A, Johnson RA. Cutaneous manifestations of human immunodeficiency virus disease. In: Wolff K, Goldsmith LA, Katz SI, et al. *Fitzpatrick's dermatology in general medicine.* 7th ed. New York, NY: McGraw-Hill; 2007. Available at: http://www.accessmedicine.com/content.aspx?aID=2998563.

43. Sausville EA, Longo DL. Principles of cancer treatment. In: Fauci AS, Braunwald E, Kasper DL, et al. *Harrison's principles of internal medicine.* 17th ed. 2008. Available at: http://www.accessmedicine.com/content.aspx?aID=2888811.

44. Schur PH, Gladman DD. *Overview of the clinical manifestations of systemic lupus erythematosus in adults.* Waltham, MA: UpToDate: 2012. Available at: http://www.uptodate.com/online with subscription.

45. Shen WC, Stan GL. *Immunology for pharmacy students.* Singapore: Harwood Academic Publisher; 1999.

46. Sutton SS, Hall PD, Norris LB, Bennett CL. Immune system. In: Sutton SS, Hall PD, Norris LB, Bennett CL, eds. *McGraw-Hill's NAPLEX® review guide.* New York, NY: McGraw-Hill; 2011. Available at: http://www.accesspharmacy.com/content.aspx?aID=725078.

47. Tamang DL, Redelman D, Alves BN, et al. Induction of granzyme B and T cell cytotoxic capacity by IL-2 or IL15 without antigens: multiclonal responses that are extremely lytic if triggered and short-lived after cytokine withdrawal. *Cytokine.* 2006; 36(3–4):148–159.

48. UpToDate. Waltham, MA: 2012. Available at: http://www.uptodate.com/online with subscription.

49. Wang F, Kieff E. Medical virology. In: Fauci AS, Braunwald E, Kasper DL, et al. *Harrison's principles of internal medicine.* 17th ed. New York, NY: McGraw-Hill; 2008. Available at: http://www.accessmedicine.com/content.aspx?aID=2873184.

50. White DA, Scribner AN, Huang JV. A comparison of patient acceptance of fingerstick whole blood and oral fluid rapid HIV screening in an emergency department. *J Acquir Immune Defic Syndr.* 2009; 52(1):75.

51. Williams IR, Rich BE, Kupper TS. Cytokines. In: Wolff K, Goldsmith LA, Katz SI, et al. *Fitzpatrick's dermatology in general medicine.* 7th ed. New York, NY: McGraw-Hill; 2007. Available at: http://www.accessmedicine.com/content.aspx?aID=2975315.

52. Yosipovitch G, Dawn AG, Greaves MW. Pathophysiology and clinical aspects of pruritus. In: Wolff K, Goldsmith LA, Katz SI, et al. *Fitzpatrick's dermatology in general medicine.* 7th ed. New York, NY: McGraw-Hill; 2007. Available at: http://www.accessmedicine.com/content.aspx?aID=2960463.

Introduction to Biochemistry

Reza Karimi

Fariba Safaiyan

CHAPTER 5

OBJECTIVES

1. Understand thermodynamics and its important roles in biochemical pathways and reactions.

2. Explain the nonlinear enzyme kinetics that describes saturation and competition. In addition, understand how Michaelis-Menten kinetics is applied in enzymatic reactions.

3. Describe the metabolism, synthesis, and regulatory mechanisms that occur in the glycolysis, gluconeogenesis, and pentos phosphate pathways.

4. Understand the β-oxidation pathway and biosynthesis of fatty acids.

5. Understand oxidation and biosynthesis of amino acids. In addition, learn about a series of well-known genetic diseases related to amino acid metabolism.

6. Describe the essential roles that the citric acid cycle and oxidative phosphorylation play in the metabolism of carbohydrates, fatty acids, and amino acids.

7. Describe the urea cycle and its important role in removing the toxic molecule, ammonium.

8. Understand the roles of the liver, adipocytes, muscles, and brain in the metabolism of carbohydrates, fatty acids, and amino acids.

9. Learn about the important roles that hormones play in the metabolism of carbohydrates, fatty acids, and amino acids.

10. Implement a series of Learning Bridge assignments at your experiential sites to bridge your didactic learning with your experiential experiences.

KEY TERMS AND DEFINITIONS

1. **Activation energy:** an energy barrier that must be overcome for a reaction to occur.

2. **Apolipoprotein:** a lipid-binding protein that participates in the transportation of triacylglycerols, phospholipids, cholesterol, and cholesteryl esters between different organs.

3. **ATP:** adenosine triphosphate; an energy-rich molecule.

4. **Chaperone:** a protein that—often at the expense of ATP hydrolysis—assists other proteins in maintaining the correct folding of proteins, particularly the newly synthesized proteins in the cytosol.

5. **Cori cycle:** A metabolic process that sends lactate from muscle to the liver, where lactate becomes pyruvate, and then from pyruvate to glucose (through gluconeogenesis), after which the glucose is finally returned to muscle to refill muscle glycogen.

6. **Denaturation:** structural effects that cause the biological activity of a protein to be reduced or eliminated.

7. **Enthalpy:** the heat under constant pressure; indicated by the symbol H.

8. **Entropy:** the amount of disorder in a system; indicated by the symbol S.

9. **Enzyme kinetics:** the rate of a reaction and the mathematical analysis of an enzyme activity.

(continues)

10. **Free energy:** the energy available (or required) to do work in a system.

11. **Gluconeogenesis:** synthesis of glucose from noncarbohydrate substrates such as oxaloacetate or pyruvate.

12. **Glucose–alanine cycle:** a pathway that elegantly employs alanine and pyruvate to assist the human body in removing the toxic ammonium.

13. **Glyceroneogenesis:** a pathway similar to gluconeogenesis that produces dihydroxyacetone phosphate (DHAP). DHAP is converted into glycerol-3-phosphate, which finally becomes a triacylglycerol.

14. **Glycolysis:** oxidation of a glucose molecule and production of two pyruvate molecules in a 10-step multienzyme pathway.

15. **Glycogenolysis:** breakdown of glycogen molecules.

16. **Feedback inhibition:** a multienzyme system in which the regulatory enzyme is inhibited by the end product.

17. **Fermentation:** the operation of the glycolysis pathway under anaerobic conditions.

18. **Hemoglobin:** a heme protein with four subunits (α_1, β_1, α_2, and β_2) that serves to carry oxygen from lungs to other tissues.

19. **Hormones:** effective signaling molecules that are secreted and diffuse into the blood capillaries, travel within the bloodstream, and diffuse out of the blood to affect a target cell. Often, a hormone produces a response by binding to either a membrane-bound receptor or an intracellular receptor.

20. **Induced fit:** a type of substrate binding that can induce a conformational change in an enzyme.

21. **k_{cat}:** a parameter that measures the number of substrate molecules turned over per enzyme molecule per unit time.

22. **k_{cat}/K_m:** a value that behaves as a second-order rate constant (and thereby has units of $M^{-1}s^{-1}$) for a reaction between substrate and free enzyme and indicates an enzymatic efficiency.

23. **Ketone bodies:** acetone, acetoacetate, and hydroxybutyrate; water-soluble molecules produced (particularly during starvation) from acetyl-CoA.

24. **Michaelis constant:** K_m; the substrate concentration at which the reaction's velocity is at its half-maximal point.

25. **Myoglobin:** a heme protein that is made of one subunit and serves as an oxygen storing protein.

26. **Pentose phosphate pathway:** an oxidative pathway that uses glucose to generate NADPH and precursors to nucleotides and a few other amino acids.

27. **Prosthetic group:** a nonprotein molecule that is permanently (i.e., irreversibly) associated with the protein. For instance, FAD and FMN are prosthetic groups for flavoprotein enzymes.

28. **Standard free energy change:** the free energy change that occurs under standard conditions and is indicated by the symbol, $\Delta G°'$.

29. **V_{max}:** the maximal velocity of an enzyme when all enzyme molecules are saturated with a substrate.

Introduction

Biochemistry plays a central role in pharmacy education. It is one of the major topics of which students should have a good understanding to comprehend other topics, particularly pharmacology and nutrients. The field of biochemistry is concerned with catabolism and anabolism of micromolecules and macromolecules and how the metabolism of these molecules results in gaining or losing daily energy.

In this chapter, we introduce thermodynamics in biochemistry and emphasize the essential roles that glycolysis, gluconeogenesis, and the pentos phosphate pathway play in the metabolism of carbohydrates. In addition, we briefly describe the important roles that fatty acids and amino acids oxidation play in providing energy in the form of ATP molecules. The end results of the metabolism of these fuels (carbohydrates, fatty acids, and amino acids) are described in the citric acid cycle, oxidative phosphorylation, and the urea cycle. Furthermore, we briefly address the critical roles that different tissues and hormones play in the integration and regulation of the metabolism of these fuels.

Thermodynamics in Biochemistry

Thermodynamics in living organisms is referred to as bioenergetics; bioenergetics is the study of energy, heat, and work. Thermodynamics is concerned with energy transfer either in an organized form (work) or in a disorganized form (heat).

An excellent example of how thermodynamics works in living organisms is the production of adenosine triphosphate (ATP) molecules. Our cells absorb nutrients from the components of our diet (e.g., fats, carbohydrates, proteins) and break their chemical bonds to release energy. The released energy is then captured in mitochondria. In the mitochondria, oxidative phosphorylation assists cells in synthesizing ATP molecules. These ATP molecules supply the cells and tissues with energy to maintain their biological functions.

There are three important concepts in thermodynamics: (1) the system, which is the process under study; (2) the surroundings, which are the areas outside of the system; and (3) the universe, which is the combined system and surroundings (**Figure 5.1**). Energy may be released by the system to the surroundings or it may be gained by the system from the surroundings. In other words, the system is where a reaction occurs and the surroundings are everything else around the system.

All energy can be divided into two types: (1) potential energy, which is a stored energy (i.e., objects that have the capacity to move but are not in motion have potential energy); and (2) kinetic energy, which is the energy of motion (i.e., objects that are in motion have kinetic energy). **Figure 5.2** demonstrates potential and kinetic energies. The ball at the top of the hill has a large potential energy compared with a ball the bottom of the hill. As soon as the ball rolls, the potential energy is converted into kinetic energy. Some of this kinetic energy is transferred to the ground and pebbles, which makes the pebbles move (work), and some of it is transferred as heat, which makes the pebbles be slightly warm. Similarly, water behind a dam has potential energy. However, its potential energy is converted into kinetic energy when the water goes over the dam.

Each particle or object in a system has both potential and kinetic energy. The sum of both energies in the system is referred to as an internal energy (E). Suppose you mix ethanol with water in a cup. The mixture (system) gets warm and the heat is given to the surroundings (e.g., the cup, you).

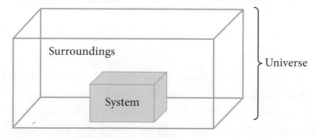

Figure 5.1 The universe includes both system and surroundings.

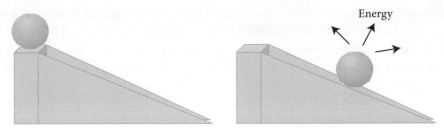

The ball has the stored potential energy.   The energy is released as kinetic energy.

Figure 5.2 Stored (potential) and released (kinetic) energy.

To measure the difference between the system's internal energy at the beginning (initial) and after a while (final), you can use delta E or ΔE (delta or its symbol, Δ, means "change in") to express the difference:

$$\Delta E = E_{final} - E_{initial} = E_{product} - E_{reactants} \tag{5.1}$$

It is obvious that a negative ΔE means E_{final} is lower than $E_{initial}$, which in turn means the internal energy has been transferred to the surroundings (or simply put, the energy has been released). In the preceding example, ΔE for the ethanol mixture will be negative. Keep in mind that the internal energy change depends only on the initial and final states of the system (which makes it easier to express Equation 5.1 to define the change), and not on the path taken from the initial state to the final state.

Energy can be transferred as heat and/or work. The total change in a system's internal energy, ΔE, is

$$\Delta E = q + w \tag{5.2}$$

where q is heat (thermal energy) and w is the work (mechanical, electrical, or chemical energy).

On one hand, energy is transferred as heat when the system and the surroundings have different temperatures. On the other hand, energy is transferred as work when an object is moved by a force. If the system does not do any work, such as when a cup of hot coffee is on your desk, and the heat is released from the system (coffee) to the surroundings (cup, desk, you), then the energy is transferred only as heat. This is because the surroundings have a lower temperature than your system. Remember energy, in the form of heat, is always transferred from a hotter area to a cooler sample until both are at the same temperature (i.e., when both samples are at thermal equilibrium). In the example, no work has been done, so w is zero and ΔE is equal to the heat, as expressed by Equation 5.3:

$$\Delta E = q \tag{5.3}$$

In contrast, when you (system) kick a ball (surroundings), the energy is transferred only as work to move the ball; that is, the object (the ball in this example) is moved by a force. Here q is zero and ΔE is expressed by Equation 5.4:

$$\Delta E = w \tag{5.4}$$

If the system loses energy as work (i.e., you lose energy by kicking the ball), the work is done by the system. Then w is negative, so ΔE becomes negative. Simply put, when the system gains energy, it is the surroundings that supply this energy; conversely, when the system loses energy, it is the surroundings that gain it (in the preceding example, the ball gets the energy from you and is able to move). This last explanation means that the energy may be converted from one form to another, but it cannot appear or disappear; that is, it cannot be either created or destroyed. This leads to a very important observation: "The total energy of the universe is constant"—the first law of thermodynamics.

$$\Delta E_{universal} = E_{system} + E_{surroundings} = 0 \tag{5.5}$$

The unit of heat and work is the joule (J). An older unit was the calorie (cal), which is the energy required to raise the temperature of 1 gram of water by 1 degree Celsius (°C). One calorie is equal to 4.184 J. The gained or lost energies in heat and work are small because they are associated with a single molecule or an atom; therefore, it is often easier to discuss the energy found in one mole of the substance (i.e., J/mol), where 1 mole represents 6.022×10^{23} molecules or atoms.

Enthalpy

All biological processes in the body, such as oxidation of a fatty acid or a glucose molecule, occur at a constant pressure. Thus, if you need to know how much heat was obtained—for instance, by oxidizing a fatty acid molecule in the body—it is the heat under constant pressure you need to know. This heat is called enthalpy and is indicated by the symbol H. Enthalpy is expressed as follows:

$$H = E + PV \tag{5.6}$$

where E is the internal energy, P is the pressure, and V is the volume. The change in enthalpy (ΔH) is the change in internal energy (ΔE) plus the product of constant pressure and the change in volume:

$$\Delta H = \Delta E + P\Delta V \tag{5.7}$$

Let's see how heat (q) under constant pressure becomes enthalpy (H). Work is expressed by Equation 5.8:

$$w = -P\Delta V \tag{5.8}$$

A combination of Equation 5.2 ($\Delta E = q + w$) and Equation 5.8 ($w = -P\Delta V$) produces Equation 5.9:

$$\Delta E = q + (-P\Delta V) = q - P\Delta V \tag{5.9}$$

Combining Equation 5.7 ($\Delta H = \Delta E + P\Delta V$) with Equation 5.9 ($\Delta E = q - P\Delta V$) gives Equation 5.10:

$$\Delta H = q - P\Delta V + P\Delta V \tag{5.10}$$

The positive and negative $P\Delta V$ terms in Equation 5.10 cancel out each other, which results in the following expression:

$$\Delta H = q \tag{5.11}$$

Equation 5.11 indicates that enthalpy is the same as the heat gained or released under a constant pressure. As was mentioned earlier, because all biological processes occur under a constant pressure and because many reactions involve little (if any) change in the volume of the reaction, $\Delta V \approx 0$ and thereby the $P\Delta V$ term becomes zero as well. The last observation means that the internal energy change expressed in Equation 5.7 ($\Delta H = \Delta E + P\Delta V$) may be expressed as follows:

$$\Delta H \approx \Delta E \tag{5.12}$$

Equation 5.12 indicates that a change in enthalpy (ΔH) is almost the same as a change in the internal energy. We will revisit this equation when we express free energy change.

To measure enthalpy, the only thing you need to know is the initial and final heat under constant pressure:

$$\Delta H = H_{final} - H_{initial} = H_{product} - H_{reactants} \tag{5.13}$$

The following example will clarify how this expression works. Suppose you mix H_2 (gas) with oxygen (gas):

$$2H_2(g) + O_2(g) \rightarrow 2H_2O(l), 485 \text{ kJ}$$

As this reaction shows, the heat is released upon water formation. This means the initial heat is higher than the final heat: $H_{final} - H_{initial}$, 0 J $-$ 485 kJ, which is -485 kJ; thus $\Delta H < 0$. This is an example of an exothermic process (i.e., when ΔH is negative).

Let's look at another example: Suppose you boil water in a pot:

$$H_2O(l) + 40.7 \text{ kJ} \rightarrow H_2O(g)$$

Obviously, the heat has been transferred from the surroundings (fire) to the system (water), with the water being vaporized into gas (g) form. Here, the system has absorbed the heat: $H_{final} - H_{initial} = 40.7 \text{ J} - 0 \text{ kJ} = +40.7\text{J}$ ($\Delta H > 0$). This is an example of an endothermic process (i.e., when ΔH is positive).

When the heat is released from the system to the surroundings, the process is exothermic. Conversely, when the system absorbs heat from the surroundings, the process is endothermic. **Figure 5.3** demonstrates exothermic and endothermic reactions in two chemical reactions.

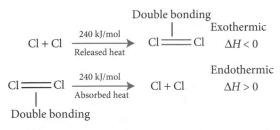

Figure 5.3 Release and gain of heat under constant pressure in exothermic and endothermic reactions, respectively.

Entropy

The amount of disorder in a system is referred to as entropy and is indicated by the symbol S. For instance, the items in **Figure 5.4A** are organized in a more orderly fashion compared with the items in **Figure 5.4B**. As a result, the items in **Figure 5.4B** have higher entropy than the items in **Figure 5.4A**. The mixture on the right (S_{final}) has more disorder than the mixture on the left, which indicates that the entropy change is positive: $\Delta S = S_{final} - S_{initial} = \Delta S > 0$.

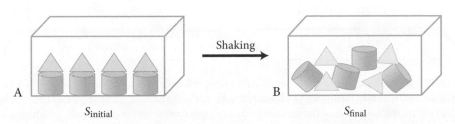

Figure 5.4 Items that are organized well (A) have lower entropy than items that are unorganized (B).

Examples of entropy are when ice melts (solid to liquid) or when water boils (liquid to gas). These disorganizations occur because there is a natural tendency toward higher entropy. Here is where the second law of thermodynamics comes from: "The universe spontaneously tends toward increasing disorder or randomness." This law states that the universe tends to have high positive entropy. Because the universe is made up of the system and the surroundings, the entropy change of the universe can be shown as follows:

$$\Delta S_{universe} = \Delta S_{system} + \Delta S_{surroundings} \tag{5.14}$$

According to the second law, the entropy change of the universe must be greater than 0. Remember either the system or the surroundings can have small disorder (low entropy). The most important point is that the sum (universe) must be a positive number. Now let's see what the relation between entropy and enthalpy is. **Figure 5.5** demonstrates the changes of entropy in the surroundings. If heat is released from the system (i.e., $-\Delta H$) to the surroundings, then obviously the entropy change (ΔS) of the surroundings increases (A) because the released heat makes the molecules in the surroundings be in more motion (in disorder). If heat is absorbed by the system ($+\Delta H$), then the ΔS of the surroundings decreases (B).

These observations in Figure 5.5 indicate that the entropy change in the surroundings is proportional to the enthalpy change in the system; that is, when ΔH_{system} increases or decreases, the $\Delta S_{surroundings}$ increases or decreases as well (see Figure 5.5). In other words:

$$\Delta S_{surroundings} \propto \Delta H_{system} \tag{5.15}$$

The symbol "$\propto$" means proportional. However, what if the temperature (T) is already high in the surroundings? A high temperature in the surroundings causes a high entropy in the surroundings. Therefore any released heat from the system cannot help so much to disorganize more molecules in the surroundings. Thus, if the temperature is high, the entropy change of the surroundings ($\Delta S_{surroundings}$) is low (or minimal), which can be expressed as follows:

$$\Delta S_{surroundings} = \frac{-H_{system}}{T} \tag{5.16}$$

The last observation leads to the rearrangement of Equation 5.15 to Equation 5.16. To know whether $\Delta S_{universe}$ for a reaction is positive (a spontaneous reaction), you have to know both $\Delta S_{surroundings}$ and ΔS_{system} (see Equation 5.14), which is a complicated process. Generally, you are interested in what happens to the system, not to the surroundings. For instance, when you boil water in a pot, you are interested in knowing what happens to the water (system) rather than in seeing what happens to the entropy or energy change of your kitchen or your house

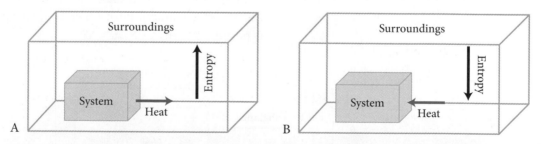

Figure 5.5 A. The heat released from the system ($-\Delta H$) makes the molecules in the surroundings be in more motion (in disorder), which in turn results in higher entropy of the surroundings. B. The heat absorbed by the system ($+\Delta H$) makes the molecules in the surroundings be in less motion (more organized), which results in a reduced entropy of the surroundings.

(surroundings). For this reason, you need something else to connect enthalpy and entropy only to the system while excluding the surroundings. Let's see what this magic "something else" is.

Let's go back to Equations 5.14 and 5.16. Combining these two equations will give Equation 5.17:

$$\Delta S_{universe} = \Delta S_{system} + \frac{-H_{system}}{T} \tag{5.17}$$

Multiplying both sides of Equation 5.17 by $-T$ assists us in expressing Equation 5.18:

$$-T\Delta S_{universe} = -T\Delta S_{system} + \Delta H_{system} \tag{5.18}$$

Equation 5.18 can also be written as Equation 5.19:

$$-T\Delta S_{universe} = \Delta H_{system} - T\Delta S_{system} \tag{5.19}$$

As can be seen from Equation 5.19, the entropy change in the universe is related to both the enthalpy and the entropy of the system. Equation 5.19 will help us to explain free energy.

Free Energy

The free energy is defined as the freed energy available (or required) to do work in any system. This freed energy can be used to make things work (happen) that otherwise wouldn't happen. In our cells, "work" involves synthesis, growth, and reproduction. In a molecule within the cell where the pressure and volume are constant, the free energy is called Gibb's free energy and is indicated by the symbol G.

To make Equation 5.19 easier to understand and to relate it to a free energy change, we can change the $-T\Delta S_{universe}$ term to ΔG, which is called free energy change. The free energy change is a measure of spontaneity of a reaction and the useful energy available from it to do work. The free energy change can now be expressed as follows:

$$\Delta G = \Delta H - T\Delta S \tag{5.20}$$

As Equation 5.20 shows, to measure the free energy change, we have to take into consideration the changes of enthalpy and entropy. In other words, we have to know two important changes about the system: the change in enthalpy (ΔH), which is almost the same as the internal energy (ΔE; see Equation 5.12), and the change in entropy (ΔS). Keep in mind that knowing only one of these values will not help you to measure ΔG.

To predict the spontaneity of a process, we need to know whether ΔG is negative or positive. **Figure 5.6** demonstrates that any process, but particularly any chemical reaction, can be classified as one of the following thermodynamic conditions:

1. If the free energy change is positive, the process ("moving the box") is not a spontaneous process (i.e., it will not occur of itself and needs continuous external influence).

2. If the free energy change is negative, once the process begins, it takes place spontaneously (i.e., doing work without any external influence).

3. If the free energy change of the process is zero, then the system is at equilibrium (i.e., no energy will be released or absorbed).

In a spontaneous reaction where ΔG is negative, the product has a lower energy than the reactants. In a nonspontaneous reaction, the reactants have lower energy than the product.

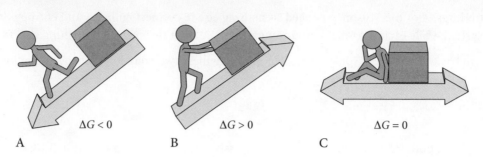

A $\Delta G < 0$ B $\Delta G > 0$ C $\Delta G = 0$

Figure 5.6 The value for the free energy change (ΔG) indicates whether a reaction occurs spontaneously (A), occurs nonspontaneously (B), or is at equilibrium (C).

The former process is depicted in **Figure 5.7**. Of course, just because a reaction has a positive ΔG, it does not mean that the reaction will never occur. There are many biochemical reactions for which ΔG is positive, yet these vital reactions still occur. The reason is that these reactions receive energy from other sources.

Standard Free Energy

If all components of the system are in their standard states (i.e., at 25°C, 1 atm pressure, 1 M molar concentration of reactants and products, and pH 7), we should be able to measure the standard free energy change ($\Delta G^{o\prime}$). In other words, the standard free energy ($\Delta G^{o\prime}$) is the free energy that occurs under standard conditions, and $\Delta G^{o\prime}$ is the difference in free energies of the products and reactants at standard conditions. This is not physiologically relevant, however, because no reaction in the body is actually carried out at 1 M, at a pH of 7.0, or at a temperature of 25°C. Nevertheless, ΔG is a physiologically applicable measure because its value for any reaction depends on the actual conditions in which the reaction takes place, including the temperature and the concentrations of the reactants or products. Thus ΔG is essentially a variable that depends on $\Delta G^{o\prime}$, the temperature, and the concentrations of all reactants and products at any given concentrations. These relationships are shown in Equation 5.21:

$$\Delta G = \Delta G^{o\prime} + RT \ln \frac{[\text{Product}]}{[\text{Reactant}]} \tag{5.21}$$

where R is the gas constant and T is the absolute temperature of the reaction. $R = 8.315$ J/(mol × K) and $T = 298$ K, so the unit for ΔG or $\Delta G^{o\prime}$ will be J/mol.

Suppose you have a reaction where A mixes with B to produce C and D:

$$A + B \leftrightarrow C + D$$

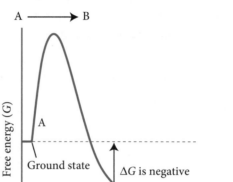

Exergonic reaction

A $\longrightarrow$ B

Figure 5.7 For a reaction to occur spontaneously, the product must have a lower energy than the reactants.

For measuring $\Delta G^{o\prime}$ you will need to start the reaction at standard conditions. However, under nonstandard conditions, ΔG should be employed rather than $\Delta G^{o\prime}$ to predict the direction of the reaction. Equation 5.21 can be used to find ΔG at any concentration of the reactants and products. At equilibrium, the free energy change (ΔG) of the process is zero (see also Figure 5.6). This means at equilibrium, Equation 5.21 becomes Equation 5.22:

$$\Delta G^{o\prime} = -RT \ \text{In} \ \frac{[C][D]}{[A][B]} \tag{5.22}$$

[A], [B], [C], and [D] are the molar concentrations of the reactants and products. Because the system is at equilibrium, the concentration ratio—that is, [C][D]/[A][B]—is actually the equilibrium constant (K'_{eq}) of the process. Therefore, Equation 5.22 can be expressed as Equation 5.23:

$$\Delta G^{o\prime} = -RT \ \text{In} \ K'_{eq} \tag{5.23}$$

Equation 5.23 is one of the most important equations in thermodynamics because it enables you to find the equilibrium constant of a reaction if you know the change in the standard free energy, and vice versa (because both R and T are constant and known).

When $\Delta G^{o\prime}$ for a reaction is positive, that reaction can also proceed under conditions in which ΔG is negative. According to Equation 5.21, if the concentration of the product is kept very low (for instance, by its removal in a subsequent metabolic step), the natural logarithmic term becomes negative and ΔG then has a negative value. Indeed, this phenomenon explains why the standard free energy change for the last reaction in the citric cycle (malate → oxaloacetate) has a positive value (30 kJ/mol) but the reaction still moves forward. The oxaloacetate (product) reacts immediately with the acetate in a subsequent step in the citric acid cycle. We will return to this important biochemical reaction when we describe the citric acid cycle later in this chapter.

Additive Standard Free Energy

Many of biochemical reactions, such as the synthesis of proteins or nucleic acids, are nonspontaneous (i.e., have positive $\Delta G^{o\prime}$). In the living system, these reactions are coupled to an energetically favorable process that has a negative $\Delta G^{o\prime}$. This kind of coupled reaction is essential to our survival. For instance, glucose is converted to carbon dioxide and water during metabolism with an enormous energy release:

$$C_6H_{12}O_6(s) + 6O_2(g) \rightarrow 6CO_2(g) + 6H_2O(l) \qquad \Delta G^{o\prime} = -2880 \ \text{kJ/mol}$$

Much of the released energy is used to synthesize ATP molecules from adenosine diphosphate (ADP). ATP is an energy-rich molecule that stores the captured energy until it is needed by the cells. Evolution has created a series of enzymes that are capable of preferentially binding and hydrolyzing ATP and using its free energy to drive endergonic reactions. In the ATP molecules, phosphoric anhydride linkages appear between the phosphate groups (**Figure 5.8**). Hydrolysis of the linkage between the second and third phosphate groups is a highly exergonic reaction that results in the release of a large amount of free energy (**Figure 5.9**). For instance, when 1 mol of ATP is hydrolyzed, 30.5 kJ of energy is released. It is important to emphasize that some other cellular molecules have even more energy-rich phosphate groups than ATP. For instance, hydrolysis of one mole of phosphoenolpyruvate (PEP) releases 62 kJ of energy. However, PEP is not used to any significant extent to drive endergonic reactions.

$$ATP \longrightarrow ADP + Pi, \Delta G^{\circ\prime} = -30.5 \text{ kJ}$$

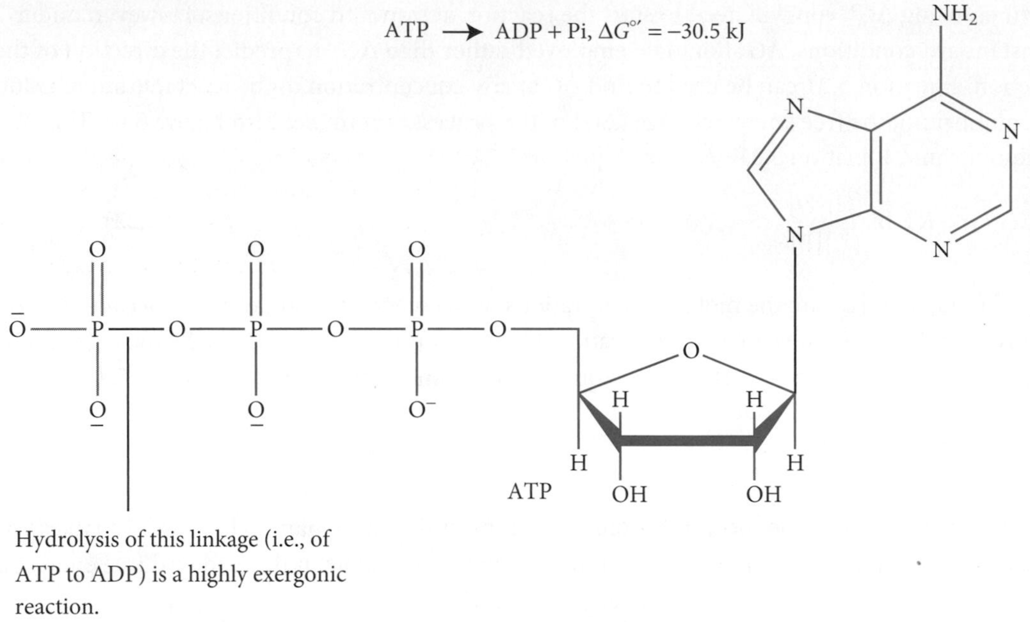
ATP
Hydrolysis of this linkage (i.e., of ATP to ADP) is a highly exergonic reaction.

Figure 5.8 Structure of an energy-rich molecule, adenosine triphosphate (ATP).

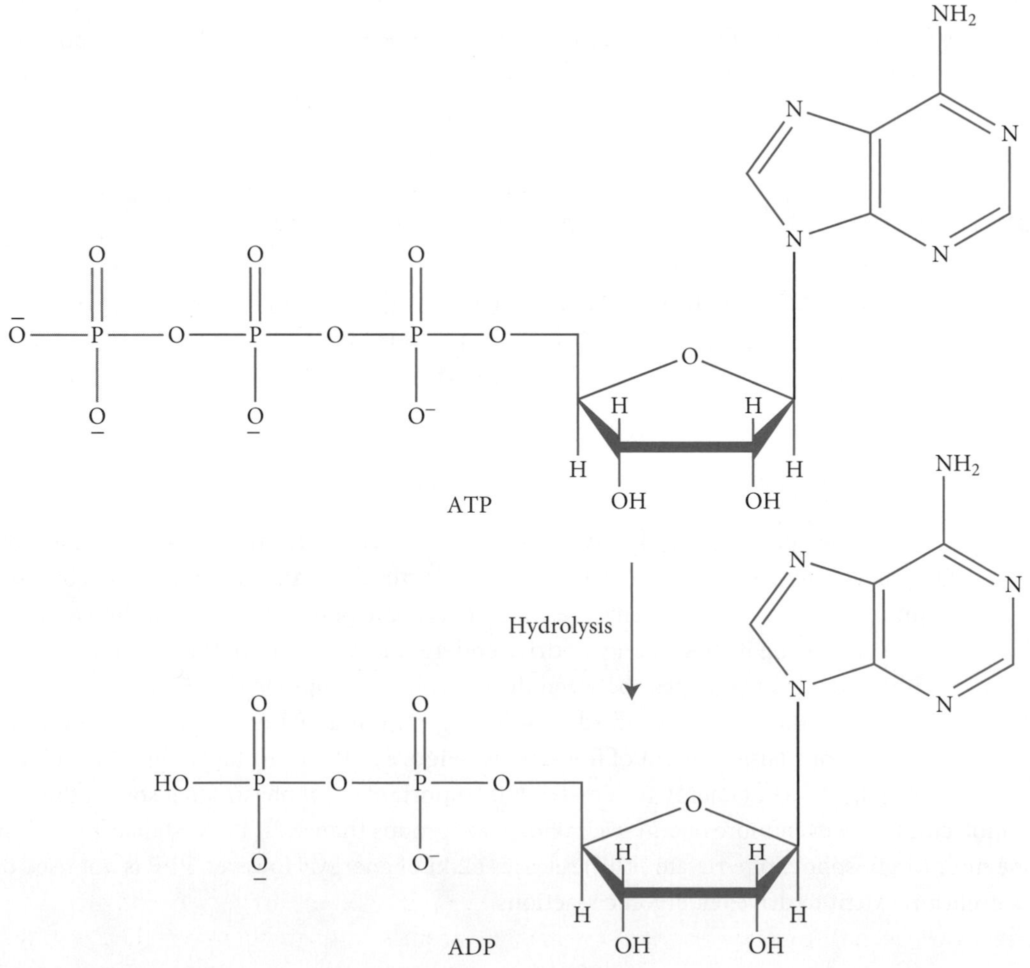
ATP
Hydrolysis
ADP

Figure 5.9 Hydrolysis of 1 mol of ATP produces ADP and releases 30.5 kJ of energy.

Reaction 1:   A → B $\Delta G_1^{\circ\prime}$

Reaction 2:   B → C $\Delta G_2^{\circ\prime}$

Sum   A → C $\Delta G_1^{\circ\prime} + \Delta G_2^{\circ\prime}$

Figure 5.10 When two chemical reactions are added to give a third reaction, $\Delta G^{\circ\prime}$ for the third reaction is the sum of the $\Delta G^{\circ\prime}$ values of the other two reactions.

When two chemical reactions are added to give a third reaction, the $\Delta G^{\circ\prime}$ value for the third reaction is the sum of the $\Delta G^{\circ\prime}$ values of the other two reactions (**Figure 5.10**). For instance, the first reaction in glycolysis—that is, phosphorylation of one glucose molecule to produce one molecule of glucose-6-phospate—includes hydrolysis of one ATP molecule. Phosphorylation of the glucose molecule also represents a coupled reaction because the ATP molecule provides the necessary energy to drive the phosphorylation reaction forward.

ATP + H_2O → ADP + Pi $\Delta G^{\circ\prime} = -30.5$ kJ/mol

Glucose + Pi → glucose-6-phosphate $\Delta G^{\circ\prime} = +13.8$ kJ/mol

Sum = ATP + glucose → ADP + glucose-6-phosphate

Sum = 13.8 + (−30.5) = −16.7 kJ/mol

Keep in mind that hydrolysis of the ATP molecules would result in the loss of most of the free energy as heat. To avoid this expensive loss, the gamma (third) phosphate of the ATP molecule is transferred (in most cases) to the reaction substrate to produce an energy-rich phosphorylated intermediate, which ultimately will form the product in an exergonic reaction.

Learning Bridge 5.1

Joe is a 17-year-old high school student who comes to your pharmacy for some advice about buying an OTC product. He complains about the muscle cramps that he has been experiencing since he started to exercise in the high school gym yesterday. In addition, he mentions that he is planning to attend the high school prom tonight and he does not want to miss this end-of-the-year school celebration. Joe has heard from his friends that an OTC product, Bengay, can relieve his muscle cramps and asks you about the effectiveness of Bengay.

Based on the information Joe provided, you suggest that Joe buy "hot packs" rather than Bengay.

A. What is your advice for Joe in regard to the OTC product Bengay?
B. Why are you suggesting the "hot packs"?
C. How do "hot packs" work?
D. How do "cold packs" work?

Oxidation and Reduction in Biochemistry

As was mentioned in the *Introduction to Biological Chemistry* chapter, oxidation is the loss of electrons and reduction is the gain of electrons. Free electrons do not actually float around; rather, whenever they are released, other molecules accept them. If a carbon atom, in an organic compound, forms a bond to an oxygen atom, the carbon becomes oxidized because of the electronegativity difference that exists between these two atoms. By the same token, if the same carbon bonds to hydrogen, the carbon atom is reduced (**Figure 5.11**).

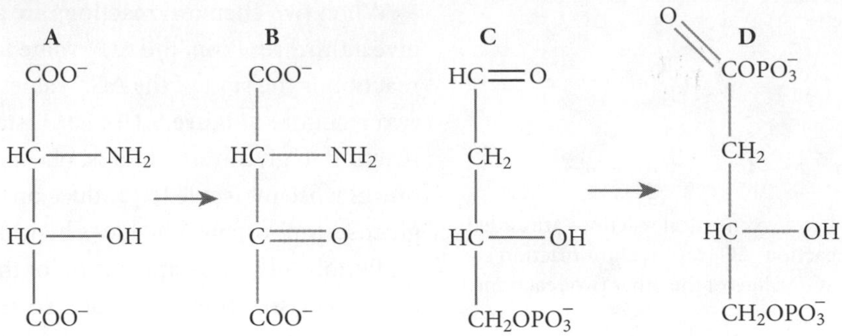

A	B	C	D

$$
\begin{array}{cccc}
\text{A} & \text{B} & \text{C} & \text{D}
\end{array}
$$

Figure 5.11 While A and C are reduced forms, B and D are oxidized forms in two different oxidation–reduction reactions.

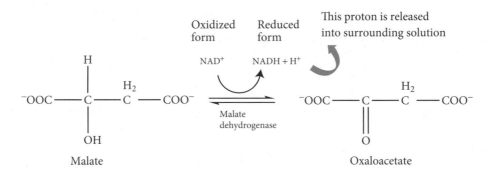

Figure 5.12 NAD$^+$ and NADH play important roles in the oxidation–reduction reactions involving many biochemical molecules.

Coenzymes as Electron Carriers

Coenzymes are organic molecules that facilitate the catalytic activity of enzymes. Examples include NAD$^+$ and NADP$^+$. Cofactors, in contrast, are inorganic substances that facilitate the catalytic activity of enzymes. Examples include Zn^{2+} and Mg^{2+}. If the coenzyme or cofactor is irreversibly bound to an enzyme, it is also called a prosthetic group. In biological systems, electrons from oxidation are generally transferred to electron-carrying coenzymes, such as NAD$^+$ or FAD to form NADH and FADH$_2$, respectively. These electron carrier coenzymes donate their electrons to acceptor molecules and become re-oxidized in the process. Enzymes that catalyze biological oxidation–reduction reactions are often referred to as "dehydrogenases." An example is the role of malate dehydrogenase in the metabolism of malate (**Figure 5.12**).

In the oxidation–reduction pathways that occur in many biochemical reactions, often two hydrogen atoms are stripped from a reduced molecule (see malate in Figure 5.12). However, one of the hydrogen atoms, as a proton, is released into surrounding solution. This indicates a total of two electrons and one proton (H$^+$) are transferred from a reduced molecule (malate in Figure 5.12) to an oxidized molecule (NAD$^+$ in Figure 5.12).

Electrons have stored energy (potential energy) and are ready to do work. Oxidative phosphorylation is a mitochondrial ATP-producing machinery that accommodates transfer of electrons along a series of carrier molecules to release energy so as to synthesize ATP molecules (**Figure 5.13**). We will return to the essential role that oxidative phosphorylation plays in biochemistry in another section of this chapter.

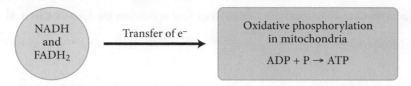

Figure 5.13 Oxidative phosphorylation takes place in an ATP-producing complex that utilizes electron carrier coenzymes to capture energy from released electrons to synthesize ATP molecules.

The important roles of electron carrier coenzymes are described next.

- *NAD⁺:* Nicotinamide adenine dinucleotide participates in many oxidation–reduction reactions where dehydrogenases reduce it to NADH. There are two forms that exist in the cells depending on whether they are carrying electrons: NADH is the reduced form of the molecule (i.e., it carries electrons and a hydrogen) and NAD⁺ is the oxidized form of NADH (i.e., it lacks electrons).

- *NADP⁺:* Nicotinamide adenine dinucleotide phosphate is another carrier coenzyme. The reduced form of NADP⁺ is NADPH. One major difference between NADH and NADPH is that NADPH donates electrons primarily for biosynthetic reactions (in particular, biosynthesis of lipids), whereas NADH donates electrons primarily to the electron transport chain for the synthesis of ATP molecules. Niacin (vitamin B_3; see also the *Introduction to Nutrients* chapter) is the source for NAD⁺ and NADP⁺.

- *FMN and FAD:* The flavin mononucleotide (FMN) and flavin adenine dinucleotide (FAD) are coenzymes that are attached to the flavoprotein enzymes that catalyze biochemical oxidation–reduction reactions. Riboflavin (vitamin B_2; see also the *Introduction to Nutrients* chapter) is the precursor for both FMN and FAD.

The attachment between a dehydrogenase enzyme and NAD⁺ or NADP⁺ is quite loose. As a result, these coenzymes move readily from one enzyme to another and carry electrons from one metabolite to another. In contrast, FMN and FAD are tightly bound to flavoprotein enzymes.

Standard Reduction Potential

To transfer electrons from a reductant to an oxidant, the oxidant must have a greater affinity for electrons than the reductant. The affinity of a substance for electrons is its standard reduction potential ($E^{\circ\prime}$), which has the units of volts (V). As the name indicates, this value is measured under standard conditions such as pH 7 and 25°C where all species are present at concentrations 1 M. The greater the $E^{\circ\prime}$ value, the greater the tendency of an oxidant to accept electrons and become reduced. **Table 5.1** indicates the standard reduction potentials for a series of biochemical reactions.

We can use the standard reduction potential to understand in which direction electrons will flow in an oxidation–reduction reaction. For instance, as shown in Table 5.1, we have:

1. Ubiquinone + $2H^+$ + $2e^-$ → ubiquinol (0.045 V)

2. Fumarate + $2H^+$ + $2e^-$ → succinate (0.031 V)

During the oxidative phosphorylation, the electrons will flow from reaction 2 to reaction 1 because reaction 1 has a larger $E^{\circ\prime}$ value, meaning a higher tendency to accept electrons. Therefore, the flow of electrons during oxidative phosphorylation will be in the direction of reaction 2 to reaction 1 (this, indeed, is what happens in complex III of the oxidative phosphorylation that we will discuss further in this chapter). As there is a relationship between the standard

Table 5.1 **Standard Reduction Potential for a Series of Biochemical Reactions**

Biochemical Reaction	Standard Reduction Potential ($E^{o'}$) in Volts
$\frac{1}{2}O_2 + 2H + 2e^- \rightarrow H_2O$	0.816
$Fe^{3+} + e^- \rightarrow Fe^{2+}$	0.771
$O_2 + 2H + 2e^- \rightarrow H_2O_2$	0.295
Ubiquinone $+ 2H + 2e^- \rightarrow$ ubiquinol	0.045
Fumarate $+ 2H + 2e^- \rightarrow$ xuccinate	0.031
$2H + 2e^- \rightarrow H_2$ (standard conditions, pH 0)	0.000
Oxaloacetate $2H + 2e^- \rightarrow$ malate	−0.166
Pyruvate $+ 2H + 2e^- \rightarrow$ lactate	−0.185
$FAD + 2H + 2e^- \rightarrow FADH_2$ (free solution)	−0.219
Glutathione dimer $+ 2H + 2e^- \rightarrow 2$ reduced glutathione	−0.23
Lipoic acid $+ 2H + 2e^- \rightarrow$ dihydrolipoic acid	−0.29
$NAD^+ + 2H + 2e^- \rightarrow NADH$	−0.320
$NADP^+ + 2H + 2e^- \rightarrow NADPH$	−0.324
Acetoacetate $+ 2H + 2e^- \rightarrow \beta$-hydroxybutyrate	−0.346
α-Ketoglutarate $+ CO_2 + 2H + 2e^- \rightarrow$ isocitrate	−0.38
$2H + 2e^- \rightarrow H_2$ (pH 7.0)	−0.414

Reproduced from: Woodbury CP. *Biochemistry for the pharmaceutical sciences.* Burlington, MA: Jones & Bartlett Learning; 2012: Chapter 1.

reduction potential and standard free energy, we can understand whether a reaction occurs spontaneously.

The change in the standard reduction potential for the preceding reaction can be written as follows:

$\Delta E^{o'} = E^{o'}$ (electron acceptor) $- E^{o'}$ (electron donor) $= (0.045 - 0.031) = 0.014$

The $\Delta E^{o'}$ value is related to $\Delta G^{o'}$ by the following equation:

$$\Delta G^{o'} = -nF \Delta E^{o'} \tag{5.24}$$

where $\Delta G^{o'}$ is the standard free energy change of a reaction (in J/mol); $\Delta E^{o'}$ is the change in the standard reduction potential of a reaction (in volts); n is the number of electrons transferred in the reaction; and F is Faraday's constant (96,500 J/V/mol).

As Equation 5.24 indicates, a spontaneous oxidation–reduction reaction is indicated by either a positive $E^{o'}$ or a negative $\Delta G^{o'}$. If $E^{o'}$ for an electron acceptor is larger than $E^{o'}$ for an electron donor, $\Delta E^{o'}$ will be a positive number (as indicated in the preceding reaction). This means there is a greater tendency of electrons to flow from the electron donor to the electron acceptor. Based on Equation 5.24, a positive value for $\Delta E^{o'}$ means a negative value for the standard free energy change, $\Delta G^{o'}$, which in turn means energy will be released and the reaction is a spontaneous reaction.

Structure of Proteins

Functions of proteins strictly depend on the structure of proteins, which in turn depends on the sequence of amino acid residues. In addition to the amino acid residues, other molecules that attach to proteins play important roles in the functions of proteins. For instance, lipids and carbohydrates can attach to proteins to build lipoproteins and glycoproteins, respectively. Other examples are myoglobin, hemoglobin, and many proteases that have iron or other elements (e.g., Mg^{2+}, Zn^{2+}) covalently attached to their structures and are essential for the functions of proteins.

Upon synthesis of proteins (i.e., post-translation), proteins fold into their native (active) conformation by twisting and turning into different structures that may include helices, sheets, turns, and loops. It is, however, the primary structure of a protein that indicates the exact order of the amino acid residues in the protein. In addition, the primary structure dictates the final form a protein will take as the structures twist and fold. Keep in mind that while the peptide bond is a covalent bond and, therefore, the most stable bond in proteins, many weak interactions such as van der Waals attractions, hydrogen bonds, ionic bonds, and hydrophobic interactions exist within the structure of proteins. These weak interactions play important roles in shaping and maintaining the structural integrity of proteins.

The native conformation ensures that the protein is in its biologically active form. In an aqueous solution, the native conformation is determined by two major factors: (1) formation of the maximum number of hydrogen bonds with the aqueous solution and (2) placement of hydrophobic amino acid residues away from the aqueous solution (i.e., positioned within the protein). As a result, the most important contribution to the stability of a protein's conformation—that is, the tendency to maintain the native conformation—is the increase in the disorder (entropy) of the water molecules surrounding the protein (**Figure 5.14**). In other words, the increased entropy forces the hydrophobic amino acids to reside inside the protein (away from the hydrophilic aqueous solution) to maintain its native functional structure.

Keep in mind that a peptide bond is built between every linked amino acid in a protein chain involving each amino acid's carbonyl carbon and the nitrogen atom of the next amino acid. Due to the delocalization of electrons over the peptide bond, only two bonds per amino acid are able to rotate (**Figure 5.15**).

There are four different protein structures: primary structure, secondary structure, tertiary structure, and quaternary structure.

Primary Structure

Primary structure defines the linear sequence of amino acids that are linked by many peptide bonds (**Figure 5.16**). One can compare the evolutionary relationships between two proteins by looking at their primary structures and sequences. The primary structure of a protein is predicted by the gene that encodes that particular protein. As a result, information about the amino acid residues assist scientists in learning more about the genetic information.

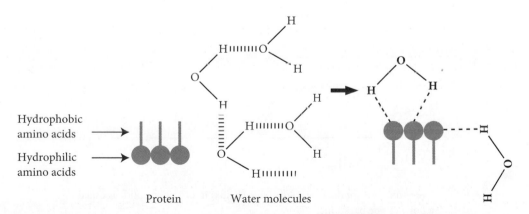

Hydrophobic amino acids →

Hydrophilic amino acids →

Protein   Water molecules

Figure 5.14 Increasing entropy in the water molecules surrounding a protein significantly contributes to the stability of a protein's conformation.

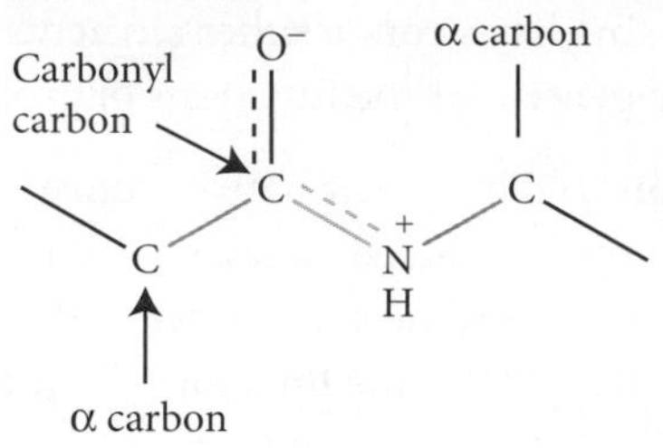

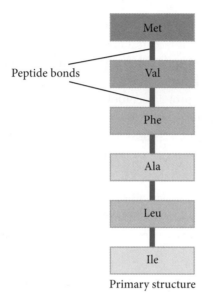

Figure 5.15 Because of delocalization of electrons between carbonyl carbon and the nitrogen atom, the peptide bond cannot rotate freely, whereas other bonds can rotate.

Met

Val

Phe

Ala

Leu

Ile

Peptide bonds

Primary structure

Figure 5.16 The linear sequence of amino acids determines the primary structure of a protein.

Secondary Structure

Secondary structure refers to a structure of a protein that assumes regular and repeated patterns of folding of the protein's backbone (**Figure 5.17**). The two most common folding patterns in the secondary structure of proteins are the α-helix and β-sheet.

α-Helix

The α-helix can be imagined as a ribbon of amino acids wrapped around a tube to form a secondary structure (**Figure 5.18**). Since the inside diameter of the α-helix leaves no room for side chains, all of the side chains of an α-helix project outward. Keep in mind that while the α-helix has a stable arrangement, it is a flexible helix.

Several factors can disrupt the structure of an α-helix, including (1) electrostatic repulsion or attraction with ionizable side chains such as Asp or Arg; (2) bulkiness of adjacent side chains such as Thr or Leu; (3) the inflexibility of the amino acid Pro within the helix; and (4) too much flexibility of the glycine amino acid. For instance, the nitrogen of proline in the peptide bond does not have any free hydrogen with which to participate in hydrogen bonding with other amino acids. In addition, the rigid $N—C_{\alpha}$ bond (see **Figure 5.19**) does not allow the $N—C_{\alpha}$ bond to rotate (recall the delocalization of electrons shown in Figure 5.15), which encourages proline to kink or bend in an α-helix. In addition, due to the lack of any hydrogen bonds, proline makes the α-helix assume a less stable structure (Figure 5.19). Glycine, however, is the only amino acid that does not have

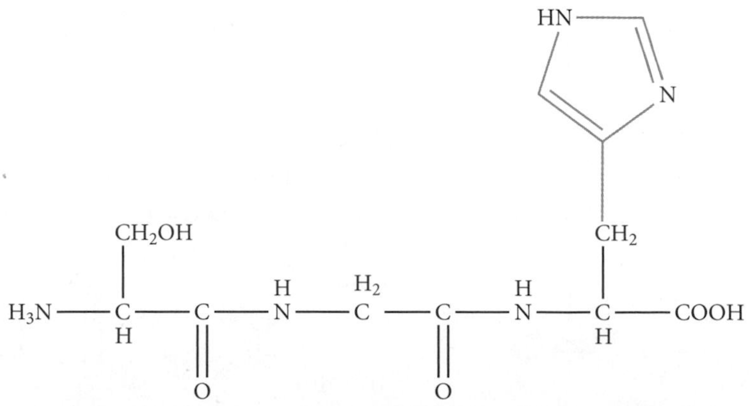

Everything except the blue colors (side chains) in this polypeptide is called a polypeptide backbone.

Figure 5.17 The sequence of amino acid residues includes both side chains and backbones of a protein.

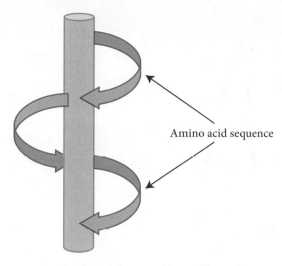

Figure 5.18 The α-helix resembles a ribbon of amino acid residues wrapped around a tube.

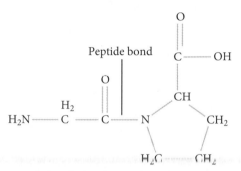

Peptide bond of proline and another amino acid

Figure 5.19 The nitrogen atom of the proline amino acid cannot make any hydrogen bonds with the other amino acid side chains.

A protein, entirely made of β-sheets

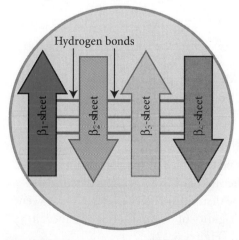

Figure 5.20 Two regions of the same polypeptide in a β-sheet structure can position themselves next to each other in parallel or antiparallel formats.

a side chain (it has only a hydrogen atom; see also the *Introduction to Cell Biology* chapter). As a result, glycine has a high tendency to form a coiled form, a structure that is not desirable in an α-helix.

β-Sheet

In contrast to the α-helix, two regions of the same polypeptide in a β-sheet structure can position themselves next to each other in a side-by-side format (parallel or antiparallel sheets; **Figure 5.20**). Similar to the structure of an α-helix, the structure of a β-sheet is stabilized by hydrogen bonding between adjacent chains. In addition and similar to the α-helix, the β-sheet projects its side chains outward. The side chains of the β-sheet are often small and protrude from either side of the β-sheet.

Tertiary Structure

In contrast to the secondary structure of a protein, in which the amino acid residues are often close to one another, the structure of a tertiary protein may be significantly influenced by amino acid residues that are very far from one another. The hydrophobic interactions or hydrogen, ionic, and disulfide bonds that occur between the side chains play important roles in the tertiary structure (**Figure 5.21**). These bonding interactions can cause the protein to twist, bend, fold, or make loops.

Quaternary Structure

Many proteins are formed when multiple polypeptide chains or subunits associate with one another. The quaternary structure describes how different subunits of a protein are attached to one another and shape the overall protein. In a quaternary structure, the attachment of subunits is critical for the overall function of the protein. For instance, hemoglobin is made of four subunits. Only when these subunits interact with each other to build the quaternary structure is hemoglobin capable of transporting oxygen in the blood.

Proteins can be classified into two major groups with respect to the tertiary or secondary structure: fibrous proteins and globular proteins.

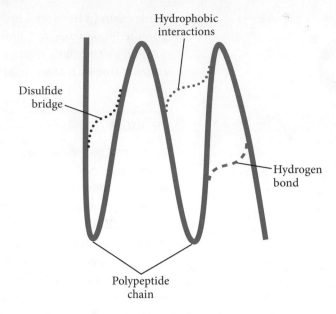

Figure 5.21 Many interactions and bonds between the side chains determine the tertiary structure of a protein.

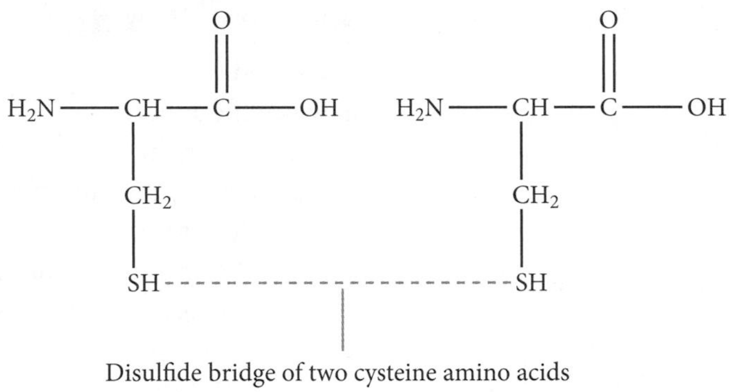

Disulfide bridge of two cysteine amino acids

Figure 5.22 A disulfide bridge is built when two cysteine amino acid residues interact with each other.

Fibrous Proteins

Fibrous proteins have long strands or sheets of polypeptide. They are insoluble in water because they contain a large number of hydrophobic amino acids. Mechanically, they provide a strong support, shape, and external protection to vertebrates. There are three subclasses in this group: α-keratin, β-fibroin, and collagen.

- *α-keratin:* In α-keratin, the polypeptides are mainly in the α-helix conformation. These proteins are found in hair, fingernails, horns, beaks, and other structures. Two strands of keratin oriented in parallel can wrap around each other to form a super-twisted coil. The strength and stability of α-keratin are enhanced by the disulfide bridges that occur between two cysteine amino acid residues, which explains the rigidity of α-keratin (for instance, it explains why a hair strand or nail is not easily broken) (**Figure 5 22**).

- *β-fibroin:* Silk fibroin that is produced by insects and spiders is a protein in which the polypeptide is almost entirely in the β-conformation.

- *Collagen:* Collagen is the most abundant protein in mammals (an estimated 30% of total body proteins) and its functions are to provide structure to, protect, and support the softer tissues and to connect these tissues with the skeleton. Collagen plays an important role in cellular adhesion and migration as well because it is able to interact with cells through integrins (see the *Introduction to Cell Biology* chapter).

Collagen can be found in bones, tendons, skin, blood vessels, and the cornea of the eye. It is built when three polypeptide chains wrap around each other in a tight triple-helix format, forming many hydrogen bonds, which makes the overall structure of collagen strong and compact. Each polypeptide chain is more than 1,000 amino acids long. One can find a repeated sequence of three amino acid residues in which every third amino acid is glycine. Glycine is a small amino acid that fits very well within these polypeptides. Collagen is one of the few proteins that has a significant amount of hydroxyproline and hydroxylysine residues. Vitamin C is important for the formation of these latter two modified amino acids and, as a result, vitamin C is an important vitamin for the formation of collagen (see also the *Introduction to Nutrients* chapter).

Globular Proteins

Globular proteins have polypeptide chains that are folded into a globular shape. The hydrophobic amino acid residues are embedded within the proteins, and hydrophilic amino acid residues are found at the surface of the proteins. As a result, globular proteins are water-soluble. Globular proteins are the workhorses of the cell; that is, they are involved in many metabolic, catabolic, and transport reactions. Two typical globular proteins are myoglobin and hemoglobin, which are able to bind and transport oxygen.

Denatured Proteins

Denaturation occurs when the biological activity of a protein that is folded properly is reduced or eliminated. A change in the pH of a solution that has dissolved a protein can influence the overall structure of the protein and results in complete denaturation. For instance, a change in the net charge on the protein can result in electrostatic attractions or repulsions between differently charged polypeptides or even charged amino acid residues, resulting in complete denaturation. Likewise, salts or organic solvents, when added to a protein solution, can disrupt hydrogen bonds and hydrophobic interactions within the protein. While some proteins are denatured permanently, others may be able to return to their native structures and functions upon a change in the solution they are dissolved in. For instance, when the salt or the organic solvent is removed from a protein solution, that particular protein may be able to resume its native structure and function.

A chaperone is a protein that—often at the expense of ATP hydrolysis—assists other proteins in maintaining the correct folding of proteins, particularly the newly synthesized proteins in the cytosol. A chaperone binds to the exposed hydrophobic surfaces of proteins and thereby blocks proteins' aggregation. Once the folding is complete, the chaperone leaves the folded protein to support folding of another protein.

Function of Proteins

Proteins are macromolecules with, on average, 200–300 amino acids, though some are bigger (hemoglobin has more than 500 amino acids) and some are smaller (insulin has fewer than 60 amino acids). Proteins are able to perform many functions based on their amino acid constitution and flexibility. Almost every cellular function in the living cell depends on proteins. For instance, motion of cells and organisms depends on contractile proteins (an example is myosin).

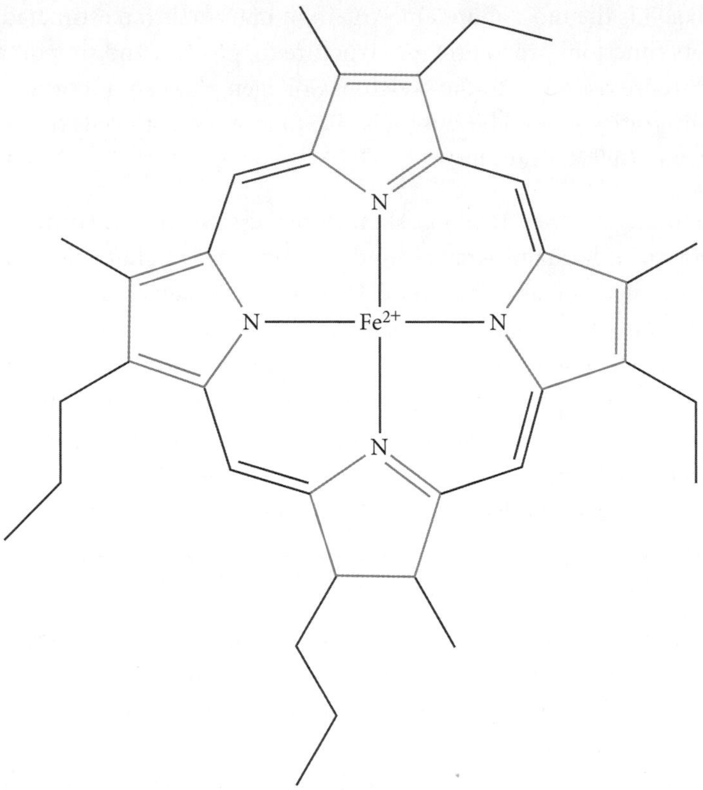

Figure 5.23 Structure of heme. All four pyrrole rings (blue) play important roles in the function of heme in both myoglobin and hemoglobin.

Catalysis of all biochemical reactions is carried out by enzymes (an example is ATPase). The structure of cells and the extracellular matrix in which they are embedded are mainly made of proteins (an example is collagen). The transport of materials in body fluids depends on proteins (an example is hemoglobin). Receptors, many transport channels, and other signaling molecules are proteins as well (an example is transmembrane proteins).

Sometimes the function of a protein depends on the prosthetic group that is a nonprotein structure. The prosthetic group is permanently (i.e., irreversibly) associated with the protein. As mentioned elsewhere, FAD and FMN are prosthetic groups for flavoprotein enzymes. Another example is the hemoglobin protein, which contains a porphyrin molecule consisting of four pyrrole rings and a central iron atom. The complex of porphyrin and iron is called heme; it is a prosthetic group of hemoglobin and myoglobin (**Figure 5.23**). The iron atom can have six coordination bonds: four attach the porphyrin molecule to the central nitrogen atoms, the fifth binding establishes a link to myoglobin or hemoglobin via the nitrogen atom of a histidine residue (proximal His) right below the porphyrin ring, and the sixth coordination bond is available to bind O_2.

The functions of two important proteins, myoglobin and hemoglobin, are described in the following sections.

Myoglobin

Myoglobin has only one subunit. This heme globular protein is largely found in the muscle tissue, where it serves as a storage unit for oxygen. While myoglobin has only one subunit, it has a heme prosthetic group, similar to hemoglobin, that is able to attach one oxygen molecule. Muscle tissues have a high oxygen demand and, as a result, myoglobin provides significant oxygen reserves to meet the oxygen demand. Myoglobin releases its oxygen (ligand), which is then used for many metabolic reactions. Accordingly, myoglobin should have an ability to bind and dissociate oxygen. As a globular protein, myoglobin has hydrophilic amino acids on the surface and hydrophobic amino acids in the interior of the protein. Therefore, the interior is rich in the Leu, Val, Phe, and Met amino acids.

Hemoglobin

In contrast to myoglobin, hemoglobin (Hb) is a protein with four subunits: α_1, β_1, α_2, and β_2. This globular protein is largely found in erythrocytes (it occupies more than 95% of an erythrocyte), where it is responsible for binding oxygen in the lung and carrying it throughout the body to sites where the oxygen is required for aerobic metabolic pathways. When the erythrocytes are destroyed and broken down, the protein moiety (globin) of hemoglobin is degraded into amino acids that are used for energy production or are recycled into other proteins. The iron is recovered and returned into the bone marrow, while the porphyrin moiety is broken down and excreted by the liver into bile forms, such as bilirubin and biliverdin, that contribute to the color of feces.

Each hemoglobin subunit contains a heme prosthetic group. Proteins that are evolutionarily related to one another are included within the same family. For instance, myoglobin and the β subunit of hemoglobin are members of the same family. The quaternary structure of hemoglobin leads to the physiologically important role of allosteric proteins. In allosteric proteins, the binding of a ligand to one site changes the ligand-binding affinity for the other sites on the same protein, a property that is lacking in the single-subunit myoglobin molecule. It is not necessary to have identical ligands for these multiple sites on an allosteric protein. However, the four oxygen molecules (ligands) are identical for the four subunits of the hemoglobin molecule.

The geometries of binding of an oxygen molecule (O_2) and a carbon monoxide molecule (CO) to heme are slightly different. In myoglobin and hemoglobin, there is a histidine residue, called distal His, that does not interact directly with the heme iron; rather, this residue interacts with the ligand (i.e., oxygen). CO binds 20,000 times more tightly than oxygen to a free heme. However, when heme is attached to myoglobin and hemoglobin, a steric hindrance reduces this strength to 200 (i.e., CO has 200 times higher affinity than oxygen for binding to myoglobin and hemoglobin). CO still has a higher affinity than oxygen for myoglobin and hemoglobin, so it is a very toxic molecule (gas) because it excludes oxygen from binding to these two important globular proteins.

All leukocytes and erythrocytes in the blood are formed from red bone marrow cells known as stem cells. A stem cell divides continually and differentiates into specific types of cells throughout the life of an organism. In the cell maturation process, some of the stem cells produce daughter cells that contain large amounts of hemoglobin. These daughter cells gradually lose their intracellular organelles such as the nucleus, mitochondria, and endoplasmic reticulum (ER) and differentiate into erythrocytes (mature erythrocytes do not have mitochondria, Golgi apparatus, ER, or a nucleus and, as a result, have more space for hemoglobin). One single erythrocyte contains approximately 200 million hemoglobin molecules. Because erythrocytes do not have nuclei, they have a short life, living for only 90–120 days.

There are two major conformations of hemoglobin: the T (tense) state and the R (relaxed) state. The T conformation has a low affinity for oxygen, whereas the R conformation has a high affinity for oxygen. In hemoglobin, the transition from T state to R state (i.e., from low to high affinity) is triggered by oxygen binding. The interplay between the T and R states is typical of an allosteric protein.

An interesting question is why the structure of myoglobin fits so well with its function as an oxygen-storage protein, whereas the multisubunit structure of hemoglobin fits so well with its role as an oxygen carrier protein. The binding of oxygen to a single binding site of myoglobin results in a high affinity even in tissues where the concentration of oxygen is low. In contrast, the allosteric binding of O_2 to the multiple binding sites of hemoglobin results in high affinity at a high concentration of O_2, like that found in the lungs, and low affinity when the oxygen concentration is low, as in tissues. The conformational changes of hemoglobin also explain why oxygen is released from their sites in the tissues. The pH in the tissues is slightly lower (more acidic) than the pH in the lungs. At a lower pH (i.e., a higher H^+ concentration), a few amino acid residues, including histidine, become protonated, which stabilizes the T-state conformation of the hemoglobin subunits. This condition explains why hemoglobin releases oxygen in the tissues.

The reversible binding of oxygen to hemoglobin is also affected by other molecules such as CO_2 and 2,3-bisphosphoglycerate. These molecules are called allosteric effectors because their binding at one subunit on the hemoglobin affects the binding of oxygen to the heme groups at other subunits within the same hemoglobin molecule.

In addition to carrying oxygen from lungs to peripheral tissues, hemoglobin plays an important role in carrying CO_2 in the opposite direction—that is, from the tissues to the lungs. Hemoglobin transports approximately 20% of the total H^+ and CO_2 produced in tissues to the lungs and kidneys. The binding of H^+ and CO_2 to hemoglobin is inversely related to the binding of oxygen, a phenomenon known as the Bohr effect.

Bisphosphoglycerate and Hemoglobin

The allosteric effector known as 2,3-bisphosphoglycerate (2,3-BPG) is present in high concentrations in erythrocytes. Binding of 2,3-BPG to hemoglobin decreases hemoglobin's affinity for oxygen. This occurs because 2,3-BPG (through its negative charges and by electrostatic interactions) binds to the positively charged environment created in a cavity between the β subunits. The 2,3-BPG molecule binds selectively to hemoglobin in the low-affinity T state, thereby stabilizing hemoglobin's conformation. As a result, the binding of oxygen to hemoglobin is regulated by 2,3-BPG. The concentration 2,3-BPG in erythrocytes increases in conditions such as chronic hypoxia (i.e., insufficient functioning of lungs or circulatory system) or at high altitudes where it is difficult to obtain sufficient oxygen. The large amount of 2,3-BPG present in this scenario ensures that hemoglobin releases oxygen in the tissues.

Sickle cell anemia is an inherited disorder involving hemoglobin. There are hundreds variants of hemoglobin, which differ in their amino acid composition. One of the well-known variants is hemoglobin S. In hemoglobin S, a single amino acid residue, Glu, is replaced by another residue, Val, in the sixth amino acid position of the β chain of this mutant hemoglobin. This amino acid substitution leads to aggregation and thereby the typical sickle shape of erythrocytes, which in turn leads to obstruction of blood flow, intense pain, and loss of erythrocytes. The aggregation problem does not occur during oxygenation, but rather after the hemoglobin has released its oxygen— that is, during deoxygenation. Sickle cell anemia is quite prevalent in individuals of African, Mediterranean, Middle Eastern, and Asian Indian ancestry.

Enzyme Kinetics in Biochemistry

Many of the biochemical reactions (catabolism or metabolism) occur spontaneously (i.e., they have a negative ΔG). However, these reactions may proceed forward so slowly that they are of no value for our survival. If cells did not evolve to generate enzymes to speed up biochemical reactions, life would not have been possible. With exception of catalytic RNAs, all enzymes are proteins. Enzymes are found both inside cells (intracellular enzymes) and outside cells (extracellular enzymes).

Enzymes convert a target molecule, known as a substrate, into a different molecule, or product. An enzyme accelerates a reaction rate usually to such an extent that the reaction nearly does not take place in the absence of the enzyme. Keep in mind that at equilibrium and in the presence of an enzyme, the concentrations of reactants and products are not different from the concentrations of reactants and products in the absence of the enzyme. An example that will help you appreciate the role of an enzyme is the reaction that takes millions of years (approximately 900 million years) to break down one molecule of urea (substrate) in the absence of the urease enzyme. By comparison, in the presence of urease at 37°C, it takes seconds to break down the urea molecule.

All of the biochemical reactions that occur in the human body are catalyzed by enzymes. As a result, the malfunction of a single enzyme can result in physiological abnormalities, disease, or even death. Both synthesis and functioning of enzymes are regulated. While the former type of regulation occurs at the level of transcription or translation (which may take hours), the latter one takes place at the level of catalytic efficiency affected by the binding of substrate (which may take only seconds).

Many enzyme names are based on their functions. For instance, transferases are enzymes that catalyze the transfer of a particular functional group from one molecule to another. Examples are transaminases, which transfer amino groups from amino acids, and decarboxylases, which remove carboxyl groups from neurotransmitters or hormones. **Table 5.2** summarizes six major classes of enzymes that catalyze many biochemical reactions.

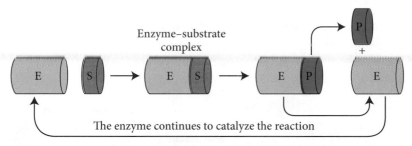

Figure 5.24 An enzyme (E) binds to a substrate (S) and forms an enzyme–substrate complex, which immediately is catalyzed to produce a product (P).

Table 5.2 Six Major Classes of Enzymes That Catalyze Many Biochemical Reactions

Enzyme Class	Type of Reaction	Examples
Oxidoreductases	Reduction–oxidation (redox)	Glucose-6-phosphate dehydrogenase, dihydrofolate reductase
Transferases	Move chemical group	Pyruvate kinase, hexokinase
Hydrolases	Hydrolysis; bond cleavage with transfer of functional group to water	Chmotrypsin, lysozyme, RNase A
Lyases	Nonhydrolytic bond cleavage	Fumarase
Isomerases	Intramolecular group transfer (isomerization)	Triose phosphate isomerase, methylmalonyl-CoA mutase
Ligases	Synthesis of new covalent bond between substrates, using ATP hydrolysis	RNA polymerase, pyruvate carboxylase

Reproduced from: Woodbury, CP. *Biochemistry for the pharmaceutical sciences.* **Burlington, MA: Jones & Bartlett Learning; 2012: Chapter 6.**

Enzymes have an area such as a pocket-shaped gap that is called an active site. The molecule that binds to the active site and is catalyzed by the enzyme is referred to as a substrate. Indeed, the binding of substrate to enzyme stabilizes the structure of an enzyme. Although the enzyme (E) joins the substrate (S) for a short time to make the product (P), the enzyme and product split apart immediately afterward, releasing the enzyme (**Figure 5.24**). Unlike the substrate, the enzyme is not consumed in the process. Therefore, the enzyme continues to react if more substrate is available.

To explore how this process works, let's start with a simple enzymatic reaction (compare it with Figure 5.24):

$$E + S \rightleftharpoons ES \rightleftharpoons EP \rightleftharpoons E + P$$

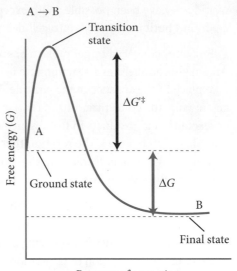

Figure 5.25 The rate of a reaction depends on the activation energy of the reaction, $\Delta G'^{\ddagger}$.

Keep in mind that an enzyme cannot alter the laws of thermodynamics. This means enzymes simply influence the rate of a reaction; they do not change the equilibrium for a reaction. Most biochemical reactions have an energy barrier that must be overcome before the reaction can happen, known as the activation energy ($G'^{\ddagger}$).

While ΔG is the difference between the free energy in S and P, $\Delta G'^{\ddagger}$ is the difference between free energy in S and the transition state (**Figure 5.25**). As shown in Figure 5.25, the ground state is the starting point for the forward reaction. The rate of conversion from a substrate (A) to a product (B)

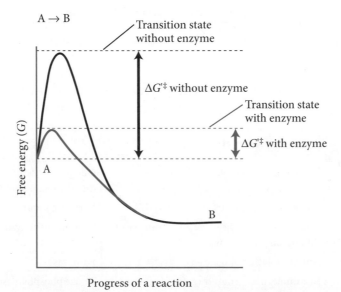

Figure 5.26 An enzyme lowers the activation energy by making a new transition state.

Adapted from: Nelson DL, Cox MM. *Lehninger principles of biochemistry*, 5th ed. New York: W. H. Freeman and Company; 2008: Chapter 6.

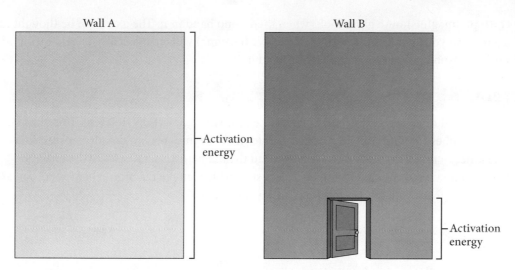

Figure 5.27 (A) Activation energy can resemble a wall that a substrate has to jump over to get to the other side of the wall. (B) An enzyme can resemble a door that can lower the activation energy by permitting the substrate to easily get to the other side.

does not depend on the free-energy difference between them, but rather the activation energy change of the reaction, $\Delta G'^{\ddagger}$. Enzymes (including catalysts) speed up reactions by lowering the activation energy for a particular reaction (**Figure 5.26**).

In the absence of an enzyme, the substrate goes through a transition state that has a higher free energy than S alone (Figure 5.26). Conversely, in the presence of an enzyme, the free energy to reach the transition state is lower. The free energy change between the ground state and the state when the product is formed remains the same regardless of an enzyme's involvement (Figure 5.26). In other words, the rate of conversion from substrate to product does not depend on the free energy difference between them. The rate of the reaction depends on the activation energy of the reaction, $\Delta G'^{\ddagger}$; thus, the lower activation energy, the more rapidly a reaction can proceed.

Let's use an analogy to explain the role of an enzyme and the activation energy in a reaction. Suppose there are two tall walls in front of your friend (A) and you (B) (**Figure 5.27**). Your wall has a door; your friend's wall doesn't. Suppose also that both of you have been asked to go to the other side of the wall. You, by going through the door, will get to the other side in seconds, while your friend first has to climb up to the top of the wall (transition state) to get to the other side, which may take several minutes. Here the door acts as an enzyme (E) that helps you (S) to bypass the tall wall (activation energy, $\Delta G'^{\ddagger}$) to get to the other side (P).

The activation energy is a barrier to the reaction. The higher the activation energy, the more slowly a reaction will occur. In other words, the old bonds in the substrate must be broken so that new bonds can be formed. In every catalytic pathway where several steps occur in a reaction, the overall rate is determined by the step that has the highest activation energy (the slowest reaction rate). This step is called the rate-limiting step in the pathway because it dictates the rate at which the entire reaction can proceed.

Enzymes are not rigid molecules; instead, an enzyme changes its shape when the substrate binds at the active site of the enzyme. The concept of induced fit refers to the flexibility of the enzyme—that is, when the substrate, by binding to the active site, can induce a conformational change in the enzyme. This change may bring catalytic groups of the enzyme into a "fit" position. To envision this concept, imagine how a glove looks when there is no hand in it. The glove can be thought of as an enzyme and your hand as a substrate. The glove (enzyme) will change its shape and form to fit to your hand (substrate) when you put your hand in it.

Enzyme Kinetics

The biochemical reactions that occur in a living cell (*in vivo*) are virtifually different from those that occur in test tubes (*in vitro*) due to the unique roles that enzymes play in the former reactions. Enzyme kinetics refers to the rate of a reaction and the mathematical analysis of the enzyme activity. To understand the enzyme kinetics, let's start with a simple reaction scheme between an enzyme and a substrate that proceeds reversibly at a fast rate:

$$E + S \underset{k_{-1}}{\overset{k_1}{\rightleftharpoons}} ES \qquad\qquad \text{(Scheme a)}$$

The parameters k_1 *and* k_{-1} are rate constants.

The ES complex can also break down into the enzyme and product (P) at a much slower rate:

$$ES \underset{k_{-2}}{\overset{k_2}{\rightleftharpoons}} E + P \qquad\qquad \text{(Scheme b)}$$

The Michaelis-Menten equation includes these reactions schemes and rate constants and explains well how a change in the substrate concentration can change the velocity of a catalytic reaction. However, first let's see how we can express the Michaelis-Menten equation.

For measuring the Michaelis-Menten equation, we can begin with the whole reaction scheme for the enzyme and substrate interaction:

$$E + S \underset{k_{-1}}{\overset{k_1}{\rightleftharpoons}} ES \underset{k_{-2}}{\overset{k_2}{\rightleftharpoons}} E + P \qquad\qquad \text{(Scheme c)}$$

Here k_1 is the rate constant for ES formation and k_{-1} and k_2 are the rate constants for ES breakdown.

Often, kinetic measurements in enzymology are made in the beginning of a reaction when less than 10% of substrate has been used, which leads to very small amount of product formation. Therefore, one can neglect [P]. This results in canceling the reverse rate constant, k_{-2}, as well. As a result, scheme c can be written as follows:

$$E + S \underset{k_{-1}}{\overset{k_1}{\rightleftharpoons}} ES \underset{\cancel{k_{-2}}}{\overset{k_2}{\rightleftharpoons}} E + P \qquad\qquad \text{(Scheme d)}$$

Because the second step in scheme d is the slowest step (i.e., it is a rate-limiting step), k_2 determines the overall rate of the entire reaction. One can determine V_0 by using the rate of the breakdown of ES to form product as follows:

$$V_0 = k_2[ES] \qquad\qquad (5.25)$$

This expression shows the initial velocity (V_0) can be calculated by knowing the rate constant k_2 and the concentration of the enzyme–substrate complex (ES). In other words, we are focusing on the second step in scheme d:

$$ES \xrightarrow{k_2} E + P$$

To calculate V_0, we must know the exact concentration of ES. Keep in mind that when the enzyme is saturated with S, $[E_t]$ (total enzyme concentration) is equal to ES. This means Equation 5.25 can be expressed as follows:

$$V_{max} = k_2[E_t] \tag{5.26}$$

However, we are also interested in measuring V_0 (i.e., the beginning of the reaction) and for that reason, we must use ES. It is very difficult to measure the concentration of ES at the beginning of a reaction (experimentally, it is difficult to know how much of an enzyme is in complex with its substrate). As a result, one can express ES in this way:

$$[ES] = \frac{[E_t][S]}{K_m + [S]} \tag{5.27}$$

where [ES] is the concentration of enzyme–substrate complex, E_t is the total enzyme concentration, [S] is the concentration of substrate, and K_m is the Michaelis constant (which we will explain shortly). The important feature of Equation 5.27 is that it includes all parameters and rate constants in measuring the concentration of the enzyme–substrate complex. For instance, K_m is measured as a result of three rate constants that are involved in scheme d:

$$K_m = \frac{k_{-1} + k_2}{k_1} \tag{5.28}$$

If you replace [ES] in Equation 5.25 (i.e., $V_0 = k_2$ [ES]) with Equation 5.27, you will be able to express Equation 5.29:

$$V_0 = \frac{k_2[E_t][S]}{K_m + [S]} \tag{5.29}$$

As you noticed (from Equation 5.26), when the enzyme is saturated with S, the value of $k_2[E_t]$ will be equal to V_{max}. In other words, the maximal velocity (V_{max}) is achieved when the enzyme is saturated with the substrate and is fully engaged in catalyzing the substrate. Now we can express the Michaelis-Menten equation by rewriting Equation 5.29:

$$V_0 = \frac{V_{max}[S]}{K_m + [S]} \tag{5.30}$$

K_m has the unit of concentration. Because it is a ratio of three rate constants—$(k_{-1} + k_2)/k_1$ of a reaction—K_m is the characteristic of that reaction. A given enzyme that catalyzes a given substrate has a distinct K_m. In fact, K_m is one of the most important kinetic parameters in enzymology. Simply put, K_m represents the substrate concentration at which the reaction velocity is half-maximal.

According to the Michaelis-Menten equation (Equation 5.30), when [S] becomes very high, the active site of the enzyme becomes occupied with a new substrate molecule as soon as the product is released from the enzyme. Accordingly, the enzyme becomes "saturated" with substrate, so that further increases in [S] will not change the velocity to any significant extent. In principle, there are three simple scenarios that one can encounter during an enzymatic reaction.

Scenario A

In this scenario, the concentration of substrate is much higher (100 times or more) than K_m (i.e., [S] >> K_m). Let's use Equation 5.30 to see what actually happens. If [S] is 100 times higher than K_m, then K_m is neglected and the two [S] values cancel each other. As a result, Equation 5.30 becomes Equation 5.30A:

$$V_0 = V_{max} \qquad (5.30A)$$

which means the enzyme is saturated with substrate. Scenario A is also illustrated in **Figure 5.28**.

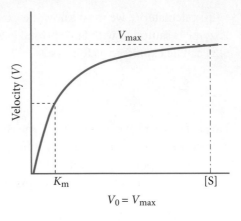

$$V_0 = V_{max}$$

Figure 5.28 When [S] >> K_m, V_0 equals V_{max} (see the dashed blue line), which in turn means the enzyme is catalyzing the substrate with its full maximal velocity.

Scenario B

In this scenario, the concentration of substrate is much lower (100 times or more) than K_m (i.e., [S] << K_m). Let's use Equation 5.30 to see what happens. If [S] is 100 times lower than K_m, then [S] in the denominator of Equation 5.30 becomes neglected, which leads to Equation 5.30B:

$$V_0 = \frac{V_{max}}{K_m} \, [S] \qquad (5.30B)$$

which means the initial velocity will change when the concentration of substrate is changed. This scenario is illustrated in **Figure 5.29**.

Scenario C

In this last scenario, [S] = K_m; K_m is equal to the substrate concentration at which the velocity is half of its maximal value. Let's use Equation 5.30 again to see what happens. If [S] is equal to K_m, Equation 5.30 becomes

$$V_0 = \frac{V_{max}[1]}{1+[1]} = 0.5 V_{max} \qquad (5.30C)$$

Scenario C is illustrated in **Figure 5.30**.

Simply put, the Michaelis-Menten equation tells us that V_0 is the initial velocity; V_{max} is the maximal velocity when all enzyme molecules are saturated with substrate; [S] is the concentration of substrate; and K_m is a constant characteristic for the enzyme. In the following example you will see how useful the Michaelis-Menten parameters are.

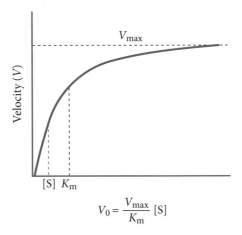

$$V_0 = \frac{V_{max}}{K_m} \, [S]$$

Figure 5.29 When [S] << K_m, V_0 changes as a result of changes in substrate concentrations.

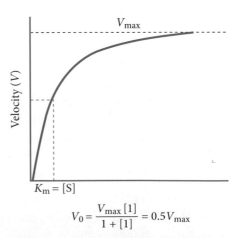

$$V_0 = \frac{V_{max}\,[1]}{1+[1]} = 0.5 V_{max}$$

Figure 5.30 When [S] = K_m, the enzyme's velocity is half of its maximal value.

Example 5.1: An enzyme that follows Michaelis-Menten kinetics catalyzes a substrate with the velocities shown in **Table 5.3**. Calculate the K_m and V_{max} values for this enzyme.

Table 5.3 Catalysis of a Reaction by an Enzyme at Different Concentrations of a Substrate

Substrate (µM)	Velocity (µmol/min)
4	1
15	5
38	20
70	38
700	40

Answer: As is shown in Table 5.3, 40 µmol/min must be V_{max} because when the concentration of substrate increases by a factor of 10 (from 70 µM to 700 µM), the velocity does not change to any significant extent. This indicates that the enzyme is saturated with its substrate; in other words, the enzyme has reached its maximal velocity. In addition, we know that K_m is the concentration of the substrate that gives $0.5V_{max}$. Therefore, ½V_{max} = 20 µmol/min and K_m is 38 µM.

Catalytic Rate Constant

Since the rate-limiting step is from ES to P (see scheme d), k_2 will be the catalytic rate of the overall reaction in scheme d. Therefore, k_2 can be called k_{cat} ("cat" stands for "catalytic rate"). Replacing k_2 by k_{cat} in Equation 5.29 will give Equation 5.31:

$$V_0 = \frac{k_{cat}[E_t][S]}{k_m + [S]} \tag{5.31}$$

The k_{cat} parameter measures the number of substrate molecules turned over per enzyme molecule, when the enzyme is saturated with the substrate, per unit time. Thus k_{cat} is interchangeably referred to as a turnover number. For the two-step reaction in reaction scheme d, $k_{cat} = k_2$. For more complex reactions, k_{cat} depends on which step in the process is the rate-limiting step. The unit of k_{cat} is seconds^{-1} (first order). For instance, k_{cat} for catalase enzyme is 4×10^7/s (or 4×10^7 s^{-1}). This number indicates that one catalase enzyme catalyzes the degradation of 4×10^7 H_2O_2 molecules in 1 second.

When $[S] \ll K_m$ (in diluted solutions), Equation 5.31 will be converted to Equation 5.32:

$$V_0 = \frac{k_{cat}}{k_m}[E_t][S] \tag{5.32}$$

The value of K_m reveals the enzyme's affinity for the substrates, while the value of k_{cat}/K_m indicates the enzyme's catalytic efficiency. Also, k_{cat}/K_m is read and said as "k_{cat} over K_m." The k_{cat}/K_m ratio behaves as a second-order rate constant (and, therefore, has units of M^{-1}s^{-1}; see also the *Introduction to Pharmaceutics* chapter) for the reaction between substrate and free enzyme. This ratio is important, as we can compare efficiencies between different enzymes by comparing their k_{cat}/K_m values. The higher the value of k_{cat}/K_m, the more efficient an enzyme is.

Example 5.2: Enzyme A has a turnover rate (k_{cat}) of 1×10^3/s at which it catalyzes a reaction. Enzyme B has a turnover rate (k_{cat}) of 0.5×10^3/s at which it catalyzes another reaction. While enzyme A has a K_m of 0.05 M, enzyme B has a K_m of 0.01 M. Which enzyme, A or B, has the highest efficiency in catalyzing its reaction?

Answer: While the turnover rate for A seems faster than that for B, because A has a higher K_m than B has, the k_{cat}/K_m for A is 0.02 $M^{-1}s^{-1}$ and the k_{cat}/K_m for B is 0.05 $M^{-1}s^{-1}$. Accordingly, B has a higher efficiency in catalyzing its reaction. Simply put, just knowing the k_{cat} will not help you determine which enzyme is more efficient.

Enzyme Inhibition

There are two classes of enzyme inhibitors (**Figure 5.31**): those causing reversible inactivation of enzymes and those whose inhibitory effects are irreversible. Inhibitors of the second class usually cause inactivation of the enzyme structure. One can find a few classes of inhibitors within the reversible inhibition category.

Competitive Inhibitors

A competitive inhibitor closely mimics the substrate so that the enzyme can accept the inhibitor to the substrate binding site. In the presence of a competitive inhibitor, the Michaelis-Menten equation (Equation 5.30) will be

$$V_0 = \frac{V_{max}[S]}{\alpha K_m + [S]} \tag{5.33}$$

in which α is

$$\alpha = 1 + \frac{[I]}{K_I} \tag{5.34}$$

αK_m is called apparent K_m, where α is equal to Equation 5.34. The concentration of the inhibitor is [I], and K_I is the dissociation constant (or inhibition constant) for the enzyme–inhibitor complex (EI). The inhibitory measurement is often expressed as K_I and is the concentration of the inhibitor that causes 50% inhibition of the enzyme. Similar to the case for K_m from Michaelis-Menten kinetics, the unit for K_I is mol/L, and a lower K_I indicates a more potent inhibitor. Substances for which the value of K_I is smaller than 1 mM are often considered potent inhibitors. As any other dissociation constant, a smaller K_I indicates a tighter binding of the inhibitor to the enzyme.

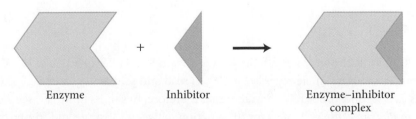

Enzyme   Inhibitor   Enzyme–inhibitor
                                              complex

Figure 5.31 An inhibitor binds to an enzyme and inhibits the catalytic activity of that enzyme.

A high concentration of [I] results in an increase in the apparent K_m. Increasing [I] causes the affinity for the substrate to decrease, simply because the inhibitor is occupying the binding site for substrate.

When a competitive inhibitor inhibits an enzyme, the V_{max} or k_{cat} value will not change, because when [S] increases relative to a fixed [I] (i.e., when [S] >> [I]), the enzyme is more likely to bind S than I (the substrate molecule outcompetes the inhibitor for the enzyme's active site). This observation is also apparent in Equation 5.33; at very large [S], V_0 approaches V_{max}, so the inhibitor cannot affect the value of V_{max} or k_{cat}.

Neostigmine (Prostigmin) is a competitive inhibitor of acetylcholine esterase (AchE), the enzyme that is responsible for hydrolysis of acetylcholine (as discussed in the *Introduction to Pharmacology and Pathophysiology* chapter). This medication is used in the symptomatic treatment of myasthenia gravis, a neuromuscular disease. Acetylcholine plays an important role in the transmission of impulses across the neuromuscular junction to stimulate a muscular contraction.

Uncompetitive Inhibitors

Uncompetitive inhibitors do not bind to the active site, but rather to other parts of the enzyme that can be far away from the substrate binding site; such binding modifies V_{max}. Equation 5.30 may be rearranged to express the enzyme kinetics for an uncompetitive inhibitor:

$$V_0 = \frac{V_{max}[S]}{K_m + \alpha'[S]} \tag{5.35}$$

in which α' is

$$\alpha' = 1 + \frac{[I]}{K_I'} \tag{5.36}$$

Uncompetitive inhibitors, unlike competitive inhibitor, bind only to the ES complex and disable the enzyme from catalyzing the desired reaction. As can be seen in Equation 5.35, at a high concentration of [S], K_m is canceled; the [S] values will cancel each other, too, so that V_0 will approach V_{max}/α'. The last observation means that no matter how large [S] is, you cannot reverse the inhibition effect on V_{max}. As a result, the value of V_{max} is affected. In addition, the binding of inhibitor distorts the active site, so K_m is also affected. This type of inhibition is rare with single-substrate enzymes but occurs more frequently when multiple substrates are present. **Table 5.4** summarizes the changes in Michaelis-Menten kinetics for uncompetitive inhibitors.

Donepezil (Aricept) is an uncompetitive inhibitor of the acetylcholine esterase enzyme, which is known to inactivate acetylcholine. As a result of such inhibition, the concentration of acetylcholine increases in the central nervous system (CNS). Donepezil is used to prevent progress of Alzheimer's disease, as patients with this disease have a deficiency of cholinergic neurons in their CNS (see also the *Introduction to Pharmacology and Pathophysiology* chapter).

Irreversible Inhibitors

Irreversible inhibition occurs when an inhibitor combines covalently with an enzyme to inactivate it irreversibly. Because an irreversible enzyme inhibitor inactivates an enzyme permanently, many of the irreversible enzyme inhibitors are toxic substances. Simply put, an inhibitor that permanently changes an amino acid side chain in the active site of an enzyme can serve as an irreversible enzyme inhibitor.

Table 5.4 Michaelis-Menten Kinetics Parameters That Are Affected by Different Reversible Enzyme Inhibitors

Inhibition	K_m	V_{max} (and k_{cat})
Competitive	Changes	Does not change
Uncompetitive	Changes	Changes
Mixed	Changes	Changes

Learning Bridge 5.2

In one of your community pharmacy rotations, a patient comes to the counter and complains about swollen and red gums. He wants to buy an OTC product that can help with his gums. You and your preceptor notice that the patient seems to be intoxicated and smells of alcohol. Your preceptor asks the patient to describe his daily diet. The patient admits that he does not eat regularly and that most of his money is spent on alcohol.

Your preceptor recommends a vitamin C supplement, Asco-Caps-500, to be taken once a day for two weeks.

A. What has caused the swollen and red gums for this patient?
B. Why can vitamin C help treat his gum problem?
C. What advice do you have for the patient?

Omeprazole (Prilosec) is known to irreversibly inhibit the gastric H^+/K^+–ATPase pump that is responsible for transporting H^+ from the parietal cells into the stomach (it reduces acid reflux). Omeprazole, despite covalently binding to the H^+/K^+–ATPase pump, is not toxic to the cell because of continuing cellular expression of the H^+/K^+-ATPase gene (see also the *Introduction to Medicinal Chemistry* chapter). A few examples of therapeutic agents with reversible and irreversible inhibitory mechanisms are discussed in the *Introduction to Medicinal Chemistry* chapter.

Regulatory Enzymes

Regulatory enzymes are essential for an efficient functioning of extracellular and intracellular biochemical pathways. Many regulatory enzymes display kinetic behaviors that do not fit into the Michaelis-Menten equation. This means a graph of V_0 versus [S] would produce a sigmoidal curve rather than a hyperbolic curve because the enzyme kinetics would be affected by molecules other than the substrate(s).

Regulation of enzymes is often carried out by allosteric enzymes, many of which are composed of multiple subunits. They are larger than nonallosteric enzymes. The subunits exhibit cooperativity in substrate binding. In addition, allosteric modulators (or allosteric effectors) are molecules (often small metabolites or cofactors) that bind to a secondary site and induce conformational changes. A positive modulator can enhance an allosteric enzyme's activity by binding to a regulatory site that is different from the catalytic site.

A typical example of an allosteric enzyme is pyruvate kinase. Pyruvate kinase (in the last step of glycolysis) is allosterically inhibited by a few molecules, particularly, by a high concentration

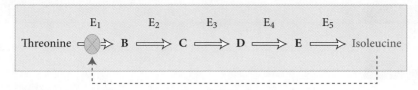

Figure 5.32 During the synthesis of the Ile amino acid, if too much Ile accumulates, Ile provides a negative feedback mechanism and inhibits the first enzyme that is involved in the synthesis of Ile.

Adapted from Nelson DL, Cox MM, and Lehninger AL. Principle of biochemistry. 5th ed. W.H. Freeman and Company; 2008, Chapter 6.

of ATP and acetyl-CoA molecules. Thus, whenever the cellular level of ATP and acetyl-CoA increases, pyruvate kinase enzyme is inhibited.

Feedback inhibition is often employed in a multienzyme system where the regulatory enzyme is inhibited by the end product. For instance, if a cell accumulates too many isoleucine amino acid molecules, the first enzyme will be inhibited by the end product, isoleucine (**Figure 5.32**).

Metabolism of Glucose

Carbohydrates are important structural and nutritional components of all living organisms. They are the most abundant energy-rich molecules that are found in nature, particularly in plants. Carbohydrates are chemical components that contain carbon, hydrogen, and oxygen. Many have the empiric formula $(CH_2O)_n$; for instance, the molecular formula of glucose is $C_6H_{12}O_6$. We can make carbohydrate from lipids and protein but the majority of carbohydrate in our bodies comes from plants.

Three classes of carbohydrates are distinguished: monosaccharides, oligosaccharides, and polysaccharides (see the *Introduction to Cell Biology* chapter). Glucose is a typical example of a monosaccharide. It is a very important molecule for life and one of the main sources used to produce energy in the form of ATP molecules. The brain consumes approximately 80% of the body's total glucose consumption per day. Glycogen and starch are the major forms of carbohydrate storage in animals and plants, respectively.

Glycolysis

Glucose is the most precious carbohydrate and the most abundant organic molecule on the earth. It is the only fuel that is used by all cells in the human body. Indeed, in some organisms, glucose is the only source of energy (e.g., in parasitic trypanosomes; see the *Introduction to Microbiology* chapter). It is also precursor for many biomolecules such as RNA, DNA, fatty acids, and amino acids.

Glycolysis is the metabolic pathway in which glucose is oxidized to produce energy in the form of ATP. Glycolysis is a universal pathway that is basically identical in the cytoplasm of prokaryotic, eukaryotic, aerobic, and anaerobic organisms. The fact that anaerobes use glycolysis indicates that glycolysis evolved before oxygen became abundant on earth (more than 3 billion years ago). In anaerobes, glycolysis is the only significant source of energy from carbohydrates. As you will see, in eukaryotes and aerobes, significantly more energy can be produced by the subsequent steps that occur in the citric acid cycle and the oxidative phosphorylation pathway.

The glycolysis pathway begins when one molecule of the six-carbon glucose breaks down over the course of 10 enzyme-catalyzed steps and ends when two molecules of a three-carbon compound, pyruvate, are produced (**Figure 5.33**). Additional products of glycolysis include two ATP molecules and two NADH molecules. Glycolysis is divided into two phases:

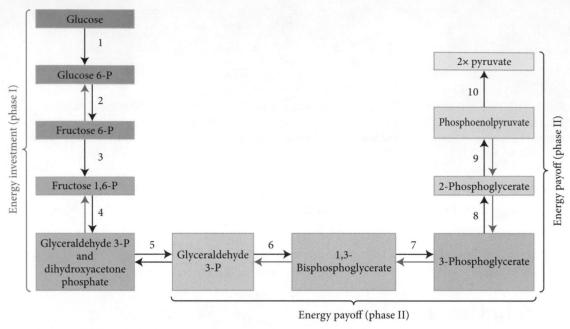

Figure 5.33 Ten steps are involved in the glycolysis pathway (black arrows). Many of the reversible reactions in glycolysis are used in gluconeogenesis (blue arrows).

1. Energy investment—when ATP molecules are invested (phase I).

2. Energy payoff—when ATP molecules are produced (phase II).

Phase I

During phase I, four enzymatic reactions take place that oxidize one glucose molecule into two 3-carbon molecules (i.e., glyceraldehyde 3-phosphate and dihydroxyacetone phosphate) (Figure 5.33). Two reactions require one ATP molecule each: hexokinase catalyzes the first reaction, and phosphofructokinase-1 catalyzes the third reaction. Both of the two reactions that consume ATP occur at the level of hexoses (six-carbon compounds).

Phase II

The two 3-carbon molecules, glyceraldehyde 3-phosphate, that are produced during phase I serve as the starting point for initiation of phase II. Phase II includes six enzymatic reactions. In this phase, two reactions produce ATP molecules. The first enzyme is phosphoglycerate kinase, which catalyzes the seventh reaction, and the second enzyme is pyruvate kinase, which catalyzes the last reaction in glycolysis (Figure 5.33).

Overall, the conversion of one molecule of glucose to two molecules of pyruvate by the glycolytic pathway results in a payoff of two molecules of NADH and four molecules of ATP. In other words, two ATP molecules are used (invested) and four ATP molecules are produced (paid off) when one glucose molecule is converted to two pyruvate molecules, resulting in a net yield of two ATP molecules.

Figure 5.34 demonstrates the metabolic fates of the end product of glycolysis, pyruvate, in the anaerobic and aerobic conditions that subsequently follow glycolysis. In other words, it is the availability of oxygen that determines the fate of the pyruvate molecules.

As Figure 5.34 demonstrates, under aerobic conditions, pyruvate is oxidized to acetyl-CoA and then moves to the citric acid cycle for further oxidation. In this cycle, in a series of reactions,

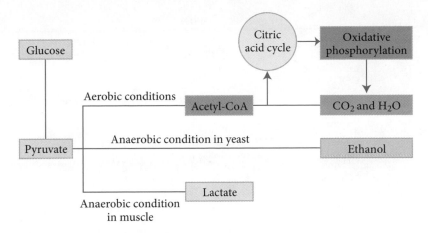

Figure 5.34 Pyruvate can take different paths after glycolysis.

CO_2, NADH, and $FADH_2$ are produced. NADH and $FADH_2$, in turn, are funneled into a chain of reactions in the mitochondria to reduce O_2 to water and to assist in the synthesis of ATP by the ATP synthase enzyme. As the name "aerobic" indicates, oxygen must be present to make this fate feasible.

In anaerobic glycolysis, glycolysis takes place under conditions in the absence of oxygen. This pathway occurs either when there is no oxygen at all (anaerobic organisms) or when the oxygen level is low (in animals experiencing extensive muscle activity). Under conditions of extensive muscle activity, ATP is consumed faster than it is produced, simply because the blood flow cannot provide enough oxygen to tissues to enable them to produce a sufficient amount of ATP. The NADH molecules that have been produced during glycolysis must be recycled (re-oxidized) to NAD^+ to allow glycolysis to continue (glycolysis is strictly dependent on the availability of NAD^+). As a result, the NADH that is produced during glycolysis will be re-oxidized to NAD^+ to produce ATP by the oxidative phosphorylation pathway, a mechanism that uses oxygen and occurs only in the mitochondria of eukaryotic organisms.

The puzzling question is what happens to this crucial re-oxidation process when a cell does not have a mitochondrion (i.e., erythrocytes), the oxygen level is low (extensive muscle activity), or the organism does not use oxygen (anaerobic organisms). In the absence of oxygen, the cell has evolved a mechanism to regenerate NAD^+. Under conditions of extensive muscle activity or where there are no mitochondria, the end product of glycolysis, pyruvate, is converted to lactate by lactate dehydrogenase enzyme to regenerate NAD^+ (**Figure 5.35**). The lactate produced in this way is sent to the blood and then to the liver. This phenomenon explains why under extensive muscle activity, the pH of human blood decreases (lactate or lactic acid is an acidic molecule). However, by using this pathway, we do not waste the glucose molecule. The produced lactate in the liver can be used, as a substrate, for gluconeogenesis (i.e., for the synthesis of glucose).

Fermentation is the operation of the glycolytic pathway under anaerobic conditions. Fermentation occurs via two pathways: (1) fermentation to lactate by lactate dehydrogenase (as described earlier) and (2) fermentation to ethanol and CO_2 in yeast (animals do not support this pathway). Yeast and a few other microorganisms convert glucose to pyruvate, and then pyruvate to ethanol and CO_2 rather than to lactate (Figure 5.34). Pyruvate decarboxylase (mammals lack this enzyme) catalyzes the removal of the carboxyl group of pyruvate to produce CO_2 and acetaldehyde. Next, alcohol dehydrogenase reduces acetaldehyde to ethanol to regenerate NAD^+.

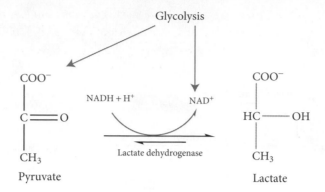

Figure 5.35 To regenerate (re-oxidize) NAD⁺, lactate is formed—an essential pathway during anaerobic conditions.

When glucose is converted to two pyruvate molecules, 146 kJ/mol of energy is released (negative $\Delta G°'$); when glucose is converted to CO_2 and H_2O, the energy released is 2,840 kJ/mol. This indicates that only 5% (146/2,840) of energy is released from glucose to pyruvate, while 95% remains to be released when pyruvate is oxidized further into CO_2 and H_2O through the citric acid cycle and the oxidative phosphorylation pathway.

Important Facts About Glycolysis

The first glycolytic reaction attaches a phosphate group to glucose, to yield glucose 6-phosphate in an irreversible reaction. This reaction is catalyzed by the enzyme hexokinase. The conversion of glucose into glucose 6-phosphate is thermodynamically unfavorable; that is, it is endergonic. As mentioned elsewhere, the kinase protein is an enzyme that catalyzes the transfer of a phosphoryl group to or from ATP. Here the phosphoryl group is transferred from ATP to glucose to produce glucose 6-phosphate.

Glucose 6-phosphate is converted to fructose-6-phosphate by the enzyme phosphohexose isomerase. This reaction is the first isomerization product (there are two isomerization reactions in glycolysis, in which step 8 is the second reaction). Isomers have the same chemical formula, meaning they are composed of the same atoms but have different arrangements of their bonds.

Fructose 6-phosphate in the fourth step is phosphorylated by the enzyme phosphofructokinase-1 (PFK-1) to produce fructose 1,6-bisphosphate. This irreversible step requires an ATP molecule (energy investment) and is highly regulated by PFK-1. The conversion of fructose 6-phosphate to fructose 1,6-bisphosphate is a biochemical key to understanding how the regulation of glycolysis occurs. PFK-1 is an allosteric and regulatory enzyme that plays a major role in glycolysis. It has the same binding site for both stimulator and inhibitor. The activity of PFK-1 increases whenever the amount of ATP is low or the amount of ADP is high. Conversely, the activity of PFK-1 decreases when the cell has a sufficient number of ATP molecules to meet its needs. Thus PFK-1 is a regulatory enzyme that responds to the amount of ADP present. It has been suggested that the conformation of the enzyme changes when ADP binds to it, which in turn increases the affinity of the enzyme for its substrate (fructose 6-phosphate). PFK-1 is a good site for regulation of glycolysis because as soon as the product is formed by this enzyme, the glycolysis process is committed to continue to the subsequent steps.

For the reactions that take place during the investment phase (the first five steps) of glycolysis, the six-carbon glucose is split into two 3-carbon molecules. Therefore, there are two glyceraldehyde 3-phosphate molecules produced at the end of the fifth step.

Interestingly, in none of the 10 enzyme-catalyzed reactions does the glucose molecule react with oxygen. Oxygen is, however, necessary later on in the mitochondria to assist the cells in producing ATP molecules. In other words, if oxygen was necessary for glycolysis to occur, anaerobic organisms would not have survived.

In the sixth reaction, glyceraldehyde 3-phosphate is both oxidized and phosphorylated to produce 1,3-bisphosphoglycerate. The enzyme that catalyzes this reaction is glyceraldehyde 3-phosphate dehydrogenase. This enzyme, unlike the kinases that catalyzed reactions 1 and 3, does not use any ATP molecule as the source of its phosphate. Instead, it adds an inorganic phosphate directly to the substrate. Inorganic phosphate (PPi) is absolutely required for glycolysis to proceed because it is an essential substrate in this step. Given that the glyceraldehyde 3-phosphate is oxidized, something (NAD^+) must be reduced (NADH). It is very important for NAD^+ to be present to accept electrons from the substrate. It has been shown that glyceraldehyde 3-phosphate dehydrogenase, beside fulfilling its important role in glycolysis, has a wide variety of cellular roles, such as in translational control (protein synthesis), tRNA export from the nucleus, and DNA repair.

The final step of glycolysis is catalyzed by a regulatory enzyme, pyruvate kinase. This enzyme catalyzes phosphoenolpyruvate (PEP) to pyruvate and concurrently transfers a phosphoryl group to ADP to form one ATP molecule in the presence of K^+ and either Mg^{2+} or Mn^{2+}. The tenth step is also a rate-limiting step (the other rate-limiting step is step 3), so it is a good candidate site for regulation. The reason that this step (last step) is slow is because under normal conditions the amount of PEP (substrate) available to bind pyruvate kinase (enzyme) is low, so the enzyme does not reach the saturation level needed to provide the maximum velocity (recall V_{max}). However, because this regulatory enzyme participates at the end of the glycolysis process, it is not one of the primary regulatory enzymes in glycolysis.

Three irreversible enzymes all serve regulatory purposes in glycolysis. Hexokinase catalyzes step 1, phosphofructokinase-1 (PFK-1) catalyzes step 3, and pyruvate kinase catalyzes step 10.

Hexokinase belongs to a hexokinase enzyme family. This family includes a variety of hexokinases that differ in their regulatory mechanisms, tissue localization, and molecular forms. These hexokinases are known as isozymes because they catalyze the same reaction but have different molecular forms and are expressed by different genes. For instance, hexokinases catalyze glucose to glucose 6-phosphate.

The liver of human has evolved a few different mechanisms to regulate the blood glucose level. One mechanism focuses on an isozyme of hexokinase with a high K_m for glucose. The hexokinase that catalyzes phosphorylation of glucose in the liver is known as glucokinase and differs from the hexokinase that acts in the muscle. As a result, these two different organs play different roles in carbohydrate metabolism. Simply put, the liver maintains blood glucose levels, whereas muscle, which lacks this ability, oxidizes glucose for production of energy. Because one of the roles of the liver is to regulate the blood glucose level, it is important for the liver to not experience a saturated condition. In other words, it is important to have a K_m in the range of 5–10 mM, which is close to the concentration of the substrate (the concentration of glucose in the blood is approximately 5 mM). As a consequence, the glucokinase enzyme does not catalyze the reaction at its maximum velocity and is sensitive to relatively small changes of glucose concentration in the blood. **Figure 5.36** illustrates the difference in K_m for hexokinase and glucokinase isozymes that are found in the muscle and liver, respectively.

The role of glucokinase in the liver is to phosphorylate glucose to glucose 6-phosphate for the synthesis of glycogen only when glucose is abundant (i.e., when the blood glucose level is high). This task is accomplished owing to the high K_m that glucokinase has. Because glucokinase has at least a

50 times higher K_m (lower affinity) for glucose compared to hexokinase (see Figure 5.36), it can bind to its substrate (glucose) whenever the blood glucose level is high.

The last enzyme in glycolysis, pyruvate kinase, is also a regulatory enzyme. ATP allosterically inhibits this enzyme to slow glycolysis when the formation of ATP molecules is unnecessary. This enzyme is also inhibited by acetyl-CoA. Acetyl-CoA is produced not only from pyruvate, but also from fatty acids and ketogenic amino acids (i.e., amino acids that can be metabolized to acetyl-CoA). In either case, a high level of acetyl-CoA leads to a high level of ATP formation. Once again, one way to slow down glycolysis is to inhibit pyruvate kinase. In addition, the glucagon hormone (a peptide hormone involved in increasing blood levels of glucose) suppresses synthesis of pyruvate kinase to slow down the glycolysis pathway. This mechanism favors gluconeogenesis over glycolysis as a means to produce glucose.

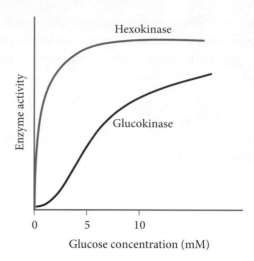

Figure 5.36 The fact that glucokinase has a K_m similar to its substrate (glucose) concentration in the blood makes the liver and glucokinase sensitive to even small changes in the glucose level in the blood.

Adapted from: Nelson DL, Cox MM. *Lehninger principles of biochemistry*, 5th ed. New York: W. H. Freeman and Company; 2008.

Gluconeogenesis

Most body tissues (e.g., brain, erythrocytes, testis, kidney, medulla) require glucose as a carbon source (a total of 160 g/day). The brain alone requires 120 g of glucose per day (75% of the body's total available glucose on a daily basis), because it cannot use the body's major energy source, fatty acids, for its survival. The amount of glucose that can be released from the body's glycogen is approximately 190 g/day, compared to 20 g/day released from body fluids. The human body stores 210 g of glucose in total, of which 160 g is used each day. Thus fasting for one day will deplete the entire glucose reserve derived from glycogen.

Gluconeogenesis entails synthesis of glucose from noncarbohydrate sources such as oxaloacetate or pyruvate. It is one of the pathways by which mammals maintain normal blood glucose levels between meals—that is, by converting pyruvate to PEP. Gluconeogenesis occurs mainly in the liver and kidney and, like glycolysis, is basically identical in all organisms. This unique biochemical process uses carbon skeletons derived from certain amino acids (also called glucogenic amino acids). However, gluconeogenesis is an expensive pathway, because it requires energy such as ATP or GTP molecules. It requires four ATP molecules, two GTP molecules, and two NADH molecules to synthesize one glucose molecule. By comparison, oxidation of glucose in glycolysis produces a net of two ATP molecules and two NADH molecules. Given these outcomes, gluconeogenesis and glycolysis are reciprocally regulated to avoid futile cycling in cells. Many of the reversible enzymatic steps of glycolysis are employed in gluconeogenesis to synthesize glucose molecules (Figure 5.33). However, three irreversible steps in glycolysis are not used in gluconeogenesis:

1. Phosphorylation of glucose to glucose 6-phosphate by hexokinase

2. Phosphorylation of fructose 6-phosphate to fructose 1,6-bisphosphate by PFK-1

3. Conversion of phosphoenolpyruvate to pyruvate by pyruvate kinase

In gluconeogenesis, two molecules of pyruvate are used to synthesize one molecule of glucose. This pathway incorporates several unique enzymes that bypass the three irreversible steps in glycolysis. For instance, pyruvate cannot directly be converted to PEP; instead, it must be carboxylated first to form oxaloacetate. For this reason, pyruvate travels to mitochondria where it is catalyzed by an enzyme called pyruvate carboxylase that requires biotin (vitamin B_7):

$$Pyruvate + HCO_3^- + ATP \rightarrow oxaloacetate + ADP + Pi$$

Pentose Phosphate Pathway

The pentose phosphate pathway is an oxidative pathway that uses glucose to generate other essential molecules. Indeed, the pentose phosphate pathway is a significant pathway for glucose oxidation because approximately 30% of the glucose in the human liver is oxidized by the pentose phosphate pathway. Two important functions are carried out by the pentose phosphate pathway: (1) generation of reducing agents, in the form of NADPH, for reductive biosynthesis process (fatty acids, steroids) within cells and (2) provision of ribose 5-phosphate (R5P) to the cell for the synthesis of nucleotides and nucleic acids.

One of the major differences between glycolysis and the pentose phosphate pathway is that glycolysis generates NADH, whereas the pentose phosphate pathway generates NADPH. NADH is used in oxidative phosphorylation to provide ATP (as discussed later in this chapter) and NADPH is used to synthesize fatty acids and steroids. Because the pentose phosphate pathway generates NADPH, tissues that are highly active in the synthesis of fatty acids and steroids (such as adipose tissue, the mammary glands, the liver, and the adrenal cortex) actively employ the pentose phosphate pathway.

The first reaction in the pentose phosphate pathway is dehydrogenation of glucose-6-phosphate to 6-phosphoglucono-δ-lactone by the enzyme glucose-6-phosphate dehydrogenase. Because this enzyme is a dehydrogenase, it oxidizes glucose and reduces NADP⁺ to NADPH (**Figure 5.37**).

Interestingly, the *E. coli* bacterium can grow in a medium in which the only carbon source is glucose. The reason is that *E. coli* obtains ribose 5-phosphate for the synthesis of nucleic acids (DNA and RNA) by utilizing the pentose phosphate pathway. Similar to the case for glycolysis and gluconeogenesis, the cytoplasm is the site for the pentose phosphate pathway.

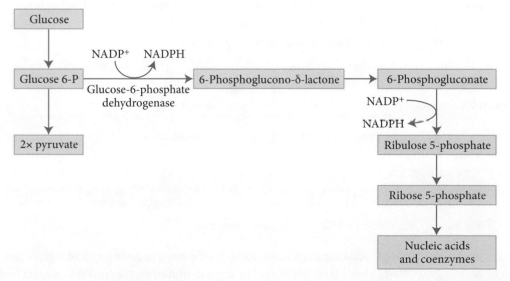

Figure 5.37 The pentose phosphate pathway generates NADPH and precursors for the synthesis of nucleic acids.

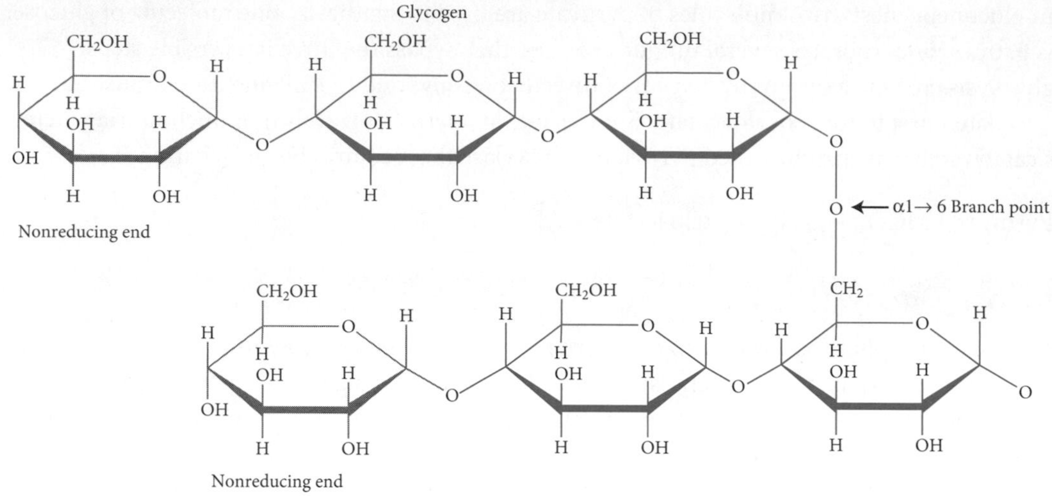

Figure 5.38 Glycogen consists of linear polymers of ($\alpha 1 \rightarrow 4$) linked D-glucose, with many branches formed by ($\alpha 1 \rightarrow 6$) glycosidic linkages to glucose.

Glucose 6-phosphate is used in both glycolysis (as a substrate in step 2) and in the pentose phosphate pathway (as a substrate in the first reaction). Which path the glucose 6-phosphate takes depends on the cellular need for NADPH in the cytoplasm. If NADPH is forming faster than it is being used for biosynthesis of fatty acids, steroids, or glutathione reduction, the first pathway in the pentose phosphate pathway is inhibited by the excess of NADPH; in turn, the glycolysis pathway will be the major fate for the glucose 6-phosphate. NADPH plays a critical role in protecting erythrocytes from hemolysis that occurs by reactive oxygen derivatives, H_2O_2, ·O2, and ·OH (see also the *Introduction to Microbiology* chapter). Consequently, patients with glucose 6-phosphate dehydrogenase deficiency should avoid any kind of stress that might trigger production of reactive oxygen derivatives.

Regulations of Glycogen Synthesis and Degradation

Humans obtain glucose either directly from ingested carbohydrates or from other resources such as pyruvate, amino acids, lactate, or glycerol via gluconeogenesis. Glucose obtained from these resources either remains soluble in the blood or is stored in a polymeric and a complex form, glycogen. Glycogen consists of linear polymers of ($\alpha 1 \rightarrow 4$) linked D-glucose, with many branches formed by ($\alpha 1 \rightarrow 6$) glycosidic linkages to glucose (**Figure 5.38**).

Glycogen Biosynthesis

Glycogen biosynthesis is a complex and sequential process that employs four enzymes:

1. Glucose + ATP $\rightarrow$ glucose-6-phosphate + ADP, by hexokinase (in muscle) or glucokinase (in liver)

2. Glucose 6-phosphate $\rightarrow$ glucose 1-phosphate, by phosphoglucomutase

3. Glucose 1-phosphate + UTP $\rightarrow$ UDP-glucose + PPi, by UDP-glucose pyrophosphorylase

4. UDP-glucose $\rightarrow$ glycogen + UDP, by glycogen synthase

Glycogen synthase catalyzes addition of glucose residues to the nonreducing end of a glycogen chain by forming ($\alpha 1 \rightarrow 4$) bonds (recall that for the degradation of glycogen you also start from the nonreducing end).

Glycogen Degradation

The glycogen phosphorylase enzyme catalyzes phosphorolytic cleavage of the terminal residue at the nonreducing ends, producing glucose 1-phosphate. In the mammalian liver, glucose 1-phosphate can either enter glycolysis or supply the blood with glucose. In glycolysis, however, glucose 1-phosphate must first undergo isomerization to glucose 6-phosphate by the enzyme phosphoglucomutase.

The glycogen phosphorylase that degrades glycogen into glucose monomers (glucose 1-phosphate) is present in two forms: glycogen phosphorylase *a* (the active form) and glycogen phosphorylase *b* (the inactive form). The glucagon hormone increases the rate of glycogen breakdown in the liver by converting glycogen phosphorylase *b* to glycogen phosphorylase *a* so as to initiate the release of glucose into the blood.

Glycogen synthase also exists in two forms: *a* (the active form) and *b* (the inactive form). Unlike glycogen phosphorylase, the glycogen synthase *a* form is not phosphorylated, whereas the *b* form is phosphorylated. The insulin hormone, by binding to insulin receptor, launches a series of enzymes that assist in blocking the phosphorylation pathway of glycogen synthase, thereby making glycogen synthase *a* available for the synthesis of glycogen.

Diseases Related to Glycogen

Under normal and healthy conditions, humans synthesize and degrade glycogen every day. A deficiency in glycogen degradation, however, can cause cells to become pathologically enlarged. It can also lead to a functional loss of glycogen as a source of cell energy. Most of the glycogen storage diseases are consequences of a specific enzyme deficiency. A few diseases (types 0–X) are related to glycogen, most of which are inherited in an autosomal recessive manner. A few of them are described here and listed in **Table 5.5**.

Type Ia (von Gierke's) Disease

Type Ia disease is caused by a deficiency in glucose 6-phosphatase, a unique enzyme found only in the liver and kidneys. This deficiency leads to the accumulation of glucose 6-phosphate, which is converted to glucose 1-phosphate by the enzyme phosphoglucomutase and results in the enlargement of glycogen. The deficiency in glucose 6-phosphatase inhibits both glycogen usage and gluconeogenesis. Metabolic symptoms range from hypoglycemia and lactic acidosis (both hypoglycemia and lactic acidosis can develop after a short fasting period) to increased levels of cholesterol, triacylglycerols, and uric acid. In addition, there is an increased risk of bleeding (during menstrual cycles) and pancreatitis.

Type Ib Disease

In type Ib disease, an enzyme, translocase, is deficient. The role of the translocase enzyme is to transport glucose 6-phosphate across the microsomal membrane. However, because patients with type Ia or Ib disease cannot effectively convert glucose 6-phosphate to glucose, they are susceptible to severe fasting hypoglycemia.

Type V (McArdle's) Disease

Type V is the most common adult glycogen storage disease, characterized by a deficiency in the muscle glycogen phosphorylase. This deficiency leads to muscle weakness, pain, and cramping during exercise, but does not cause any long-term health problem because fats are used for providing energy. Exercise causes myoglobinuria secondary to rhabdomyolysis in 50% of patients

Table 5.5 Glycogen Storage Diseases

Name	Type	Enzyme Deficiency	Affected Tissues	Clinical Presentations
	0	Glycogen synthase	Liver, muscle	Hypoglycemia and hyperketonemia
Von Gierke's disease	Ia	Glucose 6-phosphatase	Liver, kidney	Severely enlarged liver, severe hypoglycemia, lactic acidosis, ketosis, hyperuricemia, hyperlipidemia
	Ib	Endoplasmic reticulum glucose 6-phosphate transporter	Liver, kidney	Same as type Ia; impaired neutrophil function causing frequent infections
Pompe's disease	II	1,4 D-Glucosidase (lysosomal)	Liver, muscle	Cardiac failure in infancy
Cori's disease	III	Amylo 1,6-glucosidase ("debranching" enzyme)	Liver, muscle	Similar to type I but milder
Andersen's disease	IV	"Branching" enzyme	Liver	Liver cirrhosis, death usually before age 24 months
McArdle's disease	V	Phosphorylase	Muscle	Muscle cramps, easily fatigued
Hers's disease	VI	Phosphorylase	Liver	Similar to type I but milder
Tarui's disease	VII	Phosphofructokinase	Muscle	Muscle cramps, easily fatigued
	VIII	Phosphorylase kinase	Liver	Enlarged liver, hypoglycemia
	IX	Glycogen synthase	Liver	
	X	cAMP-dependent protein kinase A	Liver	Hepatomegaly, accumulation of glycogen in liver

Modified from: Woodbury CP. *Biochemistry for the pharmaceutical sciences.* Burlington, MA: Jones & Bartlett Learning; 2012: Chapter 9.

with type V disease, which explains why the urine of the affected individuals has a characteristic burgundy color. Supplements such as creatine and vitamin B_6 have been shown to benefit some patients by improving their muscle functions.

Type VI (Hers's) Disease

In type VI disease, there is a deficiency in the liver glycogen phosphorylase. Metabolic symptoms range from hepatomegaly and mild hypoglycemia to hyperlipidemia and ketosis. These symptoms may improve with age (by puberty and later).

Fatty Acid Metabolism

Oxidation of Fatty Acids

Fatty acids are energy-rich storage molecules that contain much more energy when compared with carbohydrates of similar molecular weight. Fatty acids are stored as triacylglycerols in adipose tissue. The brain cannot use fats for energy; instead, this tissue has a specific demand for glucose. However, under conditions of starvation—that is, when blood glucose levels are low (starvation) or cellular access to glucose is limited (untreated diabetes)—the brain is able to use ketone bodies that mostly are synthesized from fatty acid oxidation.

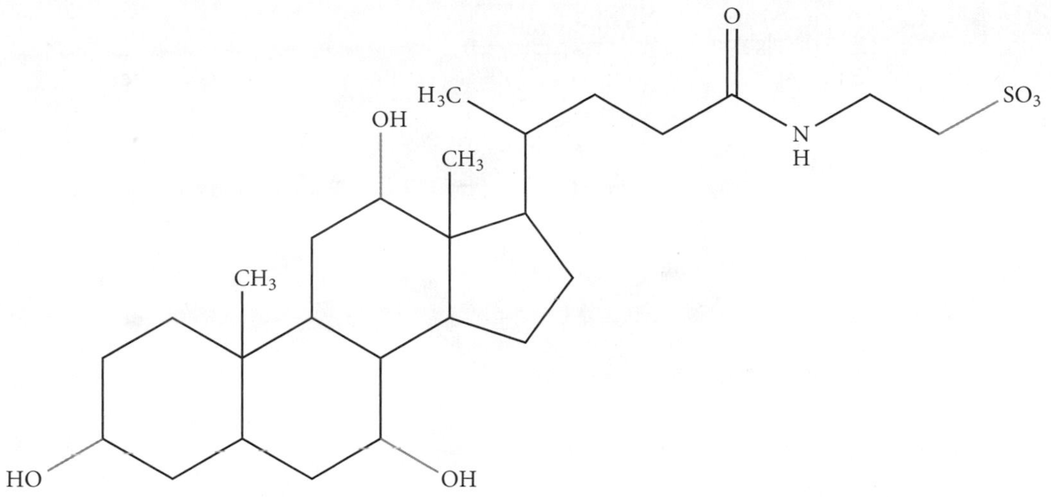

Taurocholic acid

Figure 5.39 Structure of taurocholic acid, an amphipathic molecule. The colored functional groups indicate the hydrophilic moieties of taurocholic acid.

Taurocholic acid is a bile acid that is an amphipathic compound, meaning it contains both hydrophobic and hydrophilic components (**Figure 5.39**). Bile acids are synthesized from cholesterol in the liver and are stored in the gallbladder. The hydrophobic components of a bile acid associate with the lipid, and the hydrophilic components associate with water molecules, serving to solubilize (emulsify) the insoluble lipid.

Lipids are widely distributed and are present in all cells. There are two major groups of lipids: simple and complex lipids. Simple lipids include (1) triacylglycerols, fatty acids attached to a glycerol backbone (an example is butter); (2) waxes, long-chain fatty acid esters of alcohol (an example is beeswax); and (3) steroids (an example is cholesterol). Complex lipids include (1) phospholipids, membrane lipids having long-chain fatty acids attached to a glycerol backbone as well as a phosphate group (an example is lecithin); (2) glycolipids, membrane lipids having long-chain fatty acids attached to a glycerol backbone as well as attached oligosaccharides (an example is galactolipids); and (3) sphingolipids, membrane lipids having a long-chain fatty acid attached to sphingosine, but no glycerol backbone (an example is ceramides). While adipose tissue is rich in triacylglycerols and serves as a site for lipid storage, the complex lipids are embedded in the cell membranes.

Lipids are large molecules that must first be degraded into smaller molecules before they can pass through the intestinal wall. Bile acids are amphipathic molecules (Figure 5.39) that are released from the gallbladder into the small intestine upon ingestion of a meal that is rich in lipids. The bile acids' function is to convert fats into mixed micelles that are prone to hydrolysis by a pancreatic lipase. Pancreatic lipase hydrolyzes triacylglycerols into glycerol (by removing all three fatty acids), monoacylglycerols (by removing two fatty acids), and diacylglycerols (by removing one fatty acid). Upon entering a cell, the hydrolysis products of this digestion can be combined back into triacylglycerols in the ER and Golgi complexes of the intestinal mucosa cells.

Apolipoprotein is a lipid-binding protein that participates in the transportation of triacylglycerols, phospholipids, cholesterol, and cholesteryl esters between different organs. In addition, it may function as a ligand to a few receptors involved in the lipid uptake from the GI tract. When an apolipoprotein is attached to a lipid, it produces a plasma lipoprotein (**Figure 5.40**). At least 10 human apolipoproteins are found in the plasma lipoproteins. Based on the density of a lipoprotein, one can characterize lipoproteins as chylomicrons, very-low-density lipoproteins (VLDL),

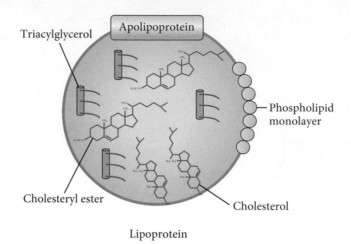

Lipoprotein

Figure 5.40 Structure of a lipoprotein.

Adapted from: Nelson DL, Cox MM. *Lehninger principles of biochemistry*, 5th ed. New York: W. H. Freeman and Company; 2008: Chapter 21.

Table 5.6 Characteristics and Functions of Plasma Lipoproteins

Lipoprotein	Size (nm)	Density Range (g/mL)	Cholesterol Ester (Weight %)	Major Function
Chylomicron	100–1,000	<0.94	3	Dietary triacylglycerol transport
Very low density (VLDL)	30–80	0.94–1.006	14	Endogenous triacylglycerol transport
Intermediate density (IDL)	25–30	1.006–1.019	30	Endogenous cholesterol transport, triacylglycerol transport, LDL precursor
Low density (LDL)	20–25	1.019–1.063	38	Endogenous cholesterol transport
High density (HDL)	5–12	1.063–1.21	15–20	Removal of cholesterol from tissue outside the liver

Reproduced from: Woodbury CP. *Biochemistry for the pharmaceutical sciences.* Burlington, MA: Jones & Bartlett Learning; 2012: Chapter 13.

intermediate-density lipoproteins (IDL), low-density lipoproteins (LDL), and high-density lipoproteins (HDL). Cholesterol and triacylglycerols are the major plasma lipids. **Table 5.6** summarizes the characteristics and functions of plasma lipoproteins.

Ingested lipids from our diet are combined with apolipoproteins (such as Apo A-I and Apo A-II; see **Table 5.7**) to form chylomicrons that transport lipids through the blood and lymphatic system to the tissues. In the capillaries, a specific apolipoprotein, Apo C-II, activates lipoprotein lipase. Lipoprotein lipase hydrolyzes triacylglycerols into fatty acids and glycerol so as to supply fatty acids to various tissues. In the muscle cells, these fatty acids are oxidized for energy (via the β-oxidation pathway); in adipose tissue, they are re-esterified to triacylglycerols for storage. The remnants of chylomicrons travel through the blood to the liver, where they are taken up by endocytosis and the remaining triacylglycerols are oxidized to provide energy. A deficiency of Apo C-II in human causes elevated triacylglycerol levels in the blood, whereas production of Apo E4 has been linked to the development of Alzheimer's disease.

Table 5.7 Lipoproteins and Their Major Apolipoproteins

Lipoprotein Class	Major Apolipoproteins	Major Lipid Components
Chylomicrons	Apo A-I, Apo A-II, Apo A-IV, Apo B-48, Apo C-I, Apo C-II, Apo C-III, Apo E	Triacylglycerols and phospholipids
VLDL	Apo B-100, Apo C-I, Apo C-II, Apo C-III, Apo E	Triacylglycerols, phospholipids, cholesterol, and cholesterol esters
IDL	Apo B-100, Apo C-I, Apo C-II, Apo C-III, Apo E	Composition intermediate between VLDL and LDL; triacylglycerols notably depleted
LDL	Apo B-100	Cholesterol esters, phospholipids, triacylglycerols, cholesterol
HDL	Apo A-I, Apo A-II, Apo A-IV, Apo C-I, Apo C-II, Apo C-III, Apo D, Apo E	Phospholipids and cholesterol esters

Reproduced from: Woodbury CP. *Biochemistry for the pharmaceutical sciences.* Burlington, MA: Jones & Bartlett Learning; 2012: Chapter 13.

In addition to receiving fatty acids from the diet, humans' adipose tissue, which approximately makes up 15% of a young adult, supplies fatty acids to other tissues. When glucose levels are low during long periods between meals, two hormones—glucagon and epinephrine—stimulate the adenylate cyclase enzyme to produce cyclic AMP (cAMP; see also the *Introduction to Pharmacodynamics* chapter). The cAMP molecule activates protein kinase A (PKA) to phosphorylate a protein called preilipin. Preilipin, in turn, activates adipose lipase to hydrolyze triacylglycerols stored in the adipose tissue into fatty acids and glycerol. The released and free fatty acids enter the bloodstream. Due to free fatty acids' chemical structures (which leads to water insolubility), these compounds are rarely found in the bloodstream as independent entities. Instead, they are bound and carried by the water-soluble protein albumin, an abundant plasma protein. Each albumin molecule can noncovalently bind as many as 10 fatty acids. The serum albumin transports fatty acids to other tissues where the fatty acids enter the β-oxidation pathway to provide energy in the form of ATP molecules.

β Oxidation of Fatty Acids

Before fatty acids undergo oxidation, they have to be activated. The activation is a two-step mechanism that is catalyzed by an enzyme, acyl-CoA synthetase. A fatty acid reacts first with an ATP molecule, which results in the release of inorganic phosphate (PPi). In a subsequent step, the fatty acid is transferred to a large molecule, coenzyme A.

Fatty acid + CoA +ATP → Fatty acyl-CoA + AMP + PPi

The hydrolysis of ATP by inorganic pyrophosphatase makes the overall $\Delta G^{\circ\prime}$ more negative (spontaneous). Keep in mind that the fatty acid activation occurs in the outer mitochondrial membrane, whereas the β-oxidation pathway occurs in the mitochondrial matrix. A shuttle system transports fatty acids into the mitochondria; this shuttle system requires carnitine. The enzyme carnitine acyltransferase I catalyzes the formation of fatty acyl-carnitine, which readily crosses the mitochondrial inner membrane. In contrast, the fatty acyl-CoA alone cannot pass through the inner membrane (**Figure 5.41**).

The enzyme carnitine acyltransferase II, which is located on the inner face of the inner membrane, regenerates fatty acyl-CoA and carnitine (Figure 5.41). Abnormal fatty acid metabolism is associated with clinical disorders caused by lack of carnitine or carnitine acyltransferase I or II

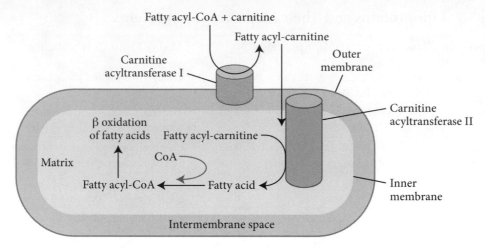

Figure 5.41 Carnitine plays an important role in transporting fatty acid into the matrix of the mitochondrion.

enzymes; such a deficiency results in muscle pain during exercise. L-Carnitine (Carnitor) can be used to treat carnitine deficiencies.

The energy that is stored in fatty acids is released through the β-oxidation pathway in the mitochondria. This pathway includes four reactions that occur in repeating cycles until the entire fatty acid is oxidized into many acetyl-CoA molecules. In other words, in each cycle, a fatty acid is successively oxidized and shortened by two carbons and its released energy is captured by the reduced energy carriers NADH and FADH$_2$. Both of these electron carrier coenzymes move into the next pathway—oxidative phosphorylation—to produce ATP molecules.

Each cycle of the β-oxidation pathway involves four reactions: dehydrogenation, hydration, dehydrogenation, and thiolytic cleavage. During each cycle, a coenzyme A is used. As a result, one acetyl-CoA molecule is produced at the end of each cycle of these four reactions. The rest of the fatty acids go through another round of β oxidation until they are entirely converted to many acetyl-CoA molecules. The number of acetyl-CoA molecules produced from β oxidation of a fatty acid depends on the number of carbon atoms in that particular fatty acid (see the following reaction).

The overall products of the β oxidation of palmitoyl-CoA, a saturated fatty acid with 16 carbons, is shown in the following reaction scheme:

Palmitoyl-CoA + 7CoA-SH + 7FAD + 7NAD$^+$ + 7H$_2$O → 8 acetyl-CoA + 7FADH$_2$ + 7NADH + 7H$^+$

Simply put, if you start with a 16-carbon fatty acid, you can produce 8 acetyl-CoA molecules. The oxidation of fatty acids is tightly regulated. Fatty acyl-CoA formation as well as the carnitine acyltransferases are involved in the regulation of the β oxidation.

In the liver, fatty acids have two major roles: (1) β oxidation in the mitochondria and (2) conversion of fatty acids into triacylglycerol in the cytosol. Keep in mind that β oxidation of fatty acids can occur in peroxisomes as well. In peroxisomes, electrons are passed to the coenzyme FAD to produce FADH$_2$. To regenerate FAD, the electrons from FADH$_2$ are donated to oxygen, which then forms the toxic molecule hydrogen peroxide (H$_2$O$_2$). Although H$_2$O$_2$ is a potent and damaging oxidant, the catalase enzyme breaks down H$_2$O$_2$ into water and oxygen. Because there is

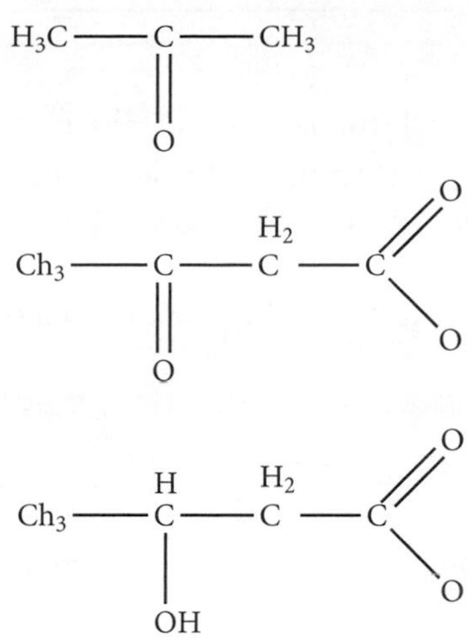

Figure 5.42 Structures of ketone bodies.

no respiratory chain in the peroxisome, no ATP molecules are generated there. (The β oxidation of all yeasts' fatty acids occurs only in peroxisomes.)

When acetyl-CoA molecules are in excess (i.e., when they are beyond their capacity to be oxidized or used for fatty acid synthesis), they are converted into ketone bodies, including acetone, acetoacetate, and hydroxybutyrate. **Figure 5.42** shows the structures of these three ketone bodies.

Ketone bodies are overproduced during prolonged fasting, particularly when glycogen is depleted and fatty acids from stored triacylglycerols become the principal fuel for daily energy. In addition, untreated diabetes mellitus leads to overproduction of ketone bodies. Because the brain prefers to use glucose as its energy source, oxaloacetate from the citric acid cycle is used in the gluconeogenesis pathway to produce glucose. The use of oxaloacetate slows down the citric acid cycle. As a consequence, the acetyl-CoA that is produced by β oxidation cannot be oxidized via the citric acid cycle; in turn, it begins to accumulate. Eventually, the accumulation of acetyl-CoA promotes the formation of ketone bodies.

Diabetic ketoacidosis (DKA) is an uncontrolled form of ketosis (elevated ketone bodies levels in the blood) and, if not treated, is fatal. In DKA, the blood glucose concentration is greater than 300 mg/dL, the blood pH is less than 7.2 (ketone bodies are acidic molecules), and the concentration of ketone bodies is greater than 90 mg/dL (the normal serum concentration of ketone bodies is less than 3 mg/dL).

Other minor pathways can also oxidize fatty acids. For instance, the α oxidation that occurs in peroxisomes is effective in shortening fatty acids that cannot be oxidized by the mitochondrial β oxidation. A typical example is oxidation of phytanic acid. Refsum's disease is caused by nonfunctional α oxidation in peroxisomes, and is characterized by an accumulation of phytanic acid in both the central and peripheral nervous systems. Patients with Refsum's disease develop distal and proximal sensory loss in a progressive fashion; these losses lead to weaknesses in the legs and arm muscles, respectively. To counteract these effects, patients must restrict their consumption of phytanic precursors such as fish oils and ruminant fats.

Another minor oxidation pathway is omega oxidation (ω oxidation), which oxidizes medium- and long-chain fatty acids in the ER. As the name indicates, oxidation begins from the other end (the end opposite to the carboxyl group) of a fatty acid—that is, the ω carbon.

The Citric Acid Cycle

The citric acid cycle plays a central role in humans' daily metabolism because the end product of glycolysis, fatty acid oxidation, and amino acid oxidation can produce acetyl-CoA, which serves as the first substrate for the citric acid cycle (**Figure 5.43**). A number of coenzymes are produced in the cycle's reactions (**Figure 5.44**). These coenzymes deliver electrons to the oxidative phosphorylation process, resulting in a significant payoff of energy (i.e., production of many ATP molecules; **Figure 5.45**).

To have a functional citric acid cycle, the metabolism of carbohydrates, fats, and proteins must lead to the synthesis of acetyl-CoA. Acetyl-CoA is synthesized directly either from the β oxidation

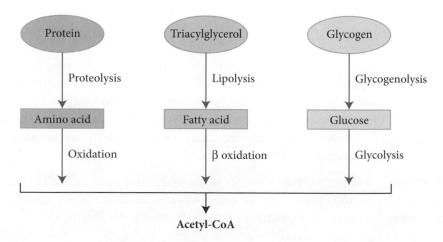

Figure 5.43 Acetyl-CoA is produced from oxidation of fatty acids, amino acids, and glucose.

of fatty acids or from a pyruvate molecule. In the latter case, pyruvate molecules move out of the cytosol in which glycolysis took place and enter the matrix of the mitochondria. In the mitochondria, the pyruvate molecule undergoes a reaction in which it is converted to an acetyl-CoA molecule. Acetyl-CoA, as a two-carbon molecule, enters the citric acid cycle and leaves the cycle as CO_2.

Production of Acetyl-CoA

Acetyl-CoA consists of an acetyl group (CH_3—C=O) attached to a coenzyme A molecule. Coenzyme A is a large complex molecule that contains ADP, pantothenic acid (vitamin B_5), and a reactive thiol group (SH). The

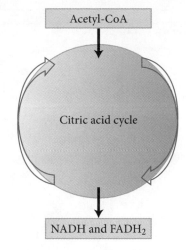

Figure 5.44 Electron carrier coenzymes, NADH and FADH$_2$, are produced in the citric acid cycle.

acetyl group is covalently bound to the thiol group. Pyruvate dehydrogenase complex is a multienzyme complex (it includes three enzymes) that removes a carboxyl group from pyruvate to form acetyl-CoA, as part of a mechanism that occurs in the mitochondrial matrix. In addition to NAD$^+$ and FAD, which serve as electron carriers, two different SH-containing molecules—coenzyme A and lipoic acid—and a cofactor, thiamine pyrophosphate (TPP), are involved. Thiamine (vitamin B$_1$) is essential for the synthesis of TPP. Three enzymes and the coenzymes are clustered together to ensure that the synthesis of an acetyl-CoA molecule occurs quickly.

The human disease beriberi is caused by a deficiency of thiamine in the diet (see also the *Introduction to Nutrients* chapter). Without TPP, the pyruvate dehydrogenase complex cannot

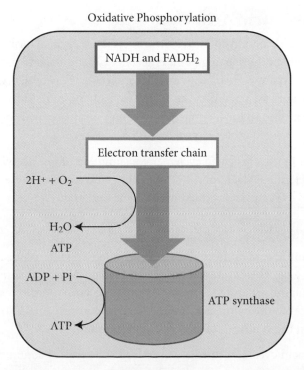

Figure 5.45 The electron transport chain in the oxidative phosphorylation reduces oxygen to water and captures energy from the electron carrier coenzymes to synthesize ATP molecules.

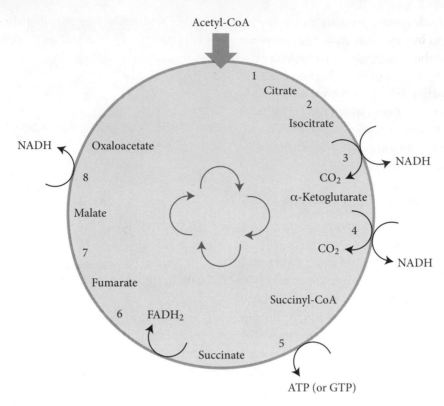

Figure 5.46 Reactions of the citric acid cycle.

convert pyruvate into acetyl-CoA, which leads to accumulation of the pyruvate molecules and inadequate synthesis of ATP molecules.

Reactions of the Citric Acid Cycle

As the name indicates, the reactions of the citric acid cycle are cyclic. During this cycle, a series of reactions occurs in which the starting point is acetyl-CoA and the end product is oxaloacetate. This oxaloacetate is then ready to react with another molecule of acetyl-CoA. During each round of the cycle, one acetyl-CoA enters the cycle, two CO_2 molecules leave the cycle, and one oxaloacetate molecule is used to form citrate. Interestingly, oxaloacetate is used as substrate but is not consumed in the citric acid cycle (**Figure 5.46**).

The overall production in the citric acid cycle per consumption of one acetyl-CoA molecule comprises three NADH, one $FADH_2$, one ATP (or GTP), and two CO_2 molecules. Similar to the case with glycolysis, no oxygen is consumed in the citric acid cycle.

Important Facts About the Citric Acid Cycle

In the first step of the citric acid cycle, acetyl-CoA is condensed with oxaloacetate to form citrate by citrate synthase enzyme. The citrate synthase is up-regulated by ADP and is inhibited by citrate, NADH, and ATP. When more citrate is produced than is necessary, the excess citrate is transported from the mitochondrion to the cytoplasm, where it can be converted back to acetyl-CoA and subsequently participate in the synthesis of fatty acid and steroids.

Isocitrate is a citric acid cycle intermediate produced as a result of action of the enzyme aconitase on citrate. Fluorocitrate, a potent inhibitor of the enzyme aconitase, is a deadly poison. By inhibiting aconitase, fluorocitrate prevents the citric acid cycle from operating.

CO_2 is produced in two reactions in the citric acid cycle: in step 3 by isocitrate dehydrogenase and in step 4 by α-ketoglutarate dehydrogenase reactions. The two CO_2 molecules produced in the first turn of the citric acid cycle originate from the two carboxyl groups found in the oxaloacetate.

The concentration of the citric acid cycle intermediates remains constant because the intermediates that leave the cycle to join other pathways are balanced by the intermediates that join the cycle, a process called anaplerotic reaction.

The citric acid cycle is regulated by four factors: conversion of pyruvate to acetyl-CoA by pyruvate dehydrogenase complex; entry of acetyl-CoA into the cycle by citrate synthase (step 1); formation of α-ketoglutarate by isocitrate dehydrogenase (step 3); and formation of succinyl-CoA by α-ketoglutarate dehydrogenase (step 4).

Lipid Biosynthesis

Most of the fatty acids are synthesized from dietary glucose because humans are able to use glucose in glycolysis to synthesize pyruvate, which in turn can be converted to acetyl-CoA. Acetyl-CoA is the initial molecule used in fatty acid synthesis. In contrast to the fatty acid β oxidation that occurs in the mitochondria, the synthesis of fatty acids occurs in cytoplasm. The liver is the major site for fatty acid synthesis in the human body.

The major source of acetyl-CoA is the mitochondria, where the oxidation of pyruvate (recall the pyruvate dehydrogenase complex) produces acetyl-CoA. However, this acetyl-CoA source is not directly available for fatty acid biosynthesis because the mitochondrial inner membrane is impermeable to acetyl-CoA. Cells, however, have developed a shuttle system to transfer acetyl-CoA from mitochondria to the cytoplasm where the biosynthesis of fatty acids occurs. When acetyl-CoA interacts with oxaloacetate (recall the first step in the citric acid cycle), citrate is produced. This citrate is able to pass through the mitochondrial inner membrane to reach the cytoplasm because of the mitochondrial citrate transporter. Upon reaching the cytoplasm, citrate is cleaved by an enzyme called citrate lyase to produce acetyl-CoA and oxaloacetate. This unique shuttle system allows acetyl-CoA to be available in the cytoplasm so that it can participate in the biosynthesis of fatty acids. Similar to glycolysis and gluconeogenesis and the glycogen synthesis and degradation mechanisms, the biosynthesis and degradation of lipids are carried out by two different pathways.

The key contributor to fatty acid synthesis is acetyl-CoA that is carboxylated to malonyl-CoA catalyzed by the enzyme acetyl-CoA carboxylase. One ATP molecule is used in this reaction. Acetyl-CoA carboxylase has three functional regions: biotin carboxylase, a biotin carrier protein, and transcarboxylase. As is true in the majority of carboxylation reactions, this enzyme's prosthetic group is biotin (vitamin B_7). Carboxylation of acetyl-CoA to malonyl-CoA is both irreversible and a committed step; in other words, once it occurs, the biosynthesis of fatty acids is committed to occur. This carboxylation step is also the rate-limiting step in fatty acid synthesis.

All of the reactions in the synthesis of fatty acids are catalyzed by a multiple-enzyme complex called fatty acid synthase (FAS). This complex is built by seven proteins. Except for one, all of these proteins have catalytic activity and serve as enzymes that work closely together to catalyze the formation of fatty acids.

The biosynthesis of fatty acids such as palmitate requires acetyl-CoA and the input of energy in two forms: ATP (7 molecules), which is required to attach CO_2 to acetyl-CoA to make malonyl-CoA, and NADPH (14 molecules), which serves as the reducing power. The NADPH/NAD ratio is very high in the hepatocytes, which explains why these cells work as a site for reductive reactions such as the biosynthesis of fatty acids and steroids.

Fatty acid biosynthesis is regulated by hormonal mechanisms. Epinephrine, glucagon, and insulin are all involved in this regulation process. The first enzyme in the fatty acid synthesis, acetyl-CoA carboxylase, plays a key role in the regulation process. For instance, phosphorylation of acetyl-CoA carboxylase by kinases inactivates acetyl-CoA carboxylase, in a process triggered by epinephrine and glucagon. This hormonal regulatory mechanism is explained well by the fact that epinephrine and glucagon play important roles in the degradation of glycogen to increase blood glucose levels. Thus, when these two hormones are released, it indicates that the body requires energy in the form of ATP as opposed to needing to store energy in the form of lipids.

In contrast to epinephrine and glucagon, insulin stimulates the biosynthesis of fatty acids. For instance, insulin increases the entry of glucose into cells (particularly myocytes and adipocytes), which in turn leads to the production of NADPH via the pentose phosphate pathway. In addition, insulin activates the pyruvate dehydrogenase complex, which promotes synthesis of acetyl-CoA. Furthermore, it stimulates dephosphorylation of acetyl-CoA carboxylase to stimulate the biosynthesis of fatty acids. The overall message associated with insulin release is that the body needs to store energy in the form of glycogen or lipids.

As mentioned, a reciprocally regulated mechanism is necessary to avoid futile cycling between fatty acid oxidation and biosynthesis. The concentration of malonyl-CoA inhibits the oxidation of fatty acids by inhibiting the activity of carnitine acyltransferase I (see Figure 5.41). This inhibition process blocks the entry of acetyl-CoA into the mitochondrial matrix. As a result, when the synthesis of fatty acid is under way, no acetyl groups are transported to the mitochondria to undergo β oxidation.

Essential Fatty Acids

Because humans lack the necessary enzymes to make double bonds in fatty acids with more than 9 carbon atoms, they must consume essential fatty acids such as linoleic acid (double bonds at carbons 9 and 12) and linolenic acid (double bonds at carbons 9, 12, and 15) as part of their diets (**Figure 5.47**). Both linoleic acid and linolenic acid are found in large amounts in fish and plants and are precursors to arachidonyl-CoA. Most of the arachidonyl-CoA is used for phospholipid synthesis, including arachidonic acid. Arachidonic acid is characterized by a 20-carbon fatty acid and is released from the cell membrane upon activation of phospholipase A_2 (**Figure 5.48**).

Arachidonic acid is a precursor for a class of hormone-like molecules known as eicosanoids (prostaglandins, thromboxanes, and leukotrienes). Eicosanoids are a family of very potent biological signaling molecules that even at very diluted concentrations produce profound cellular effects. All mammalian cells, except erythrocytes, can synthesize eicosanoids. Eicosanoids differ from other signaling molecules such as epinephrine or glucagon in that they do not travel long distances between their points of release and their points of action.

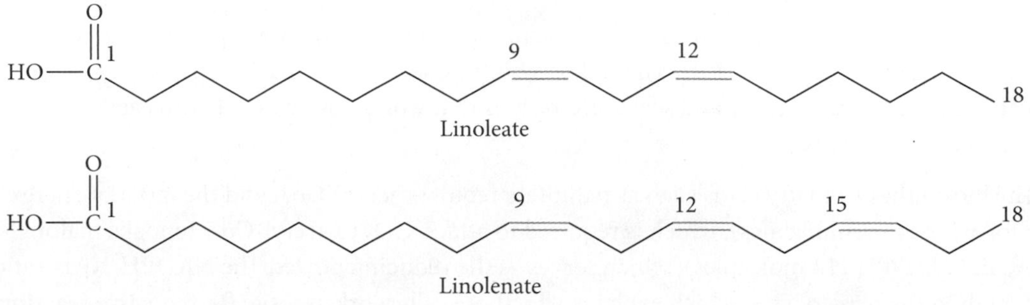

Figure 5.47 Structures of two essential fatty acids: linoleic acid (linoleate) and linolenic acid (linolenate).

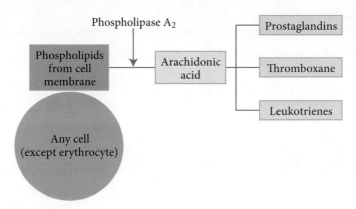

Figure 5.48 Phospholipase A$_2$ catalyzes the release of arachidonic acid from the cell membrane. Prednisone and prednisolone are steroid drugs that inhibit this catalytic activity, which results in the inhibition of eicosanoids (prostaglandins, thromboxanes, and leukotrienes).

Several different prostaglandins have been identified. Prostaglandin H synthase (PGHS) is a heme-containing enzyme bound to smooth endoplasmic reticulum membranes that catalyzes the "cyclic" pathway that leads to the production of prostaglandins and thromboxanes. This enzyme has two catalytic activities: as oxygenase and as peroxidase. The enzyme that has both catalytic activities is called cyclooxygenase (COX). Nonsteroidal anti-inflammatory drugs (NSAIDs) such as acetyl salicylic acid (adult aspirin), ibuprofen (Advil), and naproxen (Aleve) inhibit cyclooxygenase enzyme activity.

Acetyl salicylic acid acetylates the serine group of cyclooxygenases, thereby inhibiting the synthesis of both prostaglandins and thromboxanes. In mammals, there are two isozymes of prostaglandin H synthase: COX-1 (or PGHS-1) and COX-2 (or PGHS-2).

COX-1 is expressed at low levels in gastric mucosa, kidney, platelets, and vascular endothelial cells. This isozyme is known to be essential for the synthesis of prostaglandins that regulate the secretion of gastric mucin so as to protect gastric mucosa from the low pH and proteolytic enzymes in the stomach. As a result, drugs that inhibit COX-1 (such as NSAIDs) can leave the stomach vulnerable to the effects of gastric acid, which in turn can result in stomach pain and gastrointestinal ulceration (see also the *Introduction to Pharmacology and Pathophysiology* chapter).

COX-2 expression is stimulated by growth factors and cytokines. This isozyme has a similar structure to COX-1. COX-2 levels increase in inflammatory diseases such as arthritis. It has been suggested that ibuprofen acts more specifically on COX-2, although ibuprofen is a less effective inhibitor compared with acetyl salicylic acid. Flurbiprofen (Ansaid, from Canada) appears to inhibit COX-2 more selectively than COX-1, which makes this drug a good choice over other NSAIDs when irritation of the stomach is a factor in selecting a medication. Flurbiprofen also has a carboxyl group, which indicates that the acidic part of acetyl salicylic acid is not responsible for the stomach pain. Celecoxib (Celebrex) acts 10–20 times more selectively on COX-2 than on COX-1. This drug is used to inhibit inflammation and does not have a significant effect on the production of gastric mucin in stomach. However, because it contains sulfonamide, it may cause rashes in some patients. Celecoxib may also increase patients' risk of cardiovascular events, including myocardial infarction and stroke. The structures of celecoxib, acetyl salicylic acid, ibuprofen, and flurbiprofen are shown in **Figure 5.49**.

Thromboxane synthase converts prostaglandin H$_2$ (PGH$_2$) to thromboxane, which in turn induces the blood clotting process. A daily low dose (81 mg) of acetyl salicylic acid may reduce individuals' risk of myocardial infarction and stroke by reducing the synthesis of thromboxane.

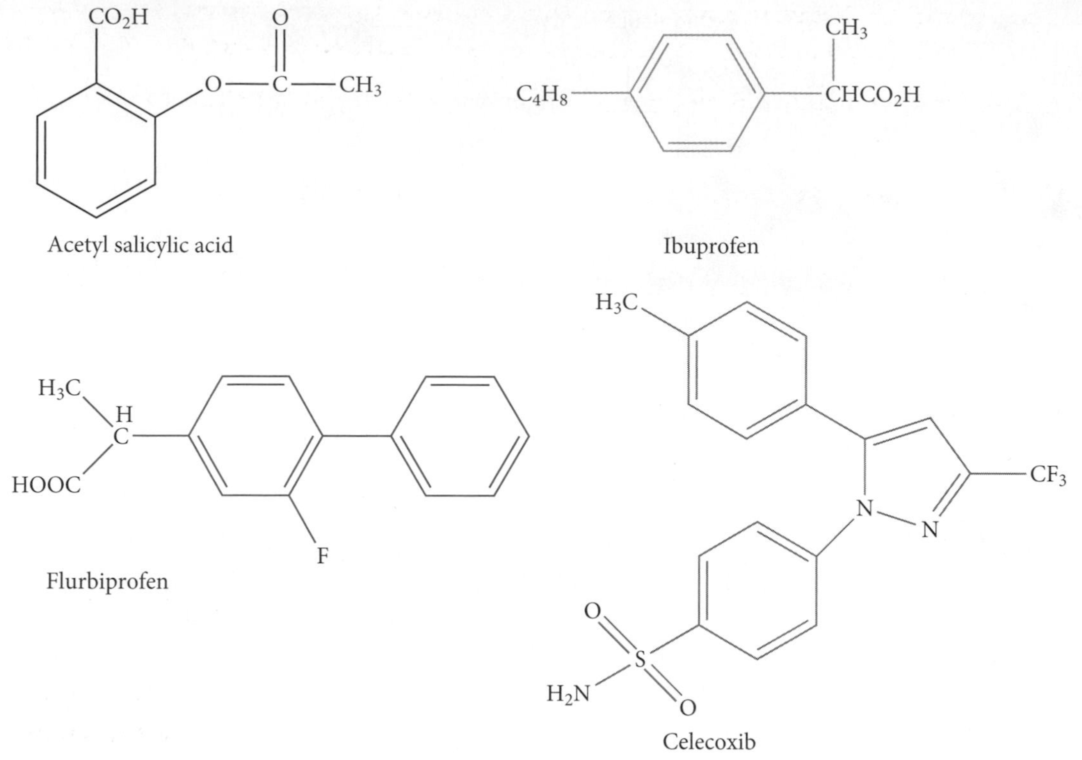

Figure 5.49 Structures of a few NSAIDs used to inhibit COX-1 and COX-2 isozymes.

Leukotrienes are potent inflammatory mediators that are synthesized when lipoxygenases act on arachidonic acids. This pathway is recognized as a "linear pathway" because leukotrienes are linear molecules compared to prostaglandins or thromboxanes, which are cyclic pathways. Leukotriene D_4 is known to induce contraction of the muscles lining the airways to the lung; as a result, it is a good target for agents used in the treatment of respiratory problems (see also the *Introduction to Pharmacology and Pathophysiology* chapter).

Steroid agents such as prednisolone (Orapred) and prednisone (Prednisone Intensol), both of which have potent anti-inflammatory activities, can inhibit phospholipase A_2, thereby decreasing the production of leukotrienes and reducing the synthesis of prostaglandins and thromboxanes. This inhibition explains why steroids have far more adverse effects compared with NSAIDs.

Synthesis of Triacylglycerol

There are two possible fates for newly synthesized fatty acids: being stored as metabolic energy and being incorporated into membrane lipids. When cells are not growing and have extra fatty acids, the former fate predominates. In contrast, during rapid cell growth, the latter is the predominant form.

Both fatty acyl-CoA and glycerol 3-phosphate are precursors to triacylglycerols. Glycerol 3-phosphate can be produced either by reduction of dihydroxyacetone phosphate (DHAP; recall step 4 in glycolysis—Figure 5.33), which is catalyzed by glycerol 3-phosphate dehydrogenase, or by the ATP-dependent phosphorylation of glycerol, which is catalyzed by the glycerol kinase enzyme. The two hydroxyl groups of glycerol 3-phosphate are joined by two fatty acyl-CoA molecules to form diacylglycerol 3-phosphate, which is also called phosphatidic acid (**Figure 5.50**). Phosphatidic acid is a precursor to both phospholipids and triacylglycerols. Synthesis of each fatty acyl-CoA molecule requires one ATP molecule. The enzyme phosphatidic acid phosphatase catalyzes the removal of the phosphate group of phosphatidic acid to produce 1,2-diacylglycerol, which in turn is converted to triacylglycerol by the acyl transferase enzyme.

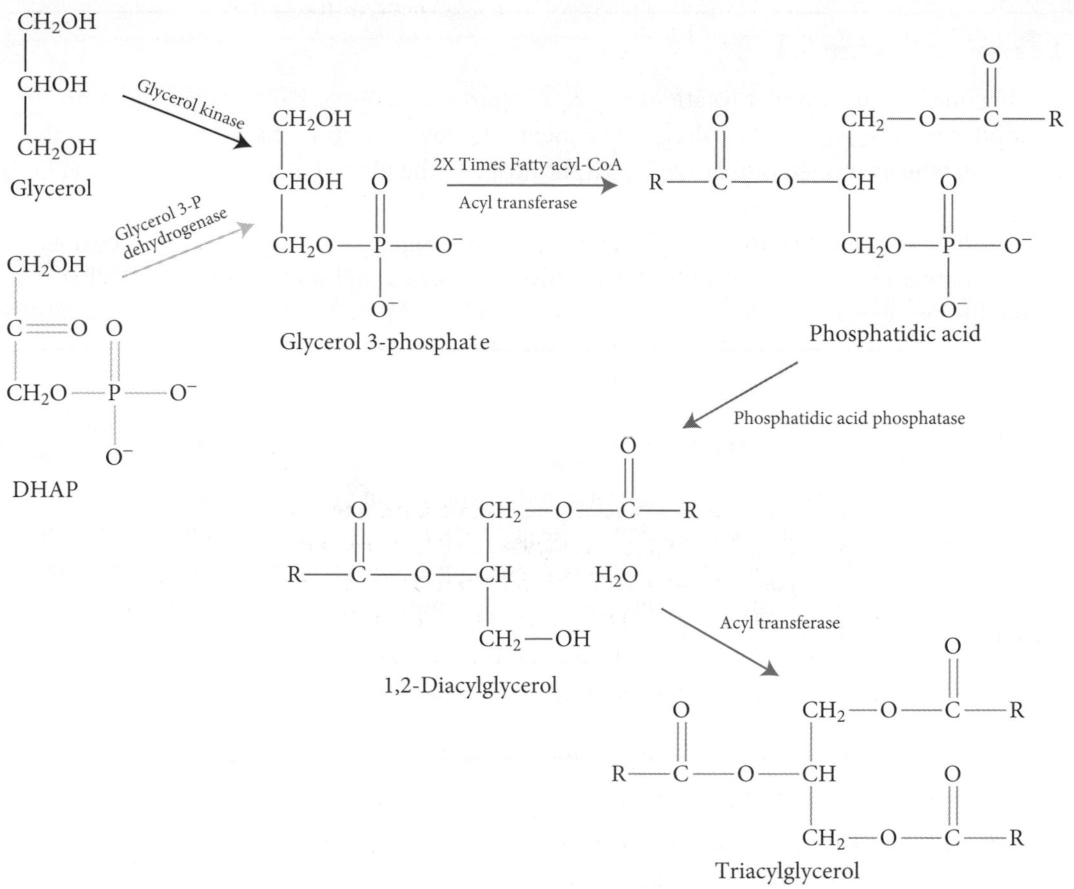

Figure 5.50 Synthesis of phosphatidic acid, a precursor to triacylglycerol, occurs by two different pathways and is catalyzed by two different enzymes, glycerol-3-phosphate dehydrogenase and glycerol kinase.

The rate of triacylglycerol biosynthesis is affected by insulin. Insulin promotes the conversion of carbohydrates into triacylglycerols. As a result, a lack of insulin hormone reduces the biosynthesis of triacylglycerol, which may explain the weight loss that occurs in patients with type 1 diabetes.

The glyceroneogenesis process that is responsible for the synthesis of triacylglycerol follows the same pathway as gluconeogenesis up to the formation of DHAP. From that point, DHAP is converted into glycerol 3-phosphate, which then follows the phosphatidic acid synthesis pathway (Figure 5.50) to become triacylglycerol.

Rosiglitazone (Avandia) belongs to the class of thiazolidinedione antidiabetic agents, which reduce the levels of circulating fatty acids in the blood. It has been suggested that a high level of fatty acids in the blood interferes with glucose utilization in muscle, which in turn promotes insulin resistance. Rosiglitazone activates a nuclear receptor, which then activates PEP carboxykinase (recall the process of gluconeogenesis) in the adipose tissue. PEP carboxykinase is a regulatory enzyme that is important in the conversion of pyruvate to PEP. More PEP means more substrate for the formation of DHAP (and stimulation of glyceroneogenesis), which in turn means more production of glycerol 3-phosphate. Because the latter molecule, together with three fatty acids, is involved in the synthesis of triacylglycerol, the levels of circulating free fatty acids are reduced. To prescribe Avandia, the FDA requires both the physician and the patient enroll in the Avandia–Rosiglitazone Medicines Access Program™, as this agent has been shown to cause edema that could result in cardiovascular problems.

Learning Bridge 5.4

During one of your summer rotations in a retail pharmacy, a 50-year-old patient comes to your pharmacy to buy an OTC drug. The patient asks you a question that he forgot to ask the physician who examined him last week. At the hospital, the physician told the patient that he had a high amount of plasma VLDL. He wonders why he should have this abnormality. He admits that he drinks two to three glasses of wine every night with his friends and is curious about whether his alcohol consumption has anything to do with his elevated VLDL. What would be your explanation?

Amino Acid Oxidation

The major fate of amino acids is to be recycled in the synthesis of proteins. However, amino acid oxidation makes a significant contribution to the generation of energy as well. Dietary protein intake is necessary because the amino acids are needed for oxidative degradation, synthesis of cellular proteins, and synthesis of neurotransmitters, hormones, heme, nucleotides, and other molecules important for the body's function.

Three different sources supply the amino acids that undergo oxidative degradation:

- Utilization of amino acids produced during normal cellular protein degradation (endogenous proteins)

- After digesting a protein-rich meal, when the amount of amino acids present exceeds the need for protein synthesis (exogenous proteins)

- During starvation, when glycogen is depleted and carbohydrates are not available (endogenous proteins)

Proteins must be degraded before their building blocks, amino acids, are released for oxidation. The human GI tract contains many proteases that facilitate protein degradation (see also the *Introduction to Nutrients* chapter). Briefly, gastrin is a hormone released from the gastric mucosa that stimulates secretion of HCl from parietal cells and the release of pepsinogen from the chief cells into the stomach. Pepsinogen is a zymogen that, after its conversion to the proteolytic enzyme pepsin, degrades proteins within the acidic milieu of the stomach. When the gasteric content travels from the stomach to the small intestine, the higher pH of the small intestine stimulates secretion of another hormone from the duodenum, secretin, into the blood. Secretin stimulates the pancreas to release bicarbonate to neutralize the acidic pH, which is optimal for the activity of many proteases that can degrade proteins in the GI tract.

Amino acids can arrive to the liver from several different sources: from digested proteins (as any amino acid), from muscles (as alanine and glutamine), and from the brain (as glutamine). In the cytoplasm of liver cells, amino groups from the degraded amino acids bind to α-ketoglutarate to form glutamate. These reactions are catalyzed by a series of enzymes called aminotransferases (**Figure 5.51**). The glutamate is transported into the mitochondria, where it undergoes oxidative deamination.

All of the aminotransferases require the prosthetic group pyridoxal phosphate (PLP), which transiently accepts the amino group. PLP is derived from pyridoxine (also known as vitamin B_6). PLP is also important for many decarboxylase enzymes that produce neurotransmitters. For instance, the decarboxylases that convert histidine to histamine, glutamate to GABA, tryptophan to serotonin, and dopa to dopamine, all require PLP as a coenzyme. Isoniazid (Isotamine, from

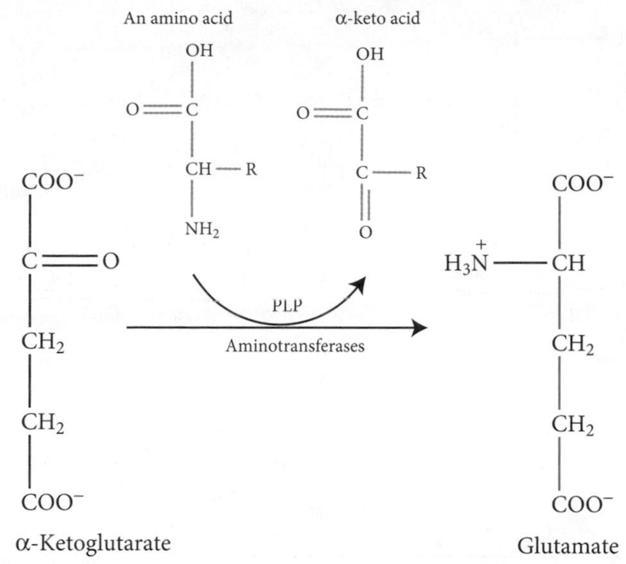

An amino acid · α-keto acid · α-Ketoglutarate · Glutamate · PLP · Aminotransferases

Figure 5.51 The amino groups of amino acids are added to α-ketoglutarate to form glutamate. These reactions are catalyzed by a series of enzymes called aminotransferases in the presence of pyridoxal phosphate (PLP). Adapted from: Nelson DL, Cox MM. *Lehninger principles of biochemistry*, 5th ed. New York: W. H. Freeman and Company; 2008: Chapter 18.

Canada), a drug used in the treatment of tuberculosis, can bind to pyridoxal phosphate and induce a vitamin B_6 deficiency (evidenced as mental confusion). Therefore, when isoniazid treatment is prescribed, a B_6 supplement is needed (see also the *Introduction to Nutrients* chapter).

As mentioned earlier, the glutamate that has been produced by aminotransferases/PLP travels from the cytoplasm to the mitochondria of the liver cells, where it undergoes oxidative deamination catalyzed by the glutamate dehydrogenase enzyme. This enzyme is unique in that it can use either NAD^+ or $NADP^+$. In this reaction, the glutamate dehydrogenase enzyme is allosterically regulated by ADP and GTP. It is important for this enzyme to be present in the mitochondria to ensure that the toxic molecule released as part of the reaction, free ammonium (NH_4), is sequestered inside the mitochondria (**Figure 5.52**).

It has been suggested that one reason why ammonium acts as a toxic molecule is that the large amount of NH_4 present shifts the equilibrium to the left—that is, to the side of the reaction catalyzed by the glutamate dehydrogenase enzyme (Figure 5.52). This depletes the citric acid cycle of α-ketoglutarate, which ultimately leads to less ATP production. Confusion, coma, and death may all result from a deficiency of ATP molecules. The toxic free ammonium molecules that are produced in the brain (for instance, by a nucleotide or an amino acid degradation) must be sent to the liver (as part of the urea cycle) to be converted into the nontoxic form, urea.

The ammonium molecules produced through oxidative deamination in the extrahepatic tissues (e.g., muscles, brain) are transferred by transamination to glutamate, thereby forming glutamine. This reaction is catalyzed by glutamine synthetase and requires one ATP molecule. The glutamine, which now carries the toxic ammonium, travels through the blood from the extrahepatic tissues to the liver, where the amino group is released by the mitochondrial glutaminase to produce glutamate and ammonium. The ammonium, when delivered in this way to the liver, is converted to urea and then excreted. Through the action of this effective pathway, the toxic free ammonium does not contaminate the blood.

The glucose–alanine cycle is another pathway that assists the body in removing toxic ammonium from the body. Toxic ammonium formed by amino acid degradation in the muscles is

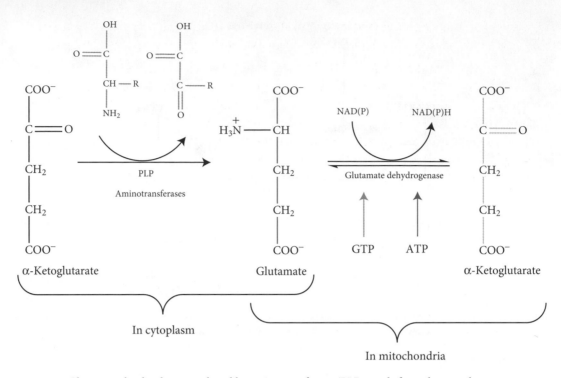

Figure 5.52 Glutamate that has been produced by aminotransferases/PLP travels from the cytoplasm to the mitochondria of the liver cells, where it undergoes oxidative deamination catalyzed by the glutamate dehydrogenase enzyme. While GTP is decreases, ATP stimulates the enzyme activity of glutamate dehydrogenase.

collected in the form of glutamate by the transamination process. Glutamate can transfer its amino group to the end product of glycolysis, pyruvate. The addition of this amino group results in the formation of alanine. Next, alanine, as the carrier for ammonium, travels to the liver. In the liver, alanine is converted back to pyruvate by a transamination process. Its amino group is eventually converted to urea through the urea cycle, and the pyruvate is converted to glucose through the gluconeogenesis pathway. The glucose is exported from the liver, returning to the muscle for use in glycolysis and energy production. In essence, this process not only takes care of the toxic ammonium in the muscle but also utilizes the glucose–alanine cycle to produce glucose.

Although amino acids provide a significant amount of energy, under normal circumstances they do not undergo the oxidation process. However, after 24 hours of starvation, the liver glycogen is depleted. Because the brain still needs glucose, expendable muscle proteins are degraded at that point and the glucogenic amino acids are oxidized to provide glucose (by gluconeogenesis).

Amino acids are classified as glucogenic, ketogenic, or both. The glucogenic amino acids are converted to intermediates (such as pyruvate and α-ketoglutarate) that can serve as substrates for gluconeogenesis. In contrast, the ketogenic amino acids (such as leucine and isoleucine) are catabolized to yield acetyl-CoA or acetoacetyl-CoA, the precursors for ketone bodies.

Biosynthesis of Amino Acids

Amino acids are synthesized by a transamination (recall the role of aminotransferases) process that combines a carbon skeleton with an amino group in the presence of PLP. Many amino acids are derived from intermediates in glycolysis (3-phosphoglycerate and pyruvate), the citric acid cycle (oxaloacetate and α-ketoglutarate), and the pentose phosphate pathway (ribose 5-phosphate and erythrose-4-phosphate). For instance, 3-phosphoglycerate is a precursor to serine and pyruvate is a precursor to alanine, valine, and leucine; oxaloacetate and α-ketoglutarate are precursors to aspartate and glutamate, respectively; ribose 5-phosphate is a precursor to histidine; and erythrose 4-phosphate is a precursor to aromatic amino acids.

Based on their ability to synthesize amino acids, amino acids are divided into two groups: essential and nonessential. The essential amino acids include amino acids that humans cannot synthesize and, therefore, they must be consumed as part of the diet. The nine essential amino acids are histidine, isoleucine, leucine, lysine, methionine, phenylalanine, threonine, tryptophan, and valine (see also the *Introduction to Cell Biology* chapter). Arginine is also an essential amino acid for juveniles. All other amino acids are nonessential amino acids—that is, humans are able to synthesize them in our bodies.

Tyrosine and cysteine are classified as nonessential amino acids, but both are synthesized from essential amino acids. Tyrosine is synthesized from the essential amino acid, phenylalanine; the phenylalanine hydroxylase enzyme catalyzes hydroxylation at carbon 4 of the phenyl group of phenylalanine. A deficiency of this enzyme results in the devastating disease known as phenylketonuria (discussed later in this chapter). Cysteine is synthesized from the essential amino acid methionine. Given their means of synthesis, consumption of cysteine and tyrosine can affect the requirements for methionine and phenylalanine, respectively.

The Urea Cycle

Urea is a molecule with two nitrogen atoms (**Figure 5.53**). As a result of the efficient urea cycle in the liver, approximately 80% of the body's nitrogen is excreted as urea. During starvation, urea production is high because cellular proteins are degraded and their carbon skeletons are oxidized to provide energy. Both mitochondria and cytosol are necessary for the urea cycle to occur. Notably, orinithine and citrulline play important roles in both the mitochondria and the cytosol to convert the toxic ammonium into urea.

Figure 5.54 identifies the enzymes and molecules that are involved in the synthesis of urea. Urea synthesis in human takes place in the liver. The ammonium that is generated in the hepatic mitochondria is mixed with CO_2 (derived from mitochondrial HCO_3^- in the respiration process) to build carbamoyl phosphate. This reaction occurs in the mitochondrial matrix and is catalyzed by a regulatory enzyme, carbamoyl phosphate synthetase I. At that point, carbamoyl phosphate is ready to enter the urea cycle. Carbamoyl phosphate synthetase I, which is found in high concentration in the mitochondrial matrix of hepatocytes, regulates the production of urea; a deficiency of this enzyme leads to high blood concentration of ammonium, thereby causing toxicity to the cells.

The starting point of the urea cycle is ornithine, which interacts with carbamoyl phosphate to form citrulline. This reaction is catalyzed by ornithine transcarbamylase. Citrulline then interacts with aspartate to form argininosuccinate, in a reaction catalyzed by argininosuccinate synthetase. Argininosuccinate is metabolized to arginine and fumarate by argininosuccinase. Fumarate enters the citric acid cycle, whereas arginine is cleaved by arginase to yield urea and ornithine.

As part of this synthesis process, the two nitrogen atoms in the urea molecules come from the toxic ammonium and aspartate amino acid. When we have too many amino acids in our cells, however, two biochemical reactions occur:

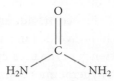

Figure 5.53 Structure of urea.

- Transamination of the amino acids in the cytoplasm (α-ketoglutarate + amino acid), which produces

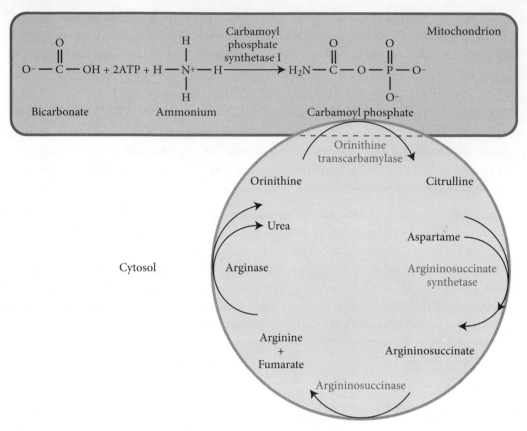

Figure 5.54 Reactions and enzymes involved in the urea cycle.

glutamate and a carbon skeleton. The latter molecule is used in different metabolic products to produce energy.

- Oxidative deamination of glutamate in the mitochondria to give α-ketoglutarate $+ NH_4^+$, in which α-ketoglutarate joins the citric acid cycle (Figure 5.52).

Hyperammonemia is a disease characterized by the accumulation of toxic ammonium in the body. This disease may have several causes, including a shortage of the enzymes needed for the formation of urea (e.g., carbamoyl phosphate synthetase I, arginase) and mutation in a binding site for GTP on the glutamate dehydrogenase enzyme (Figure 5.52). In the latter pathway, GTP serves as a negative regulator for the glutamate dehydrogenase enzyme, and impaired binding of the GTP molecule results in uncontrolled oxidative deamination. Awareness of hyperammonemia is important because failure to promptly recognize this disease can result in permanent brain damage or death.

Serum ammonium concentrations as low as 100–200 µM can result in lethargy, confusion, and vomiting. Conversely, higher concentrations may result in coma and high cranial pressure. Treatments for such imbalances often rely on a combination of restriction of protein intake, use of medications, and hemodialysis to remove nitrogen. In addition, glucocorticoids are known to increase protein degradation; for this reason, their use should be avoided in patients with hyperammonemia. Another drug that can interfere with the efficiency of the urea cycle is valproic acid (Depakote), which should not be used in patients with hyperammonemia. It has been suggested that valproic acid inhibits the regulatory enzyme carbamoyl phosphate synthetase I.

Learning Bridge 5.5

Amy Johnson comes to your pharmacy to fill her husband's prescription for valproic acid (Depakote). The prescription reads as follows:

> Depakote ER, 500 mg
>
> 1 tablet in the morning for 30 days for seizure
>
> Refill: 2

When the medication is filled and checked by your preceptor, you go to the counter to provide counseling to Amy. When you ask if her husband is taking any other medications, Amy says no, but she explains what happened earlier that morning. Her husband, Joe, was in the hospital in the morning and was diagnosed with cirrhosis (a chronic disease of the liver in which the liver cells are not functional). Joe was confused and was not oriented to time and place. In addition, Amy mentions that one of the nurses told her that Joe may have been poisoned with his own ammonium.

A. What advice do you have for Amy's husband?

B. Your preceptor believes you need to contact the patient's prescriber as soon as possible. Why?

Learning Bridge 5.6

During your introductory pharmacy practice experience in a health system rotation, you see a prescription for a neonatal patient that has been faxed to the hospital's pharmacy. The prescription reads as follows:

> Ammonul, 2.5 mL/kg, I.V. Administer as a loading dose 1.5–2 hours and then continue with the same dose as an infusion over 24 hours.

Your preceptor has never seen this medication before and asks you what ammonul is good for.

A. Different doses of ammonul are used for different enzyme deficiencies. Which enzyme deficiency has been diagnosed in this patient?

B. Explain why ammonul has been prescribed for the neonatal patient.

C. Use biochemical terms to explain the mechanism of action of ammonul to your preceptor.

Metabolic Deficiency of Amino Acids

In many countries, a small amount of newborn blood (and sometimes urine) is collected to check for inherited diseases. These diseases are often related to amino acid metabolism that leads to the accumulation of toxic molecules. The accumulation of these toxic molecules, in turn, results in permanent brain damage or death.

The following well-known inherited diseases are all caused by deficiencies in amino acid metabolism.

Phenylketonuria

Phenylketonuria (PKU) results from a defect in either phenylalanine hydroxylase or the enzyme dihydrobiopterin reductase that catalyzes regeneration of tetrahydrobiopterin. In patients with

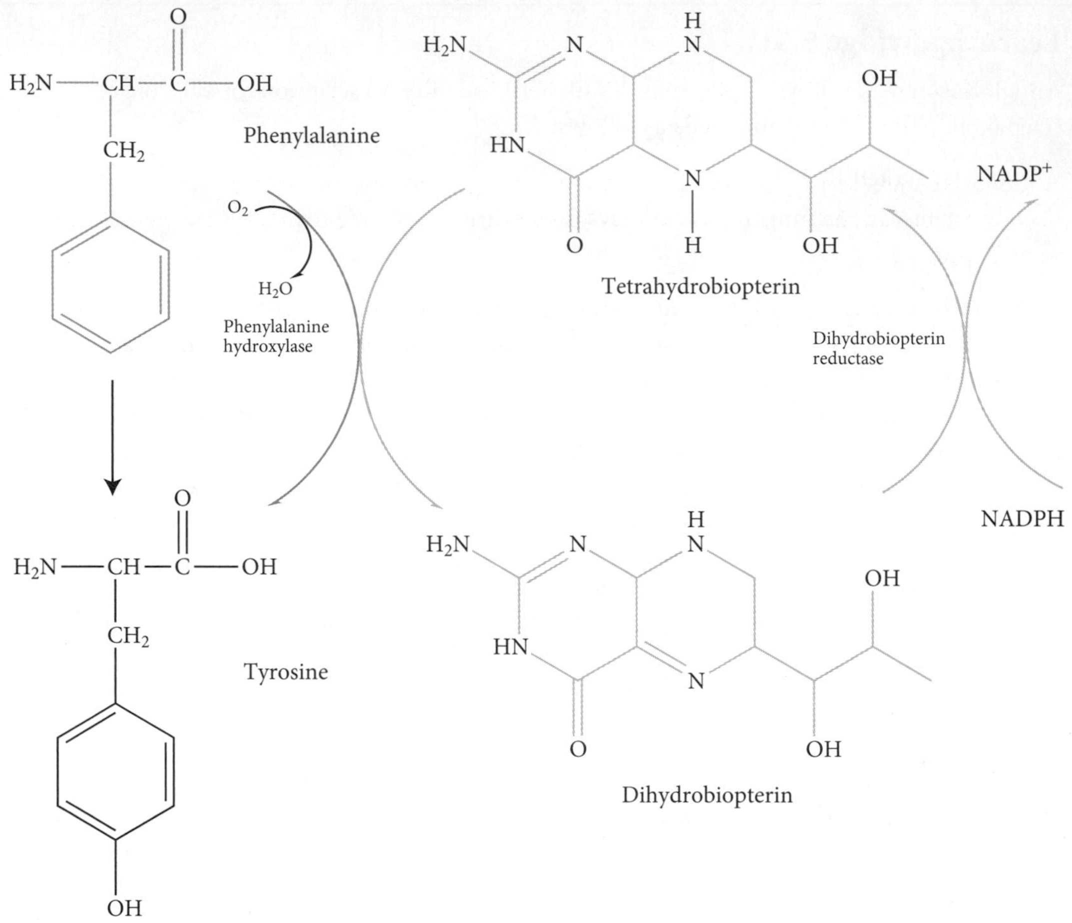

Figure 5.55 Synthesis of tyrosine from phenylalanine.
Modified from: Woodbury CP. *Biochemistry for the pharmaceutical sciences.* Burlington, MA: Jones & Bartlett Learning; 2012: Chapter 14.

PKU, phenylalanine, upon transamination, is converted to phenylpyruvate, which then accumulates in tissues, blood, and urine. The majority of phenylpyruvate is metabolized into phenylacetate and phenyllactate. It is phenylacetate that gives the musty odor to the urine of PKU patients (**Figure 5.55**).

Maple Syrup Urine Disease

Maple syrup urine disease (MSUD) affects metabolism of the branched-chain amino acids (BCAAs) leucine, isoleucine, and valine. In the extrahepatic tissues of patients with MSUD, after transamination, the α-keto acids of these amino acids accumulate in the blood and finally spill over into urine because of a deficient branched-chain α-keto acid dehydrogenase complex. Muscles extensively use the BCAAs for energy and synthesis of alanine. A lack of alanine results in a deficient glucose–alanine cycle.

Infants with MSUD become lethargic and uninterested in feeding within four to five days after their birth. As in other genetic diseases, it is critical to treat the affected infants; if they remain untreated, they may die or suffer from severe neurological impairment. A major treatment option is dietary management of MSUD to maintain blood levels of leucine, isoleucine, and valine within their normal ranges. Because these amino acids are essential amino acids, they should not be excluded from the diet, however.

Albinism

A genetic defect associated with the tyrosinase enzyme leads to albinism. As a consequence of this defect, melanin (a black pigment synthesized from tyrosine, normally found in the skin, hair, and eyes) is not produced. In the melanocytes in the skin, the tyrosinase enzyme converts tyrosine first to dopa and then to dopaquinone; dopaquinone is a highly reactive molecule that is finally condensed to produce melanin. Because of a lack of melanin, affected patients are extremely sensitive to sunlight.

Methylmalonic Acidemia

Methylmalonic acidemia (MMA) is a fetal disease that results in the accumulation of methylmalonic acid in the blood and leads to severe metabolic acidosis. A defect in the enzyme methylmalonyl-CoA mutase or a deficiency in vitamin B_{12} is the underlying cause. Lowering the amount of protein consumed in the diet or the amount of odd-numbered fatty acids is essential in these patients. Some affected individuals are treated with large daily injection doses of vitamin B_{12}.

The metabolism of the amino acids methionine, threonine, valine, and isoleucine, and of odd-numbered fatty acids, leads to the formation of propionyl-CoA. The methylmalonyl-CoA mutase is responsible for conversion of L-methylmalonyl-CoA to succinyl-CoA. Another consequence of an ineffective methylmalonyl-CoA mutase is a lack of succinyl-CoA synthesis. Succinyl-CoA is one of the intermediates in the citric acid cycle, and deficiencies in this compound affect the effectiveness of the citric acid cycle, ultimately resulting in a lower rate of ATP production.

Alkaptonuria

Alkaptonuria is caused by a deficiency in the metabolism of the tyrosine and phenylalanine amino acids. The enzyme homogentisate dioxygenase (HGD) cannot effectively metabolize these two amino acids, which results in the accumulation of homogentisic acid in the urine. As a result of this molecule's presence in excess amounts, the urine has a characteristic brownish-black color. Alkaptonuria often does not produce any symptoms until middle life (40 years of age or older), when joint disease or low back pain develops. However, the risk of cardiovascular disease is increased in older patients.

Oxidative Phosphorylation

Oxidative phosphorylation is an ATP-producing machinery, located inside of mitochondria, that employs a series of enzymes and electron carrier coenzymes, in an electron transport chain (ETC) process, to synthesize ATP molecules. The mitochondrial matrix contains pyruvate dehydrogenase complex and the enzymes necessary to support the citric acid cycle, β-oxidation, and amino acid oxidation pathways. Acetyl-CoA, produced from the oxidation of glucose, fatty acids, and amino acids, enters the citric acid cycle and becomes oxidized to produce CO_2 and NADH and $FADH_2$. In the mitochondrial matrix, both NADH and $FADH_2$ are oxidized to give up protons (H^+) and electrons. In the outer membranes of mitochondria, porins allow small molecules and ions to readily move through the membrane. In contrast, the inner membrane is impermeable to most small molecules and ions, including protons (**Figure 5.56**).

Components of the Oxidative Phosphorylation Machinery

Ubiquinone

Commonly known as coenzyme Q (CoQ), ubiquinone is a mobile component of the inner mitochondrial membrane that can gather electrons from NADH and pass them along to other

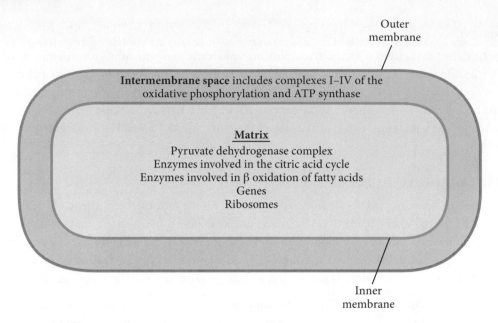

Figure 5.56 The structure of a mitochondrion and its contents.

electron carriers of the ETC. CoQ is made of 10 isoprenoid molecules. As a result, it is highly hydrophobic and can freely diffuse through the mitochondrial inner membrane. The natural product coenzyme Q10, which consists of ubiquinone, has been prescribed in doses of as much as 30–200 mg/day to patients to improve the effectiveness of the ETC in producing energy (ATP molecules).

Iron–Sulfur Proteins

Iron–sulfur proteins are involved in one-electron transfer when one iron atom of the iron–sulfur molecule is oxidized or reduced. Several important redox proteins contain iron–sulfur, including the NADH dehydrogenase complex (complex I) and cytochromes.

Cytochromes

Cytochromes are brown heme-containing proteins. Indeed, a mitochondrion has a characteristic brown color due to the color of its rich cytochromes. The major respiratory cytochromes are classified as *a*, *b*, and *c*. While cytochromes *a* and *b* are not soluble proteins, cytochrome *c* is a soluble protein of the inter membrane that accepts electrons from complex III.

ETC Complexes (I–IV)

- *Complex I*: NADH that enters the ETC is re-oxidized to NAD$^+$ by complex I, also known as NADH dehydrogenase. The electrons from NADH are transferred to the prosthetic group, FMN. Recall from Table 5.1 that the difference in the standard reduction potentials dictates which reaction donates electrons and which reaction accepts electrons.

- *Complex II*: At this site, electrons enter from FADH$_2$ that are produced by the enzyme succinate dehydrogenase in the citric acid cycle. Both complex I (NADH dehydrogenase) and complex II (succinate dehydrogenase) donate their electrons to the same electron acceptor,

CoQ. In addition, both complexes I and II contain iron–sulfur proteins, which participate in the electron transfer mechanism. This electron transfer is also explained by differences in the reactions' standard reduction potentials (see Table 5.1).

- *Complex III*: Complex III (also called cytochrome bc_1) contains a functional core that is made of cytochromes b and c_1, plus an iron–sulfur protein. Complex III transfers electrons from ubiquinol (QH_2) to the soluble cytochrome c, which is able to travel to complex IV.

- *Complex IV*: Complex IV is the final step of the ETC. It is also known as cytochrome oxidase, because it accepts electrons from cytochrome c. Complex IV contains cytochromes a and a_3. Each electron goes from cytochrome c to the copper center (Cu_A) and then to a heme group a. From there, the electron travels to an iron–copper center consisting of an iron atom, heme a_3, and a copper ion (Cu_B). It is in complex IV that electrons are finally transferred to the molecular oxygen to reduce it to water.

ATP Synthase

ATP synthase is a multiple-subunit enzyme that has two active components: F_0, which is an integral membrane protein, and F_1, which is peripheral membrane protein that faces the matrix. ATP synthase binds its substrates (ADP and inorganic phosphate) at its catalytic site inside the matrix. The ATP molecules, upon synthesis, are released from the ATP synthase enzyme.

Synthesis of ATP

During the oxidative phosphorylation, both NADH and $FADH_2$ release their H atoms. The electrons are removed from the H atoms (H becomes H^+ ion or simply a proton) and flow down the ETC within the intermembrane space, whereas the protons remain in the matrix. When the electrons travel through the ETC, the free energy released is used by each complex (complexes

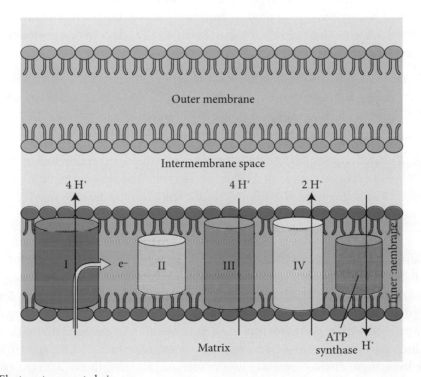

Figure 5.57 Electron transport chain.

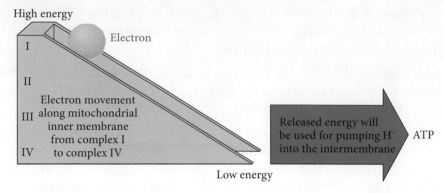

Figure 5.58 Electron release from one complex to another within the mitochondrial inner membrane.

I through IV) to pump protons from the matrix into the intermembrane space. These protons can enter only in one way from their high-concentration site, the intermembrane space, into the matrix—namely, by a mechanism that is coupled to the ATP synthase enzyme. The energy received from this proton movement is captured by the ATP synthase enzyme to synthesize ATP molecules (**Figure 5.57**).

Moving from left to right in the inner membrane, as shown in Figure 5.57, can be described as moving from the top to the bottom of a hypothetical set of electron stairs, as shown in **Figure 5.58**. More and more energy is released because of moving from a high energy level to a low energy level; in other words, electrons move down an energy gradient (recall that free energy always moves from a high energy level to a low energy level). This energy release is used to pump H^+ from the matrix to the intermembrane space, as the electron movement changes the shape of complexes I, III, and IV to transport protons across the inner membrane.

Two important conditions must be met in the oxidative phosphorylation process to have an efficient ETC. First, a large number of protons must be present in the intermembrane space. Second, the inner mitochondrial membrane must be physically intact so that protons cannot enter the matrix from locations other than the ATP synthase sites.

A few toxic molecules may potentially block the electron transfer process. Rotenone is an insecticide that blocks electron transfer from the iron–sulfur center of complex I to ubiquinone. Antimycin A blocks the electron transport from cytochrome b to cytochrome c_1 in complex III. Cyanide, azide, and carbon monoxide block electrons that pass through complex IV.

Regulation of oxidative phosphorylation is influenced by the electron flow and by the concentration of ADP. When the concentration of ADP is low, electron flow slows; when it is high, electron flow is promoted. The ultimate regulatory goal is achieved when the demand for ATP is low, preventing unnecessary oxidation of glucose, fatty acids, and amino acids.

A leak in the inner mitochondrial membrane destroys the proton gradient; in turn, no proton gradient means no driving force to stimulate the ATP synthase enzyme. In other words, uncoupling the ETC from the oxidative phosphorylation system results in the release of energy as heat rather than as ATP molecules. In this uncoupling process, electrons continue to pass through the ETC to reduce oxygen to water, but no ATP molecule is produced. The uncoupling process explains why patients with hyperthyroidism are heat intolerant. An excess of thyroid hormone is known to increase the level of expression of two uncoupling proteins, UCP2 and UCP3. Most patients with hyperthyroidism complain of heat intolerance and sweatiness, with the excessive perspiration being a result of dissipation of the excess heat through evaporation from the skin surface.

Metabolism of Nucleotides

Nitrogen Metabolism

Nitrogen is an important and necessary element of biological molecules such as amino acids, nucleotides, porphyrin, and some phospholipids (recall sphingolipids). Despite plentiful nitrogen gas (N_2, which constitutes 80% of the air we breathe) in our atmosphere, we are unable to incorporate these atoms directly into our biological molecules. Converting N_2 into its reduced form, NH_4^+, requires a large energy investment—which could be an evolutionary reason why humans are not able to reduce N_2 gas. A total of 16 ATP molecules are required to reduce one N_2 molecule to two ammonium molecules, because it requires a significant energy investment to break the $N \equiv N$ triple bond that exists in N_2.

The reduction of N_2 to NH_4^+, through the pathway called nitrogen fixation, can be carried out by only a few organisms such as bacteria and cyanobacteria. For instance, *Rhizobium*, which lives in a symbiotic relationship within the roots of a few plants, is able to carry out nitrogen fixation for those plants. Soil bacteria synthesize NO_3^- and NH_4^+, which are absorbed by some plants such as corn (many plants can perform this process by themselves as well).

Reduced nitrogen, from plants, enters the human body as amino acids and proteins. Once amino acid molecules enter a cell, the amino group is available for many synthetic reactions. For example, plants, after absorption of NH_4^+ molecules, incorporate them into glutamine, an amino acid. The nitrogen from the amide functional group of glutamine is a source of the amino group in many biosynthetic processes (**Figure 5.59**). Both glutamate and glutamine are key amino acids that serve as nitrogen donors to many other molecules. These two amino acids also played critical roles in amino acid oxidation and the removal of toxic ammonium.

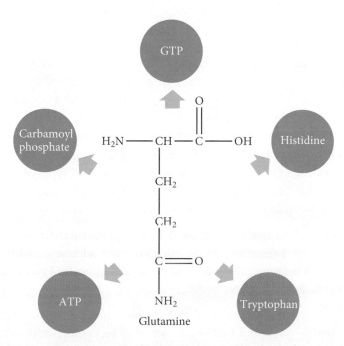

Figure 5.59 The nitrogen from the amide functional group of glutamine is a source of the amino group found in many nitrogen-containing molecules.

Adapted from Nelson DL, Cox MM, and Lehninger AL. Principle of biochemistry. 5th ed. W.H. Freeman and Company; 2008. Chapter 22.

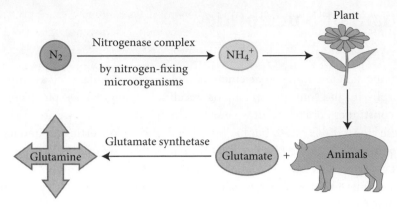

Figure 5.60 The biochemical path from N_2 to the amino acids glutamate and glutamine.

Glutamine synthetase is found in all organisms and is involved in the conversion of NH_4^+ to the amino acid glutamate to produce glutamine. **Figure 5.60** illustrates the path taken by nitrogen gas as it is converted into amino acids in animals.

As shown in Figure 5.60, first, molecular nitrogen (N_2) is reduced to ammonia in a reaction that is catalyzed by the nitrogenase complex. Second, ammonia is incorporated into glutamine by glutamine synthetase, which is found in all organisms. However, access to glutamate is required to make glutamine. In bacteria and plants, glutamate synthase produces glutamate—but animals do not have this enzyme. Consequently, animals use a transamination mechanism to synthesize glutamate. Another minor route from ammonia to glutamate occurs in the mitochondria, where glutamate dehydrogenase catalyzes formation of glutamate (recall Figure 5.52): α-Ketoglutarate + NH_4^+ + NADPH $\rightarrow$ Glutamate + $NADP^+$ + H_2O.

Important Nitrogen-Containing Molecules

Heme

Glycine amino acid and succinyl-CoA combine to form α-amino β-ketoadipate, which in turn is decarboxylated to form δ-aminolevulinate. The entire process is catalyzed by δ-aminolevulinate synthase. Two molecules of δ-aminolevulinate merge together to form a five-membered ring of porphobilinogen. Similarly, four porphobilinogen molecules combine to produce porphyrin (heme), which is an important component of hemoglobin. Folic acid (vitamin B_9; see also the *Introduction to Nutrients* chapter) is required to synthesize the amino acid glycine. Indeed, this mechanism explains why folic acid is an important vitamin for patients with some specific types of anemia.

Nitric Oxide

Nitric oxide (NO) is a hormone that is synthesized from oxygen and the amino acid arginine. The enzyme that catalyzes this reaction is nitric oxide synthase, a heme-containing enzyme. Both NADPH and FAD, as well as tetrahydrobiopterin (recall the synthesis of tyrosine from phenylalanine), are involved in the synthesis of NO.

Nitric oxide participates in many physiological reactions. However, it is an unstable molecule that cannot be stored. Its synthesis is stimulated by interaction of NO synthase with Ca^{2+}-calmodulin. A large amount of NO is synthesized in the central nervous system. Nitric oxide stimulates the soluble guanylyl cyclase to synthesize cGMP (see also the *Introduction to Pharmacodynamics* chapter). In addition, NO is involved in the regulation of blood pressure, the inhibition of blood clotting, and the destruction of damaged cells by macrophages. An inadequate amount of NO has been associated with male impotence, migraine headache, and Parkinson's disease. Furthermore, NO is known to inhibit the citric acid cycle enzyme aconitase, which catalyzes the conversion of citrate to isocitrate (recall step 2 in the citric acid cycle), and the cytochrome oxidase enzyme, which is involved in oxidative phosphorylation. In this way, NO may play a role in the regulation of fuel metabolism.

Neurotransmitters

Many neurotransmitters are derived from amino acids and, as a result, they contain nitrogen atoms. For instance, tyrosine is a precursor to dopa, dopamine, norepinephrine and epinephrine; glutamate is a precursor to GABA; histidine is a precursor to histamine; and tryptophan is a precursor to serotonin. The biosynthesis of these neurotransmitters is described in the *Introduction to Nutrients* chapter.

Learning Bridge 5.7

During one of your community pharmacy rotations, Jennifer, who is the manager of a hardware store, comes to your pharmacy with her daughter, Amy. Amy is an 8-year-old student who just finished second grade. Jennifer asks you where she can find an OTC product called aspartame. She explains that aspartame has been recommended by one of her friends as a way to cut down on the amount of sugar in Amy's diet, as Jennifer is concerned about Amy's weight. You notice that Amy has pale skin, blond hair, and blue eyes.

While you are directing Jennifer to the OTC department, you ask her if Amy has been diagnosed with any diseases. Jennifer mentions that Amy was diagnosed with PKU soon after her birth. You advise Jennifer to not buy any aspartame products for Amy.

A. What is PKU?
B. Why does Amy have pale skin, blond hair, and blue eyes?
C. Why shouldn't Amy use aspartame?
D. What advice do you have for Jennifer?

Biosynthesis and Degradation of Nucleotides

Nucleotides play important roles in many biochemical processes, including (1) serving as precursors for nucleic acids (DNA and RNA); (2) assisting in building intermediates such as UDP-glucose and CDP-diacylglycerol, which are used in the biosynthesis of glycogen and phospholipids, respectively; (3) synthesis of ATP and GTP as energy sources; (4) synthesis of electron carrier coenzymes; and (5) synthesis of second messengers such as cAMP and cGMP.

Most organisms can synthesize purine and pyrimidine nucleotides from other molecules such as amino acids and CO_2 (**Figure 5.61**). These pathways are almost identical in all organisms. Nucleotides can also be recycled from the breakdown of previously synthesized DNA or RNA—that is, from so-called salvage pathways. For instance, it is known that pancreatic ribonuclease or DNase in the small intestine cleaves the phosphodiester bonds of RNA or DNA that are derived from foods.

Glutamine plays a major role in the synthesis of inosine-5-monophosphate (IMP, also known as inosinate). IMP is a purine nucleotide that is important for the synthesis of guanosine monophosphate (GMP) and adenosine monophosphate (AMP). Interestingly, the energy requirements for the AMP pathway are met by GTP molecules, whereas the energy requirements for the GMP pathway are met by ATP molecules.

A series of molecules can inhibit the synthesis of nucleotides. For instance, azaserine is a structural analog of glutamine. Because of its similarity to this amino acid, it competitively inhibits the enzymes involved in the transfer of the amide group of glutamine to nucleotides and tryptophan. While azaserine is a toxic molecule, its presence in the body would not immediately be fatal because it takes time for replication, transcription, and translation to be effected and to cause death. The structure of azaserine is shown in **Figure 5.62**.

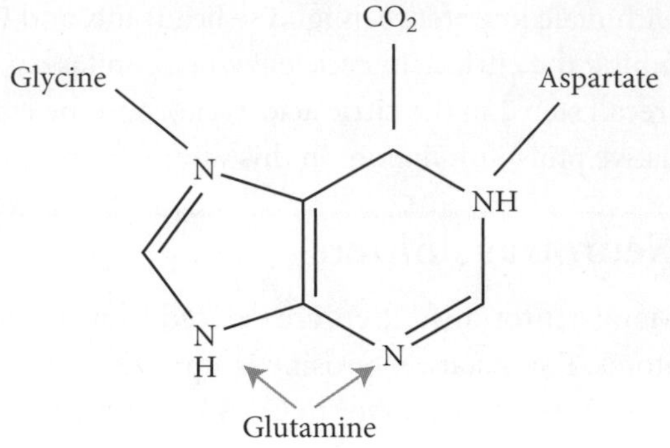

Figure 5.61 A few molecules contribute to the carbon and nitrogen atoms of nucleotides.

Hormonal Regulation of Mammalian Metabolism

In differentiated and complex organisms such as mammals, many tissues work together to maintain a constant level of fuel for their cells. These tissues must be able to meet everyday challenges in the form of fasting, obesity, fear, stress, muscular activity, and illness. To do so, these tissues must successfully coordinate different metabolic pathways to meet the body's needs. Hormones play a major role in the coordination between these tissues.

The liver plays a central role in anabolism and catabolism as well as in processing and distributing nutrients to other tissues. Metabolism is a biochemical process that encompasses both catabolism and anabolism. Catabolism comprises exothermic pathways that facilitate the breakdown of large and complex molecules into smaller molecules to produce energy. An example is the oxidation of fatty acids to CO_2 and H_2O. Anabolism, in contrast, comprises endothermic pathways that facilitate the synthesis of large and complex molecules from smaller precursors. An example is the synthesis of glycogen from glucose.

In many metabolic pathways, the availability of the substrate plays an essential role in the regulation of the metabolism. The concentration of substrate usually falls below the saturation level (e.g., when [S] is equal to K_m), so that regulation of the enzyme can be achieved by varying the amount of substrate. An example is the role played by glucokinase in the liver, which was explained elsewhere in this chapter.

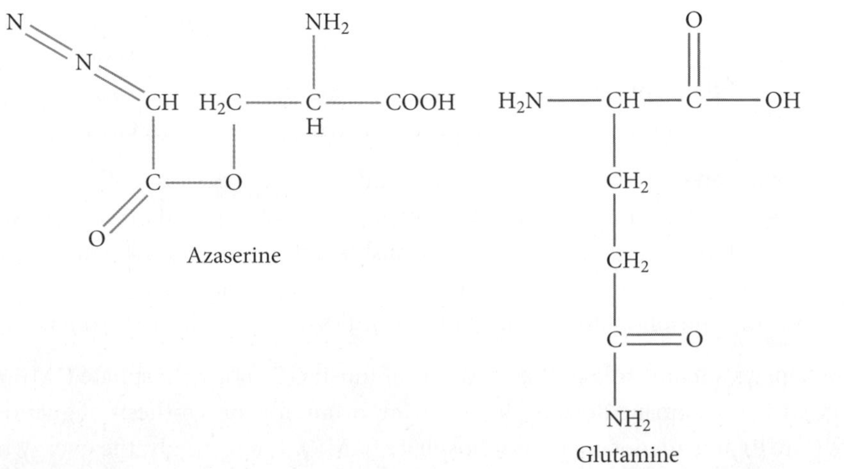

Figure 5.62 Due to the structural similarity between azaserine and glutamine, azaserine is toxic to cells.

Before describing the roles of hormones in the regulation of mammalian metabolism, it is imperative to introduce a few tissues that play central roles in the metabolism of fuels.

Liver

The liver is the largest solid organ in humans. Venous blood from the intestine, and to a lesser extent from the stomach and spleen, moves through the portal vein and then to the liver. As a result, many drugs and nutrients that are absorbed by the GI tract go through the portal vein to the liver before they are distributed into the circulation. The liver has a remarkable metabolic flexibility that determines the fate of glucose, amino acids, and fatty acids within the body.

Interestingly, the concentration of glucose in the liver is almost identical to the concentration of glucose in the blood (i.e., approximately 5 mM). This results in an effective phosphorylation mechanism of glucose to glucose-6-phosphate. Glucose-6-phosphate may take five different routes in the liver depending on the needs of other tissues: (1) dephosphorylation and release of glucose into the bloodstream; (2) conversion to liver glycogen; (3) oxidation via glycolysis and the citric acid cycle; (4) oxidation to acetyl-CoA, which then serves as a precursor for the synthesis of triacylglycerols, phospholipids, and cholesterol; and (5) oxidation via the pentose phosphate pathway for the production of NADPH and precursors to the formation of nucleotides.

The liver also plays a major role in the metabolism of amino acids. There are many possible fates for the amino acids that arrive in the liver after their intestinal uptake. These fates include (1) synthesis of proteins, particularly for the liver, as it has a high turnover of proteins; (2) transmission, via the blood, to other organs for the synthesis of tissue proteins; (3) synthesis of nucleotides, hormones, and heme; (4) deamination, followed by degradation, to yield pyruvate; (5) involvement of pyruvate in gluconeogenesis for the synthesis of glucose; (6) oxidation of pyruvate to acetyl-CoA; (7) conversion of acetyl-CoA into lipids; and (8) providing an effective glucose–alanine cycle to reduce the amount of toxic ammonium in the body.

Fatty acids also undergo different metabolic fates in the liver: (1) conversion into hepatocytes' membrane phospholipids; (2) β oxidation to acetyl-CoA, followed by the synthesis of cholesterol; (3) oxidation and conversion to ketone bodies for export to the brain; and (4) conversion to triacylglycerol for export in plasma lipoproteins.

Adipose Tissue

Adipose tissue is metabolically active and is specialized to take up lipids from the blood and store lipids in large fat droplets within its cells. Two types of adipose cells are distinguished: white and brown. White adipose cells are more common in humans. In a white adipose cell, a large single fat droplet occupies a significant portion of the adipocyte. Adipose tissue is distributed throughout the body, being found under the skin (due to lipids' poor ability to signal heat, they serve as heat barriers), in the palms of the hands, around the deep blood vessels, and in the abdominal cavity.

Because it contains energy-rich molecules (triacylglycerols), adipose tissue responds rapidly to hormonal signals in the metabolic communications that take place within the liver, skeletal muscles, and heart. Indeed, the largest energy store in a well-nourished human is not glycogen, but rather triacylglycerols. Adipose tissue has the capacity to store enough energy to support an adult human for 2 months, whereas the liver's glycogen supply can provide energy sufficient to maintain the body for only 24 hours.

When the body needs energy, triacylglycerols stored in the adipose tissue are broken down by hormone-sensitive lipase. Epinephrine, norepinephrine, adrenocorticotropic, and glucagon hormones all have the ability to activate adenylate cyclase in the adipose plasma membrane to produce cAMP. cAMP-dependent protein kinase phosphorylates triacylglycerol lipase, which in turn activates the lipolysis process. The lipolysis process then causes the degradation of each triacylglycerol molecule into three fatty acids and one glycerol molecule. The fatty acids are bound to serum albumin so that they can be transported to other tissues, such as skeletal muscles, the heart, and the renal cortex, in the β-oxidation pathway and ultimately used for energy production. The other part of triacylglycerol—that is, glycerol—is sent to the liver, where it is phosphorylated by glycerol kinase to glycerol-3-phosphate and then to dihydroxyacetone phosphate (recall DHAP in Figure 5.50). DHAP is an intermediate in the processes of glycolysis, gluconeogenesis, and glyceroneogenesis.

Simply put, you can make energy from both parts of a triacylglycerol molecule. It is estimated that fatty acids' β oxidation accounts for 95% of the energy available to the body, whereas conversion of glycerol into pyruvate accounts for 5% of the available energy from a triacylglycerol molecule.

Muscles

Muscles are able to metabolize glucose, fatty acids, and ketone bodies. In a resting muscle, fatty acids are the major energy source; in contrast, during exercise, glucose from the muscle glycogen is the major energy source. Skeletal muscle consumes more than 50% of total O_2 in resting conditions but more than 90% of this total during extensive muscle activity. The higher rate of oxygen consumption in the latter case occurs because extensive muscle activity consumes large quantities of ATP. Because the blood flow cannot provide O_2 fast enough to the oxidative phosphorylation pathway to produce the large amount of ATP molecules needed, muscle glycogen begins to undergo anaerobic glycolysis to produce lactate. This lactate is transported by the blood to the liver, where the gluconeogenesis process produces first pyruvate and then glucose. The conversion of lactate to pyruvate is catalyzed by the lactate dehydrogenase enzyme. The energy source (ATP) that drives the gluconeogenesis is provided by fatty acids' β oxidation. Finally, the glucose, once synthesized in the liver, is returned to muscle to refill the muscle's glycogen store, a biochemical process known as the Cori cycle.

Creatine is a natural product found in abundant amounts in meat and fish. The body also makes creatine by using amino acids—namely, glycine and arginine. Creatine is transported to the muscle and nerves, where it interacts with a phosphate group to produce phosphocreatine, in a reaction catalyzed by the creatine kinase enzyme (**Figure 5.63**). Because phosphocreatine is a hydrophilic molecule, it cannot leave the cell, but rather donates its phosphate to ADP to make an ATP molecule. This type of ATP production, which is called substrate-level ATP synthesis, differs significantly from the synthesis of ATP molecules that occurs in the oxidative phosphorylation pathway.

The heart contains large amounts of creatine kinase, which explains why it is the first enzyme to appear in the blood after a myocardial infarction. Having extra phosphocreatine in muscle cells can enhance athletic performance in many sports, although this source of energy is available for just a few seconds and is restored only when the muscle rests after a prolonged exercise. Because creatine enhances athletic performance, it is a popular supplement among many athletes.

Brain

The brain has very high rate of metabolism but possesses only a very limited amount of glycogen. Additionally, the brain cannot use fatty acids as an energy source; after binding to serum albumin, fatty acids cannot cross the blood–brain barrier. Consequently, the brain needs a constant supply of glucose that is delivered on an ongoing basis, even when we are asleep. During fasting conditions, when the liver glycogen is no longer available, the brain can use ketone bodies that are

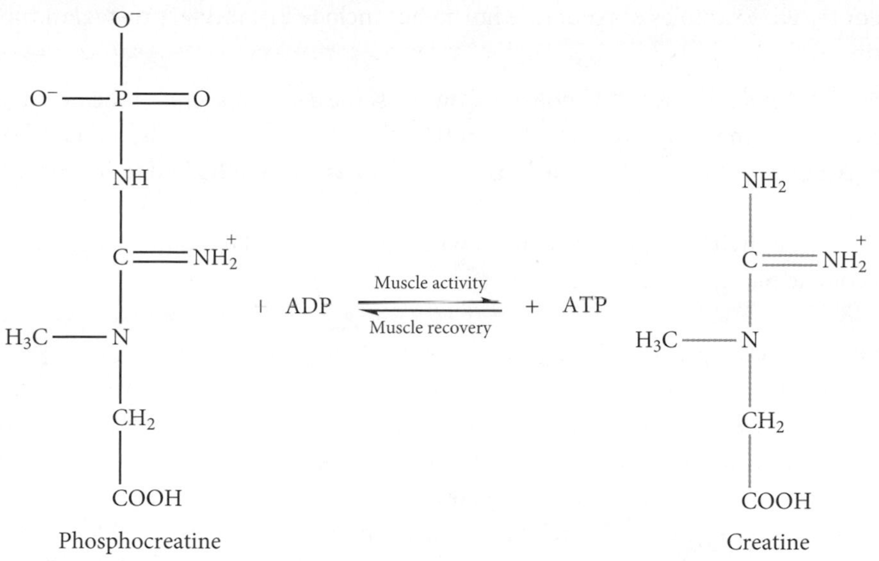

Figure 5.63 Synthesis and use of phosphocreatine in muscle.

synthesized from acetyl-CoA as its energy source. Ketone bodies, in contrast to fatty acids, have free carboxyl groups that make them soluble in the blood; thus they can readily cross the blood–brain barrier to reach the brain. The unique pathway of using ketone bodies allows the body to avoid muscle proteins' degradation, at least in the short term. Nevertheless, when the two other energy resources—glycogen and triacylglycerols—are exhausted, the brain turns to muscle proteins' degradation as its ultimate source of glucose (via gluconeogenesis).

The brain uses a significant amount of ATP molecules (approximately 60% of the glucose utilization of a human at rest) to fuel the Na^+/K^+ pumps necessary to maintain neuron membrane potentials. Even though the brain represents only 2% of the total body weight, it consumes nearly 20% of the total consumed oxygen. Such oxygen, even while a person is at rest or asleep, is important to produce ATP molecules in an uninterrupted fashion. The high demand for oxygen and ATP synthesis explains why a loss of oxygen during cardiac arrest results in loss of consciousness within 10 seconds and irreversible brain damage within a few minutes.

Hormones

As mentioned earlier, hormones regulate and coordinate mammalian metabolism by communicating with the tissues described earlier in this section. Hormones are secreted into the extracellular fluid, from which they diffuse into the blood capillaries, travel with the bloodstream, and diffuse out to interact with the target cells or tissues. Generally, hormones are polypeptides (insulin, glucagon), amino acid derivatives (epinephrine, nitric oxide), proteins (anterior pituitary hormones), or steroids (aldosterone, estrogen). Based on the means of hormonal release and the cells that they act on, hormones can be classified as endocrine, paracrine, or autocrine hormones.

- *Endocrine Hormones:* These hormones are secreted by specific tissues, called endocrine glands (e.g., thyroid, pituitary, testis), into the bloodstream and affect far-reaching cells. Examples of endocrine hormones include insulin, glucagon, thyroid hormones, aldosterone, and epinephrine.

- *Paracrine Hormones:* These hormones act on cells that are in the immediate vicinity or local environment where the hormones are released. Usually the two cells (i.e., the cell that releases the hormone and the cell that receives the hormone) are adjacent to each other in the same organ or tissue. Examples of paracrine hormones include histamine, prostaglandins, and gasterin.

- *Autocrine Hormones:* These hormones act on the same cell that secreted the hormones. Autocrine signaling is tightly controlled; if the control mechanism fails, it could lead to cancer. An example of an autocrine hormone is human growth hormone (hGH), which is produced by the glandular cells of the endometrium during the menstrual cycle. An elevated level of hGH has been associated with the presence of endometrial carcinoma cells, a gynecologic malignancy.

A few hormones are produced during conditions of stress. Stress can arise not only from a stressful situation but also from trauma, injury, surgery, burns, and infections. Regardless of the underlying cause, stress can lead to enhanced oxygen consumption and hypermetabolism. It is known that epinephrine and cortisol are released upon stress. These hormones cause an increase in the blood glucose level: epinephrine stimulates adenylate cyclase to produce cAMP, while cortisol stimulates gluconeogenesis. The release of glucagon can also increase the blood glucose level. However, epinephrine is released when a higher than normal level of glucose is required, whereas glucagon kicks in when the level of glucose is abnormally low.

Epinephrine and glucagon activate breakdown of glycogen and inactivate glycogen synthase. This is a typical example of how the anabolic and catabolic pathway for glycogen is reciprocally regulated. Despite the fact that epinephrine and glucagon exert similar actions, both are released from different tissues at different times. For instance, epinephrine is released from the adrenal medulla when we are confronted with a stressful situation (see also the *Introduction to Pharmacology and Pathophysiology* chapter). As a result of this epinephrine secretion, glycogenolysis, lipolysis, and the release of glucagon from pancreas are promoted. Glucagon is released in response to a low blood glucose level. It stimulates gluconeogenesis in the liver by inhibiting the pyruvate kinase enzyme (the last enzyme in glycolysis). Consequently, the amount of PEP increases, which results in the stimulation of gluconeogenesis. Commercial synthesized glucagon (GlucaGen, 1 mg) is available to treat severe hypoglycemia in diabetic patients.

Muscle cells do not express a glucagon receptor, so they do not respond to glucagon. Moreover, because glucagon simultaneously stimulates glycogen degradation and gluconeogenesis, the glucose from these pathways will not be consumed by the liver, but rather is sent to the blood to maintain the normal level of glucose and to supply glucose to other tissues.

The insulin hormone also plays an important role in the regulation of fuel metabolism, as described both in this chapter and in the *Introduction to Pharmacology and Pathophysiology* chapter. Insulin reduces the blood glucose level (in contrast to the effects from epinephrine, glucagon, and cortisol), but its release is not associated with any stress. During starvation, glucose utilization is low because of an inadequate glucose supply. Similarly, in untreated diabetes, glucose utilization is low. The latter effect is caused by a lack or an inadequate amount of insulin to promote glucose uptake by myocytes and adipocytes.

Steroid Hormones

Steroid hormones are involved in signal transduction by changing the expression of specific genes. All of the steroid hormones are synthesized from cholesterol. Although they always have the same complex of four carbon rings, each steroid has a different side chain (**Figure 5.64**). All or some of the carbons that are projected from carbon 17 (Figure 5.64) are removed during the synthesis of steroid hormones. Only three organs can convert cholesterol into steroid hormones: the adrenal cortex, the testis, and the ovary.

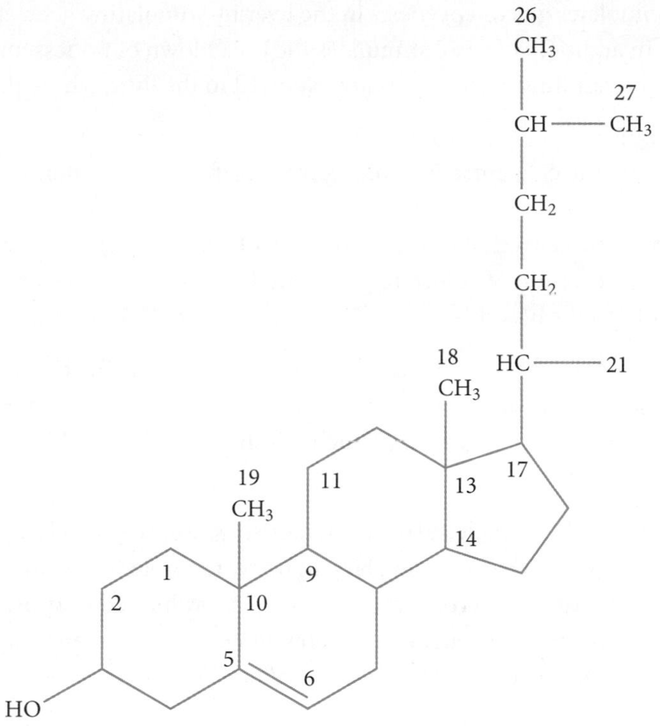

Figure 5.64 General structure of steroid hormones.

Because steroid hormones are water insoluble, transport proteins are needed to assist these hormones in reaching their target cells. Among these proteins are transcortin, androgen-binding proteins, sex-hormone-binding proteins, and, to a lesser extent, albumin. Once the steroid hormones reach their target cells, they dissociate from their transport proteins, span the cell membrane, enter the cytoplasm, and bind to their nuclear receptors to affect a specific gene expression.

Mammalian cells are unable to completely degrade steroid compounds. As a result, steroid hormones undergo a few reactions in the liver, including a reduction mechanism that reduces their unsaturated bonds and adds hydroxyl groups. These hydroxyl groups assist steroid hormones in binding to glucuronic acid or sulforic acid (conjugation mechanism; see also the *Introduction to Medicinal Chemistry* chapter). A significant portion (70–80%) of these metabolites are released into the blood (they are no longer water insoluble), filtered within the kidney, and finally released into the urine.

Steroid hormones are categorized into five major classes: progesterone, cortisol (glucocorticoid), aldosterone (mineralocorticoid), testosterone (androgen), and estradiol (estrogen). While cortisol and aldosterone are synthesized in the cortex of the adrenal gland, progesterone, testosterone, and estradiol are produced in the male and female gonads (i.e., testes in males and ovaries in females) and in the placenta of females.

Progesterone regulates the female reproductive cycle; it controls the movement of the egg within the lumen of the fallopian tube and during labor regulates uterine contraction. Males also produce progesterone, albeit in smaller amounts than in females. Progesterone may be associated with the emotional and physical changes that occur during premenstrual syndrome (PMS). PMS symptoms, which include abdominal bloating, headache, fatigue, anxiety, and depression, usually occur a few days before menstruation begins.

Cortisol is the most potent glucocorticoid produced by the cortex of the adrenal gland. As a steroid hormone that affects gene expression, it acts much more slowly than epinephrine and glucagon. Cortisol stimulates gluconeogenesis in the liver by stimulating gene expression for PEP carboxykinase. In addition, cortisol stimulates the breakdown of nonessential (expendable) proteins in muscle. The resulting amino acids are exported to the liver, where they can be converted to glucose by gluconeogenesis.

Aldosterone regulates the concentrations of electrolytes in the blood; that is, it controls the reabsorption of inorganic ions by the kidney. Aldosterone binds to its receptor and activates specific genes to express proteins that change the influx of Na^+, K^+, Mg^{2+}, and water across the target cell's membrane. Secretion of aldosterone is stimulated by a decreased amount of Na^+ and an increased amount of K^+ in the blood.

Both the testis and the ovary synthesize androgens and estrogens. The testes predominantly secrete androgens (such as testosterone), which are also known as male sex hormones. In contrast, the ovaries predominantly produce estrogens (such as estradiol), which are also known as female sex hormones.

Testosterone is responsible for male sexual characteristics. Approximately 95% of all testosterone is produced in the testis, where testosterone plays an important role in spermatogenesis (i.e., production of sperm). Use of testosterone and its analogs is prohibited in sports because they can bind to testosterone receptor and stimulate the expression of genes that enhance the development of lean muscle mass, which may consequently (and unfairly) improve athletic performance.

Estradiol is an estrogen hormone that promotes development of sexual characteristics in females. It is directly involved in the growth and development of the vagina, uterus, and fallopian tubes. Estrogen affects lipid metabolism by decreasing serum lipoprotein and triacylglycerol levels. As a result, the HDL level increases and the LDL level decreases—effects that make estrogen an attractive therapeutic agent in postmenopausal women.

Learning Bridge 5.8

During one of your rotations in a health system, a patient is brought to your site. This patient is suspected to have overdosed with a beta blocker that caused severe bradycardia and profound hypotension. The attending physician prescribes an intravenous injection of glucagon (5 mg), to be followed by continuous IV infusion glucagon as an antidote.

A. Why is glucagon recommended in this case?
B. Is this dose (5 mg) the same as the glucagon dose used to treat hypoglycemia? Why?
C. Why didn't the physician prescribe epinephrine as an antidote?

Learning Bridge 5.9

Amy is a 32-year-old teacher who works for a well-known high school in Portland, Oregon. Amy is pregnant; her baby is due in 7 months. Over the past 2 weeks, Amy has noted heavy sweating and she constantly feels hot. She feels like she has an "endless fever." Amy visited her physician last week and mentioned her excessively sweating skin, which has caused her embarrassment at her school. She has lost weight, despite the fact she has an excessive appetite. On the physical examination, Amy's heart rate was rapid (115 beats/min) and she appeared restless. A laboratory test was ordered and indicated hyperthyroidism.

Amy comes to your pharmacy to have her prescriptions filled and to buy aspirin for her fever. While she is waiting to have her medications dispensed, she asks you a few questions about her medical problems.

A. Why is Amy so hot?

B. Is her "endless fever" caused by an infection?

C. Why is Amy losing weight despite having a good appetite?

Golden Keys for Pharmacy Students

1. Thermodynamics is the study of energy, heat, and work. This field is concerned with energy transfer either in an organized form (work) or in a disorganized form (heat).

2. There are three important concepts in thermodynamics: (a) the system, which is the process under study; (b) the surroundings, which are the areas outside of the system; and (c) the universe, which is the system and surroundings combined.

3. The first law in thermodynamics states that the total energy change of the universe is constant.

4. The second law in thermodynamics states that the universe tends spontaneously toward disorder and randomness.

5. Energy can be divided into two terms: potential energy, which is stored energy, and kinetic energy, which is the energy of motion.

6. Any chemical reaction can be classified as meeting one of three thermodynamic conditions: (a) if the free energy change is positive, the process does not occur spontaneously; (b) if the free energy change is negative, once the process begins, it takes place spontaneously; and (c) if the free energy change of the process is zero, the system is at equilibrium.

7. Coenzymes are organic molecules that facilitate the catalytic activity of enzymes; examples include NAD^+ and $NADP^+$. Cofactors are inorganic molecules that facilitate the catalytic activity of enzymes; examples include Zn^{2+} and Mg^{2+}.

8. In the oxidation–reduction pathways that occur in many biochemical reactions, two hydrogen atoms are often stripped from a reduced molecule. One of these hydrogen atoms, as a proton, is then released into the surrounding solution.

9. While vitamin B_2 is important for the synthesis of FMN and FAD, vitamin B_3 is important for the synthesis of NAD and NADP.

10. Proteins can be classified into two major groups with respect to their tertiary or secondary structure: fibrous (water-insoluble proteins) and globular (water-soluble proteins).

11. Carbon monoxide has a higher affinity than oxygen for myoglobin and hemoglobin. It is a very toxic gas because it excludes oxygen from binding to these two important globular proteins.

12. Sickle cell anemia is an inherited disorder of hemoglobin. There are hundreds of variants of hemoglobin, which differ in their amino acid composition. One well-known variant is hemoglobin S.

13   An enzyme cannot alter the laws of thermodynamics. Thus enzymes can influence the rate of a reaction, but they cannot change the equilibrium for a reaction.

14.   The Michaelis-Menten equation is the most important equation in nonlinear kinetics:

$$V_0 = \frac{V_{max}[S]}{K_m + [S]}$$

15.   The k_{cat}/K_m ratio is important because it enables you to compare efficiencies between different enzymes. The higher the value of k_{cat}/K_m, the more efficient an enzyme is.

16.   There are two classes of enzyme inhibitors: reversible and irreversible. Irreversible inhibitors usually cause inactivation of the enzyme's structure.

17.   Glycolysis is a metabolic pathway in which glucose is oxidized to produce energy in the form of ATP. This universal pathway is identical in all organisms.

18.   The net gain from glycolysis is two pyruvate molecules, two ATP molecules, and two NADH molecules.

19.   In anaerobic glycolysis, glycolysis occurs in the absence of oxygen. This pathway is activated either when there is no oxygen available (anaerobic organisms) or when the oxygen level is low (animals engaging in extensive muscle activity).

20.   Glycolysis generates NADH, whereas the pentose phosphate pathway generates NADPH.

21.   Fatty acids are energy-rich molecules that store much more energy than carbohydrates of similar molecular size.

22.   Fatty acids are stored as triacylglycerols in adipose tissue. The brain cannot use fats for energy, but rather has a specific demand for glucose.

23.   Carnitine plays an important role in transporting fatty acids into the matrix of a mitochondrion.

24.   Ketone bodies are overproduced during prolonged fasting, particularly when glycogen is depleted and fatty acids from stored triacylglycerols become the principal fuel.

25.   Diabetic ketoacidosis is an uncontrolled form of ketosis (i.e., elevated ketone body levels in the blood) and, if not treated, is fatal.

26.   The citric acid cycle plays a central role in fuel metabolism because glycolysis, fatty acid oxidation, and amino acid oxidation can all produce acetyl-CoA, which then serves as an input to the citric acid cycle.

27.   Most of the body's fatty acids are synthesized from dietary glucose; the body is able to use glucose during glycolysis to synthesize pyruvate, which in turn can be converted to acetyl-CoA.

28.   All of the reactions in the synthesis of fatty acids are catalyzed by the multiple-enzyme complex called fatty acid synthase (FAS).

29.   Both linoleic acid and linolenic acid are found in large amounts in fish and plants, and both are important for the synthesis of arachidonic acid, which is a precursor for eicosanoids.

30.   Insulin promotes the conversion of carbohydrates into triacylglycerols.

31.   Intake of protein through the diet is necessary because the amino acids are needed for oxidative degradation, synthesis of cellular protein, and synthesis of neurotransmitters, hormones, heme, nucleotides, and other molecules.

32. All of the aminotransferases require the prosthetic group pyridoxal phosphate (PLP). PLP is derived from pyridoxine (vitamin B_6).

33. Ammonium acts as a toxic molecule when the presence of a large amount of NH_4 shifts the equilibrium to the left in the reaction catalyzed by the glutamate dehydrogenase enzyme. This depletes the citric acid cycle of α-ketoglutarate, which in turn leads to less ATP production.

34. The heart contains large amounts of creatine kinase, which explains why it is the first enzyme that appears in the blood after myocardial infarction.

35. The brain uses a significant number of ATP molecules (approximately 60% of the total amount of glucose utilized by a human at rest) to meet the Na^+/K^+ pumps' needs and maintain the neuron membrane potentials.

36. Hormones include polypeptides (insulin, glucagon), amino acid derivatives (epinephrine, nitric oxide), proteins (anterior pituitary hormones), and steroids (aldosterone, estrogen).

37. Steroid hormones are involved in signal transduction by changing the expression of specific genes. All of the steroid hormones are synthesized from cholesterol, and all have the same structure of four carbon rings but different side chains.

38. The five major classes of steroid hormones are progesterone, cortisol (glucocorticoid), aldosterone (mineralocorticoid), testosterone (androgen), and estradiol (estrogen).

Learning Bridge Answers

5.1 **A.** Bengay will temporarily relieve his muscle pain. It contains methyl salicylate, menthol, and camphor. Methyl salicylate is an analgesic but has a characteristic wintergreen odor that may not be appropriate for the patient because he is attending his prom tonight. While it is important to share this information, it is prudent to let the patient decide about Bengay.

B. "Hot packs", upon squeezing, produce heat that can assist the patient in relieving his muscle cramps and providing some muscle relaxation.

C. Hot packs contain a solid salt, $CaCl_2$, separated by a wall from water (all located inside the package). The package is activated when it is hit hard or squeezed hard to break the wall, with the $CaCl_2$ then becoming dissolved in the water. This exothermic reaction releases approximately −70 kJ/mol of heat.

D. Cold packs contain a solid salt, NH_4NO_3, separated by a wall from water (all located inside the package). The package is activated when it is hit hard enough to break the wall, with the NH_4NO_3 then becoming dissolved in the water. This endothermic reaction absorbs 25 kJ/mol of heat and, as a result, lowers the temperature to treat athletic injuries or a temporary headache.

5.2 **A.** The presence of uncommon amino acids in proteins usually is a result of chemical modifications of common amino acid side chains that occur in the post-translation process. For instance, hydroxylation of proline and lysine leads to formation of 4-hydroxyproline and 5-hydroxylysine, respectively. Collagen is rich in 4-hydroxyproline (the other common amino acid in collagen is glycine, which accounts for every third amino acid) and 5-hydroxylysine. There are two enzymes that hydroxylate proline and lysine, both of which require vitamin C as a coenzyme. Lack of vitamin C results in a fragile collagen, which in turn leads to fragile blood vessels, osteoporosis, and, in infants and children, abnormal bone development (this is one reason why infant food should contain vitamin C).

B. For a patient with red or swollen gums, bleeding gums, or a bleeding problem due to a small cut anywhere on the body (caused by fragile blood vessels), vitamin C is a good supplement to recommend. Obviously, the patient in this case spends his money on alcohol, so he has a poor diet (which means poor intake of vitamin C).

C. Make sure that the patient has no allergy to ascorbic acid. Counsel him to take Asco-Caps-500 with food if it upsets his stomach and to take the tablet with a full glass of water.

5.3 A. The wild-type enzyme has a lower K_m value, so it should have a higher affinity for the substrate (there is an inverse relationship between the affinity of a substrate and K_m).

B. The wild-type enzyme. The efficiency of an enzyme is indicated by its k_{cat}/K_m value. Despite the fact that the mutant enzyme has a higher k_{cat}, the k_{cat}/K_m ratio for the wild-type enzyme is large.

C. Neither enzyme will influence the equilibrium constant. Recall that enzymes influence the rate of a reaction by lowering the activation energy; they do not change the equilibrium constant. Thus the presence of an enzyme does not affect the amount of product generated.

5.4 Because the patient is drinking large amounts of alcohol, he must also have a problem with his diet. High consumption of ethanol results in high production of NADH (recall that the alcohol dehydrogenase enzyme oxidizes ethanol and, for that reason, reduces NAD to NADH). A lower level of NAD means a slower citric acid cycle because the citric acid cycle needs NAD to operate maximally (recall steps 4 and 8 in the citric acid cycle). This in turn leads to accumulation of acetyl-CoA, which may stop β oxidation of fatty acids. The excess of fatty acids, together with the glycerol presence, will lead to formation of many triacylglycerols. Large amounts of triacylglycerols means that the patient's blood must contain a large amount of either chylomicrons or very-low-density lipoprotein (VLDL). This patient is unlikely to have a large amount of chylomicrons because these usually come from dietary fats (in contrast to VLDL, which is produced by endogenous synthesis/biosynthesis of fats).

5.5 A. Joe is confused and has cirrhosis, and it is likely that he is poisoned by his own ammonium; thus the urea cycle in his liver is not functioning normally. The high concentration of ammonium could arise because one or more of the enzymes involved in the urea cycle are not working very well. A low-protein diet should reduce the amount of amino acid degradation, thereby reducing the amount of ammonium present.

B. You should contact the prescriber to change valproic acid to another antiepileptic drug. Valproic acid inhibits the regulatory enzyme carbamoyl phosphate synthetase I, thereby decreasing urea cycle function. Thus use of valproic acid increases the toxic ammonium level and causes hyperammonemia—a problem that Joe already has.

5.6 A. The indicated dose is used for a deficiency in the urea cycle enzymes carbamoyl phosphate synthetase I and ornithine transcarbamylase.

B. The urea cycle enzyme deficiencies decrease the rate at which the toxic ammonium is converted to urea. Therefore, low urea cycle activity will lead to a high level of ammonium in the body. Ammonul is used to reduce the toxic level of ammonium.

C. Ammonul consists of a mixture of sodium salts of phenylacetate and benzoate. In the liver, benzoate is conjugated with glycine to form hippuric acid, and sodium phenylacetate is conjugated with glutamine to form phenylacetylglutamine. Sequestering both glycine and glutamine forces cells to generate more of these two amino acids by incorporating the toxic ammonium into glycine and glutamine amino acids.

5.7 **A.** Phenylketonuria (PKU) is a genetic disease. Patients with PKU have a defect in either the phenylalanine hydroxylase enzyme, which hydroxylates phenylalanine to tyrosine, or dihydrobiopterin reductase, which catalyzes regeneration of tetra-hydrobiopterin. Patients with either or both of these deficiencies cannot convert phenylalanine to tyrosine (structurally they differ only in one hydroxyl group). If PKU is not detected or not treated, it can lead to mental retardation (see also Figure 5.55).

B. Because patients with PKU cannot convert phenylalanine into tyrosine, their synthesis of melanin is reduced (compare this condition with albinism). This is why patients with PKU also have a very light skin pigmentation.

C. Aspartame is an artificial sweetener that is synthesized from aspartic acid and phenylalanine. The C terminal (the carboxyl part) of phenylalanine is esterified to a methyl group. This dipeptide is metabolized in the body to its components: aspartic acid, phenylalanine, and methanol (an ester whose hydrolysis gives a carboxylic acid and an alcohol). Because Amy has PKU, she has to watch her consumption of any food or beverage that contains phenylalanine, including diet cola and aspartame.

D. Amy does not need to use any supplement to cut down the amount of sugar in her diet. Instead, Jennifer can help Amy improve her diet and perhaps engage in short exercises on a daily basis.

5.8 **A.** The injection of glucagon increases the secretion of epinephrine and norepinephrine, which then compete with the excess of the administered beta blocker.

B. The dose used in this scenario is much higher than the dose (1 mg) used to treat hypoglycemia.

C. A dose of epinephrine (up to 0.2 mg/kg) can be used as an antidote to treat a beta-blocker overdose. However, epinephrine is often reserved for the treatment of bronchospasm, bronchial asthma, anaphylactic reaction, and cardiac arrest. Glucagon injection is expensive, and not all hospitals use glucagon as an antidote as a remedy for beta-blocker overdose.

5.9 **A.** The excess of thyroid hormone interferes with the production of ATP through the increased level of expression of two uncoupling proteins, UCP2 and UCP3. As a consequence, fewer ATP molecules are produced for a given level of O_2 and fuel consumption. The uncoupling proteins generate heat. Most patients with hyperthyroidism complain of heat intolerance and sweatiness. The excessive perspiration is a result of dissipation of the excess heat through evaporation from the skin surface.

B. An elevated WBC count (leukocytosis) is often an indication of infection, signaled by increased production of granulocytes (neutrophils, basophils, and eosinophils). The patient does not have any fever. There is no sign of infection and the excess amount of T_4 present due to her hyperthyroidism explains her hot skin.

C. Due to the large amount of thyroid hormone present, Amy is overexpressing the genes that control the citric acid cycle and oxidative phosphorylation pathways, which results in a high metabolic rate. As a result, she is experiencing a weight loss.

Problems and Solutions

Problem 5.1 Calculate $\Delta G^{\circ\prime}$ for an acetic acid solution in water at 25°C. pK_a for HAc is 4.75.

Solution 5.1 You can utilize the dissociation constant to measure the value of $\Delta G^{\circ\prime}$ in this problem. The antilog of −4.75 will give you the dissociation constant for HAc, which is 1.75×10^{-5}.

$$\Delta G^{\circ\prime} = -RT \ln K'_{eq} = (-8.315 \text{ J/mol} \cdot \text{K}) \times (298 \text{ K}) \times \ln 1.75 \times 10^{-5} = 27.1 \text{ kJ/mol}$$

Problem 5.2 Suppose you go out hiking on a Sunday morning. Somewhere along the road, you collect wood to make a fire so that you can brew a cup of coffee. Describe how the boiling water obeys the first law of thermodynamics.

Solution 5.2 First law: The total energy change of the universe is constant.

$$\Delta E_{universe} = \Delta E_{system} + \Delta E_{surroundings} = 0$$

Suppose the water initially has (artificially) 1 kJ/mol of energy; at the boiling point, it has 100 kJ/mol of energy.

Let's first calculate the energy change for the system. Here, the system (water) will gain energy from the surroundings (wood). Initially the water will have 1 kJ/mol of energy, but after gaining the energy from the wood (heat) it will have 100 kJ/mol of energy, so the initial E is 1 and the final E is 100.

$$\Delta E_{system} = E_{final} - E_{initial} = 100 - 1 = +99$$

At the same time that this happens to the system (water), the opposite process happens to the surroundings (wood). Suppose the wood initially has an initial energy as much as 100 kJ/mol (remember—these are just artificial numbers). Upon burning, all of this energy is released as heat to the system (water). Thus the initial E is 100 and the final E is 1.

$$\Delta E_{surroundings} = E_{final} - E_{initial} = 1 - 100 = -99$$

Now revisit the first equation and see what happens to the total energy change of the universe:

$$\Delta E_{universe} = \Delta E_{system} + E_{surroundings} = +99 - 99 = 0$$

Problem 5.3 Identify whether each of the following statements is correct or false, and explain why.

  A. In a reaction under standard conditions, only the reactants are at 1 M.

  B. When $\Delta G^{\circ\prime}$ is positive, K'_{eq} is less than 1.

  C. ΔG and $\Delta G^{\circ\prime}$ have the same definition.

Solution 5. 3 All of them are false.

  A. Both reactants and products are fixed at 1 M.

  B. $\Delta G^{\circ\prime} = -RT \ln K'_{eq}$, so when $\Delta G^{\circ\prime}$ is less than 0, the term $-RT \ln K'_{eq}$ has a negative value and K'_{eq} is greater than 1.

  C. $\Delta G^{\circ\prime}$ is the difference in free energies of the products and reactants at standard conditions. ΔG is a variable that depends on $\Delta G^{\circ\prime}$, the temperature, and the concentrations of all reactants and products.

Problem 5.4 Suppose you mix an 0.1 M solution of glucose 1-phosphate with a mutase enzyme that catalyzes isomerization of glucose 1-phosphate to glucose 6-phosphate at room temperature. Assume that at equilibrium, the concentration of glucose-1-phosphate is 1×10^{-3} M and the concentration of glucose 6-phosphate is 1×10^{-2} M. Based on these data, calculate K'_{eq} and $\Delta G^{0\prime}$ in the direction of glucose 6-phosphate formation. $R = 8.315$ J/mol·K.

Solution 5.4 You have the concentration of reactant and product at equilibrium and the absolute temperature at room temperature is 298 K (273 + 25), so you can calculate K'_{eq}.

$$K'_{eq} = \frac{[\text{glucose 6-phosphate}]}{[\text{glucose 1-phosphate}]} = \frac{0.01 \text{ M}}{0.001 \text{ M}} = 10$$

$$\Delta G^{0\prime} = -RT \ln K'_{eq} = (-8.315 \text{ J/mol} \cdot \text{K}) \times (298 \text{ K}) \times (\ln 10) = -5.70 \text{ kJ/mol}$$

Problem 5.5 Under standard conditions, the reaction shown in Problem 5.5:

   A. will proceed spontaneously from left to right.

   B. will never reach equilibrium.

   C. will proceed at a rapid rate.

   D. will not occur at all.

   E. will proceed from left to right in the presence of an energy source such as ATP.

Solution 5.5 A is correct.

Problem 5.6 Explain why, in enzyme competitive inhibition, K_m is increased but V_{max} is unchanged.

Solution 5.6 The presence of a competitor reduces the binding of a substrate to an enzyme. As a result, the concentration of substrate needed to reach ½V_{max} (i.e., K_m) will increase. However, the effect of the inhibitor will be completely overcome by a high substrate concentration, so V_{max} will not be changed.

Problem 5.7 In a multienzymatic process, the regulatory enzymes are usually the first enzymes in the pathway. Why?

Solution 5.7 Catalyzing even the first few reactions of a pathway that produces an unwanted product is a waste of energy and resources. As a result, the first enzyme is often an ideal place to turn on or off the whole enzymatic sequence.

Problem 5.8 Why does the Lineweaver-Burk (double reciprocal) graph provide more accurate kinetics parameters compared with a simple V_0 versus [S] graph?

Solution 5.8 A graph of V_0 as a function of [S] is hyperbolic and the exact maximum velocity can never be achieved experimentally (it is not feasible to carry out experiments at infinitely high [S]). The Lineweaver-Burk transformation of the Michaelis-Menten equation, however, gives a linear plot that allows you to readily calculate the Michaelis-Menten kinetic parameters.

The Lineweaver-Burk equation can be obtained simply by inverting the Michaelis-Menten equation:

$$V_0 = \frac{K_{max}[S]}{K_m + [S]}$$

$$1/V_0 = \frac{K_m + [S]}{V_{max}[S]}$$

$$1/V_0 = \left(\frac{K_m}{V_{max}} \times \frac{1}{[S]}\right) + \frac{[S]}{V_{max}[S]}$$

$$1/V_0 = \left(\frac{K_m}{V_{max}} \times \frac{1}{[S]}\right) + \frac{1}{V_{max}}$$

The last equation is a Lineweaver-Burk equation and follows a linear equation. In a linear equation, you have $y = kx + m$, which is similar to the last equation in the preceding sequence. Here y is the y-axis ($1/V_0$ in the figure), k is the rate constant or slope (K_m/V_{max} in the figure), x is the x-axis ($1/[S]$ in the figure), and m is the intercept on the y-axis ($1/V_{max}$ in the figure). In addition, the x-axis intercept gives $-1/K_m$.

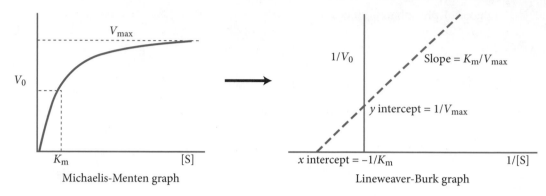

Transforming a Michaelis-Menten graph into a Lineweaver-Burk graph.

Problem 5. 9 You, as a PharmD working in a biotechnology company, obtain the following set of data for the alcohol dehydrogenase enzyme, which is known to metabolize alcohol with Michaelis-Menten kinetics.

Alcohol Concentration (μM)	Initial Velocity of Alcohol Dehydrogenase (μmol/min)
1	53
2	96
10	400
50	520
100	680
1,000	797
9,000	800

    A.   Calculate V_{max} for the alcohol dehydrogenase enzyme.

    B.   What is K_m for the enzyme?

Solution 5.9

    A. V_{max} is approximately 800 μmol/min, because when you increase the concentration of substrate (alcohol) by 9 times (from 1,000 to 9,000), the rate does not change as dramatically.

    B. K_m is 10 mM because K_m is the concentration of the substrate that gives half of the V_{max} value.

Problem 5.10 Suppose A is mixed with B to produce C and D: A + B → C + D. If the equilibrium constant for this reaction is 5,000, what sign (positive or negative) do you predict for the standard free energy change ($\Delta G^{o\prime}$) for the reaction? Is this reaction a spontaneous reaction? Why or why not?

Solution 5.10 $\Delta G^{\circ\prime} = -RT \ln K'_{eq}$. If K'_{eq} is a large (positive) number, the entire term $-RT \ln K'_{eq}$ (and therefore $\Delta G^{\circ\prime}$) has a relatively large negative value. It is a spontaneous reaction because $\Delta G^{\circ\prime}$ has a negative sign.

Problem 5.11 What is the difference between an exothermic process and an exergonic process?

Solution 5.11 In an exothermic process, the enthalpy (ΔH) is negative; in an exergonic process, the free energy change (ΔG) is negative. An exothermic process does not guarantee a spontaneous process (because of entropy, which also plays an important role). Conversely, an exergonic process means a spontaneous reaction.

Problem 5.12 Synthesis of an uncoupling protein in the mitochondrial inner membrane can:

    A. stop all mitochondrial metabolism.

    B. reduce the effectiveness of the citric acid cycle.

    C. stop mitochondrial ATP formation but still allow continued O_2 consumption.

    D. allow continued mitochondrial ATP formation but stop O_2 consumption.

Solution 5.12 C is correct.

Problem 5.13 Name four enzymes or classes of enzymes that are active in "mopping up" ammonium. (Hint: none of these enzymes is involved in the urea cycle.)

Solution 5.13 Aminotransferase enzymes, glutamate dehydrogenase, glutamine synthetase, and carbamoyl phosphate synthetase I.

Problem 5.14 Glutamine synthetase and glutaminase enzymes play an important role in removing the toxic ammonium from the body. Explain why.

Solution 5.14 The glutamine synthetase enzyme catalyzes addition of the toxic ammonium to glutamate to synthesize glutamine. Glutamine is transferred to the liver (through the blood), where its amino group is released from glutamine (by the glutaminase enzyme) to produce glutamate and ammonium. Ammonium is then used in the urea cycle to produce the harmless molecule, urea.

Problem 5.15 Why does a carbohydrate-rich food have a sleep-inducing effect?

Solution 5.15 An intake of carbohydrate-rich food increases the secretion of insulin as the body attempts to reduce the blood glucose level. However, insulin also increases the uptake of amino acids into muscles, which in turn reduces the amount of amino acids in the blood. The overall effect is to reduce competition between other amino acids and tryptophan so that tryptophan can reach the brain. In the brain, tryptophan is converted to serotonin, which in turn induces sleep. For the same reason, a protein-rich food results in a wakefulness condition.

Problem 5.16 Why does mutation in the binding site of GTP in glutamate dehydrogenase result in hyperinsulinism?

Solution 5.16 GTP works as a negative modulator for the glutamate dehydrogenase enzyme that catalyzes the oxidative deamination of glutamate in the mitochondria. When GTP cannot bind to its site on this enzyme, glutamate dehydrogenase will not be regulated. A lack of regulation increases the amounts of ammonium (which results in hyperammonemia) and α-ketoglutarate present. α-Ketoglutarate is a potential regulator of insulin secretion in pancreatic beta cells. A large amount of insulin will be released, which leads to hyperinsulinism. It has been suggested that the genetic disease known as hyperinsulinism hyperammonemia is caused by a mutation that alters the allosteric binding site for GTP.

Problem 5.17 Which of the following citric acid cycle intermediates can be converted to the inhibitory neurotransmitter GABA?

    A. α-Ketoglutarate

    B. Citrate

    C. Succinyl-CoA

    D. Malate

    E. Oxaloacetate

Solution 5.17 A is correct, because α-ketoglutarate can be converted to glutamic acid, which can then be converted to GABA.

Problem 5.18 Which of the following statements is incorrect regarding acetyl-CoA?

    A. Acetyl-CoA consists of an acetyl group (CH_3—C=O) attached to a coenzyme A molecule.

    B. Pyruvate dehydrogenase complex is a multienzyme complex (it includes three enzymes) that removes a carboxyl group from pyruvate to form acetyl-CoA.

    C. Both NAD^+ and FAD act as electron carriers in the formation of acetyl-CoA.

    D. Thiamine (vitamin B_1) is essential for the synthesis of acetyl-CoA.

    E. Glycolysis is the only pathway that produces pyruvate to synthesize acetyl-CoA.

Solution 5.18 E is incorrect, because ketogenic amino acids can also produce acetyl-CoA.

Problem 5.19 Phenylketonuria results from a defect in:

    A. phenylalanine hydroxylase.

    B. dihydrobiopterin reductase.

    C. tyrosinase.

    D. Both A and B.

    E. Bothe A and C.

Solution 5.19 D is correct.

Problem 5.20 Name the hydrophobic molecule that is a mobile component of the inner mitochondrial membrane and that collects electrons from NADH and passes them along to other electron carriers of the ETC.

Solution 5.20 Ubiquinone, which is also known as coenzyme Q (CoQ).

Problem 5.21 True or False: The nitrogen from the amide functional group of glutamine is a source of the amino group in many biosynthetic processes.

Solution 5.21 True; both glutamate and glutamine amino acids are the key amino acids that serve as nitrogen donors to many other molecules.

Problem 5.22 Which of the following molecules is *not* involved in the synthesis of nitric oxide (NO)?

    A. NADPH

    B. Arginine

    C. FAD

    D. NADH

    E. Tetrahydrobiopterin

Solution 5.22 D is correct.

Problem 5.23 Which of the following genetic diseases result(s) in a metabolic deficiency of tyrosine?

    A. Alkaptonuria

    B. Maple syrup urine disease

    C. Methylmalonic acidemia

    D. Albinism

Solution 5.23 Both A and D are correct.

Problem 5.24 A cell has a large single fat droplet that occupies a significant portion of the cell. Which type of cell is this?

    A. White adipose cell

    B. Brown adipose cell

    C. A pancreatic β cell

    D. Myocyte

    E. Hepatocye

Solution 5.24 A is correct. A brown adipose cell contains multiple small fat droplets.

Problem 5.25 Explain why during starvation and diabetes mellitus, the rate of glucose utilization is low.

Solution 5.25 During starvation, glucose utilization is low because of an inadequate glucose supply. Similarly, in untreated diabetes, glucose utilization is low because insulin is important to promote glucose uptake by myocytes and adipocytes.

Problem 5.26 An enzyme with and without an inhibitor shows different kinetics (see the table that follows). What are the values for K_m and V_{max} in the absence of the inhibitor? What kind of inhibition is it?

Substrate (µM)	Velocity (µmol/min) Without Inhibitor	Velocity (µmol/min) With Inhibitor
1	20	1
3	50	10
10	100	20
25	400	50
45	785	70
200	795	100
400	800	140

Solution 5.26 The first thing you need to do is to see whether the V_{max} is changed when the inhibitor is present. The V_{max} without the inhibitor is 800 µmol/min and half of it indicates the K_m (25 µM). The V_{max} is changed with the inhibitor. As a result, the K_m (45 µM) is changed too. This is a typical example of uncompetitive inhibition because both V_{max} and K_m are changed.

References

1. Amato AA, Barohn RJ. Peripheral neuropathy. In: Fauci AS, Kasper DL, Jameson JL, et al., eds. *Harrison's principles of internal medicine.* 18th ed. New York, NY: McGraw-Hill; 2012. Available at: http://www.accesspharmacy.com/content.aspx?aID=9148461.

2. Bender DA, Mayes PA. Metabolism of glycogen. In: Murray RK, Kennelly PJ, Rodwell VW, et al., eds. *Harper's illustrated biochemistry.* 29th ed. New York, NY: McGraw-Hill; 2011. Available at: http://www.accesspharmacy.com/content.aspx?aID=55882780.

3. Bender DA, Mayes PA. Nutrition, digestion, and absorption. In: Murray RK, Kennelly PJ, Rodwell VW, et al., eds. *Harper's illustrated biochemistry.* 29th ed. New York, NY: McGraw-Hill; 2011. Available at: http://www.accesspharmacy.com/content.aspx?aID=55885448.

4. Embury SH. Sickle cell disease. In: *AccessScience.* New York, NY: McGraw-Hill; 2008. Available at: http://www.accessscience.com.

5. Gigg RH. Lipid. In: *AccessScience.* New York, NY: McGraw-Hill; 2012. Available at: http://www.accessscience.com.

6. Horwich A, Fenton W. Molecular chaperone. In: *AccessScience.* New York, NY: McGraw-Hill; 2007. Available at: http://www.accessscience.com.

7. Interactive Chemistry Multimedia Courseware. *Solutions, solubility and precipitation, reaction rates, states of matter, bonding I and II.* Chico, CA: CyberEd, Inc.; 2001.

8. Kemp R. Thermodynamics (biology). In: *AccessScience.* New York, NY: McGraw-Hill; 2001. Available at: http://www.accessscience.com.

9. Kennelly PJ, Rodwell VW. Proteins: myoglobin and hemoglobin. In: Murray RK, Kennelly PJ, Rodwell VW, et al., eds. *Harper's illustrated biochemistry.* 29th ed. New York, NY: McGraw-Hill; 2011. Available at: http://www.accesspharmacy.com/content.aspx?aID=55881466.

10. Kishnani PS, Chen Y. Glycogen storage diseases and other inherited disorders of carbohydrate metabolism. In: Fauci AS, Kasper DL, Jameson JL, et al., eds. *Harrison's principles of internal medicine. 18th ed.* New York, NY: McGraw-Hill; 2012. Available at: http://www.accesspharmacy.com/content.aspx?aID=9144477.

11. Lee S, Lee G, Turner M. *BrainChip for biochemistry.* Williston, VT: Blackwell; 2002.

12. Longo N. Inherited disorders of amino acid metabolism in adults. In: Fauci AS, Kasper DL, Jameson JL, et al., eds. *Harrison's principles of internal medicine.* 18th ed. New York, NY: McGraw-Hill; 2012. Available at: http://www.accesspharmacy.com/content.aspx?aID=9144725.

13. Murray RK. Muscle and the cytoskeleton. In: Murray RK, Bender DA, Botham KM, et al., eds. *Harper's illustrated biochemistry.* 28th ed. New York, NY: McGraw Hill; 2009. Available at: http://www.accesspharmacy.com/content.aspx?aID=5230483.

14. Nelson DL, Cox MM. *Lehninger principles of biochemistry.* 5th ed. New York: W. H. Freeman and Company; 2008.

15. Osgood M, Ocorr K. *The absolute, ultimate guide to Lehninger principles of biochemistry.* 4th ed. New York: W. H. Freeman and Company; 2005.

16. Ouellette RJ. *Introduction to general, organic and biological chemistry.* 4th ed. Upper Saddle River: Prentice-Hall; 1997.

17. Pandey V, Perry JK, Mohankumar KM, et al. Autocrine human growth hormone stimulates oncogenicity of endometrial carcinoma cells. *Endocrinology* 2008;149(8):3909–3919.

18. Pelley JW, Goljan EF. *Biochemistry.* St. Louis: Mosby; 2003.

19. Pratt CW, Cornely K. *Essential biochemistry*, 2nd ed. Hoboken, NJ: John Wiley & Sons; 2011.

20. Raven P, Johnson G. *Biology.* 6th ed. New York: McGraw-Hill; 2002.

21. Russell RM, Suter PM. Vitamin and trace mineral deficiency and excess. In: Fauci AS, Braunwald E, Kasper DL, et al. *Harrison's principles of internal medicine.* 17th ed. New York: McGraw-Hill; 2008. Available at: http://www.accesspharmacy.com/content.aspx?aID=2865172.

22. Silberberg MS. *Chemistry: the molecular nature of matter and change.* 3rd ed. New York: McGraw-Hill; 2003.

23. Silberberg MS. *Principles of general chemistry.* New York: McGraw-Hill; 2006.

24. Smith C, Marks AD, Lieberman M. *Mark's basic medical biochemistry: a clinical approach.* 2nd ed. Baltimore, MD: LLW; 2005.

25. Talbert RL. Dyslipidemia. In: Talbert RL, DiPiro JT, Matzke GR, et al., eds. *Pharmacotherapy: a pathophysiologic approach.* 8th ed. New York, NY: McGraw-Hill; 2011. Available at: http://www.accesspharmacy.com/content.aspx?aID=7974214.

26. Timberlake KC. *Organic and biological chemistry: structures of life.* San Francisco, CA: Benjamin Cummings; 2001.

27. Tymoczko JL, Berg JM, Stryer L. *Biochemistry: a short course.* New York: W. H. Freeman and Company; 2010.

28. UpToDate. Waltham, MA: 2012. Available at: http://www.uptodate.com/online with subscription.

29. Wellner D, Royer, GP, Stellwag EJ. Enzyme. In: *AccessScience.* New York, NY: McGraw-Hill; 2008. Available at: http://www.accessscience.com.

30. Woodbury CP, Jr. *Biochemistry for the pharmaceutical sciences.* Burlington, MA: Jones & Bartlett Learning; 2012.

Introduction to Pharmacodynamics

Reza Karimi

1. Understand the physiology behind the gastrointestinal tract and the route of oral drug administration and physiological influences on pharmacodynamics.

2. Understand the dynamics and functions of the major signal transduction systems and their different biomedical and biological responses in regard to receptor–ligand interactions.

3. Learn about the dynamics and mathematical expressions behind receptor–ligand interactions.

4. Understand dose–response relationships and factors that affect a pharmacological response.

5. Learn about agonistic, antagonistic, and partial agonistic binding of drugs to receptors.

6. Learn about different concepts such as addition, synergism, and potentiation that lead to an enhancement effect of drugs.

7. List a few regulatory mechanisms for receptors.

8. Implement a series of Learning Bridge assignments at your experiential sites to bridge your didactic learning with your experiential experiences.

1. **cAMP:** cyclic adenosine 3',5"-monophosphate; a second messenger that plays an important role in signal transduction.

2. **cGMP:** cyclic guanosine 3',5"monophosphate; a second messenger that plays an important role in signal transduction.

3. **Dose–response relationship:** when an endogenous or exogenous ligand binds to a receptor and produces a pharmacological effect. The effect can approach a maximum value (also called E_{max}) in which a further increase in the ligand concentration does not produce any higher response.

4. **Efficacy:** the ability of a drug to produce a pharmacological response when it interacts with its receptor.

5. **First-pass metabolism:** a type of metabolism in which drugs that are absorbed by the gastrointestinal tract go through the portal vein to the liver and are metabolized there before they are distributed to the general circulation.

6. **Homeostasis:** a balanced physiological process that protects and maintains the integrity of the internal environment (e.g., an organ, a cell).

7. **IP_3:** inositol 1,4,5-triphosphate; it is generated from the cell membrane's phospholipids, diffuses through the cytoplasm to the endoplasmic reticulum, and binds to its receptor to stimulate Ca^{2+} channels to open and release Ca^{2+} into the cytoplasm.

8. **Isoforms:** two or more protein forms that have the same function but have been expressed by different genes.

(continues)

9. **Isozyme:** two or more enzymes that catalyze the same reaction but are expressed by different genes.

10. **MEC:** minimum effective concentration; the plasma drug concentration that produces the minimum pharmacological effect.

11. **MTC:** minimum toxic concentration; the plasma drug concentration that produces the minimum toxic effect.

12. **PDE:** a cyclic nucleotide phosphodiesterase enzyme that degrades either cAMP or cGMP.

13. **Pharmacokinetics (PK):** the study of the rate and extent of drug absorption, distribution, and elimination from the body.

14. **Pharmacodynamics (PD):** the study of the molecular interactions of drugs and receptors.

15. **Pharmacology:** the study of how drugs interact with the body to produce a biochemical or physiological effect.

16. **Physiological receptors:** receptors that can recognize and accept exogenous ligands.

17. **Potency:** a measure of the concentration (or dose) of a drug that produces 50% of the maximal effect.

18. **Protein kinases:** a class of enzymes that transfer a phosphate group from an ATP molecule to a protein.

19. **Receptors:** large intracellular or integral proteins that, by receiving chemical signals, play important roles in many physiological and cellular functions.

20. **Signal transduction:** the movement of signals from outside to inside of a cell, or vice versa.

Introduction

The field of pharmacodynamics studies how a ligand (endogenous or exogenous), such as a hormone or a neurotransmitter, binds to its receptor to produce a pharmacological response. In addition, pharmacodynamics is concerned with factors that affect the ligand–receptor binding. Signal transduction is the cornerstone of pharmacodynamics. This mechanism employs proteins in the form of enzymes or receptors that receive a specific signal and in a sensitive manner convert that signal to a series of biochemical and physiological events. As a result, the specificity and sensitivity of receptors and the concentration of ligands are of paramount importance in pharmacodynamics.

In this chapter, an introduction to physiology of homeostasis and the gastrointestinal (GI) tract is provided to lay the groundwork for appreciating how different factors affect the role of pharmacodynamics in oral absorption of drugs. The important roles that efficacy and potency play in producing a dose–response relationship are emphasized. In addition, different subtypes of ligand–receptor interactions, such as agonistic, antagonistic, and partial agonistic, and a few regulatory mechanisms for receptors are described.

Physiological Influences on Pharmacodynamics

Receptors are large proteins that play an important role in the field of pharmacodynamics. Receptors have the ability to amplify physiological signals and, as a result, they are potential targets for drugs. Receptors have two major functions: binding to their specific molecules (ligands) and sending signals (signal transduction) to a series of events. This dual function indicates that there must be at least two domains on a receptor: a ligand-binding domain and an effector domain. The unique characteristic of receptors is that they serve as proteins to recognize and accept endogenous and exogenous ligands. Exogenous ligands (xenobiotics or drug products) should, however, mimic the structures of the endogenous ligands. Receptors that can recognize and accept exogenous ligands are called physiological receptors.

Just as a drug's effect is produced after binding to a receptor, so can that effect be terminated when the drug dissociates from the receptor (although an exception exists in the form of "constitutive activity," a concept that is explained later on in this chapter). If a drug does not dissociate due to a very tight binding (such as a covalent bond), the effect continues to be produced as long as the receptor–drug complex remains intact. However, the latter process does not last too long because at some point the receptor–drug complex is degraded and eliminated, and a new free receptor is synthesized.

A drug molecule is considerably smaller in size than a receptor. The specific binding site on a receptor may be identified and studied. Intensive crystallography studies and genetic changes (mutations) in wild-type receptors have revealed important features of receptors, their binding sites, and their roles in pharmacodynamics. Because the affinity of a drug to a receptor and the chemical structure of a drug play important roles in producing a physiological effect, the effects of drugs depend on a combination of physiological and physicochemical factors. In addition, the pathophysiology may contribute to the effect of a drug. In other words, a drug may produce a different effect (or no effect at all) in an individual who does not have any abnormality in a cellular or physiological function. Conversely, a drug's effect can change due to a disease state. For instance, in patients who have cirrhosis accompanied by reduced hepatic metabolism, oral administration of drugs that extensively are metabolized by the liver will result in an increase in those drugs' systemic bioavailability (plasma level). Patients with liver cirrhosis also have a reduced glomerular filtration rate and renal plasma flow, which accounts for their decreased renal elimination of drugs such as fluconazole (Diflucan), lithium (Lithobid), and ofloxacin (Apo-Oflox, from Canada).

A variety of physiological and physicochemical factors affect pharmacodynamics, pharmacology, pharmacokinetics, biochemistry, and pharmaceutics. Often, these fields are integrated when a drug action is studied; thus it is not surprising when one finds overlapping factors that can affect all of the fields.

Physiology of Homeostasis

Higher-order eukaryotic organisms, including humans, are multicellular organisms with many unique and diverse cells. In fact, there are approximately 200 different cells in humans. Cells that are alike assemble to form a tissue. Several tissues, in turn, assemble to make an organ. An organ performs a specific function, and each organ belongs to an organ system. For instance, the heart is part of the cardiovascular system and the lungs are part of the respiratory system. Because there are many organ systems, there must be a coordination process between them to maintain the daily functions of the organism. This coordination process is carried out by the nervous system and the endocrine system.

Interestingly, nerve cells, after having grown and built a network with other nerve cells, do not divide (indeed, some nerve cells even die during embryonic deployment). In contrast, the cells of the endocrine system divide frequently, and some even adapt their growth based on a specific need. For instance, pancreatic cells are known to divide and grow as needed. To maintain homeostasis, the various organ systems work at different speeds. For instance, the autonomic nervous system rapidly adjusts to changes in the environment by releasing neurotransmitters to produce an effect. By comparison, the endocrine system acts much more slowly by releasing hormones into the systemic circulation, which can take hours and even days to produce any effect.

All organ systems (e.g., cardiovascular, respiratory, digestive, urinary) work together to maintain homeostasis. Homeostasis is a balanced physiological process that protects and maintains the integrity of the internal environment (e.g., an organ, a cell). For instance, when the digestive system breaks down proteins into amino acids, the cardiovascular system distributes those amino acids to the cells to protect the integrity of cells from starvation. Another example of homeostasis occurs when you suddenly stand up from a sitting position and your blood pressure falls (hypotension). This hypotensive effect immediately forces the nervous system to constrict your blood vessels to increase the blood pressure and return it to a normal level. Another example is when you maintain your blood glucose concentration at a constant level (at 5 mM). While your muscles take up glucose from your blood, your liver supplies more glucose to the blood to maintain the level of blood glucose at a constant 5 mM.

Through evolution, organisms have developed a remarkable collection of regulatory mechanisms for maintaining homeostasis. If the homeostasis does not work correctly, however, we become sick. In the glucose uptake example, if your muscle cells (myocytes) cannot take up sufficient glucose from your blood (because of a lack of insulin), your blood glucose level will be high (diabetes). This excess level of glucose produces many severe physiological consequences—ketoacidosis, for example, is a life-threatening condition.

Understanding drug absorption, the physiology of the GI tract, and the various factors that affect drug absorption can assist students in understanding the important role that pharmacodynamics plays when drugs interact with receptors and other macromolecules in the body. Because the majority of drugs are administered orally, a brief overview of GI physiology and oral drug absorption is provided in the following subsections.

Physiology and Routes of Oral Drug Absorption

After oral drug administration, the drug, which could be in a solid form (e.g., tablets, capsules) or a liquid dosage form (e.g., emulsion, suspension), enters the esophagus. It has only a short transit time there, which makes the esophagus a poor site for absorption of orally administered drugs. After its passage through the esophagus, the drug is dissolved in the GI tract. The GI tract includes the stomach, the small intestine (which includes the duodenum, jejunum, and ileum), and the large intestine. Finally, the GI tract ends in the rectum. The various areas of the GI tract have their own characteristics (pH, surface area, and secretions) and, therefore, differently influence drug absorption. It is from one of these areas that the drug will be absorbed into the circulation and thereby reach its site of action.

The anatomy of the GI tract includes four layers of tissues: mucosa, submucosa, muscularis external, and serosa (**Figure 6.1**).

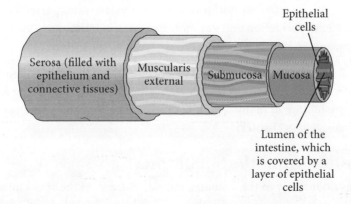

Figure 6.1 Different layers of the GI tract.

The mucosa itself is made of three layers:

- Epithelial cells, which are in contact with the intestinal content
- Lamina propria, which is the underlying supportive tissue of the epithelial cell and contains blood vessels, lymphatic vessels, and nerves
- A layer of muscle fibers (muscularis mucosa)

The absorption of drugs occurs through the epithelial cells into the blood capillaries of the lamina propria; the blood carrying these cells then travels through capillaries into the rest of the body. These epithelial cells are tightly packed (tight junction) to allow drugs (particularly un-ionized or hydrophobic drugs) to pass through a passive transcellular diffusion (see also the *Introduction to Pharmacokinetics* chapter).

Drug Absorption from the Stomach

The mucosa of the stomach wall has hundreds of gastric glands. Each gastric gland contains four major types of cells:

- *Mucous neck cells* secrete mucins. Mucins are large glycoproteins that form a mucous layer that adheres to the surface of epithelial cells of the stomach to protect those cells from gastric acid. These epithelial cells secrete HCO_3^- ions that become trapped in the mucous layer and make this layer neutral (pH = 7.0). Anything (e.g., NSAIDs, *Helicobacter pylori* bacterial infection) that destroys the mucosal integrity can cause an ulcer.

- *Parietal cells* have the H^+-K^+ ATPase enzyme on the surface of their cell membranes. The H^+-K^+ ATPase exchanges an H^+ ion (pumps it out to the stomach) for each K^+ ion (pumps it into the parietal cell). The K^+ ions that have been pumped into the cell enter the interstitial fluid by K^+ channels. It is the H^+ that makes the stomach an acidic environment. The stomach already has a high concentration of H^+, so pumping H^+ from an area of a low concentration (parietal cell) to an area of high concentration (stomach) requires an active transporter system (ATPase) and energy in the form of ATP molecules. Parietal cells also have receptors for histamine (a hormone), gastrin (a hormone), and acetylcholine (a neurotransmitter).

- *Chief cells* secrete pepsinogen. The secretion of HCl assists in converting pepsinogen (an inactive precursor or zymogen) to active pepsin. Pepsin needs to be in an acidic environment (pH of 1–3) to be in its active form. The role of pepsin is to degrade proteins into small fragments of polypeptides in the stomach. Pepsin is inactivated reversibly and irreversibly at pH 4 and 7, respectively.

- *Enteroendocrine cells* secrete four hormones: histamine (activates parietal cells), serotonin (stimulates stomach contraction and gut motility), gastrin (stimulates parietal cells to release HCl), and somatostatin (inhibits the effect of gastrin).

Due to the short transit time (less than 1 hour) of a drug in the stomach, no significant drug absorption occurs from this part of the GI tract. However, the stomach's gastric acid assists with disintegration and dissolution of many oral solid drugs, including tablets and capsules (see also the *Introduction to Pharmaceutics* chapter).

Drug Absorption from the Small Intestine

The dissolved drugs do not stay in the stomach, but rather travel to the small intestine. Due to the collectively large surface area of the villi that are lined with epithelial and goblet cells and the 4-hour transit time of drugs, many drugs are absorbed from the small intestine. Each villus of the small intestine has a supportive network of capillaries (**Figure 6.2**). Many drugs and nutrients are

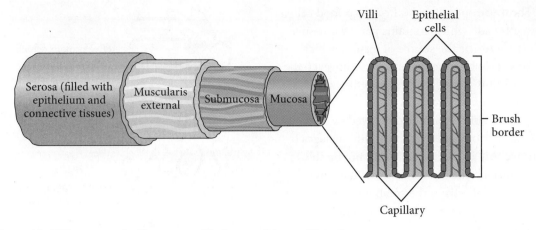

Figure 6.2 Villi occupy a significant area of the lumen of the small intestine.

absorbed into these capillaries and then move into the portal vein. The pH of the small intestine is higher due to the secretion of bicarbonate from the pancreas into the small intestine. The greatest surface areas of the small intestine are found in the duodenum and jejunum, because the villi are found in their highest concentration in these two areas. Therefore, the majority of drugs are absorbed from these two areas.

Drug Absorption from the Large Intestine

The large intestine does not have any villi, so it does not provide an adequate surface area for a drug absorption. However, the large intestine plays an important role in the absorption of water and electrolytes into the circulation. The pH of the large intestine is approximately 7. Keep in mind if a drug is not fully absorbed in the small intestine, it may be absorbed from the large intestine. However, often drugs are not absorbed in this organ, but rather are excreted in the feces.

Many factors affect the role of pharmacodynamics in oral absorption of drugs. For instance, it has been suggested that the sensitivity of β-adrenergic receptors declines as we get older. As a result, elderly patients may respond to a β-adrenergic blocker differently compared with younger patients. In addition, aging reduces the levels of testosterone, a sex hormone, in both men and women, which may in turn affect the intracellular receptor binding of steroids. Other factors that can affect the absorption of drugs (particularly orally administered drugs) include gastric acid, molecular size of drugs, first-pass metabolism, cytochrome P450 enzymes, foods, drug formulation, disintegration and dissolution rates, blood flow, solubility, pH and pK_a, intestinal microflora, efflux transporters, transcytosis, and carrier-mediated transporters. While some of these factors are discussed in this chapter, others are discussed elsewhere in this text.

Gastric Acid

Polypeptides and proteins are denatured in the acidic environment of the stomach (**Figure 6.3**). The more a drug is denatured, the more it is prone to attack by the enzyme pepsin (pepsin hydrolyzes polypeptides and proteins into small fragments). Insulin (a peptide hormone) is an example of a compound that is destroyed by the acidic milieu of the stomach. Some drugs are acid-labile (acid-sensitive). One typical example is the members of the penicillin class, which lose their effectiveness due to the acidic degradation of penicillin. Another example is erythromycin, which is destroyed by gastric acid. However, enteric-coated and esterified forms of erythromycin are stable in gastric acid.

Some Europeans and others eat a food called "sweetbread," which contains pancreas tissue. The pancreas is the source of insulin, which affects carbohydrate metabolism. However, the high insulin content in the "sweetbread" does not interfere with carbohydrate metabolism because insulin is simply destroyed by the acidic pH of the stomach. Even if insulin manages to survive this acidic milieu, it will not be able to pass through the aqueous mucus that covers the epithelial cells in the small intestine (see the discussion of the molecular size of drugs in the next subsection).

By the same token, some drugs actually need gastric acid to be effectively absorbed. One example is ferrous sulfate (Feosol), an iron supplement. Another example is oral ketoconazole (Apo-Ketoconazole, from Canada), an antifungal agent. As a result and to increase the absorption of these drugs, pharmacists should advise their patients to take these drugs with orange juice (which has citric acid) and administer them at least 2 hours before taking any antacids or acid suppressive agents.

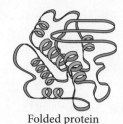

Active protein, which may resist proteolysis

Folded protein

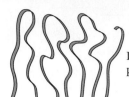

Inactive protein, which is prone to proteolysis

Denatured protein

Figure 6.3 Properly folded proteins are unfolded and denatured in the acidic milieu of the stomach.

Molecular Size of Drugs

Goblet cells are the second most abundant cells (after epithelial cells) on the villi. Goblet cells produce a mucous layer that makes a film inside the lumen of the small intestine to cover the epithelial cells. The mucous layer does not allow large drug molecules (larger than 800 daltons) to reach the epithelial cells. For instance, low-molecular-weight heparin (LMWH), also known as enoxaparin (Lovenox), is an anticoagulant that is given intravenously (IV) or subcutaneously (SC) and is used to treat thrombosis. An oral dosage form of enoxaparin will, however, have limited oral absorption because enoxaparin, due to its large molecular weight (more than 4,000 g/mol), cannot go through the mucous layer of the GI tract. Therefore, enoxaparin is administered only as an IV or SC formulation. Insulin is another example; its molecular weight is more than 5,000 g/mol, so it cannot pass through the mucous layer of the GI tract.

First-Pass Metabolism

Many drugs that are absorbed by the GI tract go through the portal vein to the liver before they are distributed to the general circulation. The reason is that all of the venous blood from the stomach, the small intestine, and the large intestine enters the portal vein and then moves to the liver. Approximately 75% of all blood that reaches the liver does so via the portal vein. In the liver, the drugs carried in this blood are metabolized (first-pass metabolism). For example, propranolol (Inderal LA), an antihypertensive agent, has a high first-pass metabolism. This effect means that a total of 100–200 mg orally administered propranolol tablets, in essence, equals 1–3 mg of an intravenous injection of propranolol.

Food

A drug may interact with a specific chemical component of a food in a manner that makes the drug–component combination an insoluble complex. For instance, absorption of digoxin

(Lanoxin), and thereby this drug's plasma concentration, is decreased by foods that contain fiber or are high in pectin. Similarly, members of the tetracycline drug class interact with calcium, magnesium, zinc, iron, and aluminum. Because these ions reduce the absorption of tetracycline, patients should take tetracycline antibiotics at least 2 hours before taking any iron supplements or antacids.

Another example of a food's effect on drug metabolism can be seen with the effect of leafy vegetables on warfarin (Coumadin). Patients who take warfarin should maintain consistency in their intake of green leafy vegetables. These vegetables contain large amounts of vitamin K; vitamin K, in turn, is important for the formation of prothrombin, a blood protein that plays a key role in the blood clotting process. Changing the amount of vitamin K (inconsistency in the intake of green leaves), therefore, changes the therapeutic effect of warfarin. For this reason, patients should be advised not to change their dietary habits once they are stabilized on warfarin.

The absorption of omeprazole is also reduced by food. Because consumption of food increases stomach acid, this drug will be released into stomach rather than at its actual site of action—that is, the parietal cells lining the stomach.

Consumption of some foods also slows gastric emptying, which in turn delays the transport of drugs from stomach to small intestine and may affect drug absorption. Conversely, consumption of fiber (fruit) and whole grains can sometimes cause diarrhea, which causes a drug to move quickly throughout the GI tract (less transition time and thereby less drug absorption). Penicillin derivatives are also known to cause diarrhea. Because the diarrhea causes a drug to move quickly throughout the GI tract, many drugs may not effectively be absorbed when they are administered concurrently with penicillin derivatives.

Effects of Age

The stomach acidity is low (achlorhydria) in infants (1 month to 1 year). This leads to an increased absorption of basic drugs (which are less ionized in a higher pH) and decreased absorption of acidic drugs (which are more ionized in a higher pH) through gastric membranes. In addition, gastric motility (gastric emptying time) is slowed in infants, which results in slow absorption of oral drugs in the small intestine. However, their gastric motility is fully developed within the first 6 to 8 months of life. Aminoglycosides (e.g., neomycin, amikacin, gentamicin) have a longer half-life ($t_{1/2}$) in children who are younger than 6 months, in part because they have a reduced renal elimination rate.

Age also affects the level of serum albumin. Serum albumin is an abundant protein in the blood that binds reversibly to many drugs. Drugs that are bound to albumin are pharmacologically inactive because only free drug can bind to receptors or act on other targets. The amount of serum albumin is low in infants, which results in higher concentrations of unbound drugs (more effect). Similarly, malnourished elderly patients have lower serum albumin, which may increase the effect (or toxicity) of certain drugs. In addition, a low serum albumin leads to a higher blood flow; in other words, the more albumin, the more viscous the blood is. Albumin has the highest affinity for weakly acidic and hydrophobic drugs.

Similar to the case for the pediatric population, members of the geriatric population tend to have decreased stomach acidity. Decreased stomach acidity leads to reduced absorption of a few drugs. As mentioned earlier, iron supplements or oral ketoconazole are best absorbed when taken with an orange juice. Atazanavir (Reyataz) and indinavir (Crixivan), two antiviral agents (see the *Introduction to Microbiology* chapter), require normal acid levels in the stomach for their optimal absorption.

The total body water (TBW) accounts for 60% of total body weight in men and 50% of total body weight in women. While two-thirds of TBW is located in the intracellular compartment, one-third is located in the extracellular compartment. TBW is reduced in elderly patients because of reduced muscle mass and increased lipid storage. Because of the higher rate of lipid storage in such individuals, the availability of hydrophobic drugs in the plasma is low (see the *Introduction to Pharmacokinetics* chapter), which results in a delay in these drugs reaching the excretory organs (e.g., liver, kidneys). The latter process results in an increased duration of action for the drugs.

Elderly individuals are also prone to be affected by physiological changes of aging or patho-physiological consequences that arise from one or more diseases. For instance, the hepatic first-pass effect is reduced in the elderly population, which results in lower hepatic metabolism and ultimately leads to increased plasma concentration of drugs. Likewise, aging reduces the density and sensitivity of receptors. For instance, it has been suggested that the sensitivity of muscarinic, β-adrenergic, α_1-adrenergic, and μ-opioid receptors declines as a consequence of aging. A change in receptors' sensitivity may cause a change in the affinity between a drug and a receptor, a change in the binding of a drug to a receptor, or a change in the structure and function of a receptor.

Obesity

Obesity affects both pharmacokinetics and pharmacodynamics by altering the volume of distribution. The more lipid storage that occurs, the higher the volume of distribution will be for hydrophobic drugs. In turn, the higher the volume of distribution, the longer the half-life of drugs (lower elimination rate; see also the *Introduction to Pharmacokinetics* chapter). For instance, hydrophobic drugs such as benzodiazepines have lower elimination rates in obese patients. Moreover, weight gain often results in insulin resistance. It has been suggested that obese individuals who are not diabetic may have the same level of insulin resistance as patients who have type 2 diabetes. One explanation for this phenomenon could be too much circulating fatty acid in the blood. Fatty acids interfere with glucose uptake into muscle (insulin resistance). This effect could also explain why pregnant women, who produce large amounts of fatty acids, are prone to develop insulin resistance (i.e., gestational diabetes).

Receptors

Many important physiological and biological functions are accomplished by chemical messengers—that is, hormones or ions that arrive via the bloodstream or neurotransmitters that are released by nerve cells. These messengers are received by receptors. Many hydrophilic hormones (e.g., peptide hormones such as insulin and glucagon) interact with receptors located in the plasma membrane and transmit signals to the cytoplasm. The entire process is called transmembrane signaling. In contrast, hydrophobic hormones (thyroid, steroid, and retinoid hormones) are able to cross the cell membrane and interact with their intracellular receptors located inside the cells. As a result, these hydrophobic ligands do not have any transmembrane receptors, but rather have intracellular receptors.

Most often the interaction between the messenger and the receptor is achieved noncovalently, similar to an enzyme–substrate interaction. Hormones are ligands that are the "first messengers," whereas Ca^{2+}, cAMP, IP_3, diacylglycerol, and cGMP are the "second messengers" that are released or synthesized when the hormone binds to its receptor. The roles of second messengers are to stimulate or inhibit a series of biochemical events in the cytoplasm or nucleus.

Many drugs mimic the endogenous ligands and, as a result, are able to bind to physiological receptors. By binding to receptors, these drugs—much like the endogenous ligands—initiate a series of events that leads to biochemical changes in a cell and ultimately results in pharmacological responses. Because receptors play important roles in receiving extracellular signals and turn those signals into intracellular signals, any alteration in receptors' affinity for their ligands can have immediate biochemical and physiological impacts.

Not all proteins in the plasma membranes are receptors. While some proteins are receptors, others serve as transporters, ion channels, or enzymes. These proteins have essential functions as well. For instance, due to the hydrophobic nature of the lipid bilayer of the plasma membrane, anions and cations cannot readily cross plasma membranes. The influx and outflow of ions are critical regulatory events in both excitable and nonexcitable cells. To maintain the electrochemical gradients required to maintain or produce a membrane potential, all cells express ion transporters for Na^+, K^+, Ca^{2+}, and Cl^-. For instance, the human body expresses more than 200 different ion channels to regulate precisely the flow of Na^+, K^+, Ca^{2+}, and Cl^- across the cell membranes.

The names of receptors are often designated based on the names of the ligands (or a class of ligands) that they bind. For instance, while insulin (ligand) binds to an insulin receptor, norepinephrine (ligand) binds to adrenergic receptors. A single cell may have different receptors for different ligands—for example, a hepatocyte has receptors for insulin and glucagon ligands. In addition, the same receptor for a ligand could be expressed in different cells. For example, insulin receptors are largely expressed on hepatocytes, myocytes, and adipocytes.

Signal transduction refers to the movement of chemical signals (e.g., hormones, neurotransmitters, second messengers) from outside a cell to inside the cell. The movement of signals can follow a simple path, like the ion channels of the plasma membrane that open and close in response to a chemical ligand, or can be more complex, like the coupling of ligand–receptor interactions that leads to a series of protein activation and phosphorylation steps that change enzyme activities and protein conformations in the cytoplasm of a cell.

Transmembrane Signaling and Signal Transduction

The terms *transmembrane signaling* and *signal transduction* have often been used interchangeably, even though there is a slight distinction between the two. Transmembrane signaling refers to sending an extracellular signal through a cell membrane receptor. Signal transduction is a much broader concept, referring to sending a signal through a cell membrane where the receptor may not be an embedded cell membrane receptor, but rather an intracellular receptor. For simplicity, the term "signal transduction" is used throughout this chapter.

Six signal transduction systems are employed by receptors:

1. Gated ion channels
2. Receptor enzymes
3. Serpentine receptors
4. Receptors for hydrophobic ligands
5. Receptors without intrinsic enzyme activity
6. Adhesion receptors

Before these receptors are described and their signaling roles are elucidated, it is necessary to explain a few important molecules that are involved in the signaling pathways.

Adenylyl Cyclase

Adenylyl cyclase (AC) is a large membrane-bound enzyme that is folded multiple times inside the cell membrane. It has 12 transmembrane regions, with two bundles of 6 transmembrane components. Adenylyl cyclase catalyzes the synthesis of cyclic adenosine-3',5'-monophosphate (cAMP) by acting on an ATP molecule. Ten isoforms have been identified to date, including a recently identified free isoform (soluble) in mammalian sperm. Each isoform has a unique tissue expression and distribution, which may indicate AC catalyzes the formation of cAMP in many different tissues. Each AC has two regulatory components—stimulatory G proteins (designated as Gs) and inhibitory G proteins (designated as Gi)—that stimulate and inactivate the catalytic activity of AC, respectively. Due to AC's involvement in many signaling pathways, certain hormones stimulate AC (e.g., calcitonin, glucagon, epinephrine, antidiuretic hormone) while others inhibit AC (e.g., acetylcholine, somatostatin, angiotensin II).

Guanylyl Cyclase

Guanylyl cyclase, similar to AC, catalyzes formation of a cyclic nucleotide, cyclic guanosine monophosphate (cGMP). Guanylyl cyclase exists in two forms: type 1 (transmembrane) and type 2 (a heme-containing soluble enzyme). There are seven isoforms of type 1 and four isoforms of type 2. Guanylyl cyclases are found in most tissues.

Cardiac atrial tissue (atrial myocytes) express a short peptide (28 amino acids) called atrial natriuretic peptide (ANP) that has important roles in natriuresis, diuresis, vasodilation, and inhibition of aldosterone secretion. The ANP activates the membrane-bound guanylyl cyclase, which results in an increased rate of synthesis of cGMP. In addition, nitric oxide hormone (and even compounds that contain NO) activates the soluble guanylyl cyclase to synthesize cGMP.

Cyclic Adenosine Monophosphate

The second messenger cAMP is synthesized by the adenylyl cyclase enzyme. Cyclic AMP plays important roles in many cellular functions, including cell growth and differentiation, regulation of gene expression, and apoptosis. While cAMP has many targets, perhaps the most relevant one in this chapter is the cyclic AMP-dependent protein kinase (PKA) that is involved in the adrenergic receptors' roles and functions (see the discussion of the role of epinephrine in serpentine receptors later in this chapter).

cAMP is rapidly degraded by an enzyme called cyclic nucleotide phosphodiesterase. As will be discussed in conjunction with serpentine receptors in this chapter, cAMP is involved in activation of glycogen phosphorylase *a* and glycogenolysis and, as a result, plays a significant role in increasing the blood glucose levels.

Cyclic Guanosine Monophosphate

The guanylyl cyclase enzyme catalyzes formation of cyclic GMP by acting on a GTP molecule. Similar to the inactivation of cAMP, cGMP phosphodiesterase (PDE) enzyme degrades cGMP. A few agents, such as sildenafil (Viagra) and tadalafil (Cialis), inhibit cGMP phosphodiesterase (PDE) to increase the level of cGMP. The cyclic GMP plays a major role in promoting smooth muscle relaxation by inhibiting calcium influx, activating potassium channels, and stimulating cGMP-dependent kinase (PKG)—mechanisms that will be discussed further later in this chapter.

Calcium

Calcium is another important second messenger that plays important roles in the signal transduction. The concentration of Ca^{2+} in the cytoplasm is very low (10^{-6} M), while the concentration outside the cell and inside the endoplasmic reticulum (ER) is 10^{-3} M. Calcium regulates a series of responses that include gene expression, contraction, secretion, and metabolism. It can enter a cell through ion channels (Ca^{2+} channels) that are located in the plasma membrane or it can be released from intercellular storage by hormones or growth factors. For instance, when the calcium channels in the ER open, Ca^{2+} is released into the cytoplasm. Intracellular Ca^{2+} levels cause skeletal muscle cells to contract and stimulate some endocrine cells to secrete hormones.

Because calcium plays an important role in many cellular functions, disruption of calcium influx or efflux can have severe physiological consequences. For instance, damage to the ligand-gated Ca^{2+} channel or voltage-gated Ca^{2+} channel (discussed later) causes Ca^{2+} to move down its concentration gradient into the cytoplasm of cells. The resulting increase in intracellular Ca^{2+} inhibits the ATPase enzyme during oxidative phosphorylation (which results in less synthesis of ATP), alters the function of microfilaments, enhances the activation of hydrolytic enzymes, and increases the generation of reactive species such as reactive nitrogen species (RNS) and reactive oxygen species (ROS), which ultimately damage many other cells.

Some of the serpentine receptors (see the discussion of serpentine receptors later in this chapter), by binding to their ligands, activate their G protein, Gq. For example, when the oxytocin or vasopressin hormones bind to their receptors, the α subunit of Gq in turn binds to and activates a plasma membrane enzyme called phospholipase C. Phospholipase C catalyzes the production of two other second messengers, inositol 1,4,5-triphosphate (IP_3) and diacylglycerol, from the phosphatidylinositol 4,5-bisphosphate found in the plasma membrane. IP_3 has its own receptor. This IP_3 receptor is a large protein and is found in high concentrations in the membrane of the ER. The role of IP_3 molecules is to diffuse through the cytoplasm to the ER and bind to the specific IP_3 receptor. The binding of IP_3 to its receptor stimulates Ca^{2+} channels to open and releases Ca^{2+} into the cytoplasm (**Figure 6.4**). The released Ca^{2+}, together with the diacylglycerol, activates another protein kinase, PKC, which in turn phosphorylates a variety of proteins to change their activities and, consequently, to mediate a wide range of signaling events.

Calcium regulates a number of enzymes, often through a Ca^{2+} binding protein called calmodulin. This small protein is found in all eukaryotic cells. Due to its unique structure, calmodulin is able

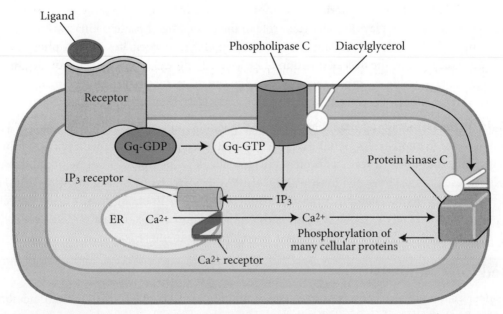

Figure 6.4 Binding of a ligand to its receptor activates phospholipase C, which in turn releases diacylglycerol and IP_3 from the phospholipids of the cell membrane. The overall results are to increase intracellular Ca^{2+} and activate protein kinase C.

Adapted from: Nelson DL, Cox MM, and Lehninger AL. *Principles of biochemistry*, 5th ed. New York: W. H. Freeman and Company; 2008: Chapter 12.

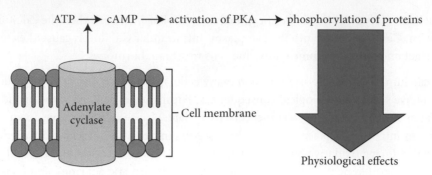

Figure 6.5 The cAMP-dependent protein kinase A (PKA) is activated by cAMP that is synthesized by the adenylate cyclase enzyme.

to bind four calcium ions and, therefore, serves as an intracellular receptor for regulatory calcium signals. An increase in cytosolic Ca^{2+} concentration allows Ca^{2+} to bind to the four binding sites on calmodulin. As a consequence of the Ca^{2+} binding, calmodulin undergoes a conformational change that allows it to interact with other cytoplasmic proteins to influence a series of cellular responses. The activation of calmodulin by Ca^{2+} is similar to the activation of PKA by cAMP, except here the Ca^{2+}–calmodulin complex has no enzymatic activity on its own, but rather activates other proteins and enzymes.

Protein Kinases

Protein kinases are a class of enzymes that transfer a phosphate group from an ATP molecule to a protein—a reversible process called protein phosphorylation. Protein phosphorylation is primarily directed at serine, threonine, and tyrosine amino acid residues in proteins (all of these amino acid residues have an OH group; see also the *Introduction to Cell Biology* chapter). Nearly one-third of our proteins inside of cells are phosphorylated by protein kinases. More than 100 protein kinases have been identified in humans; indeed, the human genome has about 500 protein kinase genes. Protein phosphorylation plays an important role in the regulation of protein kinases. For instance, protein kinase A (PKA) is not activated until a cAMP molecule participates in PKA phosphorylation (**Figure 6.5**). While the overall function of kinases is to phosphorylate other proteins, there are considerable differences among them in regard to their size, subunit composition, autophosphorylation, kinetic parameters (e.g., K_m, k_{cat}), and substrate specificity.

One of the major roles of protein kinases is the regulation of the cell cycle. The passage of a cell from one phase to another through the cell cycle is controlled by proteins called cyclins. Cyclins are regulatory subunits of a series of protein kinases called cyclin-dependent protein kinases (CDKs). These proteins have no kinase activities unless they are tightly bound to the cyclins. For instance, while CDK1 facilitates the transition from the G_2 phase to the M phase during the cell cycle, CDK2 initiates DNA synthesis in the early S phase (**Figure 6.6**). To date, 9 CDKs (referred to as CDK1 through CDK9) and 11 cyclins have been identified in humans.

Gated Ion Channels

Many drugs act on their receptors to stimulate or inhibit the influx of ions through cell membrane channels. For instance, a few drugs that cause calcium influx can affect the release of neurotransmitters and gene expression. Similarly, endogenous ligands can bind to their receptors and open ion channels. For instance, the endogenous ligand known as acetylcholine binds to acetylcholine receptor and increases the Na^+ influx from the extracellular fluid into the cells. Based on gating

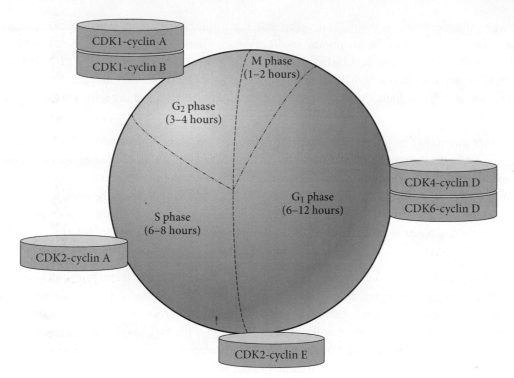

Figure 6.6 The eukaryotic cell cycle and the points where cyclin-dependent protein kinases (CDKs) are activated by different cyclins.

Adapted from: Murray RK, Jacob M, Varghese J. Cancer: an overview. In: Murray RK, Kennelly PJ, Rodwell VW, et al., eds. *Harper's illustrated biochemistry*, 29th ed. New York: McGraw-Hill; 2011. Available at: http://www.accesspharmacy.com /content.aspx?aID=55887057.

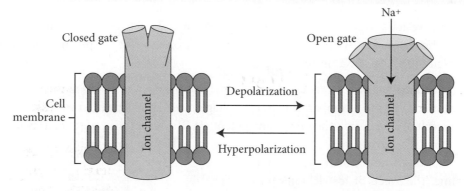

Figure 6.7 Voltage-gated ion channels open and close as a result of changes in the cell membrane potential.

mechanisms, the gated ion channels are classified as either voltage-gated ion channels or ligand-gated ion channels. The movement of ions across these two gates results in an influx of cations into the cell to cause depolarization or an influx of anions to cause hyperpolarization.

Voltage-Gated Ion Channels

Voltage-gated ion channels do not bind to their ligands directly, but rather (and as their name indicates) respond and are controlled by a change in the membrane potential. In other words, the opening probability of these channels depends on the membrane voltage (**Figure 6.7**). Voltage-gated ion channels provide a major pathway for K^+, Cl^-, Na^+, and Ca^{2+} ions in many types of cells. For example, K^+, Na^+, and Ca^{2+} gates open when the membrane potential becomes more positive inside (i.e., when the membrane potential is depolarized). For instance, the voltage-gated Na⁺ channels are closed when the voltage of the membrane is –60 mV (i.e., when the membrane is at rest), but are open when the membrane is depolarized (i.e., when the inside of the cell is positive). The depolarization effect arrives when acetylcholine binds to its receptor. These ion channels are very selective and the rate of influx is high. For instance, the Na⁺ channel is 100 times more selective for Na⁺ than for Ca^{2+} or K⁺ ions, and the rate of ion influx is more than 10 million Na⁺ ions per second.

Another example of how the voltage-gated ion channels work, and indeed communicate with other channels, is when the opening of Na⁺ channels in the previous example causes depolarization of nerve cells, which in turn opens the voltage-gated Ca^{2+} channels and results in an influx of Ca^{2+} ions. An increased entry of intracellular Ca^{2+} into the presynaptic neuron results in the release of acetylcholine neurotransmitter from the secretory vesicles containing acetylcholine into the synaptic cleft. The acetylcholine binds to its receptor on the next neuron and causes opening of voltage-gated Na⁺ channels. The entire cycle is then repeated to send the action potential from one neuron to another.

Use of the calcium-channel blocker agent, verapamil (Calan), demonstrates how blocking these channels causes a physiological change. Verapamil inhibits voltage-gated calcium channels in the vascular smooth muscle and myocardium so as to reduce blood pressure and produce antiarrhythmic effects, respectively. A series of anticonvulsant agents act through the voltage-gated sodium channels. For instance, phenytoin (Dilantin) and carbamazepine (TEGretol) decrease seizure activity by decreasing the influx of Na⁺ ions across cell membranes.

Ligand-Gated Ion Channels

To explain this class of gated ion channels, one can return to the neurotransmitter acetylcholine as an example. The acetylcholine receptor and its ligand acetylcholine, and their roles in signal transduction, have been studied extensively. The nicotinic acetylcholine receptor is found in the postsynaptic membrane of neurons at certain synapses and in myocytes at neuromuscular junctions. Synaptic vesicles in synaptic knobs contain approximately 10,000 acetylcholine molecules per vesicle. The released acetylcholine binds to its receptor on the postsynaptic neuron, which in turn results in the influx of Na⁺ into the cell.

The acetylcholine receptor serves as an ion channel and opens in response to the neurotransmitter acetylcholine (a ligand—compare it with the voltage-gated ion channel, in which the channel opens as a result of a change in the membrane potential). The receptor (ion channel) is formed from five subunits (two α subunits and one subunit each of β, γ, and δ), where the N termini of the two α subunits bind the neurotransmitter acetylcholine. The effects of acetylcholine on the postsynaptic ion channel are mainly due to protein conformational changes. By binding to its receptor, acetylcholine changes the receptor conformation from a closed to an opened form. As a result, Na⁺, Ca^{2+}, or K⁺ moves in (other ions cannot move in). The ligand binding is positively cooperative, such that binding to the first α subunit increases the binding affinity of other α subunits to acetylcholine (**Figure 6.8**).

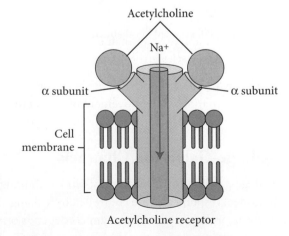

Figure 6.8 A ligand-gated ion channel reacting to its ligand, acetylcholine.

While the role of the acetylcholine receptor channel is to facilitate influx of ions and is a typical example of a ligand-gated ion channel, similar ion channels have been studied for the serotonin

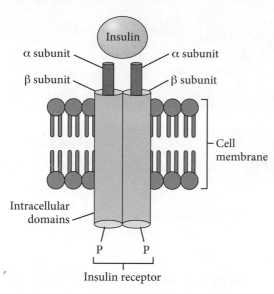

Figure 6.9 A receptor enzyme. The intercellular domains of the insulin receptor undergo auto-phosphorylation upon binding of insulin to its receptor.

neurotransmitter and amino acid ligands such as glutamate and glycine. For instance, binding of the serotonin or glutamate ligands to their receptor channels facilitates ion entry of K^+, Na^+, and Ca^{2+}; in contrast, binding of the glycine ligand to its receptor channel facilitates ion entry of Cl^-. Another example is binding of the major inhibitory neurotransmitter gamma-aminobutyric acid (GABA) to its receptor channel, which facilitates entry of Cl^- ion, causing hyperpolarization of the neuron. Because GABA has an inhibitory effect on the action potential (through entry of Cl^- and hyperpolarization of neurons), benzodiazepines have been suggested to increase the entry of Cl^- ions through the GABA receptor as well. However, benzodiazepines do not compete with GABA for the GABA's binding site, but rather bind to their own binding site on the GABA receptor.

Receptor Enzymes

Receptor enzymes have two domains: a single membrane-spanning domain that faces the extracellular environment for receiving a signal and a catalytic domain that faces the cytosol of a cell. The catalytic domain (or the intracellular domain) could be a protein tyrosine kinase, a serine kinase, or a guanylyl cyclase. The binding of the ligand activates the enzymatic domain, which in turn affects cellular metabolism by phosphorylation of different target proteins (**Figure 6.9**).

In the receptor enzyme signal transduction system, important receptors include epidermal growth factor (EGF), insulin receptor, and many other trophic hormones. Insulin receptor is a glycoprotein that has two α and two β subunits, all of which are stabilized by disulfide bonds. The intracellular domain of the β chains are the site of tyrosine kinase activity. The tyrosine kinase activity of the β subunit is triggered by auto-phosphorylation of Tyr residues in the C-terminal domain of the β subunit. This tyrosine kinase then transfers a phosphoryl group from ATP molecules to the hydroxyl group of Tyr residues of other target proteins such as insulin receptor substrate (IRS).

Because many of the tyrosine kinases are involved in signaling pathways in neoplastic diseases, some of the receptor enzymes are good targets for therapeutic agents that seek to inhibit the signaling pathways. For example, the monoclonal antibody trastuzumab (Herceptin) binds to the extracellular domain of the human epidermal growth factor receptor 2 (HER-2) and thereby produces cellular cytotoxicity by inhibiting the S phase of the cell cycle (recall from the *Introduction to Cell Biology* chapter that the S phase is where DNA, RNA, and protein synthesis occur). In doing so, it suppresses the expression of HER-2 receptors on cancerous cells. The HER-2 receptor is overexpressed in approximately 30% of patients who have developed breast cancer. In addition, this receptor is found, albeit to different degrees, in other malignancies such as ovarian, lung, and prostate cancers. Due to pharmacogenomics and genetic variations among patients, it is imperative to check whether the patient is overexpressing the gene for HER-2 to ensure that he or she will be able to benefit from a trastuzumab treatment, a process that is discussed more in detail in the *Introduction to Pharmacogenomics* chapter.

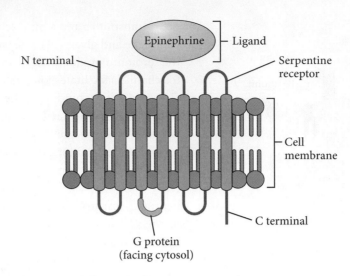

Figure 6.10 A serpentine receptor that has been folded back and forth seven times inside of the cell membrane.

Serpentine Receptors

Serpentine receptors bind to extracellular ligands and enhance intracellular concentrations of second messengers such as cAMP, Ca^{2+}, and phosphoinositides. The second messengers that are small molecules or ions bind to a variety of proteins and thereby change the shapes and functions of those proteins. Upon binding of the ligand to a serpentine receptor, a G protein that is located on the cytoplasmic face of the plasma membrane becomes activated. Consequently, these receptors are called G-protein receptors. A unique characteristic of a serpentine receptor (as indicated by its name) is that the receptor is folded and embedded back and forth seven times across the cell membrane (**Figure 6.10**).

Serpentine receptors are targets of many drugs, including antihistamines, neuroleptics, antidepressants, and antihypertensive agents. An example of a serpentine receptor is the β-adrenergic receptor. In 2012, two scientists, Brian Kobilka and Robert Lefkowitz, won the Nobel Prize in chemistry for their work elucidating the signaling mechanism for serpentine receptors.

The following discussion briefly describes the role of a serpentine receptor. Epinephrine is an adrenergic ligand that binds to its specific receptor (β-adrenergic receptor) on the cell surface. This binding promotes a conformational change in the cytosolic domain of the receptor, which in turn binds to a Gs protein. The α subunit of the Gs protein has the binding site for either GDP or GTP. The ligand-bound receptor causes GTP to replace GDP, such that the Gs protein becomes activated. The Gs protein then activates adenylate cyclase, which catalyzes the synthesis of cAMP. The cAMP-dependent protein kinase, PKA, becomes activated by cAMP. PKA activates phosphorylase *b* kinase, which in turn converts glycogen phosphorylase *b* to glycogen phosphorylase *a*, which finally leads to glycogenolysis (**Figure 6.11**). PKA is able to phosphorylate many physiological targets, including metabolic enzymes, transport proteins, regulatory proteins, other protein kinases, ion channels, and transcription factors.

Different serpentine receptors may utilize the G proteins differently. Indeed, it is known that G proteins facilitate the sending of signals for more than 500 receptors. Whereas Gs activates

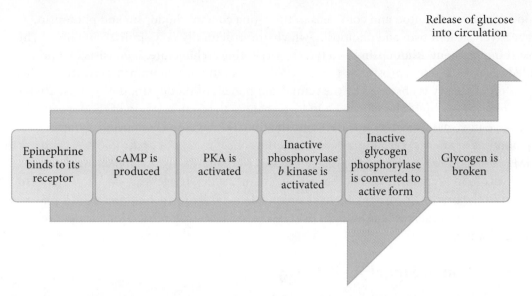

Figure 6.11 The cascade of reactions that occur when epinephrine binds to a serpentine receptor (β-adrenergic receptor).

adenylate cyclase when epinephrine binds to its β-adrenergic receptors, Gq activates phospholipase C to generate diacylglycerol and IP_3 when oxytocin or vasopressin hormones bind to their serpentine receptors. In addition, when epinephrine binds to an α_2-adrenergic receptor, the enzymatic activity of AC is inhibited because the α_2-adrenergic receptor is not coupled to Gs, but rather to Gi, which is an inhibitory G protein.

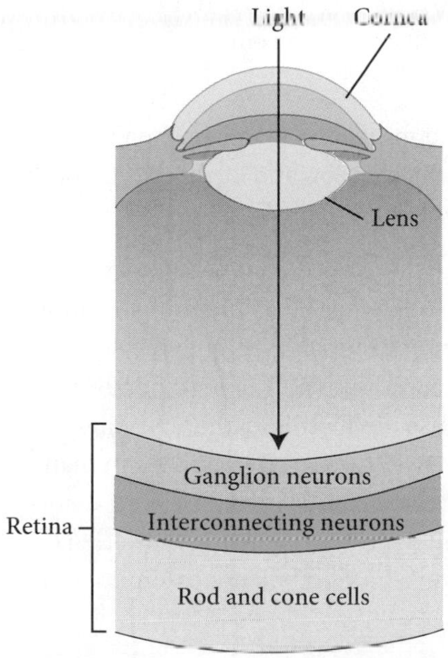

The detection of light (vision), odors (olfaction), and tastes (gustation) in vertebrates also employs serpentine receptors, which act through the G proteins to change the sensory neurons' electrical potential. The retina is made of three layers of cells: (1) rods and cones; (2) interconnecting neurons (bipolar cells); and (3) ganglion cells (**Figure 6.12**).

Cone cells function in bright light and are responsible for color vision. A human retina contains approximately 6 million cone cells. Because cones require a reasonable amount of light to be stimulated, they function only during the day. This is why we are able to see colors only during the daytime—in other words, when the light intensity is high enough to stimulate the cone receptors.

The light must first pass through both the ganglion cells and the bipolar cells before it can reach and affect the photoreceptors

Figure 6.12 The anatomy of the eye where light reaches the retina to induce a signal transduction.
Adapted from: Nelson DL, Cox MM, and Lehninger AL. *Principles of biochemistry*, 5th ed. New York: W. H. Freeman and Company; 2008; Chapter 12.

(rod and cone cells). Rod and cone cells in the retina contain rhodopsin and photopsin, respectively. Rhodopsin and photopsin, which are structurally very similar, contain a light-absorbing pigment. Rhodopsin has a typical serpentine architecture. It consists of a protein called opsin linked to a prosthetic group called 11-*cis* retinal, a vitamin A derivative. When a photon of energy is absorbed by the retinal component of rhodopsin, the conformation of the prosthetic group is altered, which in turn changes the conformation of rhodopsin—the first stage in visual transduction. The conformational changes in rhodopsin (upon receiving photons of energy) result in a decrease in the concentration of cyclic GMP. A decrease in cGMP in the outer segment of the rod cell causes Na^+- and Ca^{2+}-gated ion channels to close. This leads to hyperpolarization of the cell membrane, which triggers an electrical signal to be sent to the brain. The drugs sildenafil and tadalafil, both of which inhibit cGMP phosphodiesterase (PDE), increase the amount of cGMP and cause dose-related impairment of color discrimination.

Interruption of Signaling Pathways

Toxins produced by *Bordetella pertussis* (which causes whooping cough) and *Vibrio cholerae* (which causes cholera, a life-threatening dehydration caused by watery diarrhea) are able to increase the synthesis of cAMP and thereby interrupt many hosts' cellular functions. The cholera toxin, for example, catalyzes the addition of the ADP-ribose moiety of nicotinamide adenine dinucleotide (NAD) to the α subunit of the Gs protein and inhibits the Gs protein's GTPase activity, thereby making the Gs protein remain attached to GTP (which is the active form of Gs). The activated Gs protein stimulates adenylate cyclase to produce cAMP continuously, which in turn stimulates water, bicarbonate, and Cl^- secretion into the intestinal lumen.

Similarly, *B. pertussis* catalyzes the addition of the ADP-ribose moiety of NAD to the Gi protein and inhibits displacement of GDP by GTP. This action finally blocks the effect of Gi to inhibit adenylate cyclase.

Both Gs and Gi are active when they are in their GTP-bound forms and inactive when they are in their GDP-bound forms. Both toxins interfere with signal transduction and affect a series of the metabolic events that are dependent on the signaling pathways.

Graves's disease is another example in which the signaling pathway is interrupted. Graves's disease causes production of antibodies that serve as agonists to the thyroid-stimulating hormone (TSH) protein, a serpentine receptor. Binding of the antibodies activates the AC enzyme, leading to increased synthesis of cAMP. The cAMP stimulates the expression of the thyroglobulin and thyroid peroxidase genes. Ultimately, the overall effect is to cause the thyroid pathophysiology (excessive secretion of the thyroid hormone, T_4) evident in Graves's disease. In addition, in many patients with McCune-Albright syndrome (a rare genetic syndrome characterized by bone disorders, skin hyperpigmentation, and endocrine dysfunction), the G-protein signaling in the TSH receptor is interrupted, such that these patients produce excessive thyroid hormones similar to the case in Graves's disease.

Xanthine derivatives such as caffeine and theophylline are known to inhibit cyclic nucleotide phosphodiesterase and increase the amount of cAMP present. The elevated cAMP level stimulates activation of glycogen phosphorylase *a* and glycogenolysis; and increased blood glucose level in the body soon follows (see also **Figure 6.11**).

Learning Bridge 6.1

Joe is a 28-year-old biochemist who works for the United Nations in its International Affairs division. He just returned from a trip abroad. Joe comes to your pharmacy and complains about dehydration that has been caused by watery diarrhea. One of the attending physicians at a local clinic, which Joe visited yesterday, mentioned that he has contracted some bacterial infections overseas. To Joe's surprise, the attending physician did not prescribe any antibiotic. However, the physician asked him to contact a pharmacist and buy an oral rehydration solution (ORS). You also notice that Joe has sunken eyes and appears weak.

Joe comes to the counter and asks you a few questions:

A. Which kind of infection do I have that does not require an antibiotic?
B. Why have I been asked to buy an ORS?
C. I have a master of science in biochemistry. Can you please tell me, on the cellular level, why I have watery diarrhea?

Receptors for Hydrophobic Ligands

A few ligands are hydrophobic and, as a result, do not have any plasma membrane receptors; instead, their targeted proteins are intracellular receptors. In this class, one can find steroids (corticosteroids, mineralocorticoids, sex steroids, and vitamin D) and thyroid hormones. These receptors are involved in the expression of genes. Because these ligands are hydrophobic, they are strictly dependent on other proteins to assist them in traveling from the site of their synthesis to the site of their action through the blood circulation. For instance, transcortin, androgen-binding proteins, and sex-hormone-binding proteins assist steroid hormones in the blood to travel and reach their target cells, and transthyretin assists thyroid hormones in doing the same.

Once the steroid hormones reach their target cells, they dissociate from their transport proteins, spontaneously pass through the cell membrane and enter the cytoplasm, bind to their receptor, and then migrate to the nucleus. In the nucleus, their function is to induce (or, to a lesser extent, repress) transcription of specific genes. The receptors that bind steroid hormones have a high-affinity ligand-binding property. These receptors belong to a large family of structurally similar DNA-binding proteins. Depending on the nature of the steroid hormones, the receptor-binding complex may occur in the cytoplasm (e.g., for glucocorticoids) or in the nucleus (e.g., for estrogen and androgen).

Binding of steroids to their receptors changes the conformation of these receptors in which the hormone–receptor complex can bind to specific DNA sequences called hormone response element (HRE). The binding to HRE can either activate or repress the transcription of adjacent genes (**Figure 6.13**).

Steroid receptors share some structural similarities. All of the known steroid receptors contain a small DNA-binding domain that contains zinc, which is an essential element for the DNA binding. The zinc stabilizes the structure of the domain; without it, the domain would unfold.

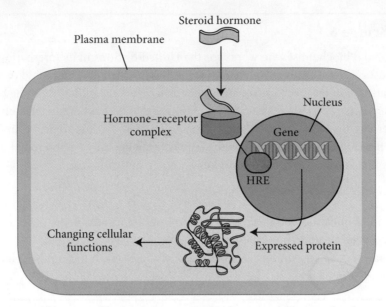

Figure 6.13 Due to steroid hormones' hydrophobic structures, they can readily span the plasma membrane so as to enter the cytoplasm or nucleus.

A hormone–receptor complex can bind to several HREs and, as a result, many gene expressions can be changed by the same hormone. Each type of HRE can influence the transcription of a large number of genes (50–100 genes). For this reason, binding of a steroid hormone–receptor complex to its HRE has a large amplified effect on cellular function.

Steroid hormones—in contrast to peptide hormones, which rapidly act on membrane receptors (recall the roles of glucagon and insulin)—are relatively slow acting. The reason for their slow action is that it takes longer (30 minutes to several hours) to activate the expression of a gene for the synthesis of an enzyme or a protein than to act directly on preexisting enzymes. The slow action partially explains why steroids (e.g., budesonide, fluticasone) are not appropriate for rapidly relieving breathing difficulty in acute bronchial asthma. However, the action of steroid hormones lasts for a longer duration (hours to days) than that of peptide hormones. The reason for the longer effect is that the turnover of most enzymes and proteins expressed by these ligands is slow.

Learning Bridge 6.2

Amy Johnson is a 48-year-old fashion designer who works for a well-known clothing company on the West Coast. Amy was diagnosed with type 2 diabetes six months ago. She comes to your pharmacy for a refill of her prescription, metformin (Glucophage), 500 mg twice daily. Upon a routine review of her medical records, you notice that despite filling her prescription for metformin since her diagnosis, Amy's blood glucose has remained high (120 mg/dL).

You decide to talk to her to learn more about her medical adherence. Amy admits that she occasionally forgets to take the second metformin tablet, although that occurs only rarely. She also mentions that she drinks three cups of tea and three cups of coffee every day.

What is your reaction to Amy's responses? Use your knowledge about signal transduction to justify your answer.

Receptors Without Intrinsic Activity

Some receptor proteins do not have any intrinsic enzyme activities. For instance, cells express cytokine receptors that respond to growth hormone, erythropoietin, and γ-interferon. The intracellular domain of these receptors binds a soluble tyrosine kinase called Janus kinase (JAK). Upon the ligand binding, JAK phosphorylates other proteins that are signal transducers and activators of transcription (STAT, for short) to regulate transcription of a gene. The entire pathway is referred to as the JAK-STAT pathway. Mammals contain four JAKs and six STATs that activate gene transcription differently in different cell types.

Perhaps the most relevant process to describe in this chapter is the binding of erythropoietin (EPO) to its receptor. Erythropoietin is a hormone built of 165 amino acid residues that is synthesized in the kidney. The binding of EPO to its receptor stimulates production of erythrocytes. The EPO receptor has no enzymatic activity. However, the intercellular domain of the EPO-bound receptor complex binds a soluble JAK, which in turn phosphorylates several of the tyrosine residues of the EPO receptor. These phosphorylated tyrosine residues bind a domain of STAT. This process brings the STAT domain close enough to JAK to be phosphorylated by JAK as well. The phosphorylated STAT domain then enters the cell nucleus and promotes expression of genes that are essential for erythrocyte maturation. An erythropoietin deficiency is the underlying cause for anemia in 90% of the patients who have end-stage renal failure and are on dialysis.

Adhesion Receptors

Adhesion molecules such as integrins, cadherins, and selectins (see also the *Introduction to Cell Biology* chapter) and immunoglobulin-like cell adhesion molecules (Ig-CAM) are involved in a variety of signaling pathways. These receptors have both extracellular and intracellular domains. While the extracellular domain is attached to macromolecule proteins such as collagen and fibronectin, the intracellular domain is attached to the cytoskeleton (largely to actin and filaments) of the cytoplasm. Upon receiving the appropriate signals, these adhesion receptors facilitate cell migration, cell–cell adhesion, and platelet aggregation at the site of tissue injury; mediate tissue repair; and perform other critical functions to restore the body to homeostasis. For instance, an integrin receptor has two subunits, α and β (the β subunit is also known as CD18). A genetic mutation that encodes a nonfunctional β subunit results in the immunological disease known as leukocyte adhesion deficiency (LAD). In this disease, the nonfunctional β subunit does not allow leukocytes to adhere to the blood vessel so that they can migrate through the blood vessel to reach the site of an infection. LAD is a genetic disease. Affected infants often suffer from recurrent infections, and many die of infections before the age of 2.

Learning Bridge 6.3

Amy works as a cashier in a grocery store in Hillsboro, Oregon. Her daughter Emily is a 7-year-old first grader who has been diagnosed with occasional bronchospasm (difficulty with breathing). Today, Amy comes to your pharmacy to receive Emily's Proventil. She mentions to you that Amy's sister, Jennifer, also has breathing difficulty. Jennifer is not using Proventil, but rather Pulmicort. Jennifer is very happy with Pulmicort and has suggested that Amy ask her physician to prescribe Pulmicort for Emily. Amy asks you to call Emily's physician and request a prescription for Pulmicort.

(continues)

(continued)

Your preceptor asks you for your reaction and also asks you to answer the following questions:

A. What would be your answer to Amy's question?
B. What is the major difference between Proventil and Pulmicort?
C. How will you explain to Amy which drug is better for Emily?

Learning Bridge 6.4

At an airport in the Midwest, while you are waiting for your flight to go home over the Christmas break, you observe that one of the pilots is very angry and is arguing with a TSA officer. The pilot claims that he does not understand why, according to the airline policy, he cannot take sildenafil (Viagra) before he flies the plane (some airlines nowadays restrict their pilots from flying for 24 hours after using sildenafil).

You notice that the pilot's argument with the TSA officer has put him in a stressful situation, and he has made what seems to be a gesture indicating chest pain. While you are approaching him, you see that the pilot takes one tablet from a tiny amber glass container and puts it under his tongue. You listen calmly to his complaint and tell him you would be happy to explain why sildenafil may not be appropriate right before his flight. What would be your explanation?

Dose–Response Relationship

Receptor–Ligand Affinity

Receptors play important roles in selecting their ligands (drugs), but it is the concentration of the ligand at a receptor site that governs a biological response. While the majority of interactions of ligands or drugs with their receptors are transient (i.e., reversible), one can find irreversible interactions as well. Here we focus first on reversible receptor–ligand binding. The binding of a receptor with its ligand produces a receptor–ligand complex (RL) that often leads to a conformational change of the receptor. This change can entail either a minor tweak or a major adjustment of the receptor's polypeptide chain.

According to the law of mass action, at equilibrium, the equilibrium constant (K_a, which here is also called the association constant) for a reaction between a receptor and a ligand (shown in the following reaction scheme) is expressed by Equation 6.1:

Receptor (R) + Ligand (L) $\leftrightarrow$ Receptor–Ligand (RL)

$$K_a = \frac{[RL]}{[R][L]} \tag{6.1}$$

K_a provides a measure of an affinity of the ligand for the receptor. The [RL] complex is directly related to the concentrations of free ligand (L), free receptor (R), and the association constant (K_a), as indicated in Equation 6.2:

$$K_a[R][L] = [RL] \tag{6.2}$$

The fraction of receptor that is bound to ligand, θ, is shown in Equation 6.3:

$$\theta = \frac{\text{Occupied binding sites}}{\text{Total binding sites}} \qquad (6.3)$$

The occupied binding site is [RL] and the total binding site is [RL] + [R]. With respect to this observation, we can rewrite Equation 6.3 as Equation 6.4:

$$\theta = \frac{[RL]}{[RL]+[R]} \qquad (6.4)$$

According to Equation 6.2, we can replace [RL] with $K_a[L][R]$ and rewrite Equation 6.4 in the form of Equation 6.5:

$$\theta = \frac{K_a[R][L]}{K_a[R][L]+[R]} \qquad (6.5)$$

If we divide all parameters in Equation 6.5 by [R], we obtain Equation 6.6:

$$\theta = \frac{K_a[L]}{K_a[L]+1} \qquad (6.6)$$

To simplify Equation 6.6 further, we can divide all parameters in Equation 6.6 by K_a, which yields Equation 6.7:

$$\theta = \frac{[L]}{[L]+\frac{1}{K_a}} \qquad (6.7)$$

K_a has units of concentration^{-1} (M^{-1}) and measures affinity; that is, the greater the value of K_a, the greater the affinity. It is, however, more practical to use the reciprocal of the association constant— the dissociation constant, K_d—which has the unit of concentration (M). Therefore Equation 6.7 can also be written as Equation 6.8:

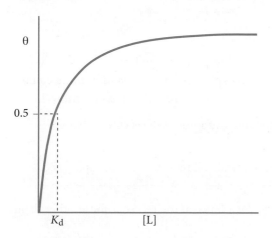

$$\theta = \frac{[L]}{[L]+K_d} \qquad (6.8)$$

If a fixed amount of a receptor is incubated with varying amounts of a ligand, the fraction of the receptors that are bound with ligand (θ) may then be determined. A plot of this fraction versus ligand concentration [L] should yield a hyperbolic curve. The concentration of L that matches to 50% of θ gives the value of K_d (**Figure 6.14**).

Now let's see if the parameters in Equation 6.8 make sense in regard to the ligand-binding affinity. When [L] is equal to K_d, half (50%) of the binding site is occupied. (Check this out: put in 1 for [L] and 1 for K_d in Equation 6.8.) Basically, K_d is the concentration of the ligand at which 50% of the available ligand-binding sites are occupied. For instance, the protein avidin has a binding affinity (K_d) of 1×10^{-15} M to biotin (which is the ligand for avidin). Insulin receptor

Figure 6.14 If a fixed amount of a receptor is incubated with varying amounts of a ligand, the fraction (θ) of the receptors that are bound with ligand can be determined. The parameter K_d represents the concentration of the ligand at which 50% of the available ligand-binding sites are occupied.

Adapted from: Nelson DL, Cox MM, and Lehninger AL. Principles of biochemistry, 5th ed. New York: W. H. Freeman and Company; 2008; Chapter 5.

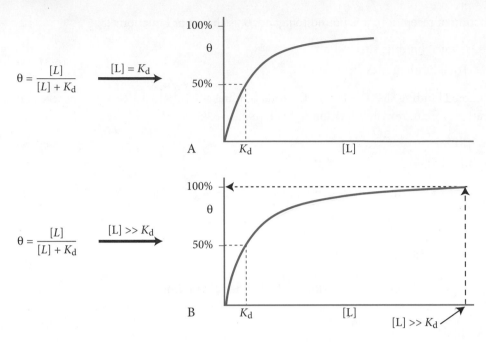

$$\theta = \frac{[L]}{[L] + K_d} \xrightarrow{\quad [L] = K_d \quad}$$

$$\theta = \frac{[L]}{[L] + K_d} \xrightarrow{\quad [L] \gg K_d \quad}$$

Figure 6.15 (A) When the concentration of a ligand is equal to its K_d, the ligand occupies 50% of the available ligand-binding sites. (B) When the concentration of a ligand is much more (at least 100 times more) than its K_d, the ligand occupies 100% of the available ligand-binding sites.

has a K_d value of 0.1 nM for insulin (ligand). Based on Equation 6.8, the concentration of insulin that is equal to its K_d (0.1 nM) occupies 50% of the insulin receptor binding sites. Based on the same equation, when the insulin concentration is much higher (100 times) than K_d (in our case, 10 nM), insulin hormone occupies 100% of the insulin receptor binding sites. These examples are also shown in **Figure 6.15**.

Plasma Drug Concentration Profile

Efficacy and Potency of Drugs

Efficacy is the ability of a drug to produce a pharmacological response when it interacts with its receptor. The same mathematic description that we used to explain receptor–ligand binding can be used to explain the efficacy of drugs. However, one has to make three important assumptions here:

1. The extent of the biological response is proportional to the amount of receptors that are bound to a ligand.

2. The maximum biological response (E_{max}) is achieved when all receptors are occupied (i.e., when there are no "spare receptors").

3. Binding of a drug to the receptor does not change the affinity of the receptor for another drug (i.e., it does not lead to cooperativity).

Spare receptors are those receptors that do not have to be occupied to produce a maximal response. One can express the binding of a drug to a receptor as follows:

$$\frac{E}{E_{max}} = \frac{[D]}{[D] + K_d} \tag{6.9}$$

Notice that Equation 6.9 is very similar to Equation 6.8 $\left(\theta = \dfrac{[L]}{[L] + K_d}\right)$.

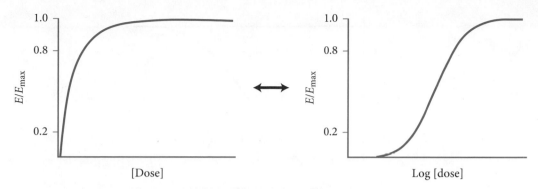

Figure 6.16 Dose–response curves. The logarithm of the dose (or drug concentration) on the *x*-axis is often used to allow the range of the drug concentrations to be more readily perceived.

Adapted from: Clark M, Finkel R, Rey J and Whalen, K. *Pharmacology*, 5th ed. Lippincott Williams and Wilkins; 2012; Chapter 2.

E is the effect of the drug at concentration [D]; E_{max} is the maximal effect of the drug (i.e., when all of the receptors are occupied by the drug); and K_d is the dissociation constant for a given drug [D]. If you plot the ratio of E/E_{max} as a function of a drug dose, you will get a hyperbolic curve. However, often the logarithm of the dose (or drug concentration) is used to allow the range of the drug concentrations to be more readily perceived (**Figure 6.16**).

Equation 6.9 and **Figure 6.17** can be used to explain two important concepts:

- If the drug concentration (or dose) is much higher than K_d, E/E_{max} becomes 1 (or 100%). This indicates the drug molecules have occupied all of the receptor sites (i.e., receptors are saturated with the drug molecules).

- If the drug concentration (or dose) is equal to its K_d, 50% of the maximum effect (EC_{50}) has been achieved by the drug. EC_{50} indicates potency. Basically, the potency is a measure of the concentration (or dose) of the drug that is necessary to produce 50% of the maximal effect (**Figure 6.18**). Keep in mind that potency and EC_{50} have a reciprocal relationship: the higher the value of EC_{50}, the lower the potency.

When EC_{50} is less than K_d, the dose that is required to produce potency is lower than the dose that is required to occupy 50% of the cell's total receptors. This indicates that the cell expresses more receptors than it needs to produce the maximal pharmacological response. In other words, the cell expresses "spare receptors." When spare receptors are present, you should not assume that

$$\frac{E}{E_{max}} = \frac{[D]}{[D] + K_d}$$

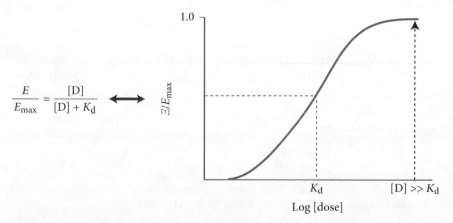

Figure 6.17 In both Equation 6.9 and this figure, when [D] is much larger (at least 100 times larger) than K_d, E/E_{max} becomes 100% and the drug molecules have occupied all of the receptor sites.

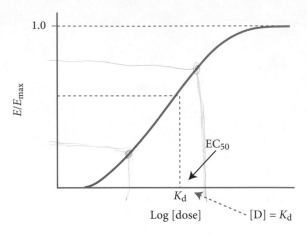

Figure 6.18 The potency of a drug is a measure of the concentration (or dose) of the drug that is necessary to produce 50% of the maximal effect.

Table 6.1 Relationship Between Affinity and Potency

Dose–Response System Without Spare Receptors	Dose–Response System with Spare Receptors
When $EC_{50} = K_d$ $EC_{50} \downarrow$; $K_d \downarrow$; Potency $\uparrow$	When $EC_{50} < K_d$ $EC_{50}\downarrow$; Potency$\uparrow$; here you don't know how K_d changes. In other words, you cannot utilize K_d to estimate potency.

EC_{50} is the same as K_d. **Table 6.1** summarizes the relationship between K_d and potency in a dose–response system with and without spare receptors.

Let's use a few examples to make these pharmacodynamic concepts clearer.

Example 6.1: Which of the antipsychotic drugs in **Table 6.2** has the lowest affinity to all three dopamine receptors? Which drug has the highest affinity to the D_3 dopamine receptors?

Table 6.2 Affinity of Different Antipsychotic Agents to Different Dopamine Receptors

Antipsychotic Drugs	K_d (nM)		
	Dopamine Receptor 2 (D_2)	Dopamine Receptor 3 (D_3)	Dopamine Receptor 4 (D_4)
Chlorpromazine	0.55	1.2	9.7
Clozapine	35	83	22
Haloperidol	0.53	2.7	2.3
Quetiapine	105	340	2,000

Modified from: Strange PG. Antipsychotic drugs: importance of dopamine receptors for mechanisms of therapeutic actions and side effects. *Pharmacol Rev.* 2001:53(1)119–134.

Answer: The affinity of a receptor for a drug is measured by its dissociation constant. The higher the K_d, the lower the affinity. Quetiapine has the lowest affinity and chlorpromazine has the highest affinity for the D_3 dopamine receptors.

Example 6.2: Suppose the drugs in Table 6.2 produce the maximal effect at certain drug concentrations and there are no spare dopamine receptors. Which of these antipsychotic drugs has the lowest potency relative to all three dopamine receptors?

Answer: The potency is the concentration of a drug that produces 50% of the maximal pharmacological response. As there are no spare receptors in this example, the potency or EC_{50} is represented by K_d. The higher the K_d, the higher the EC_{50} and the lower the potency. Quetiapine has the lowest potency for all three dopamine receptors.

Example 6.3: Based on the presented information indicated in **Figure 6.19**, which of the following statements is correct?

   A. Chlorpromazine has a higher potency than clozapine.

   B. Chlorpromazine has a lower potency than clozapine.

   C. Chlorpromazine has a higher efficacy than clozapine.

   D. Clozapine has a higher efficacy than chlorpromazine.

   E. Clozapine and chlorpromazine have the same efficacy.

Answer: Both A and E are correct. Estimate EC_{50} and you will see that the value for chlorpromazine is lower than the value for clozapine, which means chlorpromazine has a higher potency. As both drugs have the same maximal effect (plateau), both have the same efficacy.

A few parameters are affected by binding of a drug to a receptor. It is important briefly to emphasize their role in pharmacodynamics. Some of these parameters are indicated in **Figure 6.20**.

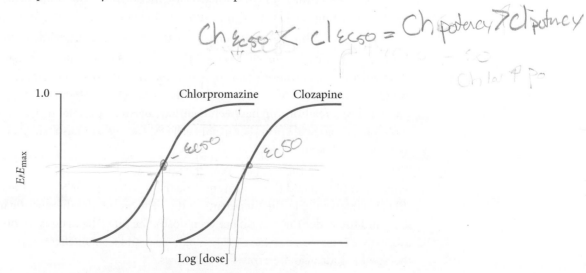

Figure 6.19 A hypothetical dose–response system for chlorpromazine and clozapine.

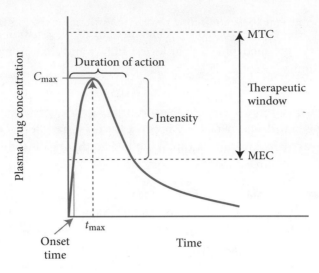

Figure 6.20 A few parameters that play important roles in a dose–response system. This plasma drug profile reflects a single oral dose administration of a drug.
Adapted from: Hedaya M. *Basic pharmacokinetics.* Boca Raton: CRC Press; 2012.

Intensity of a Response: The intensity of a pharmacological response has to do with the number of receptors occupied by a drug. The higher the plasma drug concentration, the greater the pharmacological response—at least until the maximum effect is achieved. The intensity changes in a manner paralleling the peak concentration; in other words, a high peak concentration results in a high intensity.

MEC: The minimum effective concentration is the plasma drug concentration that produces the minimum pharmacological effect.

Onset Time: The onset time is the time required for a plasma drug concentration to produce an MEC.

Duration of Effect: The duration of effect is the time for which the plasma drug concentration stays above the MEC.

Therapeutic Range: The therapeutic range identifies those points when the pharmacological effect is between the MEC and the minimum toxic concentration of the drug in plasma (MTC). Clinicians use therapeutic drug monitoring (discussed later) to maintain the plasma drug concentration within the therapeutic range.

t_{max}: The t_{max} is the time required to achieve the maximum plasma drug concentration.

Therapeutic Drug Monitoring (TDM): TDM is a process in which clinicians use plasma drug concentrations and apply pharmacokinetics and pharmacodynamics to monitor a patient's response to a drug therapy. TDM is often applied to drugs for which a direct relationship has been identified between plasma drug concentration and pharmacological effect. For instance, TDM for digoxin has resulted in a significant reduction in digoxin toxicity.

Therapeutic Index: The ratio between the minimum dose that is toxic for 50% of the population (TD_{50}) and the minimum dose that is effective for 50% of the population (ED_{50}) is referred to as the therapeutic index. The higher the therapeutic index for a drug and the wider the margin between doses, the safer the drug is. In other words, a safe drug is expected to have a large toxic dose and a small effective dose. The therapeutic index can be expressed as follows:

$$\text{Therapeutic index} = \frac{TD_{50}}{ED_{50}} \qquad (6.10)$$

For instance, one can compare warfarin with ibuprofen (Advil) to identify which drug has a higher therapeutic index (i.e., which drug is safer). The data in **Figure 6.21** apply to different doses of warfarin and ibuprofen. As shown in the figure, ibuprofen has a higher therapeutic index. Pay attention to the doses that produce the desired therapeutic effect and a toxic effect for 50% of patients.

Therapeutic Window: This parameter is clinically more useful than the therapeutic index; it describes the difference between the MEC and the MTC for a particular drug (**Figure 6.20**). For instance, the MEC for total phenytoin (Dilantin) is 10 μg/mL and the observed MTC is 20 μg/mL. Accordingly, the therapeutic window for phenytoin is 10–20 μg/mL. In other words, 10–20 μg/mL is a safe and acceptable range of plasma concentrations when designing a dosing regimen.

Keep in mind that a receptor can be in its active form even if a ligand is not bound to the receptor. Receptor activity in the absence of ligand is referred to as constitutive activity. If a higher than expected dose of a drug must be administered to produce a pharmacological response, the response is called hyporeactive or tolerance. While endogenous ligands act as the natural ligands to stimulate a receptor, many drugs available on the market either stimulate a receptor or block a receptor from binding its natural ligand. It is important to expand the roles of these drugs in pharmacodynamics.

Agonists

A drug that binds to a receptor and mimics the effects of an endogenous molecule is an agonist drug. For instance, the drug fluticasone (Flovent HFA) mimics corticoid and binds to corticoid steroid receptors to produce an anti-inflammatory effect. Not all agonists for the same receptor have the same affinity, however. For instance, fluticasone has 18 times higher affinity (18 times lower K_d) for the corticoid receptor compared to dexamethasone (Baycadron).

Partial Agonists

A drug that binds to a receptor but is not as effective as the endogenous ligands is called a partial agonist. Even if all of the receptor sites are occupied, the E_{max} will not be produced by a partial agonist. **Figure 6.22** demonstrates dose–response curves for agonist and partial agonist agents.

The reason that a partial agonist does not produce a full effect may not be related to its decreased affinity to the receptor. Instead, it may not be able to fully activate the receptor. There are two scenarios that can happen with partial agonists:

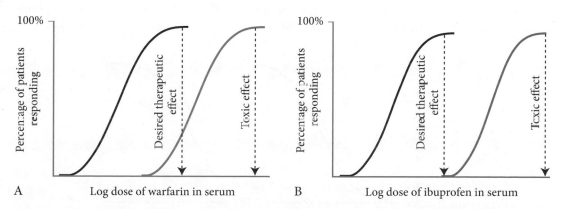

Figure 6.21 Dose–response plots for (A) warfarin and (B) ibuprofen.
Adapted from: Clark M, Finkel R, Rey J and Whalen, K. *Pharmacology*, 5th ed. Lippincott Williams and Wilkins; 2012; Chapter 2.

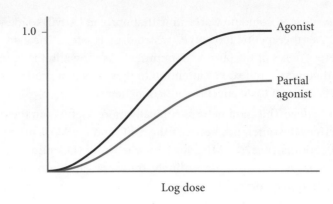

Figure 6.22 Dose–response curves for agonist and partial agonist agents.

1. A partial agonist in the absence of a full agonist serves as a partial agonist.

2. A partial agonist in the presence of a full agonist competes with the full agonist and blocks the agonist's effect.

Antagonists

A drug that binds to a receptor and blocks the binding of the endogenous ligand or another drug is called an antagonist. An antagonist has affinity for a receptor but does not have any intrinsic activity. Four classes of antagonists are distinguished: (1) competitive antagonists, (2) noncompetitive antagonists, (3) chemical antagonists, and (4) physiologic antagonists.

Competitive Antagonists

These drugs bind reversibly to a receptor and compete with an agonist seeking to bind to the same binding site. A competitive antagonist's effects, however, are diminished if the dose of the agonist is increased sufficiently. In the presence of a full agonist, a competitive antagonist shifts the agonist's dose–response curve to the right but does not change the maximum response. A typical example of this type of drug is prazosin (Minipress, an antihypertensive agent), which competes with norepinephrine for binding to α_1-adrenergic receptors. **Figure 6.23** demonstrates how the dose–response curve is shifted for an agonist with and without a competitive antagonist. At higher doses of norepinephrine, the maximum effect from the agonist is achieved.

Noncompetitive Antagonists

A noncompetitive antagonist binds to the receptor at a site different from the agonist binding site (i.e., to an allosteric binding site). It is also possible for an antagonist to bind irreversibly to the

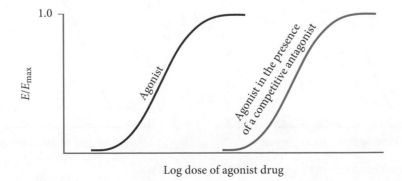

Figure 6.23 A dose–response system in the presence and the absence of a competitive antagonist.

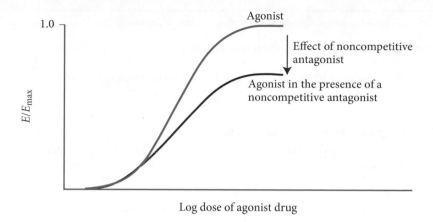

Figure 6.24 A dose–response system in the presence and the absence of a noncompetitive antagonist.

active site and thereby reduce the ability of the agonist to compete and produce a response. Thus, no matter how high the concentration of the agonist dose, the agonist cannot compete with the noncompetitive antagonist (**Figure 6.24**). Phenoxybenzamine (Dibenzyline) is a noncompetitive antagonist to adrenergic receptors that reduces the hypertension risk associated with excess release of catecholamines from an adrenal tumor (pheochromocytoma—a rare neuroendocrine tumor).

The release of a noncompetitive antagonist may be a slow process that results in a prolonged antagonistic effect. For instance, amlodipine (Norvasc) dissociates slowly from calcium channels so that it has a lengthy duration of antihypertensive action (24 hours).

Chemical Antagonists

A chemical antagonist mediates the effect of another drug by binding to and inactivating that drug. One example is protamine sulfate (an antidote for heparin), a highly positively charged molecule that binds to the negatively charged heparin molecule and makes heparin inactive. Because there is no receptor involved in a chemical antagonism process, these agents are also called nonreceptor antagonists.

Physiologic Antagonists

A physiologic antagonist acts by counteracting a regulatory pathway. For instance, propranolol (Inderal LA) is used to treat tachycardia in patients with hyperthyroidism. Although the exact mechanism is not known, an increased level of thyroid hormones (recall the hyperthyroidism observed in Graves's disease) results in an increased number of the beta-adrenergic receptors. To counter this effect, propranolol is often given to patients with hyperthyroidism.

Learning Bridge 6.5

Joe is a 71-year-old retired teacher who used to teach physics in a high school. Today, he comes to your pharmacy to ask you a few questions about his medication, tamsulosin (Flomax), which he started to take 2 days ago. This drug has been prescribed for his prostatic hyperplasia, to treat his bladder outlet obstruction symptoms. Tamsulosin is known to block α_1-receptors in the smooth muscle of the bladder and causes relaxation that reduces resistance to urinary outflow.

(continues)

Enhancement of Drug Effects

Three concepts are used to describe an enhancement effect for drugs: addition, synergism, and potentiation.

Addition

In addition, when two different drugs with the same pharmacological effect that either have the same or different strengths are combined, the combined effect is equal to the sum of the individual effect. Such an effect is seen with trimethoprim-sulfamethoxazole (Septra DS), which is used to inhibit bacterial infection. Both trimethoprim and sulfamethoxazole have antibiotic effects, but when they are combined the total effect is equal to the sum of both drugs' effects. Folic acid is reduced to dihydrofolate and then to tetrahydrofolate (THF; the active form of folic acid); sulfamethoxazole inhibits the synthesis of bacterial folic acid. In contrast, trimethoprim inhibits bacterial formation of THF. **Figure 6.25** depicts this addition effect.

Synergism

In synergism, when two different drugs with the same pharmacological effect (that either have the same or different strengths) are combined, the combined effect is greater than the sum of the individual effects (**Figure 6.26**). For example, when penicillin is combined with gentamicin, the penicillin enhances the cellular uptake of gentamicin by bacteria.

A side effect of a medication may also be affected by a synergistic mechanism. For instance, diclofenac sodium (Cambia, an NSAID used to treat osteoarthritis) produces synergistic GI bleeding effects when it is combined with warfarin. In addition, co-administration of two drugs, each with a toxic effect that is tolerable by an organ, can enhance the toxicity and result in organ damage. For instance, combining administration of two nephrotoxic drugs can result in kidney failure, even though the dose of each individual drug alone does not produce toxicity to any significant extent.

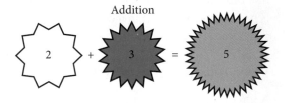

Figure 6.25 The combination of trimethoprim with sulfamethoxazole results in an effect that is equal to the total effect received from the individual trimethoprim and sulfamethoxazole antibiotics. The numbers are arbitrary here.

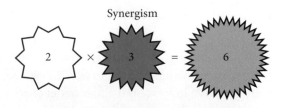

Figure 6.26 The combination of penicillin and gentamicin results in an effect that is greater than the total effect received from these two individual antibiotics. The numbers are arbitrary here.

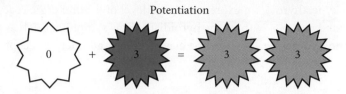

Potentiation

Figure 6.27 The combination of amoxicillin and clavulanic acid results in a better effect compared with using amoxicillin alone. In this example, clavulanic acid has no antibiotic effect. The numbers are arbitrary here.

Potentiation

In potentiation, an ineffective drug increases the effect of another effective drug. For instance, carbidopa alone does not have any significant effect in treating Parkinson's disease. When it is combined with dopa, however, the half-time of dopa is prolonged. Similarly, the agent known as Augmentin includes two drugs: amoxicillin and clavulanic acid. While Augmentin's bactericidal effect is derived from amoxicillin, clavulanic acid has no antimicrobial effect on its own. However, clavulanic acid is important for protecting amoxicillin from destruction. In this way, the effect of Augmentin is enhanced by potentiation (**Figure 6.27**). A third example involves Stribild, which includes four active ingredients: elvitegravir (a protease inhibitor), emtricitabine (a nucleotide reverse transcriptase inhibitor [NRTI]), tenofovir disoproxil fumarate (a NRTI), and cobicistat. Cobicistat has no pharmacological activity of its own, but rather is used to inhibit CYP3A4 and thereby reduce metabolic inactivation of the elvitegravir component in Stribild.

Regulation of Receptors

Because receptors play a crucial role in the signaling pathways, their number, intensity, location, and sensitivity are regulated within the body. While the regulation occurs within seconds for some receptors, it may take days for others.

If a receptor is continuously receiving a ligand (agonist), there is a chance that receptor responses might be reduced, a phenomenon referred to as tachyphylaxis. For instance, a molecule called β-arrestin binds to an intracellular component of the β-adrenergic receptors when these receptors are constantly binding to their agonistic ligands. The role of β-arrestin is to block access of the Gs protein, which might otherwise desensitize the receptor within minutes. When the agonist is removed, β-arrestin also dissociates from the intracellular component of the β-adrenergic receptors, allowing restoration of these receptors back to their full sensitivity.

Another example of regulation arises when an agonist-bound receptor is internalized by an endocytosis process. The endocytosis prevents the ligand from accessing the receptor. The removal of the receptor from the membrane may be only temporary because the internalized receptor may be relocalized into the membrane (which is the case for morphine receptors), or the receptor may be permanently degraded (which is the case for epidermal growth factor receptors). In the latter case, a new receptor will emerge upon expressing its gene, which may take anywhere from hours to a day.

In addition to these mechanisms, both down-regulation and up-regulation of receptors can occur. Down-regulation of receptor expression may take place when a receptor is continuously exposed to an agonistic ligand. Conversely, up-regulation of receptor expression may occur if the receptor is blocked by an antagonist for several days. However, these changes in receptor expressions can be caused by pathophysiological factors as well. As mentioned earlier in this chapter, approximately 30% of patients with breast cancer overexpress the HER-2 receptor. Similarly, some patients with hyperthyroidism express a higher level of β-adrenergic receptors, which explains why untreated patients with hyperthyroidism show symptoms such as palpitation and tremor. However, the underlying cause for the elevation in β-adrenergic receptors is not fully understood.

Golden Keys for Pharmacy Students

1. Receptors have two major functions: binding to their specific molecules (ligands) and sending signals (signal transduction). Thus there must be at least two domains on a receptor: a ligand-binding domain and an effector domain.

2. A change in drug sensitivity may be the result of a change in the affinity between a drug and a receptor, a change in the binding to a receptor, or a change in the structure and function of a receptor.

3. The large intestine does not have any villi, so it does not provide an adequate surface area for drug absorption.

4. Due to the large surface areas of villi that are lined with epithelial and goblet cells and the 4-hour transit time of drugs, many drugs are absorbed from the small intestine.

5. Polypeptides and proteins are denatured in the acidic environment of the stomach. The more a drug is denatured, the more it is prone to proteolytic hydrolysis.

6. Goblets cells are the second most abundant cells (after epithelial cells) on the villi. Goblet cells produce a mucous layer that makes a film inside the lumen of the small intestine to cover the epithelial cells. The mucous layer does not allow large drug molecules (larger than 800 daltons) to reach the epithelial cells.

7. Many drugs that are absorbed by the GI tract travel through the portal vein to the liver before they are distributed to the general circulation. The venous blood from the stomach, the small intestine, and the large intestine passes into the portal vein and then moves to the liver.

8. The presence of food in the stomach slows gastric emptying, which in turn delays the transport of a drug from the stomach to the small intestine.

9. The stomach acidity is low (achlorhydria) in infants (1 month to 1 year). This leads to increased absorption of basic drugs (which are less ionized in a higher pH) and decreased absorption of acidic drugs (which are more ionized in a higher pH) through the gastric membranes.

10. Drugs that are bound to albumin are pharmacologically inactive because only free drug can act on receptors or other targets. The amount of serum albumin is low in infants, which results in higher levels of unbound drugs in these patients.

11. Albumin has the highest affinity for weak acidic and hydrophobic drugs.

12. The hepatic first-pass effect is reduced in the elderly population, which results in lower hepatic metabolism and, ultimately, increased plasma concentrations of many drug products.

13. The sensitivity of muscarinic, β-adrenergic, α_1-adrenergic, and μ-opioid receptors declines as a consequence of aging.

14. The more lipid storage of hydrophobic drugs that occurs, the higher the volume of distribution, which results in a longer half-life for these drugs (lower elimination rate).

15. Hormones are ligands that are the "first messengers"; Ca^{2+}, cAMP, IP_3, diacylglycerol, and cGMP are the "second messengers" that are released or synthesized when hormones bind to their receptor.

16. Cyclic AMP plays important roles in many cellular functions, including cell growth and differentiation, regulation of gene expression, and apoptosis.

17. The concentration of Ca^{2+} in the cytoplasm is very low (10^{-6} M); the concentration of this ion outside the cell and inside the ER is 10^{-3} M.

18. The detection of light (vision), odors (olfaction), and tastes (gustation) in vertebrates relies on serpentine receptors that act through the G proteins to change the sensory neurons' electrical potential.

19. The toxins produced by *Bordetella pertussis* (which causes whooping cough) and by *Vibrio cholerae* (which causes cholera) are able to increase the synthesis of cAMP and thereby interrupt many hosts' cellular functions.

20. When steroid hormones reach their target cells, they dissociate from their transport proteins, spontaneously pass through the cell membrane and enter the cytoplasm, bind to their receptor, and then migrate to the nucleus. In the nucleus, their function is to induce (or, to a lesser extent, repress) transcription of specific genes.

21. The physiological effect from steroid hormones occurs slowly, whereas the physiological effects of peptide hormones occurs rapidly.

22. Receptors play important roles in selecting their ligands (drugs), but it is the concentration of the ligand at a receptor binding site that governs the biological response to ligand–receptor binding.

23. Spare receptors are those receptors that do not have to be occupied for a ligand or drug to produce the maximal response.

24. Potency and EC_{50} have a reciprocal relationship: the higher the EC_{50}, the lower the potency.

25. The affinity of a receptor for a drug is measured by its dissociation constant. The higher the value of K_d, the lower the affinity.

26. An agonist is a drug that binds to a receptor and mimics the effects of an endogenous molecule.

27. A partial agonist is a drug that binds to a receptor but is not as effective as the endogenous ligands.

28. An antagonist is a drug that binds to a receptor and blocks the binding of the endogenous ligand or another drug.

29. Down-regulation of receptor expression may occur when a receptor is exposed in a continuous manner to an agonist. Up-regulation of receptor expression may occur as well if the receptor is blocked by an antagonist for several days.

30. A noncompetitive antagonist binds to the receptor at a site different from the agonist binding site (i.e., to an allosteric binding site).

Learning Bridge Answers

6.1 A. Joe has most likely been infected with *Vibrio cholerae*. If not treated, this disease can cause life-threatening dehydration and electrolyte imbalance. The causative bacterium is often found in contaminated water. Patients with *V. cholerae* infection recover fairly quickly if they are appropriately treated with an ORS. Tetracyclines such as doxycycline, trimethoprim-sulfamethoxazole, and macrolide agents have been used in severe cases, but the bacterium has developed resistance against these antibiotics.

B. Joe is losing many electrolytes (of particular concern is potassium) in his watery diarrhea, so it is important to treat his electrolyte imbalance. Rapid restoration of the fluid loss should be initiated as soon as possible. It has been suggested that rice-based ORS is more efficacious than glucose-based ORS because the rice-based ORS can reduce fluid requirements.

C. Explain to Joe that the cholera toxin interrupts signal transduction by catalyzing the addition of the ADP-ribose moiety of nicotinamide adenine dinucleotide to the α subunit of the Gs protein and inhibits the Gs protein's GTPase activity; the Gs protein then becomes attached to GTP (the active form of Gs). The activated Gs protein stimulates adenylate cyclase to produce cAMP continuously, which in turn stimulates water, bicarbonate, and Cl^- secretion into the intestinal lumen.

6.2 It seems Amy is in good compliance with her metformin therapy. However, she needs to cut down on the amount of coffee and tea that she drinks. Coffee and tea contain xanthine derivatives—namely, caffeine and theophylline, respectively. These xanthine derivatives inhibit the cyclic nucleotide phosphodiesterase enzyme and increase the amount of cAMP present. The elevated cAMP activates the cAMP-dependent protein kinase (PKA). PKA activates phosphorylase *b* kinase, which in turn converts glycogen phosphorylase *b* to glycogen phosphorylase *a*, which finally initiates glycogenolysis. Consequently, Amy's blood glucose level is increased.

6.3 A. These two drugs are two different medications that are used for different reasons. While Proventil is used for acute breathing difficulty and has a rapid action (1–2 minutes), Pulmicort is not appropriate for use in acute bronchospasm but rather is typically used for chronic breathing difficulty.

B. The active ingredient in Proventil is albuterol, a $β_2$-adrenergic receptor agonist that has a rapid bronchodilation effect. It stimulates the serpentine $β_2$-receptor, which in turn activates the adenylate cyclase enzyme to synthesize more cAMP. The cyclic AMP, in turn, activates PKA, which lowers intracellular calcium concentrations. A decrease in the intracellular Ca^{2+} concentration results in smooth muscle relaxation, thereby alleviating bronchospasm. Budesonide (Pulmicort) is also used to prevent shortness of breath and difficulty with breathing associated with lung diseases. Because it is a steroid agent, it will affect nuclear receptors so as to alter expression of a few genes. As a result, it will take hours before any effect is seen with Pulmicort.

C. Although the agent in Pulmicort can help Emily to breathe better, because Pulmicort is a steroid agent it will act slowly; thus it will not assist Emily in rapidly achieving a bronchodilation effect. In addition, it may take 2–6 weeks to see the full effect from Pulmicort—which is not helpful at all for Emily's acute breathing difficulty.

6.4 Sildenafil inhibits phosphodiesterase 5 (PDE5), the enzyme that degrades cGMP. By administering this drug, the pilot will have a higher concentration of cGMP and thereby better vasodilation. However, sildenafil may also inhibit phosphodiesterase 6, the isoenzyme that breaks down cGMP in the rod cells of the retina. A higher concentration of cGMP leads to opened Na^+ and Ca^{2+} channels, and thereby an impaired response of the rod cells to light. Basically, the pilot's vision will be impaired—which is why he should avoid flying an aircraft.

Your observation also indicates that the pilot is suffering from angina pectoris and most likely is using nitroglycerin tablets to relieve his chest pain. Angina pectoris is a very painful symptom of coronary artery disease. This disease occurs when the coronary arteries in the heart become narrowed, making it difficult for oxygen to flow.

Nitroglycerin relieves the pain when it is hydrolyzed into nitric oxide (NO) in the blood. NO activates guanylate cyclase to synthesize cGMP; cGMP, in turn, sequesters Ca^{2+} and thereby enables muscle cells lining the walls of blood vessels to relax (vasodilation). It is wise to advise the pilot to avoid taking sildenafil concurrently with his nitroglycerin tablets, as sildenafil will potentiate the effect of nitroglycerin (i.e., enhance the vasodilatory effect of nitroglycerin).

6.5 A. Tamsulosin is a competitive antagonist of α_1-receptors in the smooth muscle of the bladder and peripheral vasculature that blocks the uptake of catecholamines (norepinephrine and epinephrine). As a result, it not only reduces resistance to urinary outflow, but also results in vasodilation and reduced blood pressure. The reduced blood pressure causes orthostatic hypotension, which explains his dizziness. Advise Joe to have a support handy whenever he stands up from a lying or sitting position to avoid a fall.

B. Tamsulosin binds reversibly to α_1-receptors and competes for the same site against the agonists such as the natural ligands (catecholamines).

C. The α_1-receptors, upon binding to their ligands (catecholamines), activate Gq protein, which in turn activates phospholipase C to synthesize IP_3 and diacylglycerol. Both of these molecules are second messengers that increase intracellular concentration of calcium, thereby producing smooth muscle contraction. Obviously, blocking α_1-receptors will produce the opposite effects, such as bladder relaxation and hypotension.

Problems and Solutions

Problem 6.1 Which of the following physiological conditions is a homeostatic process?

- **A.** Albumin is an abundant plasma protein that uptakes or releases hydrogen ions to maintain the blood's pH.
- **B.** Cells uptake glucose (fuel) and release CO_2 (waste).
- **C.** Termogenin proteins maintain body temperature.
- **D.** Insulin glargine is a long-acting insulin preparation that maintains a constant insulin level for 24 hours.
- **E.** Only A and B
- **F.** All of the above except C
- **G.** All of the above except D
- **H.** All of the above

Solution 6.1 G is correct.

Problem 6.2 The mucosa of the stomach wall has hundreds of gastric glands. Each gastric gland has four major cells. Name these four cells and their functions.

Solution 6.2 Mucous neck cells (secrete mucins); parietal cells (secrete HCl); chief cells (secrete pepsinogen); and enteroendocrine cells (secrete hormones).

Problem 6.3 Which of the following characteristics plays an important role in the absorption of an oral drug? (Choose all that apply.)

- **A.** The long transit time in the small intestine
- **B.** The large surface area at the ileum
- **C.** The large surface area at the duodenum
- **D.** The large surface area at the jejunum
- **E.** The large surface area of villi in the small intestine

Solution 6.3 All except B. While villi are found in the ileum, they are not concentrated there (less surface area). The transit time, which is 4 hours, provides enough time for drugs to travel through the villi and be absorbed there.

Problem 6.4 Why is gastric acid important in the synthesis of hemoglobin?

Solution 6.4 The acidic environment of the stomach converts ferric iron (Fe^{3+}) to ferrous iron (Fe^{2+}). The latter form is absorbed better and will be used to form heme for the synthesis of hemoglobin. Approximately two-thirds of the body's iron is found inside hemoglobin and myoglobin proteins, and one-third is stored in the iron-storage protein, ferritin.

Problem 6.5 True or false? Erythromycin and azithromycin belong to the class of macrolide antibiotics, all of which have a similar mechanism of action. The drug absorption rate for erythromycin and azithromycin is the same in all areas of the GI tract.

Solution 6.5 False. Different areas of the GI tract have different surface areas and different pH. Having the same mechanism of action and coming from the same class does not mean that drugs are similarly absorbed from the GI tract. For instance, while the acidic pH of stomach destroys erythromycin, the low pH does not affect azithromycin.

Problem 6.6 Haloperidol has a K_d of 0.53 nM for dopamine receptor 2. Suppose haloperidol can produce its maximum antipsychotic effect at a certain concentration. Based on the information given here, suggest an EC_{50} and a haloperidol concentration that would produce the E_{max} for haloperidol. Suppose there are no spare dopamine receptors.

Solution 6.6 Based on the given information, the concentration of haloperidol that is equal to its K_d (0.53 nM) is the EC_{50} or potency. When the drug concentration is much higher (100 times) than K_d (in our case, 53 nM), haloperidol occupies 100% of the D_2 receptor binding sites and produces an E_{max} (maximal effect). Remember, if the spare receptors exist, you cannot assume that EC_{50} and K_d are the same.

Problem 6.7 Penicillin doses are commonly given in amounts 10 times higher than penicillin's MEC. Penicillin is a typical example of a drug with: (Choose all that apply.)

    A. a large therapeutic index.
    B. a narrow therapeutic index.
    C. a large therapeutic window.
    D. a small therapeutic window.
    E. a partial agonistic effect.

Solution 6.7 A and C are correct.

Problem 6.8 Probenecid is an NSAID that is an acidic drug. Diazepam (which is used to treat anxiety disorders) is a hydrophobic drug. Which of the following statements is (are) correct?

    A. Probenecid is more free (unbound to albumin) than diazepam in the plasma.
    B. Diazepam is more free (unbound to albumin) than probenecid in the plasma.
    C. Diazepam has a lower elimination rate in obese patients.
    D. Diazepam has an increased duration of action in elderly patients.

Solution 6.8 All except B are correct. C and D are correct because while the volume of distribution is decreased for water-soluble drugs, it is increased for hydrophobic drugs. This results in an increased $t_{1/2}$ (or lower elimination rate) for diazepam.

Problem 6.9 Ranitidine is an inhibitor of histamine H_2-receptors of the gastric parietal cells that inhibits HCl secretion into the stomach. However, the presence of a large amount of histamine will overcome ranitidine's inhibitory effect. Which of the following statements is (are) correct?

   A. Histamine is a full agonist.

   B. Histamine is a partial agonist.

   C. Ranitidine is a competitive antagonist.

   D. Ranitidine is a noncompetitive antagonist.

   E. Ranitidine is a chemical antagonist.

Solution 6.9 A and C are correct. Histamine is the natural (endogenous) ligand for the H_2-receptors. Because the presence of a large amount of histamine reverses the inhibitory effect of ranitidine (i.e., histamine forces ranitidine to leave the receptor binding site), ranitidine must be a competitive antagonist.

Problem 6.10 True or false? Aripiprazole (an antipsychotic agent) is a partial agonist agent for dopamine receptors that competes with the full agonist (dopamine) for binding to D_2 receptors. An increasing concentration of aripiprazole reduces the response from dopamine to zero.

Solution 6.10 False. Remember, the characteristic in this problem is for a competitive antagonist—not for a partial agonist. A partial agonist in the presence of a full agonist acts as a partial antagonist. Therefore, increasing the concentration of aripiprazole will inhibit the response to only a certain level (a "partial" level and not to a zero level). A competitive antagonist, however, will reduce the response to zero.

Problem 6.11 Which of the following statements is correct regarding a dose–response system with no spare receptor?

   A. If the drug concentration is higher than the K_d, then E/E_{max} becomes 1 (or 100%).

   B. If the drug concentration is equal to the K_d, 50% of the maximum effect (EC_{50}) has been achieved by the drug.

   C. The higher the EC_{50}, the lower the potency.

   D. All of the above.

Solution 6.11 C is correct.

Problem 6.12 Give an example of a ligand-gated channel.

Solution 6.12 Acetylcholine receptor is an example of a ligand-gated channel.

Problem 6.13 Describe how binding of the epinephrine hormone to a β-adrenergic receptor can increase the blood glucose level.

Solution 6.13 Upon binding of the epinephrine hormone to its receptor, GTP is exchanged for GDP on a GTP-binding protein (Gs), which in turn activates adenylate cyclase to synthesize cAMP. cAMP activates the cAMP-dependent protein kinase (PKA). PKA activates phosphorylase *b* kinase, which in turn converts glycogen phosphorylase *b* to glycogen phosphorylase *a*, which finally initiates glycogenolysis.

Problem 6.14 One day when you are completing one of your rotations in a hospital, you decide to take a break and go to the cafeteria. One of the researchers at the same hospital comes to the cafeteria, too. She knows that you have finished all those basic and clinical sciences and thinks you might be able to help her with her question. She has cultured some cells from a tumor biopsy but is not sure how she should look for any oncogene in her cell culture. Using your signal transduction knowledge, how would you respond?

Solution 6.14 Because the researcher is looking for an oncogene, the fastest way to figure out if such a gene exists is to look for a G protein. When a mutation in a G protein destroys its GTPase activity, it can no longer inactivate itself by converting bound GTP to GDP. Once activated, the mutant G protein continues to send its unregulated signal. This leads to frequent activation of many protein kinases that are involved in the cell cycle. The result will be cancer.

References

1. Barrett KE, Barman SM, Boitano S, Brooks HL. Overview of cellular physiology in medical physiology. In: Barrett KE, Barman SM, Boitano S, Brooks HL, eds. *Ganong's review of medical physiology.* 24th ed. New York, NY: McGraw-Hill; 2012. Available at: http://www.accesspharmacy .com/content.aspx?aID=56260315.

2. Barrett KE, Barman SM, Boitano S, Brooks HL. Regulation of extracellular fluid composition and volume. In: Barrett KE, Barman SM, Boitano S, Brooks HL, eds. *Ganong's review of medical physiology.* 24th ed. New York, NY: McGraw-Hill; 2012. Available at: http://www.accessmedicine.com /content.aspx?aID=56265999.

3. Bauer LA. Clinical pharmacokinetics and pharmacodynamics. In: DiPiro JT, Talbert RL, Yee GC, et al., eds. *Pharmacotherapy: a pathophysiologic approach,* 7th ed. New York, NY: McGraw-Hill; 2008. Available at: http://www.accesspharmacy.com/content.aspx?aID=3197852.

4. Blumenthal DK, Garrison JC. Pharmacodynamics: molecular mechanisms of drug action. In: Brunton LL, Chabner BA, Knollmann BC, eds. *Goodman & Gilman's the pharmacological basis of therapeutics,* 12th ed. New York, NY: McGraw-Hill; 2011. Available at: http://www.accesspharmacy .com/content.aspx?aID=16658452.

5. Chapron DJ. Drug disposition and response. In: Delafuente JC, Stewart RB, eds. *Therapeutics in the elderly,* 3rd ed. Cincinnati, OH: Harvey Whitney; 2000: 257–288.

6. Clark M, Finkel R, Rey J, Whalen, K. *Pharmacology,* 5th ed. Baltimore, MD: Lippincott Williams & Wilkins; 2012.

7. Cusack BJ. Pharmacokinetics in older persons. *Am J Geriatr Pharm.* 2004;2:274–302.

8. Diez J, Simon MA, Anton F, et al. Tubular sodium handling in cirrhotic patients with ascites as analyzed by the renal lithium clearance method. *Eur J Clin Invest.* 1990;20:266–271.

9. Gough DJ, Levy DE, Johnstone RW, Clarke CJ. IFN-signaling: does it mean JAK-STAT? *Cytokine Growth Factor Rev.* 2008;19:383–394.

10. Gregus Z. Mechanisms of toxicity. In: Gregus Z, ed. *Casarett & Doull's essentials of toxicology,* 2nd ed. New York, NY: McGraw-Hill; 2010. Available at: http://www.accesspharmacy.com /content.aspx?aID=6479256.

11. Guay D, Artz MB, Hanlon JT, Schmader KE. The pharmacology of aging. In: Tallis R, Fillit H, eds. *Brocklehurst's textbook of geriatric medicine,* 6th ed. London, UK: Churchill-Livingstone; 2003:155–161.

12. Hedaya M. *Basic pharmacokinetics.* Boca Raton, FL: CRC Press, 2012.

13. Iber FL, Murphy PA, Connor ES. Age-related changes in the gastrointestinal system: effects on drug therapy. *Drugs Aging.* 1994;5:34–48.

14. Ishizu H, Shiomi S, Kawamura E, et al. Gastric emptying in patients with chronic liver diseases. *Ann Nucl Med.* 2002;16:177–182.

15. Kane RL, Ouslander JG, Abrass IB. Clinical implications of the aging process. In: *Essentials of clinical geriatrics,* 5th ed. New York, NY: McGraw-Hill; 2004:3–15.

16. Kohlmeier M, Vitamin K. In: *AccessScience.* New York, NY: McGraw-Hill; 2008. Available at: http://www.accessscience.com.

17. Martin S, Jung R. Gastrointestinal infections and enterotoxigenic poisonings. In: Talbert RL, DiPiro JT, Matzke GR, et al., eds. *Pharmacotherapy: a pathophysiologic approach,* 8th ed. New York, NY: McGraw-Hill; 2011. Available at: http://www.accesspharmacy.com/content .aspx?aID=8003383.

18. Masoro EJ. Physiology of aging. In: Tallis R, Fillit H, eds. *Brocklehurst's textbook of geriatric medicine*, 6th ed. London, UK: Churchill-Livingstone; 2003:291–299.

19. Medina PJ, Shord SS. Cancer treatment and chemotherapy. In: Talbert RL, DiPiro JT, Matzke GR, et al., eds. *Pharmacotherapy: a pathophysiologic approach*, 8th ed. New York, NY: McGraw-Hill; 2011. Available at: http://www.accesspharmacy.com/content.aspx?aID=8007280.

20. Morshed SA, Ando T, Latif R, Davies TF. Neutral antibodies to the TSH receptor are present in Graves' disease and regulate selective signaling cascades. *Endocrinology*. 2010;151(11):5537–5549.

21. Murray RK, Jacob M, Varghese J. Cancer: an overview. In: Murray RK, Kennelly PJ, Rodwell VW, et al., eds. *Harper's illustrated biochemistry*, 29th ed. New York, NY: McGraw-Hill; 2011. Available at: http://www.accesspharmacy.com/content.aspx?aID=55887057.

22. Nelson DL, Cox MM, Lehninger AL. *Principles of biochemistry*, 5th ed. New York, NY: W. H. Freeman and Company; 2008.

23. Osgood M, Ocorr K. *The absolute, ultimate guide to Lehninger principles of biochemistry*, 4th ed. New York, NY: W. H. Freeman and Company; 2005.

24. Pandit NK, Soltis RP. *Introduction to pharmaceutical sciences: an integrated approach*, 2nd ed. Baltimore, MD: Wolters Kluwer, Lippincott Williams & Wilkins; 2012.

25. Patterson RL, Boehning D, Snyder SH. Inositol 1,4,5-trisphosphate receptors as signal integrators. *Annu Rev Biochem*. 2004;73:437–465.

26. Ruhnke M, Yeates RA, Pfaff G, et al. Single-dose pharmacokinetics of fluconazole in patients with liver cirrhosis. *J Antimicrob Chemother*. 1995;35:641–647.

27. Sauer H. Cell differentiation. In: *AccessScience*. New York, NY: McGraw-Hill; 2012. Available at: http://www.accessscience.com.

28. Sotaniemi EA, Arranto AJ, Pelkonen O, Pasanen M. Age and cytochrome P450–linked drug metabolism in humans. *Clin Pharmacol Ther*. 1997;61:331–339.

29. Starner CI, Gray SL, Guay DR, et al. Geriatrics. In: DiPiro JT, Talbert RL, Yee GC, et al., eds. *Pharmacotherapy: a pathophysiologic approach*, 7th ed. New York, NY: McGraw-Hill; 2008. Available at: http://www.accesspharmacy.com/content.aspx?aID=3190958.

30. Strange PG. Antipsychotic drugs: importance of dopamine receptors for mechanisms of therapeutic actions and side effects. *Pharmacol Rev*. 2001:119–134.

31. Treish I, Schwartz R, Lindley C. Pharmacology and therapeutic use of trastuzumab in breast cancer. *Am J Health Syst Pharm*. 2000;57:2063–2076; quiz 2077–2079.

32. Trevor AJ, Katzung BG, Masters SB. Pharmacodynamics. In: Trevor AJ, Katzung BG, Masters SB, eds. *Pharmacology: examination & board review*, 9th ed. New York, NY: McGraw-Hill; 2010. Available at: http://www.accesspharmacy.com/content.aspx?aID=6543122.

33. UpToDate. Waltham, MA: 2012. Available at: http://www.uptodate.com/online with subscription.

34. von Zastrow M. Drug receptors and pharmacodynamics. In: Katzung BG, Masters SB, Trevor AJ, eds. *Basic & clinical pharmacology*, 12th ed. New York, NY: McGraw-Hill; 2012. Available at: http://www.accesspharmacy.com/content.aspx?aID=55820126.

35. Weil P. Hormone action and signal transduction. In: Murray RK, Kennelly PJ, Rodwell VW, et al., eds. *Harper's illustrated biochemistry*, 29th ed. New York, NY: McGraw-Hill; 2011. Available at: http://www.accesspharmacy.com/content.aspx?aID=55885339.

36. Westfall TC. Neurotransmission: the autonomic and somatic motor nervous systems. In: Brunton LL, Chabner BA, Knollmann BC, eds. *Goodman & Gilman's the pharmacological basis of therapeutics*, 12th ed. New York, NY: McGraw-Hill; 2011. Available at: http://www.accesspharmacy.com/content.aspx?aID=16659803.

Introduction to Medicinal Chemistry

Reza Karimi

OBJECTIVES

1. Learn how the two major metabolic phases (I and II) contribute to drug biotransformation.

2. Understand how induction and inhibition of CYP450 isozymes in the liver are affected by drugs, food, and chemicals.

3. Comprehend the principles behind the structure and function of drugs.

4. Appreciate the role that stereochemistry plays in drug actions.

5. Learn the role of lead structure–activity relationships in medicinal chemistry.

6. Learn how drugs target biological macromolecules.

7. Implement a series of Learning Bridge assignments at your experiential sites to bridge your didactic learning with your experiential experiences.

KEY TERMS AND DEFINITIONS

1. **Bioisosteres:** molecules or ions of similar size and similar chemical and physical properties that, when replaced by other bioisosteres, will not affect the biological activity of a molecule.

2. **Biological macromolecules:** proteins, carbohydrates, lipids, and nucleic acids that are essential for cellular growth and survival.

3. **Carcinogen:** a molecule that can be converted to a cancer-causing metabolite.

4. **Chiral molecule:** an organic molecule that contains a carbon atom bound to four different atoms or molecules.

5. **Compound:** a combination of two or more substances, ingredients, or elements. While the majority of drugs on the market are compounds, not all compounds are drugs.

6. **Configuration:** rearrangement of a molecule by breaking and re-forming bonds within the molecule.

7. **Conformation:** the different arrangement that occurs during the rotation around a single bond.

8. **Cytochrome P450 enzymes:** a superfamily of heme-containing enzymes in which the heme is noncovalently bound to the polypeptide chain of enzymes.

9. **Cytochrome P450 reductase:** a microsomal enzyme that is the electron donor enzyme for several oxygenase enzymes, including the cytochrome P450 isozymes.

10. **Diastereomers:** stereoisomers that are not mirror images of each other.

11. **Enantiomers:** two chiral molecules that are mirror images of each other (regardless of whether they have one or more chiral carbons).

12. **Isoforms:** two or more protein forms that have the same function but have been expressed by different genes.

(continues)

13. **Isomers:** two or more molecules with the same molecular formula (i.e., exactly the same number of carbon and hydrogen atoms) but different three-dimensional structures.

14. **Isozymes:** two or more enzymes that catalyze the same reaction but have different molecular forms and are expressed by different genes.

15. **Oxidases:** enzymes that catalyze oxidation of a substrate without incorporating an oxygen atom into the main product.

16. **Oxygenases:** enzymes that directly incorporate oxygen atoms from O_2 into substrate molecules to form a new hydroxyl or carboxyl group.

17. **Pharmacophore:** a series of functional groups that are required to exhibit a particular pharmacological activity.

18. **Phase I reactions:** oxidation, reduction, and hydrolysis reactions that occur in the smooth endoplasmic reticulum.

19. **Phase II reactions:** conjugation reactions that occur in the cytosol of cells, such as glucuronidation, sulfation, conjugation with glutathione, acetylation, and methylation.

20. **Polymorphism:** any of the genetic variations that occur at a frequency of 1% or greater in the human population and that result in altered expression or functional activity of a gene.

21. **Prodrugs:** inactive compounds that upon metabolism in the body produce active metabolites that have pharmacological effects.

22. **Racemic mixture:** a sample of a compound containing equal amounts of the two enantiomers.

Introduction

Medicinal chemistry, as its name indicates, is a scientific field that combines chemistry with the therapeutic roles that drug products fulfill. Functional groups of a drug product and their characteristics significantly contribute to the drug product's pharmacological effect. Therefore, the relationship between functional groups' characteristics and pharmacological responses is the cornerstone of medicinal chemistry. These characteristics are affected by metabolism, neighboring functional groups, and the positions that functional groups occupy in a drug product. As a result, the roles of functional groups and their characteristics are the targets for studies, research, and investigations when developing new drug products or improving drug products that are already on the market. Accordingly, knowledge about functional groups and their characteristics is of paramount importance in understanding medicinal chemistry. Students are well advised to study the functional groups described in the *Introduction to Biological Chemistry* chapter before studying the topics presented in this chapter.

This chapter begins by describing the important role that drug metabolism plays in chemical modifications and eliminations of drug products. The significance of cytochrome P450 isozymes and drug metabolism in drug–drug interactions are emphasized. In addition, factors that influence drug metabolism, such as age, sex, and food, are briefly introduced. The roles of functional groups that underlie the structure–activity relationship of drugs are briefly described. Furthermore, students are introduced to how different drug products target biological macromolecules.

Drug Metabolism

Humans are constantly exposed to xenobiotics (foreign molecules; drug products are also considered to be xenobiotics) that intentionally (e.g., use of drug products for the treatment of diseases or use of harmful substances) or unintentionally (e.g., exposure to chemicals, environmental pollution, agrochemicals, food additives, cosmetic products) enter the human body through the lungs, skin, or eyes, or simply by direct ingestion. Many of these foreign molecules provoke biological responses—some beneficial and some toxic.

Drug metabolism plays an important role in the development of drugs. Three major metabolic factors can affect the development of a drug product: (1) genetic variations to metabolize drugs (i.e., pharmacogenomics; see also the *Introduction to Pharmacogenomics* chapter); (2) drug–drug interactions; and (3) production of by-products (i.e., metabolites) that are toxic or carcinogenic. In addition, differences in expression of metabolizing enzymes among different species may limit the use of animal models for studying drug metabolism in humans.

Many drugs must be able to interact with a receptor to produce a pharmacological response (see also the *Introduction to Pharmacodynamics* chapter). To do so, they have to mimic the structures of our endogenous ligands. By the same token, drugs must be able to enter a cell if they are designed to interact with an intracellular target. Therefore, they must have a hydrophobic property that allows them to pass through the hydrophobic bilayer of a cell membrane. However, the same hydrophobic property makes it difficult for these drugs to be eliminated, as they can accumulate in the body's lipids. Drug metabolism assists in this process by increasing the water solubility of these hydrophobic drugs, allowing them to be readily removed from the body through an elimination process.

Renal excretion plays a key role in the elimination of drugs that either are small, are hydrophilic, or have functional groups that are ionizable at physiologic pH. In contrast, drugs that are large, hydrophobic, or mostly un-ionizable are not readily excreted by the kidneys. Instead, these drugs are reabsorbed from the distal tubule back to the renal vein, a mechanism known as tubular reabsorption (see also the *Introduction to Pharmacokinetics* chapter). In addition, some lipophilic molecules are strongly attached to plasma proteins, and this attachment renders them too large to be filtered at the glomerulus.

To make the foreign molecules readily available to be excreted by the kidneys, our biological system has found an alternative process, metabolism. Most drugs are metabolized in the liver, but a few are metabolized in the intestinal lumen or intestinal wall. Liver metabolism, however, is not a simple step. Multiple factors, such as hepatic blood flow, ability of the liver to extract the drug from the blood, drug affinity to plasma proteins, and hepatic diseases (e.g., cirrhosis, congestive heart failure), play important roles in the metabolism of drugs. In addition to these factors, metabolism of drugs usually occurs in the liver throughout two major metabolic pathways: Phase I and Phase II (**Figure 7.1**).

Metabolism makes drugs more hydrophilic so that they can be excreted. Due to the changes that take place during metabolism, the metabolic products (metabolites) are often pharmacologically less active or totally inactive. Nevertheless, some metabolites have enhanced activities or are unstable enough to serve as reactive molecules that target cellular compartments or components. Thus drug metabolism can lead to two very different outcomes: termination of the drug action or production of a drug action. Drugs with the latter outcome are called prodrugs. Drug-metabolizing enzymes have been intensively studied in an attempt to design prodrugs. The concept of prodrugs is described in more detail in a later section of this chapter.

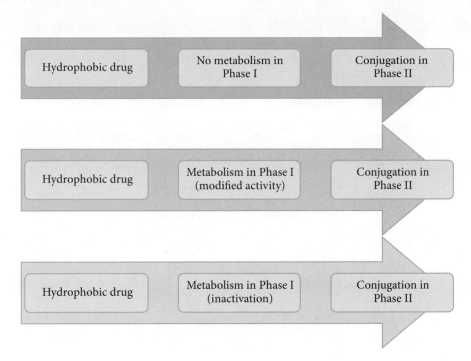

Figure 7.1 Three possible metabolic scenarios of hydrophobic drugs during Phase I and Phase II.
Adapted from: Correia MA. Drug biotransformation. In: Katzung BG, Masters SB, Trevor AJ. *Basic & clinical pharmacology*, 11th ed. New York: McGraw-Hill; 2009. Available at: http://www.accesspharmacy.com/content .aspx?aID=4515730.

All living organisms, including plants, use the same basic endogenous organic molecules for their survival. These molecules are lipids, carbohydrates, nucleic acids, and proteins. The chemistry of each of these groups is of immense interest to scientists, as these macromolecules play important roles in the living cells. Scientists are interested in learning how these organic macromolecules form, function, interact, and are metabolized in living cells. Likewise, the metabolism of xenobiotics is of particular interest because these substances can affect the function or metabolism of the endogenous macromolecules. The hepatic smooth endoplasmic reticulum (ER) is the main site of drug metabolism. Because the liver plays a crucial role in drug metabolism, both Phase I and Phase II metabolism deserve closer attention and discussion. Briefly, both phases make drugs more polar, although Phase I reactions do so by oxidation, hydrolysis, and reduction (**Figure 7.2**), and Phase II reactions do so by conjugation to form glucuronides, acetates, or sulfates. The overall goal is to inactivate the drugs and make them more prone to renal elimination.

While the liver is the major organ that plays a central role in drug metabolism, other organs contribute to many metabolic pathways of drugs. Examples include the gastrointestinal (GI) tract, lungs, kidneys, skin, and brain. Even the intestinal microorganisms come into play. For instance, oral sympathomimetics, clonazepam (Klonopin), chlorpromazine (Largactil, from Canada), and cyclosporine (Gengraf) are more extensively metabolized by the intestines than by the liver. While the intestinal metabolism complicates the overall metabolism of drugs, patients with hepatic dysfunctions may benefit from this metabolic route.

Many drugs are absorbed from the small intestine and are transported to the liver by the portal vein system (first-pass effect). Because the intestinal metabolism modifies the effect of drugs, it

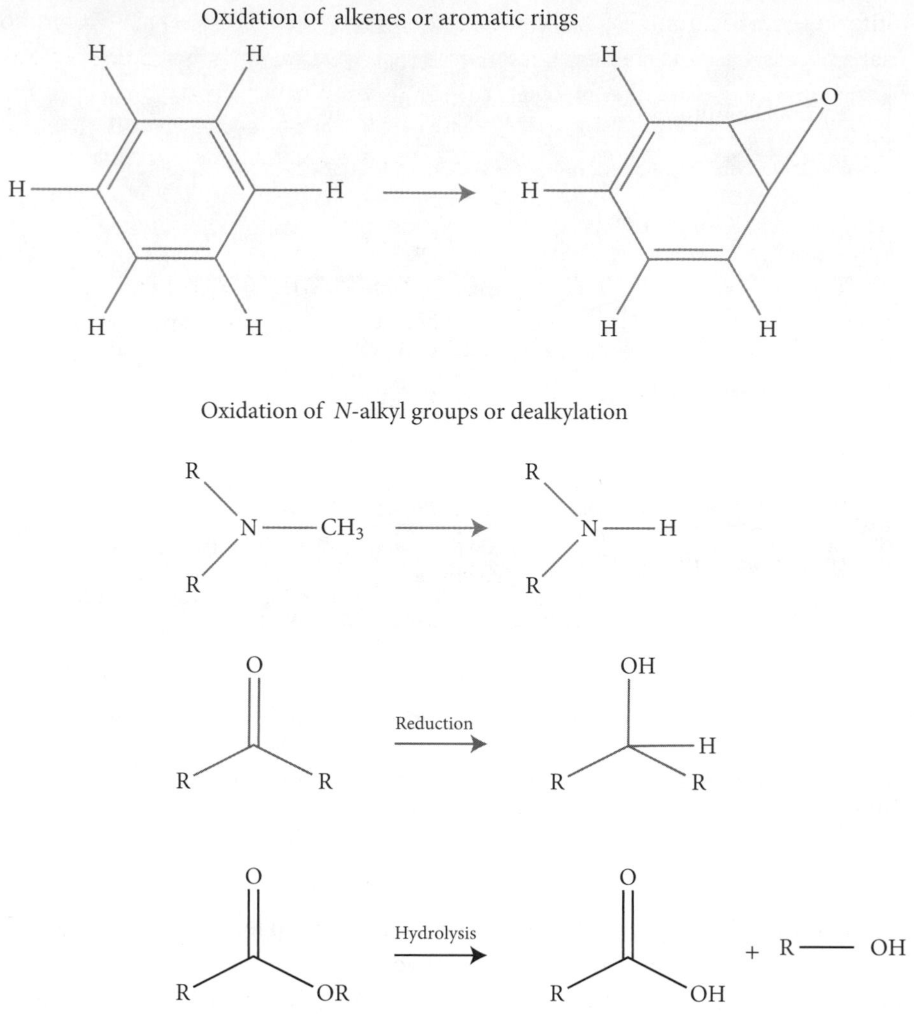

Oxidation of alkenes or aromatic rings

Oxidation of N-alkyl groups or dealkylation

Figure 7.2 Typical hepatic Phase I reactions.

contributes to the first-pass effect as well. The first-pass effect limits the bioavailability of orally administered drugs. Moreover, if a therapeutic outcome is negatively affected by the first-pass effect, alternative routes of administration must be employed to achieve an effective therapeutic outcome.

Before the important roles of Phase I and Phase II metabolism are described, it is imperative to briefly describe the cytochrome P450 proteins.

Cytochrome P450 Nomenclature and Selectivity

A cytochrome P450 enzyme can maximally absorb light at 450 nm—hence the name of these enzymes. The rapid progress made in bioinformatics and genetic information has revealed that there are 57 functional genes in humans that can be expressed to produce metabolic enzymes. Thus, as of 2013, 57 different CYP enzymes had been identified in humans. Seventy-five percent of these enzymes are known to be involved in the metabolism of xenobiotics and endogenous compounds, and 15 of these enzymes are actively involved in the metabolism of drugs. Because of the immense role that CYP450 enzymes play in the metabolism of drugs, they have been intensively studied at the genetic and molecular levels.

The multiforms of cytochrome P450 are referred to as isozymes. Isozymes are two or more enzymes that catalyze the same reaction but are expressed by different genes. Some texts use the term "isoforms" instead of "isozymes" to describe these variants. Isoforms refer to two or more protein forms that have the same function but are expressed by different genes. Because cytochrome P450 proteins have enzymatic activity, these enzymes are referred to as isozymes in this text.

CYP450 isozymes are classified into families denoted by Arabic numbers and subfamilies denoted by capital letters. For instance, in naming a CYP450 isozyme, the symbol CYP refers to a cytochrome P450; it is followed by an Arabic number denoting the family, and then a capital letter denoting the subfamily. (Cytochrome P450 isozymes are considered to belong to the same family if they have 40% or more identical amino acid sequence; they are considered to belong to the same subfamily if they have greater than 55% sequence identity.) The individual P450 isozymes are then arbitrarily numbered. Thus the well-known CYP3A4 is a cytochrome P450 that is a member of family 3 and subfamily A and is the fourth individual member of that subfamily. The same principle is applied to the nomenclature for the isozymes' genes, except that italic is used for the gene name. For instance, the gene for CYP3A4 is *CYP3A4*.

All CYP450 enzymes contain a heme molecule that is noncovalently bound to their polypeptide chain. In contrast to the significance of their catalytic activities, the specificity of the majority of these microsomal enzymes is low (which explains why the cytochrome P450 family can metabolize many different drugs) and their catalytic rate is slow (particularly when they are compared with the Phase II enzymes). Nevertheless, some isozymes act very selectively. For instance, the CYP19 subfamily has a very specific substrate (testosterone) to produce estrogen and it cannot metabolize any other xenobiotics.

A series of general practical indications and characteristics are useful in identifying isozymes. First, the hydrophobic moiety of drugs is the only known common structural feature of drugs that are metabolized by CYP450 isozymes. Second, the CYP2E subfamily is known to metabolize hydrophilic drugs that have a low molecular weight. Third, CYP3A4 has a higher affinity for hydrophobic drugs. Fourth, CYP2C9 metabolizes weakly acidic drugs, and CYP2D6 metabolizes weakly basic drugs.

Many of the CYP450 isozymes are found in the human liver, including 1A2, 2A6, 2B6, 2C8, 2C9, 2C18, 2C19, 2D6, 2E1, 3A4, 3A5, and 4A11. However, the most important are CYP1A2 (representing 15% of the total liver P450 isozymes), CYP2A6 (4%), CYP2B6 (1%), CYP2C8 (4%), CYP2C9 (20%), CYP2C19 (4%), CYP2D6 (5%), CYP2E1 (10%), and CYP3A4 (30%). Clearly, CYP2C9 and CYP3A4 are the most abundant isozymes in the liver, which explains why so many drugs are metabolized by these two isozymes. Specifically, 50% of the drugs on the market are metabolized by CYP3A4. Of course, some of these isozymes are found in other organs as well. For instance, CYP3A4 is also found, albeit to a much smaller extent, in the small intestine, kidney, nasal mucosa, lung, and stomach. CYP2C9 is also found in the small intestine, nasal mucosa, and heart.

Phase I Metabolism

As mentioned earlier, for drugs to be eliminated by the kidneys, they must be hydrophilic. The liver and Phase I metabolism play important roles in making drugs more hydrophilic by modifying the drugs' functional groups. If the drugs are not sufficiently hydrophilic after the Phase I reactions, Phase II metabolism will step in to make these drugs hydrophilic enough to be excreted by the kidneys. Not all drugs sequentially undergo metabolism by Phase I and Phase II reactions, however. Some drug products do not undergo Phase I reactions but only Phase II reactions; others undergo Phase II reactions prior to entering into Phase I reactions. For instance, the hydrazide

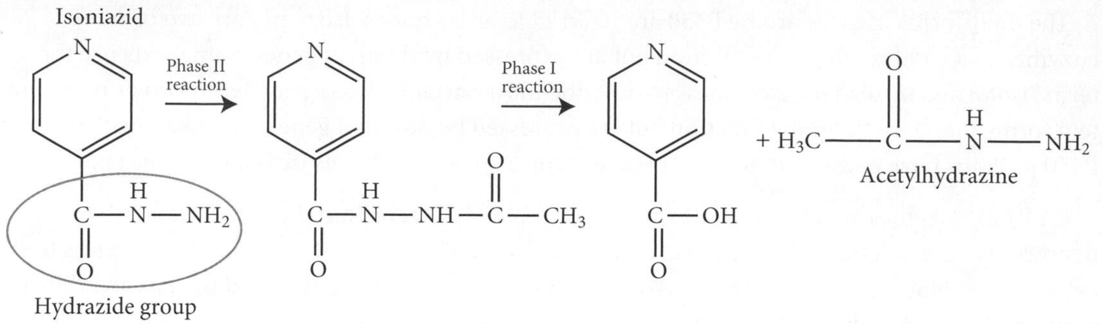

Figure 7.3 Metabolism of isoniazid by Phase I and II reactions.

group of isoniazid (Isotamine, from Canada) is first *N*-conjugated in Phase II metabolism (acetylation) without any involvement of Phase I reactions. However, after the *N*-conjugation, the isoniazid metabolite is prone to Phase I reactions. Acetylhydrazine, a by-product of isoniazid metabolism during Phase I, may accumulate in the liver to cause hepatotoxicity (**Figure 7.3**).

Most metabolic reactions are catalyzed by specific cellular enzymes, which may be located in organelles such as the endoplasmic reticulum, mitochondria, cytosol, lysosomes, or plasma membrane. The membranes of the ER, the liver, and other tissues that are involved in drug metabolism contain many metabolic enzymes. Interestingly, when the ER membranes are subjected to subcellular fractionation and isolated, they form circular compartments that are called microsomes. Microsomes are non-natural compartments that do not exist in living cells. Even so, they retain most of the morphologic and functional properties of the intact ER membranes. As a result, one can find both rough (filled with ribosomes) and smooth (no ribosomes) microsomes. The rough microsomes are rich in ribosomes and are involved with protein synthesis, while the smooth microsomes are rich in oxidative enzymes such as mixed-function oxidases or mono-oxygenases (see the following sections) and are involved with drug metabolism.

As was discussed in the *Introduction to Biochemistry* chapter, oxidative phosphorylation is an energy-producing pathway that uses oxygen to synthesize ATP molecules. Consequently, a significant amount (90%) of inhaled oxygen is used in oxidative phosphorylation. The other 10% of inhaled oxygen is consumed in a series of metabolic reactions. Indeed, more than 200 enzymes in the cell use oxygen as substrate or co-substrate. Both CYP450-dependent and -independent oxidation occur during the Phase I reactions. Let's first go through some important metabolic enzymes that use oxygen as their substrate.

Oxidases

Oxidases are enzymes that catalyze oxidation of a substrate without incorporating oxygen into the main product. Two electrons are transferred to the molecular oxygen so that the oxygen is converted to H_2O_2. Most oxidases utilize either a metal or a flavin coenzyme. For example, flavoprotein dehydrogenase is an oxidase that is involved in the oxidation of fatty acids in the peroxisomes, which results in the formation of toxic hydrogen peroxide (however, the catalase enzyme in the peroxisomes degrades hydrogen peroxide; see also the *Introduction to Cell Biology* chapter). $FADH_2$ is a reduced electron carrier coenzyme that donates its hydrogen (electrons and protons) to the molecular oxygen (O_2) to produce hydrogen peroxide (H_2O_2):

$$FADH_2 + O_2 \rightarrow FAD + H_2O_2$$

Oxygenases

Oxygenases are enzymes that incorporate oxygen atoms from O_2 directly into the substrate molecules to form a new hydroxyl or carboxyl group. These enzymes catalyze the addition of oxygen into a substrate in two steps: (1) oxygen is bound to the active site of the enzyme and (2) the bound oxygen is reduced or transferred to the substrate. Oxygenases play a crucial role in drug metabolism by adding oxygen to organic compounds; in this way, many hydrophobic compounds that are high in C and H content and low in O content can be converted to more water-soluble metabolites.

There are two forms of oxygenases: monooxygenase and dioxygenase.

Monooxygenases: Mixed-Function Oxidases and Hydroxylases

Monooxygenases catalyze addition of one atom of the molecular oxygen to an organic substrate while the second oxygen atom is released to form water. Different classes of monooxygenases may be applicable depending upon the nature of the coenzyme. Some of these enzymes use $FADH_2$, while others use NADH or NADPH to reduce the second oxygen to water. Hydroxylation of phenylalanine to tyrosine is an example of monooxygenase metabolism (**Figure 7.4**). CYP450 monooxygenases are important for the detoxification and metabolism of many drugs, including hydroxylation of steroids.

Dioxygenases

Dioxygenase enzymes incorporate both atoms of molecular oxygen into the substrate and are not widely distributed in the cell. An example of this type of metabolism is the degradation of tryptophan by tryptophan dioxygenase. The enzyme opens the indole ring of tryptophan to incorporate both oxygen atoms (molecular oxygen). Tryptophan oxygenase is induced in the liver by adrenal corticosteroids and by tryptophan itself and is feedback-inhibited by NADPH. This reaction may explain why corticosteroids lower serotonin levels, which in turn results in depression and aggression (recall that tryptophan is a precursor to serotonin) (**Figure 7.5**).

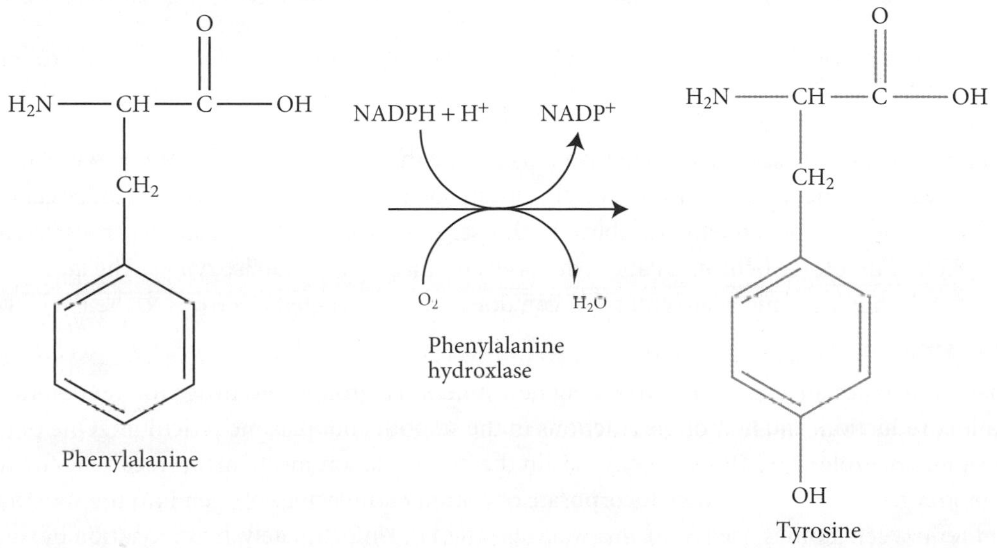

Figure 7.4 Metabolism of the amino acid phenylalanine to tyrosine amino acid by the monooxygenase enzyme phenylalanine hydroxylase.

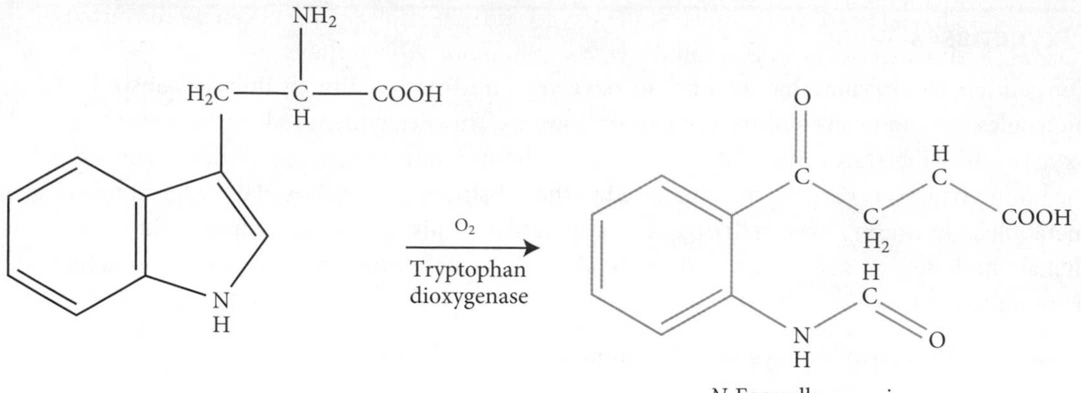

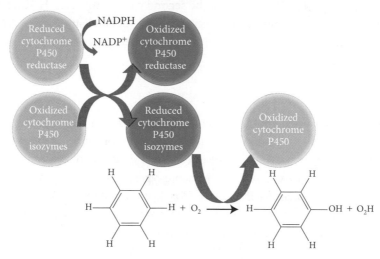

Figure 7.5 Metabolism of tryptophan by a dioxygenase enzyme that incorporates both atoms of molecular oxygen into the amino acid tryptophan.

Adapted from: Nelson DL, Cox MM, and Lehninger AL. *Principle of biochemistry*, 5th ed. W. H. Freeman and Company. 2008, chapter 21.

Figure 7.6 The interplay between cytochrome P450 reductase and cytochrome P450 in the hydroxylation of a benzene ring.

Adapted from: Nelson DL, Cox MM, and Lehninger AL. *Principle of biochemistry*, 5th ed. W. H. Freeman and Company. 2008, chapter 21.

Cytochrome P450 reductase is a microsomal enzyme that is the electron donor enzyme for several oxygenase enzymes, including cytochromes P450 and heme oxygenase (the latter catalyzes the degradation of heme to bilirubin). In this series of reactions, electrons are transferred from NADPH first to cytochrome P450 reductase, and then to CYP450 isozymes. The latter isozymes function as reduced enzymes that can donate their accepted electrons to their substrates (**Figure 7.6**).

Phase I enzymes are expert at introducing new functional groups into drugs (or xenobiotics) by oxidation, reduction, and hydrolysis reactions in the smooth endoplasmic reticulum. One of the most significant roles of CYP450 isozymes is in the hydroxylation mechanism (recall the function of monooxygenases), because they incorporate one atom of molecular oxygen into the substrate (the other oxygen atom is used to form a water molecule). Unfortunately, hydroxylation of some molecules produces toxic substances as well. For instance, the metabolic role of CYP4501A1 (CYP1A1 for short) in individuals who are smokers is significant. It has been suggested that smokers have a higher amount of CYP1A1 than nonsmokers. In the lungs of smokers, the CYP1A1 enzyme converts inactive polycyclic aromatic hydrocarbons (PAHs are procarcinogens) to active carcinogens by the hydroxylation reaction (carcinogens are molecules that can be converted to cancer-causing metabolites). In addition, it has been reported that the amount of CYP1A1 is enhanced in the placentas of pregnant women who are smokers. As a result, an increase in the hydroxylation of procarcinogens is harmful to the fetus as well.

Learning Bridge 7.1

Joe Smith is a 28-year-old professional soccer player who plays for the well-known soccer team Oregon Victory in Portland, Oregon. Recently, he has developed eczema on both of his legs, which is accompanied by a persistent itching problem. His doctor has prescribed prednisolone (Orapred), 10 mg, three times daily for 4 weeks with two refills.

Joe comes to your pharmacy to receive his second refill. While you dispense his prednisolone, he tells you that he has gained weight, feels he is no longer a good soccer player, is agitated with his team members who do not pass the ball to him when they play, and wants to quit playing professional soccer. Joe believes he has some sort of depression and asks you if there is any OTC medication to treat his depression. A review of his medical records shows that he uses only prednisolone and has not taken any other medication during the past 6 months.

A. How would you explain the cause of his depression?
B. What would you do to help Joe?

Phase II Metabolism

Many of the Phase I reactions are followed by Phase II reactions. Similar to Phase I reactions, Phase II enzymes are not very selective. During Phase II reactions, generally small polar endogenous molecules become attached to drugs or to Phase I metabolites. Most Phase II reactions result in deactivation of the drug and the production of water-soluble metabolites, which are eventually excreted in the urine or bile. During these reactions, molecules and metabolites are typically conjugated with other molecules such as glucuronic acid, sulfate, or glutathione, which makes them more water soluble. Other reactions also occur during Phase II, albeit to a much lesser extent, including glycine and glutamic acid conjugation, acetylation, and methylation.

Five reactions can occur in Phase II. While the first three make drugs more water soluble, the last two reactions do not necessarily make metabolites more polar but rather terminate their biological activity (however, methylation of pyridine-type nitrogens produces quaternary ammonium salts). Metabolites that contain functional groups such as alcohols, carboxylic acids, amines, and thiols are targets for Phase II reactions. If these functional groups are not present in a drug, they may be added by Phase I reactions.

Glucuronidation

Glucuronidation is the most frequently observed conjugation reaction. UDP-glucuronic acid acts as a glucuronyl donor, and a variety of glucuronosyltransferase enzymes (our human genome encodes at least 16 different members of this enzyme family) are present in the ER and cytosol of the liver, intestine, and kidney cells. The enzymes catalyze the glucuronidation of various endogenous and exogenous molecules and metabolites. A typical example in this category is the conjugation of many steroid drugs, particularly the conjugation of anabolic androgenic steroid metabolites into less toxic and more polar metabolites (**Figure 7.7**). Other examples of drugs that are metabolized by glucuronidation include acetaminophen (Tylenol), diazepam (Valium), and

UDG-glucuronate   Estradiol   Conjugated estradiol

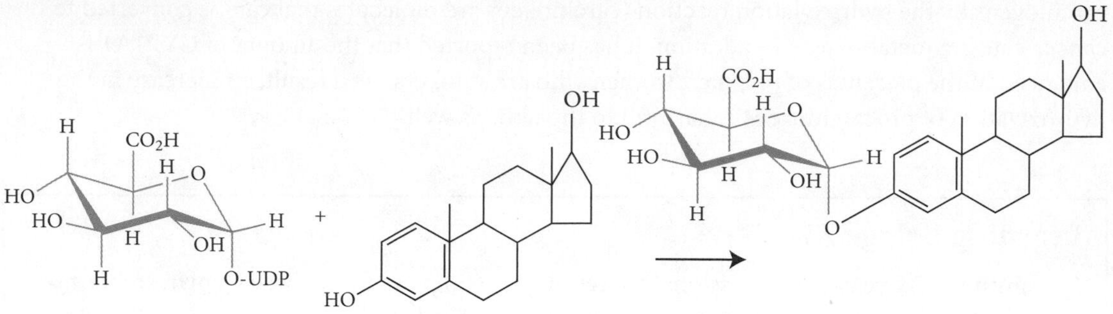

Figure 7.7 A Phase II reaction (glucuronidation) that makes steroids more hydrophilic.

digoxin (Lanoxin). Glucuronidation, however, does not always make a drug inactive. For example, the glucuronidation of morphine to morphine-6-glucuronide yields a pharmacologically active product.

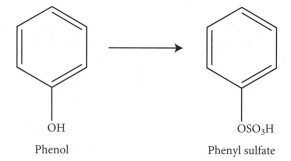

Phenol   Phenyl sulfate

Figure 7.8 Sulfation of a phenol group catalyzed by a sulfotransferase during a Phase II reaction.

Sulfation

The conjugation of the sulfate group is catalyzed by sulfotransferases that are found in platelets, brain, liver, small intestine, and kidney. Drugs that are sulfated are less active because sulfated forms are unable to bind to receptors. They usually target alcohols and phenol groups (**Figure 7.8**). Drugs that are metabolized in this way include acetaminophen and methyldopa (Apo-Methyldopa, from Canada).

Conjugation with Glutathione

Glutathione (GSH) is a tripeptide made of three amino acids: glutamic acid, cysteine, and glycine. It serves as a nucleophile (i.e., targets an electrophile group; see also the *Introduction to Biological Chemistry* chapter) to make drugs inactive (**Figure 7.9**). A typical example is ethacrynic acid (Edecrin). Glutathione *S*-transferases—the enzymes that catalyze the conjugation process—are present in large amounts in the cytosol of liver cells. GSH plays an important role in protecting DNA and RNA molecules: if toxic metabolites are not conjugated to GSH, they would covalently attach to DNA, RNA, or cell proteins. Metabolites that are conjugated to GSH are subjected to further metabolism before their excretion. GSH also plays a major role in the removal of potentially toxic hydrogen peroxide (see the *Introduction to Biochemistry* chapter).

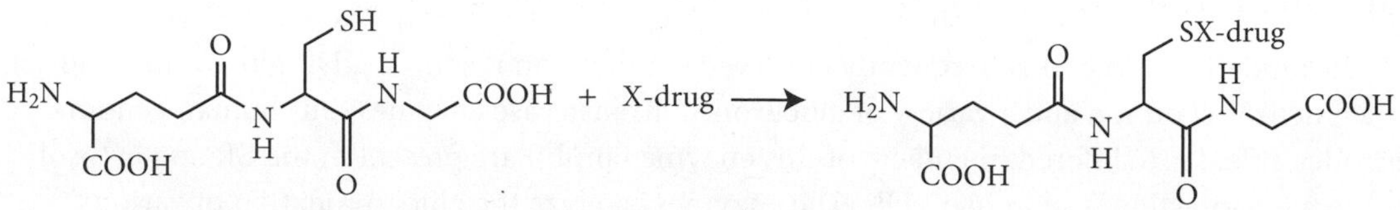

GSH   Electrophilic drug

Figure 7.9 Reaction between glutathione and an electrophilic drug inactivates the pharmacological activity of the drug during a Phase II reaction.

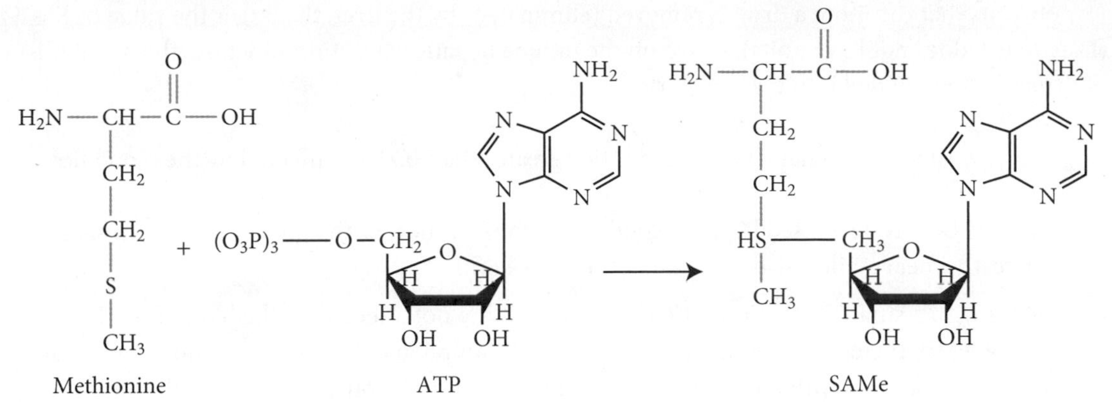

Figure 7.10 Interaction of the amino acid methionine with ATP produces *S*-adenosylmethionine (SAMe), which is a methyl donor to many reactions.

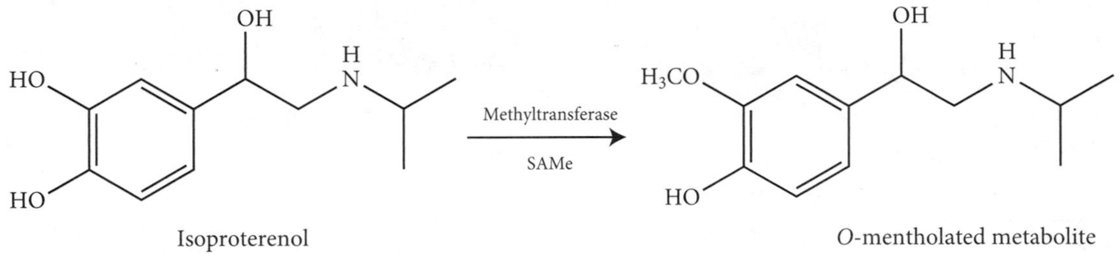

Figure 7.11 *S*-adenosylmethionine (SAMe) is used by methyltransferases as a methyl donor to metabolize drugs during Phase II reactions.

Acetylation

Acetyl-CoA is the acetyl donor in acetylation reactions. Acetylation reactions are catalyzed by acetyltransferases present in the liver. A typical example of acetylation is the metabolism of the drug isoniazid (see Figure 7.3). Similar to cytochrome P450 isozymes, polymorphisms of acetyltransferases exist, such that individuals may be classified as slow or fast acetylators. Individuals with a slow acetylation mechanism are more vulnerable to the toxic effects of isoniazid, for example, because the drug remains longer in these patients before it is metabolized. Other drugs that are metabolized by acetylation are clonazepam (KlonoPIN), dapsone, and sulfonamides.

Methylation

Methyltransferases add a methyl group to drugs and use *S*-adenosylmethionine (SAMe) as the source of the methyl group. *S*-adenosylmethionine is synthesized from the amino acid methionine and ATP (**Figure 7.10**). Despite the fact that the methylation reaction is not commonly employed during Phase II reactions, it is important for endogenous molecules such as conversion of norepinephrine to epinephrine. A typical example of drug methylation during Phase II reactions is metabolism of isoproterenol (Isuprel, a beta blocker) (**Figure 7.11**).

Hepatic Extraction Ratio

The hepatic extraction ratio (E) is a measure of how effectively a drug is removed (irreversibly) from the blood by the liver. Suppose the blood drug concentration that enters the liver is 10 mM (C_1) but when the blood leaves the liver, the concentration of the same drug is 5 mM (C_2). The extraction ratio (E) is calculated by the ratio ($C_1 - C_2$)/C_1; in our example, it is 0.5 (5 mM/10 mM).

It is obvious that the more a drug is removed (eliminated) by the liver, the larger the value of E is (note that E does not have units). Based on the unique hepatic extraction function, the metabolism of drugs can be divided into two categories.

- Drugs with a large hepatic extraction ratio (greater than 0.7) are affected by the blood flow. Drugs in this category include morphine (Kadian), meperidine (Demerol), and propranolol (Inderal LA). A decreased hepatic blood flow—for instance, in the presence of cirrhosis or congestive heart failure—decreases the clearance of these drugs.

- Drugs with a small extraction ratio (less than 0.2) are not affected by the blood flow. Drugs in this category include theophylline (Theo-24), chloramphenicol, and acetaminophen. Because these drugs are not influenced by the blood flow, their metabolism is instead affected by hepatic cellular functions. For instance, the elimination of theophylline is decreased by 45% in children with acute viral hepatitis. One has to be careful with dosing of these drugs in patients with hepatic diseases to avoid theophylline toxicity.

Pharmacogenetics and Pharmacogenomics

The terms *pharmacogenetics* and *pharmacogenomics* are often used interchangeably. Both terms have been described in different chapters (particularly in the *Introduction to Pharmacogenomics* chapter) in this text. However, a brief discussion can assist students in appreciating the roles of pharmacogenetics and pharmacogenomics in drug metabolism. Pharmacogenetics, as the name indicates, is the study of how a genetic difference accounts for variation in a drug response. Genetic variations among individuals occur in approximately every 300 to 1,000 nucleotides; in other words, any two individuals may differ by 0.1% of their more than 3 billion base pairs. In addition, a total of 10 million single-nucleotide polymorphisms (SNPs, which means a single base pair substitution) are possible. SNPs in coding regions of genes cause variations in amino acid sequences and protein functions. Pharmacogenetics investigates which of these variants or combinations of these variants account for drug effects. In contrast, pharmacogenomics is the study of genetic differences within a population and their impact on drug therapy.

Polymorphism is a common interindividual genetic variation that is caused by multiple alleles. It exists in more than 1% of the population and is known to affect patients' therapeutic response to or metabolism of a given drug. Polymorphisms that affect drug metabolism can occur in any setting, including in the enzymes that are involved in drug metabolism or in other areas such as protein transporters and receptors. Polymorphism in CYP450 isozymes is known significantly to affect drug metabolism, and the corresponding alleles in genes involved in drug metabolism have been widely studied. Today, genetic tests are available to screen for polymorphisms for CYP450 enzymes in an individual. This information is very critical when planning therapy, as knowledge about an individual's metabolic capability can assist clinicians in reducing the risk of adverse effects by adjusting the dose range to better fit a patient's metabolic capability.

One typical example of the role of polymorphism is the prescription of antihypertensive drugs for cardiovascular diseases. African American patients tend to respond better to diuretics than to angiotensin-converting enzyme (ACE) inhibitors or β-blockers (see also the *Introduction to Pharmacology and Pathophysiology* chapter). Another example focuses on the role of glucose 6-phosphate dehydrogenase (G6PD). Individuals with G6PD deficiency develop medical complications such as hemolytic anemia and kidney failure after ingestion of fava beans ("favism") or drugs such as primaquine (see also the *Introduction to Biochemistry* chapter).

A few specific cytochrome P450 genes exist in polymorphic forms, which explains the variations in drug responses that occur among many patients. Consequently, pharmacogenomics plays an important role in the study of CYP450 genes. It has been suggested that dietary differences among species during the course of evolution led to the genetic variations in producing drug-metabolizing enzymes. A good example of the polymorphic effect on drug metabolism is seen with the role of CYP2D6 in the liver. More discussion of this isozyme is provided in the next section.

CYP2D6

CYP2D6 is a large isozyme family that is highly polymorphic—120 different alleles have been identified for the CYP2D6 gene. Approximately 10% of people in the total population arc poor CYP2D6 metabolizers (7% of whites, 3% of African Americans, and 1% of Asian Americans). CYP2D6 is involved in the metabolism of nicotine. Two alleles of CYP2D6 are inactive in some individuals, which results in them having impaired metabolism of nicotine. The latter effect protects these individuals from becoming tobacco-dependent smokers owing to a higher plasma concentration of nicotine.

The metabolism of tricyclic antidepressants such as amitriptyline (Elavil, from Canada), desipramine (Norpramin), imipramine (Tofranil), and nortriptyline (Pamelor) is also affected by CYP2D6 alleles. In addition, the CYP2D6 family is responsible for a large interindividual variation in the metabolism of analgesics and anticancer drugs. While some patients are poor metabolizers, others are fast metabolizers. *O*-demethylation is also affected in patients with polymorphism of CYP2D6. For instance, the *O*-demethylation of codeine is significantly affected, as approximately 10% of codeine is *O*-demethylated by CYP2D6 to morphine to produce an analgesic effect (**Figure 7.12**). Poor metabolizers, then, do not experience the analgesic effect from codeine. As another example, tramadol (Ultram) is metabolized to *O*-desmethyltramadol by CYP2D6. A poor CYP2D6 metabolizer would not experience the analgesic effect that is produced by the metabolite, *O*-desmethyltramadol. However, it is important to recognize that such genetic variation does not account for all side effects or therapeutic variations.

To determine whether a patient is a fast or poor metabolizer, a known substrate for the particular metabolizing enzyme is given to a patient, and the patient's clearance (Cl; see the *Introduction to Pharmacokinetics* chapter) is measured. In addition, *in vitro* verification of enzyme level is undertaken.

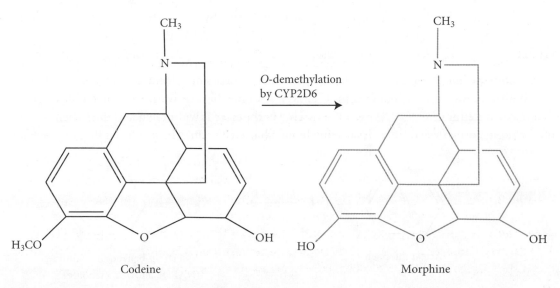

Figure 7.12 Codeine is metabolized to morphine by CYP2D6. Less CYP2D6 activity results in less product (morphine) and, as a result, less analgesic effect.

Sometimes, however, it is necessary to bypass a catalytic activity by a cytochrome enzyme to maintain the activity of a drug. For instance, desvenlafaxine (Pristiq), which is used for the treatment of major depression disorder (approved in 2011 in the United States), already contains the active metabolite. Venlafaxine requires CYP2D6 to produce an active metabolite. Desvenlafaxine, therefore, does not require the presence of CYP2D6.

Both enzyme induction and inhibition play important roles in the metabolism of drugs. A brief description of both processes is provided here to emphasize the key roles that drug metabolism and interaction play in pharmacology (see the *Introduction to Pharmacology and Pathophysiology* chapter) and toxicology (see the *Introduction to Toxicology* chapter).

Induction of CYP450 Isozymes

Drug interactions occur when the effect of one drug is changed by another drug that has already been administered, or is co-administered, or will be administered after the administration of the first drug. In most cases, induction of CYP450 isozymes results in enhanced elimination of drugs and, if a prodrug is involved, increased activity of the prodrug. Keep in mind that only the following subfamilies are inducible by xenobiotics: CYP2A, CYP2B, CYP2C, CYP2E, and CYP3A.

Different mechanisms may be employed to induce a CYP subfamily. However, the most common one is an increase in gene expression through the nuclear receptors (NRs). These receptors have considerable involvement in the transcription of genes, as they can activate a large number of CYP genes in the liver and other tissues. As a result, they play an important role by being stimulated or inhibited to regulate the expression of affected CYP subfamilies. When gene expression is involved, one must take into consideration that transcription and translation have to occur to produce more members of the CYP subfamily, which may take a few days—and hence several days may pass before any drug interaction effect becomes apparent. Similarly, if a drug is withdrawn, it may take a few days before the inducible effect from the withdrawal of the xenobiotic is abolished. For example, phenobarbital causes hypertrophy of the smooth ER and a threefold to fourfold increase in the expression of CYP450 within 4 to 6 days. By comparison, it takes 7 days to produce an inducible effect from rifampin (Rifadin) to verapamil (Calan). Not all inductions result in an increase in the gene expression, however: in some cases, induction may result in the stabilization of the transcript (mRNAs) or the gene products (isozymes).

The role of ethanol's inducing effect is apparent when the metabolism of acetaminophen is affected by ethanol. Acetaminophen is partially metabolized by the CYP2E1 isozyme to the toxic metabolite N-acetyl-p-benzoquinoneimine (NAPQI) (**Figure 7.13**). Ethanol is known to induce CYP2E1, which may lead to increased susceptibility to acetaminophen poisoning after an overdose.

As another example of enzyme induction, therapeutic doses of barbiturates accelerate the metabolism of warfarin by inducing the CYP2C9 isozyme. Because warfarin is metabolized (it is a major substrate for CYP2C9), if the administered barbiturate is withdrawn and the patient remains on the same dose of warfarin, a devastating hemorrhagic effect may be produced that can be fatal.

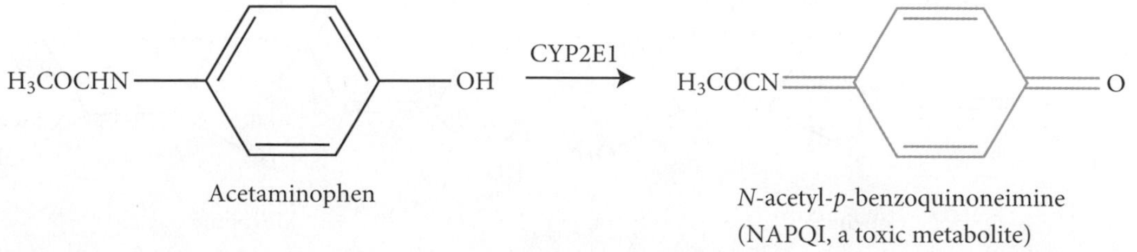

Acetaminophen

N-acetyl-p-benzoquinoneimine
(NAPQI, a toxic metabolite)

Figure 7.13 CYP2E1 can be induced by ethanol to metabolize acetaminophen to the toxic molecule, NAPQI.

Consequently, not only is it important to review a patient's current risk for drug interactions, but it is also essential to know when a drug termination may have a profound effect on other drugs that the patient is currently using.

Learning Bridge 7.2

Amy Johnson was involved with a recent minor car accident that has caused her persistent back and neck pain. She has lost her driving license due to a traffic violation and a charge of driving under the influence (DUI) that apparently caused the car accident. Her physician has prescribed a combination of hydrocodone and acetaminophen (Vicodin), 2 tablets every 6 hours, to treat Amy's intense back pain.

Amy comes to your pharmacy to fill her Vicodin prescription. Upon filling her medication, you notice that Amy smells of alcohol. Why should you counsel Amy to avoid alcohol while using Vicodin?

Inhibition of CYP450 Isozymes

Similar to the induction of CYP450 isozymes, inhibition of these isozymes can affect the levels of many drugs in the body. Inhibition of CYP450 isozymes can occur reversibly or irreversibly and, in either way, can increase the toxic level of a drug or reduce the activity of a prodrug. In addition, the inhibition mechanism can be competitive or noncompetitive. Competitive inhibition can be overcome if other xenobiotics are available that also act as substrates for the same isozyme. Inhibition of CYP450 isozymes, however, is known to cause the most common drug interactions. Another reaction that further complicates the inhibition process is when the product (metabolite) of an isozyme metabolism is able to inhibit the same isozyme. For example, erythromycin (Erythrocin) is metabolized by CYP3A4 to a metabolite that also inhibits CYP3A4.

As was mentioned in the *Introduction to Biochemistry* chapter, the inhibitory measurement is often expressed as K_i (the inhibition constant) and is defined as the concentration of the inhibitor that causes 50% inhibition of the enzyme. Similar to the K_m value from Michaelis-Menten kinetics (see also the *Introduction to Biochemistry* chapter), the unit for K_i is mol/L and a lower K_i value indicates a more potent inhibitor. Drugs with K_i values smaller than 1 mM are often considered potent inhibitors. For instance, the azole antifungal itraconazole has a K_i value of 0.02 mM and is considered a potent inhibitor of CYP3A4.

The more selectively a drug inhibits an isozyme, the more potent the drug interaction that occurs. For instance, simvastatin is mainly metabolized by CYP3A4, and the antifungal itraconazole can selectively inhibit CYP3A4. The serious complication known as rhabdomyolysis can occur when simvastatin and itraconazole are taken concurrently.

Approximately 15% of a patient population will be considered poor metabolizers in regard to CYP1A2 polymorphism. For instance, fluvoxamine (Luvox CR), an antidepressant drug that relies on the selective serotonin reuptake inhibition mechanism for its activity, is a potent inhibitor of CYP1A2. As other antidepressant drugs such as amitriptyline and imipramine are partly metabolized by CYP1A2, concurrent administration of fluvoxamine with these agents enhances the effects of amitriptyline and imipramine.

The CYP3A4 enzyme is irreversibly inhibited by grapefruit juice. In November 2012, Canadian researchers published in the *Canadian Medical Association Journal* a list of new drugs that cause serious side effects when taken with grapefruit juice. Among this list, one can find anticancer agents, antibiotics, antidiabetic agents, antibiotics, and cardiovascular agents, among others (a complete list is available at http://www.cmaj.ca/content/suppl/2012/11/26/cmaj.120951.DC1 /grape-bailey-1-at.pdf). For instance, the levels of drugs such as atorvastatin (Lipitor), dronedarone (Multaq), ergotamine (Ergomar), and halofantrine (Selzentry) are significantly increased if patients drink grapefruit juice together with their medications. Given this risk, it is important to counsel patients about potential food–drug interactions. Grapefruit juice, in addition to its effect on CYP450 isozymes, can inhibit other enzymatic systems. For instance, the absorption of fexofenadine (Allegra) is significantly reduced by grapefruit juice. Fexofenadine's absorption is dependent on a drug transporter organic anion protein, and this transporter protein is inhibited by grapefruit juice.

Clopidogrel (Plavix) is a prodrug and a major substrate for the CYP2C19 isozyme. Clopidogrel needs to be metabolized by CYP2C19 to be in an active metabolite form. Omeprazole (Prilosec) is a proton pump inhibitor that is known to inhibit this isozyme moderately, in turn potentially reducing the plasma level of the active metabolite of clopidogrel. Because clopidogrel is a critical drug to prevent myocardial infarction (MI) and stroke, pharmacists should counsel patients about this possible drug interaction. In contrast, ranitidine (Zantac, which is another type of acid-lowering agent) does not cause any drug interaction with clopidogrel.

CYP1A2, CYP2C9, and CYP3A4 are all heavily involved in drug interactions and are abundant in the human liver; thus it is important to summarize xenobiotics that induce or inhibit these subfamilies (**Tables 7.1, 7.2, and 7.3**). Interestingly, barbiturates, carbamazepine, phenobarbital, phenytoin, primidone, and rifampin are inducers for all three of these CYP subfamilies.

Table 7.1 Xenobiotics That Induce or Inhibit the Metabolic Activity of the CYP3A4 Subfamily

Xenobiotics That Induce CYP3A4	Xenobiotics That Inhibit CYP3A4	Drugs Whose Metabolism Is Affected by CYP3A4
• Carbamazepine • Garlic supplements • Oxcarbamazpine • Phenobarbital • Phenytoin • Primidone • Rifampin • St. John's wort • Topiramate	• Amiodarone • Cimetidine • Cyclosporine • Diltiazem • Fluoxetine • Grapefruit juice • Itraconazole • Ketoconazole • Macrolides • Nifedipine • Oral contraceptives • Paroxetine • Protease inhibitors • Quinidine • Steroids • Tamoxifen • Verapamil • Zafirlukast	• Atorvastatin • Benzodiazepines • Buprenorphine • Buspirone • Carbamazepine • Citalopram • Corticosteroids • Donepezil • Eszopicolone • Galantamine • Naloxone • Nifedipine • Pioglitazone (Actos) • Propranolol • (R)-Warfarin • Sildenafil • Solifenacin • Terbinafine • Theophylline • Tolterodine • Trazodone

Adapted from: Bauer LA. Clinical pharmacokinetic and pharmacodynamic concepts. In: Bauer LA, ed. *Applied clinical pharmacokinetics*, 2nd ed. New York, NY: McGraw-Hill; 2008: Chapter 1. Available at: http://www.accesspharmacy.com/content.aspx?aID=3517000.

Table 7.2 Xenobiotics That Induce or Inhibit the Metabolic Activity of the CYP2C9 Subfamily

Xenobiotics That Induce CYP2C9	Xenobiotics That Inhibit CYP2C9	Drugs Whose Metabolism Is Affected by CYP2C9
• Barbiturates • Carbamazepine • Phenobarbital • Phenytoin • Primidone • Rifampin	• Amiodarone • Atazanavir • Clopidogrel • Disulfiram • Efavirenz • Fluconazole • Fluvastatin • Isoniazid • Metronidazole • Zafirlukast	• Candesartan • Celecoxib • Chlorpropamide • Diclofenac • Glipizide • Glyburide • Ibuprofen • Losartan • Naproxen • Phenytoin • Valsartan • (S)-Warfarin

Adapted from: Bauer LA. Clinical pharmacokinetic and pharmacodynamic concepts. In: Bauer LA, ed. *Applied clinical pharmacokinetics*, 2nd ed. New York, NY: McGraw-Hill; 2008: Chapter 1. Available at: http://www.accesspharmacy.com/content.aspx?aID=3517000.

Table 7.3 Xenobiotics That Induce or Inhibit the Metabolic Activity of the CYP1A2 Subfamily

Xenobiotics That Induce CYP1A2	Xenobiotics That Inhibit CYP1A2	Drugs Whose Metabolism Is Affected by CYP1A2
• Barbiturates • Carbamazepine • Omeprazole • Phenobarbital • Phenytoin • Primidone • Rifampin	• Itraconazole • Atazanavir • Cimetidine • Ciprofloxacin • Erythromycin • Fluvoxamine • Interferon • Mexiletine • Zileuton	• Acetaminophen • Clomipramine • Imipramine • Nortriptyline • Ondansetron • Theophylline • (R)-Warfarin • Zileuton

Adapted from: Bauer LA. Clinical pharmacokinetic and pharmacodynamic concepts. In: Bauer LA, ed. *Applied clinical pharmacokinetics*, 2nd ed. New York, NY: McGraw-Hill; 2008: Chapter 1. Available at: http://www.accesspharmacy.com/content.aspx?aID=3517000.

Learning Bridge 7.3

Joe Smith has recently felt nocturnal chest pain a few times per week, particularly after eating spicy food. Upon contacting a clinic in Portland, Oregon, he was asked to immediately visit the clinic for a checkup that would include an x-ray and an electrocardiogram. The routine medical procedures did not show any cardiovascular problem. The physician diagnosed a mild form of gastroesophageal reflux disease (GERD) and explained to Joe that his chest pain was caused by heartburn rather than his past medical conditions. The physician prescribed omeprazole, 20 mg, once daily for 60 days. Joe comes to your pharmacy and asks you to fill his

(continues)

(*continued*)

prescription. During a drug review of his past medication, you notice that Joe is also currently taking clopidogrel.

Is there any drug interaction between omeprazole and clopidogrel? Why or why not? Which counseling points do you have for Joe when filling his omeprazole?

The Role of Age and Sex in Drug Metabolism

A variety of factors affect the activities of the enzymes involved in the metabolism of drugs. As mentioned earlier, because genetic variations may affect these enzymes, interindividual differences can result in a different extent of toxicity or carcinogenicity for specific drugs. However, age and sex seem to play important roles in the activities of these enzymes as well. Also, because drugs and food can change the activities of some metabolizing enzymes, it is important to review past and current medications for patients to provide effective counseling and assist them in achieving a better therapeutic outcome. In addition, various diseases (such as cirrhosis of the liver) can affect the activities of drug-metabolizing enzymes.

Age

Age is an important factor in drug interactions, but especially for pediatric patients, who are affected by both Phase I and Phase II reactions. The total amount of CYP450 in the pediatric liver is between 30% and 60% of the amount found in an adult. By the age of 10 years, however, this level is almost equal to the adult level. Expressions of metabolizing enzymes are affected by age and are a risk factor in producing adverse effects or toxicity in fetuses and children. For instance, the CYP3A7 isozyme is expressed at its highest level during the first trimester of pregnancy but its expression decreases within one year after birth.

The Phase I oxidation pathway is impaired in infants. As a result, the oxidation of theophylline, phenobarbital, phenytoin (Dilantin), and diazepam (Valium) is affected; in turn, doses of these drugs should be decreased in infants. Of particular concern is theophylline, as metabolism of this drug is slower compared to the other three drugs.

Some of the major Phase II reactions are also affected by age. For instance, while the sulfation pathway during Phase II metabolism is fully functional, the glucuronidation pathway is not fully developed in infants. The so-called gray baby syndrome is caused by decreased effectiveness of the glucuronidation pathway through glucuronyltransferases, which would otherwise metabolize chloramphenicol antibiotic. The glucuronidation pathway in infants also affects their ability to metabolize morphine. A higher morphine dose is required to achieve adequate efficacy in infants than is needed in adults, because infants are not able fully to utilize the glucuronidation pathway to produce the 6-glucuronide metabolite (6-glucuronide is 20 times more active than morphine). Sometimes a reduced enzyme activity provokes other enzymatic reactions. For instance, the metabolism of acetaminophen by glucuronidation is impaired in infants, but this effect is partly offset by the sulfation pathway.

Sex

Sex differences can cause variations in the expression of hepatic enzymes involved in both Phase I and Phase II reactions. It has been known for a long time that gender can explain differences in pharmacokinetics (bioavailability, distribution, metabolism, and excretion) and differences in pharmacology. Often these differences reflect drug metabolism that indirectly affects pharmaco-kinetics and pharmacology. For instance, it has been suggested that acetaminophen's elimination rate is 20% higher in males than in females because of a higher glucuronidation rate in males. Similarly, acetyl salicylic acid (aspirin) has a decreased rate of conjugation with amino acids during Phase II reactions in females compared with males; as a result, aspirin has a higher bioavailability in females than in males.

In addition, females express CYP3A4 in the liver more effectively than males do. The anti-cancer prodrug ifosfamide (Ifex) is metabolized by CYP3A4. Because females have a higher amount of CYP3A4, this drug is metabolized faster in females than in males, resulting in female patients being more prone to the CNS toxicity or encephalopathy adverse effects associated with ifosfamide.

The CYP1A2 isozyme also shows differences in drug metabolism based on sex. For instance, this isozyme has a faster metabolic activity in males than in females when it comes to metaboliz-ing olanzapine (Zyprexa) and clozapine (Clozaril). This explains why female patients show a better response to these antipsychotic agents in the treatment of psychotic symptoms.

Learning Bridge 7.4

At one of your introductory pharmacy practice experiences sites, you receive a prescription for atorvastatin (40 mg, once daily at bedtime) for Joe, a 53-year-old patient who has recently been diagnosed with hypercholesterolemia.

In reviewing Joe's past medication records and the drugs that he has been using, you see that atorvastatin is the only drug he has used during the past 10 months. Joe had been taking atorvastatin at a lower dose (10 mg, once daily) for 6 months, but 4 months ago his physician increased the dose to 20 mg. A further review of his medical records shows that his cholesterol level did not change at all during the past 10 months.

Apparently, the medication was not effective during the past 10 months, and you suspect that there could be a patient noncompliance issue. You decide to counsel Joe on his new prescription. After asking him about how he was taking his medication, you are convinced that the lack of therapeutic effect has nothing to do with a compliance issue. When you ask Joe whether he is using any supplements, he mentions that he takes multivitamins as well as St. John's wort to deal with his occasional depression.

A. Did your discussion with Joe about his medications reveal anything about atorvastatin's lack of therapeutic outcome?

B. How will you help Joe to achieve the full therapeutic benefit from atorvastatin?

Structure and Function of Drugs

Drug and Target Interactions

To design a new drug, one has to take into consideration the chemical structure, physical and chemical properties, and biological function of the drug. The majority of drugs are designed to be small molecules that can bind their target so as to exert a pharmacological effect. During the drug design process, a compound is synthesized or identified that has an interesting functional effect.

Investigators subsequently assess the activity profile and chemical structure until all aspects of the structure and function of the drug are assessed and optimized. For instance, structural concerns such as water solubility, acidic or basic properties, the nature and number of functional groups, and physical and chemical stabilities are reviewed, explored, and investigated by researchers. Similarly, functional concerns such as drug and target interaction and pharmacological and toxicologic effects are assayed and assessed.

Molecular modeling, which employs theoretical methods and utilizes computational techniques, assists researchers and scientists in mimicking the structural and functional properties of identified molecules. Modeling techniques include creating two- and three-dimensional (3D) structures to see a model of drug–target interaction and to estimate physiochemical properties. The three-dimensional placement of the compound's functional groups into a receptor is a critical step in displaying its functional effect. For instance, techniques such as x-ray crystallography and nuclear magnetic resonance (NMR) spectroscopy display the 3D structure of a compound in a manner that can visualize the binding of a compound to its target. Molecular modeling has helped researchers build computer models of new compounds to estimate the structure and function of newly synthesized (or identified) compounds.

Researchers must take a series of stages and challenges into consideration when developing a new drug:

- Selecting a disease or disorder that needs a drug versus improving a drug already available on the market. Economic factors play important roles here in this decision-making process (i.e., is it profitable or does it provide a financial return?).

- Selecting a drug target. Is the target a receptor, an enzyme, a protein, a DNA, or an RNA? Is it an intracellular target or an extracellular target? Does the target have a regulatory role in maintaining a specific function of a cell? Should the drug stimulate or inhibit the target? Should it act as an agonist or an antagonist for that particular target?

- Identifying a reliable experiment or a bioassay. Which experiments might effectively and efficiently be used to identify the drug target and the interaction between the drug and its target? Are these experiments simple, reliable, cost-effective, and relevant to the designed study? Which techniques and tools can be employed to separate and purify a molecule from sources such as plant extracts or other complex reactions? The separation of identical mixtures with similar physicochemical properties also requires effective and sensitive experimental methods. For instance, crystallization and distillation both require substantial amounts of material.

- Identifying and isolating a lead compound. Does the compound have any biological or pharmacological activity? Can one use an existing drug, an identified natural compound, or even medical folklore? For instance, captopril (Capoten, from Canada), an agent that is used for reducing the blood pressure, was initially a lead compound in the development of other ACE inhibitors.

- Determining the structure and its functional groups. Can x-ray crystallography and NMR spectroscopy be used to identify how many bonds are present in a compound, what the functional groups are, or what the 3D structure of the entire compound looks like? Which technical tools can be used to identify the pharmacophore (see the next section)?

- Modifying functional groups to improve drug–target interaction. Can the functional groups be modified to increase the pharmacological response or to reduce the adverse or toxic effects?

- Investigating drug metabolism, pharmacology, and toxicity. Will the drug survive the first-pass effect or contact with various metabolic enzymes of the liver or the GI tract? Will it induce liver enzymes that affect the breakdown of other drugs, causing drug–drug interactions?

- Designing a dosage form. Does the dosage form make the drug available for its site of action?

- Implementing clinical trials. Do the research and clinical trials adhere to the principles of good clinical practices (GCPs) and human subject protection (HSP)? Do the clinical trial procedures follow the FDA's guidance and regulations?

The *Introduction to Pharmaceutics* chapter provides a more detailed examination of what happens during different phases of a clinical trial when investigating and testing a newly developed drug.

Pharmacophore

A pharmacophore comprises a series of functional groups that are required to exhibit a particular pharmacological activity. According to the International Union of Pure and Applied Chemistry (IUPAC), a pharmacophore is "an ensemble of steric and electronic features that is necessary to ensure the optimal supramolecular interactions with a specific biological target and to trigger (or block) its biological response." For instance, the pharmacophore for acetylcholine (Ach) is the oxygen from the carbonyl group (to make the molecule a hydrogen bond acceptor) and the tertiary nitrogen that is important for its binding to Ach receptors (**Figure 7.14**). Removal of any of these two functional groups will reduce the effect of Ach. Once a pharmacophore is identified, it can be used for the design of other compounds that can exert the same pharmacological activity.

The pharmacophore and crystallography play important roles in finding other pharmacologically active compounds. Molecular modeling has significantly assisted medicinal chemists in identifying compounds that have the desired functional groups of the pharmacophore. As soon as a compound and its functional groups are identified, a series of chemical modifications of the functional groups can be undertaken in an attempt to enhance the potency and selectivity of the newly identified compound.

Three-Dimensional Structure of Drugs

The pharmacological activities of drugs depend mainly on how they interact with their biological targets, such as proteins (receptors, enzymes, and transporters), nucleic acids (DNA and RNA), and biological membranes (phospholipids and glycolipids). These large molecules have complex three-dimensional structures that are able to recognize and bind selectively to a ligand (drug) in only one of the many possible three-dimensional structures that they form. In other words, conformation, configuration, and isomers play important roles in drug–target interaction.

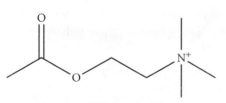

Acetylcholine (Ach)
The blue shading represents the pharmacophore of Ach.

Figure 7.14 Pharmacophore of acetylcholine. Both oxygen and the tertiary amine are important to receive a full effect from the acetylcholine neurotransmitter.

Conformation

The different arrangement of atoms that occurs during the rotation around a single bond is referred to as conformation. Hydrogen atoms on two carbon atoms can be "eclipsed," "staggered," or "skewed," for example (see also the *Introduction to Biological Chemistry* chapter). Different conformations differ slightly in energy, and, as discussed in the *Introduction to Biological Chemistry* chapter, the form that has the least energy represents the most stable form of the molecule. In the eclipsed conformation of ethane, the three hydrogen atoms that are in the back part of the molecule (rare) are unseen because they are lined up exactly in a parallel fashion behind the front three hydrogen atoms. In the staggered conformation, all six hydrogen atoms are visible because their hydrogen atoms are not similarly lined up (**Figure 7.15**). Thus the staggered conformation of ethane is more stable than the eclipsed form. The skewed form is any conformation between the eclipsed and staggered forms.

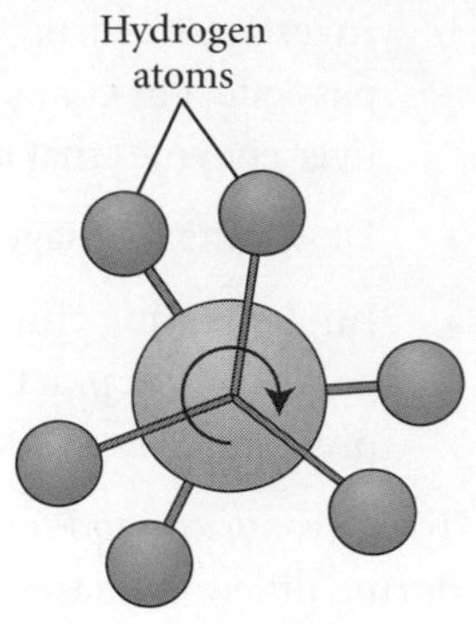

Hydrogen atoms

Ethane

Figure 7.15 Conformation of an ethane molecule in a staggered form.

Configuration

The configuration of a molecule cannot be changed unless the existing chemical bonds are broken and re-formed. The difference between configuration and confirmation is that a change in configuration cannot occur by the simple rotation of a bond. In an alkene, for example, rotation around the carbon–carbon bond does not occur. *Cis*- and *trans*-isomers are examples of compounds with different configurations (**Figure 7.16**).

Isomers

Isomers are two or more molecules that have the same molecular formula (i.e., exactly the same number of carbons and hydrogens) but assume different three-dimensional structures. There are two main types of isomerism: structural isomerism and stereoisomerism.

In structural isomerism, the isomers differ in terms of the arrangement in which the atoms are joined. For example, there are two structural isomers of C_2H_6O. Ethanol is an alcohol and has the structure CH_3CH_2OH, whereas its isomer, dimethyl ether, has the structure CH_3OCH_3. Obviously, the two isomers have different physical and chemical characteristics.

There are two kinds of stereoisomerism:

- *Geometrical isomerism* (or *cis-trans* isomers). This type of isomerism occurs in structurally rigid molecules such as alkenes, in which rotation around a particular bond is restricted (see the *cis* and *trans* structures of fumaric acid in Figure 7.16). Only one form of the geometrical isomer (i.e., only the *cis* or *trans* form) can bind to an enzyme or a receptor, which explains why *cis* and *trans* isomers have distinct biological functions.

- *Chiral molecules.* An organic molecule that contains a carbon atom to which four different atoms or molecules are joined is called a chiral molecule, with the carbon being referred to as a chiral carbon (**Figure 7.17**). If there is only one chiral carbon, there will be only two stereoisomers. If there are more chiral carbons within the same molecule, there will be

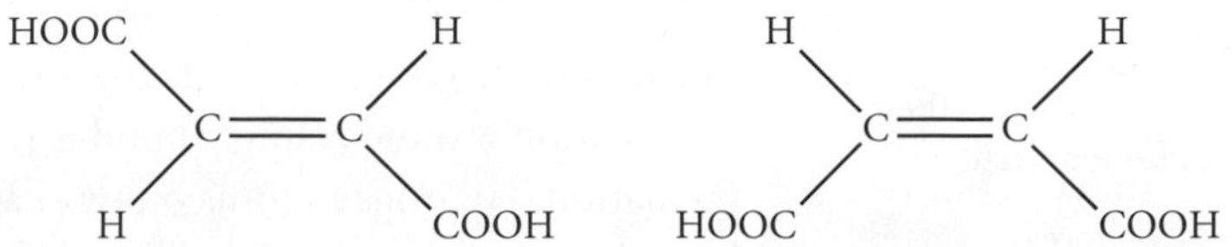

Fumaric acid (*trans*)   Fumaric acid (*cis*)

Figure 7.16 Two configurations of fumaric acid. Note that a change in either configuration cannot occur by a simple rotation of the double bond.

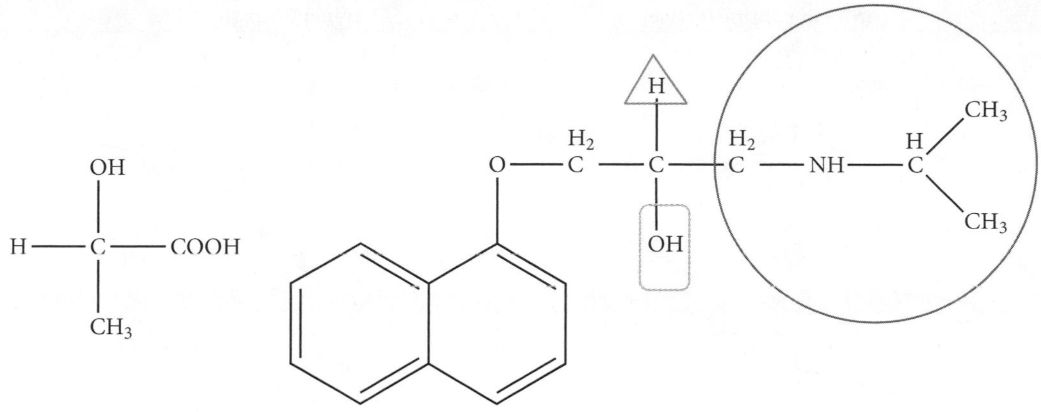

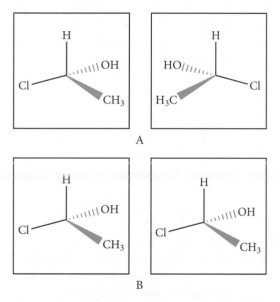

A chiral molecule   Propranolol

Figure 7.17 (A) Structure of a chiral molecule that has a chiral carbon. (B) Propranolol is a chiral compound.

A

B

Figure 7.18 (A) Structures of two enantiomers that can be mirror images of each other. (B) Structures of two diastereomers that cannot be mirror images of each other.

more than two stereoisomers. Stereoisomers that are not mirror images of each other are called diastereomers (**Figure 7.18**).

When the two chiral molecules are mirror images of each other (no matter whether they have one or more chiral carbons), they are called enantiomers (Figure 7.18). The most important way in which enantiomers differ is that they rotate a plane of polarized light in opposite directions. Polarized light is waves that by passing through special filters vibrate in a single plane.

Racemic Mixture

A sample of compound containing equal amounts of two enantiomers is called a racemic mixture. If the enantiomer rotates a plane of polarized light to the left, it is designated with the L- or (*S*)- symbol; if it rotates a plane of polarized light to the right, it is designated with the D- or (*R*)- symbol. In other words, the way one can tell which molecule is L or D is dictated by the directions in which the molecules rotate a plane of polarized light. When molecules can rotate a plane of polarized light, they are referred to as optically active isomers. Molecules that do not have chiral carbons cannot rotate a plane of polarized light.

A racemic mixture will be produced when chemical synthesis of a chiral drug results in a mixture of equal parts of the two enantiomers. Chiral drugs play an important role in pharmacology and medicinal chemistry because the two enantiomers may have different pharmacological (or toxicologic) actions. For instance, enantiomers may produce different pharmacological and physiological effects or demonstrate differences in absorption rates, transport rates, or metabolic rates. Effects of agonists and antagonists on beta-adrenergic receptors are stereoselective. For instance, all beta blockers are active when they take the form of (*S*)-enantiomers. **Figure 7.19** demonstrates that (*R*)-epinephrine cannot bind properly to its adrenergic receptor to produce any pharmacological effect.

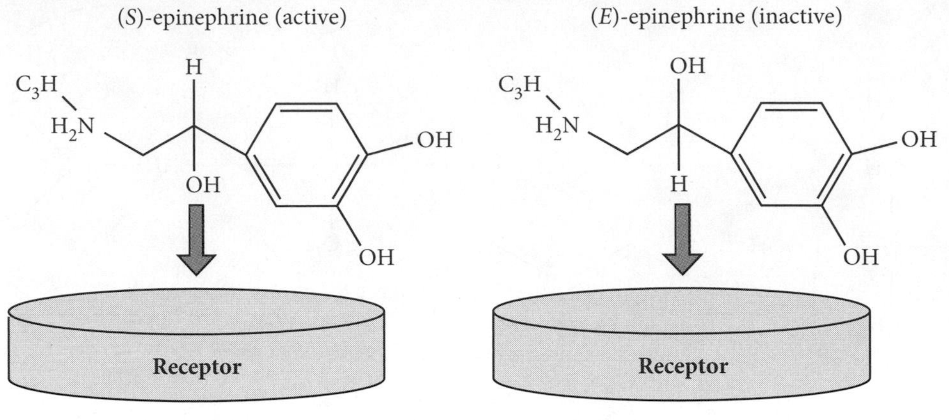

Figure 7.19 Racemic epinephrine. While (S)-epinephrine is active, (R)-epinephrine is inactive.

In 1992, the FDA issued a policy statement concerned with the development of new chiral drugs. This policy stated that in the development of racemic mixtures, researchers should use proper precautions. Certain chemical techniques may help to separate racemic mixtures, and specific analytical methods are available that can detect the presence of enantiomers during the preparation of a compound. In addition, advanced techniques can isolate mixtures of enantiomers. As a result, many drugs are available as pure enantiomers.

Penicillin works by stereoisomeric means. This antibiotic works only on peptide links of (R)-alanine that occur in the cell walls of bacteria (see also the *Introduction to Microbiology* chapter) but not in humans. Thus penicillin can kill only the bacteria because humans do not have (R)-amino acids.

Another well-known example involving stereoisomerism is thalidomide, an agent that was once used to counteract nausea in pregnancy. One enantiomer of thalidomide produced a mild sedative effect to treat morning sickness, but the other enantiomer caused devastating birth defects. This drug was responsible for some 10,000 cases of phocomelia (a birth defect in which limbs are missing) in Western Europe when it was administered as a racemic mixture to pregnant women in the late 1950s. The sedative action was caused by the (R)-enantiomer, while the (S)-enantiomer produced the devastating teratogenic effect. One of the major problems with thalidomide is that this drug undergoes racemization under physiological conditions. However, due to its other pharmacological actions, such as inhibition of inflammatory mediators, antiangiogenic activity, and T-cell-modulating activity, the racemic thalidomide (Thalomid) has been approved by the FDA for use under restricted conditions, which seek to limit any access to this drug by pregnant women. Of particular interest is thalidomide's immunomodulatory effect as a treatment for the rare disease, leprosy.

Interestingly, ibuprofen (Advil)—an NSAID that possesses anti-inflammatory, analgesic, and antipyretic effects—has a single chiral center and has been sold as a racemic mixture under many trade names. The (S)-enantiomer of ibuprofen is more active than the (R)-enantiomer. However, after absorption of the racemic ibuprofen, the (R)-enantiomer converts to the (S)-enantiomer. While the (S)-enantiomer is sold as a prescription drug in Austria and Switzerland, the FDA has rejected the approval of this enantiomer in the United States (**Figure 7.20**).

Another example of a drug that demonstrates stereoisomerism is albuterol (Proventil HFA). Albuterol is available as a racemic mixture. While (R)-albuterol causes bronchodilation,

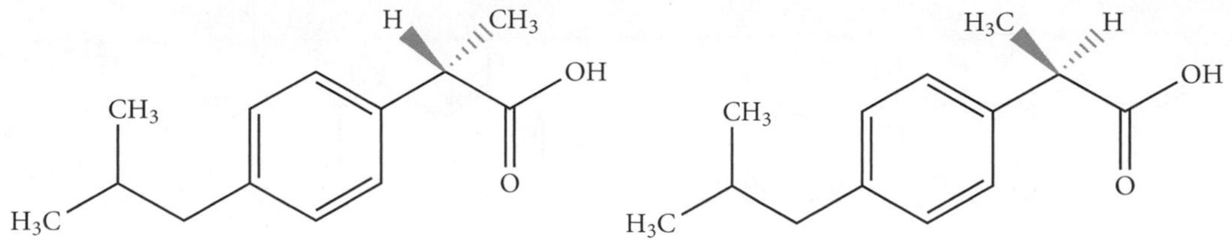

(*S*)-ibuprofen (*R*)-ibuprofen

Figure 7.20 Racemic ibuprofen. While (*R*)-ibuprofen has been approved by the FDA, (*S*)-ibuprofen is not available in the United States.

(*S*)-albuterol has no therapeutic effect. In contrast, levalbuterol (Xopenex) is not a racemic mixture and contains only (*R*)-albuterol.

Enantiomers can also affect metabolism differently or be metabolized differently by different enzymes. For instance, endogenous thyroid hormone is present in the (*S*) form, but synthetic versions of this hormone are in the (*R*) form. The (*S*) form can stimulate the basal metabolic rate to a greater extent than the (*R*) form. Another example is warfarin. The version of this drug available on the market is in a racemic mixture. (*R*)-warfarin has been suggested to be oxidized to 6-hydroxywarfarin by CYP1A2, whereas (*S*)-warfarin is oxidized to 7-hydroxywarfarin by CYP2C9. (*S*)-warfarin is known to have five times more anticoagulant activity compared with (*R*)-warfarin.

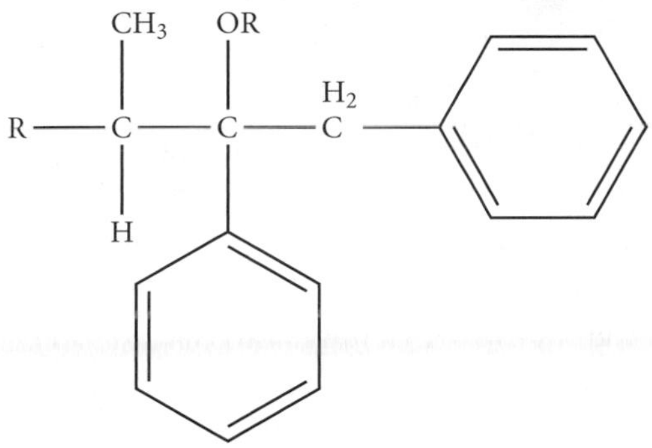

Propoxyphene

Figure 7.21 Structure of propoxyphene. As there are two chiral carbons, there are more than two enantiomers.

A drug with more than two enantiomers (two chiral centers) may behave differently, however. For example, propoxyphene (no longer available in the United States) has two chiral centers. While the (2*S*,3*R*) enantiomer has analgesic properties, the enantiomeric (2*R*,3*S*) version has a totally different pharmacological action—namely, an antitussive effect (**Figure 7.21**).

Learning Bridge 7.5

Joe is a 65-year-old patient with breathing difficulty who has been prescribed albuterol (Proventil), 2 puffs as needed, every 4–6 hours. He comes to your pharmacy to obtain a refill of his medication. You notice that he has tremor and ask him if he has seen his physician recently. Joe admits that he has noticed the tremor and some additional nervousness issues, but states that during his most recent visit his physician did not find any health problems other than his respiratory problem.

In reviewing his current and past medical records, you notice that Joe has not been on any drugs except for albuterol during the past 4 months. Joe mentions that he began to have tremor and nervousness problems after he initiated use of the albuterol inhaler.

Is there any way you can help Joe with the troublesome adverse effects from albuterol? Justify your answer.

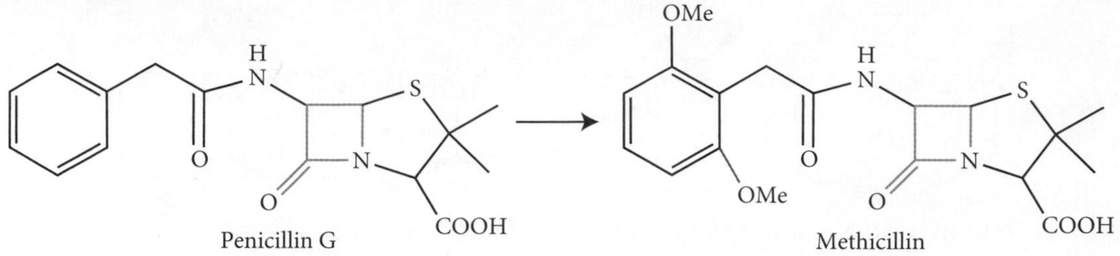

Figure 7.22 A steric shield (the gray methoxyl groups) protects methicillin from bacterial hydrolysis by β-lactamase.

Adapted from: Patrick GL. *An introduction to medicinal chemistry*, 2nd ed. New York: Oxford University Press; 2001: Chapter 14.

Stability of Drugs

Hydrolysis is a potential problem for the stability of many drugs. A few mechanisms can be used to make drugs more resistant to hydrolysis: (1) steric shields, (2) bioisosteres—electronic effects, and (3) stereoelectronic modifications.

Steric Shields

Esters and amides are prone to hydrolysis. One way to protect these functional groups is to add a steric shield to the drug. In this way, one can block a nucleophilic (electron-pair donor) or enzymatic attack (degradation) on the susceptible esters and amides. For instance, adding an alkyl group close to the functional group will protect the hydrolysis of these functional groups. For example, penicillin G is broken down by bacterial β-lactamases (enzymatic degradation that opens the β-lactam rings of penicillin). Addition of two $-OCH_3$ groups in the vicinity of the lactam ring produces methicillin, which is resistant to lactamase. The $-OCH_3$ groups prevent contact between the antibiotic and the active site of the β-lactamase (**Figure 7.22**). Keep in mind that the steric shield should not block the access of the antibiotic to its target (i.e., to bacterial transpeptidases, see also the *Introduction to Microbiology* chapter).

β-Lactam belongs to a family of antibiotics that is characterized by a unique β-lactam ring structure. Penicillin is a member of this family. An intact β-lactam ring is required for this family to demonstrate antibiotic activity, which results in the inactivation of a set of transpeptidases that catalyze the final cell membrane cross-link formation. Because viruses do not have cell walls, they are not susceptible to penicillin. Bacteria that develop resistance to the β-lactams are able to hydrolyze the β-lactam ring of the antibiotic through a β-lactamase (**Figure 7.23**).

Bioisosteres

Bioisosteres are molecules or ions of similar size and similar chemical and physical properties that, when replaced by other bioisosteres, will not affect the biological activity of a molecule. For example, CH_3 is the bioisostere of OH, and CH_2 is the bioisostere of O. It is the retention of important biological activity that determines whether two molecules are bioisosteres. Carbachol (Isopto), for example, is protected by bioisosteres' (resonance) effects from hydrolysis (**Figure 7.24**). The longer

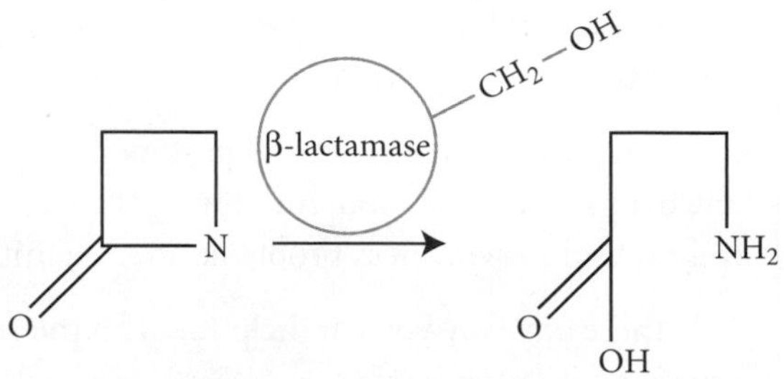

Figure 7.23 Opening (hydrolysis) of the β-lactam ring by bacterial β-lactamase.

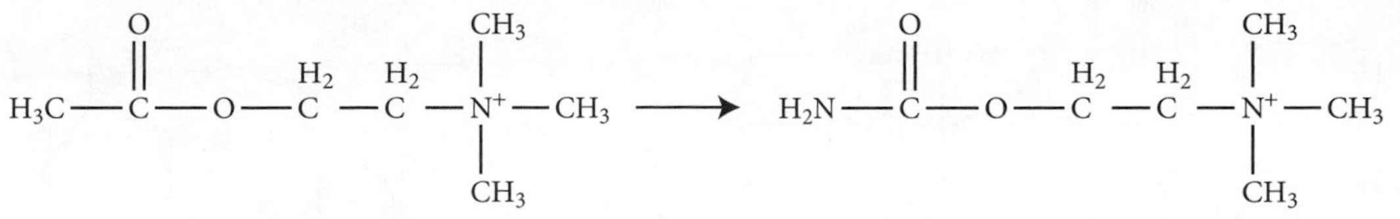

Figure 7.24 Function of bioisosteres: replacement of a methyl group by an amino group protects carbachol from hydrolysis.

duration of action of carbachol, as compared to acetylcholine, is due to the lack of hydrolysis of carbachol by the acetylcholinesterase enzyme (see also the *Introduction to Pharmacology and Pathophysiology* chapter).

Another example is propranolol (Figure 7.17), in which a replacement of the OCH_2 with $CH=CH$ or $CH_2—CH_2$ on the benzene ring eliminates the activity of propranolol, whereas replacement of OCH_2 with $NHCH_2$ does not.

Stereoelectronic Modifications

As the stereoelectronic name indicates, with this technique, both steric hindrance and electronic stabilization are used together to stabilize an unstable functional group. Procaine is a good local anesthetic, but its rapid hydrolysis makes the anesthetic effect to be very short. However, addition of two methyl groups to procaine's benzene ring causes a steric hindrance from the endogenous hydrolytic enzymes. In addition, introducing an amide group into the lidocaine (Xylocaine) structure makes lidocaine more stable than the ester group that is present in the procaine molecule (**Figure 7.25**). As a result, the anesthetic effect of lidocaine is longer than that of procaine (due to procaine's low potency and short duration of action, it has largely been replaced by other anesthetics).

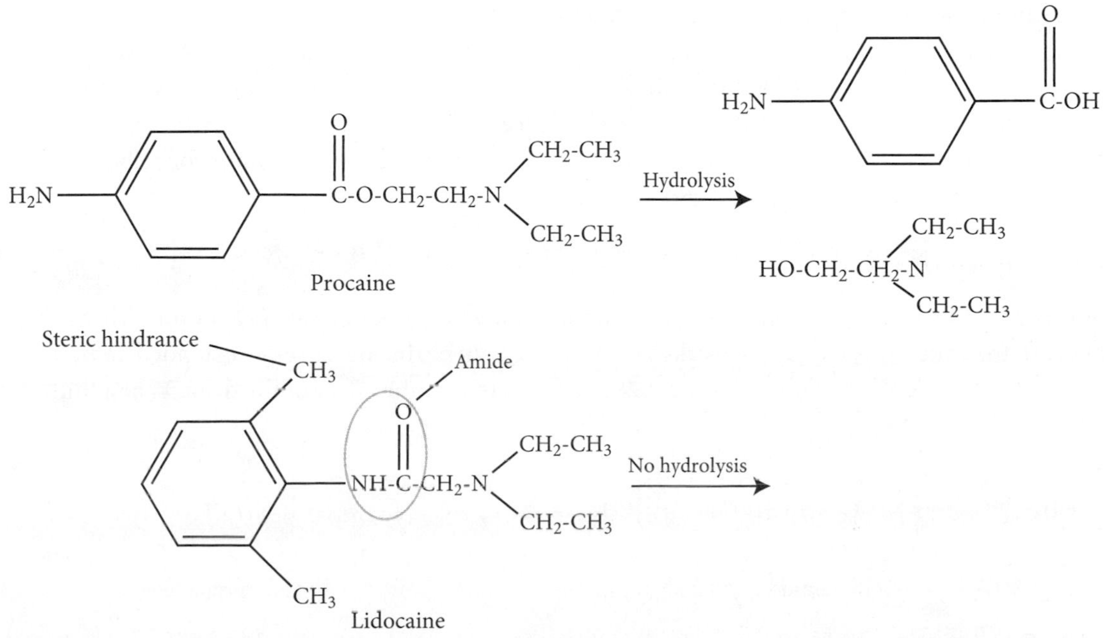

Figure 7.25 The roles of steric hindrance and the amide group are to protect lidocaine from hydrolysis.
Adapted from: Patrick GL. *An introduction to medicinal chemistry*, 2nd ed. New York: Oxford University Press; 2001: Chapter 10.

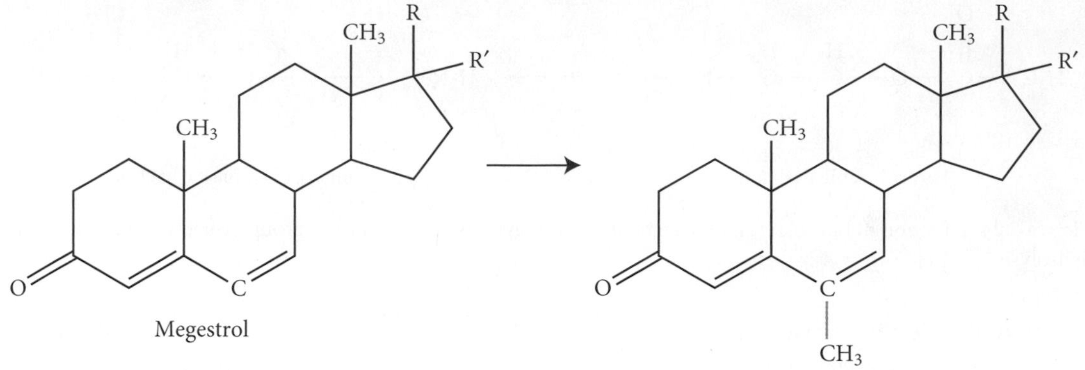

Figure 7.26 The methyl group on carbon 6 of megestrol blocks its rapid metabolism during both Phase I and II reactions.

Adapted from: Patrick GL. *An introduction to medicinal chemistry*, 2nd ed. New York: Oxford University Press; 2001: Chapter 10.

Other mechanisms can also increase the stability of the chemical structure of drugs, thereby extending the pharmacological actions of those drugs. These mechanisms include (1) metabolic blockers, (2) removal of susceptible metabolic groups, (3) group shifts, (4) ring variation, and (5) metabolic blockers.

Drugs that become polar (gaining OH by oxidation) in the metabolic process are easily excreted from the kidney. One way to overcome this fast metabolic problem is to introduce a methyl group at the site of oxidation. For instance, introduction of a methyl group works as metabolic blocker for megestrol (Megace), thereby extending the pharmacological effect of this drug (**Figure 7.26**).

Removal of Susceptible Metabolic Groups

The methyl group on an aromatic ring is susceptible to oxidation (conversion to a carboxyl group), which in turn makes the ring more hydrophilic—a characteristic that facilitates its excretion by the kidney. The susceptible group can be removed or replaced by other functional groups that are more stable in the face of oxidation. For instance, by replacing the chemically reactive methyl group on tolbutamide (Apo-Tolbutamide, from Canada) with a bioisosteric and metabolically resistant chlorine substituent, the metabolic resistance of the antidiabetic agent chlorpropamide (Apo-Chlorpropamide, from Canada) is improved ($t_{1/2}$ is increased from 6 hours for tolbutamide to 36 hours for chlorpropamide) (**Figure 7.27**).

Group Shifts

Shifting a group is a reasonable approach to implement when other pathways are diminishing the effect of the drug. This technique works very well for epinephrine because the extended carbon group (the teal alcohol group in **Figure 7.28**) does not reduce the effect of the drug. When thinking

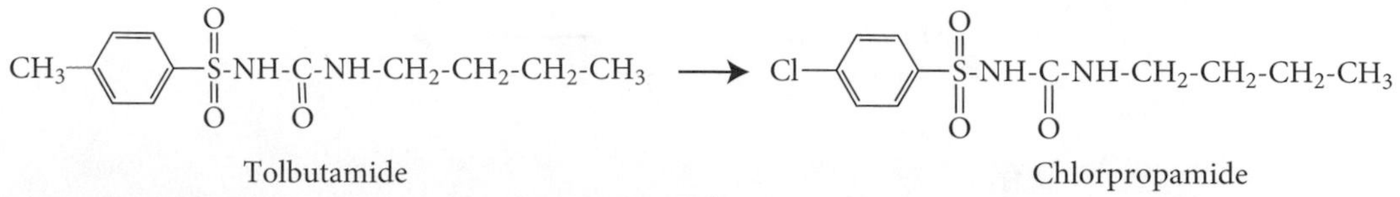

Figure 7.27 Oxidation of tolbutamide during Phase I reactions is blocked by replacing the methyl group with a chloride group.

Adapted from: Patrick GL. *An introduction to medicinal chemistry*, 2nd ed. New York: Oxford University Press; 2001: Chapter 10.

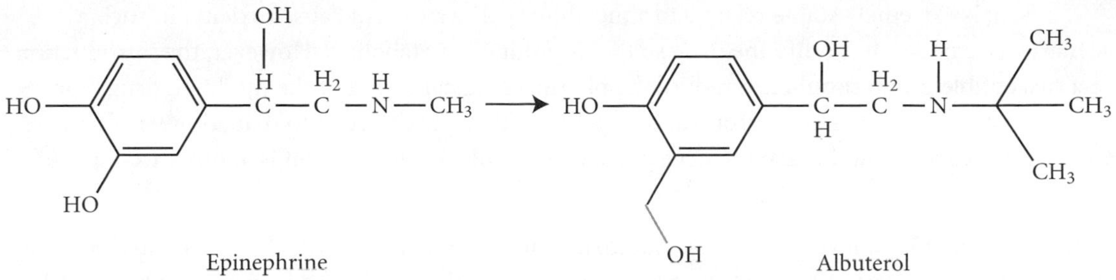

Figure 7.28 The effect of a group shift in epinephrine results in albuterol, which is more stable than epinephrine.

of the shifting group, one has to take into consideration the need to have the same binding of the functional group and to maintain the same ligand bonding to the receptor (i.e., in the case of epinephrine and albuterol, the hydrogen bonding between the drug and adrenergic receptors should remain intact).

Ring Variation

Many of the organic rings are susceptible to metabolism. Therefore, modifying the ring leads to a more stable drug. Consider the synthesis of fluconazole. Ticonazole's imidazole ring is modified to produce a more stable drug in regard to metabolism (**Figure 7.29**). While ticonazole is not available on the U.S. market, fluconazole is highly effective and is frequently prescribed as an antifungal agent. This drug interferes with fungal cytochrome P450 activity and decreases the synthesis of ergosterol, which in turn changes the integrity of the cell membrane. Ergosterol is the principal sterol in the fungal cell membrane; humans do not have ergosterol in their cell membranes, but rather cholesterol.

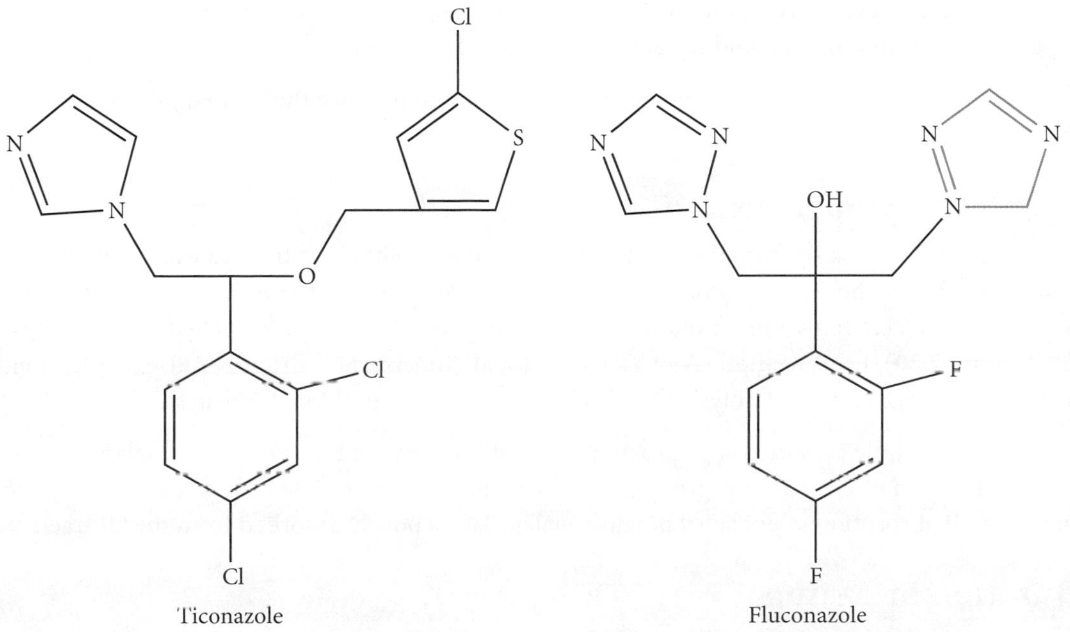

Figure 7.29 Modification of the imidazole ring results in a longer effect for the antifungal agent fluconazole.
Adapted from: Patrick GL. *An introduction to medicinal chemistry*, 2nd ed. New York: Oxford University Press; 2001: Chapter 10.

If a drug is extremely stable relative to a metabolic pathway, it can cause toxicity; in such a scenario, one needs to modify the drug so that it produces metabolites. However, the introduction of a susceptible group should not reduce the pharmacological action of the modified drug. For instance, introducing a methyl group and thereby making a drug prone to oxidation will facilitate the Phase I reactions and make the drug more hydrophilic. Hydroxylation is another example of a characteristic that can be introduced into benzene rings.

If a drug has a high level of toxicity, that toxicity must be reduced if the drug is to have utility in patients. Many of the clinical trials that fail to progress further are halted because of a high level of toxicity in the candidate drug. One effective way to reduce the toxicity of drugs is to modify the structure of the drug. For instance, the drug that preceded fluconazole in development was a compound that had a high level of toxicity. Replacing its halogen atom chlorine with another halogen atom, fluorine, reduced the toxicity and resulted in the effective drug, fluconazole.

Prodrugs

Oral drug delivery is the preferable route of administering drugs to human patients. Unfortunately, not all drugs will have the desired physicochemical and pharmacokinetic properties that allow them to be administered orally: lack of bioavailability, water insolubility, or an intolerable taste can serve as barriers to use of an oral dosage form. Unfortunately, these barriers may lead to the selection of other administration routes, which may compromise the pharmacological effect of a drug.

Prodrugs are very useful approaches to avoid these barriers and other physiochemical problems such as acid sensitivity, chemical instability, toxicity, and short $t_{1/2}$. Prodrugs are inactive compounds that, upon metabolism in the body, produce active metabolites that have pharmacological effects. While it is important to make sure that the compound is metabolized at the right time and the right place, the metabolite(s) should not produce any toxicity. Examples of well-known prodrugs include ACE inhibitors, which are used as antihypertensive agents; mesalamine (Asacol), which is used in inflammatory bowel disease; the antihypertensive minoxidil (Loniten, from Canada); the angiotensin receptor blocker losartan (Cozaar); the anticancer drug tamoxifen (Apo-Tamox, from Canada); and the antiplatelet drug clopidogrel.

Some of the barriers that can be overcome by prodrugs to produce the desired pharmacological effect are reviewed next.

Membrane Impermeability

It is important to mask hydrophilic functional groups that might block the entry of a drug through the hydrophobic moiety of the cell membrane. For instance, the ACE inhibitor enalapril (Vasotec), which contains a functional carboxyl group, is esterified to mask its hydrophilic property (**Figure 7.30**). Esterification is not a solution for all impermeable drugs because, as mentioned elsewhere in this chapter, hydrolysis of esters is often a stability problem for drugs.

Enalapril has little pharmacological activity until it is hydrolyzed in the liver to enalaprilate. The esterification of the carboxyl group (see the structure of enalaprilate in Figure 7.30) results in increased GI absorption of enalapril because enalaprilate is poorly absorbed from the GI tract.

Duration of Action

It is important for some drugs to be metabolized to the active metabolite slowly to produce a full effect. One example is mercaptopurine (Purinethol), an agent that is used to suppress immunological responses in donor grafts. This drug has a short half-life, so it is necessary to prolong its effect

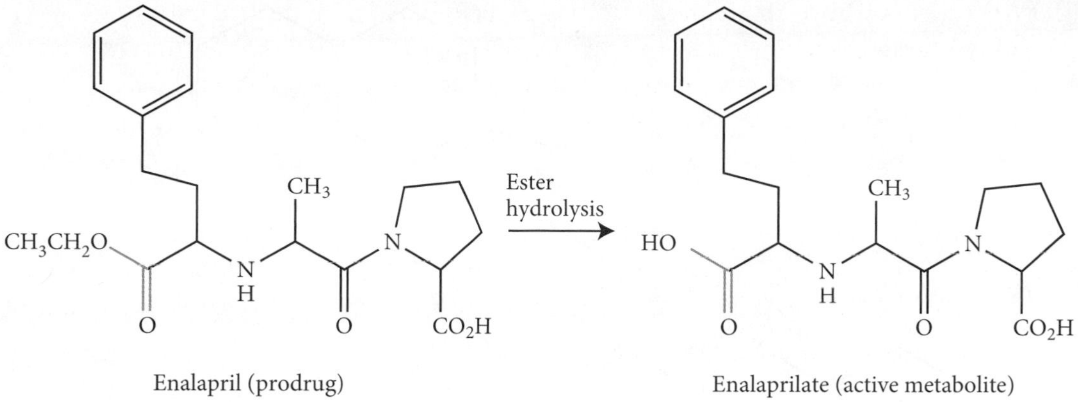

Figure 7.30 The hydrophilic moiety (carboxyl group) of the active compound, enalaprilate, is masked by converting the carboxyl group into an ester group.

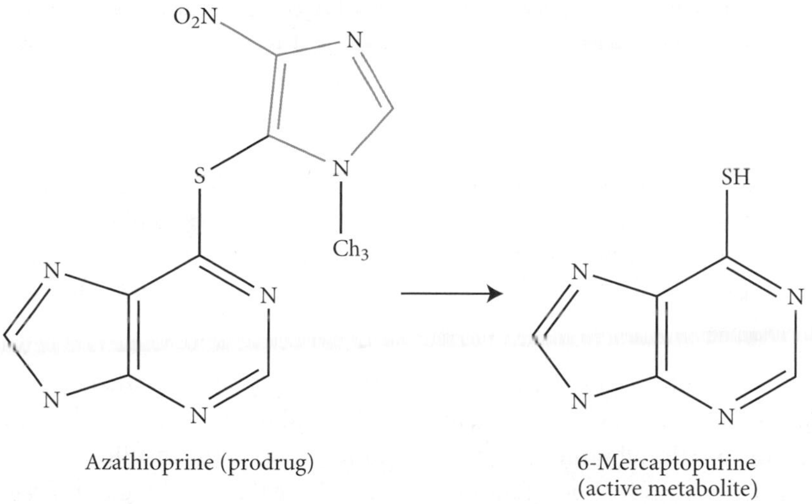

Figure 7.31 Addition of an electron-withdrawing group, NO_2, and a heterocyclic group extends the duration of action of 6-mercaptopurine.

Adapted from: Patrick GL. *An introduction to medicinal chemistry*, 2nd ed. New York: Oxford University Press; 2001: Chapter 10.

by producing a prodrug, azathioprine (Imuran), which is slowly converted to 6-mercaptopurine. The latter conversion is required because of addition of electron-withdrawing groups (in this case, an NO_2 group and a heterocyclic group) that are chemically removed to produce the active metabolite 6-mercaptopurine (**Figure 7.31**).

A drug might also be made more hydrophobic so that it can be stored in the adipocytes and then released gradually to prolong its effects. For instance, the antipsychotic drug fluphenazine (Apo-Fluphenazine Decanoate, from Canada) carries a fatty acid so that it can be stored in the adipocytes for slow release into the blood (**Figure 7.32**). A fluphenazine decanoate injection is available as a sterile solution for intramuscular (IM) administration. Esterification of fluphenazine with a fatty acid reduces the release rate of the drug from adipocytes, which in turn prolongs the drug's duration of action (the onset of action occurs within 24–72 hours and the duration of action is usually 2 weeks).

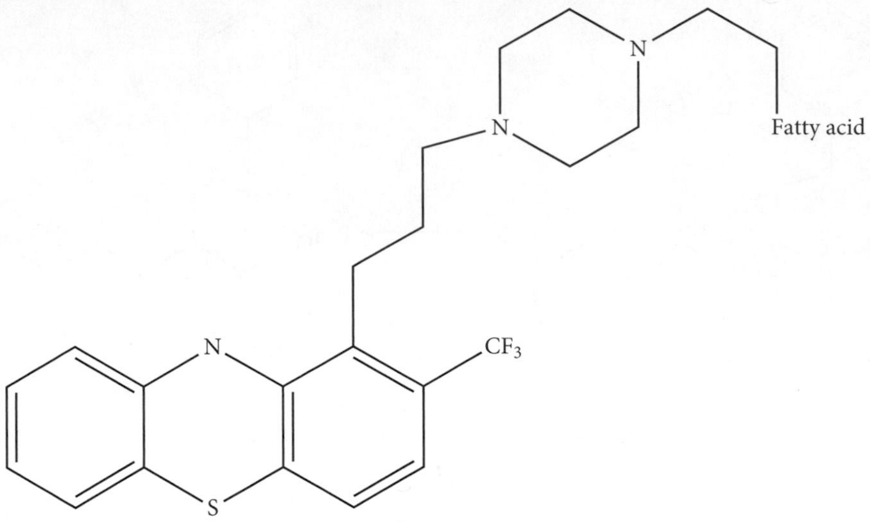

Fluphenazine decanoate

Figure 7.32 Addition of a fatty acid to fluphenazine results in a longer duration of action.
Adapted from: Patrick GL. *An introduction to medicinal chemistry*, 2nd ed. New York: Oxford University Press; 2001: Chapter 10.

Such slow release from adipose tissue can sometimes cause additive drug interactions with other concurrently administered drugs. One typical example that is frequently observed in the retail setting is the concurrent administration of methadone and a diazepam-type agent; this combination can enhance adverse effects of the drugs such as respiratory depression, drowsiness, hypotension, and sedation.

Similar to fluphenazine, insulin detemir (Levemir) has a fatty acid attached to the 29th amino acid, lysine, in the B chain of the insulin agent. The fatty acid binds to serum albumin. Collectively, the self-association and the albumin binding delay distribution of the insulin detemir to the target tissues, generating an 18- to 24-hour duration of action. Note that insulin glargine's long duration of action (24 hours) is attributable to a completely different mechanism. Glargine (Lantus) is in an acidic (pH 4.0) solution that stabilizes the hexamer structure of the insulin molecule; the hexamer structure results in a slow absorption.

One can also make a drug act more rapidly. For example, insulin lispro (Humalog) has a faster action than regular insulin because lispro is a hexamer molecule that, upon injection, dissociates into a monomer. This monomer has a higher absorption rate than regular insulin. The rapid action is made possible by the reversal of the amino acids lysine and proline of the B chain (hence the name lispro). Similarly, insulin aspart (Novolog) has a fast action (less than 15 minutes) and has one structural change: proline is changed to aspartic acid. This modification does not allow insulin to self-associate, so it remains in a monomer form.

Reducing Drug Toxicity or Adverse Effects

The development of a prodrug is a good way to reduce or eliminate an adverse effect or drug toxicity. Consider the conversion of salicylic acid to acetyl salicylic acid. Salicylic acid is known to cause GI bleeding, but the prodrug acetyl salicylic acid reduces the GI bleeding adverse effect (**Figure 7.33**).

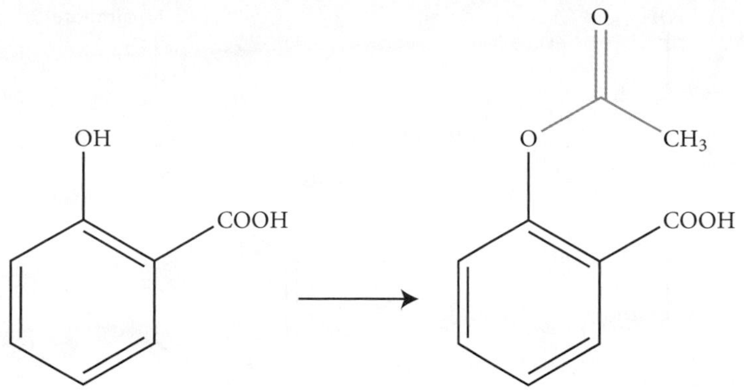

Figure 7.33 Acetyl salicylic acid has an ester group that reduces the GI bleeding associated with salicylic acid.

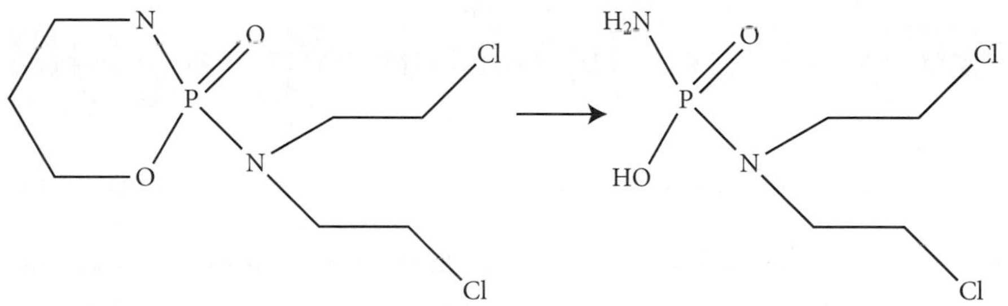

Salicylic acid

Acetyl salicylic acid

Cyclophosphamide (prodrug)

Phosphoramide mustard (toxic metabolite)

Figure 7.34 Cyclophosphamide is nontoxic as a prodrug but becomes a toxic compound upon its metabolism in cancerous cells.

Adapted from: Patrick GL. *An introduction to medicinal chemistry*, 2nd ed. New York: Oxford University Press; 2001: Chapter 10.

In other cases, it is important to mask the toxicity of a drug so that upon activation the drug becomes toxic. This approach is particularly useful for anticancer agents. For instance, cyclophosphamide (Procytox, from Canada) is nontoxic but becomes a toxic compound upon metabolism by the enzyme phosphoramidase, which is present in high concentrations in cancerous cells (**Figure 7.34**).

Increasing or Reducing Water Solubility

While increasing water solubility is often an important way to enhance a drug's dosage preparation and pharmacological effect, it is important to reduce water solubility if one needs to avoid a bitter taste. For instance, one can change the bitter taste of the antibacterial agent chloramphenicol (Chloromycetin, from Canada) by addition of a palmitate ester to the hydroxyl group (**Figure 7.35**). The ester is quickly hydrolyzed to the active metabolite upon digestion of the antibiotic.

Conversely, increasing water solubility is useful to make a drug more concentrated with less volume, particularly for drugs that will be administered via the IV route. In addition, the more water soluble an injection is, the less pain it will cause at the site of the injection. Clindamycin phosphate injection (an antibiotic drug), for example, is more water soluble than clindamycin.

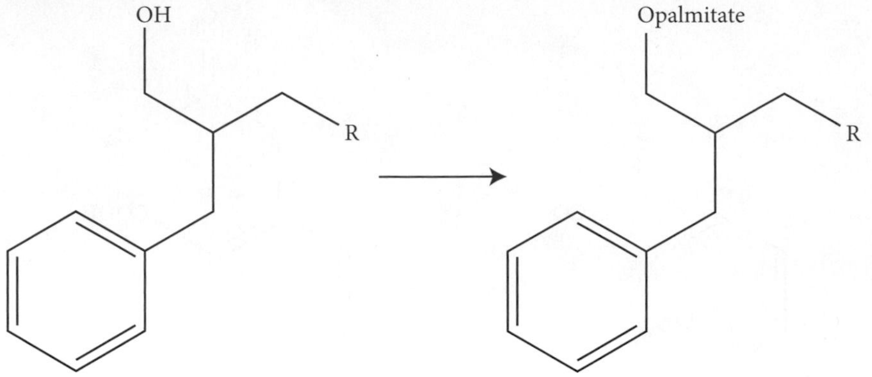

Figure 7.35 Esterification of the hydroxyl group with a fatty acid masks the bitter taste of chloramphenicol.

Lead Structure–Activity Relationships in Medicinal Chemistry

Discovery of new drugs has been associated with both luck and well-designed research and investigation. Many of the drugs that are available in the market have been produced from their parental compound or lead compound that either was naturally found from animals, plants, or microorganisms or was synthesized in a laboratory after a well-designed research study. Medicinal chemists recognize that if the initial natural or synthetic drug has good pharmacological activity, a large set of related analogs can be synthesized and screened to build a database of structure–activity relationships (SAR). Similarly, it is clear that incorporation of new functional groups could lead to more analogs with even better pharmacological results, a longer or shorter duration of action, a smaller or higher absorption or metabolic rate, or fewer or less serious adverse effects.

A typical example of a lead SAR is seen with the insulin hormone. Insulin is a polypeptide hormone that is synthesized in the pancreatic rough ER of the beta cells. Upon synthesis, the insulin hormone moves into the Golgi apparatus so that it can be packaged into membrane-bound granules. With the help of cytoplasmic microtubules, these insulin-filled granules move to the plasma membrane, where they release their insulin content by exocytosis upon receiving a few signaling pathways (see the *Introduction to Pharmacology and Pathophysiology* chapter).

Many analogs of insulin are available in the market. The fact that insulin's structure and amino acid sequence do not change significantly among a few species (e.g., humans, dogs, pigs, cows) indicates that there is a structural flexibility that does not affect the biochemical and pharmacological effects of insulin. However, even some very minor structural differences (e.g., bovine insulin differs from human insulin by only three amino acids) can cause immunological reactions or contamination problems. DNA recombinant technology can be employed to avoid these problems (see also the *Introduction to Cell Biology* chapter).

The structural flexibility of insulin has been utilized to produce other insulin analogs. For example, insulin aspart has a short-acting mechanism because the amino acid proline is changed to aspartic acid; similarly, the long-acting insulin detemir is generated by replacing the amino acid threonine in position of the B chain (amino acid number 30) with a fatty acid.

Another example of utilizing a lead SAR in finding other useful drugs is apparent with opioids. Morphine is a natural compound with profound analgesic activity. When the hydroxyl group

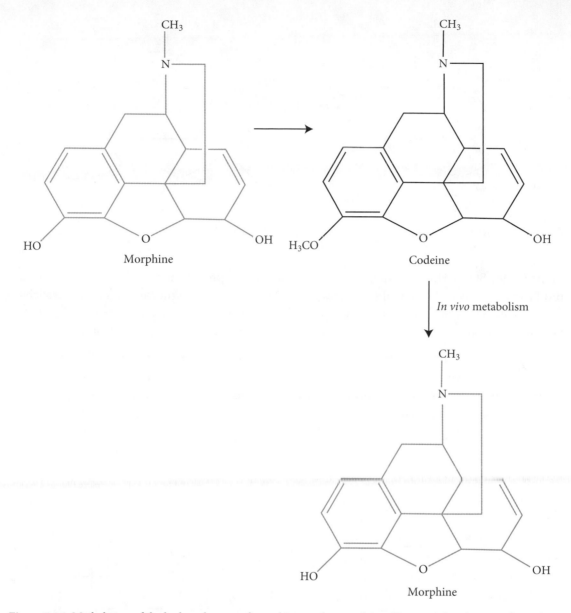

Figure 7.36 Methylation of the hydroxyl group of morphine produces codeine. However, this change reduces the analgesic effect of morphine by five times.

of morphine was methylated, a new synthetic analgesic, codeine, was discovered (**Figure 7.36**). However, when the analgesic effect of codeine was checked *in vitro*, it showed only 0.1% analgesic effectiveness compared with morphine. Later, it was discovered that the *in vivo* metabolism actually converted codeine back to morphine, which explained why codeine had 20% of morphine's effect in the *in vivo* study and only 0.1% of morphine's effect in the *in vitro* study.

Esterification of morphine's hydroxyl groups, however, produces diamorphine (commonly known as heroin; **Figure 7.37**), which produces a greater euphoric effect (although in double-blind trials it did not show superior effect compared with another potent opioid, hydromorphone [Dilaudid]). The more potent effect is due to heroin's ester groups; this compound is less hydrophilic than morphine and can more easily pass through the blood–brain barrier to reach the brain. Due to its potential for abuse, tendency to produce strong physical dependence, and devastating withdrawal symptoms, heroin is not used as a pharmacological agent in many countries, including

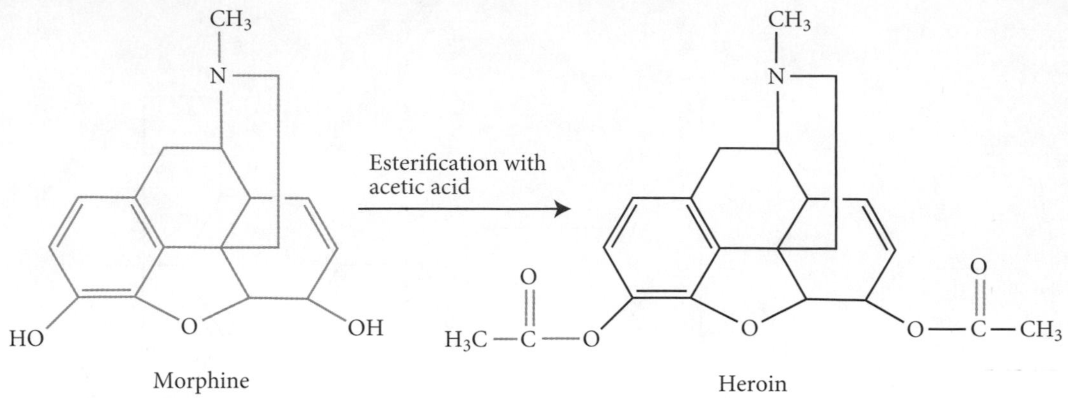

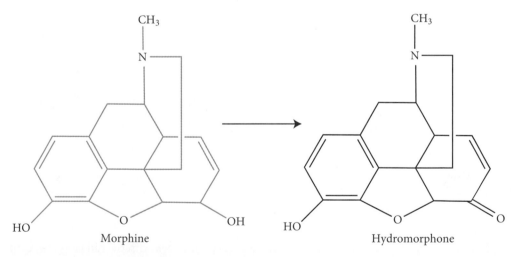

Figure 7.37 Esterification of morphine's hydroxyl groups produces heroin.

in the United States. However, due to heroin's pronounced euphoric effect, and the fact that illegal producers have been able to make it highly pure (10 times purer than the heroin that was available in the 1960s and 1970s), drug abusers can administer it nasally rather than injecting it. As a result, heroin is back on the illicit market and used by some young adults in the United States.

Similar to heroin, hydromorphone has a greater analgesic effect than morphine (it has been suggested that hydromorphone's effect is 10 times more potent than that of morphine). One of the hydroxyl groups of morphine is replaced with a carbonyl group, which makes hydromorphone less polar and enables it to pass through the blood–brain barrier with ease (**Figures 7.38** and **7.39**).

Figure 7.38 When the hydroxyl group of morphine is replaced by a ketone group, hydromorphone is produced. It has a much more potent analgesic effect than morphine.

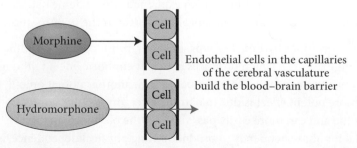

Figure 7.39 Endothelial cells in the capillaries of the cerebral vasculature allow hydrophobic drugs readily to reach the brain.

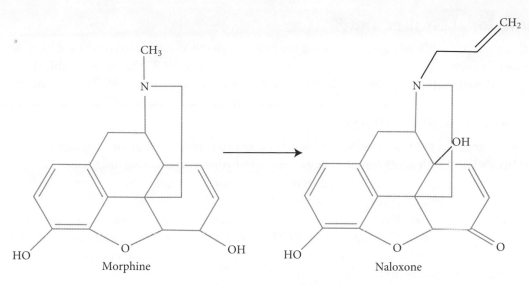

Figure 7.40 When the nitrogen group is extended, naloxone shows an antagonistic effect to opioid receptors.
Adapted from: Patrick GL. *An introduction to medicinal chemistry*, 2nd ed. New York: Oxford University Press; 2001: Chapter 17.

The search for other analogs to morphine also led to the discovery of naloxone and naltrexone. Both of these drugs are analogs to morphine, but they do not show any analgesic effect. It has been suggested that these analogs act as antagonists to opioid receptors (see also the *Introduction to Pharmacology and Pathophysiology* chapter). While they do not exert any analgesic effect, they are very useful as antidotes (because they can readily displace opioids at opioid receptors) and are also used as agents to treat opioid addiction (**Figure 7.40**).

Cimetidine (Tagamet HB 200) is a histamine H_2-receptor blocker (H_2 blocker) and selectively binds to H_2 while avoiding binding to the histamine H_1 receptor. Its effect is to reduce gastric acid secretion. Cimetidine has been the lead compound for other H_2 blockers such as ranitidine (Zantac), famotidine (Pepcid), and nizatidine (Axid). Indeed, it has been shown that when the imidazole molecule of cimetidine is replaced by a furan ring, ranitidine is synthesized in a form that has fewer side effects, much greater effectiveness (10 times more effective), and a longer duration of action compared with cimetidine (**Figure 7.41**). All four H_2 blockers are available as oral OTC products due to their nontoxic effect.

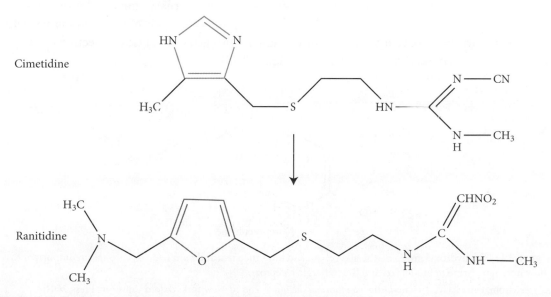

Figure 7.41 Replacement of the imidazole ring with furan produced a much better H_2 blocker.

Functional Groups and SAR

In this section, the binding roles of some of the most frequently encountered functional groups are discussed to appreciate the important role they play in producing SAR. The physiochemical properties of these functional groups are described in the *Introduction to Biological Chemistry* chapter.

Binding Role of Hydroxyl Groups

The most important physicochemical property of a hydroxyl functional group is its ability to form a hydrogen bond with another molecule. Accordingly, hydroxyl-containing drugs can hydrogen-bond to water, receptors, transporters, enzymes, or any other molecules that can form a hydrogen bond with those drugs. Many factors may contribute to the water solubility of a drug, but the presence of a hydroxyl group has a significant impact on enhancing water solubility. Conversion of the hydroxyl group to a methyl group (OH → —CH$_3$) or esterification of the hydroxyl group (OH → —O—OC—CH$_3$) will disrupt the hydrogen bonding. An example of the latter effect is seen when morphine is modified to heroin (Figure 7.37).

The strength of the interactions between the ligand (drug) and the receptor will determine recognition and affinity. For instance, the higher the chance of forming a hydrogen bond, the more specific the interaction and the greater the potency of the pharmacologically active molecule. In addition, there is a smaller likelihood that the new molecule will have reduced adverse effects (because it will not dissociate and bind to other receptors). For instance, it is known that the three hydroxyl groups on the norepinephrine (NE) molecule are important for binding of NE to adrenergic receptors (**Figure 7.42**).

Binding Role of Amino Groups

Amino groups have basic property (except the tertiary amino group). As a result, one can find this important functional group on many drug products. The presence of an amino group can help medicinal chemists make a salt version of a compound so as to increase its water solubility (recall from the *Introduction to Biological Chemistry* chapter that combining a weak base with a strong acid such as HCl can produce a salt). Amino groups can also be used to form amide groups, although the amino group must be a primary (RNH$_2$) or a secondary (R—NH—R) amine. The tertiary amine (R—NR—R) cannot form an amide because there is no proton on the nitrogen atom that can be replaced by an alkyl group. Dealkylation and then amide formation of an amine group disrupts the hydrogen bonding between drugs and its target. Quaternary amines are also important in distorting the electron cloud of aromatic rings to produce a dipole moment on the aromatic ring—that is, the positive charged end of the quaternary nitrogen can attract the electrons and induce two partial poles in the aromatic rings (**Figure 7.43**).

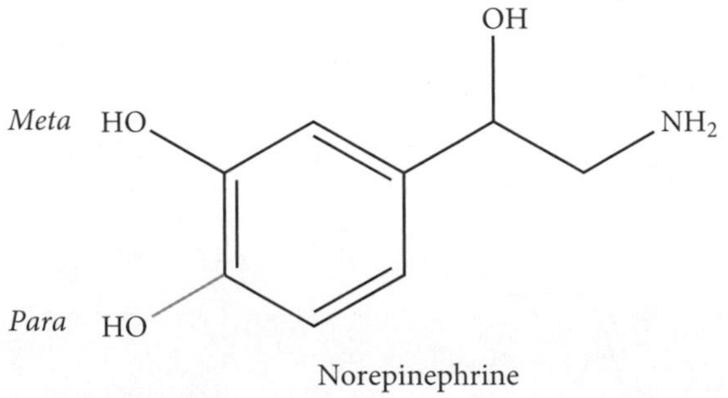

Figure 7.42 The hydroxyl group on the alkyl chain and both the *meta* and *para* hydroxyl groups are important to allow norepinephrine to bind its α- and β-adrenergic receptors.

Adapted from: Patrick GL. *An introduction to medicinal chemistry*, 2nd ed. New York: Oxford University Press; 2001: Chapter 16.

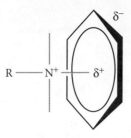

Figure 7.43 Quaternary amines are able to turn aromatic rings into dipole molecules.

The amino group shown in Figure 7.42 also plays an important role in the binding of norepinephrine to its receptors. For instance, both replacing the nitrogen atom with a carbon atom and adding carbon atoms to the hydrogen atoms of the amino group reduce the adrenergic selectivity. Indeed, when epinephrine's structure is compared with norepinephrine, one can understand why norepinephrine is more selective to α receptors than to β receptors. The extra methyl group on the structure of epinephrine plays an important role in this molecule being nonselective to adrenergic receptors. When further alkyl groups are added to the nitrogen atom, the effect on α receptors is lost. For instance, isoproterenol (Isuprel; an injection that is used in emergency situations to counteract cardiac arrest until electric shock is available) has no α-adrenergic effect because of the alkyl group that is added to the nitrogen atom of norepinephrine (**Figure 7.44**).

Binding Role of Aromatic Rings

Aromatic rings are involved in van der Waals forces because of their flat hydrophobic property (**Figure 7.45**). Hydrogenation (a reduction mechanism) of the aromatic rings leads to a decrease in the binding affinity of a drug to its target. However, hydrogenation (reduction) of an aromatic ring is a cumbersome chemical process. It is known that the aromatic ring of epinephrine or norepinephrine has an affinity to phenylalanine 290 of the adrenergic receptors. In turn, a reduction of the aromatic ring can reduce the affinity of epinephrine or norepinephrine for the adrenergic receptors. Note that one of the common metabolic problems with drugs containing a benzene ring is that they can participate in an epoxidation process that produces a reactive carcinogenic intermediate metabolite during their hydroxylation (see also the *Introduction to Biological Chemistry* chapter).

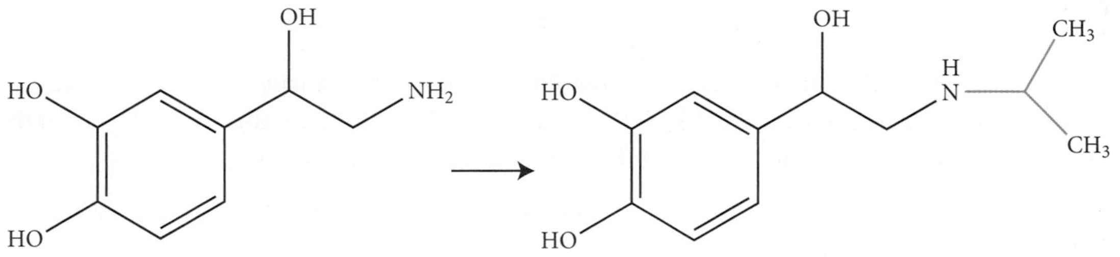

Norepinephrine

Isoproterenol

Figure 7.44 *N*-alkyl substitution on the nitrogen atom of norepinephrine eliminates any α selectivity effect on the adrenergic receptors.

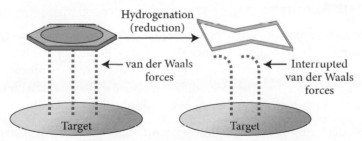

Figure 7.45 The flatness of aromatic rings plays an important role in the van der Waals forces created with a target molecule.

Adapted from: Patrick GL. *An introduction to medicinal chemistry*, 2nd ed. New York: Oxford University Press; 2001: Chapter 8.

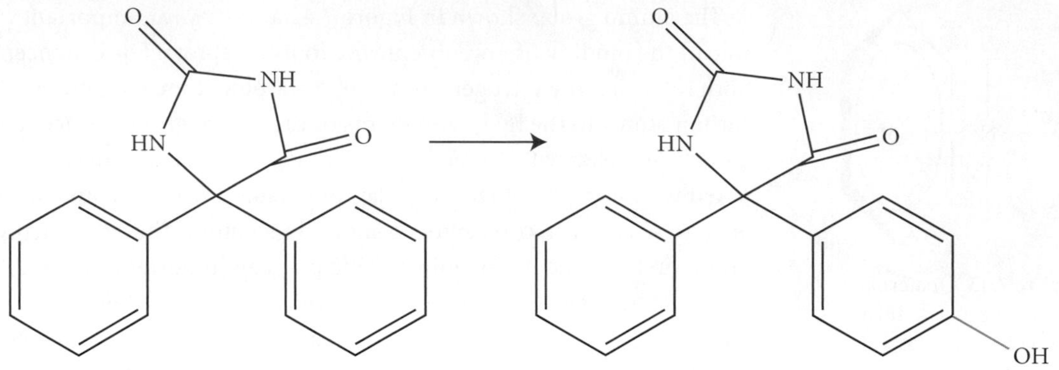

Phenytoin

Figure 7.46 Hydroxylation at the *para* position of aromatic rings is a common metabolic pathway during Phase I reactions.

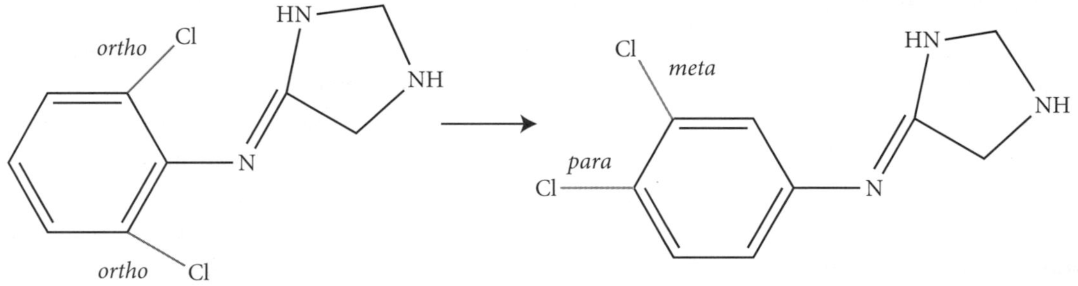

Clonidine

Figure 7.47 Changing chloride atoms from *ortho* positions to *meta* and *para* positions significantly reduces the antihypertensive effect of clonidine.

Hydroxylation of aromatic rings is a very commonly used pathway during Phase I metabolism. In humans, hydroxylation occurs always at the *para* position. For instance, the *para* position on the benzene ring of phenytoin is hydroxylated (**Figure 7.46**).

Due to the unique physical and chemical properties of aromatic rings, not only are substitutions important, but the positions in which the substitutions occur are also critical. For instance, if the two chloride atoms that are in the *ortho* position of the benzene ring of clonidine (Catapres) are changed to *meta* and *para* positions, the antihypertensive effect of clonidine is significantly reduced (**Figure 7.47**).

Binding Role of Alkenes

Hydrogenation (reduction mechanism) of an alkene group can reduce the binding affinity of an alkene drug to its target by reducing the van der Waals forces. Reduction of an alkene, however, is not as cumbersome as reduction an aromatic ring. In addition, isomers of alkenes are expected to have different binding potency and, therefore, different pharmacological activities (**Figure 7.48**). Drugs that have an alkene functional group are metabolically stable molecules.

Similar to the benzene ring epoxidation process, however, epoxidation of alkenes can occur as well. The epoxide is a chemically unstable structure because it is prone to a nucleophilic attack that causes ring opening of the epoxide. For instance, during Phase I metabolism, carbamazepine (Tegretol) is prone to epoxidation due to the alkene group in its structure. The epoxide ring immediately opens to produce carbamazepine-10,11-diol (**Figure 7.49**).

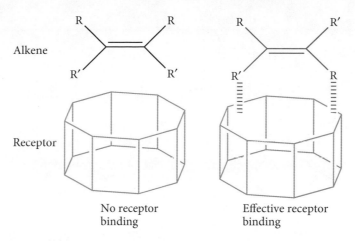

Figure 7.48 The isomers (*cis* and *trans*) of an alkene group can play important roles in receptor binding.

Adapted from: Patrick GL. *An introduction to medicinal chemistry*, 2nd ed. New York: Oxford University Press; 2001: Chapter 8.

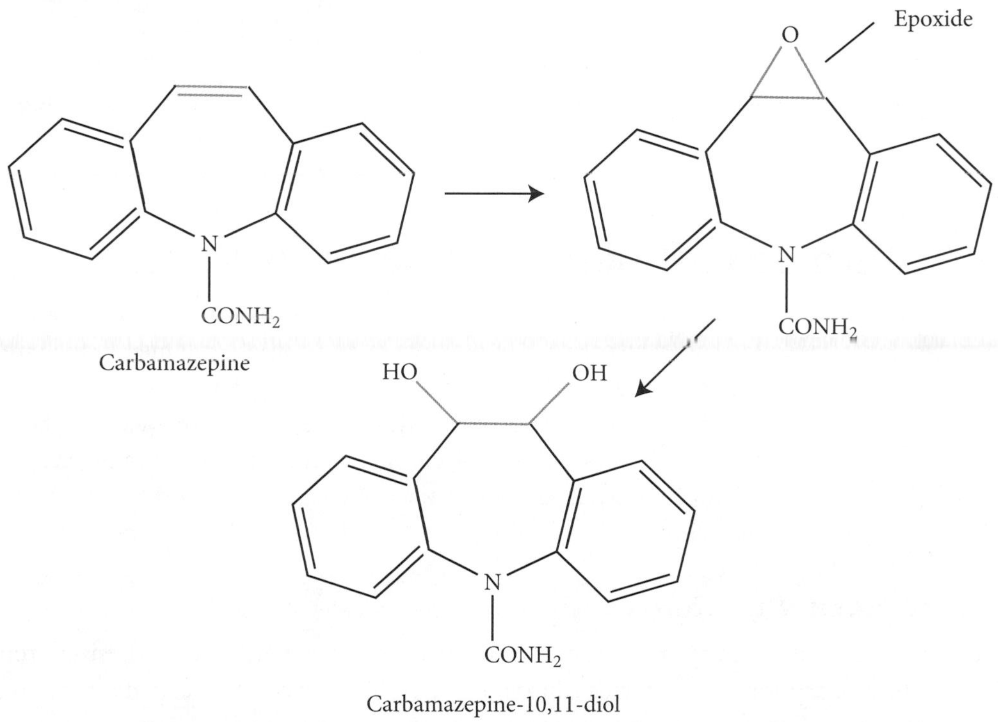

Figure 7.49 The alkene group of carbamazepine is prone to epoxide formation, which is followed by ring opening that produces carbamazepine-10,11-diol.

Adapted from: Nogrady T, Weaver DF. *Medicinal chemistry: a molecular and biochemical approach*, 3rd ed. New York: Oxford University Press; 2005: Chapter 3.

Binding Role of Ketones

Ketone groups are found on the structures of many drugs. They are readily reduced to alcohol groups. Indeed, conversion of a ketone group to an alcohol group can change the geometry of the ketone: A ketone has a flat structure, whereas an alcohol has a tetrahedral structure, which may disrupt the unique hydrogen bond of ketone groups (see **Figure 7.50**). An alcohol group can create a hydrogen bond, but the tetrahedral structure will weaken a hydrogen bond compared with the flat structure of a ketone. Reduction of ketone to alcohol is seen, for example, when cortisone is metabolically reduced to tetrahydrocortisone.

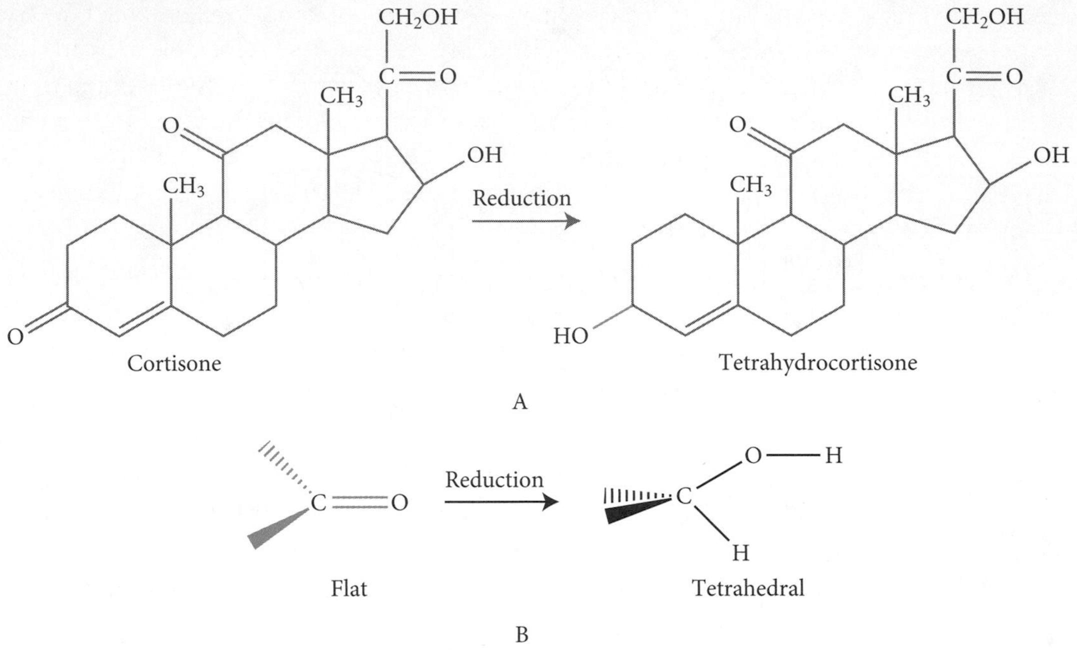

Figure 7.50 (A) Ketones are able to make hydrogen bonds with their target group, but they are prone to being reduced to an alcohol group. (B) Ketones have a flat geometry, whereas alcohols have a tetrahedral geometry.

Drugs Targeting Biological Macromolecules

Biological macromolecules are proteins, carbohydrates, lipids, and nucleic acids. All of these macromolecules are essential for cellular growth and survival. In addition, cell membranes are large molecules that are important in protecting cells and allowing for entry or exit of ions and molecules. However, because they are built from the first three types of macromolecules, they do not belong to the class of macromolecules. Macromolecules, including cell membranes, are essential for many organisms including bacteria. As a result, these molecules are good targets for drugs geared toward fighting foreign organisms.

Drugs Targeting Proteins

Molecules that have catalytic activities are enzymes, the majority of which are synthesized from amino acids (one exception arises when a ribozyme—an RNA—has catalytic activity; see also the *Introduction to Cell Biology* chapter). Because many enzymes are involved in the regulation of biochemical pathways and reactions (intracellular and extracellular), they are not only good targets for clearing bacterial infections (intracellular), but also effective targets for speeding up, slowing down, or simply blocking an endogenous biochemical pathway or a reaction in animals, including humans. Likewise, receptors and other proteins are good targets for drugs.

Drugs that block an enzymatic function may be either reversible or irreversible inhibitors. While many examples of the former can be cited, only a few irreversible inhibitors are available in the market. How strongly an inhibitor binds to an enzyme depends on the intermolecular interaction that occurs between the drug and the enzyme, which takes the form of hydrogen bonds, hydrophobic interactions, electrostatic interactions, van der Waals forces, or covalent bonds. While one or more of these interactions (except covalent binding) may be employed by reversible inhibitors, irreversible inhibitors typically rely on covalent binding.

Drugs that inhibit the transition state of an enzyme (transition-state analogs) or inhibit the catalytic site of the enzymes (mechanism-based inhibitors) are also available. Reversible inhibitors are also divided into competitive, noncompetitive, and uncompetitive inhibitors. The reversible inhibitors are time dependent; that is, as time goes by, we synthesize more of the free enzyme (unbound) such that it eventually exceeds the number of inhibited enzymes.

Drugs as Reversible Inhibitors

A drug that acts as a competitive inhibitor resembles the actual substrate for an enzyme and, as a result, is able to bind to the active site of the enzyme. It forms an enzyme–inhibitor complex and thereby blocks the binding of the substrate (see also the *Introduction to Biochemistry* chapter). It is not surprising, then, that many drugs that act as competitive inhibitors mimic the structures of endogenous substrates.

If a drug inhibits a biochemical or metabolic pathway that is essential for a cell to survive, the drug is called an antimetabolite. Antimetabolites are S-phase specific (recall that the S phase is one of the cell cycle processes in which DNA, RNA, and protein synthesis occurs; see also the *Introduction to Cell Biology* chapter). Many of the currently available antitumor drugs are classified as antimetabolites. This class also includes folic acid antagonists, which do not allow folic acid to participate in the synthesis of purine and thymine, and drugs that mimic purines and pyrimidines and thereby block synthesis of RNA and DNA molecules. For example, the folic acid antagonist known as methotrexate (Rheumatrex) structurally resembles folic acid (**Figure 7.51**). One of the

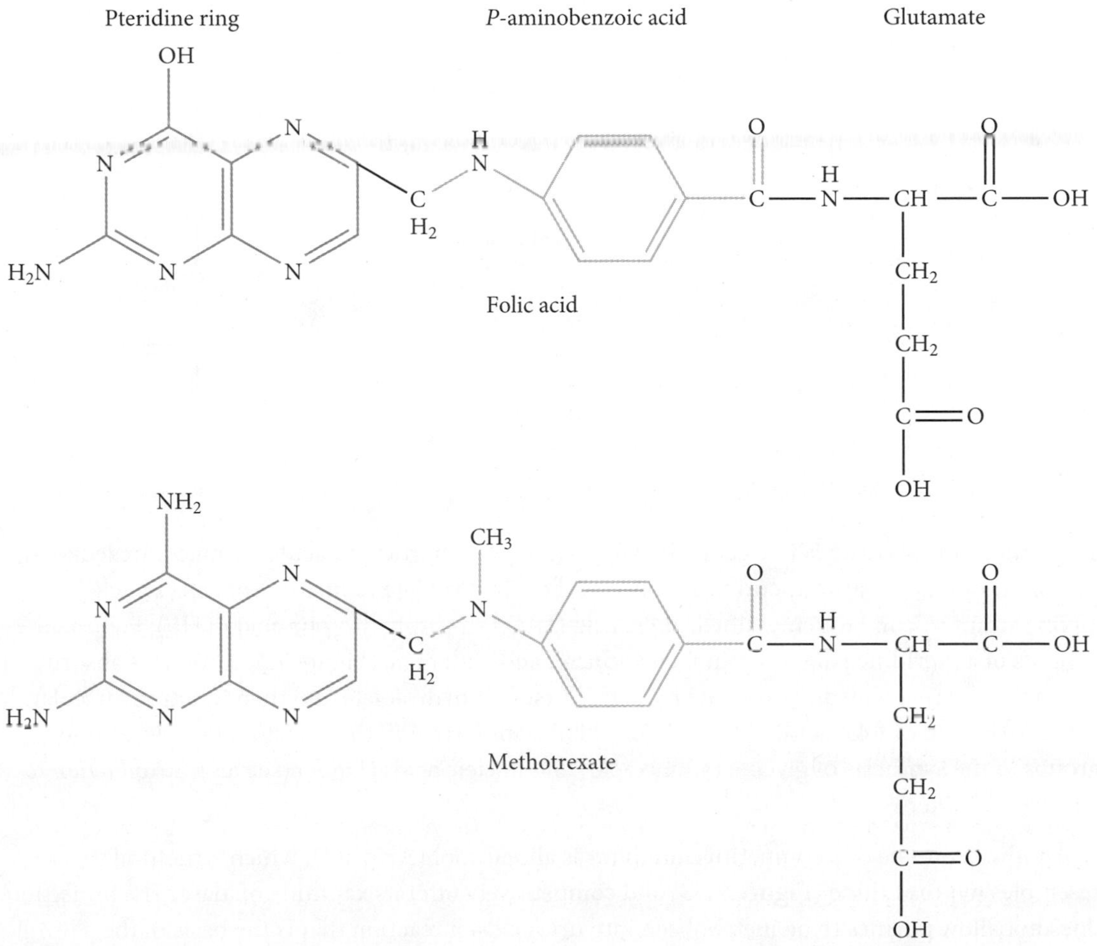

Figure 7.51 Structures of folic acid and methotrexate.

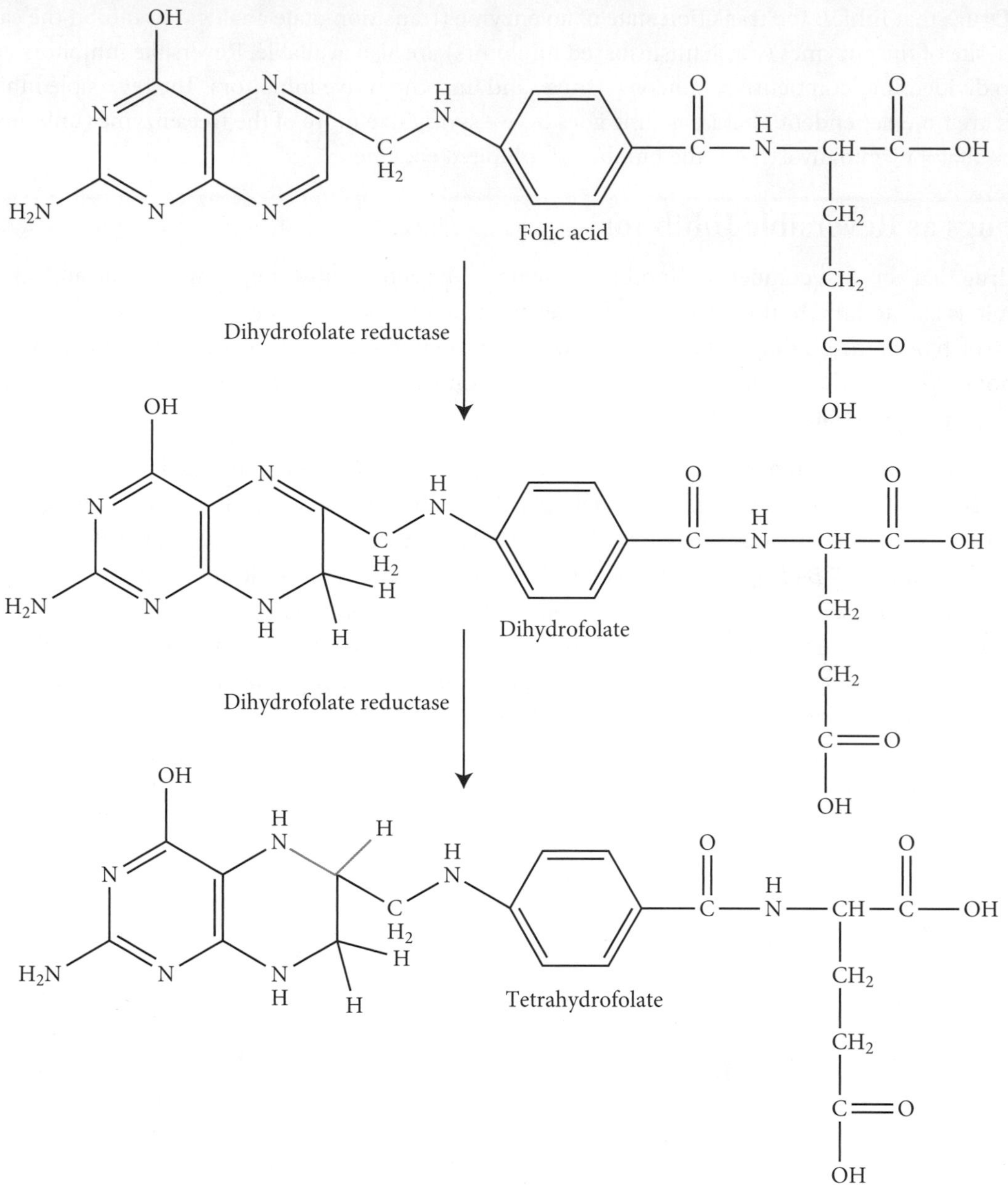

Figure 7.52 Synthesis of folic acid.

applications of this drug is to treat malignant diseases—in particular, acute lymphocytic leuke-mia. Methotrexate is a competitive inhibitor of the dihydrofolate reductase enzyme, which plays an important role in reducing dihydrofolic acid (DHF) to tetrahydrofolic acid (THF). Folic acid consists of a pteridine ring, *P*-aminobenzoic acid, and glutamate (Figure 7.51). After its absorption, folic acid is reduced by dihydrofolate reductase first to dihydrofolate and then to tetrahydrofolate (the active form of folic acid) (**Figure 7.52**). THF is important in the transfer of single carbon groups in the synthesis of glycine (amino acid) and nucleic acids (DNA) (see also *Introduction to Nutrients* chapter).

Another example of a competitive inhibitor is allopurinol (Aloprim), which structurally resembles hypoxanthine (**Figure 7.53**) and competitively inhibits xanthine oxidase. The inhibition does not allow purines to be metabolized into uric acid—a reaction that is the basis of the painful disease known as gout.

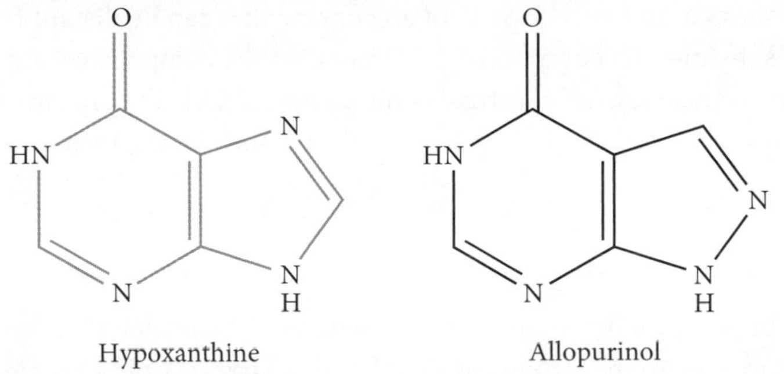

Figure 7.53 Allopurinol resembles hypoxanthine in terms of its structure, which enables it competitively to inhibit the xanthine oxidase enzyme.

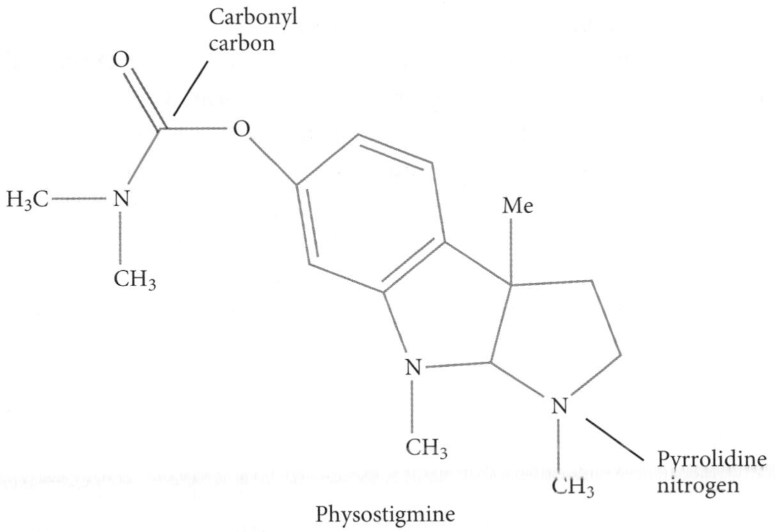

Figure 7.54 Structure of physostigmine, which is a competitive reversible inhibitor of the acetylcholinesterase enzyme.

Adapted from: Patrick GL. *An introduction to medicinal chemistry*, 2nd ed. New York: Oxford University Press; 2001: Chapter 15.

Physostigmine reversibly inhibits the activity of acetylcholinesterase and thereby stops the hydrolysis of the neurotransmitter acetylcholine. Due to its numerous side effects, this drug is often used as an antidote to toxic doses of anticholinergic drugs (i.e., life-threatening disorientation caused by atropine, diphenhydramine, and other anticholinergics). The heteroatom (nitrogen) of pyrrolidine (**Figure 7.54**) serves as a base and is positively charged at the blood's pH. The positively charged nitrogen ion interacts with the negative charge of the acetylcholinesterase enzyme to make an enzyme–substrate complex. However, the main inhibitory effect is derived from a general acid–base catalytic mechanism. Briefly, in general acid–base catalysis, the histidine part of acetylcholinesterase attracts a proton from the hydroxyl group of a serine amino acid of the same enzyme, thereby making the hydroxyl group a strong nucleophile. This nucleophile then attacks the carbonyl carbon of physostigmine (Figure 7.54). The complex formation changes the structure of the enzyme, which finally leads to inactivation of the acetylcholinesterase enzyme.

In noncompetitive inhibition, the inhibitor binds to a site on the enzyme but does not block the binding of the substrate to its active binding site on the enzyme. In other words, the substrate and the inhibitor bind to different sites on the enzyme. Given this behavior, it is difficult to use the structure of the substrate as a designing point to develop a noncompetitive inhibitor. In contrast, uncompetitive inhibitors bind to other parts of an enzyme that can be distant from the active binding site for the substrate. Uncompetitive inhibitors, unlike competitive and noncompetitive inhibitors, bind only to the enzyme–substrate complex and disable the enzyme so that it cannot catalyze its desired reaction. Relatively few therapeutic agents take the form of noncompetitive or uncompetitive inhibitors.

Drugs as Irreversible Inhibitors

An irreversible inhibitor covalently attaches to an enzyme and irreversibly inhibits the catalytic activity of the enzyme. Due to the strong covalent bond, an irreversible enzyme inhibitor can be a toxic molecule, particularly if a new enzyme is not synthesized. Simply put, any inhibitor that permanently changes an amino acid side chain that is important for the catalytic activity of an enzyme can serve as an irreversible enzyme inhibitor.

One example of an irreversible inhibitor class comprises proton pump inhibitors (PPIs) such as omeprazole, lansoprazole, and pantoprazole. Omeprazole (PriLOSEC) and other PPIs are known to inhibit irreversibly the gastric H^+/K^+-ATPase pump, which normally pumps H^+ from the parietal cells into the stomach. Omeprazole, despite its covalent bond to the H^+/K^+-ATPase pump, is not a toxic drug for the parietal cells because of continuing cellular expression of the H^+/K^+-ATPase gene. Thus the effect of omeprazole is determined by the H^+/K^+-ATPase pump's synthesis and inactivation. Consequently, there is no direct relationship between the plasma concentration of omeprazole and its pharmacological effect. In turn, while $t_{1/2}$ for omeprazole is 1 hour, its pharmacological effect lasts at least 24 hours (because it takes 24 hours to express a new H^+/K^+-ATPase, which justifies the "once daily" dose).

Another example of an irreversible inhibitor is acetyl salicylic acid (aspirin). It inhibits the cyclooxygenase enzyme and thereby irreversibly inhibits the synthesis of prostaglandin.

In addition to target enzymes, the synthesis of proteins is a major site of action for many antibiotics. One reason is that the protein synthetic machinery (particularly the structures of ribosomes) is different in eukaryotic and prokaryotic organisms, which renders it a good target to clear many infectious bacteria. Indeed, almost 50% of all available antibiotics attack protein synthesis (translation) of microorganisms (see also the *Introduction to Microbiology* chapter for a list of these antibiotics and their mechanisms).

Drugs Targeting Receptors

This class of drugs mimics the structure of a ligand and thereby either stimulates or blocks specific receptors. Many drugs target receptors, as discussed in the *Introduction to Pharmacology and Pathophysiology* chapter. For instance, sympathomimetic agents that mimic the endogenous adrenergic neurotransmitters are able to interact with and stimulate adrenergic α and β receptors. For example, clonidine is a selective α_2 agonist and salmeterol (Serevent) is a selective β_2-receptor agonist. In contrast, prazosin (Minipress), doxazosin (Cardura), and tamsulosin (Flomax) selectively block α_1 receptors.

Drugs Targeting Carbohydrates

Carbohydrates are central to recognition, adhesion, and signaling processes, particularly in cell–cell interactions. For example, many bacteria and viruses recognize host cells' carbohydrates as a means to infect host cells. In addition, carbohydrates are involved in both cellular and extracellular support and protection. Although developing drugs that can block recognition, adhesion, and signaling processes may prove to be useful, rarely will a drug effectively alter the carbohydrate-related

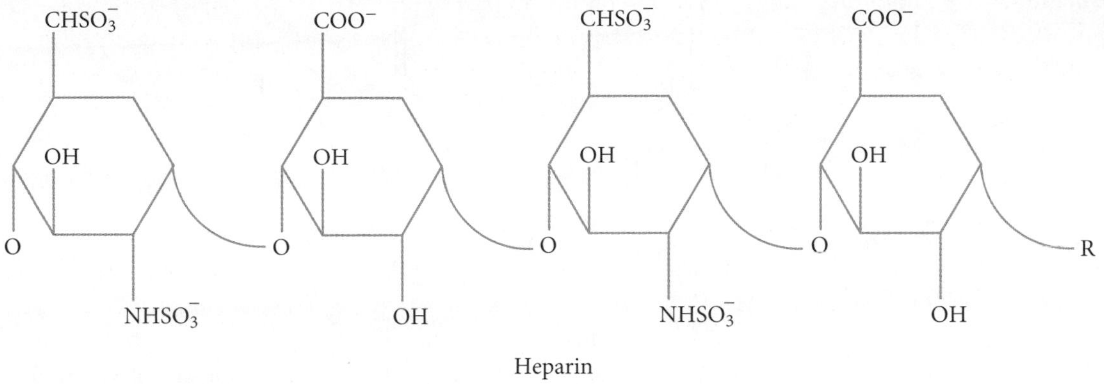

Heparin

Figure 7.55 Structure of heparin. Heparin is a polysaccharide with many negative charges that are important for its anticoagulant effect.

mechanisms. In contrast, carbohydrate-based drugs are already available with a wide range of pharmacological actions. For instance, many antibiotics, such as aminoglycosides and macrolides, contain carbohydrate moieties that are essential for their antibacterial effects.

One notable drug that contains carbohydrate is heparin (Hep-Lock). Heparin is a proteoglycan that has a distinct function in preventing coagulation of the blood by activating antithrombin III. This polysaccharide agent is a highly negatively charged compound. Its four sulfate groups are important to maintain the anticoagulant activity of heparin (**Figure 7.55**). The overall negative charge of heparin results in the drug having a high affinity for antithrombin III.

Drugs that target the bacterial cell wall and protein synthetic machinery are discussed in the *Introduction to Microbiology* chapter.

Drugs Targeting Nucleic Acids

DNA is the cellular target of many carcinogens, radiation, and antitumor drugs that are intended to impair DNA replication and transcription. The drugs that act on nucleic acids are classified as follows: (1) antimetabolites, (2) intercalating drugs, (3) alkylating drugs, (4) anthracyclines, and (5) antisense RNA.

Antimetabolites

As mentioned earlier, antimetabolites structurally resemble endogenous molecules and inhibit the S phase of the cell cycle. For example, methotrexate acts as an antagonist to folic acid; mercaptopurine (Purinethol) acts as an antagonist to purines; and fluorouracil (Adrucil) acts as an antagonist to pyrimidines. Many of the antimetabolites also have immunosuppressant actions. For instance, methotrexate is used to treat active rheumatoid arthritis in adult patients.

The structure of fluorouracil mimics the structure of uracil (which is a pyrimidine base). In the carbon-5 position of uracil, fluorouracil has a fluorine atom (**Figure 7.56**). However, fluorouracil in the cells is metabolized to 5-fluoro-2'-deoxyuridine-5'-monophosphate (5-FdUMP), which inhibits thymidylate synthase enzyme; this action results in a "thymineless death" inhibition of the DNA synthesis. In addition, fluorouracil is metabolized to 5-fluorouridine-5'-triphosphate (FUTP) and inhibits RNA processing and function. Fluorouracil is used to neutralize cancerous cells in the breast, colon, rectum, pancreas, and stomach. A topical dosage form of fluorouracil is also available to treat keratoses (a growth of keratin on the skin that often is caused by exposure of the skin to excessive sunlight).

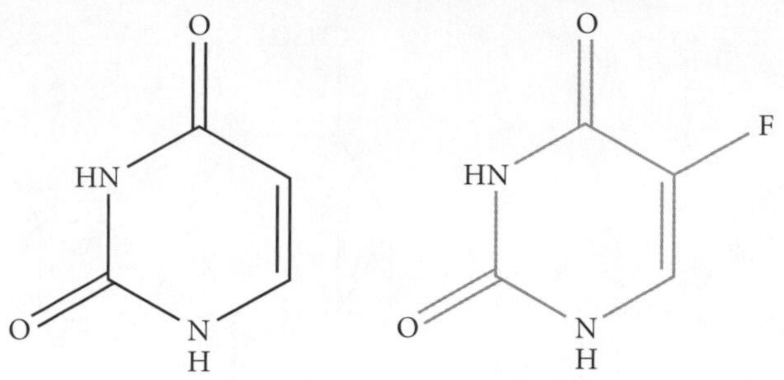

Uracil Fluorouracil

Figure 7.56 Addition of a fluoride atom at carbon number 5 of uracil produces the anticancer drug fluorouracil.

Intercalating Drugs

Many synthetic and naturally occurring drugs in this class are known to intercalate themselves between the bases of DNA through noncovalent (reversible) or covalent (irreversible) bonds. They bind in the minor or major grooves of the DNA duplex. Their binding inhibits both transcription and replication of DNA.

Drugs that serve as intercalating agents should be flat so that they can intercalate between stacked base pairs and, therefore, should have aromatic or heteroaromatic structure. Mitoxantrone (Novantrone) is an intercalating anticancer drug. It is used to treat acute nonlymphocytic leukemias, advanced prostate cancer, and relapsing–remitting multiple sclerosis. The structure of mitoxantrone is shown in **Figure 7.57**.

Alkylating Drugs

Alkylating agents are highly electrophilic drugs that react with nucleophiles (nitrogen 7 and oxygen 6 of guanine are particularly susceptible). Two type of alkylating agents are distinguished:

- Monofunctional agents (one reactive group): These agents cause DNA damage by inducing abnormal base pairing.
- Bifunctional agents (two reactive groups): These agents can form cross-links (a bridge between DNA strands, as in mechlorethamine).

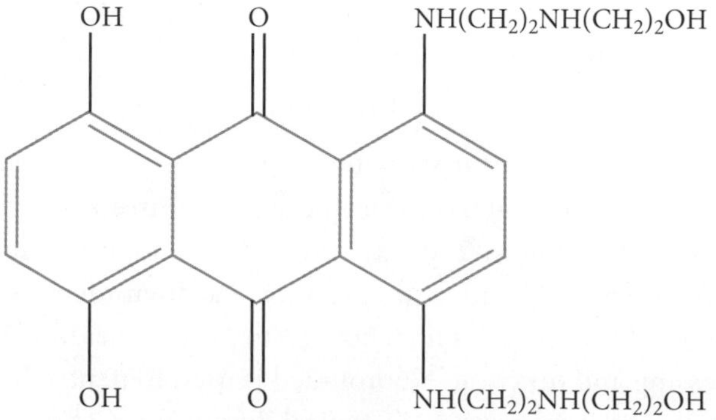

Mitoxantrone

Figure 7.57 The heteroaromatic structure of mitoxantrone makes a flat form so that it can be easily stacked between DNA bases.

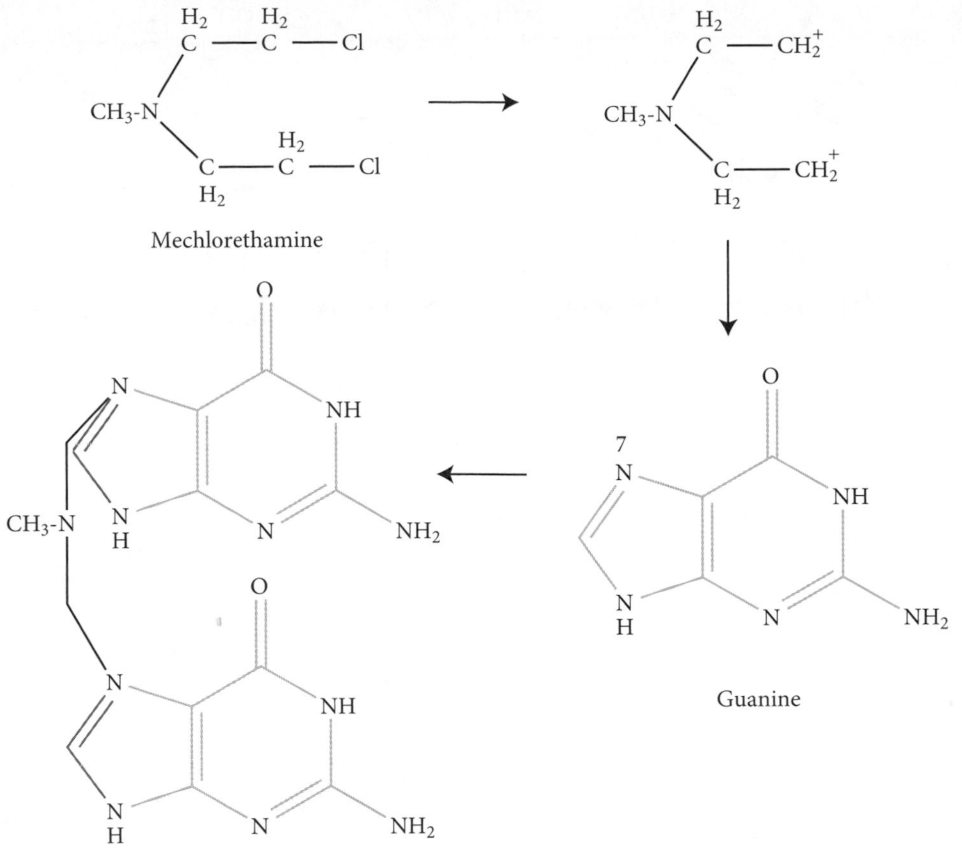

Figure 7.58 Mechlorethamine binds to nitrogen 6 or 7 of guanine and builds a bridge between two parts of the same DNA strand.

Adapted from: Patrick GL. *An introduction to medicinal chemistry*, 2nd ed. New York: Oxford University Press; 2001: Chapter 15.

Mechlorethamine (Mustargen) is a bifunctional alkylating agent that inhibits both the S and G_2 phases of the cell cycle. It inhibits DNA and RNA synthesis by cross-linking strands of nucleic acids (**Figure 7.58**). Mechlorethamine is used to treat Hodgkin's disease and non-Hodgkin's lymphoma.

Anthracyclines (DNA Cutters)

The anthracycline agents are known to inhibit topoisomerase II and generate free radicals, which ultimately result in a DNA strand scission (they are also known as DNA cutters). For instance, similar to mitoxantrone, doxorubicin (Adriamycin) has a flat structure that can intercalate between DNA base pairs (**Figure 7.59**). Doxorubicin is used to treat acute lymphocytic leukemia, Hodgkin's disease, malignant lymphoma, ovarian cancer, and bladder cancer.

Antisense RNA

Development of antisense drugs is a relatively new approach to fighting viral and microbial infections. An antisense RNA is a short (20–30 nucleotides) complementary strand of a small segment of an mRNA. Each antisense drug is designed to bind to a specific sequence of mRNA target, thereby inhibiting the protein synthetic machinery (**Figure 7.60**). An antisense RNA must enter the cells to bind to an mRNA. However, because it is an RNA molecule, it must be protected from the cell's nucleases. To achieve these properties, the antisense fragment must be chemically modified. One way to do so is to attach the antisense RNA to a ligand so that it can be recognized by cell

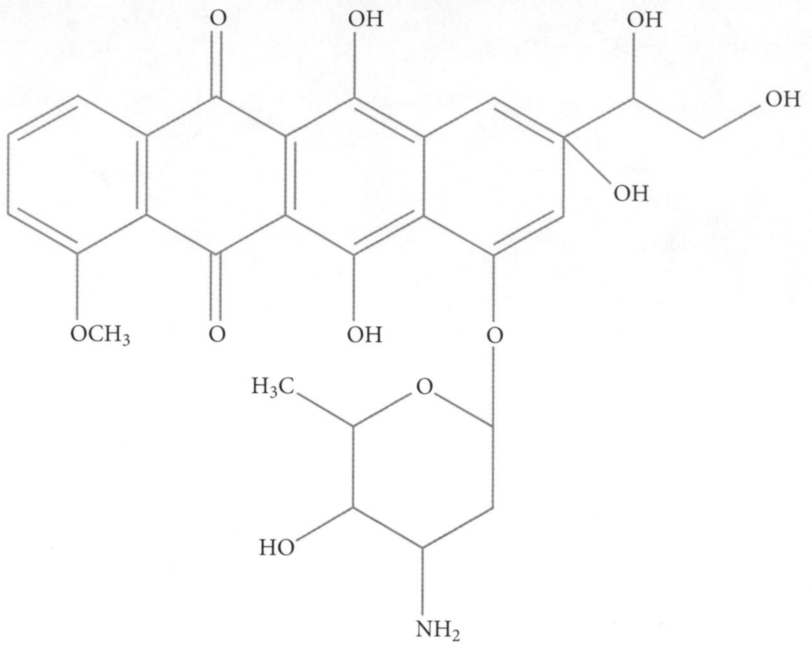

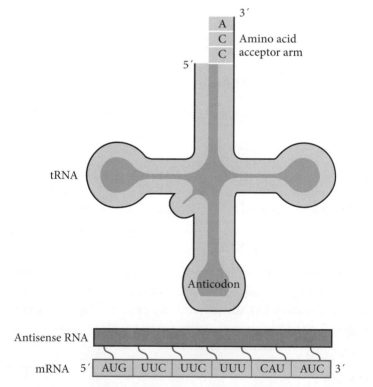

Figure 7.59 Doxorubicin has a flat structure that is able to cut DNA.

Figure 7.60 Binding of an antisense RNA to an mRNA does not allow ribosomes and tRNA to gain access to the nucleotides (codons) in the mRNA.

surface receptors and undergo endocytosis to enter the cells. One example of a synthetic antisense drug is fomivirsen (Vitravene, the first FDA-approved antisense RNA; it is no longer available in the United States). Fomivirsen contains 21 nucleotides and inhibits human cytomegalovirus (HCMV) replication; when available in the U.S. market, it was used to treat HCMV infection in patients with advanced-stage AIDS.

Learning Bridge 7.6

In one of your introductory pharmacy practice experiences, you notice that a 42-year-old female patient is anxiously waiting for her prescriptions to be filled. To assist her, you look at her patient profile and notice that she has two prescriptions: methadone (Dolophine) for chronic pain and diazepam (Valium) for ethanol withdrawal and anxiety management.

A. Do you see any drug interactions between these two agents? Justify your answer.

B. Which counseling points should you offer to this patient in regard to these two agents?

Golden Keys for Pharmacy Students

1. Phase I enzymes are found in the ER; Phase II enzymes are found in the cytosol.

2. Hepatic Phase I and Phase II reactions make drugs more polar. The overall goal is to inactivate the drugs and make them more water soluble so that they can be eliminated by the kidney.

3. The majority of metabolic pathways are catalyzed by specific cellular enzymes that may be found in organelles such as the endoplasmic reticulum (ER), mitochondria, cytosol, lysosomes, or plasma membrane.

4. The majority (90%) of molecular oxygen (O_2) is used in the oxidative phosphorylation pathway. The other 10% is used in a series of metabolic reactions.

5. Phase I enzymes are expert at introducing new functional groups into drugs (or xenobiotics) by oxidation, reduction, and hydrolysis reactions in the smooth endoplasmic reticulum.

6. Cytochrome P450 reductase is a membrane-bound microsomal enzyme that plays a central role in donating electrons to several oxygenase enzymes, including the CYP450 isozymes.

7. A hydrophobic moiety is the only known common structural feature of drugs that are metabolized by CYP450 isozymes.

8. CYP2E is known to metabolize low-molecular-weight hydrophilic drugs; CYP3A4 has a higher affinity for lipophilic drugs; CYP2C9 metabolizes weakly acidic drugs; and CYP2D6 metabolizes basic drugs.

9. The CYP2D6 isozyme is highly polymorphic—120 different alleles have been identified. Approximately 10% of the human population are poor CYP2D6 metabolizers.

10. Drugs with a high hepatic extraction ratio (greater than 0.7) are affected by blood flow. Drugs in this category include morphine (Kadian), meperidine (Demerol), and propranolol (Inderal LA).

11. Drugs with a low extraction ratio (less than 0.2) are not affected by blood flow. Drugs in this category include theophylline (Theo-24), chloramphenicol, and acetaminophen.

12. The only CYP450 isozymes that are inducible are CYP2A, CYP2B, CYP2C, CYP2E, and CYP3A.

13. The most common CYP450 induction is an increase in gene expression through the nuclear receptors. These receptors are significantly involved in the transcription of genes to regulate the expression of CYP subfamilies.

14. Acetaminophen is partially metabolized by CYP2E1 to the toxic metabolite NAPQI; ethanol is known to induce CYP2E1.

15. The inhibition of CYP450 isozymes causes the most common drug–drug interactions.

16. The CYP3A4 isozyme is irreversibly inhibited by grapefruit juice. Thus drugs that are metabolized by CYP3A4 are affected by grapefruit juice.

17. The inhibitory measurement is often expressed in the form of K_i (the inhibition constant) and identifies the concentration of the inhibitor that causes 50% inhibition of the enzyme.

18. Age, sex, and food are all factors that play important roles in the activities of metabolic enzymes during Phase I and Phase II reactions.

19. Acetaminophen's elimination rate is 20% higher in males than in females because of a higher glucuronidation rate in males.

20. Females express CYP3A4 isozyme more effectively in the liver than males do.

21. When two chiral molecules are mirror images of each other (no matter whether they have one or more chiral carbons), they are referred to as enantiomers.

22. If enantiomers rotate a plane of polarized light to the left, they are designated using the L- or (S)- symbol; if they rotate a plane of polarized light to the right, they are designated using the D- or (R)- symbol.

23. Hydrolysis is one of the greatest threats to the stability of drugs.

24. The most important physicochemical property of the hydroxyl group is its ability to form a hydrogen bond.

25. Amino groups have basic property (except a quaternary amino group). As a result, one can find this important functional group on many drug products.

26. Quaternary amines are capable of turning aromatic rings into dipole molecules.

27. Aromatic rings are involved in inducing van der Waals forces because of their flat hydrophobic property.

28. Hydrogenation (reduction mechanism) of aromatic rings leads to a decrease of the binding affinity of a drug to its target.

29. Drugs that contain the alkene functional group are metabolically stable molecules.

30. Ketone groups are commonly found in the structure of many drugs and are readily reduced to alcohol groups.

31. Drugs that act on nucleic acids may be classified as antimetabolites, intercalating drugs, alkylating drugs, anthracyclines, or antisense RNA.

Learning Bridge Answers

7.1 **A.** Prednisolone stimulates the tryptophan dioxygenase enzyme in the liver; this enzyme metabolizes tryptophan to an inactive molecule. Explains to Joe that tryptophan is an amino acid that is important for the synthesis of the neurotransmitter serotonin. A lower concentration of tryptophan means a lower concentration of serotonin, which in turn may result in depression and aggression.

B. First, ask Joe if he has experienced any significant life-changing event. If nothing significant has occurred, the depression problem is likely caused by prednisolone. Depression requires professional help from a healthcare provider, so an OTC product would not be a helpful choice to begin with. However, you should also tell Joe that after the course of prednisolone therapy is finished, his depression may disappear. In addition, tell him that prednisolone interferes with many metabolic pathways and thereby leads to weight gain, a side effect that will disappear when he finishes taking his medication. Finally, ask him to contact his healthcare provider if he still feels depressed 2 weeks after finishing his prednisolone.

7.2 It is critical to tell Amy to avoid alcohol, because acetaminophen is partially metabolized by CYP2E1 to the toxic metabolite NAPQI. Ethanol is known to induce CYP2E1 to produce more NAPQI, which may lead to an increased susceptibility to acetaminophen poisoning. Because Amy is using the maximum allowable dose of acetaminophen (4.0 g), it is likely that she will experience the hepatotoxicity effect of acetaminophen if she continues to consume alcohol. Another option would be to ask her physician to switch her medication to hydrocodone and ibuprofen, 5/200 mg (Vicoprofen), 1 tablet every 6 hours, or to reduce the dose of Vicodin.

7.3 Clopidogrel is a prodrug and a major substrate for the CYP2C19 isozyme, allowing it to be metabolized to an active metabolite form. Omeprazole is a proton pump inhibitor (PPI) and is known moderately to inhibit CYP2C19 isozyme; thus its use means that the plasma level of the active metabolite of clopidogrel may be reduced. The fact that Joe is taking clopidogrel is an indication of some cardiovascular problem, which necessitates that he continue his use of clopidogrel.

You should counsel Joe that there is a possible drug interaction between clopidogrel and omeprazole. There are a few options that you can employ: (1) suggest to his physician to switch omeprazole to ranitidine—another type of acid-lowering agent that does not cause any drug interaction with clopidogrel; or (2) suggest to his physician to switch omeprazole to another PPI that weakly inhibits CYP2C19. Pantoprazole is a weak CYP2C19 inhibitor that is unlikely to cause any significant drug interaction with clopidogrel. In addition, advise Joe to elevate the head of the bed during sleep; to avoid fatty, rich, and spicy foods (orange juice, tomato juice, and coffee have a direct irritant effect on the esophageal mucosa); to avoid smoking; to avoid lying down within 3 hours of eating, and to eat smaller meals. Obesity is associated with GERD, and losing weight can help patients to reduce the symptoms of GERD.

7.4 **A.** Yes, it did. No vitamin is known to interact with atorvastatin. However, St. John's wort is known to induce metabolism of atorvastatin by inducing CYP3A4. This could explain why Joe was not seeing any effect from atorvastatin.

B. Suggest that Joe stop using St. John's wort. When he stops using this supplement, a lower dose of atorvastatin may suffice. As a result, it is important to contact his physician and inform him of your finding and ask him to reduce the dose to the original 10 mg daily for 3 months, as Joe may not need a higher dose of atorvastatin. In addition, ask Joe to seek professional help to deal with his depression rather than taking self-care medications.

7.5 Albuterol is a racemic mixture. The (*R*)-albuterol causes bronchodilation, but the (*S*)-albuterol has no therapeutic effect. There is some controversy regarding whether (*S*)-albuterol may cause some of the adverse effects associated with albuterol. Suggest to the patient's physician that Joe switch from albuterol to levalbuterol (Xopenex) for 3 months (2 puffs every 4 6 hours as needed) to see if the adverse effects will be reduced. Levalbuterol is not a racemic mixture, but rather contains only (*R*)-albuterol; its use may reduce some of the side effects experienced by Joe. However, be aware that levalbuterol is more expensive than albuterol.

7.6 **A.** While there is no direct drug interaction between methadone and diazepam, both are CNS depressants, so there is a risk that their concomitant use will produce additive adverse effects. This is particularly true for methadone, as this agent is a hydrophobic compound that has the potential to accumulate in the adipose tissue. The methadone-storing adipose tissue releases the drug slowly into the circulation. As a result, methadone has a long half-life (8–59 hours, depending on the size of the adipose tissue) during which it remains available in the plasma; this long residence may, in turn, increase its potential for interacting with other agents. In addition, due to its adipose-storing capability, methadone puts patients at higher risk for toxicity. Concurrent use of diazepam with methadone may lead to severe adverse reactions including respiratory depression, drowsiness, hypotension, and sedation.

B. Counsel your patient that taking both of these two agents increases her risk of adverse effects. She should be careful with the number of tablets she takes for both drugs (as methadone is an analgesic agent, there is a risk that the patient may take more when she is in greater pain). The number of pills consumed should not exceed the physician's directions. In addition, because ethanol may increase the CNS depression effects of both methadone and diazepam, the patient should avoid alcohol. Furthermore, advise her to not drink any grapefruit juice, as it may elevate the plasma concentrations of both methadone and diazepam.

Problems and Solutions

Problem 7.1 Which of the following drugs can be metabolized by CYP3A4?

A. Amidarone (Cordarone), which is a hydrophobic drug

B. Amphetamine (Adderall), which is a basic drug

C. Acetyl salicylic acid (aspirin), which is an acidic drug

D. Baclofen (Lioresal), which is a hydrophilic drug

Solution 7.1 A is correct. CYP3A4 is known mostly to metabolize hydrophobic drugs.

Problem 7.2 Amy Johnson is on an anticoagulant drug, warfarin, to prevent blood coagulation. Warfarin is metabolized by the CYP2C9 enzyme. Amy is also taking rifampin, an antibiotic that is known to induce the CYP2C9 enzyme. What effect will concomitant administration of rifampin and warfarin have?

A. Increases the plasma level of warfarin

B. Increases the plasma level of rifampin

C. Reduces the plasma level of warfarin

D. Reduces the plasma level of rifampin

E. Reduces the effect of both drugs

Solution 7.2 C is correct. Warfarin will be metabolized much faster and, as a result, the warfarin dose must be increased to achieve an adequate effect. Keep in mind that when rifampin is discontinued, the amount of warfarin must be reduced as well.

Problem 7.3 A patient upon discharge from a hospital was prescribed warfarin and carbamazepine. However, the patient is advised to stop taking carbamazepine 2 weeks after he has been discharged from the hospital. It is known that carbamazepine induces CYP2C9, which is responsible for warfarin metabolism. Which of the following dose adjustments is needed to avoid any serious hemorrhagic effect?

A. When carbamazepine use is stopped, the dose of warfarin needs to be increased.

B. When carbamazepine use is stopped, the dose of warfarin needs to be decreased.

C. Continue with the same dose of warfarin.

D. When carbamazepine use is stopped, stop taking warfarin as well.

Solution 7.3 B is correct. Warfarin is known to be a major substrate for the CYP2C9 isozyme and, as a result, it is important to reduce the dose of warfarin.

Problem 7.4 A patient is prescribed rifampin as prophylaxis for *Haemophilus influenzae*, 600 mg every day for 4 days. His physician has also prescribed verapamil, 80 mg twice daily for 30 days. You as an intern believe that there may be a drug interaction between these two medications. If there is any drug interaction, what would you tell the physician to avoid any drug interaction?

Solution 7.4 It takes 7 days for an inducible effect from rifampin to verapamil to become evident. As it is important for the patient to take rifampin, it would be wise to ask his physician to wait to prescribe verapamil at least 2 weeks after he takes the last rifampin tablet.

Problem 7.5 Joe Smith smokes 10 cigarettes per day. The CYP2E1 subfamily is known to induce metabolism of tobacco to produce metabolites that are carcinogens. Explain what will happen if Joe also drinks alcohol daily.

A. Ethanol inhibits the activity of CYP2E1, which in turn increases the risk of carcinogenicity.

B. Ethanol reduces the gene expression of CYP2E1, which in turn increases the risk of carcinogenicity.

C. Ethanol increases the activity of CYP2E1, which in turn increases the risk of carcinogenicity.

Solution 7.5 C is correct.

Problem 7.6 Why is it important to separate the two enantiomers in a racemic mixture and test their biological activity?

Solution 7.6 The two enantiomers may produce very different responses. For instance, one could be beneficial and the other could be toxic. In addition, they may compete with each other and exclude or reduce each other's effects.

Problem 7.7 Which of the following molecules has the least α-adrenergic effect? Why?

A. Norepinephrine

B. Epinephrine

C. Norepinephrine with *N*-alkyl group

D. Norepinephrine with no substituent methyl group attached to the nitrogen atom

Solution 7.7 C is correct. While B has a nonselective effect, A has a smaller effect than B. D is the same as B. The nitrogen atom on the norepinephrine molecule plays an important role in the binding of norepinephrine to α receptors. The more alkylated the nitrogen group, the less affinity it has to the α receptors.

Problem 7.8 The drugs carbidopa and levodopa, which may be combined in one tablet (Sinemet), have phenol groups. Carbamazepine has a heterocyclic aromatic structure with no phenol group. Which of these drugs will undergo Phase I reactions? Why?

Solution 7.8 Carbamazepine. During Phase I reactions, hydroxylation of benzene rings occurs. Both carbidopa and levodopa already have phenol groups (or hydroxyl groups attached to their benzene rings), so they are unlikely to add another hydroxyl group during their metabolism.

Problem 7.9 In the late 1950s, thalidomide was used as a sedative to treat nausea in pregnancy. However, while this drug effectively assisted pregnant women in managing their nausea, it caused phocomelia (a birth defect in which limbs are missing) in a few European countries. Explain why thalidomide caused two totally different effects.

Solution 7.9 The sedative action was caused by the (*R*)-enantiomer. However, thalidomide was a racemic mixture, and it was shown that the (*S*)-enantiomer caused the devastating teratogenicity. One of the major problems with thalidomide is that this drug undergoes racemization under physiological conditions. As a result, this drug (which is available in the United States under restricted conditions) should not be used anywhere, under any circumstance, by any woman who is pregnant or plans to become pregnant.

Problem 7.10 Which of the following mechanisms causes insulin detemir to have a long-lasting effect?

A. Addition of a fatty acid to the 29th amino acid, lysine, in the B chain of insulin

B. Addition of a carboxyl group to the 29th amino acid, lysine, in the B chain of insulin

C. Preparation of detemir in an acidic (pH 4.0) solution, which stabilizes the hexamer structure of the insulin molecule

D. Changing the amino acid proline to aspartic acid, which does not allow insulin to self-associate and thus remains in a monomer form

Solution 7.10 A is correct. The fatty acid binds to the serum albumin. Through its self-association and albumin binding, it delays distribution of the active agent to the target tissues, which produces a duration of action of 18–24 hours.

Problem 7.11 Write one disadvantage and one advantage of antisense drugs.

Solution 7.11 Disadvantage: a high amount of antisense RNA is required to bind to all target RNA molecules in the cell. Another one is that an antisense RNA may be prone to be attacked by cellular RNases. Advantage: antisense RNA lacks immunogenicity (i.e., the cell will not be destroyed by the host immune system).

References

1. Abrams Y, Krasowski MD. Pharmacogenomics. In: South-Paul JE, Matheny SC, Lewis EL. *Current diagnosis & treatment in family medicine*, 3th ed. New York, NY: McGraw-Hill; 2011. Available at: http://www.accessmedicine.com/content.aspx?aID=8157174.

2. Bailey DG, Dresser G, Arnold JMA. Grapefruit and medication interactions: forbidden fruit or avoidable consequences? *CMAJ*. November 2012. Available at: DOI:10.1503/cmaj.120951. Copyright © 2012 Canadian Medical Association or its licensors.

3. Bauer LA. Clinical pharmacokinetic and pharmacodynamic concepts. In: Bauer LA, ed. *Applied clinical pharmacokinetics*, 2nd ed. New York, NY: McGraw-Hill; 2008. Available at: http://www.accesspharmacy.com/content.aspx?aID=3517000.

4. Bentley R. Chiral drugs. In: *AccessScience*. New York, NY: McGraw-Hill; 2000. Available at: http://www.accessscience.com.

5. Botham KM, Mayes PA. Biologic oxidation. In: Murray RK, Bender DA, Botham KM, et al. *Harper's illustrated biochemistry*, 28th ed. New York, NY: McGraw-Hill; 2009. Available at: http://www.accessmedicine.com/content.aspx?aID=5226463.

6. Bresnick S. Columbia review: high-yield organic chemistry. Baltimore, MD: Williams and Wilkins; 1996.

7. Cavallari LH, Lam YF. Pharmacogenetics. In: Wells BG, ed. *Pharmacotherapy: a pathophysiologic approach*. 8th ed. New York: McGraw-Hill; 2011. Chapter 9. http://www.accesspharmacy.com /content.aspx?aID=7966967. Accessed November 9, 2013.

8. Calvey TN. Isomerism and anaesthetic drugs. *Acta Anaesthesiol Scand*. 1995;39(106):83–90.

9. Che Y, Xiang Z. Molecular modeling for drug design. In: *AccessScience*, New York, NY: McGraw-Hill; 2008. Available at: http://www.accessscience.com.

10. Correia MA. Drug biotransformation. In: Katzung BG, Masters SB, Trevor AJ. *Basic & clinical pharmacology*, 11th ed. New York, NY: McGraw-Hill; 2009. Available at: http://www .accesspharmacy.com/content.aspx?aID=4515730.

11. Dart RC, Erdman AR, Olson KR, et al. Acetaminophen poisoning: an evidence-based consensus guideline for out-of-hospital management. *Clin Toxicol*. 2006;44:1–18.

12. Dewick PM. *Essentials of organic chemistry*. Hoboken, NJ: John Wiley & Sons; 2006.

13. Eichelbaum M, Gross AS. The genetic polymorphism of debrisoquine/sparteine metabolism: clinical aspects. *Pharmacol Ther*. 1990;46:377–394.

14. Fauci AS, Braunwald E, Kasper DL, et al. Principles of clinical pharmacology. In: Fauci AS, Braunwald E, Kasper DL, et al. *Harrison's principles of internal medicine*, 17th ed. New York, NY: McGraw-Hill; 2009. Available at: http://www.accesspharmacy.com/content.aspx?aID=9092427.

15. Feinstein RA, Miles MV. The effect of acute viral hepatitis on theophylline clearance. *Clin Pediatr*. 1985;24:357–358.

16. Franconi F, Brunelleschi S, Steardo L, Cuomo V. Gender differences in drug responses. *Pharmacol Res*. 2007;55:81–95.

17. Gonzalez FJ, Coughtrie M, Tukey RH. Drug metabolism. In: Brunton LL, Chabner BA, Knollmann BC. *Goodman & Gilman's the pharmacological basis of therapeutics*, 12th ed. New York, NY: McGraw-Hill; 2010. Available at: http://www.accesspharmacy.com/content. aspx?aID=16659426.

18. *Interactive chemistry multimedia courseware: solutions, solubility and precipitation, reaction rates, states of matter, bonding I and II*. Chico, CA: CyberEd; 2001.

19. Lemke TL, Roche VF, Zito SW. *Review of organic functional groups: introduction to medicinal organic chemistry*, 5th ed. Baltimore, MD: Lippincott Williams & Wilkins; 2011.

20. Lemke TL, Williams DA, Roche VF, Zito SW. *Foye's principles of medicinal chemistry*, 7th ed. New York, NY: Wolters Kluwer/Lippincott Williams & Wilkins; 2012.

21. Lin JH. CYP induction-mediated drug interactions: in vitro assessment and clinical implications. *Pharm Res*. 2006;23:1089–1116.

22. Mcguire TR. Multiple myeloma. In: DiPiro JT, Talbert RL, Yee GC, et al. *Pharmacotherapy: a pathophysiologic approach*, 7th ed. New York, NY: McGraw-Hill; 2008. Available at: http://www .accesspharmacy.com/content.aspx?aID=3221142.

23. Murray RK. Metabolism of xenobiotics. In: Murray RK, Bender DA, Botham KM, et al. *Harper's illustrated biochemistry*, 28th ed. New York, NY: McGraw-Hill; 2009. Available at: http://www .accessmedicine.com/content.aspx?aID=5231104.

24. Nahata MC, Taketomo C. Pediatrics. In: DiPiro JT, Talbert RL, Yee GC, et al. *Pharmacotherapy: a pathophysiologic approach*, 7th ed. New York, NY: McGraw-Hill; 2008. Available at: http://www .accesspharmacy.com/content.aspx?aID=3183519.

25. Nelson DL, Cox MM. *Lehninger principles of biochemistry*, 5th ed. New York, NY: W. H. Freeman and Company; 2008.

26. Nogrady T, Weaver DF. *Medicinal chemistry: a molecular and biochemical approach*, 3rd ed. New York, NY: Oxford University Press; 2005.

27. Osterhoudt KC, Penning TM. Drug toxicity and poisoning. In: Brunton LL, Chabner BA, Knollmann BC. *Goodman & Gilman's the pharmacological basis of therapeutics*, 12th ed. New York, NY: McGraw-Hill; 2010. Available at: http://www.accesspharmacy.com/content.aspx?aID=16658740.

28. Ouellette RJ. *Introduction to general, organic and biological chemistry*, 4th ed. Upper Saddle River, NJ: Prentice-Hall; 1997.

29. Patrick GL. *An introduction to medicinal chemistry*, 2nd ed. New York, NY: Oxford University Press; 2001.

30. Relling MV, Giacomini KM. Pharmacogenetics. In: Brunton LL, Chabner BA, Knollmann BC. *Goodman & Gilman's the pharmacological basis of therapeutics*, 12th ed. New York, NY: McGraw-Hill; 2010. Available at: http://www.accesspharmacy.com/content.aspx?aID=16659580.

31. Remington. *The science and practice of pharmacy*, 21st ed. Baltimore, MD: Lippincott Williams & Wilkins; 2005.

32. Rodwell VW. Catabolism of the carbon skeletons of amino acids. In: Murray RK, Bender DA, Botham KM, et al. *Harper's illustrated biochemistry*, 28th ed. New York, NY: McGraw-Hill; 2009. Available at: http://www.accessmedicine.com/content.aspx?aID=5227764.

33. Shargel L, Mutnick AH, Souney PF, Swanson LN. *Comprehensive pharmacy review*, 7th ed. Philadelphia, PA: Lippincott William & Wilkins; 2009.

34. Shargel L, Wu-Pong S, Yu AB. Pharmacogenetics. In: Shargel L, Wu-Pong S, Yu AB. *Applied biopharmaceutics & pharmacokinetics*, 5th ed. New York, NY: McGraw-Hill; 2005. Available at: http://www.accesspharmacy.com/content.aspx?aID=2481039.

35. Stamer UM, Lehnen K, Hothker F, et al. Impact of CYP2D6 genotype on postoperative tramadol analgesia. *Pain.* 2003;105:231–238.

36. Thomas G. *Fundamentals of medicinal chemistry*. London, UK: John Wiley & Sons; 2004.

37. Trevor AJ, Katzung BG, Masters SB. Cancer chemotherapy. In: Trevor AJ, Katzung BG, Masters SB. *Pharmacology: examination & board review*, 9th ed. New York, NY: McGraw-Hill; 2010. Available at: http://www.accesspharmacy.com/content.aspx?aID=6547085.

38. Trevor AJ, Katzung BG, Masters SB. Introduction. In: Trevor AJ, Katzung BG, Masters SB. *Pharmacology: examination & board review*, 9th ed. New York, NY: McGraw-Hill; 2010. Available at: http://www.accesspharmacy.com/content.aspx?aID=6543001; 2010.

39. UpToDate. Waltham, MA: 2012. Available at: http://www.uptodate.com/online with subscription.

40. Waxman DJ, Holloway MG. Sex differences in the expression of hepatic drug metabolizing enzymes. *Mol Pharmacol.* 2009;76:215–228.

41. Wermuth CG, Ganellin CR, Lindberg P, Mitscher LA. Glossary of terms used in medicinal chemistry (IUPAC Recommendations 1998). *Pure Applied Chem.* 1998;70(5):1129–1143.

42. Yu AB, Shargel L, Wu-Pong S. Hepatic elimination of drugs. In: Shargel L, Wu-Pong S, Yu AB. *Applied biopharmaceutics & pharmacokinetics*, 5th ed. New York, NY: McGraw-Hill; 2005. Available at: http://www.accesspharmacy.com/content.aspx?aID=2480547.

Introduction to Pharmaceutics

Reza Karimi
Susan M. Stein

OBJECTIVES

1. Understand the role of regulatory requirements in bringing a drug product to the market.

2. Comprehend basic physical pharmacy by learning the roles of physicochemical properties of drugs in designing dosage forms and drug absorption.

3. Describe different dosage forms, their characteristics, and the potential routes of drug delivery with these dosage forms.

4. Appreciate the use of drug substitution as implemented with the codes in the "Orange Book."

5. Gain basic knowledge about reaction rates and different reaction orders to understand the concepts of shelf life and half-life in the context of the drug degradation process.

6. Implement a series of Learning Bridge assignments at your experiential sites to bridge your didactic learning with your experiential experiences.

KEY TERMS AND DEFINITIONS

1. **Amorphous:** drugs in the solid state lacking a defined shape and form.

2. **Bioequivalence:** when a generic product has the same rate and extent of drug absorption (i.e., bioavailability) as the innovator product.

3. **Colligative properties:** properties of a solution that depend on the number of species in solution rather than on the chemical identity of the solute.

4. **Colloids:** a dispersion of two immiscible phases.

5. **Compound:** a combination of two or more substances, ingredients, or elements.

6. **Dissolution rate:** the rate at which a solid solute dissolves in a solvent.

7. **Dosage form:** the combination of a drug and any excipients used in a drug delivery system.

8. **Emulsion:** a liquid dispersed in an immiscible liquid.

9. **FDA:** U.S. Food and Drug Administration.

10. **First-order reaction:** a reaction for which the rate is directly proportional to the concentration of one of the reactants.

11. **Hydrophilic:** water-loving.

12. **Hydrophobic:** water-fearing.

13. **Hypertonic solution:** a solution that has a higher osmotic pressure than biological fluids.

14. **Hypotonic solution:** a solution that has a lower osmotic pressure than biological fluids.

15. **IND:** investigational new drug.

(continues)

16. **Interfacial tension:** a situation in which the intermolecular forces in two immiscible liquids cause their interface to resist expansion, which in turn brings a tension to the interface.

17. **Isotonic solution:** a solution that has the same osmotic pressure as erythrocytes.

18. **Modified-release dosage form:** any solid dosage form that has been designed to release a drug in a predetermined manner.

19. **Molecular dispersion:** a true solution; a homogeneous one-phase system.

20. **NDA:** new drug application.

21. **Orange Book:** a reference document that indicates drug products approved by the FDA based on safety and effectiveness.

22. **Partition coefficient:** the distribution of a drug molecule between organic and aqueous phases.

23. **Permeability constant:** the flux of molecules across a biological membrane.

24. **Pharmaceutics:** the study of dosage form design.

25. **Polymorphism:** the existence of multiple crystalline forms of the same drug.

26. **Rate law:** the mathematical description of the rate of a chemical reaction.

27. **Reaction rate:** the amount of change in reactants per unit time.

28. **Rheology:** the science that describes the flow of fluids (even solids and semisolids).

29. **Semisolid dosage form:** a dosage form that is not considered a solid or liquid dosage form and is often intended for topical use.

30. **Solute:** a compound or substance dissolved in another substance (typically a solvent).

31. **Solvent:** a substance (typically a solution) that is capable of dissolving a solute.

32. **Surface tension:** the force of the cohesiveness between liquid molecules when they come in contact with air.

33. **Surfactants:** the resistance of a liquid to spread out and expand its surface area when it is in contact with air.

34. **Suspension:** a solid dispersed in an immiscible liquid.

35. **Viscosity:** the resistance of a liquid to flow.

36. **Zero-order reaction:** a reaction in which the rate is independent of the concentrations of the reactants.

Introduction

Pharmaceutics is a basic science that closely studies the physiochemical properties of the active and inactive molecules that exist in a drug formulation. These physiochemical properties include stability or degradation, ionization, salt formation, and water solubility. In addition, pharmaceutics studies how a drug's various dosage forms, such as capsules, tablets, and suppositories, are formulated to not only maintain the integrity of their contents but also produce a desirable effect upon release of those contents. Biopharmaceutics is a basic science that combines pharmaceutics with factors such as the route of administration and the rate of drug release from a dosage form, studying how these factors affect a biological response upon administration of the dosage form. As a result, biopharmaceutics is concerned with (1) the physicochemical stability of the active and inactive ingredients within a drug product, (2) the route of administration, (3) the release of the drug from the dosage form, (4) the rate of disintegration and dissolution, and (5) the systemic absorption of the drug.

In this chapter we begin by examining the drug development process and the different phases involved in a clinical trial during the drug development process. To introduce basic elements of physical pharmacy, the important roles of states of matter, vapor pressure, and colligative properties are emphasized. In addition, the paramount roles that solutions and solids play in pharmaceutics and biopharmaceutics are addressed. Factors affecting solids, such as dissolution rate and diffusion coefficient, and factors affecting solutions, such as rheology, viscosity, and osmolarity, are described. Different solid and semisolid dosage forms and the roles of different pharmaceutical solutions are emphasized. Drug delivery systems form the cornerstone of biopharmaceutics and are briefly described in this chapter as well. Finally, we consider the important roles that drug degradation and reaction orders play in the shelf life of drugs.

Physical and Chemical Principles in Pharmaceutics

Physical properties are properties of an element or molecule that can be observed without the molecule undergoing any sort of chemical change—for example, boiling point, melting point, and color. For instance, a nitroglycerin molecule melts at 13°C, while a glucose molecule melts at 150°C. Chemical properties of an element or compound, in contrast to physical properties, are observed only with a chemical change of the substance. A nitroglycerin molecule is made of glycerin and nitric acid, which explains why nitroglycerin is prone to hydrolysis. For example, hydrolysis of nitroglycerin (because of its three-ester bond; **Figure 8.1**) is a chemical property of this molecule. Another example of a chemical property is the weak intermolecular interaction that occurs between nitroglycerin molecules, which explains why nitroglycerin tablets are volatile. As a result, such tablets must be stored in a tightly closed glass container. To increase the stability of nitroglycerin tablets, cotton or paper, as a filler, should not be added to the glass container. In addition, patients should avoid unnecessary and frequent opening and closing of the container to avoid a loss of the nitroglycerin ingredient from tablets.

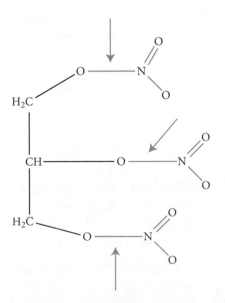

Figure 8.1 The chemical structure of a nitroglycerin molecule. The areas that are prone to hydrolysis are shown by arrows.

There are three general routes of drug administration: enteral (oral, rectal, sublingual), parenteral (intravascular [IV], intramuscular [IM], subcutaneous [SC or SQ]), and other (topical, inhalation, intranasal, transdermal). These administration routes are discussed in more detail in this chapter.

Throughout this chapter, you will encounter the names of many active and inactive ingredients. Simply put, an active ingredient is the drug substance that produces a pharmacological action. The active ingredient is rarely administered alone, but rather is typically mixed with inactive ingredients (often referred to as excipients) in a drug formulation. Excipients have many pharmaceutical roles, such as thickening, suspending, diluting, emulsifying, coloring, flavoring, and preserving agents. Some of these excipients are discussed further in this chapter. Before considering physical pharmacy and its role in drug formulation, let's briefly discuss the process of a drug development.

Drug Development

Specific steps are completed to ensure that a safe and effective drug is developed to achieve a desired therapeutic outcome. Many factors play crucial roles in the development of a drug, such as physicochemical properties of the active and inactive ingredients, effectiveness and safety of the ingredients, appropriate dosage forms, and route of administration. The drug development process is also influenced by the targeted populations and disease states that the drug is intended to treat.

In addition, physiological factors need to be addressed when developing a drug, from when a patient takes the drug to when the drug reaches its site of action. Engagement with the administration route (e.g., oral, intravenous, subcutaneous, transdermal, rectal) is the first physiological event that occurs upon administering a drug to the body. Subsequently, the drug is released from its dosage form. The physicochemical properties of the active and inactive ingredients play very important roles in determining both of these steps. In the steps that follow the release of a drug, the absorption and elimination of the drug determine the therapeutic effect. Therefore, physiological factors such as the patient's age and disease state, body mass, volume of distribution, absorption, and elimination rates play important roles as well. These physiological factors are addressed in the *Introduction to Pharmacodynamics* and *Introduction to Pharmacokinetics* chapters.

Pharmaceutical scientists or investigators carry out both *in vitro* and *in vivo* experiments during the development of a drug. *In vitro* studies (think of a lab environment) are used to investigate physiochemical properties, stability of drugs, and large-scale production of the drug. Conversely, *in vivo* studies (think of a live environment) are used to study how well animals and human subjects respond to experiments that have been carefully and ethically designed by scientists and drug investigators.

Specific stages and phases of the drug development process must be successful for the drug to receive a full review and approval from the U.S. Food and Drug Administration (FDA). Preclinical research generally involves *in vitro* lab testing and *in vivo* animal testing. When a drug is ready to be studied in humans, an investigational new drug (IND) application is submitted to the FDA. The IND application should include the following elements: (1) information about the source of the drug, (2) chemical properties and manufacturing information, (3) all available data from animals (i.e., *in vivo* studies), (4) proposed clinical plans and protocols, (5) a list of physicians who will carry out the clinical trials, and (6) an approval from the FDA review board and the investigator's home institutional review board (IRB). The IRB is responsible for reviewing the planned *in vivo* studies from an ethical standpoint. Both review boards should include experienced members who are both scientists and nonscientists, and who are mandated to evaluate any potential harm to the human subjects from the proposed clinical trial.

Clinical trials proceed through a series of phases. It is critical that in the first three phases, participants (who may be either healthy individuals or patients) are informed of the investigational status of the drug and any possible side effects that may be caused by the study. In addition, these individuals (healthy or ill, targeted population) must be informed that they can decline participation at any time during the course of the study. These strict regulations (based on the ethical principles set forth in the *Declaration of Helsinki*) are intended to protect the individuals who are subjects of the study.

Phase I Study

Phase I is designed to establish the dosing parameters of the drug. In this phase, which takes place promptly after the IND submission, the compound is administered to a small number (20–100) of healthy individuals to establish the maximum tolerated dose that does not produce severe toxicity.

In addition, drug absorption, half-life ($t_{1/2}$) of the drug in the plasma, and drug metabolism are often assessed in this phase. This clinical study phase is conducted in research centers by clinical pharmacologists. Although rare, it may be necessary to include patients in this phase as well. For example, if the drug displays a high toxicity profile, such as is often the case with cancer treatment, volunteer patients in that targeted population—rather than healthy individuals—are more appropriate and practical to include in this phase.

Phase I studies may be designed to include blinded (i.e., to avoid any biases by investigators and the human subjects, both the investigators and the human subjects do not know which drug is being administered to which subjects), nonblinded (both the investigators and the human subjects know which drug is being given), and/or placebo (healthy controlled) cohorts. The study design is based on factors such as properties of the drug, the targeted disease state, goals of investigators, and ethical considerations.

Phase II Study

During Phase II, a small population (100–200 individuals) with the targeted disease state is studied to measure the drug's therapeutic index (see the *Introduction to Pharmacodynamics* chapter), a broader range of toxicities (see the *Introduction to Toxicology* chapter), and drug formulation. The dosing regimen is selected to produce the desirable therapeutic result. In this phase, investigators may use a single-blind study design that includes a placebo medication and an established active drug (i.e., positive control) in addition to the study drug. These clinical trials are often implemented in hospitals associated with universities. Due to unsuccessful outcomes, a significant number of investigated drugs do not progress beyond Phase II. In fact, only 25% of investigated drugs progress to the next phase (Phase III).

Phase III Study

In Phase III, a much larger patient population (about 1,000 patients) is studied to confirm the drug's efficacy and side effects. Double-blind studies are often conducted in Phase III to minimize errors due to placebo effect. A Phase III clinical trial is an expensive study: a larger patient population is involved, including multiple study sites, and many specialists are involved with the study. Submission of a new drug application (NDA) to the FDA occurs after Phase III is complete.

Despite a study population size of 1,000 patients, the data from Phase III may not reveal adequate safety information. Some specific side effects may emerge only during the postmarketing period. Consequently, postmarketing analysis is as essential as premarketing analysis to confirm and complete the safety profile of the drug that has been developed during Phase III.

Phase IV Study

In Phase IV, the scale-up of batch size and the drug formulation may slightly be modified. It is also hoped that any additional side effects will be detected in this phase. While the Phase IV requirements are not as strict as those governing the previous three phases, manufacturers are required to report to the FDA any new side effects that are noticed during Phase IV.

Patent Application

While a drug is being tested on animals, a patent application is submitted to protect the compound from being synthesized by other pharmaceutical companies or investigators for a period of 20 years (i.e., 20 years from the patent approval date). After 20 years, any company or investigator may apply to the FDA for permission to make a similar drug (generic) with the same requirements for content, purity, and bioavailability as the brand-name drug. Indeed, upon expiration of the patent time frame, many manufacturers of the brand-name drugs will apply to the FDA for permission to produce generic-name drugs of their own brand-name drugs. As pharmacy students and pharmacists, it is prudent to learn about the concept of generic drugs and their impact on patient care outcomes.

Generic Drugs

The FDA requires any company that proposes to manufacture a generic drug to provide evidence that the proposed generic drug has the same active ingredient, strength, dosage form, and route of administration as the brand-name drug. However, it is not necessary for the generic drug to contain inactive ingredients identical to those found in the brand-name drug. Despite a rigorous investigation from the FDA and a thorough and evidence-based data analysis from the investigators, there is still concern among patients (and to a lesser extent among healthcare providers) that generic drugs may be less effective than the brand-name drugs from which they are derived. In a systematic review and meta-analysis study conducted by Kesselheim et al., 38 published clinical trials were analyzed to compare the clinical efficacy of generic drugs with that of their corresponding brand-name drugs in the cardiovascular disease realm. The study revealed that the generic drugs were as effective as the brand-name drugs.

The FDA describes a generic drug as "identical, or bioequivalent to a brand name drug in dosage form, safety, strength, route of administration, quality, performance characteristics and intended use. Although generic drugs are chemically identical to their branded counterparts, they are typically sold at substantial discounts from the branded price."

As noted by the FDA, one of the most attractive aspects of generic drugs is their lower cost compared with the brand-name drugs. The FDA has estimated that the cost of a generic drug's production is 80% to 85% lower than the brand-name drug's production. As a result, a generic manufacturer is able to sell its product at a lower price, which in turn results in a lower cost for patients.

Three equivalencies play important roles in establishing how a generic drug is assessed:

1. Pharmaceutical equivalent: These drugs have the same active ingredient, chemical form, dosage form, route of administration, strength and concentration, and salt forms as the corresponding brand-name drugs.

2. Therapeutic equivalent: These pharmaceutical equivalents have the same therapeutic effect and safety as the corresponding brand-name drugs.

3. Bioequivalent: These pharmaceutical equivalents have a similar rate and extent of absorption in reaching the systemic circulation (bioavailability) as the corresponding brand-name drugs.

Two drugs that are bioequivalent may not necessarily be therapeutically equivalent. An example of drugs that pharmaceutical equivalence, therapeutic equivalence, and bioequivalence is the cholesterol-reducing agent simvastatin (generic) and Zocor (brand) in 10 mg tablet form.

In addition to the above equivalencies, there is also a term called biosimilar, which is related to biological products. Biological products are purified from human and/or animal materials and include vaccines, blood and blood components, enzymes, and antibodies. Biological products are regulated differently by the FDA, and most of them are licensed under the Public Health Service Act (PHS Act). A biosimilar is a drug product that is similar to a licensed biological product and has demonstrated similarity in physicochemical and biological characteristics, safety, purity, and potency.

The reference *FDA Approved Drug Products with Therapeutic Equivalence Evaluations*, also known as the "Orange Book," lists FDA-approved drugs and their comparative equivalency status. The Orange Book and its monthly supplements are available at www.fda.gov/cder/ob. Every state in the United States has enacted a generic substitution law that allows pharmacists to substitute a generic drug for the corresponding prescribed brand-name drug, albeit under specific restrictions. It is the responsibility of pharmacists to make sure that the generic drug is pharmaceutically equivalent and has similar bioavailability to the brand-name drug. Therefore, the Orange Book is a practical tool to select an appropriate generic drug for a patient. Note, however, that the Orange Book does not include drugs approved by the FDA prior to 1938 (known as the "grandfather clause").

The Orange Book uses a two-letter coding system. The first letter is either A or B. If a product's code has the first letter A, it means the product is pharmaceutically and therapeutically equivalent to the brand-name drug product with the same bioavailability. Conversely, if a product's code has the first letter B, it means the product is not therapeutically equivalent or the product has inadequate quality standards compared to the brand-name drug product. In some states, pharmacists cannot substitute a tablet dosage form for a capsule dosage form even if the Orange Book identifies them as being therapeutically equivalent. The B letter could also mean that the product is under FDA review and a final decision has not yet been made regarding FDA approval. In any case, pharmacists should not select a product that has the first letter B in their Orange Book code as a substitute for the brand-name product. The second letter in the code indicates the dosage form or the nature of the product. **Table 8.1** explains the coding system and corresponding indications established by the FDA.

An abbreviated new drug application (ANDA) must be submitted to the FDA to approve a new generic drug. As part of this approval process, healthy humans must participate in bioequivalence studies for generic drug development (i.e., similar to a Phase I clinical trial). Investigators submit

Table 8.1 FDA's Coding System of Drugs for Drug Substitutions

Two-Letter Code	Description
AA	Drugs that are available in conventional dosage forms and are therapeutically equivalent.
AB	Drugs that have had therapeutic equivalency problems but now are therapeutically equivalent.
AN	Solutions and powders that are used for aerosolization and are therapeutically equivalent.
AO	Injectable oil solutions that are therapeutically equivalent.
AP	Injectable aqueous solutions that are therapeutically equivalent.
AT	Topical drugs that are therapeutically equivalent, assuming they have the same dosage forms.
BC	Extended-release drugs that are not therapeutically equivalent.
BD	Active ingredients that are not therapeutically equivalent.
BE	Delayed-release drugs that are not therapeutically equivalent.
BT	Topical drugs that are not therapeutically equivalent.
BX	Drugs that are likely to lose their FDA approval.
B*	Drugs for which there is serious concern about their therapeutic equivalency that needs to be resolved.

Adapted from: Abood R. *Pharmacy practice and law*, 6th ed. Sudbury, MA: Jones & Bartlett; 2011: Chapter 3.

the ANDA to FDA's Center for Drug Evaluation and Research for its review and a decision about the generic drug. Because the animal studies (Phase I) and patient studies (Phases II and III) were conducted and documented as part of the original drug's development, it is not necessary to duplicate these studies or include their results for the ANDA.

If a pharmaceutical company desires to develop a new dosage form, such as an extended-release form in addition to the already marketed immediate-release form, the new therapeutic indication requires an NDA that is subject to the same rigorous requirements as the NDA submitted for the original brand-name drug.

Rigorous compliance with regulated practices is of paramount importance to meet the FDA's requirements for manufacturing or compounding and to minimize the risk of contamination, adulteration, or misbranding of the compound. The Good Manufacturing Practice (GMP) standards have been established to ensure that manufacturers maintain an adequate and feasible level of infrastructure, equipment, and raw materials to produce a compound. Additional standards must be met regarding documentation and labeling to avoid any issue concerning the efficacy and safety of a compound. In other words, the GMP standards are quality standards that designate minimum requirements in manufacturing, processing, or packaging processes. They include both quality control (QC) and quality assurance (QA) considerations. QC tests the product and confirms that solid dosage forms have been subjected to dissolution study. This process also confirms that raw materials, packaging materials, drug products, and storage containers are not contaminated with microorganisms or other chemicals, and that the environmental systems (e.g., water system, heating system) meet expectations. QA confirms that the facility and its written policies, procedures, and protocols are adequate and effective.

Learning Bridge 8.1

On a Monday morning, a patient comes to your pharmacy with two prescriptions to be filled:

Prescription #1

Verapamil (from Abbot), 120 mg

Sig: one tablet (120 mg) by mouth once daily

Disp: 60 tablets

Refills: 1

Prescription #2

Phenytoin (from Alpharma), 125 mg/5 mL oral suspension

Sig: 5 mL by mouth once daily

Disp: 100 mL

Refills: 2

A. You do not have either of these drugs available in your store. Your preceptor advises you to look up the drugs in the Orange Book and find alternatives for them. Suppose you find **Table 8.2** in the Orange Book.

Table 8.2 Different Drugs with Different "Two-Letter Codes"

Number	Two-Letter Code	Active Ingredient	Dosage Form	Strength	Applicant
I	AB	Diltiazem	Tablet	120 mg	WestCoast Pharm
II	BC	Diltiazem	Tablet; extended release	120 mg	WestCoast Pharm
III	AB	Diltiazem	Tablet	120 mg	Oregon BioPharm
IV	AB	Phenytoin	Oral suspension	125 mg	WestCoast BioPharm
V	AP	Phenytoin	Injection	125 mg	Oregon BioPharm

Select generic drugs that are therapeutically equivalent to the brand-name drugs specified in the patient's prescriptions.

B. Suppose you selected two drugs from Table 8.2 to substitute the prescription drugs. Which of the factor(s) listed here influenced your selection for substitution? Why?

1. Efficacy

2. Bioavailability

3. Safety

4. Reaching the liver at the same rate

5. Reaching the stomach at the same rate

6. Reaching the systemic circulation at the same rate

Intramolecular and Intermolecular Forces

Intramolecular and intermolecular forces play important roles in the design of new drugs and their formulations, preparations, and stability. Intramolecular forces hold atoms together to build a molecule. Returning to our nitroglycerin example, a nitroglycerin molecule exists because of intramolecular forces between carbon, hydrogen, and nitrogen atoms. Intermolecular forces are forces that exist between molecules that define how molecules interact. For example, two nitroglycerin molecules bind to each other because of weak intermolecular forces (in this case van der Waals forces; see the *Introduction to Biological Chemistry* chapter). While the intramolecular forces explain the stability of a molecule, the intermolecular forces explain boiling points, melting point, and solubility of a molecule. The intramolecular forces consist of covalent bonds, ionic bonds, and metallic bonds; the intermolecular forces include ion-dipole bonds, hydrogen bonds, and van der Waals forces (**Figure 8.2**).

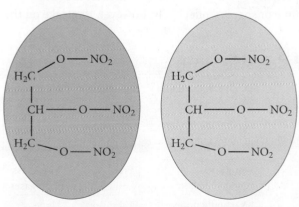

Figure 8.2 Van der Waals forces explain the intermolecular interaction between two nitroglycerin molecules.

Intermolecular forces are much weaker than intramolecular forces, so it requires much less energy to overcome an intermolecular force. For instance, it requires 46 kJ of energy to break the hydrogen bonding (intermolecular force) of 1 mole of water to vaporize water. By comparison, it requires 930 kJ of energy to break the covalent bond between O—H (intramolecular force) in 1 mole of water.

States of Matter

Everything that exists around you consists of matter. Matter is anything that has mass and is able to occupy a space. Matter exists in one of three states:

- Gas. The oxygen that you inhale or the carbon dioxide that you exhale is gaseous matter.
- Liquid. A glass of water you drink is liquid matter.
- Solid. The pen you use to write is solid matter.

Each state of matter has its own unique characteristics. The potential energy (see the *Introduction to Biochemistry* chapter) of a state of matter increases when a solid changes to a liquid or when a liquid changes to a gas state. A colloidal system is built when one of these states of matter is finely dispersed in another state of matter.

Before discussing each state of matter, let's examine a theory in physical pharmacy known as kinetic molecular theory. This theory states that:

1. All matter is made up of extremely tiny particles (i.e., ions, atoms, or molecules) that have kinetic energy and, as a result, are in continuous motion. In a solid, the motion of the particles consists of vibration and rotation; in a liquid or a gas, the particles not only vibrate and rotate but also can freely pass by each other.

2. As the temperature of matter increases, the rate of particles' movement in that substance increases as well.

3. The collisions that occur between particles are elastic. In other words, the particles do not lose energy when they collide with each other, but rather exchange energy; therefore, their total kinetic energy remains constant.

Table 8.3 indicates a few physical characteristics for the states of matter.

Gases

Due to the large space that exists between gas particles and the fact that gas particles move extremely fast, gases do not have a defined volume or shape. Collectively, however, they take on the

Table 8.3 Physical Characteristics of States of Matter

State of Matter	Volume	Density (Mass/Volume)	Compressibility	Motion	Pressure
Gas	Conforms to the shape of the container it occupies	Very low	High	Very free	High
Liquid	Has definite shape and form	High	Slightly	Free	Much less than gases
Solid	Has definite shape and form	High	Virtually none	Vibration and rotation	None

shape of the container they occupy (for instance, when oxygen molecules in a balloon take on the shape of the balloon that they occupy). Gases do not concentrate in any specific area, but rather become distributed homogeneously inside of the container because gas molecules are widely separated from one another. Gases have four major characteristics:

1. Compressibility: Because a large space separates gas particles, gases have a high compressibility.

2. Density: The large space between gas particles causes gases to have very low density.

3. Diffusion: The high kinetic energy and speed among gas particles allow gases to diffuse rapidly.

4. Pressure: Particles in a gas collide randomly and at high speed both with each other and with the walls of a container they occupy. Consequently, gases are able to produce pressure.

The ideal gas law correlates the pressure generated by a gas to the volume it occupies:

$$P = \frac{nRT}{V} \tag{8.1}$$

where P is the pressure, n is the number of particles, R is the molar gas constant, T is the absolute temperature, and V is the volume of the gas. As Equation 8.1 shows, a smaller volume (V) results in a higher pressure (P) at a constant given temperature.

It is important to emphasize the differences between two most commonly used temperatures (Kelvin and Celsius) in pharmaceutics. On the Celsius scale, 0 degrees is the point at which water molecules freeze and 100 degrees is the point at which water molecules begin to boil at sea level with an atmospheric pressure of 760 mm Hg (we will return to atmospheric pressure later in this chapter). The abbreviation for Celsius degree is °C.

The concept of absolute temperature is also important in pharmaceutics. To calculate the Kelvin temperature, indicated by the symbol K, you add 273 to the number of Celsius degrees. For example, a room temperature of 25°C equals 298 K. On the Kelvin scale, 0 K is called absolute zero because it corresponds to the temperature at which all motions of particles stop. Simply, at absolute zero (which corresponds to −273°C), there is no kinetic energy. Because temperature is based on the movement of particles, there can be no temperature lower than absolute zero. The temperature, however, is a measure of the *average* kinetic energy in a sample. Therefore, it is more scientifically valid to measure the temperature on the Kelvin scale because at 0°C there is some kinetic energy in a sample, whereas at absolute zero (−273°C) there is no kinetic energy. The variable T is used to indicate the absolute (Kelvin) temperature, while t is used to indicate temperature on the Celsius scale. Table 8.4 demonstrates differences in Celsius and Kelvin temperatures.

Table 8.4 A Few Physical Properties for Water Measured at Both Celsius and Kelvin Temperatures

Temperature of Water	K	°C
Absolute zero	0	−273
Freezing point	273	0
At room temperature	298	25
Boiling point	373	100

Blood gases, such as O_2 and CO_2, are typical gases used in clinical settings. When a few gases are mixed together, each gas is able to make a specific contribution, known as partial pressure, to the total pressure. This partial pressure is directly proportional to the gas's concentration. Most often, you will see pO_2, which is the partial pressure of oxygen, instead of the concentration of oxygen. Similarly, pCO_2 is the partial pressure of carbon dioxide in the blood. The arterial blood gas measurement describes the levels of oxygen and carbon dioxide in the blood to determine how effectively the lungs are working. The pO_2 determines tissue oxygen supply. Drugs such as barbiturates and opioids and disease states such as asthma, chronic obstructive pulmonary disease (COPD), cyanosis, breathlessness, and pulmonary embolism are known to decrease pO_2. For instance, the atmospheric pressure is 760 mm Hg (equals 1 mM or 101.3 kPa) where the pO_2 is 150 mm Hg, which means air contains 20% oxygen (150/750). The pressure of O_2 in arterial blood is approximately 100 mm Hg; that is, pO_2 is 13% (100/760), or 0.13 mM oxygen is dissolved in the blood.

While an increase in temperature increases the solubility of most solid solutes in water (see the discussion in the next section on solids), it reduces the solubility of gases in water. A high temperature (greater kinetic energy) overcomes the interaction between the solvent (water) and the gas such that the gas molecules are able to escape the solvent and reenter the gas phase existing above the solvent. An example of the effect of temperature on a gas's solubility can be seen with fish, which need to have access to dissolved oxygen in water to survive. When the temperature of the water in a fish tank increases, oxygen becomes less water soluble, which means a lower concentration of oxygen is present in the water. Lower concentration of oxygen can negatively affect the life span and survival of the fish.

Another interesting phenomenon associated with gases is their different water solubilities. For instance, CO_2 is 20 times more soluble than O_2 in water. In turn, O_2 is 2 times more soluble than nitrogen gas (N_2) in water. Henry's law (Equation 8.2) indicates that the solubility of a gas in a given liquid under a constant temperature is proportional to its pressure:

$$C = k \times P_{gas} \tag{8.2}$$

where C is the solubility of a gas at a fixed temperature in a particular solvent (g/L or M), k is the Henry's law constant (M/atm), and P_{gas} (atm) is the pressure of the gas.

The solubility of gases plays an important role in pharmaceutics. Inhalation is a valuable administration route, particularly for patients with respiratory problems. Inhaled gases such as nitrous oxide (N_2O) and halothane are used as anesthetics. N_2O is insoluble in blood and tissues (particularly in muscle and fat), so it can produce a rapid anesthetic effect. Some pharmaceutical products are aerosols, which are tiny drug particles mixed with liquefied gases. Halogenated hydrocarbons (such as hydrofluoroalkanes) are liquefiable gases that are used as propellants in inhalation devices.

Drug delivery through the large mucous membrane of the respiratory tract can be as rapid as an IV injection, owing to the large surface area of the respiratory tract (30 m²) and the large number of capillaries in the lungs (an estimated 2,000 km of capillaries exists in the lungs). In addition, if the site of action is the respiratory system, inhaled products, such as those used to treat asthma, may produce fewer systemic side effects. The *Introduction to Pharmacology and Pathophysiology* chapter describes the roles of inhaled products in treating patients with pulmonary problems. We will return to aerosols later in this chapter.

Learning Bridge 8.2

You are counseling a patient about using her new metered-dose inhaler, which is designed to deliver fluticasone (Flovent HFA). Her new inhaler contains hydrofluoroalkane propellant, in addition to the drug.

A. Describe some characteristics of hydrofluoroalkane and the drug that are necessary for the medication to be delivered correctly.

B. The inhaler must be shaken well prior to administration. Explain why this is necessary.

Solids

The intermolecular forces in solids are stronger than the corresponding forces in gases and liquids. As a result, particles in a solid state do not move freely and do not diffuse. However, particles in a solid, although not visible to the naked eye, can vibrate and rotate. The majority of drugs available in the market are in the form of solids due to their longer storage stability compared with gases and liquids. A few inherited characteristics affect the absorption of a solid drug formulation—namely, the solid's dissolution rate, diffusion coefficient, partition coefficient, permeability constant, particle size and forms, and solubility.

Dissolution Rate

Dissolution of a solid drug plays an important role in the absorption of the drug: a drug that is not dissolved generally cannot be absorbed. If the rate of dissolution is slower than the rate of absorption, the dissolution process becomes a rate limiting factor. This can happen when the drug has a low solubility in the gastrointestinal (GI) system. Poor dissolution results in poor bioavailability. In fact, in 1960, when the lifesaving antibiotics tetracycline (Apo-Tetra) and chloramphenicol (Chloromycetin, in Canada) were discovered to have low bioavailability, drug companies were forced, when developing solid dosage forms, to carry out a required dissolution test. Drugs with poor bioavailability may be useful if the intended site of drug action is the GI tract. For instance, oral vancomycin is not absorbed well and remains in the GI tract, thereby providing a local effect in treating *Clostridium difficile* infection. The United States Pharmacopeia (USP) states that the dissolution study is an extremely important quality control for solid dosage forms.

The rate of solid dissolution can be expressed by the Noyes-Whitney equation:

$$\frac{dw}{dt} = \frac{DA}{\delta}(C_s - C) \tag{8.3}$$

where

dw/dt = rate of dissolution
D = diffusion coefficient
A = surface area of the solvent particles
δ = thickness of the diffusion layer
C_s = concentration of the drug at the diffusion layer surrounding the solid
C = concentration of the drug in the bulk medium

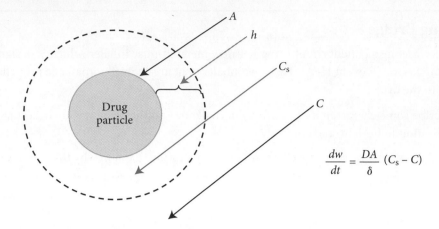

$$\frac{dw}{dt} = \frac{DA}{\delta}(C_s - C)$$

Figure 8.3 The Noyes-Whitney equation describes how different parameters can change the rate of a solid drug's dissolution.

Data from Pandit NK, Soltis RP. *Introduction to pharmaceutical sciences: an integrated approach,* 2nd ed. Philadelphia: Wolters Kluwer/Lippincott Williams & Wilkins; 2012: Chapter 7.

Figure 8.3 illustrates how the parameters in the Noyes-Whitney equation play important roles in the dissolution rate.

As the Noyes-Whitney equation indicates, the larger the surface area (A), the higher the dissolution rate. In turn, the more the particle size is reduced (by micronization), the larger the surface area (A) and the higher the dissolution rate. If the dissolution rate is the rate-limiting factor in the drug absorption, anything that can change the parameters in the Noyes-Whitney equation can change the dissolution rate, thereby changing the absorption rate. For instance, agitation (in a flask or GI tract) will result in lower δ and, in turn, a higher dissolution rate. Likewise, the presence of food in the GI tract increases the viscosity of the GI fluid, which in turn reduces the diffusion coefficient (D) and, therefore, the dissolution rate of a drug.

If a drug has little solubility in the diffusion layer, it has a low C_s value as well and, therefore, a low dissolution rate. For instance, the dissolution rate of a weakly acidic drug in the GI tract with a pH 1–3 is low. Conversely, if the pH increases, the solubility of the weakly acidic drug increases (C_s increases), which results in an increase in the dissolution rate. One method to manipulate the value of C_s for a drug is to form a potassium or sodium salt of a weakly acidic drug, which will have high solubility at an increased pH in the diffusion layer.

Diffusion Coefficient

Diffusion has been simply described as the movement of molecules within a substance. Because diffusion plays an important role in the Noyes-Whitney equation, it is important to explain Fick's law (Equation 8.4), which describes the rate of diffusion. Keep in mind that diffusion also means transfer of a drug particle through different barriers (such as different physiological layers of skin or the GI tract), and even transfer of gases through different tissues or diffusion of a drug from the blood into tissues (i.e., in an IV route of administration).

$$\text{Rate of diffusion} = \frac{DSK(C_d - C_r)}{h} \qquad (8.4)$$

where

> D = diffusion coefficient (varies for different drugs)
>
> S = surface area of the cross-sectional area of barrier (membrane)

K = partition coefficient

C_d = concentration of the drug particle in the donor side

C_r = concentration of the drug particle in the receiver side

h = thickness of the membrane

The diffusion coefficient (D) is a particle's ability to diffuse in a particular solution. Note that D is a coefficient rather than a constant—that means D can change. The diffusion coefficient depends on the molecular weight (i.e., size) of the drug particle (the larger the molecule, the smaller the value of D; see the Stokes-Einstein equation described later in this section), the solution in which the drug particle is diffusing, and the temperature. A change in the molecular size also means a change in the structure of the drug. As a result, because it alters the diffusion coefficient, changing the size of the drug is the least favorable process. If the drug concentration on the donor side (i.e., where the diffusion begins) is higher than the concentration on the receiver side (i.e., where the diffusion ends), the term ($C_d - C_r$) becomes larger, which in turn increases the diffusion rate for a passive transport system (i.e., no external energy is needed to drive the diffusion process). According to Equation 8.4, the larger the value of h, the lower the diffusion rate; the larger the value of C_d, the higher the diffusion rate; the larger the value of K, the higher the diffusion rate; and the larger the value of S, the higher the diffusion rate.

The Stokes-Einstein equation (Equation 8.5) elegantly relates the diffusion coefficient (D) to different parameters to elucidate its paramount role in both the Noyes-Whitney equation and Fick's law.

$$D = \frac{kT}{6\pi\eta r} \tag{8.5}$$

where

D = diffusion coefficient (varies for different drugs)

k = Boltzmann's constant, 1.28×10^{-23} J/K (already known from the literature)

T = absolute temperature

η = viscosity

r = radius of the drug particle

The Stokes-Einstein equation is very practical for drug particles that have a molecular weight of 1,000 g/mole or less. As Equation 8.5 indicates, the higher the temperature (T), the larger the value of D, because the system has more kinetic energy to diffuse. In addition, if the viscosity (η) is high or when the radius of the drug particle increases as a result of an increase in molecular weight, the value of D decreases.

Partition Coefficient

As stated earlier, the dissolution rate of a drug is directly related to the absorption of that drug into the body. The diffusion coefficient describes the ability of a drug to diffuse in a solution. The solubility of the drug in different solutions or across barriers will vary. Of particular interest is the solubility difference in a hydrophobic environment compared to a hydrophilic environment. The partition coefficient or partition constant (designated as P) is the ratio of concentration, or distribution, of an un-ionized drug molecule between two immiscible environments. Often, the immiscible environments or solutions are aqueous (hydrophilic) and organic (hydrophobic).

The partition coefficient may be calculated by dividing the concentration of the drug molecule in each solution:

$$P = \frac{C_o}{C_w}$$

(8.6)

where

P = partition coefficient

C_o = concentration of the drug in an organic solvent phase (typically hydrophobic)

C_w = concentration of the drug in an aqueous solvent phase (typically water)

If a drug particle has $P = 1$, then it has an equal concentration in both hydrophobic and hydrophilic environments. When designing a drug, a drug with a high hydrophobic attraction will be able to partition into the lipid bilayer; its partition coefficient will be high. A drug that is highly hydrophilic (water loving) will be found in the blood. The ideal design is a balance where the drug can pass through the lipid bilayers to be absorbed, yet is hydrophilic enough to be eliminated.

For convenience, the partition coefficient is given as a logarithmic number (i.e., as log P). The log P values for many compounds are known and can be found in the literature. As a rule of thumb, one can draw conclusions based on the value of log P:

- If a compound has log $P < 0$, the compound is highly hydrophilic. It is not a good candidate for a drug formulation because it will not be able to go through the hydrophobic bilayer of the cell membrane.

- If a compound has log $P > 3.5$, the compound is highly hydrophobic. It is most likely not a good candidate for a drug formulation because it is not soluble into the hydrophilic compartments of the body (e.g., blood, semen, saliva).

Permeability Coefficient

The permeability coefficient describes the movement or flux of drug molecules across biological barriers, such as intestinal tissue, and is expressed in Equation 8.7.

$$\text{Permeability coefficient} = \frac{PD}{h}$$

(8.7)

where

P = partition coefficient

D = diffusion coefficient

h = membrane thickness

As Equation 8.7 indicates, a larger partition coefficient (a higher hydrophobic property) or a larger diffusion coefficient (a smaller size) results in a larger permeability coefficient. Conversely, a greater membrane thickness results in a smaller permeability coefficient. In an oral form, the drug is swallowed and, ideally, will be dissolved by the time it reaches the expected area of absorption. The permeability coefficient estimates how far the drug will "permeate" across biological barriers to reach the intended site of action. In short, this calculation is vital to the success of drug action. Based on the parameters included in Equation 8.7, different epithelia from different organ systems may have different permeability coefficients for the same drug.

Types of Solids

There are three major types of solids: crystalline, amorphous, and polymeric. Polymorphs are solids that can switch between the crystalline and amorphous types.

Crystalline

Crystalline solids have a well-defined shape because the particles (ions, atoms, or molecules) are organized in an orderly repeated arrangement known as a unit cell (**Figure 8.4**). Crystals of table salt are a typical example. If you were able to see the arrangement of Na^+ and Cl^- ions (unit cells) inside a salt crystal, you would observe a symmetrical arrangement of all Na^+ and Cl^- ions within the salt. This uniform pattern is known as a crystal lattice.

Amorphous

Amorphous solids are solids that are not crystalline and, therefore, do not have any defined shape or form (**Figure 8.5**). (The word *amorphous* means "without form" in Greek.) Because amorphous solids do not have a strong crystal arrangement or strong forces among their molecules, they are more water soluble than crystalline solids. Therefore, drugs in the amorphous form have a higher solubility, which may result in a higher bioavailability. For instance, the antibiotics novobiocin and chloramphenicol in amorphous form have a higher dissolution rate than the same drugs in crystalline form. Research studies have indicated that these antibiotics, when administered in crystalline form, have almost no bioavailability; in contrast, when they are administered in amorphous form, they are absorbed rapidly from the GI tract with a high therapeutic effect.

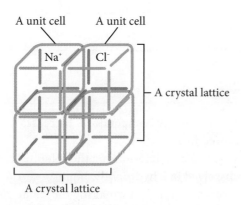

Figure 8.4 Na^+ and Cl^- ions arrangement in a salt crystal.

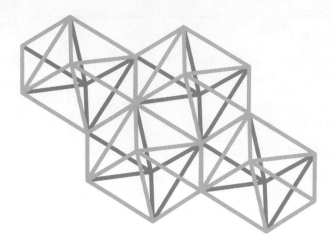

Figure 8.5 Amorphous solids do not have any defined shape or form.

Polymorphs

Many pharmaceutical compounds exist in more than one crystalline or amorphous form and, therefore, are called polymorphs. Polymorphs have different physical properties, such as different melting points and different solubility. Approximately one-third of all organic molecules exhibit polymorphism, but it is almost impossible to predict whether a drug will do so. A dosage form that has polymorphs can present storage problems because the drug may change from one form to another during the storage time; such polymorphism can result in caking of a suspension or making a cream gritty, for example (see the discussion of suspensions and creams later in this chapter). Under specific conditions, the polymorphic form that has the lowest free energy tends to be the most stable form, so other polymorphic forms will tend to be transformed into the stable form.

Polymeric

Polymeric solids are the carbon-based polymers that are often used in compounding procedures. An example is methylcellulose, a nonionic molecule that increases the viscosity of a solution. Another example is polyethylene glycol (PEG), a water-soluble polymer that is often used in suppository preparations. Due to the versatile role that PEG plays, it is discussed in detail later in this chapter.

Solubility of Solutes

The following factors affect the solubility of a solute in a given solution:

- Temperature: The rate of collisions increases when the kinetic energy (temperature) increases for a solution, which will cause more particles to be dissolved in a solution.
- Functional groups: The functional groups play an important role in determining the solubility of solutes. For instance, hydrophilic solutes are readily dissolved in a hydrophilic liquid.
- pH: The pH of a solution can change the ionization state of a solute, thereby making the solute either more soluble or insoluble.
- Surface area: The surface area of particles plays an important role in the solubility of solid particles. As indicated in the Noyes-Whitney equation (Equation 8.3), a larger A results in a higher dissolution rate.

Liquids

Liquids maintain a constant volume and have particles that are free to move. Because a liquid can pack more particles in a given volume compared to gases, liquids are much denser than gases (recall that density is defined as mass divided by volume). Also, because the space between a liquid's molecules is smaller compared with the space separating the molecules of a gas under the same temperature, liquids produce much less pressure than gases. Liquids have many unique properties: they can become solid (frozen; have freezing points), become gases (have boiling points), and have vapor pressure. Important liquid characteristics that have implications for pharmaceutics are interfacial tension, surface tension, viscosity, and wetting tendency. We will first consider vapor pressure and boiling point before focusing on these characteristics to understand how liquids occupy an important role in pharmaceutics and compounding labs.

Vapor Pressure

Vapor pressure is a physical property of pure liquids and is measured in millimeters of mercury (mm Hg). A vapor is defined as the gas phase of a substance above a liquid. All pure liquid (or even solid) substances can exist in equilibrium with the vapor that is produced above the substance. The equilibrium pressure of the saturated vapor that exists above a liquid in a sealed container is known as the vapor pressure of the liquid.

The molecules of any liquid have a variety of kinetic energies. Those molecules with the highest kinetic energy are able to escape the liquid state and enter the gas state above the liquid. The vapor pressure of a liquid ultimately depends on two important factors: the identity of the liquid (i.e., intermolecular forces) and the temperature (i.e., kinetic energy). Thus, for every liquid, the vapor pressure increases as the temperature increases. The simple mechanism behind this relationship is that at a higher temperature, the liquid's molecules have a higher kinetic energy that enables them to overcome the intermolecular forces that hold the liquid's molecules together. As a result, more molecules are able to enter the gas phase. For instance, most of the water molecules at 25°C do not have enough kinetic energy to overcome the hydrogen bonding that keeps water molecules in the liquid state. However, those molecules with the highest kinetic energy are able to make it to the surface of the liquid and enter the gas phase. This phenomenon explains why when you add flavoring agents to your compounded products, you will smell a flavoring agent in the compounding lab despite the fact that the agent is a liquid. This change of state (from liquid to gas) is called evaporation.

Any liquid that is contained in an evacuated vessel, such as an inhaler, has a vaporization tendency, and the pressure of the vapor that is produced above the liquid will reach a maximum vapor pressure. Nevertheless, the amount of liquid will not change, because a dynamic equilibrium will be established between the molecules that leave the liquid phase and those that return to the liquid back from the vapor phase. The concentration of drug particles in an inhaler remains constant because the volume of the liquid remains constant.

Sublimation

Sublimation is a process where a solid, rather than entering a liquid phase, is converted directly into a gas (i.e., it bypasses the liquid matter). Dry ice (solid) is a typical example—it is a solid form of carbon dioxide (which is normally a gas). At 760 mm Hg (atmospheric pressure), carbon dioxide does not exist as a liquid matter. Therefore, when dry ice is heated, it goes directly from the solid phase to the gas phase. This sublimation process occurs because the dry ice has a vapor pressure that is high enough to allow the carbon dioxide to vaporize rapidly. The reverse process (i.e., conversion from gas to solid) is called deposition.

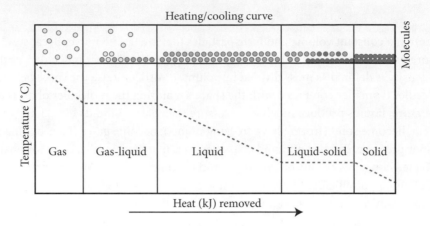

Figure 8.6 The heating and cooling curve indicates what happens to the cohesiveness of molecules in different state of matters. Kinetic energy decreases as temperature (dashed line) decreases.
Adapted from: Silberberg MS. *Principles of general chemistry*. New York: McGraw-Hill Higher Education; 2006: Chapter 12.

Figure 8.6 indicates the condensation of molecules at different state of matters.

Boiling Point

Boiling point is the temperature at which the vapor pressure of a liquid reaches 1 atm (760 mm Hg). The boiling point of each liquid depends on the intermolecular forces holding the molecules of that substance together in a liquid state. Thus the boiling point is higher for liquids that have strong intermolecular attractions than for liquids that have weak intermolecular attractions. For instance, the boiling point of a given volume of ethanol is lower (78°C) than the boiling point of the same volume of water (100°C)—a difference explained by the intermolecular attractions between ethanol and water molecules, respectively.

When the temperature of water reaches 100°C, the vapor pressure equals the atmospheric pressure (i.e., 760 mm Hg). This explains why it takes a longer time to cook an egg at a high altitude (e.g., Denver, Colorado) than at a lower altitude (e.g., a kitchen at sea level). The pressure of the atmosphere at a high altitude is lower than that at sea level. Consequently, water reaches its vapor pressure at less than 760 mm Hg, which causes water to boil at, say, 90°C instead of 100°C. Obviously, cooking an egg at a higher altitude (at 90°C) takes longer than cooking one at sea level (100°C).

Colligative Properties

Four properties of a solution depend on the number of solutes, but not the chemical identity of the solutes; these properties are referred to as colligative properties. For example, when 1 mole of NaCl is dissolved in water, it dissociates into 1 mole of Na^+ ions and 1 mole of Cl^- ions. This occurs because one molecule of NaCl can dissociate in the solution to form two ions. Conversely, glucose does not dissociate at all upon dissolving in water. Consequently, when 1 mole of glucose dissolves in water, only 1 mole of glucose is present in the solution. A molecule that dissociates in solution is called an electrolyte (e.g., NaCl), while one that does not dissociate is called a nonelectrolyte (e.g., glucose).

The four colligative properties of solutions are

1. Vapor pressure reduction

2. Boiling-point elevation

3. Freezing-point depression

4. Osmotic pressure

Let's go through each of them and discuss the important roles they play in pharmaceutics.

Vapor Pressure Reduction

A nonelectrolyte solute (sucrose [sugar]) is a solute that does not evaporate at the boiling point of the solvent (e.g., water). Generally speaking, a solute with a boiling point of less than 100°C is considered a volatile solvent. Even though a nonvolatile solute dissolves in the solution, it is mainly the solvent molecules (i.e., water molecules) at the surface of the solution that affect the vapor pressure. The larger the number of solute species that are dissolved, the lower the vapor pressure generated by the solvent molecules. This relationship arises because some of the dissolved solute species will displace some of the solvent molecules at the surface of the liquid. As a result, fewer solvent molecules can escape the solution to enter the gas phase above the solution. Addition of solutes reduces the vapor pressure in the container because fewer solvent molecules can escape the liquid to join the gas phase above the solution (**Figure 8.7**).

A practical example of reduction of the vapor pressure is the use of polyethylene glycol (PEG). PEG is added as a solution in the formulation of nitroglycerin (Nitrostat) tablets because nitroglycerin molecules diffuse and vaporize easily from tablets owing to the weak intermolecular force (van der Waals force) that exists among the nitroglycerin molecules.

Boiling-Point Elevation

As mentioned earlier, adding a nonvolatile solute to a solvent can reduce the vapor pressure. This reduction in the vapor pressure affects the boiling point as well, because now a higher

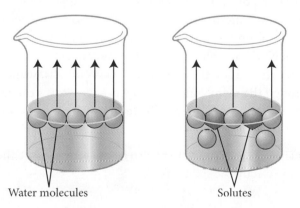

Water molecules   Solutes

Figure 8.7 Water molecules at the surface have a tendency to escape from the water. The number of solute species at the water surface (gray) decreases the number of solvent molecules that can escape into the vapor phase, resulting in a reduced vapor pressure for the solution.

Adapted from: Nelson DL, Cox MM. *Lehninger principles of biochemistry*, 4th ed. New York: W. H. Freeman; 2005: Chapter 2.

temperature is required to increase the vapor pressure to match the atmospheric pressure and thereby cause the liquid to boil. Consequently, a higher temperature is required to boil the solvent. The boiling-point elevation explains why a solute such as ethylene glycol (a "coolant"), when added to the water in the radiator of a car, prevents overheating of the engine during summer.

Freezing-Point Depression

The freezing point is the temperature at which a liquid changes its state to a solid. As a substance changes from a liquid to a solid state, the entropy of the liquid decreases; that is, molecules of the liquid go from a disorganized form to an organized form. In turn, the intermolecular attractions between molecules increase. The addition of a nonvolatile solute to a solvent increases the entropy and inhibits the ability of the solvent molecules to build an organized structure, which in turn promotes a slower freezing process for the solution (in other words, it causes a freezing-point depression). The same ethylene glycol "coolant" that was mentioned in the previous example serves as "antifreeze" on a cold winter day by reducing the freezing point of the water inside of a car's radiator. Similarly, salt (NaCl) is added to icy roads during winter to depress the freezing point of ice and prevent formation of "black ice."

Osmotic Pressure

Osmosis is simply the transport of a solvent (usually water) through a semipermeable membrane that separates two solutions with different solute concentrations. A semipermeable membrane does not allow the solute to diffuse, but the solvent can move freely across the membrane. To reach equilibrium, the solvent diffuses from the less concentrated solution to the more concentrated solution across the semipermeable membrane. Pressure is applied to the more concentrated solution to prevent water flow to the more concentrated solution. The pressure needed to stop the flow of water from the less concentrated solution to the more concentrated solution is known as the osmotic pressure.

Let's use an example to visualize the osmosis and osmotic pressure. Suppose you dissolve one tablespoon of salt (NaCl) into one glass of water (240 mL). Suppose you also dissolve two tablespoonsful of the same salt into another glass containing the same volume of water (240 mL). If you place these two solutions on either side of a semipermeable membrane, you will notice that water molecules go through the membrane from the less concentrated solution (one tablespoon of salt) to the more concentrated solution (two tablespoons of salt), while the solutes (NaCl or Na^+, Cl^-) do not go through the membrane. This water movement is called osmosis, and the pressure necessary to prevent the movement of water through the membrane is the osmotic pressure.

The ideal gas law equation (Equation 8.1) can also be used to calculate the osmotic pressure for nonelectrolyte and diluted electrolyte solutions:

$$P = \frac{nRT}{V}$$

Here P is the osmotic pressure, n is the number of moles of the solute, R is the gas constant, T is the absolute temperature, and V is the volume. Note that the ideal gas law becomes less accurate at very high temperatures that can cause a chemical reaction to occur.

Example 8.1: What is the osmotic pressure of 1 g NaCl in 1 liter of water at room temperature (25°C)? The molecular weight of NaCl is 58.5 g/mole.

Answer:

$$n = 1 \text{ g}/(58.5 \text{ g/mole}) \times 2 \text{ (ions)} = 0.034 \text{ mole}$$
$$R = 0.082 \text{ L atm/mole}$$
$$T = 273 + 25 = 298$$
$$V = 1 \text{ L}$$
$$P = (0.034 \times 0.082 \times 298)/1 \text{ L} = 0.84 \text{ atm}$$

A cell in a fluid environment can be in any of three osmotic states: isotonic, hypertonic, and hypotonic.

Isotonic Solutions

All living cells live and function in a fluid environment. Not surprisingly, then, the ionic concentrations of the intracellular and extracellular fluids have significant physiological effects on the survival of the living cells. The maintenance of a constant level of osmotic pressure for the intracellular and extracellular fluids within and around the cells plays an important role in the physiology of the entire organism. Consequently and evolutionarily, an architectural change of the cell membrane was required to provide a selective cell membrane to regulate the entry of water and solutes in and out of a cell.

A solution that has the same "tone" (osmotic pressure) as body fluids will not cause any change in the tissue or cells. An 0.9% NaCl solution (so-called normal saline) is isotonic to our blood cells. When a cell, like an erythrocyte, is exposed to fluids that are isotonic, hypertonic, or hypotonic, the water movement (osmosis) causes physiological changes that can result in detrimental changes in the cell.

In an isotonic solution, the osmotic pressure of the solution (e.g., extracellular fluid [ECF]) is the same as that of the cell cytoplasm (e.g., intracellular fluid [ICF]). This balance results in zero net water movement because the number of solutes on either side of the biological membrane is exactly the same (**Figure 8.8**). One practical example of an isotonic solution is seen with subcutaneous injections. It is critical to have isotonic solutions for subcutaneous injections because a

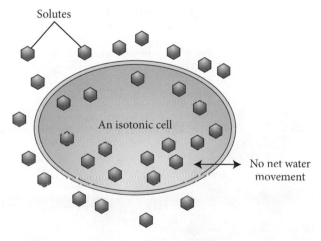

Figure 8.8 An isotonic cell. When the amount of solutes is exactly the same on either side of a cell, there will not be any movement of water into or out of the cell.

subcutaneous injection reaches many nerve terminals (nerve ending) and its content remains at the site of administration for a long period of time. If the injected solution is not isotonic, it will damage the nerve terminals and cause pain.

Hypertonic Solutions

A hypertonic solution is a solution that has a higher ("hyper") "tone"—that is, a higher osmotic pressure—than a living cell. Thus, such a solution has a higher concentration of solute than is found inside the cell. In a hypertonic solution, water moves out of the cell and dilutes the solute in the ECF, which causes the cell to shrink (**Figure 8.9**). For instance, if an erythrocyte is placed into a solution of greater concentration than 0.9% NaCl, the water moves out of the erythrocyte, causing the red blood cell to shrink. This shrinking process in an erythrocyte is known as crenation.

Hypotonic Solutions

A hypotonic solution is a solution that has lower ("hypo") "tone"—that is, a lower osmotic pressure—than a living cell. Thus, a hypotonic solution has a lower solute concentration than the cell. In a hypotonic solution, the concentration of the solution is less than that found inside of a cell (**Figure 8.10**). As a result, water moves into the cell, causing the cell to swell and burst. If you place an erythrocyte into pure water, for example, the cell swells and bursts. This swelling and bursting process in the red blood cell upon exposure to a hypotonic solution is called hemolysis.

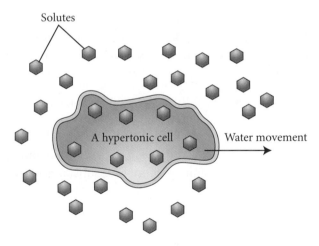

Figure 8.9 A hypertonic cell. When the amount of solute is higher outside the cell than inside the cell, water moves from inside to outside the cell, which causes the cell to shrink.

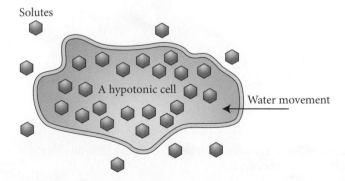

Figure 8.10 A hypotonic cell. When the amount of solute is lower outside the cell than inside the cell, water moves from outside to inside the cell, which causes the cell to burst.

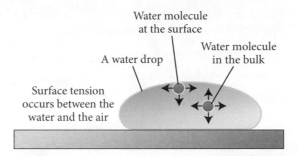

Water molecule
at the surface

Water molecule
in the bulk

A water drop

Surface tension
occurs between the
water and the air

Figure 8.11 The globular shape of a water drop depends on the surface tension between the water and the air.

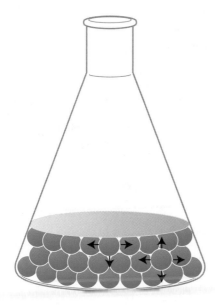

Figure 8.12 Water molecules at the surface of water make significant contributions to the surface tension phenomenon.

Surface Tension

The resistance of a liquid to spreading out and expanding its surface area when it is in contact with air brings a tension to the surface—known as, aptly enough, surface tension. Surface tension is a physical property of liquids that is caused by intermolecular forces. A liquid with strong intermolecular forces has a higher surface tension, whereas a liquid with weak intermolecular forces has a lower surface tension. For instance, a solution of benzene has a lower surface tension compared with pure water because benzene molecules are characterized by van der Waals forces, which are much weaker than the hydrogen bonds found in water. It is the surface tension that causes a drop of water to form a globular shape (**Figure 8.11**).

In Figure 8.11, notice the difference between a molecule in the center (bulk) of a droplet of water and a molecule at the surface. The water molecule in the center of the droplet is equally attracted to other water molecules via intermolecular forces created by the existing hydrogen bonds. In contrast, a molecule at the surface of the droplet is attracted to water molecules only to the sides and center because there is no molecule outside; that is, no intermolecular forces are generated with the air. Thus, the molecules at the surface are more strongly attracted to the center of the droplet and, in turn, they form a thin film around the water.

Figure 8.12 depicts another example of surface tension. Notice the intermolecular forces for molecules (e.g., water) at the top (surface) of the solution and in the middle (bulk) of the solution.

Interfacial Tension

If water molecules are mixed with oil molecules, more of the water molecules will spontaneously move to the bulk (inside) of the water, which in turn leaves fewer water molecules per unit area at the interface. The same process happens to the oil molecules. The intermolecular forces in these two immiscible liquids cause the interface to resist expansion. This brings a tension to the interface, a phenomenon known as interfacial tension (**Figure 8.13**).

Surfactants

A surfactant is a molecule that has both hydrophobic and hydrophilic properties (**Figure 8.14**). Surfactants are classified based on the nature of the hydrophilic groups they contain—that is, as anionic surfactant, cationic surfactant, non-ionic surfactant, and zwitterionic.

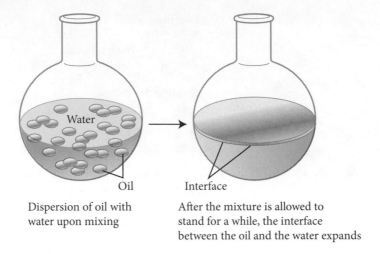

Dispersion of oil with
water upon mixing

After the mixture is allowed to
stand for a while, the interface
between the oil and the water expands

Figure 8.13 When two immiscible liquids are placed in the same container, interfacial tension is experienced by the two liquids at the boundary where they come in contact with each other.

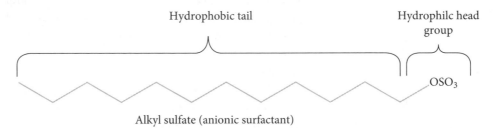

Figure 8.14 A typical structure of an anionic surfactant. Notice the hydrophilic (head) and hydrophobic (tail) components.

Because of surfactants' amphiphilic characteristic (i.e., they have both hydrophobic and hydrophilic properties), they are able to reduce interfacial or surface tension. (Other names have also been used to describe surfactant, such as surface-active agent and tenside.) **Figure 8.15** indicates how the hydrophilic head of a surfactant is placed into contact with a polar medium (water) and how the tail is placed in contact (i.e., has an affinity) with a nonpolar medium (oil).

The body contains numerous physiological surfactants. For instance, many phospholipids and a few lipoproteins in the lungs serve as surfactants that assist the lungs in maintaining a low

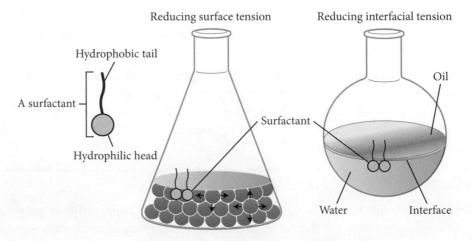

Figure 8.15 The role of a surfactant in reducing surface and interfacial tensions.

interfacial tension at the alveolar air–water interface. The role of the alveoli is to capture oxygen from inhaled air and let the oxygen be absorbed into the bloodstream. Without surfactants, alveoli would stick together and collapse during the breathing cycle.

Because of the hydrophilic and hydrophobic properties of surfactants, they are able to serve as emulsifier agents, solubilizing agents, or wetting agents. One of the most commonly used surfactants in parenteral solutions and oral suspensions is polysorbate 80 (Tween 80). This surfactant has a light brownish color, is viscous, and has a bitter taste. Polysorbate 80 has the unique property of being adsorbed on a drug particle to decrease the particle's zeta potential; in addition, it is non-ionic (so it does not change the pH of a solution), has no toxicity, and is compatible with most other inert ingredients. The zeta potential determines how particles in a colloidal system repel each other. The higher the zeta potential, the greater the chance that particles will repel each other. A pH change of the colloidal system can change the zeta potential. For example, if particles become negatively charged, they will have a higher zeta potential, which in turn will mean that the particles repel each other.

Viscosity

The resistance of a liquid to flow is called viscosity. The higher the viscosity, the more slowly the substance will flow. Blood, for instance, is more viscous than water.

The concept of viscosity was first proposed by Isaac Newton in 1687. He described viscosity as a resistance to flow and pointed out that viscosity was related to the velocity of separating parts of a solution because of their flow. Many solutions, such as low-molecular-weight liquids, follow Newton's principal description of viscosity. Other solutions, such as polymer solutions, blood, and colloidal suspensions, are not described well by Newton's law; they are referred to as non-Newtonian solutions. We will examine Newtonian and non-Newtonian solutions more closely in the rheology section of this chapter.

The viscosity of a liquid is related to its intermolecular forces and the molecular weight (size) of the molecules. The viscosity decreases as the temperature increases because the molecules have more kinetic energy with which to overcome the intermolecular forces among themselves in a viscous solution. For example, glycerol, because of its large number of hydrogen bonds, has a high viscosity (**Figure 8.16**). Molecules with the same intermolecular forces (such as water and glycerol) but different molecular sizes, however, have different viscosities. Larger molecules in a solution have a higher tendency to become entangled with one another, thereby increasing the viscosity of the solution.

Glycerol (also known as glycerin) has a valuable place in pharmaceutics. It is an excellent solvent (although not to the same extent as water and alcohol) and, in high concentration, has a preservative effect. It is used to dissolve alkalis, many salts, vegetable acids, and carbohydrates such as starch. In research labs, to avoid freezing proteins, which otherwise would inactivate enzymes, many purified proteins are stored in solutions that contain 20%–50% glycerol.

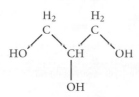

Figure 8.16 Due to its three hydroxyl groups, glycerol can produce extensive intermolecular forces (in this case, many hydrogen bonds) to increase the viscosity of a solution.

Viscosity plays important roles in rheology and drug formulations: it assists a suspension in holding its drug particles in place (i.e., the rate of sedimentation decreases when viscosity increases), increases the stability of emulsions, and modifies the release rate of a drug at its site of application. As explained earlier in this chapter, viscosity affects both the diffusion coefficient and the dissolution of drug particles (see Equations 8.3 and 8.5). A few examples of pharmaceutical agents that increase viscosity of a formulation are 0.5–5% methylcellulose USP, 0.5–1.5% carboxymethylcellulose USP, and 2–5% acacia NF.

Wetting Phenomena

When the air on the surface of solid molecules is replaced by a liquid, the solid molecules are said to be "wetted." Any molecule that reduces the surface tension of a liquid has a wetting property. However, to be called a wetting agent, the molecule must have a hydrophil–lipophil balance (HLB) number between 7 and 9 (**Figure 8.17**). HLB numbers have been generated for many surfactant molecules. The more hydrophilic an agent is, the higher its HLB value. The maximum HLB number that has been assigned is 40, but most surfactants that are commonly used in pharmaceutics have HLB numbers in the range of 1 to 20.

Non-ionic surfactants are commonly used as wetting agents. An inability to engage wetting results from a high interfacial tension between a particle and the liquid. Conversely, a reduction in the interfacial tension facilitates the wetting process. All surfactants reduce the surface/interfacial tension between two immiscible phases. **Table 8.5** indicates the roles of different HLB numbers in manufacturing of drugs.

As is shown in Figure 8.17, the dispersibility of a particle is affected by a wetting process. The poorly wetted particle has a contact angle of 180°; when the wetting process is complete (well-dispersed particles), the contact angle becomes 0°. A particle that has a 90° or greater contact angle causes a wetting problem. The wetting process facilitates drug absorption. For instance, upon disintegration of a tablet or capsule in the stomach, the particles must come in contact (be wetted) with the stomach solution to be dissolved.

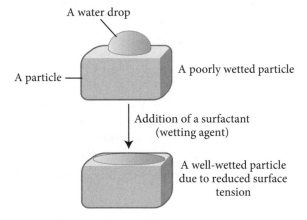

Figure 8.17 A wetting agent with a hydrophil–lipophil balance in the range 7–9 can assist in wetting a solid particle.

Table 8.5 Role of Hydrophil–Lipophil Balance (HLB) in Drug Formulation

HLB Range	Function	Agent
1–3.5	Antifoam	Ethylene glycol distearate; sorbitan tristearate (Span 65)
3.5–8	W/O* emulsifier	Sorbitan mono-oleate; sorbitan monostearate
7–9	Wetting agent	Acacia; sucrose dioleate
8–16	O/W† emulsifier	Methylcellulose; polyoxyethylene (Tween 60)
13–16	Detergent	Triton X-100; polyoxyethylene sorbitan mono-oleate (Tween 60)
15–40	Solubilizer	Sodium oleate; sodium lauryl sulfate

*Water-in-oil.

†Oil-in-water.

Adapted from: Allen LV, Popovich NG, Ansel HC. *Ansel's pharmaceutical dosage forms and drug delivery systems,* 8th ed. Philadelphia, PA: Lippincott Williams & Wilkins; 2005: Chapter 14.

Osmolarity and Osmolality

The knowledge of osmolarity and osmolality is important for pharmacists. Both osmolality and osmolarity can be calculated if you know the unit osmole. One osmole is equivalent to one mole of a dissolved nonelectrolyte solute. The osmolality of a solution is equal to the number of moles of dissolved solutes (ions or molecules) per weight (kilogram) of water. The osmolarity of a solution is equal to the number of moles of dissolved solutes (ions or molecules) per volume (liter) of water. At low concentrations of solutes, such as in human body fluids, these two terms are almost identical. Therefore, pharmacists often use these two units interchangeably.

Three solutes largely determine serum osmolality:

- Sodium, measured in mEq/L, with a normal range of 135–145 mEq/L
- Glucose, measured in mg/dL, with a normal range of 70–90 mg/dL
- Urea, measured in mg/dL, with a normal range of 5–20 mg/dL

The human body's serum osmolality varies between 275 and 310 mOsm (the average is 300 mOsm). An increase or decrease in milliosmoles is a sign of a physiological change. For this reason, measurement of serum osmolality serves as a diagnostic tool to reveal some physiological changes. One can roughly calculate the serum osmolality by the following formula:

$$\text{Serum osmolality} = 2 \times [\text{sodium}] + [\text{glucose}]/18 + [\text{urea}]/2.8 \qquad (8.8)$$

In Equation 8.8, the units of measurement for serum osmolality are mOsm/kg, as the equation accommodates conversion of mEq sodium, mg glucose, and mg blood urea (nitrogen) to milliosmoles. Glucose is an effective osmole that under normal and healthy conditions is trapped inside the cells (upon phosphorylation during the glycolysis pathway; see the *Introduction to Biochemistry* chapter), so it does not contribute greatly to the serum osmolality. However, in untreated diabetes, a severely elevated serum glucose concentration leads to hypertonicity and, in turn, water movement into the ECF. In contrast to glucose, urea is not an ionizable molecule and is not an effective osmole because it can freely cross the cell membrane and so becomes distributed equally in all body compartments. Thus, by itself, urea cannot be a contributing factor in moving water from one compartment to another. The blood urea nitrogen (BUN) value is a measure of the amount of nitrogen in the blood in the form of urea and an indicator of renal function (see the *Introduction to Nutrients* chapter).

Example 8.2: A 45-year-old man with renal failure is admitted to the hospital with weakness, sweating, and stress symptoms. His blood sample shows the following data:

Na^+ = 135 mEq/L

Glucose = 100 mg/dL

Blood urea nitrogen (BUN) = 140 mg/dL

Calculate the total serum osmolality for this patient. Does his serum osmolality explain his symptoms?

Answer: Based on Equation 8.8, osmolality = $2 \times 135 + 100/18 + 140/2.8 = 326$ mOsm/kg. The concentrations of sodium and glucose are normal. However, the concentration of urea is abnormally high. This estimated number is above the normal range of the serum osmolality, which explains the weakness, sweating, and stress symptoms (a value greater than 330 mOsm/kg will lead to disorientation, severe weakness, and fainting).

Learning Bridge 8.4

During one of your introductory pharmacy practice experiences, Amy comes to your pharmacy for advice on buying an OTC product for her acute constipation. After reviewing her medical records, you notice that her constipation is caused by her pain medication, morphine sulfate 15 mg (twice daily for 7 days). After determining that she is not pregnant and is not nursing, you suggest that she purchase sorbitol solution (70% concentration solution), 16 oz bottle, and drink 30 mL twice daily for 7 days.

Amy mentions that she is a biology teacher and knows about sorbitol as a sweetener but did not know that it also works as a laxative. Explain to Amy how sorbitol works as a hyperosmotic laxative.

Example 8.3: Calculate the unit osmole for 1 g of sucrose and NaCl. The molecular weight of sucrose is 342 g and that of NaCl is 58.5 g/mol.

Answer: A sucrose molecule does not ionize, so the moles of sucrose should be the same as the osmoles.

$$\frac{g}{g/mole} = mole$$

1 g/(342 g/mole) = 2.92 mmole = 2.92 mOsm

However, because NaCl dissociates into two ions (two solutes: Na^+ and Cl^-) and because both of these ions affect osmosis, moles are not equal to osmoles for this electrolyte.

1 g/(58.5 g/mole) = 17.1 mmole; $2 \times 17.1 = 34.2$ mOsm

Example 8.4: What is the osmolarity of a solution that contains 0.9% NaCl? (Molecular weight = 58.5 g/mole.)

Answer: An 0.9% solution means there is 0.9 g NaCl per 100 mL water, which is equal to 9 g/L. To determine the molar concentration, divide this number by the molecular weight. As two ions (two solutes) will be in the solution, the osmolarity will be 0.308, or simply 308 mOsm/L.

$$\frac{g/L}{g/mole} = \frac{9g/L}{58.5g/mole} \times 2 = 0.308 Osm/L = 308 mOsm/L$$

Example 8.5: What is the osmolality of a solution that contains 0.9% NaCl? (Molecular weight = 58.5 g/mole.)

Answer: A 100-mL volume of water weight 99.65 g. Here we need to find values with respect to weight rather than volume. An 0.9% solution means 0.9 g NaCl/99.65 g water, or 9 g/0.9965 kg. Similar to the case in Example 8.4, because two ions (two solutes) will be in the solution, the osmolality will be 0.309 or simply 309 mOsm/kg.

> ## Learning Bridge 8.5
>
> **A.** In the compounding lab, your preceptor asks you to make an oral rehydration solution (ORS) for a 5-year-old child. The following ions and sugar are added to 1 liter of water. Your preceptor asks you to calculate the osmolarity of the ORS to make sure that it will not hurt the child. What is the osmolarity of the proposed ORS?
>
> Na^+ = 0.20%; molecular weight = 23 g/mole
>
> K^+ = 0.07%; molecular weight = 39 g/mole
>
> Cl^- = 0.35%; molecular weight = 35.5 g/mole
>
> Glucose = 2%; molecular weight = 180 g/mole
>
> **B.** Your preceptor has also shown you different intravenous dextrose solutions with the following strengths: 0.5%, 5%, 10%, and 25%. He asks you to identify the intravenous dextrose solution that is isotonic. Justify your answer. (Molecular weight for dextrose = 180 g/mole.)
>
> **C.** Your preceptor asks you whether a soft drink should be advised in the treatment of dehydration while you prepare the ORS. Justify your answer.

Solutions

A solution is a homogeneous mixture of two or more components (solids, liquids) whose properties change with varying proportions of the components. A solution contains solutes that are dispersed (dissolved) uniformly in a solvent. A solute is any molecule or ion that dissolves in a medium when making a solution. The medium is called a solvent. When water serves as a solvent for a solution, the result is referred to as an aqueous solution. If the solvent is not water, it is called a liquid solution. Intramolecular forces (e.g., covalent boding, ionic bonding) play an important role in a solution. Solutions are not confined to just liquids; they may include any mixed combination of gases, liquids, or solids.

Three types of solutions are described as: saturated, unsaturated, or supersaturated. Changes in both the solvent and the solute's number (of particles) and physicochemical properties can change the type of solution. At a given temperature, in a saturated solution, the dissolved solute is at equilibrium with the solid phase (i.e., the solvent cannot dissolve any more solute). In an unsaturated solution, more solute can still be dissolved. A supersaturated solution contains more of the dissolved solute than it would normally be able to hold at a given temperature. **Figure 8.18** demonstrates the three types of solutions. We will return to the concept of solutions and its application in drug formulations later in this chapter.

There are three terms that one has to recognize when describing mixtures in pharmaceutics:

- Dispersed phase (or internal phase): The substance that is distributed in a solution.

- Continuous phase (or external phase): The vehicle of the solution. A dispersed phase plus a dispersed medium is called a dispersed system.

- Homogenous mixture: A mixture that is built when a solid, liquid, or gas is dissolved in a dispersed medium. The size of dispersed particles plays an important role in making a solution.

Figure 8.19 shows the internal (dispersed) and external (continuous) phases of a solution.

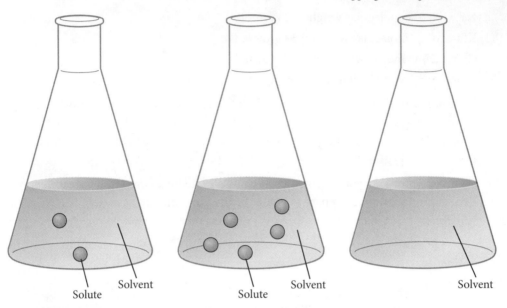

Unsaturated solution: At a given temperature, the solvent has the capacity to dissolve more solute.

Saturated solution: At a given temperature, the solvent is saturated with the solute and it cannot dissolve any additional solute.

Supersaturated solution: At a given temperature, the solvent holds more solute than it is normally capable of dissolving. A supersaturated solution can be made by raising the temperature to increase the dissolving process for the solute and then slowly dropping the temperature.

Figure 8.18 A solution can be saturated, unsaturated, or supersaturated. The least stable solution is supersaturated, as there is a risk of precipitation.

Because the viscosity affects the properties of solutions in different ways, it is important to describe rheology and its effects on solutions.

Rheology and Solutions

The word *rheology* comes from the Greek words *rheo*, which means "flow," and *logy*, which means "science of." The science of rheology, however, describes the flow of fluids (even solids and semisolids) and deformation of solids under an applied stress. Although rheology is pertinent to all states of matter (gases, liquids, and solids), its main application is to solutions and semisolid dosage forms, because the viscosity characteristics affect these solutions. As we will see in the following sections, rheology can affect patient compliance, physical stability, and even bioavailability of a drug.

Rheology can assist in predicting whether a suspension or emulsion will exhibit flocculation (when particles of an internal phase form large clusters) or coalescence (when two particles assimilate into one larger particle), resulting in undesired physical instability such as caking in a suspension and phase separation in an emulsion (**Figure 8.20**). Two major systems exist in rheology: Newtonian systems and non-Newtonian systems.

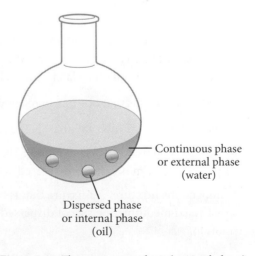

Figure 8.19 The continuous phase (external phase) and the dispersed phase (internal phase) of a solution.

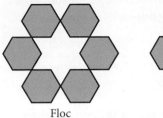

Floc   Cake

Figure 8.20 The structural difference between a floc and a cake. A floc, which often forms in a suspension, represents particles that have a weak network and is easy to resuspend (i.e., it has a loose structure). A cake, which often forms in an emulsion, has a strong network and is not easy to resuspend (i.e., it has a packed structure).

Newtonian Systems

A Newtonian system is characterized by having a constant viscosity, regardless of the shear rates applied. It can be explained by Newton's law of flow:

$$\frac{F'}{A} = \eta \times \frac{d_v}{d_r} \tag{8.9}$$

where

F'/A = shearing stress—that is, the force per unit area that brings about flow to a solution (such as shaking). Agitation is an example of shearing stress.

η = viscosity

dv/dr = rate of shearing

Equation 8.9 describes viscosity. According to Newton's law, layers of liquid are present within a flow. While the bottom layer is stationary (fixed), the other layers are mobile (not fixed). When a force (shearing stress) is applied to the top layer, this liquid moves at a constant velocity. The lower layers move with a velocity (dv) that is directly proportional to their distances (dr) from the stationary layer. The rate of shearing depends on the velocity (dv) and distance (dr) between two layers of liquids, or simply dv/dr. In a Newtonian system (a solution that contains a significant amount of water or low-molecular-weight liquids), viscosity is constant and the rate of shearing is directly proportional to the shearing stress (**Figure 8.21A**). The slope of the line in Figure 8.21A is viscosity (η).

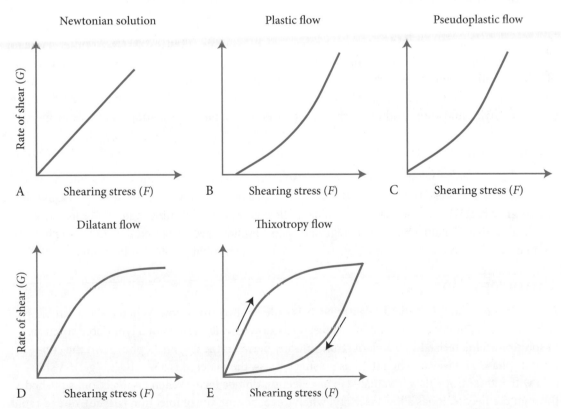

Figure 8.21 The shear rate as a function of shear stress is illustrated for Newtonian (A) and non-Newtonian (B–E) systems.

Adapted from: Allen LV, Popovich NG, Ansel HC. *Ansel's pharmaceutical dosage forms and drug delivery systems*, 8th ed. Philadelphia: Lippincott Williams & Wilkins; 2005: Chapter 14.

Other solutions, such as suspensions, emulsions, ointments, and even foods (e.g., mayonnaise, peanut butter, egg whites), represent non-Newtonian systems; their viscosity will change with a change in the rate of shearing.

Non-Newtonian Systems

In a non-Newtonian system, the viscosity can change with an increase in the shear rate (**Figure 8.21**). Newton's law of flow (Equation 8.9) cannot be applied to such a system. A unique characteristic of non-Newtonian systems is that the molecular-level structures of the solution can be rearranged reversibly in the flow. For instance, if a semisolid or solid compound is changed or rearranged through the action of a force, it will revert to its original form and shape when the force is removed.

Next, we consider the four possible non-Newtonian flows and their applications in pharmaceutics.

Plastic Flow

Newton's law of flow does not apply to most pharmaceutical solutions, such as colloidal dispersions, emulsions, and suspensions. The reason is because the viscosity of the fluid varies with the rate of a shear stress. For instance, a suspension is a typical plastic flow (**Figure 8.21B**); that is, the flow begins after a shearing stress is applied to the system (there is a yield value, as the flow does not cross the origin of the graph). This often indicates flocculated solids in the solutions. An example of plastic flow is ketchup: the ketchup does not readily flow until the system has been "sheared" by shaking the bottle.

Pseudoplastic Flow

When a solution has pseudoplastic flow, a polymer is present in the solution. The viscosity of a solution with pseudoplastic flow decreases with increasing shear rate (**Figure 8.21C**). Another name for a pseudoplastic flow is shear-thinning system. It has been suggested that the polymers in a pseudoplastic flow align themselves in such a way that they are able to slide past one another. An example of pseudoplastic flow is paint. Many inert pharmaceutical products, including natural and synthetic gums (methylcellulose and sodium carboxymethylcellulose), possess pseudoplastic flow properties.

Dilatant Flow

With a dilatant flow, applying a shear stress to a solution increases the volume of the solution. As a result of the shear stress, the viscosity of a solution with a dilatant flow increases with increasing shear rate (**Figure 8.21D**). Another name for a dilatant flow is a shear-thickening system. For instance, suspensions that contain a high percentage of dispersed solids have decreased flow following increasing rates of shear. Whipping cream is an example; it usually has a high (50%) solid content.

Thixotropy Flow

A mixture of pseudoplastic and dilatant flows is called a thixotropy flow. When a shear stress is applied, weak bonds among the molecules break down, which results in a lyophobic solution (a solution characterized by a lack of strong affinity between the dispersed phase and the continuous phase). However, when there is no shear stress, the material is a semisolid (gel). A solution with a thixotropy flow is valuable in an injection dosage form. When an injection is pushed through the needle, it has a low viscosity; when it reaches the site of injection (tissue), due to rapid formation of the gel structure, it has a higher viscosity (semisolid). Thus it stays longer at the tissue site. **Figure 8.21E** illustrates a thixotropy flow.

Table 8.6 summarizes the characteristics of non-Newtonian solutions.

Table 8.6 Characteristics and Examples of Non-Newtonian Solutions

Flow	Viscosity	Example
Plastic	Decreases at first, but reaches a constant level after the shear rate reaches a specific point (imagine how ketchup behaves when you shake it rigorously)	Suspension, ketchup, toothpaste
Pseudoplastic	Decreases with an increasing shear rate because the shear rate deforms or rearranges particles to have a lower flow resistance	Methylcellulose, paint
Dilatant	Increases with an increasing shear rate; the volume of the solution increases as well	Concentrated starch suspensions, whipping cream
Thixotropy	Decreases with an increasing shear rate	Yogurt, mayonnaise

Pharmaceutical Solutions

As described earlier, an increase in the surface area of a particle's size will increase the solubility rate of a particle in a solution. Three types of solutions are possible based on the particle size:

- True solution: a solution that is a homogenous molecular dispersion despite the fact there are two or more components; also called a one-phase system. The particle size in a true solution is less than 1 nm. Particles of a true solution are not visible to the naked eye. An example of a true solution is one in which sugar is fully dissolved in water.
- Coarse solution: a solution that has a large particle size (larger than 0.5 mm) and in which particles are visible under light microscopy. Examples of coarse solutions include emulsions and suspensions.
- Colloidal solution: a solution that has a particle size in the range of 1 nm to 0.5 mm—a size between that of a true solution and a coarse solution. The particles are visible under electron microscopy. Examples include solutions containing natural or synthetic polymers.

A liquid dosage form involves a solvent. The solvent could be water, a specific solvent, or even an oil. Liquid dosage forms include solutions, suspensions, and emulsions. These forms can be administered orally, given via IV or IM injection, or applied locally/topically. Liquid dosage forms are of particular interest in pediatric populations. Pediatric patients are not always able to chew or swallow solid dosage forms (capsules, tablets) and may refuse to accept the medication. Liquid dosage forms can also mask the bitter taste of a medication and can be administered to pediatric patients by using a syringe, which also assists parents in measuring the solution accurately. Additionally, many drugs are not originally available in a suitable dosage form, so dilution of highly concentrated drugs that are intended for adult patients may be necessary for the pediatric population. However, such a dilution may influence the stability or compatibility of the concentrated drug (see the discussion of half-life and degradation in this chapter). Another challenge with dilution of concentrated drugs is the need to identify the best solvent for that particular medication. To mask a bitter taste, pharmacists can mix medications in applesauce, syrup, or other solvents prior to dispensing the drug.

The most common causes of chemical degradation among liquid dosage forms are hydrolysis and oxidation of the dosage form's ingredients, particularly of the active ingredient. To avoid the oxidation problem, ascorbic acid (vitamin C)—an antioxidant—is often added to drug formulations. Next, we discuss a series of commonly dispensed pharmaceutical solutions.

Syrups

Syrups are solutions that contain high concentrations of sucrose or other sugars. For the pediatric population, little or no alcohol is added. The sugar is added to preserve the medication, to mask any bitter taste, and to improve the flavor. Examples are cough and antacid syrups. Syrups are either sugar based or are prepared by addition of artificial sweeteners.

Elixirs

Elixirs are solutions that contain alcohol, which may make up as much as 30% of the total solution. Because elixirs contain alcohol and water, different ingredients are initially dissolved in alcohol or water depending on the solubility of the ingredients. When making an elixir, it is imperative to add the aqueous solution to the alcoholic solution to maintain the high percentage of alcohol and to avoid precipitation of the ingredients originally dissolved in the alcoholic solution.

Elixirs have a sweet taste and should be stored in tightly sealed, amber containers away from heat or sunlight. Examples of elixirs include acetaminophen plus hydrocodone (Lortab Elixir), which is used for pain relief, and the steroid agent dexamethasone, which is mainly used for rheumatoid arthritis and allergies.

Tinctures

Tinctures also contain alcohol, but typically in smaller amounts than in an elixir (15–20% alcohol). Tinctures are prepared from vegetable materials or chemical substances. For example, a tincture of opium is used to decrease intestinal muscle contractions so as to reduce diarrhea; it may also be used as an analgesic medication. Tincture of opium contains morphine 10 mg/mL and 19% ethanol.

Aromatic Waters

Aromatic waters are saturated solutions of volatile oils (e.g., rose oil, peppermint oil) or other aromatic materials. Aromatic waters are often used for flavoring. An example is orange flower water.

Ophthalmic Solutions

Ophthalmic solutions allow instillation directly into the eyes to produce a local effect. Pharmaceutical eye drops are also included in this category. An example is the antibiotic gentamicin sulfate ophthalmic solution (Garamycin), which is used a few times per day as a topical treatment for eye infections.

Otic Solutions

Otic solutions allow direct administration of a drug into the ear to produce a local effect. These solutions may be used to remove earwax, treat ear infection, discharge material from an ear infection, or remove foreign agents from the ear. An example of an otic solution is the antibiotic ciprofloxacin (Cetraxal), which is used twice daily for 7 days to treat ear infection. Significant medication errors have occurred when an otic solution was inadvertently dispensed for ophthalmic administration. The potential for patient harm is significant, as the pH is dramatically different for each type of solution.

Topical Solutions

Topical solutions are not intended for oral use, but rather are applied on intact skin or mucous membranes. Ointments, creams, and lotions belong to this category of topical solutions. These pharmaceutically important solutions will be discussed further in the semisolids section of this chapter.

Liquids other than water are also used as solvents to make pharmaceutical solutions. Drugs that are poorly soluble in water may first be mixed with a cosolvent (alcohol or PEG) and then added to a hydrophilic solution. Dilution of the drugs in a cosolvent may result in precipitation. The following liquids are a few typical examples that are routinely used in compounding pharmacies.

Alcohol USP

Alcohol USP is available in different concentrations (94.9–99.5%) and is a good solvent for many organic compounds. For instance, dehydrated alcohol is 99.5% absolute alcohol and is almost free from water; it is useful when a water-free solvent is desired to make a solution. Due to the toxicity of alcohol, particularly for children, the FDA has recommended that the amount of alcohol in over-the-counter (OTC) products be minimized. For instance, OTC products that are intended for children younger than 6 years old and 6–12 years old should not contain more than 0.5% and 5% alcohol in a solution, respectively.

Glycerin USP (Glycerol)

Glycerin is a viscous, odorless, and colorless liquid with a sweet taste. It has a high viscosity and is largely used in pharmaceutical formulations. As mentioned elsewhere in this chapter, the names glycerol and glycerin may be used interchangeably; however, glycerol generally refers to the pure chemical form and glycerin refers to the commercially available product. Because of its hydrophilic property, glycerin is soluble in water and alcohol and is insoluble in hydrocarbons. It has a very low toxicity and, as a result, is used widely in pharmaceuticals. Because of glycerin's osmotic effect on the colon and low toxicity effect, it is also administered as a suppository (2–3 g) and has a rapid effect on bowel movement (within 30 minutes), particularly in the pediatric population.

Polyethylene Glycol

Polyethylene glycol is miscible in water and alcohol. A numbering system is used to describe the properties of PEG. For instance, "PEG 3350" reflects the actual molecular weight of PEG. The lower the PEG number, the lower the melting point and the more water-soluble the PEG base. PEG, with and without electrolytes, is also used for colon cleansing to facilitate colorectal procedures and operations. For example, GoLytely contains PEG and electrolytes in powder form. It is dispensed to the patient in a large container; the patient later adds a liquid, such as water, to dissolve the powder to make a laxative solution. A 4-liter solution can be consumed over 3 hours to have an effective evacuation of the GI tract. While low doses of PEG are used as a laxative for treatment of constipation, larger doses (4-L solution) are not recommended for routine treatment of constipation. Miralax, available on the market as a laxative OTC, is PEG 3350.

Parenteral Solutions

Parenteral solutions of drugs produce rapid, accurate, and predictable therapeutic outcomes in a very short time frame. Within this group one can find drugs intended to be delivered by the IV, IM, SC, intradermal (ID), and intrathecal (IT) routes. Some drug formulations must be given as parenteral injections because the drug needs to be delivered in its active form. An example is infliximab (Remicade), an injectable monoclonal antibody that acts against tumor necrosis factor (TNF) in the treatment of rheumatoid arthritis, Crohn's disease, and some other conditions. A parenteral drug is also the best choice in an emergency situation when a patient is unconscious or unable to absorb or retain a medication orally. However, a parenteral injection also has drawbacks, such as the potential for infection, pain upon injection, and the need for a skilled healthcare provider to administer the drug.

While the IV route is very valuable in emergency situations to produce a rapid onset, the rate of administration of the drug through the IV must be confirmed as appropriate for each drug. Some drugs may be administered rapidly, such as epinephrine, whereas others must be administered at a slow constant rate, such as nitroglycerin. The risk of adverse effects is greater with this delivery route because the solution is being directly administered intravenously. Oily solutions or insoluble drugs are not suitable for IV injections. In many cases, the SC route is suitable for poorly soluble solutions or suspensions. However, SC injections can cause pain or necrosis and are not suitable for large-volume injection. By comparison, IM injections are suitable for larger volumes, oily solutions, and some irritating substances. Of note, some SC injections, such as insulin, and some IM injections, such as EpiPen (auto-injector), are conveniently self-administered by patients.

The intradermal route of administration is suitable for injections into the corium of the skin. This route is used for many vaccinations and tuberculin and allergy skin tests. For example, the influenza virus vaccine (Fluzone), which has a small volume (e.g., 0.1 mL/dose), may be given by the ID route. Because the epidermis and dermis are almost at the surface of the skin, the needle used for ID injections is very short (26 or 27 gauge).

Stability and compatibility of the drug solution are of paramount importance for parenteral solutions. For instance, ampicillin Na (Apo-Ampi, in Canada) is stable for 72 hours in a refrigerator but when it is mixed in a D_5W solution (D_5W solution is an acidic solution that has a pH between 3.5 and 6.5, is isotonic, and contains 5% D-glucose), its stability is reduced to 4 hours. Regarding compatibility, if you add the sodium salt of a weak acid to an acidic IV solution (or a salt of a weak base to a basic IV solution), or if you add a negatively charged drug (such as heparin to flush an IV line) to a solution that contains a positively charged drug (such as an aminoglycoside antibiotic), precipitation can occur in the solution. To avoid significant patient harm, solutions that have precipitated should not be administered parenterally.

Intrathecal (IT) administration occurs via a spinal needle or an indwelling intrathecal catheter into the spinal canal. The IT route is useful to bypass the blood–brain barrier and the blood–cerebrospinal fluid (CSF) barrier and allow the drug to rapidly reach the CNS. This consideration is particularly important when treating life-threatening meningitis and other acute CNS infections. Benefits of IT administration include lower doses and the production of fewer systemic effects. Many drugs, such as anesthetics, opioids, and antibiotics, can be given intrathecally.

With parenteral solutions, the type of container holding the drug is also important. For instance, containers made of plastic polyvinyl chloride (PVC) should be avoided with nitroglycerin (because nitroglycerin migrates into PVC) or lipid-soluble drugs. Polypropylene containers are better choices because they contain only a limited amount of plastic. Photolysis (i.e., degradation of a drug by light) is a challenge for drugs such as amphotericin B (Fungizone, in Canada) and furosemide (Lasix). As a precaution, these drugs are usually packaged and stored in amber containers.

It is important to be familiar with the gauge size of needles used to deliver parenteral solutions. The gauge size refers to the outer diameter of the needle. As a rule, the smaller the gauge size number, the larger the needle. Therefore, a 20-gauge needle is larger than a 25-gauge needle. Needles of gauges 25 and 22 are used for SC and IM injections, respectively. A 16- or 18-gauge needle is used to deliver parenteral solutions.

> ### Learning Bridge 8.6
>
> Dr. Amy Johnson, the attending physician at the Northwest Clinic, calls you to prepare a pain medication. She wants to prescribe Lortab Elixir for her patient David, who is a 36-year-old carpenter. David has experienced back pain for the past 3 days—pain that has significantly interfered with his daily physical activities. The prescription reads:
>
> > Lortab Elixir: 7.5/500 mg per 15 mL
> >
> > Sig: One tablespoonful every 4 hours; if the patient experiences more pain, take extra 2 tablespoonsful prn.
> >
> > Disp: 480 mL
> >
> > Refills: 7
>
> Dr. Johnson explains that the elixir has acetaminophen as an ingredient and can help the patient if he experiences more pain. She states that she has already explained to the patient why he might need to take the extra 2 tablespoonsful.
>
> There are a few problems associated with this prescription. Try to answer and justify the following questions and then discuss your responses with your preceptor.
>
> **A.** Is this medication in the right dosage form for this patient?
>
> **B.** Is there any problem with the prescription?
>
> **C.** How much alcohol does the elixir contain?

Water for Pharmaceutical Preparations

Water has a valuable place in pharmaceutical solutions, as it is inexpensive and is a good solvent for most inorganic and organic compounds. The following is a discussion of useful water preparations.

Purified Water USP

Purified Water USP is prepared by distillation (vaporization and then condensation of vaporized water into liquid water) or ion exchange (a de-ionization process where cation and anion particles are removed from water). Most of the solid particles (contaminants) in the water are removed. Purified Water should have total solids (contaminants) in concentrations less than 10 parts per million (10 ppm; i.e., for every 10 million water molecules, there should not be more than 10 particles of solids). Purified Water should have a pH in the range of 5–7. This solvent is not a good choice for parenteral or ophthalmic products because it is not considered sterilized.

Water for Injection USP

Water for Injection USP is prepared by distillation or reverse osmosis with the same restriction as purified water—that is, no more than 10 ppm contaminants. In addition, it is pyrogen free (particularly the reverse osmosis effectively removes viruses and bacteria). Water for Injection is primarily used by manufacturers of parenteral solutions that will be sterilized after their preparation. It should be stored at the appropriate temperature to avoid any microbial growth and should be used within 24 hours of preparation.

Sterile Water for Injection USP

Sterile Water for Injection USP is similar to Water for Injection, but the water is sterilized first and then packaged in a single-dose container of 1 liter or smaller. Sterile Water for Injection USP is not isotonic and, as a result, is used only as a diluent or a vehicle when reconstituting already sterilized injectable drugs. Sterilization of water and an accurate sterility testing method are of paramount importance. Indeed, microbiological instability (or growth of microbes in products) is the biggest problem in sterile and injectable dosage forms. In September 2012, a tragic meningitis outbreak was traced to contaminated products prepared at the New England Compounding Center (NECC) in Massachusetts. Inadequate sterility testing methods may have caused the contamination. Unfortunately, products from this compounding facility were dispensed in many states and as of June 2013, 50 patients had lost their lives.

Bacteriostatic Water for Injection USP

As the name indicates, Bacteriostatic Water for Injection USP contains one or more antibacterial agents. The container must specify the name and concentration of the antibacterial agents present in the water. In addition, because of the presence of antibacterial agents, Bacteriostatic Water for Injection USP should not be used to deliver large volumes of parenteral solution. Generally if more than 5 mL water is required for a parenteral preparation, Sterile Water for Injection should be used.

Sterile Purified Water USP

Sterile Purified Water USP is sterilized and purified, but it is not used in parenteral preparations. To use water for parenteral solutions, the word "injection" must be associated with the water (such as Sterile Water for Injection or Bacteriostatic Water for Injection).

Sulfites are used as preservatives in injections, such as lidocaine hydrochloride and epinephrine injections. As approximately 0.2% of the U.S. population is vulnerable to allergy reaction to sulfites, use of these preparations warrants caution if an allergy is suspected.

Methods of Sterilization

Sterilization is the process by which contaminants, especially microorganisms, are removed from or destroyed within a solution. Technically, absolute sterility is not possible, but the methods described here accomplish a significant level of sterility to ensure safety. Sterilization can be performed using various methods, depending on the volume of fluid to be sterilized and the resources available.

To sterilize small volumes of solution, specific filters can be implemented. Filters are identified by the size of particulate that is allowed to pass through the filter. Typically, a filter membrane with a pore size of 0.22 micron or smaller is utilized. Filters should be wetted and tested prior to use to confirm their viability. The solution is then drawn into a syringe, the appropriate filter is screwed onto the end of the syringe, and a needle is attached to the opposite end of the filter. The solution is filtered as it passes through the syringe, through the filter, and into an empty sterile vial.

Larger volumes of solutions can be sterilized using steam sterilization in an autoclave, where products are exposed for approximately 15 minutes to heat in the range of 121–124°C. The temperature and pressure ensure denaturation of proteins and enzymes, thereby rendering any microorganisms destroyed.

Electrolytes and Nonelectrolyte Solutions

Similar to pharmaceutical solutions, the fluid of our body contains water plus dissolved molecules such as glucose and urea and ions such as Na^+, Cl^-, K^+, Mg_2^+, HCO_3^-, and $HPO4_2^-$. We have to maintain the appropriate concentrations of each electrolyte because even a small change may lead to serious consequences for specific extracellular or intracellular processes. Electrolytes and nonelectrolyte solutions are administered to reestablish the balance necessary to maintain bodily functions. If the patient's condition is critical, the solutions are administered parenterally. If the patient's condition is not critical, oral solutions may be prepared. The concentration of the dissolved molecules (such as glucose or urea) is measured in units of mg/dL (milligrams per deciliter). The concentrations of the electrolytes in the body fluids and in intravenous solutions are often expressed in units of mEq/L (milliequivalents per liter). An exception is phosphate. Because a phosphate injection contains a mixture of phosphate salts (monobasic potassium phosphate, KH_2PO_4, and dipotassium phosphate, K_2HPO_4), it is more convenient to express the concentration of phosphate in units of mmol/L (millimoles per liter).

Dispersed systems are solutions that contain undissolved or immiscible solutes. These solutions include suspensions, emulsions, gels, and aerosols.

Suspensions

Suspensions are dispersed systems created by suspending a finely divided solid (dispersed phase) in a liquid (continuous phase). Suspensions are used for topical, oral, and injectable solutions. When a drug is insoluble or poorly soluble, a suspension dosage formulation is warranted. Some suspensions are available in ready-to-use forms, in which particles are dispersed through a liquid vehicle. Other suspensions are provided in dried form (powder) as unit dose and multidose formulations that, upon reconstitution with a liquid (often purified water, in the case of an oral suspension), form a suspension. A typical example is azithromycin (Zithromax) powder for suspension for children. A suspension may increase the storage stability of the medications for weeks, but no suspension is really stable.

When measuring a suspension, it is important to use a syringe rather than a cylinder to measure the liquid. In addition, if less than 1 mL of liquid will be administered, use a small syringe rather than a cylinder to avoid losing any amount of the suspension. This consideration is particularly important when you dispense a suspension that includes a controlled substance.

In a suspension, if the undissolved particles are dispersed in a liquid that has lower density than the particles, the particles will settle out. In contrast, if the particles are dispersed in a liquid that has a higher density than the particles, the particles will rise to the surface and form a "cream."

Suspensions are coarse dispersions in which a dispersed phase (internal phase), which consists of insoluble particles, is dispersed uniformly throughout a continuous phase (an external phase). Particle size plays an important role in the formation of a suspension. The particle size of a suspension should be small to minimize sedimentation, yet larger than 1 μm (often in the range of 1 to 50 μm). Settling and aggregation may result in a cake formation. Caking (see Figure 8.20) is a problem with suspension dosage forms, although addition of a surface active agent facilitates dispersion of a suspension.

Suspensions are conveniently administered to infants, children, and elderly patients who have difficulty digesting tablet or capsule dosage forms. Use of a suspension dosage form may produce a higher rate of bioavailability of drugs than administration via capsules or tablets. Other advantages of suspensions are their ability to mask a bitter taste and to control the release rate of a drug. The selection of the right inert ingredients such as surfactants and viscosity-enhancing agents is important. As mentioned earlier, particle size also influences the bioavailability and pharma-cokinetics of the product. As a result, analytical experiments (e.g., using a particle size meter or viscometer) are undertaken by manufacturers to characterize the suspension formulation. A suspension is properly formulated when the dispersed phase is easily resuspended and able to settle rapidly after shaking the suspension.

In making a suspension, it is important to add a suspending agent to increase the viscosity and reduce the sedimentation of particles. Potential suspending agents include methylcellulose (a synthetic agent), acacia (a natural agent), gelatin, sugars (glucose, fructose), powdered cellulose, and veegum.

There are some challenges with suspensions. For instance, these formulations can be difficult to prepare. In addition, when their viscosity is high, they can prolong gastric emptying time and slow drug dissolution, which may result in slower drug absorption. The suspension may also be difficult to pour. As a result, it is important to maintain the viscosity within an optimal range.

Flocculation is an aggregation process that causes the dispersed particles to adhere to each other and form larger-size aggregates. The large surface area of particles in a suspension is thermodynamically unstable, which causes particles to clump together. Flocculation is not a precipitation process because it is established when particles are suspended, while precipitation is established when particles are dissolved in a solution. However, flocculation is a desirable phenomenon in a suspension because it is a reversible process. In contrast, caking of suspensions and precipitation in suspension are not desirable processes. The caking process (a deflocculation process) causes particles to form a closed aggregated structure in which the smaller particles fill the void volumes between the larger particles (see Figure 8.20). It is very difficult to resuspend particles after caking has occurred. Increasing the viscosity or reducing the particle size will not assist in preventing the caking process; instead, addition of a flocculating agent is the best way to prevent the caking process. Some flocculating agents (e.g., KCl and NaCl electrolytes, ionic and non-ionic surfactants, citrates) decrease the zeta potential of the suspended charged particles and promote flocculation.

The particles in an ideal suspension will have the following properties:

- Uniform size of particles
- Remain separated (to minimize sedimentation)
- Avoid interacting with each other
- Resuspend easily upon shaking and settle down slowly
- Physically and chemically stable during the storage shelf life
- Easy to pour

To make an ideal suspension, select a particle size that is as small as possible and a disperse medium that is as viscous as possible while maintaining the properties identified above. Suspensions for parenteral injection (which include many vaccines) must be stable upon sterilization.

The sedimentation rate can be calculated to determine a successful suspension formulation. Stokes's equation is used to calculate the sedimentation rate:

$$V = \frac{d^2(p_s - p_o)g}{18\eta} \qquad (8.10)$$

where

V = sedimentation rate (in cm/s)

d = diameter of particles

p_s = density of the disperse phase

p_o = density of the continuous phase

g = gravity

η = viscosity of the disperse phase

As Equation 8.10 indicates, assuming other parameters are unchanged, a higher viscosity leads to a lower sedimentation rate, and a higher density of the dispersed phase (p_s) results in a higher sedimentation rate. Because the density of the particles (p_s) remains constant, it is more practical to change the density of the continuous phase to reduce or increase the sedimentation rate. As Equation 8.10 indicates, if the densities of the dispersed phase and the continuous phase are equal, the rate of sedimentation becomes zero.

Many physicochemical properties are involved in the formulation of a suspension; in turn, many ingredients are added to maintain a good-quality suspension. These ingredients include surfactants, an optimal continuous phase, suspending agents, sweetening or flavoring agents, flocculating agents, and preservatives. Always counsel your patients to shake a suspension before administering it.

Thixotropic Suspensions

A thixotropic suspension has the ability to be viscous when it is stored on the shelf but becomes a fluid liquid upon shaking. Interestingly, a thixotropic suspension remains fluid long enough to be administered but slowly reverts to its original viscosity.

Sustained-Release Suspensions

Sustained-release suspensions are created when the duration of effect of an insoluble drug must be extended after its administration. Typically, this can be accomplished by encapsulating the drug in a coating to slow its absorption and extend the drug effect. An extended drug effect can result in less frequent dosing and increased adherence. For example, methylphenidate extended-release suspension for oral administration (Quillivant XR) provides once-daily dosing for treatment of attention-deficit/hyperactivity disorder. Exenetide extended-release suspension for SC injection (Bydureon) provides once every 7 days dosing for treatment of type 2 diabetes.

Otic Suspensions

Most otic preparations are solutions. Otic suspensions are formulated when an insoluble drug formulation is needed specifically for otic use. Steroid and antibiotic combinations, such as Cortisporin (neomycin, polymyxin B, and hydrocortisone), are suspension formulations because of the insolubility of the corticosteroid. Administration is typically completed with the patient's head at an uncomfortable angle, so it is prudent to administer the suspension promptly after shaking to ensure a consistent dose.

Rectal Suspensions

Rectal suspensions are generally administered in an enema formulation. The bioavailability in the rectal area can be significant but is typically poor with suspension enemas. The rectal route of administration is more useful if the drug action is intended locally and absorption is important for effectiveness. Mesalamine rectal suspension enema (Rowasa), for example, is used to treat ulcerative colitis.

Learning Bridge 8.7

On Monday, September 1, at 10:30 AM, Amy brings a prescription to your pharmacy for her son Nick. Nick is a 3-year-old boy who for the past 3 days has been complaining of sore throat and pain in his throat, particularly when he tries to eat food. Nick's pediatrician believes the sore throat is caused by a bacterium called *Streptococcus pyogenes* and has prescribed azithromycin suspension, immediate release (Zithromax) for Nick. The prescription is as follows:

> Azithromycin 200 mg/5 mL suspension
> Sig: give 10 mL daily × 5 days

Your preceptor directs you to the azithromycin powder and asks you to reconstitute the powder with distilled water to make this concentration. You have no idea how you should reconstitute the medication, but you find a package insert inside the azithromycin cardboard package.

A. Read the package insert and find out how much distilled water you should add to make the 200 mg/5 mL suspension. The bottle has 1,200 mg azithromycin powder.

B. After doing an accurate calculation, you realize that your final volume will not be enough for the stated course of therapy (10 mL × 5 days). You discuss this issue with your preceptor and suggest asking Amy to let you know how much Nick weighs. Amy tells you that Nick weighs 37 lb. Use the package insert to see how much distilled water you need to add and how many mL/day Nick should take. Show your calculation and an accurate suggested dose (if any) to your preceptor.

C. Amy tells your preceptor that Nick has also been using Mylanta since August 23 and needs to take this medication until September 8 for his upset stomach that is accompanied by gas. She asks your preceptor whether there would be any potential interaction between these two drugs. Would it be any problem for Nick to take both azithromycin and Mylanta simultaneously? Do a literature search (online or hard copy) at your site and justify your answer to your preceptor.

Emulsions

An emulsion is formed when a liquid is dispersed in an immiscible liquid. Because the two liquids are immiscible, there will be small droplets in the continuous phase. There are two forms of emulsions: oil-in-water emulsions (o/w) and water-in-oil (w/o) emulsions (**Figure 8.22**). An o/w emulsion includes a hydrophilic continuous phase and a hydrophobic dispersed phase; it is miscible with hydrophilic liquids. A w/o emulsion includes a hydrophobic continuous phase and a hydrophilic dispersed phase; it is miscible with hydrophobic liquids. An emulsion is physically unstable, so there is a risk that the two phases in an emulsion might separate from each other—a phenomenon referred to as "breaking" (an irreversible process). The breaking process occurs because the disperse phase tends to coalesce into larger and larger droplets, which finally leads to separation of the phases. The function of an emulsifier is to prevent the breaking process.

Because bacteria are capable of degrading non-ionic and anionic emulsifying agents, it is important to prevent any microbial growth by adding a preservative, such as benzoic acid (benzoate), to emulsions. Typical emulsifying agents include acacia and polysorbate 20 and 80. Acacia is a natural emulsifying agent that provides a stable emulsion with low viscosity; it is used in o/w emulsions, particularly those intended for internal use. Polysorbate 20 and 80 are synthetic emulsifiers.

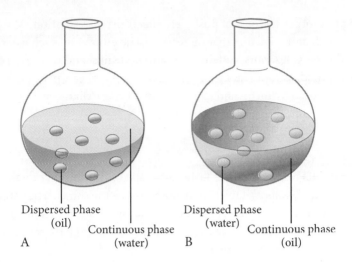

Figure 8.22 Two forms of emulsions. (A) Oil-in-water (o/w) emulsion. (B) Water-in-oil (w/o) emulsion.

Mechanisms to stabilize emulsions either lower interfacial tension or add charges on ions so that they repel each other and thereby minimize the coalescing (joining) process. For an o/w emulsion, one can use a hydrophilic emulsifier (e.g., sodium lauryl sulfate, triethanolamine stearate, sodium oleate, glyceryl monostearate). A hydrophobic emulsifier (e.g., calcium palmitate, sorbitan esters, cholesterol, wool fats) is useful for a w/o emulsion. Non-ionic emulsifiers (e.g., polysorbate and sorbitan) are used often, as they are nontoxic and are less sensitive to electrolytes and pH.

Methylcellulose is a thickening agent that is added to an emulsion to reduce a creaming process (recall that creaming is a reversible process). It is possible to reverse an o/w emulsion to a w/o emulsion. For example, adding sodium stearate stabilizes an o/w emulsion. Adding calcium chloride (or calcium stearate) then reverses this process, converting the product back to a w/o emulsion. One method for making an emulsion is the dry gum method, which combines ingredients in a 4:2:1 ratio (i.e., 4 × oil: 2 × water: 1 × dry gum emulsifier). When dispensing an emulsion formulation, a "shake well" direction should be prominently displayed on the container and the patient should be instructed to shake the product prior to measuring each dose.

Solid Dosage Forms

Many physiological and chemical factors affect absorption of a solid dosage form. Physiological factors include surface area at the site of absorption (i.e., small intestine versus large intestine), blood flow to the site of absorption (i.e., blood flow to the brain and liver as opposed to skeletal muscles), and gastric emptying rate. In addition, factors such as water solubility, drug concentration at the site of absorption, ionization states, and disintegration and dissolution rates are crucial if the product is to achieve a maximum absorption.

Passive diffusion from the GI tract significantly facilitates drug absorption for most drugs. As a result, absorption of drugs is favored for products that exhibit a hydrophobic property, minimal ionization state, and preference for absorption at a site with a larger surface area. For instance, drugs that are more hydrophobic and less ionized are better absorbed than hydrophilic or ionized drugs. By the same token, acidic drugs are better absorbed from an acidic environment (stomach, with pH 1–2) than from an alkaline environment (large intestine, with pH 8–9). Similarly, drugs are better absorbed from the small intestine, which has a larger surface area, than from the stomach or large intestine, which have smaller surface areas. Even if a drug is hydrophobic or less ionized in the stomach, increased absorption of that agent in the small intestine is possible due to the significant role that surface area plays in drug absorption.

Gastric emptying is another factor that positively affects drug absorption. The gastric emptying rate is affected by many factors. Factors that increase gastric emptying, such as presence of certain foods (raw fruits and vegetables, nuts, caffeine-containing drinks, and whole-wheat bread facilitate gastric emptying), medications (many antibiotics cause diarrhea), pH of ingested fluid (acidic foods such as tomato or orange juice), and exercise, can all cause diarrhea. Conversely, foods with high viscosity (high fiber) prolong gastric emptying time.

Tablets

Tablets contain ingredients to maintain the taste and shape of the pills. While the active ingredients may be the same in two tablets, both tablets may not produce the same therapeutic outcome in a given time. For instance, a chewable tablet has a different formulation than a controlled-release tablet, even if both contain the same active ingredient. As a result, the therapeutic effect may arrive more rapidly with a chewable tablet compared with a controlled-release tablet. Tablets are preferred dosage forms because they increase patients' compliance and have better drug stability, yet may pose significant challenges including poor water solubility, local irritation of the GI mucosa, and decreased absorption or bioavailability.

Multiple ingredients are packed inside a tablet, so the following nomenclature is used to describe a defect in making tablets:

- Picking: excessive moisture in the granulation
- Mottling: degraded drug
- Capping: air entrapped in a tablet
- Sticking: excessive moisture in the granulation
- Comminution of a powder: breaking powder particles into small pieces

It is important to perform a quality check on manufactured tablets. The following tests are carried out to ensure the quality of tablets:

- Weight uniformity and content uniformity tests ensure that each tablet contains the intended amount of drug substances.
- Disintegration and dissolution tests address whether the active ingredient will be able to be released from the tablet.
- Hardness and friability tests consider whether the tablet will be able to withstand fracture during manufacturing, packaging, and shipping.
- The elegant appearance and microbial quality of the tablet are assessed.
- The tablet should be packed in a safe manner.

Chewable Tablets

When a faster dissolution rate is desired, chewable tablets are manufactured. With this formulation, a physical and mechanical disruption such as chewing disintegrates and releases the active ingredient from the tablet. Examples include antacid tablets that upon chewing produce quick relief of heartburn. Sugars such as glucose, sorbitol, maltose, and lactose are used in the manufacturing of chewable tablets. One sugar frequently used in chewable tablets is mannitol, which, upon dissolving in the mouth, produces a sweet and cool taste. Many vitamins and antacids are available as chewable tablets. For instance, the combined antacid calcium carbonate and magnesium hydroxide (700/300 mg; Mylanta Ultra) is a chewable tablet. It is important to counsel patients to chew the tablet, rather than swallow it, to receive the full pharmacological effect.

Coated Tablets

Coated tablets are formulated to protect tablets from disintegration or dissolution caused by humidity or from a physiological site in which it is not desirable to have the active ingredient released. Several types of coated tablets are available, including film-coated, sugar-coated, and enteric-coated versions. Enteric-coated tablets (the most commonly used forms) protect the active ingredient from decomposition in the stomach. The coating is sometimes used to exclusively protect others who are not using the medication. For instance, the 5-alpha-reductase inhibitor finasteride (Proscar), used to treat symptomatic benign prostatic hyperplasia (BPH), has coating to protect a pregnant woman who inadvertently comes in contact with finasteride. Another enteric-coated tablet is acetyl salicylic acid (Ecotrin), in which the coating is intended to decrease gastrointestinal discomfort.

Capsules

Similar to tablets, capsules contain multiple ingredients encompassed within a gelatin cover. Two general forms of capsules exist: (1) hard gelatin capsules (HGCs), which are used for solid formulations, and (2) soft gelatin capsules (SGCs), which are used for liquid or semisolid formulations. SGCs are made of 30% glycerol, and glycerol or sorbitol is used to plasticize the shell of this type of capsule to make it soft. The high glycerol content, however, leads to a high hygroscopic problem. Oxygen-sensitive drugs or emulsions should not be packed inside the SGC due to potential instability. HGCs are used more often than SGCs both by pharmaceutical companies and in compounding centers. During a clinical trial, a drug product is also manufactured with hard gelatin so that the investigators can compare it with other available capsules in the market.

Gelatin is produced by partial hydrolysis of collagen proteins obtained from animals. It is odorless, tasteless, colorless, and insoluble in most organic solvents. Gelatin can swell and absorb water in amounts up to 10 times its weight. Thus one of the issues with using gelatin is that it can absorb water; when it does, capsules may stick to each other and provide an environment for microbial growth. To protect the capsule's shell from mold growth, preservatives such as benzoate are added. In addition, most capsule formulations contain a desiccant (an agent that maintains a state of dryness). However, when water is lost from the gelatin, the capsule becomes brittle and can crack. Retaining water in capsule shells, in contrast, can ensure stability for the capsules.

The acidity or basicity of their ingredients may also affect capsules. For instance, a low or high pH is known to hydrolyze gelatin. Examples of ingredients with these characteristics include vitamin A, vitamin E, and digoxin. One notable advantage of SGCs is their ability to contain poorly water-soluble drugs because of their good absorption by the GI tract. While capsules are often more expensive than tablets, capsules mask the taste and odor of the ingredients and protect light-sensitive ingredients. Capsules also use surfactants to increase the bioavailability of water-insoluble drugs. Surfactants used in capsules include sodium lauryl sulfate and sodium docusate.

Different sizes of empty gelatin capsules are available on the market to be filled at compounding pharmacies. These sizes range from 000 (largest) to 5 (smallest). The following empty gelatin capsule sizes can hold the volume indicated within parentheses: 000 (1.4 mL); 00 (0.95 mL); 0 (0.68 mL); 1 (0.50 mL); 2 (0.37 mL); 3 (0.30 mL); 4 (0.21 mL); and 5 (0.13 mL).

Semisolid Dosage Forms

Semisolid dosage forms are widely used by prescribers and patients to achieve the most desirable pharmacologic effect. Semisolids are applied to an affected area to produce a therapeutic outcome, a protective action, or a cosmetic function. They are used in the delivery of drugs through the skin, eye and ear, rectum, nasal mucosa, vagina, and urethral membranes. The application area plays an important role in the drug's absorption because of the physiological variations in the epidermal layers. Different topical vehicles, as explained in the next section, exert local effects by releasing their active ingredients onto the skin's surface. The drug then diffuses and is absorbed through the skin's different physiological layers.

Depending on the semisolid's physiochemical properties, the vehicle may remain attached to the application area for an extended time period before it is removed by washing or by other means. In such a case, the drug delivery at the application area is prolonged. However, semisolid dosage forms should be elegant in appearance, should not be gritty, and should not irritate skin. The vehicle that represents the base in which the drug is delivered plays a crucial role in achieving a successful therapeutic outcome.

Semisolid dosage forms are often preferred over other dosage forms because of their unique topical delivery method, easy application, rapid formulation or compounding, and bypassing of first-pass metabolism in the liver or drug degradation in the gastrointestinal tract. Vehicles for semisolid dosage forms include ointments, creams, gels, pastes, and lotions.

Ointments

Ointments are used for external application to skin or mucous membranes. While they serve as vehicles to deliver a drug, they also function as skin protection and emollients (i.e., to soften the skin). An ointment's characteristics include having more oil than water, being "sticky" or "greasy," staying longer on the skin (slow skin absorption), and melting at body temperature. Despite the fact that ointments are the most potent vehicles because of their occlusive nature, most patients do not like ointments because they are "greasy." Four different types of ointment bases may be used:

- Oleaginous bases (hydrocarbon bases)
- Absorption bases
- Water-removable bases
- Water-soluble bases

Oleaginous Bases (Hydrocarbon Bases)

Due to the hydrocarbon properties of oleaginous bases, they increase skin hydration by reducing the rate of water loss from the skin. Such products absorb less than 5% water and, as a result, they do not become rancid. However, they are difficult to wash off with water. Examples include petrolatum USP and white petrolatum USP. Vaseline is made of petrolatum USP. Many antibiotics that are suitable for topical applications are compatible with petrolatum.

Absorption Bases

Absorption bases are difficult to wash off, but they are less "greasy" than oleaginous bases. They do not provide the same occlusion (skin hydration) as oleaginous bases. Absorption bases are useful because one can incorporate a small volume of a drug solution and then further incorporate this mixture with an oleaginous base (that is why they are called absorption bases). Examples include lanolin oil and cold creams, which are used in topical and cosmetic preparations.

Water-Removable Bases

These o/w emulsions resemble creams. As their name indicates, water-removable bases are easily washed with water and can be diluted with water or aqueous solutions. Examples include hydrophilic ointments and vanishing creams.

Water-Soluble Bases

These bases are easily washable (do not contain any water-insoluble components) and are good choices for both water-soluble and-water insoluble drugs. Often a mixture of different percentages of polyethylene glycol with different molecular weights is used. For instance, PEG with a molecular weight less than 600 is a liquid; PEG with a molecular weight greater than 1,000 is a wax-like material; and PEG with a molecular weight between 600 and 1,000 is a semisolid. Examples of water-soluble bases include 40% PEG 3350 (solid) and 60% PEG 400 (liquid), which makes a suitable ointment.

Creams

Creams, similar to ointments, are used for external application to skin or mucous membranes and serve as emollients to soften or sooth the affected areas. The drugs are dispersed in a suitable base, often in an o/w emulsion or in alcohol if the drug is water soluble. Creams have more water than oil (most creams are o/w emulsions), and they are less "sticky" or "greasy" and less viscous than ointments. Creams do not provide the same effective occlusive effects that ointments provide, however.

After application to the affected area, the water in a cream evaporates and, as a result, the cream's active ingredients can relieve inflamed skin. Creams spread easily on the skin, so they are suitable for covering larger surface areas. In addition, creams are quickly absorbed in the skin. Many patients prefer creams over ointments because creams are easier to apply, spread better, and are removed by water.

Gels

Gels are suspensions (with a particle size in the range of 1 nm to 0.5 μm) made of macromolecules (often large organic molecules) interpenetrated by a solvent to produce a high degree of three-dimensional cross-linking structure. Two forms of gels are available: water based and organic solvent based. These formulations are transparent or semitransparent, are nongreasy, and are particularly useful for application to hairy areas. Gels that are formed by creation of covalent bonds between their macromolecules are irreversible gels, whereas gels that are formed by creation of hydrogen bonds between their macromolecules are heat-reversible gels.

Pastes

Pastes are very thick and stiff and are intended for external application to skin. They are actually ointments to which a high concentration of an insoluble solid has been added; as a consequence, they are less penetrating than ointments. Pastes are less greasy than ointments because the solid particles in pastes absorb the fluid hydrocarbon material in the preparation. The high viscosity makes pastes adhere to the skin surface for a longer period of time. Similar to ointments, they form a smooth water-impermeable film at the site of application. Levigation, in which the drug is ground to a fine powder and incorporated into a base with or without the addition of a liquid, is often used to produce pastes.

Lotions

Lotions are commonly used for topical application on the hands, body, and face. These products are usually o/w emulsions, although w/o lotions are sometimes compounded. Lotions are the least potent vehicle for topical application but are useful in hairy and large application areas. Because they take the form of powder-in-water, it is important to counsel patients to shake the container before each application to apply a desirable therapeutic concentration at the affected area.

Suppositories

Utilizing the chemical properties of a suppository base, suppositories dissolve or melt at body temperature. These products have a series of advantages over other dosage forms. Notably, they bypass the first-pass effect (to avoid hepatic degradation), and the active ingredient is absorbed through the rectal mucosa and into the circulation through the rectal veins. Suppositories are also useful when drugs cannot be administered orally (e.g., for infants, patients in coma, patients with a vomiting condition, patients with GI problems). Approximately 50% of the drug that is absorbed from the rectum will avoid the first-pass metabolism because a major drug metabolism enzyme, CYP3A4, is present in the upper intestine but not in the lower intestine. For this reason, it is important to counsel patients to not insert the suppository very far in the rectum. Disadvantages of suppositories include irregular or incomplete rectal absorption and potential irritation of the rectal mucosa (the latter point has to do with the suppository's base). Forms of suppositories vary based on the site of application.

It is relatively easy to compound suppositories. First, clean the mold with soap and water, and then dry the mold. Mineral oil is often used to lubricate a mold in the fusion method of making suppositories. The total weight of a suppository for adult patients should be 2,000 mg (including the drug). A specific amount of a base—for instance, cocoa butter—is used and melted at 35°C. The melted base is mixed with a specific drug and is poured into the mold cavities. It is important to slightly overfill the cavities, as some shrinking will occur upon cooling of the base. In addition, it is wise to calculate the amount of base and drug with 1–2 extra suppositories in case there is a loss of material during the compounding procedures.

Rectal Use

Rectal suppositories are cylindrical and have bullet-like shape; the finished products weigh 2 g for adults and less for children. Rectal suppositories can be used by patients who cannot take oral medications or for pediatric patients to stimulate bowel movement. As mentioned earlier, rectal absorption can be irregular. Moreover, certain suppository bases such as PEG can cause irritation of the rectal mucosa—PEG is water soluble and can draw water from the rectum and, as a result, can cause irritation.

Vaginal Use

Vaginal suppositories are oval and weigh 3–5 g. They are often used for local effects to treat bacterial or fungal infections (although systemic effects may occur as well), to reinstate the vaginal mucosa, or as contraceptives. An example is triaconazole (Terazol 3). Vaginal suppositories should be inserted as far as possible without causing any pain or discomfort. Because the vaginal pH is acidic (around 4.5), most vaginal suppositories are buffered at a pH of 4.5. The water-soluble PEG is the base most commonly used in vaginal suppositories. Vaginal tablets (vaginal inserts) are more common than vaginal suppositories due to their stability and ease of manufacturing.

Urethral Use

Urethral suppositories are approximately 5 cm (female) or 12 cm (male) in length and are pellet shaped. They are often used for local infections in the male urethra and, to a much lesser extent, for erectile dysfunction. For example, alprostadil (Muse Pellet) is used to achieve an erection.

Suppository Bases

The suppository base plays an important role in the release of the drug into rectum. Similar to the case with different ointment bases, selection of the right suppository base is crucial to produce an optimal therapeutic outcome. A good suppository base should not melt at temperatures less than 30°C and should be compatible with a variety of drugs, be inert (harmless and inactive), and be easily compounded in a pharmacy. Rectal fluid is neutral (pH 7) with no buffer capacity; the vaginal pH is 4.5. The latter pH ensures that most of the microbial organisms do not grow at this acidic pH.

Cocoa Butter

Cocoa butter is a fat-soluble, hydrophobic base that melts at a temperature between 33°C and 35°C (ideal for suppositories). It is a mixture of glycerides and must be stored in the refrigerator. This base is a good choice for rectal suppositories but less ideal for vaginal or urethral formulations. Cocoa butter is very useful for hydrophilic drugs because its hydrophobic nature allows for faster release of hydrophilic drugs—a beneficial characteristic when a rapid effect is desired. A formulation of sodium valproate suppositories, used to treat epilepsy, has rapid drug absorption.

Polyethylene Glycol

Polyethylene glycol is a water-soluble, hydrophilic base. As mentioned earlier, a series of PEG bases with different molecular weights is available. Generally, a combination of solid and liquid PEG is preferred to make suppositories. The PEG base does not melt at body temperature; instead, it dissolves in the body. As a result, it can be stored without refrigeration. PEG may cause rectal irritation because it draws water from the rectum. In contrast to cocoa butter, it causes hydrophobic drugs to be released more rapidly. A typical example involves compounding of diazepam suppositories to treat epilepsy in children. Selecting a PEG with a melting point that is higher than the body temperature is not a problem in this indication because the suppositories dissolve rather than melt inside the body.

Other Dosage Forms

Transdermal Drug Delivery Systems

In contrast to semisolid dosage forms that produce local effects, transdermal drug delivery systems (TDDSs) produce systematic effects. An ideal drug for transdermal drug delivery should be potent (i.e., doses should be small), of low molecular weight (400 Da or less), water soluble to be released from a membrane, lipid soluble to be absorbed through the skin, and have a relatively short half-life (10 hours or less).

Two types of transdermal patches are currently available: reservoir/membrane controlled and matrix controlled. The underlying principle for both types is that the active ingredient is held within a reservoir, the patch has a membrane that facilitates the release of the active ingredient, and an adhesive layer attaches the patch to the skin. It has been suggested that among the various types of patches, the drug-in-adhesive (DIA) system is a preferred TDDS due to its avoidance of leakage and "dose-dumping" problems. However, one emerging concern about the DIA system is that crystallization of drug particles can affect the release of the drug from the patch.

A TDDS offers some significant benefits to patients. Transdermal delivery is useful when the first-pass effect is high (and the drug can avoid being metabolized when it is absorbed through the skin) or the patient has difficulty ingesting an oral dosage form. In addition, because the TDDS delivers a drug through the skin over an extended period of time, it is popular among patients and may assist patients in medication adherence. For instance, many patients prefer transdermal nitroglycerin over the sublingual version because the former provides hours of protection against angina (the patch is placed over the chest area and can protect the patient for 12 hours against angina pectoris).

Transdermal patches can also be used for nonhuman animals (dogs, cats, cows, and horses). The drawback of using a TDDS is that it cannot be used to deliver a rapid effect or in acute situations (because of slow diffusion of the active ingredients). Examples of TDDS products include methylphenidate (Daytrana) patches used in children with attention-deficit/hyperactivity disorder. However, not all drugs can easily diffuse through different layers of the skin. Factors that affect drug absorption include the surface area of the affected area, the nature of the vehicle, the hydrophobic nature of the drug, and inflammation of the skin (because the cutaneous blood flow is increased by skin inflammation).

Because the drug diffuses into the dermal layers of the skin slowly, there is a lag time before the onset of the drug action is observed. Conversely, upon removal of the patch, diffusion of the drug continues through the different layers of the skin into the systemic circulation. This factor explains why a fentanyl-overdosed patient needs to be watched over 24 hours after the removal of the patch. Because the size of the patch plays an important role in the dose–response relationship, a larger transdermal patch has a higher dose–response profile than a smaller patch. The solubility of the drug in the skin is the most important factor that dictates the rate of drug absorption through the skin. In addition, the drug's concentration plays an essential role in the drug absorption per unit of surface area—the higher the concentration, the higher the drug absorption rate.

A more advanced transdermal dosage form, known as a controlled-released patch, is now available on the market. Examples of drugs provided in such formulations include nicotine (NicoDerm), for smoking cessation; scopolamine (Transderm Scop), for motion sickness; nitroglycerin (Nitro-Dur), for angina pectoris; various steroids for birth control; and fentanyl (Duragesic), a synthetic opioid used for pain management. Another example is oxybutynin (Oxytrol), which competitively inhibits acetylcholine, resulting in the relaxation of the bladder's smooth muscle.

Sublingual Dosage Forms

Relatively few sublingual dosage formulations are available. Perhaps the most commonly encountered sublingual products are the nitroglycerin tablets (Nitrostat) that are used to treat angina pectoris. The venous drainage from the mouth and the unique absorption from the oral mucosa make this route of administration attractive for certain drugs. One major advantage of sublingual formulations over oral tablets is that a sublingual tablet bypasses the portal circulation, which protects the drug from intestinal degradation and from the hepatic first-pass metabolism. Thus, a major reason for creating a sublingual (and buccal) dosage form is to countermand an extensive first-pass effect.

To maintain an effective dissolution rate, the sublingual dosage form does not contain a disintegrant and is compressed lightly (soft tablet). The sublingual nitroglycerin tablet response becomes apparent after 2 minutes (because it has high lipid solubility) and the effect lasts for at least 20 minutes.

Aerosols

Aerosol formulations are useful to deliver the intended drug directly into the lungs for absorption and for direct action. Typically, the drug must tolerate aerosolization. Delivery vehicles include metered-dose inhalers, dry-powder inhalers, nebulizers, and sprays (skin and dental sprays). The drug formulation may be a suspension prior to aerosolization, in which case surfactants are employed to maintain dispersion of the particles.

Propellants are utilized to aid in drug delivery and have recently been switched from chlorofluorocarbons to hydrofluorocarbons due to environmental concerns. Adoption of the new propellants required drug formulation revisions for some drugs, such as albuterol. Albuterol sulfate, used to treat bronchospasm, is a widely used inhalation product. The albuterol particles are delivered directly to the lungs via a metered-dose inhaler. As the name implies, each pump of such an inhaler releases a measured dose of drug directly into the patient's lungs. For accurate dose delivery, patients must follow very specific instructions, (i.e., shake the inhaler well, hold it 1–2 inches from the mouth, exhale, and press the inhaler with the next inhalation).

Powder Dosage Forms

Powder is a unique dosage form that is infrequently dispensed. However, due to its physicochemical properties and the fact that many other dosage forms are compounded using a powder, it is important to explore its roles and characteristics in pharmaceutics. The United States Pharmacopeia has divided powders into different categories based on their ability to pass through standard sieves; they range from very coarse, coarse, moderately coarse, to fine and very fine. A very coarse powder passes through a #8 sieve (2.36 mm), while a very fine powder completely passes through a #80 sieve (180 μm).

Three types of powders are used: (1) bulk powders for internal use, (2) bulk powders for external use, and (3) divided (single dose) powders. One should be cautious with bulk powders for internal use. If the drug is potent, the quantity of the powder can be quite small, and obtaining accurate measurements can be a challenging task. Powders for oral use can be dispensed by dividing them into premeasured doses in glassine or waxed paper.

Powders are particularly useful when it is not feasible to prepare a suspension or emulsion or when the desired dosage form is not chemically stable. In addition, powders are useful when the patient has difficulty in swallowing a tablet or a capsule. Another advantage of powders over tablets and capsules is that powders bypass concerns about the disintegration rate. Hygroscopic and volatile powders are best protected by a waxed paper that is waterproof. The following techniques are routinely used in a compounding pharmacy to prepare a powder.

Trituration

Trituration is a technique by which a mortar and pestle are used to grind and combine one or more coarse powders into smaller particles.

Pulverization by Intervention

Pulverization by intervention is a grinding technique used for drug substances that resist grinding by physical means (i.e., are gummy or soft). In this case, intervention means adding a small amount of a volatile liquid that aids in the milling process. The liquid is then easily removed or evaporated when the pulverization is complete. For instance, camphor can be pulverized readily if a small amount of alcohol is added.

Geometric Dilution

Geometric dilution is a process by which different quantities of drugs can be combined together to obtain a homogeneous mixture. Often drug quantities are much smaller than the amount of diluents used to dispense an accurate dose. When compounding these types of powders, the drug is mixed with an equal quantity of diluent and blended. Subsequent additions of the diluents are added to the prior mixture in equal quantities until all of the diluent has been mixed in. Diluents have multiple roles in compounding a medication. They are often used to promote granulation or compaction, serve as fillers, facilitate disintegration in the GI tract, and serve as lubricants, antiadherents, and glidants to reduce friction or adhesion between particles. Interestingly, starch has multiple ingredient roles: it is used as a filler, diluent, disintegrant, glidant, binding agent, and flocculating agent.

Levigation

Levigation is a process of blending and grinding a particle to reduce the particle's size, while using a small quantity of a solvent in which the drug is not soluble. The liquid is called a levigating agent. In addition to the levigating agent's function to reduce a particle's size, it displaces the air at the solid–air interface with a liquid that is miscible with an external phase. The external phase can be a syrup in suspensions or a cream for topical dosage forms. Glycerin is an example of a levigating agent. In general, the quantity of a levigating agent should not exceed 5% of the final dosage form's weight or volume.

Milling of Powder

Milling is the process of mechanically reducing the particle size of solids before they are formulated into the final product. For this process, one needs to add a lubricant to coat the surface of powder. Drug particles that are temperature sensitive may undergo degradation, however, because the milling procedure can generate heat.

Some powders are liquefied (i.e., becoming eutectic mixtures) upon mixing with other powders or materials. In this case, an additional substance is required to insulate the powder particles. For instance, starch, bentonite, magnesium oxide, and magnesium carbonate are used to protect a mixture of acetyl salicylic acid and camphor from becoming a eutectic mixture.

Glass mortars are good choices for milling chemotherapeutic and cytotoxic agents, and porcelains, which have a smooth surface, are ideal for blending powders. A ceramic mortar that has a rough inner surface is preferred for comminution of a powder. Always use plastic spatulas for chemicals (such as iodine) that may interact with stainless steel.

Granules

Granules have larger mass than powder particles, as well as a diameter that may be as large as 2–4 mm. Granules, however, are produced when powder particles aggregate with each other. Granulation is useful to avoid segregation of different particle sizes during storage or drug administration. Because many granules are derived from powders, granules and powders behave similarly. To facilitate effective absorption of a drug that is in granule form, it is important that the granule disintegrates into particles prior to its absorption.

Balances are used to weigh powders and granules. Two balances are used routinely in a compounding lab: torsion (which is inside a glass box) and electronic balance.

Learning Bridge 8.8

Dr. Fettner, a dermatologist, has contacted you to ask for clarification regarding a topical formulation for treating a patient with severe psoriasis. He has prescribed various commercially available forms of coal tar without success. He would like you to prepare Coal Tar USP but he cannot recall the formulation and would like to know which vehicle is used and why. By definition, Coal Tar USP contains coal tar, polysorbate 80, and zinc oxide paste. Describe the type of vehicle you would recommend and why.

Modified-Release Dosage Forms

Modified-release dosage forms include extended release (granules, capsules, and tablets), delayed release (granules, capsules, and tablets), and repeat action (tablets) with a slow and consistent release profile of the active ingredient that occurs within 8 hours or longer.

Generally speaking, the dissolution rate of a tablet in the GI fluids determines the rate of absorption, which is the cornerstone principle for modified-release dosage forms. The matrix that envelops the active (and inactive) ingredient of such forms is an inert solid vehicle that plays an important role in the dissolution, permeation, and diffusion of the product's content. It is critical to have a water permeation matrix to control the rate of water influx into the product, which in turn governs the rate of drug dissolution inside the matrix. Once the active ingredient is dissolved inside the matrix, one can control the rate of drug diffusion and ensure that a desirable rate is achieved.

As the term "release" indicates in their names, the dissolution rate of these tablets and capsules in the GI tract is an important factor contributing to the rate of drug absorption. Such dosage forms provide myriad benefits, including less frequency of administration, improved patient compliance, maintenance of a constant release over a specific time frame, and decreased side effects. The last advantage is associated with a reduction in an immediate achievement of C_{max} (see the *Introduction to Pharmacokinetics* chapter). However, one has to be careful with these dosage forms before administration, particularly when they are not supposed to be chewed or crushed, to avoid "dose dumping." The high concentration of the active ingredient in these dosage forms, upon immediate release (i.e., by chewing or crushing), can cause toxicity. Another potential problem is the misuse of the slow-release process in these dosage forms. For instance, oxycodone (OxyContin), which is a controlled-release dosage form, can be misused for its slow and lengthy release.

Extended Release

Extended release, also referred to sustained release, produces a prolonged and consistent therapeutic response. As a result, such formulations minimize the fluctuation of drug levels in the blood and can increase patient adherence. Extended-release dosage forms are not suitable for drugs that have a long half-life, such as chlorpheniramine (Aller-Chlor), which has a half-life of 24 hours. These forms have the unique characteristics of extending the therapeutic effect of a drug by releasing it slowly (ideally through a zero-order reaction rate, as discussed later in this chapter) and reducing the side effects that often are caused by fluctuating plasma drug levels. In addition, a drug formulated for extended release should be absorbed similarly to an IV drug infusion. Because the release of the drug is slow, it represents a rate-limiting factor in the drug's absorption.

Many pathophysiological factors can influence the absorption of an extended-release drug and, as a result, the absorption may not follow a zero-order rate. Because the extended-release product remains longer in the GI tract, the characteristics of the GI tract (e.g., pH, blood flow, site of absorption, presence of food, GI motility) can affect the release and absorption of the active ingredient. The physicochemical properties of a drug as well as the required dose are other factors to consider when formulating an extended-release drug. For instance, it is difficult to create an extended-release form if the drug is water soluble in an acidic environment (stomach) and water insoluble in the small intestine. If a drug is susceptible to degradation by gastric acid, it must be protected from stomach acidity. Cellulose acetate phthalate is a good choice to coat tablets because it resists stomach acidity—it dissolves at pH 6 or higher. Excessive drug coating can decrease bioavailability, however, whereas too little protection may result in degradation of the drug in

Table 8.7 Characteristics of Modified-Release Dosage Forms

Extended Release	Delayed Release	Repeat Action
Extends the therapeutic effect of a drug by slowly releasing the drug, thereby reducing the dose frequency and side effects.	Does not release the drug at the administration time; rather, the release is delayed at the site of action. Enteric-coated drugs belong to this category.	A multidose system that contains two layers and, therefore, two phases of release—immediate release followed by a delayed release. Suitable for chronic treatments that require frequent dosing.

the stomach and cause toxicity. An example of an extended-release tablet is methylphenidate (Metadate ER), which is used as a CNS stimulant. While extended-release drugs are more expensive on a per-tablet basis than the corresponding immediate-release dosage forms, their overall cost of use is less because they produce fewer side effects and require less frequent doses.

Delayed Release

A delayed-release tablet slows release of the active ingredient to ensure that it reaches the site of action. The delayed release allows the drug to avoid being destroyed or inactivated by physiological factors. A typical example of a delayed-release tablet is the OTC medication omeprazole delayed-release (Prilosec OTC), used to treat gastric or duodenal ulcers.

Repeat Action Tablets (Repetabs)

These dosage forms consist of compression-coated tablets with an outer immediate-release (IR) tablet and an inner time-dependent (enteric-type) coated tablet. An example is albuterol tablets (VoSpire ER, also known as Proventil Repetabs), which are used to relieve bronchospasm. Repetabs contain one IR dose and one delayed-release dose. These dosage forms offer the convenience of having two doses in one tablet, which in turn improves patient compliance.

Table 8.7 indicates the differences between the various modified-release dosage forms.

Learning Bridge 8.9

Mrs. Chowdrey, a 68-year-old female, has been diagnosed with non-Hodgkin's lymphoma and has been receiving various pain medications. The physician has called you and would like to know which forms of morphine are available. Make a list of the available nonparenteral dosage forms, and identify the advantages of each formulation for Ms. Chowdrey.

Novel Drug Delivery and Dosage Forms

New drug dosage formulations and new drug delivery systems are under continual research and development. If a drug is targeted directly to the intended site of action, then fewer adverse effects, lower doses, less frequent dosing, and more consistent drug levels may result. Additionally, targeted drug delivery may allow extended drug exposure and maximize the drug effect.

Formulations gaining favor include liposomes, in which the drug is encapsulated in a hydrophobic ball of phospholipids. The drug, often hydrophilic, is protected from damage and disintegration while traveling to the site of action. Amphotericin B liposome (AmBisome) is available as a suspension to be reconstituted upon use. The liposome formulation dramatically decreases the adverse effects of this drug while improving its efficacy.

Another newer formulation is rapid-dissolving tablets. The rapid drug absorption via the tongue is especially useful for drugs that must bypass the gastrointestinal tract to remain active. Rizatriptan (Maxalt) and zolmitriptan (Zomig) both come in orally disintegrating tablet formulations. Migraine suffers often experience disabling pain and severe nausea when seeking treatment. Orally disintegrating tablets are placed on the tongue and quickly dissolve, removing the necessity of swallowing a drug to receive the therapeutic benefit.

Implantable pumps are innovative drug delivery systems that allow a drug to be delivered via a pump implanted in the patient's subcutaneous tissue. An osmotic pump releases the drug, such as insulin, directly to the site of action and is powered by osmotic pressure within the pump itself. Other implantable pumps are quite sophisticated and can be programmed to deliver drug at variable rates. Depending on the drug, the implantable pump's drug administration rate may be adjusted after implantation.

Excipients in Pharmaceutics

Excipients are incorporated into drug formulations to support and stabilize drugs. These materials are generally inactive ingredients, and the wide selection available allows manufacturers and drug compounders to identify options that have the best compatibility with the intended drug. **Table 8.8** lists some commonly used excipients in pharmaceuticals.

Reaction Kinetics

As a pharmacist, you must be able to calculate the right dose of a medication for your patient. Regardless of the dosage form for the drug—that is, whether the drug is in a solution, tablet, or ointment—the rate of degradation of the drug should be known. By the same token, the rate of absorption, distribution, and elimination of the drug should be known. Therefore, it is important for pharmacists to understand the concept of reaction kinetics.

Table 8.8 Commonly Used Excipients in the Formulation of Different Dosage Forms

Type	Purpose	Examples
Binders	Provide cohesive qualities to enhance compressibility and hold tablets together	Cellulose, lactose, acacia gum
Fillers	Increase the bulk of the intended tablets	Cellulose, lactose, calcium phosphate
Lubricants	Allow tablets to be easily removed from molds	Stearates
Disintegrants	Increase disintegration of formulations in the gastrointestinal tract	Carboxymethyl cellulose
Emulsifiers	Provide stabilization of an emulsion and increase suspendability	Acacia, Span 40 (sorbitan monopalmitate)
Coating	Protect tablets from deterioration prior to administration; can improve flavor	HPMC, gelatin
Preservative	Improve stability and extend the time before expiration	Citric acid, parabens
Flavors, sweeteners	Improve flavor	Fructose, artificial flavors
Stabilizers	For o/w emulsions for specific lotions and ointments	Stearyl alcohol, glyceryl monostearate

The study of reaction rates and the factors that influence reaction rates—such as temperature, concentration, and enzymes (catalysts), which are often described in mathematical terms—is known as reaction kinetics. The terms *chemical kinetics, reaction kinetics,* or simply *kinetics* have the same meaning and are used interchangeably. Before we go into details of reaction kinetics, let's examine the term *rate*.

A rate is defined as change in a process or an amount of an object per unit of time. Rates of chemical reactions can be tremendously fast; for example, the initial reactions in photosynthesis may occur in periods as short as 1×10^{-6} second. Reaction rates can also be extremely slow. For instance, it takes 950 million years to hydrolyze one urea molecule in the absence of a urase enzyme. Understanding reaction rates gives pharmacists an idea of what happens at the molecular level during chemical or biochemical reactions.

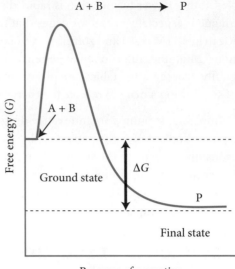

Figure 8.23 The energy change that occurs during an exergonic reaction process. The product has a smaller free energy (*G*) value than the reactants.

In studying reaction rates, one question is of particular concern: why do some chemical or biochemical reactions occur slowly while others occur quickly? First, the reaction needs to be physically possible. Sometimes, even if molecules are mixed together, they will not necessarily react with each other. The probability that a chemical reaction will occur is determined by thermodynamics. For instance, for a reaction to have a high probability of occurring (i.e., an exergonic reaction; see the *Introduction to Biochemistry* chapter), the free energy of the product should be less than the free energy of the reactants (i.e., when the reactants are converted into a product, the energy stored in the reactants is released) (**Figure 8.23**). However, if the reaction is endergonic, the product will have a higher free energy than the reactants.

When the product has less free energy than the reactants, the free energy change (ΔG) becomes negative, which means the reaction is thermodynamically favorable and, therefore, has a high probability of occurring (Figure 8.23; see also the *Introduction to Biochemistry* chapter). Keep in mind that ΔG does not give you any information about how fast a reaction occurs. To know why some reactions are faster than others, one has to consider factors such as catalysts/enzymology (described in the *Introduction to Biochemistry* chapter), temperature, and surface area of a reactant.

One goal of kinetics is to measure the rates of specific chemical reactions—that is, to determine how fast products are made when specific reactants are mixed together. Many pharmaceutical companies are interested in speeding up the rate of a reaction rather than maximizing the amount of product created in the reaction. The expression that describes the speed of a chemical reaction is called a rate law.

Before we describe the rate law, we will briefly review how to measure reaction rates. A simple reaction can be represented by a general reaction:

$$R \rightarrow P$$

where R is the reactant and P is the product. Looking at this reaction scheme, we can see that as the reactant R is consumed, the product P is formed. We can then analyze the reaction by measuring either the amount of lost reactant or the amount of gained product over a specific time frame. Let's put these words into equation form:

$$\text{Rate} = -\frac{[\Delta R]}{\Delta t} \tag{8.11}$$

$$\text{Rate} = \frac{[\Delta P]}{\Delta t} \tag{8.12}$$

Recall that the concentration of the reactant becomes smaller and smaller as it is used up to form more and more product. As a consequence, the overall expression for the reaction rate will be negative. Because the reaction rate itself cannot be reported with a negative sign, we can simply multiply the value found for the rate by –1 to obtain a positive sign for the calculated rate. To feel confident about removing the negative sign, remember that you are a making—rather than losing—a product in a reaction.

Let's put Equations 8.11 and 8.12 into a "colorful" experiment to visualize how these equations can be useful for expressing when the "colorful" experiment becomes "colorless." Assume that bromine reacts with formic acid in the following reaction:

$$Br_2\,(aq) + HCOOH\,(aq) \rightarrow 2\ Br^-\,(aq) + 2\ H^+\,(aq) + CO_2\,(g)$$

The color of bromine (Br_2) is brown and all other species in the reaction are colorless. The more Br_2 that reacts with the formic acid, the less Br_2 that remains in the solution, and the less brown color that remains (i.e., after a given time, there is no brown color left in the reaction mixture). We can measure the change in Br_2 concentration (for instance, by spectroscopy, which analyzes the light passing through the solution) at some initial time (0 time) and again at a final time (let's say after 60 seconds) to measure the rate of the reaction. Suppose at the initial time the concentration of Br_2 is 10 mM, and at the final time the concentration is 1 mM. Because the rate is calculated based on measurements taken at two points in time, the rate will represent the average rate during the interval time. In this case, the rate is 0.15 mM/s.

$$\text{Rate} = \frac{[\Delta Br_2]}{\Delta t} = -\frac{[Br_2]_f - [Br_2]_i}{t_f - t_i} = \frac{9\ \text{mM}}{60\ \text{s}} = 0.15\ \text{mM/s} \tag{8.13}$$

where the subscript "f" means "final" and the subscript "i" means "initial" (concentration or time).

In fact, the reaction rate for the bromine reaction is proportional to the concentration of Br_2 (Equation 8.14). Thus, as the concentration of Br_2 increases, the rate of the reaction also increases. In such a condition, one can express the reaction rate as follows:

$$\text{Rate } \alpha \ [Br_2] \tag{8.14}$$

$$\text{Rate} = k[Br_2] \tag{8.15}$$

The term k in Equation 8.15 is known as the rate constant and is specific to a particular reaction at a given temperature. We can rewrite Equation 8.15 as follows:

$$k = \frac{\text{Rate}}{[Br_2]} \tag{8.16}$$

To understand what kind of unit the rate constant has, we can look at the unit that was calculated in Equation 8.13—that is, mM/s. The unit for $[Br_2]$ is mM, so the unit for k is s^{-1} or "per second."

Rate Law

Pharmacists and scientists in a pharmaceutical company often want to know how fast products are made when specific reactants are mixed together. Accordingly, they apply an expression that describes the speed of a chemical reaction, known as the rate law. Most reactions progress more rapidly when the concentrations of the reactants increase (this is also apparent from Equation 8.15—when you increase the concentration of Br_2, the rate increases as well). It has been suggested that for the majority of reactions, one can express an equation (rate law) in which the reaction rate is proportional to the reactant's concentration raised to a power. Thus the rate is equal to a rate constant (k) multiplied by the concentration of each reactant raised to a power. Equation 8.15 is an example of a rate law.

Knowing a reaction's rate law is important because it enables us to determine how fast a given product will be produced when known concentrations of reactants react with each other. You can calculate the rate constant, k, of a reaction if you know the rate law for a reaction and the concentrations of the reactants. Similarly, you can calculate the rate if you know the rate law and the rate constant. Note that the rate and the rate constant are two different parameters. While a rate is a changing parameter (variable), the rate constant, as the name indicates, is constant and does not change for a given reaction.

One important factor to consider when calculating rates and rate constants is that the reactant concentrations are generally those concentrations present at the beginning of the experiment (i.e., the initial concentrations). An initial concentration is preferred because as the reaction progresses, the concentrations of the reactants decrease to a point that it is difficult to experimentally and accurately measure them.

For a reaction to occur, atoms, molecules, or ions must collide with each other in the correct orientations and with sufficient speed. If the molecules are not facing each other correctly, the likelihood that they will form new bonds is low. Similarly, if the reactants are moving too slowly, the available energy is too small to break existing bonds. Because the reactants have to physically contact one another for a chemical reaction to occur, it is obvious that the more concentrated the reactants are (i.e., the more molecules that are present in a solution), the greater the chance that the molecules will react with each other to form a product.

An example will serve to illustrate the effects of concentration on the rate of a reaction. Suppose there are only 2 students in the lecture hall A and 100 students in the lecture hall B. All of the students, in both lecture halls, are walking around the room with the same rate constant (i.e., with the same k). Obviously, the students in lecture hall B are more likely to bump into one another than the students in lecture hall A. Because the rate constant (k) is the same for both movements in A and B, the rate at which students run into each other in lecture hall B per unit of time should be higher than the corresponding rate for the students in lecture hall A.

The unit of the rate constant may differ for different reactions depending on the reaction order. A reaction order is the sum of powers of the reactants' concentrations that are expressed in a rate law. The three different reaction orders are referred to as zero, first, and second. For instance, the rate law expressed in Equation 8.15 describes how the reaction rate depends directly on the concentration of Br_2. Because the power of the reactant's concentration (Br_2) is 1 ("first"), the reaction order for the rate constant for Equation 8.15 is a first-order rate. If the rate law had been Rate $= k$ $[Br_2]^2$, the reaction order for the rate constant would have been a second-order rate because the power of the reactant's concentration would be 2 ("second").

The slowest step in a reaction dictates the rate at which the entire reaction can proceed; hence it is known as the rate-limiting step. In designing and developing a drug that stimulates or inhibits an enzyme, it is critical to identify which step in the stimulation or inhibition process is the rate-limiting step. Rate-limiting steps are often regulatory steps in reactions (many examples are provided in the *Introduction to Biochemistry* chapter). As a result, if you manipulate the regulatory step(s), you most likely will be able to influence the entire reaction.

To further explain the important role that a rate-limiting step plays, let's consider the following scenario. Three students have been asked to write a report about a drug. One writes the introduction to the report, one writes the part dealing with the drug's mechanism of action, and one writes the overall conclusion. If the student who writes the introduction works slowly, then no matter how quickly the other two students complete their parts, the report will be ready only when the introduction is written. In this example, the speed of the student who writes the introduction governs the overall speed of the entire assignment. As a result, anything that discourages (inhibits) or encourages (stimulates) this student will have a profound effect on the overall speed of the progress of the assignment (reaction).

Reaction Order

It is imperative to understand how the reaction orders occur and are calculated. Many drugs' absorption and elimination rates are related to these orders (both concepts are discussed in more detail in the *Introduction to Pharmacokinetics* chapter). For instance, when a full dose of a drug is dissolved in the gastrointestinal fluids, the rate of absorption and the elimination of oral dosage drugs often follow first-order kinetics. The three reaction orders are explained in the following sections to clarify how the degradation of drugs is related to their storage lifetime.

Zero-Order Reaction

The rate in a zero-order reaction is independent of the concentrations of the reactants. The plateaus in **Figure 8.24** depict a typical zero-order reaction rate. No matter how much you increase the concentration of the reactant, you do not increase the reaction rate. In graph A in Figure 8.24, which depicts a nonlinear reaction, the plateau represents an enzyme that is saturated with its substrate; as a result, the enzyme has reached its maximum velocity (V_{max}; see the *Introduction to Biochemistry* chapter).

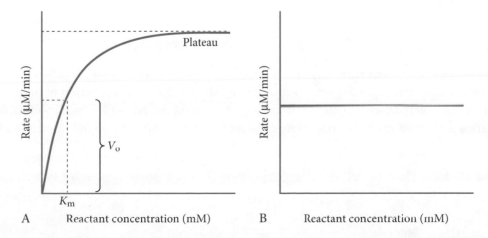

Figure 8.24 (A) A zero-order reaction rate in a nonlinear enzymatic reaction process. (B) A zero-order reaction rate in a chemical reaction. The plateaus in both A and B represent zero-order reactions that do not change when the concentration of the reactant is increased.

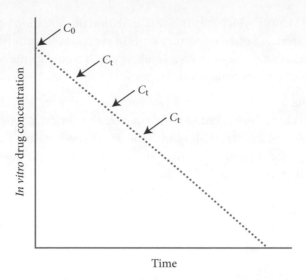

Figure 8.25 A zero-order reaction rate that indicates how fast a drug degrades in a solution at room temperature. C_0 is the concentration of the drug at time 0, and C_t is the concentration of the drug at a given time.

Another example of a zero-order reaction rate is a situation in which a drug is degraded at a constant rate. For instance, if you dissolve 1 mole of a drug that is not stable at room temperature in 1 liter of water, the initial drug concentration (C_0) is 1 M. If you leave this drug solution at room temperature and take samples at different times to measure the drug concentrations, you will notice that the drug concentrations (C_t) decline over time (in other words, the drug degrades more as it stays at room temperature for a longer time). If the drug degradation follows a zero-order reaction rate, the graph of this reaction will be a straight line whose slope represents the zero-order rate (**Figure 8.25**).

As mentioned earlier, a zero-order rate means that the rate of the reaction is not dependent on the concentration of the reactants. We can express the zero-order reaction rate for the straight line in Figure 8.25 as follows:

$$\frac{dC_t}{dt} = -k_0 \tag{8.17}$$

Integration of Equation 8.17 gives Equation 8.18:

$$C_t = -k_0 t + C_0 \tag{8.18}$$

C_t is the concentration that remains in the solution, and C_0 is the initial concentration of the drug that has not been degraded yet. If we graph the data for $C_t - C_0$ as a function of time, we can build a straight degradation line in which the slope represents the zero-order rate constant (k_0). To determine the unit for a zero-order rate constant (i.e., for k_0), we can rewrite Equation 8.18 as follows:

$$C_0 - C_t = -k_0 t \tag{8.19}$$

$$k_0 = \frac{(C_0 - C_t)}{t} = \frac{M}{second} \tag{8.20}$$

Half-life

The greatest degradation threat to most drug solutions is hydrolysis, a reaction that is accelerated by increasing temperature (i.e., hydrolysis occurs more rapidly at room temperature compared to storing the drug solution in a refrigerator). However, other factors such as light, air, and moisture can also expedite drug degradation. A degradation process can lead to detrimental effects such as a loss of drug activity (or loss of potency), production of toxic by-products, and changes in the color and taste of the drug that can significantly affect the patient's compliance. Drug degradation occurs to the greatest extent in solutions, followed by suspensions and solid dosage forms (tablets, capsules). For this reason, pharmacy staff members who work with drug solutions should receive training regarding why a specific storage temperature is important to maintain the full activity of a drug solution.

In pharmaceutics, the half-life ($t_{1/2}$) of a drug is the time required for 50% (half) of the initial concentration (or amount) of the drug to be degraded during its storage time frame. The $t_{1/2}$ parameter is an important concept that assists pharmacists in calculating the shelf life of a drug. The shelf life of a drug in a given dosage form is the time during which at least 90% of the product remains intact and active while being stored; it is also called t_{90}. The 10% (or less) cutoff for loss of activity is acceptable by the FDA. Accordingly, drug manufacturers use the t_{90} value as the basis for the expiration dates placed on the packaging of their products. A few drugs have a more restricted FDA requirement. For instance, the cutoff for loss of activity for levothyroxine (Levothroid) is 5%.

Let's first calculate $t_{1/2}$ before explaining how one can calculate t_{90}. Keep in mind that C_t at the end of one half-life is equal to 50% of C_0. We can calculate $t_{1/2}$ for a zero-order reaction by utilizing Equation 8.19 to express Equations 8.21 and 8.22:

$$C_0 - 0.5C_0 = -k_0 t_{1/2} \tag{8.21}$$

$$t_{1/2} = \frac{1/2 C_0}{k_0} \tag{8.22}$$

Similarly, to calculate t_{90}, we observe that C_t during the drug's shelf life is equal to 90% of C_0 (i.e., $C_t = 0.9C_0$). To calculate the shelf life of a drug, we can use Equation 8.21 to express Equation 8.23:

$$C_0 - 0.9C_0 = -k_0 t_{90\%} \tag{8.23}$$

This expression is equivalent to

$$0.1C_0 = k_0 t_{90\%} \tag{8.24}$$

and

$$t_{90\%} = 0.1C_0/k_0 \tag{8.25}$$

There are a few key points about the zero-order degradation rate that are important to remember:

- This rate is independent of the concentration.
- A graph of concentration versus time on a linear paper yields a straight line.
- The half-life is a changing parameter (because C_0 is changing).
- The shelf life (90%) of the drug ($t_{90\%}$) depends on the concentration (see Equation 8.25).

Keep in mind that $t_{1/2}$ is calculated differently for different reaction orders.

Example 8.6: A drug solution that has an initial drug concentration of 100 mM undergoes a zero-order reaction (decomposition) with a rate constant of 10 mM/day at room temperature in a pharmacy. Calculate the half-life for this drug.

Answer: According to Equation 8.22, $t_{1/2}$ will be 5 days.

$$t_{1/2} = \frac{\frac{1}{2}\,100 \text{ mM}}{10 \text{ mM/day}}$$

According to Equation 8.25, the shelf life is

$$t_{90\%} = \frac{0.1 \times 100 \text{ mM}}{10 \text{ mM/day}} = 1 \text{ day}$$

This means that a drug solution that remains at the counter for more than 1 day in the pharmacy will contain less than 90% active drug.

First-Order Reaction

In a first-order reaction, the reaction rate is directly proportional to the concentration of one of the reactants. The order of the reaction can be determined experimentally. For example, a quick review of data presented in **Table 8.9** reveals that the breakdown of hydrogen peroxide to oxygen and water is a first-order reaction:

$$2 \text{ H}_2\text{O}_2 \rightarrow \text{O}_2 + 2 \text{ H}_2\text{O}$$

For each initial concentration of hydrogen peroxide, the initial rate of hydrogen peroxide breakdown was measured. To determine the order of the reaction rate, similar to Equation 8.15, begin by writing the general rate law equation (see Equation 8.26) for the reaction. In this case, the rate equals k multiplied by the concentration of hydrogen peroxide (S) raised to an unknown

Table 8.9 Degradation Rate of Hydrogen Peroxide Is Directly Proportional to Its concentration

Experiment Number	Initial H_2O_2 (M)	Initial Rate of Degradation (M/s)
1	0.01	2.2×10^{-5}
2	0.02	4.4×10^{-5}
3	0.03	6.6×10^{-5}

power (x). When the unknown x becomes known, it gives you information about the order of the reaction (or the order of the rate constant in this reaction).

$$\text{Rate} = k[S]^x \tag{8.26}$$

To determine the power, which in turn will tell you the reaction order, the experimental relationship between the increase in the reactant's concentration and the increase in the initial rate is very helpful (as explained earlier, it is important to measure the initial rate). As Table 8.9 indicates, when the initial concentration of hydrogen peroxide is increased 100% (i.e., by a factor of 2), as occurs between the first and second experiments, the reaction rate also increases 100% (i.e., by a factor of 2). By the same token, when the initial concentration is increased three times, the reaction rate is increased three times as well. Because of the one-to-one correlation that exists between the changes in concentrations and in rates, the reaction follows first-order kinetics. Basically, the unknown power (x) in Equation 8.26 is 1, so the rate constant will be first order.

Now let's see what the unit for a first-order rate constant (k) is. This is important because as soon as you see the unit, you should be able to determine whether the reaction is a first- or second-order reaction. The rate, as mentioned earlier, will have the unit M s^{-1} and the units for [S] will be M. Returning to Equation 8.26, you will see that the unit is s^{-1} ("per second") because of Equation 8.27:

$$\text{Rate} = k[S]^1 \tag{8.27}$$

$$k = \text{rate} / [S] = M \text{ s}^{-1} / M = s^{-1}$$

The M units will cancel each other, leaving s^{-1} as the unit for the first-order rate constant. Depending on the time used in the experiment, the unit could be per minute, per hour, per day, or something else.

Figure 8.26 shows a typical first-order reaction graph for degradation of a drug solution at room temperature (compare it with the zero-order reaction). Notice that the drug degradation rate is not a linear process, but rather is exponential. If you graph the drug concentration that remains

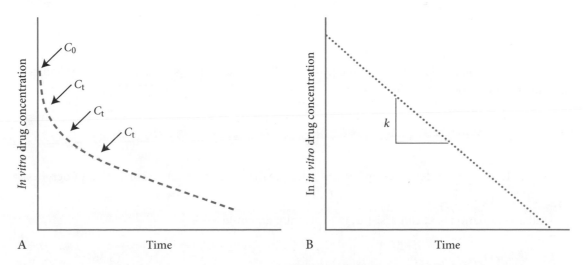

Figure 8.26 (A) A first-order reaction in which a drug is degraded with a first-order rate constant. C_0 is the concentration of the drug at time 0, and C_t is the concentration of the drug at a given time. (B) The same data shown on a natural logarithm scale (the slope of the line is the reaction rate constant, k).

active at different times on a semi-log graph paper, it will yield a straight line with a slope that is the first-order rate constant.

In a first-order reaction, the concentration of a drug decreases with a rate that is proportional to the concentration of the remaining drug. We can express this process by using Equation 8.28:

$$\frac{dC_t}{dt} = -kC_t \tag{8.28}$$

The integration of Equation 8.28 gives Equation 8.29:

$$\ln(C_t/C_0) = -kt \tag{8.29}$$

To remove the negative sign, we can use the following expression:

$$\ln(C_0/C_t) = kt \tag{8.30}$$

The anti-natural logarithm of Equation 8.30 yields the Equation 8.31 (which is an exponential equation).

$$C_t = C_0 e^{-kt} \tag{8.31}$$

C_t is the concentration remaining to be degraded at a given time, and C_0 is the initial concentration of the drug at time 0 (Figure 8.26A). You can calculate the rate constant by plotting the natural logarithm of C_t/C_0 (i.e., $\ln C_t/C_0$) as a function of time, which yields a straight line. The slope of the straight line represents the rate constant.

We can also calculate the half-life ($t_{1/2}$) for the first-order reaction. Set C_t equal to one-half of C_0 to calculate the half-life. Equation 8.31 can then be written as follows:

$$\ln \frac{C_0}{1/2C_0} = kt_{1/2} \tag{8.32}$$

which yields Equation 8.33:

$$\ln 2 = kt_{1/2} \tag{8.33}$$

By using Equation 8.33 (where ln2 is equal to 0.693), we can express Equation 8.34 to calculate half-life for a first-order reaction:

$$t_{1/2} = \frac{0.693}{k} \tag{8.34}$$

Similar to the zero-order reaction, we can calculate the shelf life ($t_{90\%}$) of a drug that undergoes first-order degradation (i.e., when $C_t = 0.9C_0$).

Utilizing Equation 8.32 can assist us in expressing Equation 8.35:

$$\ln \frac{C_0}{0.9C_0} = kt_{90\%} \tag{8.35}$$

This is equal to Equation 8.36:

$$0.105 = kt_{90\%} \text{ or } t_{90\%} = 0.105/k \tag{8.36}$$

Example 8.7: The first-order rate constant for the degradation of an antibiotic is 3.5×10^{-7}/s. What is the half-life ($t_{1/2}$) of this drug's degradation? What is the shelf life ($t_{90\%}$) of the antibiotic?

Answer: To calculate the half-life, you should use Equation 8.34. The answer is 23 days.

$$t_{1/2} = \frac{0.693}{3.5^{-7}\,\text{s}^{-1}}$$

The shelf life ($t_{90\%}$) of the drug is

$$t_{90\%} = 0.105/k = 83 \text{ hours}$$

There are a few key points for the first-order degradation rate that are important to remember:

- The rate is dependent on the concentration.
- The half-life is constant because of $0.693/k$ (i.e., both numbers are constant).
- The value of $t_{90\%}$ is independent of the concentration.

Keep in mind that while the degradation of drug solutions is often a first-order reaction process, the degradation of suspensions is often a zero-order reaction process.

Learning Bridge 8.10

During the third day of your introductory pharmacy practice experience, your preceptor asks you to reconstitute the powder of azithromycin (Zmax) with distilled water to make a single-dose azithromycin suspension (final concentration = 27 mg/mL) for a pediatric patient. In addition, she asks you to fill another antibiotic solution, azithromycin (ophthalmic, 10 mg/mL; Azasite) for another pediatric patient.

Suppose the azithromycin suspension has a half-life of decomposition of 2.5 days at room temperature and the azithromycin (ophthalmic) solution has a half-life of decomposition of 90 days at 8°C (refrigerator). To counsel the patients' parents about storing their children's medications without compromising the active ingredient in these two solutions, your preceptor asks you to answer the following questions for both antibiotics:

A. What order of degradation kinetics does the antibiotic follow in each of the dosage forms?

B. What is the degradation rate constant for the antibiotic in each of the dosage forms at the temperatures provided?

C. How long will it take for the antibiotic in each dosage form to degrade to 90% of its original labeled concentration if stored at the indicated storage temperatures?

Second-Order Reaction

Similar to the case with other reaction orders, the power of the reactant's concentration plays an important role in determining the kinetic order of a reaction. For a second-order reaction, the rate is proportional to the concentrations of two reactants, each raised to the first power, or alternatively to the concentration of one reactant raised to the second power (i.e., squared). Let's look at an example to see exactly what a second-order reaction means.

If the degradation of urea by a urease enzyme can be described by the data in **Table 8.10**, we can calculate the order of the kinetic rate constant (k).

As described earlier, to determine the order of a reaction rate, write the general rate law equation for the reaction. In this case, the rate is equal to k multiplied by the concentration of urea (C, or reactant), raised to some unknown power, x (recall that we encountered a similar situation in Equation 8.27). When the unknown x becomes known, it gives you information about the order of the reaction.

Rate = $k[C]^x$: As Table 8.10 indicates, the initial concentration increases 100% (2 times) between the first and second experiments. However, the initial reaction rate increases 4 times between the same experiments. Between the first and third experiments, the initial concentration increases 3 times but the initial rate increases 9 times (from 1.7×10^{-5} to 15.3×10^{-5}).

The data presented in Table 8.10 indicate that the rate for the urea degradation is proportional to the square of the urea's (reactant) concentration. Simply put, x must be 2, and the order of the rate constant must be second order. The rate law for a second-order reaction in our example can be expressed as follows:

$$\text{Rate} = k[C]^2 \tag{8.37}$$

Let's see what the unit for a second-order rate constant is. As usual, the unit for the rate (velocity) is M s^{-1} and the concentration of the reactant is M^2. Equation 8.37 can assist us in determining the units of a second-order rate constant:

$$k = \text{Rate}/[C]^2 = \text{M s}^{-1}/\text{M}^2 = \text{s}^{-1}\,\text{M}^{-1}$$

In a second-order reaction, the concentration of a drug decreases at a rate that is proportional to the square of the concentration of the remaining drug:

$$\frac{dC_t}{dt} = -k[C_t]^2 \tag{8.38}$$

Table 8.10 Degradation of Urea by a Urease Enzyme Follows a Second-Order Kinetic Rate

Experiment Number	Initial Urea Concentration (C)	Initial Degradation Rate
1	0.01 M	1.7×10^{-5} M/s
2	0.02 M	6.8×10^{-5} M/s
3	0.03 M	15.3×10^{-5} M/s

The integration of Equation 8.38 gives Equation 8.39:

$$\frac{1}{[C_t]} - \frac{1}{[C_0]} = kt \tag{8.39}$$

This expression can be rearranged to give Equation 8.40:

$$\frac{1}{[C_t]} = kt + \frac{1}{[C_0]} \tag{8.40}$$

From Equation 8.40, we can see that if we graph $1/[C_t]$ as a function of time, it yields a linear slope where the slope is k and the y-intercept is $1/[C_0]$ (**Figure 8.27**).

We can also calculate the half-life for a second-order reaction. C_t at the first half-life will be $[C_t] = [C_0]/2$. Substituting this expression into Equation 8.40 gives Equation 8.41:

$$\frac{1}{[C_0]/2} = kt_{1/2} + \frac{1}{[C_0]} \tag{8.41}$$

Solving for $t_{1/2}$, we have

$$\frac{2}{[C_0]} - \frac{1}{[C_0]} = kt_{1/2} \tag{8.42}$$

$$t_{1/2} = \frac{1}{k[C_0]} \tag{8.43}$$

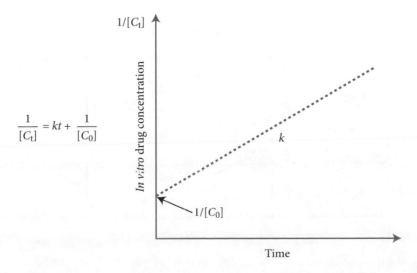

Figure 8.27 The second-order rate constant can be calculated by using the equation and the slope of a graph that depicts the inverse of drug concentrations ($1/C_t$) as a function of time.

Example 8.8: Two iodine atoms can react with each other to form the molecular gas, iodine. This reaction is known to be carried out at a second-order rate. The second-order rate constant is known: 6.93×10^{10} M^{-1} s^{-1}. The initial concentration of iodine was 0.09 M.

A. Calculate the concentration of iodine atom after 3 minutes.

B. Calculate the half-life of the reaction.

Answer: According to Equation 8.40, we have $[C_t] = 8.02 \times 10^{-14}$ M; according to Equation 8.43, the half-life will be 1.60×10^{-10} second.

$$\frac{1}{[C_t]} = kt + \frac{1}{[C_0]}$$

$$\frac{1}{[C_t]} = 6.93 \times 10^{10} \text{ M}^{-1} \text{ s}^{-1} \times 180 \text{ s} + \frac{1}{0.09 \text{ M}} = 8.02 \times 10^{-14} \text{ M}$$

$$t_{1/2} = \frac{1}{k[C_0]} = 1.60 \times 10^{-10} \text{s}$$

Notice that the calculated concentration after 3 minutes (180 seconds) is very low (8.02×10^{-14} M), which will be almost impossible to detect in the solution. Because of the very fast rate constant, almost none of the reactant (iodine atoms) will be left after 180 seconds. In addition, notice that the half-life is inversely proportional to the initial concentration of reactant. The more reactant present, the shorter the half-time—at a high concentration of reactant, more iodine atoms are found in the solution and collide with each other to produce the iodine molecule.

Figure 8.28 summarizes different degradation rate orders for a drug.

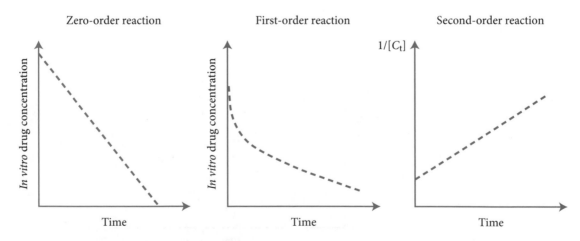

Figure 8.28 *In vitro* degradation of a drug by three different reaction orders C_t is the *in vitro* drug concentration..

Reaching Equilibrium in a Reaction

The majority of reactions do not reach a complete end; in other words, a reaction rarely reaches the point at which all reactants have been converted to a product. Instead, an incomplete point—that is, equilibrium—will be reached. At the equilibrium, the rate of product formation (the forward rate) and the rate of product breakdown (the reverse rate) are equal. The equilibrium constant, K_{eq}, can be expressed by Equation 8.44 and is the ratio of product concentrations to reactant concentrations when the reaction is at equilibrium.

$$A + B \rightleftharpoons C + D$$

$$K_{eq} = \frac{[C][D]}{[A][B]} \tag{8.44}$$

A reaction at equilibrium does not stop. Once a reaction has reached equilibrium, the overall ratio of products to reactants does not change—but that does not mean equal concentrations of all reactants and products will be present. In addition, K_{eq} is entirely different from the rate or rate constant for a reaction, and it will not be affected by the reaction rate constant. The relationship between the equilibrium and rate constants can also be expressed. We can write the rate law for the forward and reverse reactions at equilibrium. For the previous reaction, in which A and B reacted to produce C and D, we can write the rate law for the forward (f) and reverse (r) reactions as follows:

$$V = k_f[A][B] = k_r[C][D] \tag{8.45}$$

where V is the velocity and k_f and k_r are the forward and reverse rate constants, respectively. At equilibrium, the rate of the forward reaction exactly balances the rate of the reverse reaction. Accordingly, we can rewrite Equation 8.45 as Equation 8.46:

$$\frac{k_f}{k_r} = \frac{[C][D]}{[A][B]} = K_{eq} \tag{8.46}$$

If the forward rate goes up, the reverse rate goes up as well, which makes K_{eq} a constant and unchanged parameter.

Golden Keys for Pharmacy Students

1. While it is the active ingredient in a drug that produces the pharmacological effect, the inactive ingredients (excipients) play essential pharmaceutical roles through their thickening, suspending, diluting, emulsifying, coloring, flavoring, or preserving properties.

2. When a drug is ready to be studied in humans, its developer submits an investigational new drug (IND) application to the FDA.

3. A clinical trial of a drug proceeds through four well-established phases.

   - Phase I: The investigational compound is given to a small healthy population (20–100) to establish the maximum tolerated dose and the limits of its toxicity.

- Phase II: A small patient population (100–200) with the targeted disease state is given the drug to study its therapeutic index, a broader range of toxicities, and drug formulation.
- Phase III: Approximately 1,000 patients receive the drug to confirm its efficacy and side effects.
- Phase IV: A scale-up of the batch size occurs.

4. The FDA requires that any generic drug have the same active ingredient, strength, dosage form, and route of administration as the brand-name drug.

5. Good Manufacturing Practice (GMP) is a quality standard that specifies the minimum requirements in manufacturing, processing, packaging, and storing processes.

6. Inhalation is an important administration route for patients with respiratory problems. Drug delivery through the large mucous membranes of the respiratory tract occurs as rapidly as drug delivery through IV injection thanks to the large surface area of the respiratory tract and the enriched capillaries in the lungs.

7. Dissolution plays an important role in the absorption of a solid drug. If the dissolution rate is slower than the absorption rate, the dissolution rate becomes a rate-limiting factor.

8. The vapor pressure of a liquid is a unique property of the liquid and depends on two important factors: the identity of the liquid (intermolecular forces) and the temperature (kinetic energy).

9. Colligative properties of solutions include vapor pressure reduction, boiling-point elevation, freezing-point depression, and osmotic pressure. All of these properties depend on the number (but not the chemical identity) of solute particles in a solution.

10. Osmosis is the transport of a solvent (usually water) across a semipermeable membrane that separates two solutions with different concentrations.

11. A solution that has the same "tone" (osmotic pressure) as body fluids will not cause any change in the tissue. An 0.9% NaCl solution (normal saline) is an isotonic solution to human blood cells.

12. The resistance of a liquid to spread out and expand its surface area creates surface tension. Surface tension is a physical property of liquids that is caused by intermolecular forces.

13. A surfactant is a molecule that has both hydrophobic and hydrophilic properties owing to its structure. Surfactants are classified based on the nature of their hydrophilic groups.

14. Glycerol has a valuable place in pharmaceutics. It is an excellent solvent and in a high concentration has a preservative effect.

15. Any molecule that reduces the surface tension of a liquid has a wetting property. A wetting agent has a hydrophil–lipophil balance (HLB) number between 7 and 9. Non-ionic surfactants are commonly used as wetting agents.

16. HLB numbers have been generated for many surfactant molecules. The more hydrophilic an agent is, the higher its HLB number.

17. One osmole is equal to one mole of a dissolved nonelectrolyte solute. Osmolality of a solution is equal to the number of moles of dissolved solutes (ions or molecules) per weight (kilogram) of water. Osmolarity of a solution is equal to the number of moles of dissolved solutes (ions or molecules) per volume (liter) of water.

18. In the Newtonian system, molecules have a constant viscosity, regardless of the shear rates applied. In a non-Newtonian system, the viscosity can change with an increase in the shear rate.

19. By definition, there are three types of dispersions: (1) true solutions, which have a homogenous molecular dispersion and a particle size less than 1 nm (e.g., dissolved sugar in water); (2) coarse dispersions, which have a particle size larger than 0.5 mm, with particles being visible under light microscopes (e.g., an emulsion); and (3) colloidal dispersions, which have a particle size in the range of 1 nm to 0.5 mm.

20. Polyethylene glycol (PEG) is soluble in water and alcohol. The lower the PEG number, the lower melting point and the more water-soluble the PEG base is.

21. A suspension is a coarse dispersion in which an internal phase, consisting of insoluble particles, is dispersed homogeneously within an external phase. A suspension dosage form is useful for insoluble or poorly soluble drugs, to mask the bitter taste of a drug, and to control the release rate of a drug.

22. Flocculation is an aggregation process that causes the dispersed particles to adhere to one another and form large aggregates. Flocculation is not a problem in a suspension because it is a reversible process. In contrast, caking causes particles to form a compact aggregated structure within a suspension.

23. There are two forms of emulsions: (1) oil-in-water emulsions (o/w), in which the continuous phase is hydrophilic and the dispersed phase is hydrophobic (miscible with hydrophilic liquids); and (2) water-in-oil (w/o), in which the continuous phase is hydrophobic and the dispersed phase is hydrophilic (miscible with hydrophobic liquids).

24. An emulsion is a physically unstable solution, and there is a risk that the two phases (external and internal phases) in an emulsion might separate from each other ("breaking" process).

25. In manufacturing tablets, a series of quality control tests need to be carried out, including weight and content uniformity tests; disintegration, dissolution, hardness, friability, and microbial tests; and elegant appearance and safe packing.

26. Capsules are often more expensive than tablets on a per-unit basis, but they have advantages over tablets including their ability to mask the taste and odor of the ingredients, protect any light-sensitive ingredients, and use of surfactants to increase the bioavailability of water-insoluble drugs.

27. Semisolid dosage forms should be elegant in appearance, should not be gritty, and should not irritate the skin. The vehicle—that is, the base in which the drug is delivered—plays a crucial role in achieving a successful therapeutic outcome.

28. Suppositories offer a series of advantages, such as reducing the first-pass effect, going through the rectal mucosa into the circulation through the rectal veins, and being useful when it is difficult for patients to take oral drugs.

29. The larger the size of a transdermal patch, the higher the dose–response. Similarly, the higher the drug concentration of the active ingredient, the higher the drug absorption rate.

30. In "dose dumping," the high concentration of the active ingredient in a modified-release dosage form, upon unintentional immediate release (by chewing or crushing), causes toxicity.

31. While degradation of drug solutions is often a first-order reaction process, the degradation of suspensions is often a zero-order reaction process.

32. The rate of a zero-order reaction is independent of the concentrations of the reactants.

33. In a first-order reaction, the reaction rate is directly proportional to the concentration of one of the reactants.

34. In a second-order reaction, the reaction rate is proportional to the concentration of two reactants, each raised to the first power, or alternatively to the concentration of one reactant raised to the second power (squared).

Learning Bridge Answers

8.1 **A.** For prescription 1, both drugs I and III should be fine, as both have AB codes, which indicate they are therapeutically equivalent. For prescription 2, drug IV is not therapeutically equivalent to drug V. The pharmacy store needs to order drug IV rather than replacing it with drug V.

B. B and F are correct answers. While reaching the systemic circulation is a process, the bioavailability is the fraction of a drug that reaches the systemic circulation in an unchanged form. For example, if 100 mg of a drug is given orally, but the plasma concentration of the drug is only 40 mg, the bioavailability of the drug is 0.4 (40/100), or 40%.

8.2 **A.** Ideal propellants are stable at room temperature. Both the drug and the propellant must be compatible (either as a solution or as a suspension) and remain stable for a reasonable length of time (for expiration dating purposes). The drug must tolerate the particle size for aerosolization and benefit from having a delivery site in the lung tissue or absorption in the lungs.

B. The propellant and the drug must be mixed sufficiently so an appropriate dose is delivered.

8.3 Griseofulvin's GI absorption is significantly affected by a micronization process (i.e., by decreasing the particle size) of the drug. The GI absorption of the ultramicrosize is 50% higher than the absorption of the microsize.

According to the Noyes-Whitney equation and Figure 8.3, decreasing a drug's particle size increases the dissolution rate of the drug. Griseofulvin has poor water solubility, so reducing its particle size increases the drug's surface area. This increases its dissolution rate, which in turn increases its absorption.

$$\frac{dw}{dt} = \frac{DA}{\delta}(C_s - C)$$

8.4 Sorbitol is used as a sweetening or a solubilizing agent in some liquid dosage forms, including elixirs. However, even though sorbitol is referred to as an inert agent, it can cause osmotic diarrhea. For instance, 20 g sorbitol can work as a laxative agent. In addition, some patients are intolerant to as little as 10 g sorbitol.

While sorbitol can be found in many formulations, it is frequently included in acetaminophen, ibuprofen, potassium gluconate, and pseudoephedrine formulations. In addition and because of sorbitol's sweet and pleasant taste, it is included in chewable tablets as well as chewing gums. In contrast to lactose, which is fermented by intestinal bacteria, sorbitol is not fermented to any significant extent by microorganisms. In addition, it is not readily absorbed from the GI tract. Furthermore, sorbitol is found in fruits such as apples, pears, and peaches. Both hypertonicity and the content of sorbitol contribute to the GI intolerance. The colon plays an important role in reabsorbing excess water prior to discharging water from the body. When the colon cannot reabsorb the excess of water, diarrhea occurs. Sorbitol causes diarrhea because it accumulates and, owing to its osmotic effect, draws water into the colon; this stimulates bowel movements.

Advise Amy that there may be some side effects associated with sorbitol such as dry mouth and nausea.

8.5 **A.** You have to calculate the osmolarity of all the ingredients to know the total osmolarity of the solution. The following equation can be used to calculate the osmolarity of the electrolytes in the ORS:

$(g/L)/(g/mole) \times$ number of solute species = Osm/L

For Na^+ with a molecular weight of 23 g/mole, we have

$$\frac{g/L}{g/mole} = \frac{2\,g/L}{23\,g/mole} \times 1 = 87\,mOsm/L$$

$K^+ = 0.07\%; (0.7\,g/L)/(39\,g/mol) = 18\,mOsm/L$

$Cl^- = 0.35\%; (3.5\,g/L)/(39\,g/mol) = 99\,mOsm/L$

Glucose $= 1.9\%; (19\,g/L)/(180\,g/mol) = 111\,mOsm/L$

$87 + 18 + 99 + 110 = 310\,mOsm/L$

B. The same equation can assist you in calculating the osmolarity. You have to identify and apply all the indicated strengths to identify the correct answer. The correct answer is 5% intravenous dextrose solution (5% is equal to 0.5 g/100 mL, or 50 g/L). Because dextrose is not an ionizable molecule, calculation of the concentration (mole/L) gives you the same number as osmolarity (Osm/L).

$$\frac{50\,g/L}{180\,g/mol} = 278\,mmol/L = 278\,mOsm/L$$

C. Soft drinks and sweetened fruit drinks are often nonelectrolyte solutions. They should be avoided here because they can cause osmotic diarrhea, which may worsen the dehydration problem.

8.6 **A.** Although there is nothing wrong with prescribing an elixir, this is not the right dosage form for David. If a higher dose of acetaminophen is needed (as it is for this patient), the dose of hydrocodone will increase as well. Many healthcare providers try to prescribe separate active ingredients to avoid any possible overdose risk with the ingredients that exist in an elixir. Elixirs with only one active ingredient do not cause any dosing problems.

B. Always calculate the maximum possible dose. In this case, the prescription calls for the patient to receive 4 g acetaminophen (8 × 500 mg) and 60 mg hydrocodone. Although the acetaminophen amount is the maximum allowable dose, there is a risk of acetaminophen-induced hepatotoxicity overdose due to the "prn" instruction. In addition, the maximum dose of hydrocodone is 40 mg/day, which is another reason why the prescribed elixir should be changed to two separate medications. Hydrocodone alone is not available in the United States, so the attending physician needs to change hydrocodone to another opioid pain reliever.

Use of "tablespoon" as a measurement unit is strongly discouraged in the directions section of a prescription and on the label of the medication to reduce medication errors.

One tablespoonful (tbs) contains about 15 mL, and one teaspoonful (tsp) is about 5 mL. The physician should have written 15 mL in the sig section of the prescription. In addition, a controlled substance, Schedule III (hydrocodone), cannot be refilled more than 5 times.

C. Lortab Elixir contains 7% alcohol.

8.7 A. According to the package insert, to make 200 mg/mL azithromycin, you need to add 15 mL of the distilled water, which will make a total volume of 30 mL azithromycin.

B. The suggested pediatric azithromycin dose for this infection is 12 mg/kg/day. Nick's weight is 37 lb, which is equal to 17 kg (37/2.2). This weight corresponds to 204 mg/day. Because the concentration of the reconstituted azithromycin is 200 mg/5 mL, 5 mL/day should suffice to kill the bacteria within 5 days. Your preceptor should call Nick's pediatrician and inform him of the dosing recommendation.

C. Antacids are known to slow the absorption of azithromycin because they bind to azithromycin and do not allow it to be absorbed from the intestine. Nick should take azithromycin at least 1–2 hours before taking Mylanta.

8.8 Coal Tar USP is still a widely prescribed product compounded in pharmacies for patients. This formulation, by definition of the United States Pharmacopeia, contains coal tar 1%, polysorbate 80 0.5%, and zinc oxide paste.

The vehicle in this formulation is zinc oxide paste. The zinc oxide component actually provides a preservative action, as it is an antiseptic. The paste vehicle is hydrophobic, stiff, and occlusive, providing protective qualities. The polysorbate 80 serves as an emulsifying agent, allowing the coal tar to smoothly integrate into the paste.

8.9 The list of the available nonparenteral dosage forms, including the advantages of each formulation for Ms. Chowdrey, are given here. This information can be obtained by accessing a drug formulary via a database such as *Micromedex* or *Facts and Comparisons*. Morphine is available in the following oral formulations:

- Oral capsule, extended release: good for taking doses less often, easier to swallow than a tablet
- Oral solution: good if having difficulty swallowing
- Oral tablet: good for taking more often and could adjust the dose as needed for breakthrough pain
- Oral tablet, extended release: good for taking doses less often, smaller than a capsule
- Rectal suppository: good if cannot take by mouth

8.10 A. Because suspensions and solutions often have zero-order and first-order degradation processes, respectively, the degradation rate constant for the suspension is zero order and that for the ophthalmic solution is first order.

B. To calculate the rate constants, we need to know $t_{1/2}$ for both medications. For the extended-release suspension (Zmax), $t_{1/2}$ is 2.5 days at room temperature. The following equation can be used to calculate the zero-order rate constant:

$$t_{1/2} = \frac{1/2 C_0}{k}$$

$$2.5 = \frac{0.5 \times 27 \text{ mg/mL}}{k}$$

$$k = 5.4 \text{ (mg/mL)} / \text{day}$$

For the azithromycin ophthalmic solution (Azasite), $t_{1/2}$ is 90 days at 8°C. The following equation can be used to calculate the first-order rate constant:

$$t_{1/2} = \frac{0.693}{k}$$

$$k = 7.7 \times 10^{-3}/\text{day}$$

C. To calculate $t_{90\%}$, we need to know the rate constant and the initial concentration of the drug. For the extended-release suspension (Zmax), k_0 is 5.4 (mg/mL)/day. The following equation can be used:

$$t_{90\%} = 0.1C_0/k_0$$

$$t_{90\%} = \frac{0.1 \times 27 \ \frac{\text{mg}}{\text{mL}}}{5.4 \ \frac{\text{mg}}{\text{mL}}/\text{day}} = 0.5 \text{ day} = 12 \text{ hours}$$

The shelf life at 25°C (room temperature) is 12 hours, after which the drug suspension must be discarded. For the ophthalmic solution Azasite, k is 7.7×10^{-3}/day. The following equation can be used to calculate $t_{90\%}$:

$$\ln \frac{C_0}{0.9C_0} = kt_{90\%}$$

$$t_{90\%} = 0.105/k; \ t_{90\%} = 0.105/7.7 \times 10^{-3}/\text{day} = 14 \text{ day}$$

The shelf life at 8°C (refrigerator) is 14 days, after which the solution must be discarded.

Problems and Solutions

Problem 8.1 Does a liquid in a sealed drug inhaler evaporate?

Solution 8.1 Yes, it does, but you don't see any changes in the volume of the liquid because the rates of evaporation and condensation are the same. After a while, the rate of vaporization equals the rate of condensation. The vapor molecules above the liquid (in the closed container) exert a pressure that is saturated; this pressure is called the vapor pressure.

Problem 8.2 Why does an electrolyte solute such as NaCl reduce the vapor pressure twice as much as a nonelectrolyte solute such as sucrose?

Solution 8.2 The number of solutes in a solvent affects the vapor pressure. Because NaCl is an electrolyte, it is able to dissociate in water into two ions (Na^+ and Cl^-). As a result, NaCl reduces the vapor pressure more than adding the same concentration of a nonelectrolyte solute.

Problem 8.3 You are a PharmD working in a pharmaceutical company and are in charge of formulating nitroglycerin tablets. You know that, due to intermolecular van der Waals forces, nitroglycerin diffuses and vaporizes easily from tablets. What would you do to overcome this problem?

Solution 8.3 Vapor pressure plays an important role in the stability of nitroglycerin, which is a liquid at room temperature. It is critical to reduce the vapor pressure by adding an inert solute such as polyethylene glycol.

Problem 8.4 Which of the following molecules has the highest surface tension?

   A. Benzene
   B. Naphthalene
   C. Water

Solution 8.4 C. Water, because the strong hydrogen bonds among water molecules pull the molecules more strongly to the center of a droplet. Benzene has the lowest surface tension (benzene has one aromatic ring, and naphthalene has two aromatic rings).

Problem 8.5 Why is an 0.9% NaCl solution an isotonic solution to our blood cells?

Solution 8.5 Normal saline and blood have the same freezing-point depression, $-0.52°C$. For instance, 5.9% of sodium penicillin G has the same freezing point as 0.9% NaCl, which means both are isotonic solutions to the blood cells.

Problem 8.6 Which class does white petrolatum USP belong to?

   A. Oleaginous bases
   B. Absorption bases
   C. Water-removable bases
   D. Water-soluble bases

Solution 8.6 A is correct.

Problem 8.7 Finasteride (Proscar) is used to treat symptomatic benign prostatic hyperplasia (BPH). Why are finasteride tablets available in coated dosage forms?

   A. To protect them from disintegration and dissolution in the stomach
   B. To avoid first-pass metabolism
   C. To make sure that their active ingredient is released into circulation to competitively inhibit the 5-alpha-reductase enzyme
   D. To protect any pregnant woman who inadvertently comes in contact with finasteride tablets

Solution 8.7 D is correct. This example demonstrates that there are different reasons why tablets are coated.

Problem 8.8 Match the following gelatin capsule sizes with their corresponding volume.

   Size: 000; 00; 0; 1; 2; 3; 4; 5.
   Volume: 0.13 mL; 0.68 mL; 0.95 mL; 0.30 mL; 0.21 mL; 0.37 mL; 1.4 mL.

Solution 8.8 000 (1.4 mL); 00 (0.95 mL); 0 (0.68 mL); 1 (0.50 mL); 2 (0.37 mL); 3 (0.30 mL); 4 (0.21 mL); 5 (0.13 mL).

Problem 8.9 Oil is immiscible with water-soluble solutions. For example, if you mix 1 cup of oil with 4 tablespoons of vinegar, you will see that the vinegar is not miscible in the oil. However, if you add 2 egg yolks, the vinegar will be easily mixed with the oil. By adding a little salt, you have a home-made mayonnaise. Egg yolk contains lecithin (phosphatidylcholine). What is the pharmaceutical name of lecithin in our example? What is the pharmaceutical name of this dispersion (mayonnaise)?

   A. Thickening agent; suspension
   B. Thickening agent; emulsion
   C. Surfactant; suspension
   D. Surfactant; emulsion
   E. Vehicle; cream
   F. Flavoring agent; emulsion

Solution 8.9 D is the correct answer. Lecithin (phosphatidylcholine) in the egg yolk acts as a surfactant because it has both hydrophilic (a charged head group) and hydrophobic (two hydrophobic tails) groups. The surfactant is an emulsifier agent in this case because it will help two immiscible liquids become dispersed in each other.

Problem 8.10 Which of the following suppository bases may cause irritation of the rectal mucosa?

- **A.** Cocoa butter
- **B.** Fattibase
- **C.** Polyethylene glycol

Solution 8.10 C is correct because it is a water-soluble base. Because the PEG base is water soluble, it picks up water (to be dissolved) and causes slight dehydration of the rectal mucosa, which in turn causes irritation.

Problem 8.11 In making a suspension, it is important to add a thickening agent, such as methylcellulose, to increase the:

- **A.** Viscosity and to reduce sedimentation of particles in the suspension.
- **B.** Caking process in the suspension.
- **C.** Solubility of water-insoluble ingredients.
- **D.** Stability of the active ingredient.
- **E.** Palatability of the active and inactive ingredients.

Solution 8.11 A is correct.

Problem 8.12 The particles in an ideal suspension should:

- **A.** Have a uniform size of particles.
- **B.** Remain separated (to minimize sedimentation).
- **C.** Not interact with each other.
- **D.** Resuspend easily upon shaking.
- **E.** Be physically and chemically stable during its shelf life.
- **F.** Be easy to pour.
- **G.** A, B, and D.
- **H.** All of the above.
- **I.** All of the above except E.

Solution 8.12 H is correct.

Problem 8.13 Are "A"-rated generic drugs as safe and as effective as brand-name drugs? Why?

Solution 8.13 Yes, because they have to be therapeutically equivalent.

Problem 8.14 To be considered bioequivalent, two drugs must show similarity in: (Choose all that apply.)

- **A.** Efficacy.
- **B.** Bioavailability.
- **C.** Safety.
- **D.** Reaching the liver.
- **E.** Reaching the stomach.
- **F.** Reaching the systemic circulation.

Solution 8.14 B and F are correct. While reaching the systemic circulation is a process, the bioavailability is the fraction of a drug that reaches the systemic circulation in an unchanged form. For example, if 100 mg of a drug is given orally and the plasma concentration of the drug is 40 mg, the bioavailability of the drug is 0.4 (40/100), or 40%.

Problem 8.15 True or False: Drugs A and B have the same strength, active ingredient, and salt form. However, these two drugs have different excipients (inactive ingredients). Drugs A and B are pharmaceutical equivalents by definition. If so, why?

Solution 8.15 True; pharmaceutical equivalents can have different inactive ingredients (e.g., emulsifiers, diluents).

Problem 8.16 Should a solid drug have hydrophilic or hydrophobic properties in the GI system? Why?

Solution 8.16 A solid drug should have high hydrophobic property, yet also be hydrophilic. It needs to be hydrophilic to be dissolved in the GI fluid and reach the epithelial cell lining of the small intestine to reach the systemic circulation. It needs to be highly hydrophobic to go through the cell membranes. Indeed, this is why many drugs are weakly acidic and basic drugs (i.e., have both hydrophilic and hydrophobic properties).

Problem 8.17 The antifungal drug griseofulvin absorption is significantly affected by a micronization (decreasing particle size) process of the drug. However, the absorption of potassium chloride is not affected by the micronization process. Explain why.

Solution 8.17 According to the Noyes-Whitney equation, decreasing a drug's particle size increases the drug's dissolution rate, which in turn increases the drug's absorption. Griseofulvin has poor water solubility; reducing the particle size increases the drug's surface area, thereby increasing its dissolution rate and ultimately its absorption. Potassium chloride is already highly water soluble, so an increase in its surface area will not change its absorption.

Problem 8.18. A weakly acidic drug has a low dissolution rate in the GI fluid with a pH of 1–3. By using the Noyes-Whitney equation, one can show that the C_s can be increased to enhance the dissolution rate of the weakly acidic drug in the GI fluid. Explain how this is possible.

Solution 8.18 The weakly acidic drug will be in an un-ionized form at pH 1–3, so it will show poor solubility in the GI fluid. C_s is the concentration of the drug at the diffusion layer that surrounds the solid. A low solubility results in a low C_s and, therefore, a low dissolution rate. When the weakly acidic drug is made in a salt form, the ionized form of the salt will increase C_s, thereby increasing the dissolution rate.

Problem 8.19 EyeVisible 10 mg/mL is an ophthalmic solution. The degradation rate for EyeVisible follows first-order kinetics and is 1.1×10^{-3}/hr. Calculate the half-life of the active ingredient. Also calculate the number of days after which this product can no longer be used.

Solution 8.19 Because this medication's degradation follows first-order kinetics, we can use the following equation to calculate its $t_{1/2}$:

$$t_{1/2} = 0.693/k$$

$$t_{1/2} = 0.693/1.1 \times 10^{-3}/hr = 630 \text{ hr} = 26 \text{ days}$$

To calculate $t_{90\%}$, we use the following equation for a first-order kinetic process: $t_{90\%} = 0.105/k = 95 \text{ hr} = 4 \text{ days}$. To receive a full effect of EyeVisible, a person should not use this medication beyond 4 days (because after 4 days there will be less than 90% of the active ingredient left in the solution).

Problem 8.20 Match each vehicle with the most appropriate description.

Syrup	A. Contains a lower (less than 20%) alcohol content
Elixir	B. Contains a high concentration of sucrose or sugars
Tincture	C. Applied to an affected area rather than taken orally
Topical solution	D. Contains higher (up to 30%) alcohol content

Solution 8.20 1 = B; 2 = D; 3 = A; 4 = C.

Problem 8.21 Which of the following solutions can be used to prepare sterile intravenous medications in a pharmacy environment? (Choose all that apply.)

- **A.** Sterile Water for Injection USP
- **B.** Water for Injection USP
- **C.** Bacteriostatic Water for Injection USP
- **D.** Sterile Purified Water USP
- **E.** Purified Water USP

Solution 8.21 Only solutions that have been sterilized by the manufacturer should be used to prepare sterile intravenous medications. Therefore, choices A and C are correct. Choice E is not sterile; choice B is intended for use by manufacturers to be sterilized after a drug is added; choice D is not intended for injection administration.

Problem 8.22 Match the following terminology with the most appropriate description.

1. Geometric dilution	A. Use a mortar and pestle to grind coarse powders together
2. Levigation	B. Add a small amount of volatile liquid to aid in grinding the mixture
3. Pulverization by intervention	C. Mix equal quantities of powders, slowly increasing the mixture by equal amounts with each addition
4. Trituration	D. Add a small amount of a solvent to aid in blending the mixture

Solution 8.22 1 = C, 2 = D, 3 = B, 4 = A.

Problem 8.23 Describe the difference between an extended-release dosage form and a delayed-release dosage form.

Solution 8.23 An extended-release dosage form slowly releases the drug and extends the therapeutic effect. A delayed-release dosage form does not release the drug until it reaches the site of action. Once at the site of action, the drug is released.

Problem 8.24 Which of the following methods would increase the ability of a hydrophobic or insoluble drug to successfully be incorporated into a drug formulation? (Choose all that apply.)

- **A.** Levigation
- **B.** Mixture with a cosolvent
- **C.** Liposome with a hydrophobic center
- **D.** Suspension in a liquid

Solution 8.24 All of the above would be appropriate. The method selected would be further delineated depending on the intended site of drug action. For example, levigation would be a better choice for a topical drug, whereas a liposome would be a better choice for an injectable drug.

Problem 8.25 Select the true statements regarding transdermal drug delivery. (Choose all that apply.)

- **A.** Delivers drug quickly
- **B.** Excellent choice for a drug that has poor bioavailability

    C. Excellent choice for potent drugs

    D. Improves patient adherence

    E. Excellent choice for highly hydrophilic drugs

Solution 8.25 B, C, and D are correct. Transdermal administration is an excellent drug delivery system for drugs that have poor bioavailability because topical absorption avoids first-pass metabolism; for potent drugs due to the limited formulation size; and for improving patient adherence because the dosing frequency is usually infrequent (i.e., every 24–72 hours). Transdermal delivery does not release the drug rapidly; instead, it releases the drug slowly, allowing for slow absorption and less frequent dosing intervals. Also, the drug should be a balance of hydrophilic and hydrophobic to be released from the membrane and absorbed through the skin.

    We would like to thank Dr. Deepa Rao for her review and comments on the earlier version of this chapter.

References

1. Abood H. *Pharmacy practice and the law,* 6th ed. Sudbury, MA: Jones & Bartlett; 2011.

2. Allen LV, Popovich NG, Ansel HC. *Ansel's pharmaceutical dosage forms and drug delivery systems,* 8th ed. Philadelphia, PA: Lippincott Williams & Wilkins; 2005.

3. Attwood D. Florence AT. *FASTtrack: physical pharmacy.* London, UK: Pharmaceutical Press; 2008.

4. Burzynski JA, Walsh-Chocolaad T. Myelodysplastic syndromes. In: Talbert RL, DiPiro JT, Matzke GR, et al., eds. *Pharmacotherapy: a pathophysiologic approach*, 8th ed. New York, NY: McGraw-Hill; 2011. Available at: http://www.accesspharmacy.com/content.aspx?aID=8010906.

5. Buxton IL, Benet LZ. Pharmacokinetics: the dynamics of drug absorption, distribution, metabolism, and elimination. In: Brunton LL, Chabner BA, Knollmann BC. *Goodman & Gilman's the pharmacological basis of therapeutics*, 12th ed. New York, NY: McGraw-Hill; 2010. Available at: http://www.accesspharmacy.com/content.aspx?aID=16658120.

6. Cook PH. Glycerol. In: *AccessScience*. New York, NY: McGraw-Hill; 2008. Available at: http://www.accessscience.com.

7. DailyMed current medication information. Available at: http://dailymed.nlm.nih.gov/dailymed/about.cfm. Accessed November 20, 2012.

8. Delaney KA, Vassallo SU. Thermoregulatory principles. In: Delaney KA, Vassallo SU, eds. *Goldfrank's toxicologic emergencies*, 9th ed. New York, NY: McGraw-Hill; 2011. Available at: http://www.accesspharmacy.com/content.aspx?aID=6505084.

9. Dickerson RN, Sacks GS. Medication administration considerations with specialized nutrition support. In: DiPiro JT, Talbert RL, Yee GC, et al. *Pharmacotherapy: a pathophysiologic approach*, 8th ed. New York, NY: McGraw-Hill; 2011. Available at: http://www.accesspharmacy.com/content.aspx?aID=80122402011.

10. Florence AT, Attwood D. *Physicochemical principles of pharmacy*, 4th ed. London, UK: Pharmaceutical Press; 2011.

11. Food and Drug Administration. Approved drug products: therapeutic equivalence-related terms. Available at: http://www.fda.gov/downloads/Drugs/DevelopmentApprovalProcess/UCM071436.pdf. Accessed April 5, 2013.

12. Food and Drug Administration. Facts about generic drugs. Available at: http://www.fda.gov /drugs/resourcesforyou/consumers/buyingusingmedicinesafely/understandinggenericdrugs /ucm167991.htm. Accessed November 8, 2012.

13. Food and Drug Administration. Information for Consumers (Biosimilars). Available at: http://www.fda.gov/Drugs/DevelopmentApprovalProcess/HowDrugsareDeveloped andApproved/ApprovalApplications/TherapeuticBiologicApplications/Biosimilars /ucm241718.htm. Accessed September 6, 2013.

14. *Interactive chemistry multimedia courseware: solutions, solubility and precipitation, reaction rates, states of matter, bonding I and II.* Chico, CA: CyberEd; 2001.

15. Jain P, Banga AK. Induction and inhibition of crystallization in drug-in-adhesive-type transdermal patches. *Pharma Res.* 2013:30(2):562–571.

16. Kennelly PJ, Rodwell VW. Enzymes: kinetics. In: Murray RK, Bender DA, Botham KM, et al. *Harper's illustrated biochemistry*, 28th ed. New York, NY: McGraw-Hill; 2009. Available at: http://www.accesspharmacy.com/content.aspx?aID=5226003.

17. Kesselheim AS, Misono AS, Lee JL, et al. Clinical equivalence of generic and brand name drugs used in cardiovascular disease: a systematic review and meta-analysis. *JAMA.* 2008;300(21):2514–2526.

18. Marshall WJ and Bangert SK. *Clinical chemistry: hydrogen ion homoeostasis and blood gases*, 5th ed. Edinburg, UK: Elsevier Health Sciences; 2004.

19. Nachtrieb NH. Sublimation. In: *AccessScience*. New York, NY: McGraw-Hill; 2008. Available at: http://www.accessscience.com.

20. Nahata MC, Taketomo C. Pediatrics. In: DiPiro JT, Talbert RL, Yee GC, et al. *Pharmacotherapy: a pathophysiologic approach*, 7th ed. New York, NY: McGraw-Hill; 2008. Available at: http://www.accesspharmacy.com/content.aspx?aID=3183519.

21. Nelson DL, Cox MM. *Lehninger principles of biochemistry*, 4th ed. New York, NY: W. H. Freeman and Company; 2005.

22. Nelson DL, Cox MM. *Lehninger principles of biochemistry*, 5th ed. New York, NY: W. H. Freeman and Company; 2008.

23. Nordt SP, Vivero LE. Pharmaceutical additives. In: Nordt SP, Vivero LE, eds. *Goldfrank's toxicologic emergencies*, 9th ed. New York, NY: McGraw-Hill; 2011. Available at: http://www .accesspharmacy.com/content.aspx?aID=6515332.

24. Osterhoudt KC, Penning TM. Drug toxicity and poisoning. In: Brunton LL, Chabner BA, Knollmann BC. *Goodman & Gilman's the pharmacological basis of therapeutics*, 12th ed. New York, NY: McGraw-Hill; 2010. Available at: http://www.accesspharmacy.com/content .aspx?aID=16658740.

25. Pandit NK, Soltis RP. *Introduction to pharmaceutical sciences: an integrated approach*, 2nd ed. Philadelphia, PA: Wolters Kluwer/Lippincott Williams & Wilkins; 2012.

26. Powell PH, Fleming VH. Diarrhea, constipation, and irritable bowel syndrome. In: DiPiro JT, Talbert RL, Yee GC, et al. *Pharmacotherapy: a pathophysiologic approach*, 8th ed. New York, NY: McGraw-Hill; 2011. Available at: http://www.accesspharmacy.com/content .aspx?aID=7978775.

27. Remington. *The science and practice of pharmacy*, 21st ed. New York: Lippincott Williams and Wilkins; 2005.

28. Schramm LL. Surfactant. In: *AccessScience*. New York, NY: McGraw-Hill; 2008. Available at: http://www.accessscience.com.

29. Shargel L, Mutnick AH, Souney PF, Swanson LN. *Comprehensive pharmacy review*, 7th ed. Philadelphia, PA: Lippincott Williams & Wilkins; 2009.

30. Shargel L, Wu-Pong S, Yu ABC. Introduction to biopharmaceutics and pharmacokinetics. In: *Applied biopharmaceutics & pharmacokinetics*, 5th ed. New York, NY: McGraw-Hill; 2005. Available at: http://www.accesspharmacy.com/content.aspx?aID=2480000.

31. Shargel L, Wu-Pong S, Yu ABC. Modified-release drug products. In: *Applied biopharmaceutics & pharmacokinetics*, 5th ed. New York, NY: McGraw-Hill; 2005. Available at: http://www.accesspharmacy.com/content.aspx?aID=2481984.

32. Silberberg MS. *Chemistry: the molecular nature of matter and change*, 3rd ed. New York, NY: McGraw-Hill; 2003.

33. Silberberg MS. *Principles of general chemistry*. New York, NY McGraw-Hill; 2006.

34. Trevor AJ, Katzung BG, Masters SB. Drug evaluation and regulation. In: *Pharmacology: examination & board review*, 9th ed. New York, NY: McGraw-Hill; 2010. Available at: http://www.accesspharmacy.com/content.aspx?aID=6543318.

35. UpToDate. Waltham, MA: 2012. Available at: http://www.uptodate.com/online with subscription.

36. U.S. Department of Health and Human Services, Food and Drug Administration. Available at: http://www.accessdata.fda.gov/scripts/cder/ob/default.cfm. Accessed November 8, 2012.

37. William AB, Schilb TP. Osmoregulatory mechanisms. In: *AccessScience*. New York, NY: McGraw-Hill; 2008. Available at: http://www.accessscience.com.

Introduction to Pharmacokinetics

Reza Karimi
Fawzy Elbarbry

OBJECTIVES

1. Understand the basic concepts of drug absorption, distribution, metabolism, and elimination.

2. Recognize the importance and application of bioavailability, the volume of distribution, clearance, and half-life in pharmacokinetics.

3. Describe the differences between one- and two-compartment models and their applications in pharmacokinetics.

4. Analyze plasma concentration–time graphs and calculate absorption and elimination rate constants for intravenously and extravascularly administered drugs.

5. Define the steady-state condition during constant-rate IV infusion, multiple-drug administration, and intermittent infusions.

6. Describe how changes in pharmacokinetic parameters affect the value and time to achieve steady-state concentration.

7. Describe the major pathways found in renal excretion.

8. Recommend the dosing regimen required to achieve therapeutic plasma levels of a few drug products that follow nonlinear pharmacokinetics.

9. Implement a series of Learning Bridge assignments at your experiential sites to bridge your didactic learning with your experiential experiences.

KEY TERMS AND DEFINITIONS

1. **ADME:** absorption, distribution, metabolism, and excretion of a drug.

2. **AUC:** area under the plasma concentration–time curve.

3. **Bioavailability:** the fraction of the administered dose that reaches the systemic circulation; in the range of 0–100%. Its symbol is F and it is unitless.

4. **Clearance:** a measurement of how efficiently the body can eliminate (clear) a drug from the systemic circulation per unit of time.

5. **Compartment model:** a body volume (a tissue, an organ, or the whole body) that is a valuable model to predict the drug concentrations in the plasma at single or different doses.

6. C_p: plasma drug concentration.

7. $C_{p_{ss}}$: plasma drug concentration at steady state.

8. **Extraction ratio:** the fraction of a drug that has been irreversibly removed from the blood (by an eliminating organ) as the blood passes through that specific organ. Its symbol is E and it is unitless.

(continues)

(CONTINUED)

9. **Extravascular route:** administration of a drug into a site other than a vein, such as orally, transdermally, intramuscularly, or rectally.

10. **First-pass effect:** elimination of a drug before it reaches the systemic circulation.

11. **GFR:** glomerular filtration rate.

12. **Half-life:** the time that it takes to reduce the concentration of the drug in the body by 50% after absorption and distribution of the drug are complete.

13. **Intermittent drug infusion:** repeated IV drug infusions intended to prevent a toxic effect from IV administration.

14. **Loading dose:** the amount of drug that, when distributed in V_d, will give a desired plasma drug concentration.

15. **MEC:** minimum effective concentration; the plasma drug concentration that produces the minimum pharmacological effect.

16. **MTC:** minimum toxic concentration; the plasma drug concentration that produces the minimum toxic effect.

17. **Trough plasma drug concentrations**: the minimum drug concentration found in the plasma.

18. V_d: apparent volume of distribution; the volume in the body in which a drug is distributed.

Introduction

Pharmacokinetics is the science that underpins four kinetic processes—absorption, distribution, metabolism, and excretion (ADME)—that occur after a drug has been released from its dosage form. Drug elimination is a collective term that includes metabolism and excretion.

A drug, upon administration into the body, is in a dynamic state in which it may bind cells and cellular molecules in tissues, bind to proteins in the plasma, move between tissues and body fluids, or be metabolized. Because these dynamic events create complexity in knowing exactly where the drug is and what its concentration at a given time is, mathematical and statistical models are used to assist clinicians and researchers in estimating the doses required to achieve a therapeutic outcome at a given time. Pharmacokinetics can help clinicians and researchers apply mathematical models to explain or predict the kinetics of ADME, calculate an optimal dosage regimen for patients, estimate drug accumulation in the body, find a correlation between a drug dose and its toxicity, and explain how physiological changes or pathophysiological conditions affect ADME.

This chapter introduces pharmacokinetics by discussing basic concepts in ADME and describing bioavailability, volume of distribution, clearance, and half-life—all parameters that play essential roles in pharmacokinetics. The application of one- and two-compartment models in calculating these parameters is described. A series of pharmacokinetics equations are provided to facilitate understanding and measurements of absorption and elimination rate constants for intravenously and extravascularly administered drugs. Near the end of this chapter, major mechanisms that assist the kidney in excreting drug products are addressed, and the nonlinear pharmacokinetics is briefly discussed.

Pharmacokinetics

Experimental and theoretical approaches are employed to measure or predict the kinetics of ADME after drug administration. In addition to mathematical models, statistical approaches are used to estimate parameters involved in ADME, to identify error in data analysis, and to design optimal dosing regimens for patients in different populations (e.g., pediatric, geriatric, obese, pregnant, female, and male).

For instance, the following scenario emphasizes the role of and need for understanding pharmacokinetics in the treatment of an infection. Amy is a 25-year-old female who is seen by her primary care physician for a mild urinary tract infection. Her physician prescribed an antibiotic, trimethoprim-sulfamethoxazole (Bactrim DS), one tablet twice daily for 3 days to treat her infection. How can this drug eliminate the infectious agent in the urinary tract when it is administered orally? Why did the physician prescribe a dose of one tablet twice daily for 3 days versus two tablets twice daily for 7 days? Why did the pharmacist counsel Amy to take the medication with a full glass of water and advise her to finish all the dispensed tablets even if she felt better before completing the course of therapy? Understanding the pharmacokinetics of drugs will answer these questions.

To study pharmacokinetics, students are expected to understand basic mathematics, including algebraically and graphically driven equations and exponential and logarithmic data. They should also be able to use linear and semi-log graph paper to apply experimental or theoretical data to calculate one or more pharmacokinetic parameters.

Because pharmacokinetics affects pharmacology, it is important to recognize the interrelationship that exists between pharmacokinetics and pharmacology. While pharmacokinetics describes how rapidly or slowly a drug is absorbed or eliminated, it may not affect the ultimate pharmacological effect of the drug. In other words, pharmacokinetics is affected by alterations in ADME caused by physiological deficiency, anatomical damage, or disease state, but the ADME alteration may not affect the pharmacology of the drug. For example, patients with cirrhosis (a liver disease) have delayed gastric emptying due to altered action of their gastrointestinal hormones. This delayed gastric emptying lowers the absorption rate of a drug, but the extent of drug absorption may not be changed at all. As a consequence, the pharmacological effect will be delayed but will be fully achieved. In contrast, if patients with cirrhosis have less effective liver metabolism or a reduced glomerular filtration rate in their kidneys, the bioavailability and renal elimination of the same drug may be affected.

Similarly, it is imperative to understand the interrelationship that can occur between pharmacokinetics and biochemistry. For instance, the biochemical architecture of the cell membrane may affect the pharmacokinetics of a drug. No matter whether a drug has to pass through a single layer of cells (such as the epithelial cells that line the intestinal tract) or through multiple layers of cells (such as the cells in the epidermis, dermis, and subcutaneous layer of the skin), the cell membrane and drug diffusion play major roles in drug distribution by permitting the drug to reach the blood circulation.

How effectively a drug is distributed depends on the physicochemical properties of the drug. The extent of distribution is indicated by the volume of distribution (V_d). Estimation of pharmacokinetics parameters, such as clearance (Cl) and V_d, requires making assumptions related to a specific pharmacokinetics model. Pharmacokinetics models allow quantitative (mathematical) description and calculation of rates for ADME after a drug is administered and prediction of alterations that can occur to ADME owing to physiological and pathological changes. These practical models can be compartmental, physiological, or noncompartmental (described later in this chapter). Before these models are described and their applications in pharmacokinetics are emphasized, we should first describe a few important concepts in pharmacokinetics.

Clearance

Clearance is a parameter that measures how efficient the body can eliminate (clear) a drug from the systemic circulation per unit of time. Clearance is simply calculated from the elimination rate of a drug and the plasma drug concentration:

$$Cl = \frac{\text{Elimination rate}}{\text{Plasma concentration}} \tag{9.1}$$

If a drug's elimination follows first-order kinetics (most drugs do), clearance is a constant parameter (the first-order kinetics and other reaction orders are described in the *Introduction to Pharmaceutics* chapter). If you rearrange Equation 9.1 to Equation 9.2, you can see that the drug's elimination rate is directly proportional to the drug's concentration in the plasma (i.e., the elimination exhibits a "linear" process), simply because Cl is a constant.

Drug's elimination rate = Cl × Drug's concentration in the plasma   (9.2)

Equation 9.2 indicates that a higher drug concentration in the plasma leads to a higher elimination rate, which can be considered a unique defense mechanism that enables the body to react and adjust to the plasma concentration of a drug so as to avoid any drug accumulation or toxicity. When the elimination of a drug exhibits first-order kinetics, graphing plasma drug concentration as a function of time on a Cartesian scale demonstrates an exponential relationship with a negative slope (**Figure 9.1**). Keep in mind that in mathematics (and pharmacokinetic graphs), the *x*-axis represents the independent variable (often time in pharmacokinetics) and the *y*-axis represents the dependent variable (often plasma drug concentration in pharmacokinetics).

A few drugs are eliminated with zero-order kinetics—that is, their elimination does not exhibit linear kinetics. Such drugs include heparin (HepFlush-10), omeprazol (PriLOSEC OTC), phenytoin (Dilantin), and warfarin (Coumadin). For these drugs, the clearance changes depending on the drug's concentration in the plasma. As a result, Equation 9.2 cannot be used to measure the clearance of drugs that exhibit nonlinear elimination. As explained in the *Introduction to Pharmaceutics* chapter, there are fundamental differences between zero-order and first-order kinetics; these discrepancies will be reinforced later in this chapter.

The clearance rate depends on the drug and the physiological condition(s) of the organs that eliminate the drug. If a drug is cleared by more than one organ, the clearance rates for that drug are additive. For instance, clearance of a drug from the blood may occur as a result of clearance of that particular drug by the lung, kidney, and liver. To determine the clearance of this drug from the blood, we can use the following additive equation:

$$Cl = Cl_{lung} + Cl_{hepatic} + Cl_{renal} + Cl_{other} \qquad (9.3)$$

The two main elimination sites are hepatic and renal, however. The extraction capability of an organ and the blood flow to that organ play important roles in clearing a drug from that specific organ. For instance, the blood may be completely cleared of a particular drug when the drug passes through the liver. In such a case, the total clearance from the body is dependent only on the blood flow that goes through the liver (hepatic).

To describe clearance from a physiological point of view, we can express the following equation to show the relationship between blood flow and hepatic clearance:

$$Cl_{hepatic} = Q \times E \qquad (9.4)$$

where $Cl_{hepatic}$ is the clearance of a drug from the liver as an eliminating organ, Q is the blood flow to the liver, and E is the extraction ratio. For instance, when a drug enters the liver it has concentration C_1, and when it leaves the liver it has concentration

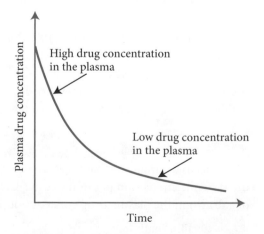

Figure 9.1 A typical drug elimination that exhibits first-order kinetics.

C_2; the extraction ratio, E, is $[(C_1 - C_2)/C_1]$. Obviously, if the elimination of a drug occurs in the liver, C_2 is smaller than C_1. The extraction ratio, then, is the fraction of the drug that is irreversibly removed from the blood (by an eliminating organ) as blood passes through that organ. In other words, a high E indicates a high extraction capability.

Equation 9.4 is not used extensively by clinicians, but it is useful when we need to know how a disease state affects the eliminating organ's clearance. Physiological conditions that alter blood flow can also alter total clearance for drugs that have a high extraction ratio (for instance, propranolol and lidocaine have a high E).

To further emphasize the roles of Q and E in clearance, let's consider the condition known as hypoalbuminemia. Elderly patients who do not eat adequate amounts of protein often suffer from hypoalbuminemia, in which levels of albumin in blood are abnormally low. This results in a lower viscosity of the blood, which in turn increases the blood flow (Q). Consequently, propranolol and lidocaine (high E values) have a higher Cl in these patients compared with healthy individuals. We will return to the important roles that clearance and its application play in pharmacokinetics later in this chapter.

Apparent Volume of Distribution

The apparent volume of distribution is the volume in the body in which a drug is distributed. V_d plays a significant role in the effects of a drug in the body and, as Equation 9.5 demonstrates, its value can be estimated if the *amount* of the drug in the body and the resulting plasma concentration are known. This condition can be met only right after an intravenous (IV) bolus dose has been administered:

$$V_d = \frac{\text{Dose}}{C_{p_0}}$$

(9.5)

where C_{p_0} is the plasma drug concentration at time 0.

Equation 9.5 indicates that if a drug is completely retained in the blood plasma, it will have a small V_d that is equal to the plasma volume (according to **Table 9.1**, V_d should be 3.5 L). In contrast, if a drug is mainly distributed to tissues, its concentration in the plasma will be low and, as a result, V_d will be large—perhaps exceeding the body's total volume. As an example, consider quinacrine, an antibiotic that is not available in the United States. Because of its high intracellular distribution, quinacrine has a V_d of 50,000 L in adult patients. Obviously, no human body can contain this large volume, which explains why V_d does not have a physical equivalent, but rather is referred to as an "apparent volume" of distribution. Such large values for V_d are possible, but are rarely seen; instead, most drugs have a V_d that is equal to or smaller than the body weight.

Upon its administration, regardless of the route of drug administration, a drug can enter the body fluid in three distinct pathways:

- Being trapped in the blood plasma due to having a large molecular size or being tightly bound to plasma proteins. Either scenario leads to a lower volume of distribution, as the drug is less able to pass through the endothelial cell junctions of the capillaries and enter other compartments of the body. Heparin follows this pathway.
- Being trapped in the extracellular fluid due to having a small molecular size but being highly hydrophilic. The small molecular size allows the drug to pass through the endothelial cell junctions of the capillaries. Due to its hydrophilic nature, however, it is not able to span the cell membrane of tissue cells; instead, the drug stays in the hydrophilic-friendly environment

Table 9.1 Normal Physical Volumes of Different Compartments in Healthy 70-kg Males

Total body water (TBW) is equal to approximately 60% of body weight in men (and 50% of body weight in women).	
Compartment	**Volume (Liters)**
Plasma	3.5
Interstitial fluid	10.5
Extracellular fluid (plasma + interstitial fluid)	14
Intracellular fluid	28
Total body water (extracellular fluid + intracellular fluid)	42
Fat	20

Adapted from: Shires G. Fluid and electrolyte management of the surgical patient. In: Brunicardi FC, Andersen DK, Billiar TR, et al., eds. *Schwartz's principles of surgery*, 9th ed. New York, NY: McGraw-Hill; 2010. Available at: http://www.accessmedicine.com/content.aspx?aID=5011700.

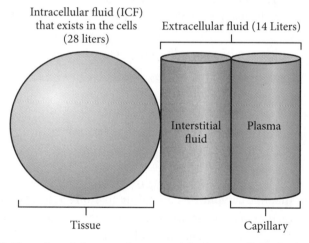

Figure 9.2 Extracellular fluid consists of plasma and interstitial fluid. Intracellular fluid refers to water inside of cells.

of the interstitial fluid (extracellular fluid comprises plasma and interstitial fluids; **Figure 9.2**). A typical example of a drug that follows this pathway is the highly charged aminoglycoside antibiotic gentamicin (gentamicin sulfate).

- Being trapped in the total body water. In this case, the drug has both a small molecular size and is hydrophobic enough to enter the intracellular fluid of the body. As a result, it will be found everywhere in the body where fluid is present. Theophylline (Elixophyllin Elixir) is an example of a drug that can reach all fluid compartments of the body and, as a result, has a volume of distribution equal to the total body water (Figure 9.2).

Simply put, the chemical structure of drugs affects V_d. When a drug is hydrophilic, it will remain in the extracellular fluid, leading to a lower value for V_d for that particular drug. In contrast, a hydrophobic drug will escape the extracellular fluid and move into tissues, which results in a higher value for V_d. The latter effect explains why obese patients have higher V_d values for hydrophobic drugs.

Except for obesity, which alters the ratio of the total body water to the total body fat (which is important to take into consideration in the distribution of highly lipid-soluble drugs), the physical volumes, presented in Table 9.1, are not as important as V_d in pharmacokinetics measurements.

As mentioned earlier, V_d is often determined by a single IV administration of a known dose of a drug, with the total concentration of drug in the plasma then being measured at different time points (to be able to extrapolate to the time 0 in a graph that has plasma concentrations as a function of time). However, this procedure is not necessary and is rarely employed. Instead, an average volume of distribution obtained from other patients with similar physical and medical conditions (e.g., age, weight, gender, renal failure, liver failure) is used to estimate the volume of distribution for a particular drug.

Approximately 55% of the blood consists of plasma, and the remaining 45% is made up of erythrocytes (red blood cells), leukocytes (white blood cells), and platelets. Plasma, in turn, is 90% water and 10% solutes, which include both organic molecules (e.g., amino acids, urea, hormones, glucose, lactic acid) and inorganic ions (e.g., Na^+, K^+, Ca^{2+}). A significant (70%) component of these solutes comprises plasma proteins such as albumin (which plays an important role in binding exogenous molecules), apolipoproteins (which play important roles in transporting lipids), transferrin (which plays an important role in transporting iron), immunoglobulin molecules (which play important roles in immunology), and fibrinogen and prothrombin (which play important roles in the blood coagulation cascade).

If blood is taken from the vein, placed in a test tube, and prevented from clotting, it separates into two phases: plasma (the upper phase) and blood cells. However, if the clotting process is not prevented, a yellowish fluid escapes the clot; it is referred to as serum. Because serum analysis is more convenient and the concentrations of most ions and molecules in both plasma and serum are almost the same, many clinical measurements are carried out using serum. As a result, the drug concentration is often interchangeably given either as plasma concentration or serum concentration; these values are almost identical.

Compartmental Systems

The simplest method to collect information and data related to ADME is to give a drug to a patient and take blood samples over time to measure the plasma concentrations of the drug in the blood samples. If we assume that the concentration of a drug in plasma is in equilibrium with concentrations in tissues, any change in plasma concentrations indicates a change in tissue concentrations as well. The compartment model can represent a body volume (a tissue, an organ, or the whole body) and is a valuable way to predict the drug concentrations in the plasma at single or different doses, calculate the extent of drug accumulation with multiple doses, and determine many parameters such as C_{max}, t_{max}, absorption, and elimination rates.

A simple plot of drug concentration versus time can identify a compartmental model, but the model that has the least statistical error in curve fitting is often considered to be the best choice of model for a pharmacokinetics study. Despite the fact that assumptions and hypothetical compartments can assist clinicians in predicting the dynamics of drugs in the body, they have to be careful to not solely rely on a model to predict the dynamic of a drug. For instance, for some drugs it is not useful to predict pharmacological effects by determining the drug concentration in the plasma. In some cases, polymorphism and pharmacogenomics (see the *Introduction to Pharmacogenomics* chapter) can make the prediction complex and unreliable.

As mentioned earlier, several different compartmental models are possible, and a review of each model can facilitate student learning in applied pharmacokinetics.

One-Compartment Model

In this simple model, the entire body is considered to be one compartment, and we assume that drug is rapidly distributed to all parts of the body. Let's first go through a single drug administration (both intravenously and extravascularly).

Single Intravenous Injection (Bolus) in a One-Compartment Model

The one-compartment model is the simplest model in pharmacokinetics measurement, in which an IV bolus dose of a drug is administered and the drug is distributed instantaneously. The full distribution of the drug is achieved immediately, although this does not mean that the drug is distributed equally to all tissues (**Figure 9.3**). The value of V_d can be readily calculated if you know the injected dose and the immediate drug concentration in the plasma.

Regarding the elimination process, the drug leaves the body (compartment) in a pattern governed by a first-order rate constant. The drug elimination process in a one-compartment model is represented as drug elimination from all eliminating organs (e.g., metabolism and excretion). Because the elimination follows first-order kinetics, the rate of change in the concentration of the drug in the plasma (i.e., dC_p/dt) can mathematically be expressed by using a differential equation:

$$\frac{dC_p}{dt} = -kC_p \tag{9.6}$$

where k is the first-order elimination rate constant and C_p is the concentration of the drug in the plasma. The negative sign reflects the fact that, due to the drug elimination, the concentration of the drug in the plasma decreases with time. Integration of Equation 9.6 with respect to time from 0 to infinity (i.e., 0 to ∞) is shown in Equation 9.7, which describes the natural logarithm of the plasma drug concentration at any given time (i.e., $\ln C_{pt}$):

$$\ln C_{pt} = \ln C_{p0} - kt \text{ (which can also be rearranged to } \ln (C_{pt}/C_{p0}) = -kt) \tag{9.7}$$

The anti-natural logarithm of Equation 9.7 yields the exponential equation:

$$C_{pt} = C_{p0} e^{-kt} \tag{9.8}$$

where C_{pt} is the plasma drug concentration at any given time, C_{p0} is the concentration of the drug at time 0 (which for an IV equals dose/V_d), and k is the elimination rate constant. A simple plot of $\ln C_{pt}$ versus time gives a straight line with a negative slope that represents the elimination rate constant of the drug from the body (**Figure 9.4**).

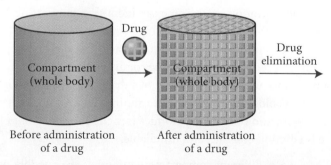

Figure 9.3 Using the whole body as one-compartment model for a single IV bolus dose.

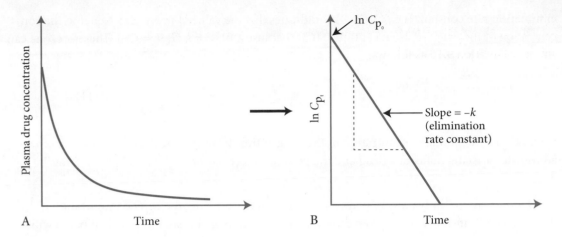

Figure 9.4 The first-order elimination rate of a single bolus dose in a one-compartment model. (A) A plot of the plasma drug concentration as a function of time. (B) The natural logarithm (ln) of C_t as a function of time. k is the elimination rate constant.

The one-compartment model can be applied to administration of a drug that rapidly equilibrates with the tissue compartment (see Figure 9.3). As Figure 9.4 demonstrates, the plasma drug concentration declines over time for an injected IV drug. This is the simplest way to determine whether a one-compartment model can be applied to an administered drug. The IV drugs that produce the straight line in the graph equilibrate rapidly between blood and various tissues. Rapid equilibrium does not mean that the concentration of the drug is the same throughout the entire compartment (body); rather, it means changes that take place in the plasma concentration are proportional to changes that occur in the drug concentration in tissues.

Equation 9.8 can also be rearranged by taking the logarithm, rather than the natural logarithm, of all terms in Equation 9.8; that logarithm yields Equation 9.9:

$$\log C_{P_t} = \frac{-kt}{2.303} + \log C_{p0} \tag{9.9}$$

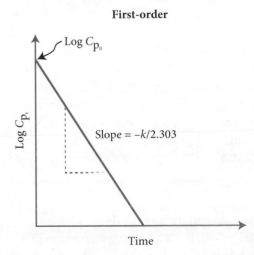

First-order

Figure 9.5 In a one-compartment model of a single bolus dose, the logarithm of C_{p_t} as a function of time gives a straight declining line whose slope is $-k/2.303$.

A simple plot of $\log C_{p_t}$ versus time gives a straight declining line whose slope is $-k/2.303$. Multiplying 2.303 and the slope of this declining line gives the elimination rate constant, k (**Figure 9.5**).

In a one-compartment model, V_d for each drug is constant and has volume units such as liters or liters per kilogram of body weight. The value of V_d is determined after IV bolus administration and is mathematically expressed as follows:

$$V_d = \frac{\text{Dose}_{IV}}{k \, \text{AUC}} \tag{9.10}$$

where the bolus dose is the intravenous dose of the drug in the body at time 0, k is the elimination rate constant, and AUC is the area under the drug concentration versus time curve. In a single administered bolus dose, AUC is calculated by dividing C_{p0} by the elimination rate constant (i.e., C_{p0}/k). This indicates that the value of (k AUC) is equal to the concentration of the drug in plasma at time 0 (C_0) (because k AUC = $k\ C_{p0}/k = C_{p0}$). Therefore, one can simplify Equation 9.10 as follows:

$$V_d = \frac{\text{Dose}_{IV}}{C_{p0}}$$

(9.11)

where C_{p0} is the plasma concentration of the drug at time 0 (see Figure 9.5). For instance, if we administer a 10 mg bolus of a drug and the plasma concentration at time 0 (C_{p0}) is 0.5 mg/L, V_d is 20 L.

As Equation 9.11 indicates, V_d plays a major role in determining the drug concentration in the plasma. For instance, for a given dose, a patient with a high V_d has a low C_{p0} compared with a patient who has a low V_d. If a minimum concentration is necessary to produce a pharmacological effect, the patient with the higher V_d will most likely not receive any effect from the drug (because of his or her lower C_{p0}). Keep in mind that an individual can have different V_d values for different drugs. By the same token, different patients can have different V_d values for the same drug. A large V_d is evidence that the drug is distributed to tissues. Conversely, a high rate of protein binding indicates that the drug is in the plasma, but not in the tissue.

Example 9.1: Calculate the IV dose of theophylline that is required to *immediately* achieve a plasma concentration of 15 mg/L if V_d for theophylline is 30 L.

Answer: According to Equation 9.11:

$$V_d = \frac{\text{Dose}_{IV}}{C_{p0}}$$

Dose = 30 L × 15 mg/L = 450 mg

Thus, 450 mg theophylline should be given as an IV bolus dose to immediately achieve a plasma concentration of 15 mg/L in this patient.

To calculate V_d in a one-compartment model when the bolus dose is known, we can plot the plasma drug concentrations as a function of time and extrapolate the regression straight line to the *y*-axis to calculate C_{p0} (see the straight line in Figure 9.5). This means C_{p0} represents the instantaneous drug concentration in the plasma. However, as mentioned earlier, we can use Equation 9.10 to calculate V_d but the AUC and elimination rate constant must be known as well. Regardless of which equations are applied, the most accurate way to calculate a V_d value is to use a bolus dose in a one-compartment model and plot a graph such as Figure 9.5.

Half-life

The half-life of a drug is the time that it takes to reduce the concentration of the drug in the body by 50% after absorption and distribution of the drug are complete. For a one-compartment model, because elimination is a first-order process, the elimination half-life ($t_{1/2}$) is calculated by utilizing Equation 9.7 to express Equations 9.12 through 9.15:

$$\ln(C_{p0}/C_{pt}) = kt$$

(9.12)

At $t_{1/2}$, plasma drug concentration is 50% of C_{p0}:

$$\ln(C_{p0} / 0.5C_{p0}) = kt_{1/2} \tag{9.13}$$

$$\ln 2 = kt_{1/2} \tag{9.14}$$

$$t_{1/2} = \frac{\ln 2}{k} = \frac{0.693}{k} \tag{9.15}$$

In first-order kinetics, the half-life is a constant parameter, and is dependent on the clearance and V_d. In a one-compartment model with a bolus dose, the clearance is equal to the elimination rate constant multiplied by V_d:

$$Cl = kV_d \tag{9.16}$$

$$k = \frac{Cl}{V_d} \tag{9.17}$$

As Equation 9.17 indicates, the elimination rate constant (k) represents how quickly serum concentrations decrease in the plasma. Inserting Equation 9.17 into Equation 9.15, we can calculate the half-life by employing the V_d and Cl parameters as shown in Equation 9.18:

$$t_{1/2} = \frac{0.693V_d}{Cl} \tag{9.18}$$

Equation 9.18 indicates that any change in either V_d or Cl will result in a change in $t_{1/2}$. For instance, for a drug with a large V_d, $t_{1/2}$ will be large as well. This result makes sense because if a drug has a large V_d, it means the drug has a large tissue concentration, which in turn indicates that the elimination process will be slow. As a result, the half-life increases for that particular drug. Note that a change in $t_{1/2}$ does not necessarily mean that Cl has changed—$t_{1/2}$ can change simply because of a change in V_d (recall that Cl is a constant when a drug is eliminated by first-order kinetics).

Example 9.2: Examine the data in **Table 9.2** and calculate the half-life of each drug.

Table 9.2 Pharmacokinetic Parameters of Theophylline and Ampicillin after Administering a Single IV Dose

Drug	V_d (L/kg)	k (hr^{-1})	$t_{1/2}$ (hr)
Theophylline	0.45	0.11	
Ampicillin	0.30	0.60	

Answer: Based on Equation 9.15, we can readily calculate the half-life for theophylline:

$$t_{1/2} = \frac{0.693}{0.11} = 6.3 \text{ hr}$$

and the half-life for ampicillin:

$$t_{1/2} = \frac{0.693}{0.60} = 1.16 \text{ hr}$$

Learning Bridge 9.1

During one of your introductory pharmacy practice experiences in a hospital, you notice that the attending physician has ordered an IV bolus dose (400 mg) of an antibiotic for a patient who acquired a serious bacterial infection. Your preceptor asks you to calculate the following parameters to estimate the half-life for the IV antibiotic. She shows you the linear plot of the plasma concentration–time profile shown in **Exhibit 9.1** and asks you to calculate the following parameters: C_{p0}, Cl, $t_{1/2}$, AUC, and V_d.

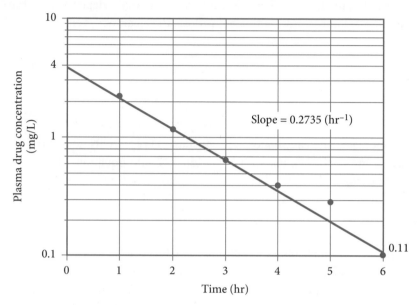

Exhibit 9.1 Plasma concentration–time graph after a single IV dose of 400 mg of an antibiotic.

Single Dose Administered Extravascularly in a One-Compartment Model

When a drug is given extravascularly (e.g., orally, transdermally, intramuscularly, rectally) to a patient, the entire dose may not be absorbed. For instance, a tablet may not be completely distributed to be absorbed, a fraction of drug may be metabolized prior to reaching the systemic circulation, or a transdermal patch may release a drug over a longer period of time.

For instance, for an orally administered drug to be absorbed, the drug needs to go through several organs and membranes before it reaches the systemic circulation. Consequently, a drug that needs to be absorbed through the gastrointestinal (GI) tract may be metabolized by cytochrome P450 enzymes (of particular concern is CYP3A4, which accounts for a significant amount of the GI tract's cytochrome 450 enzymes; see the *Introduction to Medicinal Chemistry* chapter). In addition, the same drug may be pumped back (by P-glycoprotein) into the lumen of the GI tract, which in turn reduces the drug absorption from the GI tract. Even if a drug is effectively absorbed from the GI tract, it may encounter another barrier—namely, metabolism in the liver. The latter barrier arises because a drug that enters the portal vein directly reaches the liver and may undergo another set of metabolic reactions in the liver. As a result of this metabolism, a large amount of a drug may be lost. Elimination of a drug before it reaches the systemic circulation is called the "first-pass effect" or "pre-systemic elimination."

When a drug is absorbed into the circulation upon its administration, the plasma drug concentration increases and reaches a maximum concentration referred to as C_{max}. The phase of the curve

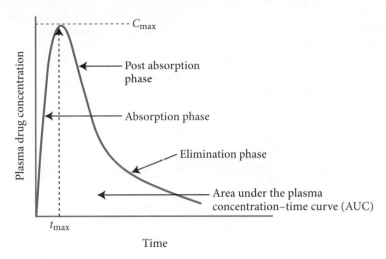

Figure 9.6 A single dose of a drug administered extravascularly in a one-compartment model. Adapted from: Hedaya M. *Basic pharmacokinetics.* Boca Raton: CRC Press; 2012: Chapter 9.

over which the absorption of the drug occurs is called the absorption phase. At the time the drug reaches C_{max} (i.e., t_{max}), the absorption rate equals the elimination rate. After this time, the drug elimination will be higher than the drug absorption, which results in a declining curve (**Figure 9.6**).

Because the drug is not instantly absorbed in an extravascularly administered route, both the administered dose and the fraction of the dose that reaches the systemic circulation play important roles in determining the bioavailability of the drug. The bioavailability of a drug (F) is the fraction of the administered dose that reaches the systemic circulation; it is in the range of 0–100%, where 0% is no absorption at all and 100% is complete drug absorption. With the intravenous route, F is 100%, as the drug instantly and completely reaches the systemic circulation. In contrast, with an extravascularly administered drug, factors such as incomplete absorption, metabolism, and distribution of the drug into other tissues prior to reaching the systemic circulation can significantly reduce the bioavailability of the drug. The absorption and elimination rates for a single extravascularly administered drug most often follow first-order kinetics.

We can calculate the bioavailability of a drug if it displays linear pharmacokinetics. The parameter F is calculated by administering a given dose both extravascularly and intravenously. A comparison between plasma concentrations achieved after both administrations in the same individual reveals the bioavailability. To make the measurement and calculation of F simple and cost-effective, instead of comparing the drug concentrations at different time points, the total area under the serum concentration–time curve (AUC) is compared for both the extravascularly and intravenously administered drug (**Figure 9.7**).

If the dose is the same for both routes, F for a given drug can be calculated by taking the ratio of the AUC for the extravascularly administered dose to the AUC for the intravenously administered dose. For instance, if 1 mg of a drug is administered orally (PO) to a patient, and then a few weeks later the same dose is given intravenously, F would be calculated by dividing AUC_{PO} by AUC_{IV}.

Sometimes, it is difficult to administer the same dose of a drug intravenously or extravascularly due to a side effect or poor absorption, or simply due to the fact that the drug concentration in the plasma is too low to measure. In this case, the bioavailability can be calculated by using different doses. Equation 9.19 takes the different doses into consideration:

$$F(\text{absolute}) = \frac{AUC_{PO}}{AUC_{IV}} \times \frac{D_{IV}}{D_{PO}} \tag{9.19}$$

where D_{IV} is the intravenous dose and D_{PO} is the oral dose.

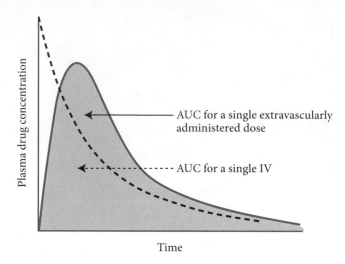

Figure 9.7 The area under the plasma concentration curve (AUC) for a single orally administered dose (closed curve) and a single intravenously administered dose (open curve).

Example 9.3: After a single oral dose of 300 mg procainamide (an antiarrhythmic drug) was given to a patient, the observed AUC was 10 mg•hr/L. What is the absolute bioavailability of oral procainamide if the observed AUC after an IV dose of 300 mg in the same patient was 12 mg•hr/L?

Answer: Using Equation 9.19 can assist you in calculating the absolute bioavailability:

$$F(\text{absolute}) = \frac{10}{12} \times \frac{300}{300} = 0.83, \text{ or } 83\%$$

Besides AUC, two other parameters are used to describe bioavailability: C_{max} and t_{max}. In contrast, $t_{1/2}$ is usually independent of the route of drug administration and is not used to measure the bioavailability of a drug. C_{max}, AUC, and t_{max} play important roles in determining whether two drugs are bioequivalent and whether a new drug has an "AB" rating in the FDA's list of "Approved Drug Products with Therapeutic Equivalence Evaluations" (see the discussion of the "Orange Book" in the *Introduction to Pharmaceutics* chapter). For instance, for a drug to be classified as bioequivalent to another drug, or simply to be called a generic version of a brand-name drug, the FDA requires the manufacturer to provide data that show C_{max}, AUC, and t_{max} for the generic and brand-name drugs' dosage forms are equal (with marginal statistical differences). The manufacturer of the generic drug has to administer a single dose or multiple doses of both the generic and brand-name drugs to a group of 20 individuals to provide evidence that these parameters are identical for both drugs. The ratio between $AUC_{generic}$ and AUC_{brand} is known as the relative bioavailability and is expressed as follows:

$$F(\text{relative}) = \frac{AUC_{generic}}{AUC_{brand}} \times \frac{D_{brand}}{D_{generic}} \tag{9.20}$$

where D indicates the brand-name and generic doses. The relative bioavailability can be multiplied by 100 to express it as a percentage.

The relative bioavailability can also be measured in terms of urinary drug excretion. It is important to detect and measure the total unchanged drug excreted in the urine for both generic and brand-name drugs. However, while urinary excretion measurement is more convenient for patients, a few factors may affect this outcome; for instance, the pH of the urine can affect the excretion rate for weakly acidic or basic drugs.

Example 9.4: Tylenol solution was used as a reference standard for the evaluation of the relative bioavailability of a new oral solid dosage form of acetaminophen called Paramol. What is the relative bioavailability of Paramol tablets based on the results shown in **Table 9.3**?

Table 9.3 Area under the Curve Data for Tylenol and Paramol after Oral Administration of 200 mg and 400 mg Doses, Respectively

Drug	Dose (mg)	AUC (mg•hr/L)
Tylenol	200	65
Paramol	400	130

Answer: According to Equation 9.20, the relative bioavailability is

$$F(\text{relative}) = \frac{400}{200} \times \frac{65}{130} = 1 \times 100 = 100\%$$

With the single bolus dose, absorption occurred instantly; in turn, the absorption rate was not taken into consideration when calculating V_d or Cl. However, the calculation of the plasma concentration of an orally administered drug is more complicated compared with the same calculation for an intravenously administered drug. In the former case, we have to take into consideration F, as well as both absorption and elimination rate constants:

$$C_p = \frac{FDk_a}{V_d(k_a - k)}\ (e^{-kt} - e^{-k_a t}) \tag{9.21}$$

where F is the bioavailability, D is the initial oral dose at time 0, k_a is the absorption rate constant, and k is the elimination rate constant. Both the absorption and elimination rate constants must be included to calculate the plasma drug concentration after oral administration.

Let's look at an example to see how we can use Equation 9.21 to calculate a few important parameters.

Example 9.5: A single dose of 1 mg/kg of an analgesic agent was given to an 80-kg patient as an oral tablet. The plasma concentration–time profile is described by the following equation:

$$C_p = 20\left(e^{-0.135t} - e^{-0.653t}\right)$$

where C_p is in mg/L and t is in hours. The drug has 100% bioavailability.

A. What is the absorption rate constant?

B. What is the plasma concentration 3 hours after the drug's administration?

C. Three weeks later, the patient starts to suffer from nausea and vomiting and becomes unable to take medication orally. If this drug is available in an IV formulation (40 mg/mL), what will be the IV dose required to achieve the same concentration as the oral formulation dose?

Answer:

A. If you compare the provided equation with Equation 9.21, which describes plasma concentration after a single oral dose, you will recognize that the absorption rate constant (k_a) and the elimination rate constant (k) are 0.635 hr^{-1} and 0.135 hr^{-1}, respectively.

B. Using the provided equation and $t = 3$ hours, the plasma concentration will be

$$C_p = 20\left(e^{-0.135 \times 3} - e^{-0.653 \times 3}\right) = 10.5 \text{ mg/L}$$

C. Because F is 100%, the IV dose should be the same as the oral dose (i.e., 80 mg). As the IV formulation is available in a 40 mg/mL formulation, a 2 mL IV dose should achieve the same concentration as an 80 mg oral dose.

Both the absorption and elimination rate constants play important roles when we want to calculate the time that it takes to reach the maximum plasma drug concentration, t_{max}.

$$t_{max} = \frac{\ln k_a - \ln k}{k_a - k} = \frac{2.303 \log(k_a / k)}{k_a - k} \tag{9.22}$$

Equation 9.22 indicates that t_{max} is not dependent on F, D, or V_d (see Equation 9.21), but rather on the absorption (k_a) and elimination (k) rate constants. The calculation of t_{max} is useful when we want to compare the rate of drug absorption for two or more drug products. In other words, a drug that has a smaller t_{max} value has a faster drug absorption.

Learning Bridge 9.2

During one of your advanced pharmacy practice experiences, your preceptor provides the following information and asks you to answer the questions and share your rationale with two other medical students who are joining you during your rounds with a medical team. Nifedipine (Adalat) is a Ca^{2+}-channel blocker that is commonly used to treat hypertension.

Table 9.4 shows some pharmacokinetic parameters after oral administration of 40 mg of this drug with and without grapefruit juice.

Table 9.4 Pharmacokinetic Parameters of Nifedipine after Oral Administration of 40 mg with and without Grapefruit Juice

Pharmacokinetic Parameter	Control (with Water)	With Grapefruit Juice
C_{max} (mg/L)	10.5	71.9
AUC (mg•hr/L)	32.5	247.8
t_{max} (hr)	3	3
Plasma-concentration–time profile equation	$C_p = 20\left(e^{-0.135t} - e^{-0.653t}\right)$	$C_p = 115\left(e^{-0.085t} - e^{-0.610t}\right)$

A. What is the effect of grapefruit juice on the oral absorption kinetics of nifedipine?

B. What is the possible mechanism (explanation) of the observed effect of grapefruit juice on nifedipine kinetics?

C. How would grapefruit juice affect the onset, intensity, and duration of action for nifedipine?

D. Calculate the nifedipine plasma concentration 3 hours after administration of a 40 mg dose in both cases.

E. What is the elimination half-life of nifedipine in both cases?

Intravenous Infusion in a One-Compartment Model

Drugs that are administered intravenously are either given as a single dose (bolus) or are infused slowly at a constant rate through a vein into the plasma (intravenous infusion). The intravenous infusion route of administration is often chosen to control plasma drug concentrations to better fit a patient's needs. For instance, when a drug (often an antibiotic) must be included in a solution of mixed electrolytes, the most effective approach is to administer the drug solution as an intravenous infusion. In addition, for drugs with a narrow therapeutic window (e.g., heparin, warfarin, theophylline, clozapine), an IV infusion helps maintain a constant plasma drug concentration, thereby eliminating fluctuations that might otherwise occur between the peak (maximum) and trough (minimum) drug concentrations. Clinicians must be careful when administering intravenous infusions, as some drugs are lethal when infused too rapidly. For example, high concentrations of potassium solutions can cause cardiac arrest. By comparison, an infusion dose of a potassium solution of as much as 10 mEq over 2–3 hours is harmless.

Figure 9.8 demonstrates a typical infusion profile for a plasma drug concentration. As shown in the figure, the plasma concentration of the drug increases gradually until it reaches a steady-state level ($C_{p_{ss}}$). At this point, the elimination rate of the drug is equal to the infusion rate of the drug entering the body.

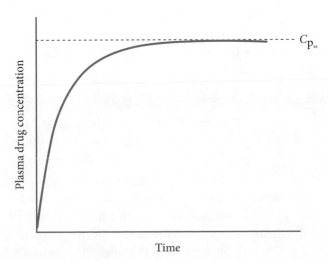

Figure 9.8 The plasma drug concentration at the steady-state level ($C_{p_{ss}}$) with an infused IV dose in a one-compartment model.

Figure 9.8 depicts a typical zero-order infusion rate. One can express the rate of drug infusion as follows:

$$R = kD_{ss} \tag{9.23}$$

where R is the infusion rate, k is the first-order elimination rate constant, and D_{ss} is the amount of the drug in the plasma at the steady state. Because D_{ss} is equal to the plasma drug concentration at steady state (C_{pss}) multiplied by V_d (or $C_{pss}V_d$), we can rearrange Equation 9.23 as follows:

$$R = kC_{pss} V_d \tag{9.24}$$

which assists us in expressing Equation 9.25:

$$C_{pss} = \frac{R}{kV_d} \tag{9.25}$$

As shown in Equation 9.25, C_{pss} is proportional to the rate of infusion. In other words, if we need to achieve a higher C_{pss}, a higher infusion rate is required. Equation 9.25 is a useful way to determine the infusion rate for a drug if we have access to values of C_{pss}, k, and V_d from the literature for a particular drug.

> **Example 9.6:** What is the steady-state concentration of theophylline during a constant-rate IV infusion of 15 mg/hr? ($V_d = 30$ L, $k = 0.1$ hr^{-1}.)
>
> *Answer:* Using Equation 9.25, we can calculate the plasma drug concentration at steady state:
>
> $$C_{pss} = \frac{15\,\text{mg}/\text{hr}}{0.1\,\text{hr}^{-1} \times 30\,\text{L}} = 5\,\text{mg}/\text{L}$$

As was mentioned elsewhere in this chapter (see Equation 9.17), the clearance is equal to the elimination rate constant (k) multiplied by V_d (i.e., $Cl = k \times V_d$). We can incorporate Equation 9.17 into Equation 9.25 to obtain Equation 9.26:

$$C_{pss} = \frac{R}{Cl} \tag{9.26}$$

In other words, the infusion rate (R) is equal to $C_{pss} \times Cl$. It should be clear that C_{pss} depends only on the infusion rate and total body clearance. Neither V_d nor k affects the value of C_{pss}.

> **Example 9.7:** What infusion rate is required to achieve a steady-state concentration of theophylline of 10 mg/L? ($V_d = 30$ L, $k = 0.1$ hr^{-1}.)
>
> *Answer:* $R = (C_{pss})(Cl) = (10\,\text{mg/L}) (0.1\,\text{hr}^{-1})(30\,\text{L}) = 30$ mg/hr
>
> (Note: In Examples 9.6 and 9.7, notice that doubling the infusion rate (from 15 mg/hr to 30 mg/hr) resulted in a twofold increase in steady-state concentration. This is one of the hallmarks of linear kinetics.)

The half-life is a useful parameter to determine the time required to reach a steady-state concentration of a drug in the body. For instance, we know that it takes three half-lives to achieve 90% of a steady-state plasma drug concentration and five to six half-lives to reach an almost complete steady-state level. The longer the half-life for a drug, the longer it takes to reach C_{pss} (**Figure 9.9**).

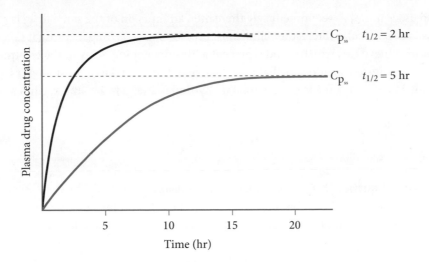

Figure 9.9 The half-life determines the time needed for the plasma drug concentration to reach the steady-state level ($C_{p_{ss}}$).

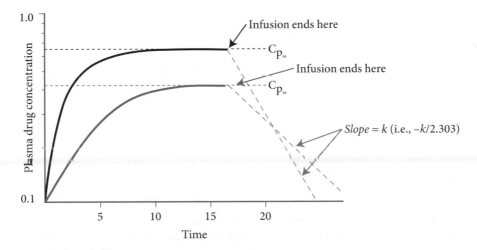

Figure 9.10 Drugs with different half-lives display different first-order elimination rates on a semi-log scale ($t_{1/2}$ for the lower curve is larger than the corresponding value for the upper curve).

Because there may be as much as a 10% error in data analysis, most clinicians consider concentrations obtained after three half-lives to be the steady-state concentration.

With an intravenous infusion route and a one-compartment model, the infused drug follows zero-order input. At the end of the infusion input, however, most drugs demonstrate a first-order elimination rate from the plasma (**Figure 9.10**). As a result, the elimination rate will be different for different infused drugs.

If the infusion is terminated (see the end of the infusion in Figure 9.10), the plasma concentration declines following first-order kinetics (the rate of elimination depends on k). The values of k and $t_{1/2}$ can be calculated from the slope of the declining line representing the elimination phase. Another important parameter that can be calculated in this case is the loading dose.

Loading Dose

The loading dose is the amount of drug that, when distributed in V_d, will give the desired plasma drug concentration. A loading dose assists clinicians in achieving $C_{p_{ss}}$ more rapidly. The loading dose is given as an initial dose; immediately thereafter, an infusion of the same drug is started. This process is of particular interest for clinicians if $t_{1/2}$ for a drug is long, because it takes five to six half-lives to achieve C_{Pss}, which could represent a life-threatening delay in the treatment of some diseases. For instance, lidocaine has a half-life of 2 hours; it takes almost 6 hours to reach C_{Pss} with this drug. When lidocaine is used to treat arrhythmias after a heart attack, clinicians inject a loading dose to reach C_{Pss} more quickly (a routine procedure in hospitals). One can calculate the loading dose as follows:

$$D_{L} = C_{Pss} \times V_{d} \qquad (9.27)$$

As expressed in Equation 9.26, C_{Pss} is equal to the infusion rate divided by Cl. We can utilize Equation 9.26 to understand the relationship between the infusion rate and the loading dose. If we merge Equation 9.26 with Equation 9.27, we can express Equations 9.28 and 9.29:

$$D_{L} = \frac{R}{Cl} V_{d} \qquad (9.28)$$

Because $Cl = kV_{d}$:

$$D_{L} = \frac{R}{k} \qquad (9.29)$$

These equations indicate that the loading dose is directly proportional to the infusion rate.

If the toxicity of a drug is high, a large loading dose may cause toxicity in the body with no apparent medical advantages. To avoid this problem, the loading dose may be divided into smaller doses and administered over a longer period of time. **Figure 9.11** summarizes several plasma drug profiles with and without loading doses. Notice that a loading dose does not alter the value of C_{Pss}, but does provide a faster way to reach the steady state.

Intermittent Drug Infusion

To prevent a toxic effect from an IV administration caused by a high drug concentration, clinicians can give repeated IV drug infusions. The underlying principle is that an IV infusion is given for a short period of time, followed by a period of drug elimination; the same short IV infusion/elimination pattern is repeated until the drug reaches the steady-state level. If the given dose,

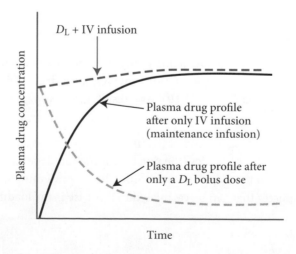

Figure 9.11 Plasma drug profiles as a function of time in the presence and absence of a loading dose.

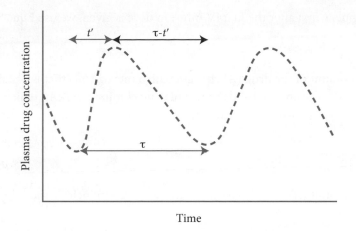

Figure 9.12 The plasma drug concentration profile for an intermittent drug infusion. t' is the time over which the drug is infused; τ is the dose interval time; and $\tau - t'$ is the time between the maximum and minimum plasma drug concentrations.

Adapted from: Hedaya M. *Basic pharmacokinetics.* Boca Raton: CRC Press; 2012: Chapter 18.

infusion rate, and dose intervals are constant at the steady-state level, the maximum and minimum plasma drug concentrations will remain constant as well. **Figure 9.12** demonstrates how the plasma drug concentrations behave in an intermittent drug infusion process.

In Figure 9.12, t' is the infusion time, and τ is the dose interval time—that is, the interval that goes from the administration of the first dose until the administration of the second dose, and so on. In addition, Figure 9.12 shows the time between the maximum and minimum plasma drug concentrations, is $\tau - t'$.

To better understand the pharmacokinetics of intermittent IV infusion, we can look at each repeated dose separately. **Figure 9.13** shows what happens after the first infusion is administered in an intermittent infusion administration.

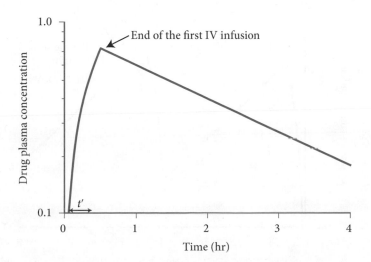

Figure 9.13 The plasma drug concentration profile after administration of the first infusion in an intermittent drug infusion.

Adapted from: Hedaya M. *Basic pharmacokinetics.* Boca Raton: CRC Press; 2012: Chapter 18.

To see what happens first after the first IV infusion dose is given, we use Equation 9.30:

$$\frac{dA}{dt} = R_0 - kA \tag{9.30}$$

That is to say, the amount of the drug (A) changes with a rate (dA/dt) that is equal to the difference between the rate of IV infusion (R_0) and the rate of drug elimination (kA), which in our one-compartment model is a first-order kinetics rate constant. The integration of Equation 9.30 gives Equation 9.31:

$$A = \frac{R_0}{k}\left(1 - e^{-kt}\right) \tag{9.31}$$

To convert the amount (A) to a plasma concentration, we can include the volume of distribution in the expression:

$$C_p = \frac{R_0}{kV_d}\left(1 - e^{-kt}\right) \tag{9.32}$$

If the infusion time is long, the exponential component of this equation equals 1, which results in a simpler equation:

$$C_p = \frac{R_0}{kV_d} \tag{9.33}$$

We can utilize Equation 9.32 to determine C_p at the end of the first IV drug infusion (see Figure 9.13) that has been administered over a time (t'):

$$C_p = \frac{R_0}{kV_d}\left(1 - e^{-kt'}\right) \tag{9.34}$$

Now let's see what happens after the second repeated IV dose is administered in an intermittent infusion administration. Here, the plasma drug concentration is the sum of the plasma drug concentration from the drug infusion plus the plasma drug concentration remaining from the first dose. In other words, when we inject the second dose, there is still some drug present in the plasma (C_{px}), which must be added to Equation 9.34. To calculate the drug concentration in the plasma at the end of the second IV dose (**Figure 9.14**), we can use the following equation:

$$C_p = \frac{R_0}{kV_d}\left(1 - e^{-kt'}\right) + C_{px}\, e^{-kt'} \tag{9.35}$$

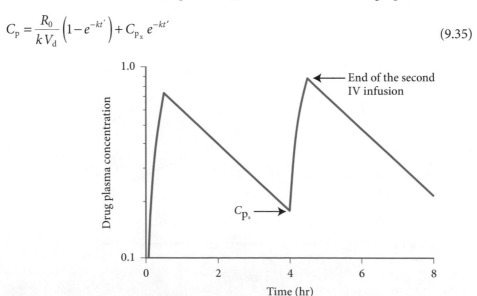

Figure 9.14 The plasma drug concentration profile after administration of the first and second infusions in an intermittent drug infusion.

Adapted from: Hedaya M. *Basic pharmacokinetics.* Boca Raton: CRC Press; 2012: Chapter 18.

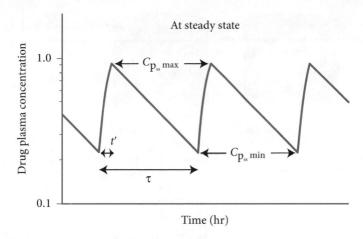

Figure 9.15 The plasma drug concentration profile after administration of repeated infusion doses in an intermittent drug infusion. $C_{p_{ss}\,max}$ and $C_{p_{ss}\,min}$ represent the maximum and minimum plasma concentrations at steady-state levels, respectively.

Adapted from: Hedaya M. *Basic pharmacokinetics*. Boca Raton: CRC Press; 2012: Chapter 18.

The repeated infusions continue until the accumulated plasma drug concentration reaches two steady-state levels: a maximum steady state ($C_{p_{ss}\,max}$) and a minimum steady state ($C_{p_{ss}\,min}$) (**Figure 9.15**). Both steady-state levels are directly proportional to the administered dose, assuming the body clearance is constant; that is, the higher the dose, the larger the $C_{p_{ss}\,max}$ and $C_{p_{ss}\,min}$. In contrast, if the dose and V_d are constant, a patient with lower body clearance will have a higher steady-state concentration.

Because there are two steady-state levels, we can calculate the average steady-state level by using Equation 9.36:

$$C_{av} = \frac{FD_0}{kV_d\tau} \tag{9.36}$$

where C_{av} is the average steady-state concentration, F is the bioavailability, D_0 is the initial given dose, k is the elimination rate, V_d is the distribution volume, and τ is the dose interval.

> **Example 9.8:** A patient was admitted to the hospital because of severe pneumonia. The physician administered 225 mg IV bolus doses of an antibiotic every 6 hours. What is the average steady-state concentration of this drug in the patient? ($V_d = 20$ L, $k = 0.1155$ hr^{-1}.)
>
> *Answer:* We use Equation 9.36 to calculate the average steady-state concentration:
>
> $$C_{av} = \frac{FD_0}{kV_d\tau} = \frac{1 \times 225\,\text{mg}}{0.1155\,\text{hr}^{-1} \times 20\,\text{L} \times 6\,\text{hr}} = 21.6\,\text{mg}/\text{L}$$

Two-Compartment Model

To determine whether a two-compartment model is appropriate for an administered drug, we can inject a bolus IV injection and plot the logarithm (or natural logarithm) of the plasma drug concentration as a function of time. If data obtained yield a biphasic curve, rather than the straight line that is characteristic of a one-compartment model, a two-compartment model must be used to measure the pharmacokinetics parameters. With a two-compartment model, the drug is

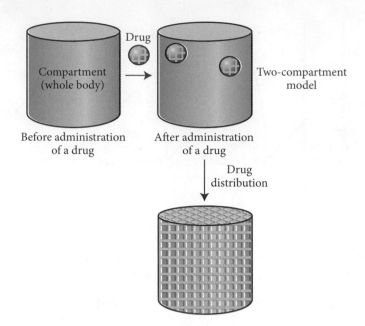

Figure 9.16 Drug distribution in a two-compartment model.

distributed into different tissues at different rates. Often, however, clinicians assume that a drug follows a one-compartment model—an assumption that makes the measurement of pharmacokinetics parameters a simpler process. Naturally, this assumption is valid only if it does not produce any error.

In a two-compartment model, the drug requires a longer time to reach equilibrium between tissue and plasma drug concentrations. After reaching equilibrium, the drug is considered to be distributed to the entire body (**Figure 9.16**).

The first-order kinetic rate plays an instrumental role in a two-compartment model. In such a model, we assume that the drug transfer rate constant between the central and peripheral compartments (k_1), the drug transfer rate constant between the peripheral and central compartments (k_2), and the elimination rate constant from the central compartment (k_3) follow first-order kinetics (**Figure 9.17**). The central compartment includes blood and well-perfused organs such as the liver, brain, and kidney; the peripheral compartment includes poorly perfused tissues such as muscle and fat.

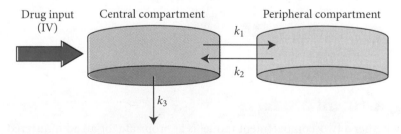

Figure 9.17 Different first-order rates are involved in a two-compartment model. k_1 represents the drug transfer rate constant between the central and peripheral compartments; k_2 represents the drug transfer rate constant between the peripheral and central compartments; and k_3 represents the elimination rate constant from the central compartment.

Adapted from: Hedaya M. *Basic pharmacokinetics.* Boca Raton: CRC Press; 2012: Chapter 17.

As mentioned earlier, a two-compartment model employing semi-log data to graph a plasma drug concentration profile depicts a biphasic curve. For instance, if a patient is given a bolus dose (A), the plasma drug concentration will show a rapid distribution rate from the central compartment to the peripheral compartment, then reaches a complete equilibrium between the central and peripheral compartments, followed by a slow elimination rate from the central compartment (Figure 9.17). This behavior can be graphed in a plasma drug concentration profile.

The amount of the drug will change as a function of time in a two-compartment model. Because the rate of this change in the central compartment, at any given time, is equal to the sum of the drug transfer from the peripheral to the central compartment, minus the rate of drug transfer from the central to the peripheral compartment, minus the elimination rate from the central compartment (see Figure 9.17), we can use a simplified equation to calculate the plasma drug concentration (C_p):

$$C_p = Ae^{-\alpha t} + Be^{-\beta t}$$

(9.37)

where C_p is the plasma drug concentration, A and B are the hybrid coefficients that have units of concentration, α is the first-order hybrid rate constant for distribution, and β is the first-order hybrid rate constant for elimination. If we plot the plasma drug concentration as a function of time, the plasma drug concentration decays according to a biphasic curve (**Figure 9.18**). We can obtain all relevant data in Equation 9.37 from this biphasic curve to calculate C_p.

An oral drug can also fit the two-compartment model if the drug is rapidly absorbed into the central component, but then slowly distributed to the peripheral component. A semi-log plot of the plasma drug concentration will result in a biphasic declining line right after the absorption phase ends (**Figure 9.19**). However, if the same drug has a slow absorption rate, it will be difficult to predict any plasma drug concentration profile.

Drug Absorption

The absorption of a drug occurs when the drug travels to the central compartment following its administration. The rate and extent of absorption depends on the route of drug administration.

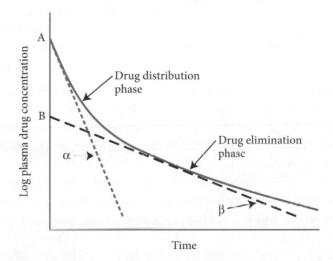

Figure 9.18 Administration of single bolus dose in a two-compartment model. In the semi-logarithmic plot, α is the first-order distribution rate constant that describes a rapid distribution of the drug from the central compartment to the peripheral compartment. β is the first-order elimination rate constant that describes the elimination of the drug from both central and peripheral compartments.

Adapted from: Hedaya M. *Basic pharmacokinetics.* Boca Raton: CRC Press; 2012: Chapter 17.

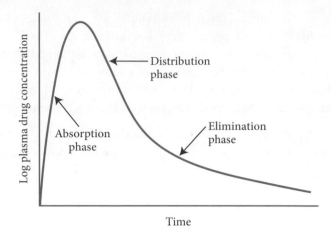

Figure 9.19 A typical plasma drug concentration profile for an oral dosage form in a two-compartment model. As long as the drug's absorption exceeds its distribution and elimination, an uphill curve (absorption phase) will hold. The plasma drug concentration will result in a biexponential declining line right after the absorption phase ends.

For instance, while an IV drug is immediately absorbed into the central compartment and has a bioavailability that is complete and rapid, an oral solid dosage form needs to be first disintegrated and distributed before it can be absorbed into the central compartment. Other factors such as the GI tract, the drug's physicochemical properties, the surface area available for absorption, blood flow to the site of absorption, intestinal metabolism, gastric acid, gastric motility, and the gastric emptying rate, which are regulated by neural feedback, gender and age, and the first-pass effect, can influence the absorption of an oral drug. We can use the term "bioavailability" to describe absorption. Bioavailability indicates the rate and extent to which the active ingredient of a drug is absorbed and becomes available to its site of action or remains in the systemic circulation, from which the drug has access to its site of action. Simply put, if the administered dose of a drug is inactivated before it reaches the systemic circulation, the bioavailability will be reduced.

Oral Absorption

For drugs given in solid forms (tablets, capsules), the rate of disintegration or dissolution in the GI tract may limit their absorption. Both the disintegration and dissolution rates, however, can be utilized to formulate controlled-release forms (see the *Introduction to Pharmaceutics* chapter) that are designed to produce a slow and consistent absorption of a drug for 8 hours or longer.

As mentioned earlier, many factors make the oral absorption of a drug a complex process. For instance, most drugs' absorption from the GI tract occurs by passive diffusion when the drug is un-ionized. Drugs that have an acidic property are un-ionized in the stomach (pH 1–2), whereas drugs that have a basic property are un-ionized in the upper intestine. The mucous neck cells secret mucins; these large glycoproteins form a mucus layer that adheres to the surface of epithelial cells of the stomach to protect those epithelial cells from gastric acid. The mucus layer does not allow large drug molecules (more than 800 Da) to reach the epithelial cells and, as a result, reduces drug absorption. The surface area of the GI tract also has a major impact on drug absorption. The villi of the upper intestine (see the *Introduction to Pharmacodynamics* chapter), particularly in the duodenum and jejunum, provide an extremely large surface area (the surface area in the stomach is comparatively small). Thus, even if a drug is predominantly ionized in the small intestine and un-ionized in the stomach, the drug absorption rate for the ionized drug from the small intestine will be higher than the drug absorption rate for the un-ionized drug from the stomach.

Absorption Kinetics after Extravascular Drug Administration

With an extravascular delivery route, drugs do not directly enter into the systemic circulation. Such delivery routes include oral, sublingual, transdermal, intramuscular, subcutaneous, inhalation, and rectal administration. Absorption of drugs administered extravascularly is complicated by many variables, such as drug degradation, disintegration/dissolution rates, and food, among others. For simplicity's sake, most pharmacokinetic models assume drugs delivered in this way demonstrate a first-order absorption rate. No matter whether a first-order or a zero-order absorption rate applies, the net rate of drug accumulation in the plasma at any given time is equal to the rate of drug absorption minus the rate of drug elimination.

During the absorption phase (see **Figure 9.20**), the rate of drug absorption must be greater than the rate of drug elimination for the drug to enter into the desired areas of the body. During the absorption phase, elimination of drug may occur despite the fact that the absorption phase predominates.

As Figure 9.20 indicates, when the plasma drug concentration reaches C_{max}, the rates of drug absorption and drug elimination are equal and there is no net change in the plasma concentration of the drug. Because the rate of drug elimination exceeds the rate of absorption (after t_{max}), the post-absorption phase appears on the plasma drug concentration graph. Finally, when absorption is complete, the elimination phase appears. The rate of the elimination phase indicates how fast a drug exits from the plasma (Figure 9.20).

Zero-Order Drug Absorption (Single Oral Dose)

On some occasions, the zero-order drug absorption occurs when the drug absorption is saturable or when a controlled-release dosage form follows a zero-order absorption process. In a zero-order absorption process, the drug is absorbed into the central compartment at a constant rate, k_0. It is then immediately eliminated from the body by a first-order rate constant, k (**Figure 9.21**). For simplicity, absorption of many drugs has been assumed to follow first-order kinetics. As a result, we will not discuss any zero-order absorption rates in this chapter.

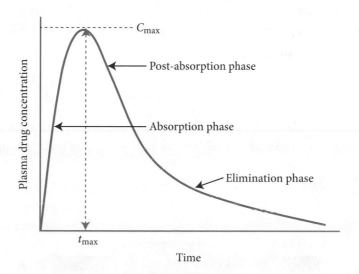

Figure 9.20 A plasma drug concentration profile for an oral dosage form. At C_{max}, the rate of absorption equals the rate of elimination. The post-absorption phase is the period in which absorption of the drug continues after t_{max} is reached. When the absorption is complete, the elimination phase begins.

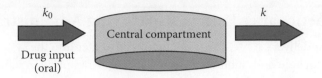

Figure 9.21 A drug with a zero-order absorption rate (k_0) can display a first-order elimination rate constant (k).

First-Order Absorption Model (Single Oral Dose)

When a drug has a first-order absorption profile, we can assume that both the absorption rate and the elimination rate follow first-order kinetics. In other words, a drug's input across the GI tract and then its elimination from the body are first-order processes. This model applies to oral drugs that are in solution, immediate-release dosage forms, tablets, capsules, and suppositories. Drugs administered intramuscularly and subcutaneously are also likely to follow a first-order absorption process. **Figure 9.22** demonstrates a one-compartment model for first-order drug absorption and first-order elimination.

As mentioned earlier, both k_a (the absorption rate constant) and k (the elimination rate constant) for these drugs follow first-order kinetics. Keep in mind that any solid dosage form must first be disintegrated before it can be distributed. Only drugs that are distributed in the GI tract will be absorbed into the body. The amount of drug in the GI tract decreases exponentially with the k_a rate constant. We can express an equation to describe this process:

$$A = \text{Dose } e^{-k_a t} \tag{9.38}$$

The rate of the change in the amount of a drug in the body depends on the rate of drug absorption and the rate of drug elimination. We can express this rate of change as follows:

$$\frac{dA}{dt} = k_a A - kA \tag{9.39}$$

Simply put, when a drug disappears from the GI tract, it is absorbed into the body. At the beginning of this process, the rate of absorption is higher than the rate of elimination. Over time, the rate of elimination becomes higher than the rate of drug absorption (**Figure 9.23**).

Integration of Equation 9.39 gives Equation 9.40:

$$A_t = \frac{Dk_a}{k_a - k_1} \left(e^{-kt} - e^{k_a t} \right) \tag{9.40}$$

However, because an extravascularly administered dose will not necessarily have 100% bioavailability, we have to take the bioavailability (F) into consideration. This leads to Equation 9.41:

$$A_t = \frac{FDk_a}{k_a - k} \left(e^{-kt} - e^{k_a t} \right) \tag{9.41}$$

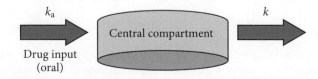

Figure 9.22 An oral drug with a first-order absorption rate constant (k_a) also displays a first-order elimination rate constant (k).

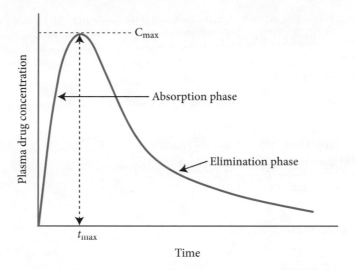

Figure 9.23 The plasma drug concentration profile for an orally administered drug with a first-order absorption rate and a first-order elimination rate.

where D is the administered dose, F is the fraction of the dose that reaches the systemic circulation (bioavailability), and A_t is the amount of the drug at any given time. To calculate the maximum plasma drug concentration, we need to incorporate the volume of distribution into Equation 9.41, which yields the following expression:

$$C_{max} = \frac{FDk_a}{V_d(k_a - k)}\left(e^{-kt_{max}} - e^{k_a t_{max}}\right) \tag{9.42}$$

where C_{max} is the maximum plasma drug concentration (also called the peak concentration) and t_{max} is the time it takes to reach C_{max}. At C_{max}, the rate of drug absorption is equal to the rate of drug elimination. As Equation 9.42 shows, C_{max} is directly proportional to the given dose (D) and the fraction of the dose that reaches the systemic circulation (F). Equation 9.42 is useful for clinicians because it is difficult to know exactly when (at which value of t_{max}) C_{max} will be measured in blood samples.

Plotting the plasma drug concentration on a semi-log scale as a function of time yields a straight declining line, which indicates that the drug has been fully absorbed and its concentration is declining because of the drug's elimination from the plasma. The slope of this declining line will give k, and the half-life can be calculated from the expression $0.693/k$ (**Figure 9.24**).

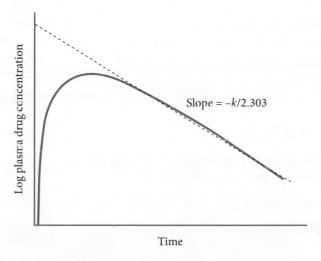

Figure 9.24 Plasma drug concentration profile for a single oral dose using a semi-log scale.

In addition, if you know the administered dose, the bioavailability, and the volume of distribution, you should be able to calculate AUC:

$$\text{AUC} = \frac{FD}{V_d k} = \frac{FD}{\text{Cl}} \tag{9.43}$$

As $V_d \times k$ equals the clearance, we can calculate Cl as well.

Example 9.9: A newly FDA-approved oral drug comes to the U.S. market as a treatment for severe infection. The pharmaceutical company provides the following data in the package insert:

> Absorption rate constant: 1.2 hr^{-1}
>
> Elimination rate constant: 0.3 hr^{-1}
>
> Volume of distribution: 15 L

A. Calculate the maximum plasma drug concentration if you know that the peak concentration is achieved 3 hours after giving a single oral dose of 20 mg. This drug achieves full absorption and is estimated to have 80% bioavailability.

B. Calculate AUC and Cl for this drug.

Answer:

A. This question asks you to calculate C_{max}. You can use Equation 9.42 to do so. It is important to identify which of the rate constants given in the problem represent k_a and k_1. F is 0.8.

$$C_{max} = \frac{FD k_a}{V_d (k_a - k)} (e^{-k t_{max}} - e^{k_a t_{max}})$$

$$C_{max} = \frac{0.8 \times 20 \text{ mg} \times 1.2 \text{ hr}^{-1}}{15 \text{ L} \times (1.2 - 0.3) \text{ hr}^{-1}} \left(e^{-0.3 \text{ hr}^{-1} \times 3 \text{ hr}} - e^{-1.2 \text{ hr}^{-1} \times 3 \text{ hr}} \right) = 0.54 \text{ mg / mL}$$

B. Using Equation 9.43, we can calculate AUC and Cl:

$$\text{AUC} = \frac{FD}{V_d k} = \frac{0.8 \times 20 \text{ mg}}{15 \text{ L} \times 0.3 \text{ hr}^{-1}} = 3.56 \left(\frac{\text{mg}}{\text{L}} \right) \text{hr}$$

Because clearance is equal to the elimination rate times V_d, Cl = 4.5 L/hr.

As noted earlier, the rate of absorption for an extravascularly administered drug will be affected by many complex factors. However, once the absorption rate constant (k_a) is determined, it identifies a general absorption rate that represents the net result of all those influential factors. For this reason, it is important to know how to calculate k_a for an extravascularly administered drug. Perhaps the simplest practical technique to calculate k_a is the method of residuals.

The Method of Residuals

In the method of residuals, we can use the elimination rate constant to calculate the absorption rate constant under the following three assumptions:

1. The absorption rate constant (k_a) is larger than the elimination rate constant (k_1).

2. The first-order pharmacokinetics can be applied to both the absorption and elimination rate constants.

3. The extravascularly administered drug follows a one-compartment model.

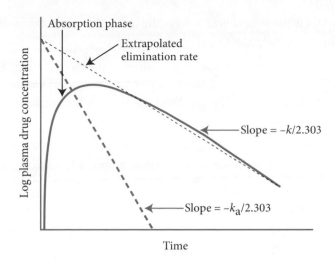

Figure 9.25 Plasma drug concentration profile for a single oral dose of metformin using a semi-log scale and the method of residuals.

To calculate k_a, we need to have access to the plasma drug concentrations. For example, suppose Joe Smith is given metformin tablets (500 mg/day) to reduce his blood glucose. After he receives the first dose, blood samples are taken and the concentration of metformin is measured at different times. The plasma concentration profile of metformin in this patient is shown in **Figure 9.25**.

We can back-extrapolate the elimination phase line to the y-intercept. We should take at least three points on the upper part of the back-extrapolated elimination rate. Subtract these points from the three corresponding points on the absorption phase curve, and then plot the differences as a function of time on the same plot. The result will be a declining straight line that represents the absorption rate. The slope of this curve is equal to $-k_a/2.303$, an expression that we can then use to calculate k_a. To reiterate, a minimum of three points should be used to generate the absorption rate for this plot.

Drug Distribution

After absorption of a drug into the blood, the drug becomes distributed into the interstitial and intracellular fluids. Similar to the absorption process, a series of factors affect drug distribution, including physicochemical properties of the drug, cardiac output, blood flow, capillary permeability, protein binding, and tissue volume. The organs that have a high blood flow are first to receive the drug (e.g., liver, kidney, brain). It may require several minutes to several hours for concentration of a drug to reach equilibrium between the various tissues and the blood. However, because of the high permeability of the capillary endothelial membrane, the distribution of drugs into the interstitial fluid occurs rapidly (unless, of course, the drug is too large to pass through this membrane or is tightly bound to a plasma protein).

Plasma proteins in the bloodstream significantly affect the distribution of a drug into tissues. Most protein binding reactions, however, are reversible. Indeed, this reversibility may lead to toxicity with a few drugs that have high protein binding affinity and capacity. Warfarin (Coumadin), for example, demonstrates 99% protein binding.

Because it is the unbound fraction of the drug that can produce a pharmacological effect, when a drug dissociates from a protein, that action increases the levels of unbound drug in the blood. The drug may then travel more to tissues, which in turn increases the volume of distribution. Therefore, drugs with a large V_d are known to have low plasma protein binding, high lipid solubility, and high tissue binding. For example, digoxin (Lanoxin) and tricyclic antidepressants have a large V_d due to their tissue binding. As a result, and in case of an overdose, these drugs are not easily removed from the body through dialysis.

Some proteins are found to a greater extent than others in the bloodstream. The most abundant protein is albumin, which serves as a major carrier for weak acidic and hydrophobic drugs. Another abundant protein is the α_1-acid glycoprotein, which binds basic drugs. Other proteins can bind drugs but are present in such small amounts in the circulation that their impact on drug distribution is not significant.

Drug concentrations in urine are much higher than in blood. A few factors that affect drug distribution are summarized here:

1. *Competition for binding to plasma proteins.* Competition for the same binding site on a plasma protein increases the amount of unbound drug in the plasma, which often results in a stronger pharmacological effect.

2. *Displacement of drugs from tissue binding sites.* Displacement from tissue binding sites can increase the blood concentration of the displaced drugs. Many drugs accumulate in tissues at higher concentrations. For instance, chronic use of the antimalarial agent quinacrine results in a concentration of this drug that is more than 1,000 times higher in the liver than in the blood. Similar to plasma protein binding, binding of drugs to tissues is reversible. Drugs that bind tightly to tissues can, therefore, produce a prolonged effect because they only gradually and slowly dissociate to reach the site of action. The tetracycline antibiotics, for example, can accumulate in bones for this reason.

   Tissue binding is of particular concern when a toxic molecule or element has a high affinity for tissues. For instance, lead (an element) has an affinity for bones. Because the bones serve as a reservoir for lead, a slow release of the lead into the blood can cause toxicity because the lead can persist in the blood even long after the lead exposure has ended.

3. *Alterations in the blood–brain barrier.* An active P-glycoprotein–mediated efflux process from the capillary endothelial cells has significant effects on the blood–brain barrier (i.e., increases the barrier). As a result, modulation of the P-glycoprotein's function will change the drug distribution into the brain.

4. *Capillary endothelium permeability.* A few transport systems, such as paracellular gaps and transcellular mechanisms, affect drug distribution. For instance, drugs with a molecular weight in the range of 20,000–30,000 Da or smaller can go through paracellular gaps in the capillary endothelium. However, the rate at which the paracellular transport system moves molecules is size dependent: the larger the molecule, the slower the rate. The concentration gradient is another factor that facilitates the paracellular transport system. Because the paracellular transport system is a passive diffusion system, Fick's law (described in the *Introduction to Pharmaceutics* chapter) applies to this system. Hydrophilic drugs cannot go through the membrane bilayer, so they need to use the paracellular pathway as well. Thus the paracellular transport system is not restricted by the hydrophobic or hydrophilic nature of a molecule. In contrast, lipophilic drugs can diffuse through the cell membrane by the transcellular pathway. In addition, drugs with large molecular weights can enter the endothelial cells by a transcytosis pathway, which involves influx via vesicles (**Figure 9.26**).

5. *Blood flow.* While blood flow plays an important role in drug distribution, if the drug transport system through the endothelial cells is slow (which is the case for the paracellular and transcytosis pathways), a change in blood flow will not affect drug distribution to any significant extent.

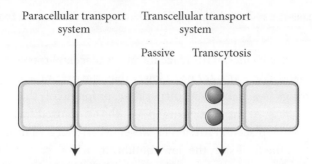

Figure 9.26 Drug transport systems that play important roles in drug distribution.
Adapted from: Pandit NK, Soltis RP. *Introduction to pharmaceutical sciences: an integrated approach*, 2nd ed. Philadelphia: Wolters Kluwer/Lippincott Williams & Wilkins; 2012: Chapter 5.

Diseases that directly affect drug distribution need to be taken into consideration as well. Of particular concern are dermatologic diseases that disrupt the stratum corneum, which in turn leads to increased percutaneous absorption of topical drugs, particularly steroids.

The central nervous system (CNS) also influences drug distribution. The capillary endothelial cells that constitute the blood–brain barrier have tight junctions that make it difficult for molecules to utilize the paracellular transport system to enter the brain. Therefore, the lipophilic property and un-ionization state of drugs play crucial roles in the distribution of drugs in the CNS. For instance, lipophilic drugs such as benzodiazepines readily cross the blood–brain barrier.

Multiple mechanisms are available to assist other drugs in crossing the blood–brain barrier. For instance, nutrient-specific transport systems in the CNS facilitate transport of glucose and amino acids into the brain. Large aromatic amino acids such as phenylalanine and tyrosine are carried across the blood–brain barrier by a transport system called System L. In turn, similar molecules, such as levodopa, can easily be transported across this barrier. Ingestion of protein-rich foods delays absorption of levodopa because System L becomes saturated with high plasma concentrations of amino acids released from the food. This process explains why patients should take levodopa at least 1 hour before eating a meal.

The blood–brain barrier can also protect the CNS from toxic hydrophilic molecules. Another important mechanism that protects us from distribution of toxic exogenous molecules is the efflux carrier proteins that are present in the brain's capillary endothelial cells. Two important efflux proteins, MDR1 (P-gp) and organic anion–transporting polypeptide (OATP), are able to remove a large number of drugs/exogenous molecules from the endothelial cells.

Sometimes, an intentional remodeling of the blood–brain barrier is utilized to transport drugs that otherwise could not cross this barrier. For instance, in the treatment of CNS lymphomas, methotrexate (Rheumatrex), an anticancer drug, cannot reach the brain and its tumor cells. To facilitate transport of this molecule, the blood–brain barrier is disrupted to treat patients with the methotrexate therapy.

Distribution of drugs across the placenta is also important, as many drugs are not recommended to be used during pregnancy. Drugs' physiochemical properties and the placenta's physiological nature play important roles in the distribution of a drug to the fetus. Because lipid-soluble drugs readily cross the placenta, ionized or water-soluble drugs are preferred for pregnant women. The efflux carrier protein P-gp is present in the placenta to protect the fetus from toxic agents. However, this carrier protein causes problems for pregnant women who are infected with HIV: viral protease inhibitor agents (see the *Introduction to Microbiology* chapter) are rejected by the fetus, which may increase the risk of vertical HIV infection (HIV infection from infected mother to fetus).

The pH of the blood on both sides of the placenta affects placental transfer of a drug as well. The pH of the blood on the fetal side is 0.1–0.2 units lower than the pH of the blood on the maternal side. As a result, basic drugs (e.g., morphine, meperidine, propranolol) that reach the fetal blood tend to be in the ionized state. At the equilibrium point, the un-ionized fraction of a drug will be the same on either side of the placental barrier. However, when a larger amount of a drug in the ionized form is present on the fetal side, the new equilibrium will force a higher amount of total (ionized plus un-ionized) drug into the fetus, which can produce toxicity in the fetus.

Hydrophobic drugs pass more freely into breast milk than do water-soluble drugs. However, because milk is more acidic than plasma, basic drugs are ionized; they become trapped in the breast milk, leading to a higher concentration of these molecules than is seen with acidic drugs.

Drug Metabolism

Drug metabolism is an important component of pharmacokinetics. Through this process, the drug is irreversibly broken into other metabolites, which may be either active or inactive molecules. Drug metabolism, which is also known as biotransformation, is an enzymatic process. The salient enzymes are mainly located in the liver, although the kidney, lung, small intestine, and skin also contain metabolic enzymes that are involved in drug metabolism.

While some drugs are excreted unchanged by the body, others are degraded by plasma or liver enzymes. In addition, while many drugs are metabolized by liver enzymes, they may be excreted by another organ—namely, the kidney. Most drugs reach liver via the portal vein and are partially metabolized in the liver before they enter the systemic circulation (recall the first-pass effect). Other drugs (for example, nitroglycerin) are hydrolyzed in the GI tract. To ensure that it achieves the desired pharmacological effect, nitroglycerin is administered sublingually. Factors that can affect drug metabolism include age, obesity, gender, pregnancy, disease states, and food, among others. In addition, variations in genes (genetic polymorphism) may lead to differing drug effects. More detailed information about drug metabolism is presented in the *Introduction to Medicinal Chemistry* chapter.

Drug Elimination

Drug elimination is an irreversible process in which the body tries to remove a drug by a particular route of elimination. It is largely divided into two major processes: excretion and biotransformation. Simply put, elimination of a drug means termination of the drug's action. When a drug is eliminated, it is not necessarily excreted. In other words, a drug may be excreted long after it has been eliminated. For drugs that are not metabolized, excretion is the same as elimination. In contrast, for drugs that produce active metabolites, elimination of the parent drug is not the same as elimination of the drug. By the same token, disappearance of a drug from the bloodstream does not necessarily mean that the drug is eliminated. Perhaps the drug has become attached irreversibly to its receptor and will continue to produce an effect, despite the fact that it cannot be found in the blood. This process explains why phenoxybenzamine (Dibenzyline; an irreversible inhibitor of α-adrenergic receptors) is rapidly (less than 1 hour) removed from the blood after its administration but its pharmacological effect persists for 2 days.

In drug excretion, the kidney plays a major role. A drug reaches the bladder after exiting from the kidney and then is excreted into the urine. As a result, the most important organ in an excretion process is the kidney. Drugs that are not excreted by the kidney are either excreted in the bile or excreted directly into the large intestinal tract and then into the feces with no absorption process. In addition, drug excretion occurs in breast milk—an important consideration when prescribing drugs to nursing mothers. A minor drug excretion route involves the lung, though it is significant only for anesthetic gases. While other routes to some extent contribute to drug elimination, renal excretion is the main process—most drugs are excreted by the kidney.

Three major pathways are involved in renal excretion, and any disease that alters renal function can alter all three pathways. While renal function is not fully developed during the first few months of a neonate's life, during adulthood there is a 1% decline in renal function each year. As a result, clinicians must be careful when calculating therapeutic doses in pediatric and geriatric patient populations.

Glomerular Filtration

Glomerular filtration (GF) is a process that filters small molecules (molecular weight less than 500 Da), including both ionized and un-ionized drugs, from the plasma. Large molecules, including protein-bound drugs, are not filtered at the glomerulus. While the filtrate contains electrolytes, amino acids, and glucose, it also contains waste products such as urea. The reabsorption process occurs at different compartments of the kidney, including the proximal tubule, loops of Henle, and distal tubules. Therefore, it is not surprising that diseases that damage the kidneys can hinder the GF process as well.

The hydrostatic pressure within the glomerular capillaries is the driving force in glomerular filtration. Approximately 25% of the cardiac output, in the form of blood supply, reaches the kidneys via the renal artery. Indeed, approximately 180 L of fluid is filtered each day through the kidneys. However, the average urine volume is 1–1.5 L, which indicates that almost 99% of the fluid volume that is filtered at the glomerulus is reabsorbed.

The rate at which many drugs are filtered by the glomerulus (GFR) can be an indication of active and healthy kidneys. A healthy and normal adult male has a GFR of 120 mL/min, which is normalized to 1.73 m^2 (the standard body surface area). The GFR has been measured by using substances such as inulin or creatinine that neither are reabsorbed. The GFR for drugs is directly related to the amount of free drug in the plasma; in other words, when the free drug concentration in the plasma increases, the GFR for that drug also increases, which results in renal drug clearance.

Measuring creatinine in the urine is not a reliable way to measure the GFR because creatinine is not only removed by GF but also secreted actively by the renal tubules (see the next section). As a result, the measured urine creatinine does not represent the true GFR. In addition, measuring creatinine in this way requires a 24-hour urine collection—an often challenging task for both patients (particularly in an outpatient setting) and clinicians. Measuring serum creatinine clearance (CrCl), in contrast, is a reliable way to estimate the GFR. Creatinine clearance comprises the volume of plasma (mL) cleared from creatinine per minute. The established and widely used Cockcroft–Gault method is used to accurately measure the GFR for males (for females, this CrCl value is multiplied by 0.85 because of their lower muscle mass compared to males):

$$\text{Creatinine clearance } (\text{CrCl}) = \frac{(140 - \text{age})(\text{weight in kg})}{\text{Serum creatinine in } \frac{\text{mg}}{\text{dL}} \times 72} \qquad (9.44)$$

As is apparent in Equation 9.44, age, weight, and gender play important roles in estimating GFR. A normal value for GFR is 90–120 mL/min. It is important to mention that GFR decreases with age. A normal value for the GFR indicates a well-functioning GF process. A low value, such as 15–29 mL/min, indicates a severe decrease in the GFR; a value less than 15 mL/min is an indication of end-stage renal disease, a severe renal failure condition.

> Example 9.10: Calculate CrCl for a 30-year-old woman with a serum creatinine of 1 mg/dL and a body weight of 132 lb.
>
> *Answer:* First calculate her weight in kilograms (132/2.2 = 60 kg). According to the Cockcroft–Gault method, we have
>
> $$\text{Creatinine clearance }(\text{CrCl}) = \frac{(140 - 30)(60 \text{ kg})}{1 \text{ mg}/\text{dL} \times 72} = 92 \text{ mL}/\text{min}$$
>
> Because this individual is female, we must multiply this result by 0.85. This patient's CrCl is 78 mL/min, which indicates that she has a mild decrease in her GFR.

Active Tubular Secretion

Active tubular secretion is a carrier-mediated system whose function depends on the energy input. Similar to other active transport systems, the carrier proteins can become saturated and drugs are transported against a concentration gradient. Drugs that have similar structures can also compete for the same carrier system.

Two active renal secretion systems exist: (1) active renal secretion of weak acids and (2) active renal secretion of weak bases. Probenecid is a weakly acidic drug that competes with penicillin for the same carrier system. PAH (*p*-amino-hippuric acid) is often used to measure active tubular secretion because it is secreted by the tubular cells at a very rapid rate.

Depending on the pathway of drug elimination, protein binding will affect the drug's elimination half-life. For instance, for drugs that are solely excreted by GF, the elimination half-life will change with a change in the plasma protein binding. By comparison, for drugs that are solely secreted by active tubular secretion, protein binding will not affect their elimination to any significant extent.

Passive Tubular Reabsorption

When a drug is filtered through GF, it can be reabsorbed in either an active or a passive process. The reabsorption process depends on the ionization of drugs. Therefore, a pH change in the fluid in the renal tubules (i.e., urine pH) and a change in the dissociation constant (pK_a) of a drug can affect the tubular reabsorption process. Food can change the urine's pH. For instance, consumption of vegetables and fruits and diets rich in carbohydrates make the urine more basic, whereas diets rich in protein make the urine more acidic.

Un-ionized drugs have a greater membrane permeability, which results in a more dramatic reabsorption process from the renal tubules back into the body. This process can be manipulated to increase excretion of a drug that is causing a toxic effect. For instance, to increase excretion of aspirin (a weakly acidic drug), one can make urine basic (e.g., through ingestion of bicarbonate),

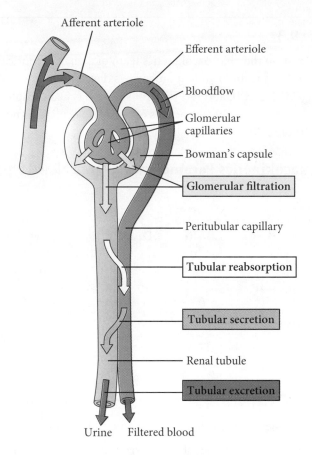

Afferent arteriole

Efferent arteriole

Bloodflow

Glomerular capillaries

Bowman's capsule

Glomerular filtration

Peritubular capillary

Tubular reabsorption

Tubular secretion

Renal tubule

Tubular excretion

Urine   Filtered blood

Figure 9.27 Three major mechanisms that assist the kidney in the excretion of drugs.

which in turn increases the ionization of aspirin. The ionized aspirin molecules cannot readily be reabsorbed, so the excretion process proceeds at a higher rate (for more examples, see the *Introduction to Toxicology* chapter).

Figure 9.27 demonstrates all three mechanisms of renal excretion.

Biliary Excretion

Biliary excretion may also occur for some drugs. This route of elimination is usually included in the hepatic clearance rate. Drugs that enter the GI tract reach the liver through the portal vein. Some of these drugs may undergo metabolism through glucuronide conjugation. The metabolites from this process are excreted into bile inside the gallbladder, emptied in the GI tract via the bile duct, and finally may be hydrolyzed by the gut's bacteria to be reabsorbed. Ethinyl estradiol—the estrogen found in many currently available oral contraceptives—follows this pathway. Upon entering the liver, estrogen forms conjugated estrogen, travels to the gallbladder, and is emptied into the duodenum of the small intestine. The intestinal microflora produce enzymes that hydrolyze conjugated estrogens to free estrogen, facilitating enterohepatic circulation of the free estrogen (see also the *Introduction to Microbiology* chapter).

Learning Bridge 9.3

You are a senior scientist on the pharmacokinetics team of a pharmaceutical company (PacifiCO). The drug design team in your company has developed three new broad-spectrum antibiotic molecules (FAEI, FAEII, and FAEIII). Your team has just completed a preliminary study examining the pharmacokinetic properties of these molecules. Some of this study's results are shown in **Table 9.5**.

Table 9.5 Pharmacokinetics Parameters of Three New Hypothetical Antibiotics

Antibiotic	Oral Bioavailability (F, %)	Elimination Half-life ($t_{1/2}$, hr)	Volume of Distribution (V_d, L/kg)	% Metabolism by Liver	% Excretion by Kidney
FAEI	100	6	4.5	20	80
FAEII	60	12	2.5	10	5
FAEIII	0	24	0.7	75	25

Carefully examine the results and answer the following questions. Provide a brief explanation for each answer.

A. Recommend a therapeutic application for an oral formulation of FAEIII.

B. Which drug will require frequent administration to maintain the drug concentration within the therapeutic range all the time?

C. If the same IV dose (normalized to body weight) of these drugs is used, which drug will produce the highest initial concentration, C_{po}?

D. If the target concentration is 5 mg/L, which drug will require the highest dose (normalized to body weight)?

E. Which drug will be more suitable (safer) for a patient who has renal failure and is taking two antiepileptic drugs that are potential inducers for the liver metabolizing enzymes?

Nonlinear Pharmacokinetics

A few drugs do not follow the rules of linear pharmacokinetics; that is, C_{pss} and AUC do not change proportionally with a change in the dose. This nonlinear process makes the prediction of plasma drug concentrations difficult. **Figure 9.28** compares linear and nonlinear pharmacokinetics. Interestingly, if C_{pss} and AUC increase less than expected after an increase in dose, it indicates that the serum proteins that bind the drug are becoming saturated. An example of a drug that follows this kind of nonlinear pattern is valproic acid (Depakote).

Because the enzymes that are involved in the metabolism and elimination of these drugs can become saturated, we might expect that C_{pss} (or AUC) would increase more compared with a linear pharmacokinetic process when the same dose is given (see drug A in Figure 9.28). As a result of this saturation process, we can apply Michaelis-Menten kinetics to the metabolism/elimination process.

Phenytoin follows typical nonlinear pharmacokinetics: when the plasma drug concentration increases, the elimination pathway for metabolism of the drug becomes saturated, which results in

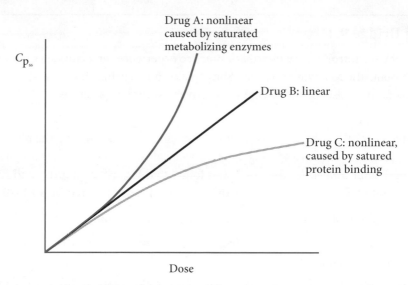

Figure 9.28 The plasma drug concentrations at steady-state level ($C_{p_{ss}}$) that increase with increasing doses of three different drugs are associated with three different profiles: linear (drug B) and nonlinear pharmacokinetics (drugs A and C).

a longer half-life. We can explain this saturation process by applying the Michaelis-Menten equation (see also the *Introduction to Biochemistry* chapter):

$$v = \frac{V_{max}C_p}{K_m + C_p} \tag{9.45}$$

where v is the rate of change of the plasma drug concentration and V_{max} is the maximum metabolic rate. K_m is the serum concentration of a drug at which the rate of metabolism is equal to 50% of V_{max} (i.e., $V_{max}/2$). Technically, K_m indicates that the serum concentration of a drug starts to be nonproportional to changes in $C_{p_{ss}}$ and AUC. Interestingly, most drugs are metabolized by hepatic enzymes but still follow linear pharmacokinetics because the therapeutic range for most drugs is well below the value of K_m for the enzymatic system. As you can see, at low C_p (when $K_m \gg C_p$), Equation 9.45 becomes Equation 9.46 and the process follows first-order kinetics:

$$v = \frac{V_{max} C_p}{K_m} \tag{9.46}$$

In contrast, at high C_p (when $K_m \ll C_p$), v becomes V_{max}, which is a typical zero-order rate (because K_m is neglected and the two C_p elements cancel each other in Equation 9.45). Most patients experience nonlinear pharmacokinetics when they take phenytoin because this drug's therapeutic range is higher than K_m (K_m for phenytoin is approximately 16 µM, but the therapeutic range clusters around 50 µM).

Example 9.11: Phenytoin is an anticonvulsant drug with an elimination process that is nonlinear. Its V_{max} and K_m values in a patient were 600 mg/day and 5 mg/L, respectively. What is the phenytoin daily dose required to achieve a steady-state plasma concentration of 15 mg/L? (Oral bioavailability of phenytoin is 100%.)

Answer: At steady state, the dosing rate should be equal to the elimination rate:

$$\text{Rate} = \frac{V_{max} \, C_p}{K_m + C_p} = \frac{(600 \text{ mg}/\text{day})(15 \text{ mg}/\text{L})}{(5 \text{ mg}/\text{L})(15 \text{ mg}/\text{L})} = 450 \text{ mg}/\text{day}$$

Learning Bridge 9.4

During one of your introductory pharmacy practice experiences at a clinic in Oregon, your preceptor presents the following scenario. She explains further that she assisted a physician to adjust the phenytoin dose for the patient to effectively control his seizures.

FA is a 70-kg male patient who is receiving 130 mg phenytoin twice daily to control his seizures. After 1 month of therapy, his serum phenytoin level was 5 mg/L. The physician increased his phenytoin dose to 480 mg daily. This new dose resulted in a serum phenytoin level of 24 mg/L after 3 weeks of therapy. It was found that V_{max} is 625 mg/day and K_m is 7 mg/L. (V_d was 46 L and F was 100%. The therapeutic range for phenytoin is 10–20 mg/L.)

    A. Why did the physician increase the phenytoin dose to 480 mg/day?

    B. What will be the therapeutic outcome (i.e., effective, not effective, or toxic) of the new recommended dose?

    C. Recommend a dosage regimen to maintain the phenytoin serum level at 15 mg/L.

Learning Bridge 9.5

Lipitor (atorvastatin) is a commonly used cholesterol-lowering drug. When examining the package insert for Lipitor, you find this statement: "Special Populations: Geriatric: Plasma concentrations of atorvastatin are higher (approximately 40% for C_{max} and 30% for AUC) in healthy elderly subjects (65 years and older) than in young adults."

Comment on this statement (i.e., why do you think this statement may be correct or incorrect) using information provided in this chapter.

Table 9.6 lists practical parameters, symbols, and units frequently used in pharmacokinetics.

Table 9.6 Practical Parameters That Are Frequently Used in Pharmacokinetics

Parameter	Symbol	Unit	Example
Absorption rate constant	k_a	1/time	hr^{-1}
Area under the curve	AUC	Concentration × time	(mg/L) · hr
Bioavailability	F	None	$F = 0.8$ (or 80%)
Clearance	Cl	Volume/time	L/hr
Concentration	C	Mass/volume	µg/L
Dose	D or X_o	Mass	mg
Extraction ratio	E	None	$E = 0.75$ (or 75%)
Half-life	$t_{1/2}$	Time	hr
Michaelis-Menten constant	K_m	Concentration	µg/L
Rate	(dX/dt)	Mass/time	mg/hr
	(dC/dt)	Concentration/time	(ng/mL) · hr
Rate constant			
• **Zero order**	k_0	Mass/time	mg/hr
• **First order**	k	1/time	hr^{-1}
Clearance	Cl	Volume/time	L/hr
Volume of distribution	V_d	Volume	L
		Volume/weight	mL/kg

Table 9.7 shows the equations commonly used when measuring different pharmacokinetic parameters at different conditions.

Table 9.7 Equations Commonly Used to Calculate Important Pharmacokinetic Parameters

Parameter	Equation	Conditions of Drug Administration
Volume of distribution (V_d)	$$V_d = \frac{\text{Dose}}{C_{p0}}$$ $$V_d = \frac{\text{Dose}_{IV}}{k\,\text{AUC}}$$	Single intravenous injection (bolus) in a one-compartment model
Measurement of the elimination rate constant (k)	$$\log C_{P_t} = \frac{-kt}{2.303} + \log C_{p0}$$ or $$\ln(C_{P_t}/C_{p0}) = -kt$$	
Plasma drug concentration at time 0	$C_{p0} = k\,\text{AUC}$	
Area under curve (AUC)	$\text{AUC} = \text{Dose/CL}$	
Time it takes to reduce the concentration of the drug in the body by 50% after absorption and distribution of the drug are complete ($t_{1/2}$)	$$t_{1/2} = \frac{\ln 2}{k} = \frac{0.693}{k}$$ or $$t_{1/2} = \frac{0.693 V_d}{Cl}$$	
Clearance	$Cl = kV_d$	
Fraction of the administered dose that reaches the systemic circulation: bioavailability (F)	$$F(\text{absolute}) = \frac{\text{AUC}_{PO}}{\text{AUC}_{IV}} \times \frac{D_{IV}}{D_{PO}}$$	Single dose administered extravascularly in a one-compartment model
Plasma drug concentration	$$C_p = \frac{FDk_a}{V_d(k_a - k)}(e^{-kt} - e^{-k_a t})$$	
Area under curve (AUC)	$$\text{AUC} = \frac{FD}{kV_d}$$ or $$\text{AUC} = \frac{FD}{Cl}$$	
Maximum plasma drug concentration (C_{Pmax})	$$C_{Pmax} = \frac{FDk_a}{V_d(k_a - k)}(e^{-kt_{max}} - e^{k_a t_{max}})$$	
Time it takes to reach the maximum plasma drug concentration (t_{max})	$$t_{max} = \frac{\ln k_a - \ln k}{k_a - k} = \frac{2.303 \log(k_a/k)}{k_a - k}$$	

(continues)

Table 9.7 Equations Commonly Used to Calculate Important Pharmacokinetic Parameters (*continued*)

Parameter	Equation	Conditions of Drug Administration
Infusion rate (R)	$R = k\, C_{P_{ss}} V_d$	Intravenous infusion in a one-compartment model
Plasma drug concentration	$C_{P_{ss}} = \dfrac{R}{Cl}$	
Loading dose	$D_L = C_{P_{ss}} \times V_d$ or $D_L = \dfrac{R}{Cl} V_d$ or $D_L = \dfrac{R}{k}$	
Plasma drug concentration with the first dose	$C_p = \dfrac{R_0}{kV_d}\left(1 - e^{-kt}\right)$	Intermittent drug infusion
Plasma drug concentration with the first dose plus the second dose	$C_p = \dfrac{R_0}{kV_d}\left(1 - e^{-kt'}\right) + C_{px}e^{-kt'}$	
Average steady state	$C_{av} = \dfrac{FD_0}{kV_d\tau}$	
Plasma drug concentration	$C_p = Ae^{-\alpha t} + Be^{-\beta t}$	Single intravenous injection (bolus) in a two-compartment model
Rate of change of plasma drug concentration	$v = \dfrac{V_{max}C_p}{K_m + C_p}$	Nonlinear pharmacokinetics

Golden Keys for Pharmacy Students

1. If a drug is eliminated with first-order kinetics (as is the case for most drugs), clearance is a constant parameter.

2. Because clearance is a constant parameter for a drug that is eliminated with first-order kinetics, a higher plasma drug concentration leads to a higher elimination rate.

3. While a drug may be eliminated in the liver, lung, kidneys, GI tract, or similar route, the two main elimination organs are the liver and kidneys.

4. If a drug is completely retained in the blood plasma, it will have a small V_d that is equal to the plasma volume (3.5 L). If a drug is mainly distributed to tissues, its V_d will be large and the plasma drug concentration low.

5. Upon administration of a drug, the drug can enter the body fluid through three distinct pathways: (1) remain in the plasma; (2) travel back and forth from the plasma to the interstitial fluid (extracellular fluid); or (3) travel back and forth in all fluid compartments (extracellular and intracellular fluids).

6. Use of serum is more convenient than plasma for measurement purposes, and the concentrations of most electrolytes and molecules are almost identical in plasma and serum.

7. In a one-compartment model, the entire body is considered as one compartment and all involved tissues have the same blood flow and drug affinity.

8. A drug is not instantly absorbed in an extravascularly administered route; as a result, both the administered dose and the fraction of the dose that reaches the systemic circulation play important roles in determining the drug's bioavailability.

9. Bioavailability is the fraction of the administered dose that reaches the systemic circulation. It is a fraction (unitless) parameter.

10. The first-pass effect is the elimination of a drug before it reaches the systemic circulation.

11. k_a is the first-order absorption rate constant, which determines the rate of drug absorption from the site of administration. k_a accounts for all the necessary steps required for drug absorption into the systemic circulation, including disintegration, dissolution, and absorption.

12. At a steady-state condition, the rates of drug administration and drug elimination are the same.

13. C_{pss} is directly proportional to the infusion rate and inversely proportional to total body clearance.

14. The time to achieve a steady-state condition depends on the half-life of the drug. It takes five to six half-lives to reach steady-state plasma drug concentrations.

15. A loading dose may be required to achieve a faster approach to a steady state, but its administration does not affect the value of C_{pss}.

16. Nonlinear pharmacokinetic behavior can result if at least one of the ADME processes is zero order.

17. Careful adjustment of the doses of drugs that have nonlinear pharmacokinetics is necessary because even small changes in a dosing rate can result in significant changes in drug concentration.

18. For drugs with a narrow therapeutic window (e.g., heparin, warfarin, theophylline), an IV infusion assists in maintaining a constant plasma drug concentration so as to eliminate fluctuations that may occur between the peak (maximum) and trough (minimum) drug concentrations.

19. Lipid-soluble drugs readily cross the placenta. Therefore, ionized or water-soluble drugs are preferred for pregnant women.

20. The capillary endothelial cells that constitute the blood–brain barrier have tight junctions that make it difficult for drugs to utilize the paracellular transport system.

21. The lipophilic property and un-ionization state of drugs play crucial roles in the CNS distribution, because lipophilic and un-ionized drugs readily cross the blood–brain barrier.

22. The pH of the blood on both sides of the placenta affects placental transfer of a drug. The pH of the blood on the fetal side is 0.1–0.2 lower than the pH of the blood on the maternal side. As a result, basic drugs (e.g., morphine, meperidine, propranolol) that reach the fetal blood tend to be in the ionized state.

23. Some drugs do not follow the rules of linear pharmacokinetics; that is, C_{pss} and AUC do not change proportionally with a change in the dose, which makes the prediction of plasma drug concentrations difficult.

24. When a drug is eliminated, it is not necessarily excreted. In other words, a drug may be excreted long after the drug has been eliminated by a metabolic route.

25. Glomerular filtration (GF) is a process that filters small molecules (molecular weight less than 500 Da), including both ionized and un-ionized drugs, from the plasma. Large molecules, including protein-bound drugs, are not filtered at the glomerulus.

26. Measuring creatinine in the urine is not a reliable way to assess GFR because creatinine is not only removed by the GF process, but also secreted actively by the renal tubules.

Learning Bridge Answers

9.1 **A.** The y-intercept in the provided graph represents C_{p0}: $C_{p0} = 4$ mg/L.

   B. The slope of the provided graph is $(-k/2.303)$: $k = 0.63$ hr^{-1}.

   C. As $t_{1/2} = (0.693/k)$, $t_{1/2} = 1.1$ hr. (Half-life can be estimated from the graph as well.)

   D. $V_d = (\text{Dose}/C_{p0}) = (400 \text{ mg}/4 \text{ mg/L}) = 100$ L.

   E. $\text{Cl} = (kV_d) = (0.63 \text{ hr}^{-1})(100 \text{ L}) = 63$ L/hr.

   F. $\text{AUC} = \text{Dose}/\text{Cl} = (400 \text{ mg}/63 \text{ L/hr}) = 6.35$ mg•hr/L.

(Note: Always check your units and make sure they match the parametrs you are looking for.)

9.2 **A.** More than a sixfold increase in maximum plasma concentration; more than a sevenfold increase in the area under the curve; no significant increase in time to reach the maximum plasma concentration; no significant change in the absorption rate constant (k_a); significant decrease in the elimination rate constant (k)

   B. k is reduced; dose is the same; AUC is increased; V_d is constant (same drug)

$$\text{AUC} = \frac{FD}{kV_d}$$

$$\text{AUC} = \frac{FD}{\text{Cl}}$$

   The observed effect may be due to increasing bioavailability (e.g., by inhibiting the first-pass effect) and/or decreasing clearance (e.g., by inhibiting liver metabolizing enzymes) by the grapefruit juice.

   D. Onset: k_a and t_{max} did not change significantly, so the onset of action may stay the same.

   Intensity: C_{max} increased significantly, so intensity may increase.

   Duration: As k decreases, half-life increases and duration of action will be longer.

   Recall from the *Introduction to Pharmacodynamics* chapter that the intensity of a pharmacological response changes in parallel to the peak concentration; that is, a high peak concentration results in a high intensity.

   D. t_{max} is 3 hours—that is, the time at which C_{max} is reached. C_p at 3 hours is 10.5 mg/L in the control group and 71.9 mg/L in the grapefruit juice–treated group.

   E. $t_{1/2} = \dfrac{0.693}{k}$

   For the control group: $k = 0.135$ hr^{-1}, so $t_{1/2} = 5.1$ hr.

   For the grapefruit juice–treated group: $k = 0.085$ hr^{-1}, so $t_{1/2} = 8.1$ hr.

9.3 **A.** Because of its 0% bioavailability after oral administration, FAEIII is not absorbed into the systemic circulation from the oral formulation. Therefore, oral FAEIII cannot be used for systemic purposes. However, it can be used to treat local (intestinal) infections; it is an intestinal antiseptic (amino glycoside is an example).

B. FAEI, with a shorter half-life (i.e., a large elimination rate constant, k) requires frequent administration to maintain the drug concentration within the therapeutic range.

C. $C_{p0} = \dfrac{\text{Dose}}{V_d}$

If the same doses are used, the drug with the lowest volume of distribution will produce the highest initial plasma concentration, C_{p0}. The correct answer is FAEIII.

D. $C_{p0} = \dfrac{\text{Dose}}{V_d}$

If the same concentration is to be achieved, the drug with the highest volume of distribution will require the highest dose. The correct answer is FAEI.

E. FAEI and FAEIII are eliminated by both liver metabolism and renal excretion to a large extent. Accordingly, renal failure and induction of liver enzymes could significantly affect their plasma concentration (renal failure results in drug accumulation and toxicity, but enzyme induction results in faster elimination and subtherapeutic concentrations). However, the extent of FAEII elimination by liver and kidney is not significant. Therefore, renal failure and induction of the metabolizing enzymes do not have significant effects on its plasma concentration. FAEII would be safer to use in this patient because it would not require frequent therapeutic drug monitoring or dose adjustment.

9.4 **A.** The 260 mg/day dose resulted in a C_{pss} of 5 mg/L, which is less than the minimum effective concentration (MEC). Accordingly, phenytoin will not show any therapeutic effect at this dose.

B. The 480 mg/day dose resulted in a C_{pss} of 24 mg/L, which is greater than the minimum toxic concentration (MTC; see the *Introduction to Pharmacodynamics* chapter). Accordingly, phenytoin will produce toxic signs at this dose. Recall from the *Introduction to Pharmacodynamics* chapter that the MTC is the plasma drug concentration that produces the minimum toxic effect.

C. A dosage regimen to maintain phenytoin serum level at 15 mg/L:

$$\frac{FD}{\tau} = \frac{V_{max}C_{pss}}{K_m + C_{pss}} = \frac{(625 \text{ mg / day})(15 \text{ mg / L})}{(7 \text{ mg / L})(15 \text{ mg / L})} = 425 \text{ mg / day}$$

9.5 $AUC = \dfrac{FD}{Cl}$

If elderly patients use the same dose as young adults, then a 30% higher AUC may result from the reduced clearance mechanism(s) in the elderly patients compared to young adults. As atorvastatin is eliminated mainly by liver metabolism, reduced liver function in geriatric subjects could potentially increase the atorvastatin exposure level (AUC) compared to subjects with normal liver functions.

$$C_{max} = \frac{FDk_a}{V_d(k_a - k_1)}\left(e^{-k_1 t_{max}} - e^{k_a t_{max}}\right)$$

Again, reducing the clearance efficiency, especially liver metabolism, in a geriatric population reduces the elimination rate constant (k), as V_d is constant. A reduced k increases C_{max}.

Problems and Solutions

Problem 9.1 Which of the following statements is correct when a drug is absorbed by a first-order process?

 A. The absorption rate is constant.
 B. The rate constant for the absorption process is constant.
 C. A linear relationship exists between the amount of the drug absorbed and time.
 D. The absorption rate constant is the same as the absorption rate.

Solution 9.1 B is correct; first-order kinetics is characterized by a rate that is proportional to the drug's amount.

Problem 9.2 Theophylline is a drug used for bronchial asthma. What is the expected initial plasma concentration (C_{p0}) after an IV theophylline dose of 10 mg/kg? (V_d of theophylline in this patient is 0.5 L/kg.)

 A. 20 mg/kg
 B. 20 mg/L
 C. 2 mg/L
 D. 200 mg/L

Solution 9.2 B is correct.

$$C_{p0} = \frac{\text{Dose}}{V_d} = \frac{10 \text{ mg} / \text{kg}}{0.5 \text{ L} / \text{kg}} = 20 \text{ mg} / \text{L}$$

Problem 9.3 Assuming the drug elimination follows first-order kinetics, which of the following pharmacokinetic parameters will change proportionally with a dose?

 A. Area under the curve (AUC)
 B. Total body clearance (Cl)
 C. Volume of distribution (V_d)
 D. Elimination rate constant (k)

Solution 9.3 A is correct. In linear kinetics, both AUC and plasma concentration are directly proportional to the dose. However, Cl, V_d, k, and half-life are dose-independent parameters.

Problem 9.4 Which of the following statements correctly describes the effect of changing V_d on the steady-state concentration (C_{ps}) during the constant rate infusion?

 A. C_{ps} is inversely proportional to V_d.
 B. V_d does not affect C_{ps}.
 C. V_d affects only the time to achieve C_{ps}.
 D. B and C are correct.
 E. None of the above is correct.

Solution 9.4 D is correct. Remember that V_d does not affect the value of C_{ps}. However, due to its effect on half-life, any change in V_d may affect the time required to achieve C_{ps}.

Problem 9.5 After administration of a constant-rate IV infusion of 1 mg/kg/hr theophylline, a steady-state concentration of 20 mg/L was achieved. What is the total body clearance of theophylline?

 A. 0.05 L/hr/kg
 B. 0.05 L/kg
 C. 0.05 L/hr
 D. 0.50 L/hr/kg

Solution 9.5 A is correct.

$$C_{ss} = \frac{R}{Cl}, \quad CL = (1 \text{ mg/kg/hr})/20 \text{ mg/L} = 0.05 \text{ L/hr/kg}$$

Problems 9.6 and 9.7 are related to the information in this table:

Drug	Elimination Rate Constant (hr^{-1})
A	4.2
B	1.2
C	0.1
D	0.5

Problem 9.6 Which of these drugs will reach a steady state faster during a constant-rate infusion?

   A. A
   B. B
   C. C
   D. D
   E. There is not enough information to calculate the time to steady state.

Solution 9.6 A is correct. Usually five to six half-lives are required to achieve a steady state. As drug A has the highest elimination rate constant, it should have the shortest half-life and, therefore, requires the shortest time to achieve a steady state.

Problem 9.7 Which of these drugs will achieve a higher steady-state concentration after a constant-rate infusion of 100 mg/hr?

   A. A
   B. B
   C. C
   D. D
   E. There is not enough information to calculate the steady-state concentration.

Solution 9.7 E is correct. We need the V_d value for each drug to be able to calculate C_{pss} after IV infusion of 100 mg/hr.

Problems 9.8 and 9.11 refer to the following case:

A patient is receiving 100 mg gentamicin every 8 hours as a constant-rate infusion over a period of 0.5 hr. The value of k for this drug is 0.2 hr^{-1} and V_d is 14 L. Gentamicin is eliminated completely by the kidney and follows linear kinetics.

Problem 9.8 What is the gentamicin infusion rate (R) in this patient?

   A. 100 mg/hr
   B. 200 mg/hr
   C. 12.5 mg/hr
   D. 50 mg/hr
   E. None of the above

Solution 9.8 B is correct.

$$R = \frac{\text{Dose}}{\text{Infusion time}} = \frac{100 \text{ mg}}{0.5 \text{ hr}} = \frac{200 \text{ mg}}{\text{hr}}$$

Problem 9.9 How long does it take for this drug to achieve a steady state in this patient?

   A. 10 hr
   B. 20 hr
   C. 30 hr
   D. 60 hr

Solution 9.9

$$t_{1/2} = \frac{0.693}{k} = \frac{0.693}{0.2} = 3.5 \text{ hr}$$

As five to six half-lives are required to achieve a steady-state condition, answer B is correct.

Problem 9.10 If the physician was to increase the dose to 200 mg while keeping the dosing interval and infusion time the same, the average steady-state concentration will:

   A. Not change.
   B. Decrease proportionally.
   C. Increase proportionally.
   D. Be the mean of the maximum and minimum concentrations.

Solution 9.10 C is correct.

$$C_{P_{ss,average}} = \frac{FD/\tau}{Cl}$$

This equation shows that the average steady-state concentration is directly proportional to the administered dose.

Problem 9.11 After 2 weeks of therapy, the patient developed acute renal failure. What will happen if the patient continues taking 200 mg gentamicin every 8 hours?

   A. Gentamicin's Cl_T will be higher and its steady-state concentration will be lower.
   B. Gentamicin's Cl_T will be lower and its steady-state concentration will be lower.
   C. Gentamicin's Cl_T will be higher and its steady-state concentration will be higher.
   D. Gentamicin's Cl_T will be lower and its steady-state concentration will be higher.

Solution 9.11 D is correct.

$$C_{P_{ss,average}} = \frac{FD/\tau}{Cl}$$

The equation shows that the average steady-state concentration is inversely proportional to clearance.

Problem 9.12 The method of residuals is used to calculate:

   A. The elimination rate constant.
   B. The volume of distribution.
   C. The absorption rate constant.
   D. The area under the curve.

Solution 9.12 C is correct. With this method, we can utilize the elimination rate constant to calculate the absorption rate constant under the following three assumptions:

1.   The absorption rate constant (k_a) is larger than the elimination rate constant (k_1).

2. The first-order pharmacokinetics can be applied to both the absorption and elimination rate constants.

3. The extravascularly administered drug follows a one-compartment model.

Problem 9.13 Which of the following statements is correct regarding oral administration of a drug?

    A. The absolute bioavailability is always 100%.
    B. The absolute bioavailability is always 0%.
    C. The absolute bioavailability can be between 0% and 100%.
    D. The absolute bioavailability can be more than 100%.

Solution 9.13 C is correct. After extravascular administration, the fraction of the dose that reaches the systemic circulation can range from 0% to 100% depending on the drug's characteristics. For example, the hydrophilic aminoglycoside antibiotics have 0% bioavailability after their oral administration.

Problem 9.14 The method of residuals was used to determine the absorption rate constant of an antibiotic after oral administration. The slope of the line that represents the relationship between the residuals and time on a semi-log scale was -0.10 hr^{-1}. What is the half-life of the absorption process of this antibiotic?

    A. 3.0 hr
    B. 0.5 hr
    C. 5.6 hr
    D. Cannot be determined from the available data

Solution 9.14 A is correct. The slope of this line is equal to $-k_a/2.303$, so

$$k_a = (2.303)(0.10) = 0.2303 \text{ hr}^{-1}$$

Half-life of the absorption process = $(0.693/k_a)$ = 3.0 hr

Problem 9.15 Which of the following statements about the zero-order kinetics is correct?

    A. In zero-order kinetics, the doses of drugs are much larger than the K_m of the enzyme involved in the reaction.
    B. In zero-order kinetics, the doses of drugs are much smaller than the K_m of the enzyme involved in the reaction.
    C. In zero-order kinetics, the enzyme involved in the reaction is saturated by a large free plasma drug concentration.

Solution 9.15 The correct answer is A and C. According to the nonlinear kinetics, when the drug concentration is much larger than the K_m, the velocity of the enzyme reaches a plateau, which is a typical trend of zero-order kinetics. See Equations 9.45 and 9.46.

Problem 9.16 True or False: In an IV infusion drug administration, the steady-state level of the plasma drug concentration is directly proportional to the infusion rate.

Solution 9.16 True; because according to Equation 9.25, if we need to achieve a higher C_{pss}, a higher infusion rate is required.

Our sincere thanks go to Dr. Mohsen Hedaya who reviewed this chapter and provided valuable comments about improving the quality of the chapter.

References

1. Angelov L, Doolittle ND, Kraemer DF, et al. Blood–brain barrier disruption and intra-arterial methotrexate-based therapy for newly diagnosed primary CNS lymphoma: a multi-institutional experience. *J Clin Oncol.* 2009;27:3503–3509.

2. Bauer LA. Clinical pharmacokinetic and pharmacodynamic concepts. In: Bauer LA. *Applied clinical pharmacokinetics*, 2nd ed. New York, NY: McGraw-Hill; 2008. Available at: http://www.accesspharmacy.com/content.aspx?aID=3517000.

3. Bauer LA. Clinical pharmacokinetics and pharmacodynamics. In: DiPiro JT, Talbert RL, Yee GC, et al. *Pharmacotherapy: a pathophysiologic approach*, 8th ed. New York, NY: McGraw-Hill; 2011. Available at: http://www.accesspharmacy.com/content.aspx?aID=7966654.

4. Bauer LA. Vancomycin. In: Bauer LA. *Applied clinical pharmacokinetics*, 2nd ed. New York, NY: McGraw-Hill; 2008. Available at: http://www.accesspharmacy.com/content.aspx?aID=3519284.

5. Burkhart C, Morrell D, Goldsmith L. Dermatological pharmacology. In: Brunton LL, Chabner BA, Knollmann BC, eds. *Goodman & Gilman's the pharmacological basis of therapeutics*, 12th ed. New York, NY: McGraw-Hill; 2011. Available at: http://www.accessmedicine.com/content.aspx?aID=16682148.

6. Buxton IL, Benet LZ. Pharmacokinetics: the dynamics of drug absorption, distribution, metabolism, and elimination. In: Brunton LL, Chabner BA, Knollmann BC, eds. *Goodman & Gilman's the pharmacological basis of therapeutics*, 12th ed. New York, NY: McGraw-Hill; 2011. Available at: http://www.accessmedicine.com/content.aspx?aID=16658120.

7. Byers JP, Sarver JG. Pharmacokinetic modeling. In: *Pharmacology principles and practice.* Amsterdam: Academic Press; 2009: Chapter 10.

8. Clark M, Finkel R, Rey J, Whalen K. *Pharmacology*, 5th ed. Philadelphia, PA: Lippincott Williams & Wilkins; 2012.

9. Fauci AS, Braunwald E, Kasper DL, et al. Principles of clinical pharmacology. In: Fauci AS, Braunwald E, Kasper DL, et al. *Harrison's principles of internal medicine*, 17th ed. New York, NY: McGraw-Hill; 2011. Available at: http://www.accesspharmacy.com/content.aspx?aID=9092427.

10. Hedaya M. *Basic pharmacokinetics*, 2nd ed. Boca Raton, FL: CRC Press, Pharmacy Education Series; 2012.

11. Holford NH, Holford NH. Pharmacokinetics and pharmacodynamics: rational dosing and the time course of drug action. In: Katzung BG, Masters SB, Trevor AJ, eds. *Basic & clinical pharmacology*, 12th ed. New York, NY: McGraw-Hill; 2012. Available at: http://www.accesspharmacy.com/content.aspx?aID=55820341.

12. Horn JR. Important drug interactions and their mechanisms. In: Katzung BG, Masters SB, Trevor AJ, eds. *Basic and clinical pharmacology*, 11th ed. New York, NY: McGraw-Hill; 2011. Available at: http://www.accessmedicine.com/content.aspx?aID=4523488.

13. Jerling M. Clinical pharmacokinetics of ranolazine. *Clin Pharmacokinetics.* 2006;45:469–491.

14. Lam YW. Drug therapy individualization in patients with hepatic disease and genetic alterations in drug metabolizing activity. In: DiPiro JT, Talbert RL, Yee GC, et al. *Pharmacotherapy: a pathophysiologic approach*, 8th ed. New York, NY: McGraw-Hill; 2011. Available at: http://www.accesspharmacy.com/content.aspx?aID=7980183.

15. Mandell GL, Mandell JE, Dolin R, Mandell D. *Bennett's principles and practice of infectious diseases*, 7th ed. Philadelphia, PA: Churchill Livingstone Elsevier; 2009.

16. Marshall WJ, Bangert SK. *Clinical chemistry: the kidneys*, 5th ed. Edinburgh, UK: Elsevier Health Sciences; 2004.

17. Marshall WJ, Bangert SK. *Clinical chemistry, water, sodium, and potassium*, 5th ed. Edinburgh, UK: Elsevier Health Sciences; 2004.

18. McDonald JS, Yarnell RW. Obstetric analgesia and anesthesia. In: DeCherney AH, Nathan L, eds. *Current diagnosis & treatment obstetrics & gynecology*, 10th ed. New York, NY: McGraw-Hill; 2011. Available at: http://www.accessmedicine.com/content.aspx?aID=2386037.

19. Nemire RE, Kier KL. *Pharmacy clerkship manual: a survival manual for students*, 2nd ed. New York, NY: McGraw-Hill; 2009: Chapter 12. Available at: http://www.accesspharmacy.com/content.aspx?aID=5258468.

20. Shargel L, Mutnick AH, Souney PF, Swanson LN. *Comprehensive pharmacy review*, 7th ed. Philadelphia, PA: Lippincott Williams & Wilkins; 2009.

21. Shargel L, Wu-Pong S, Yu A. Drug elimination and clearance. In: Shargel L, Wu-Pong S, Yu ABC. *Applied biopharmaceutics & pharmacokinetics*, 5th ed. New York, NY: McGraw-Hill; 2005. Available at: http://www.accesspharmacy.com/content.aspx?aID=2486691.

22. Shargel L, Wu-Pong S, Yu A. Intravenous infusion. In: Shargel L, Wu-Pong S, Yu ABC. *Applied biopharmaceutics & pharmacokinetics*, 5th ed. New York, NY: McGraw-Hill; 2005. Available at: http://www.accesspharmacy.com/content.aspx?aID=2486353.

23. Shargel L, Wu-Pong S, Yu A. Introduction to biopharmaceutics and pharmacokinetics. In: Shargel L, Wu-Pong S, Yu ABC. *Applied biopharmaceutics & pharmacokinetics*, 5th ed. New York, NY: McGraw-Hill; 2005. Available at: http://www.accesspharmacy.com/content.aspx?aID=2480000.

24. Shargel L, Wu-Pong S, Yu A. Pharmacokinetics of oral absorption. In: Shargel L, Wu-Pong S, Yu ABC. *Applied biopharmaceutics & pharmacokinetics*, 5th ed. New York, NY: McGraw-Hill; 2005. Available at: http://www.accesspharmacy.com/content.aspx?aID=2487124.

25. Shen DD. Toxicokinetics. In: Klaassen CD, Watkins JB III. *Casarett & Doull's essentials of toxicology*, 2nd ed. New York: McGraw-Hill; 2010. Available at: http://www.accesspharmacy.com/content.aspx?aID=6480784.

26. Shires G. Fluid and electrolyte management of the surgical patient. In: Brunicardi FC, Andersen DK, Billiar TR, et al., eds. *Schwartz's principles of surgery*, 9th ed. New York, NY: McGraw-Hill; 2010. Available at: http://www.accessmedicine.com/content.aspx?aID=5011700.

27. Trevor AJ, Katzung BG, Masters SB. Introduction. In: Trevor AJ, Katzung BG, Masters SB. *Pharmacology: examination & board review*, 9th ed. New York, NY: McGraw-Hill; 2010. Available at: http://www.accesspharmacy.com/content.aspx?aID=6543001.

28. Trevor AJ, Katzung BG, Masters SB. Pharmacokinetics. In: Trevor AJ, Katzung BG, Masters SB. *Pharmacology: examination & board review*, 9th ed. New York, NY: McGraw-Hill; 2010. Available at: http://www.accesspharmacy.com/content.aspx?aID=6543207.

29. UpToDate. Waltham, MA: 2012. Available at: http://www.uptodate.com/online with subscription.

Introduction to Pharmacology and Pathophysiology

Reza Karimi
Seher Khan

CHAPTER 10

OBJECTIVES

1. Understand the sympathetic and parasympathetic nervous system, and discuss the pharmacology of therapeutic agents that act through the autonomic nervous system.

2. Learn about the pathophysiology associated with depression and neurodegenerative diseases, and discuss the drug therapy to treat these conditions.

3. Delineate the significance of pain management, and learn about opioids and other medications used in the treatment of pain.

4. Understand the pathophysiology and pharmacological management of hypertension, heart failure, and hyperlipidemia.

5. Identify the major classes of drugs acting on the respiratory system, and differentiate between asthma and chronic obstructive pulmonary disease.

6. Describe the pathophysiology of diabetes mellitus and thyroid disorders, and list the drugs used in the treatment of these disorders and discuss their mechanisms of action.

7. Understand the pathophysiology that underlies malfunction in the gastrointestinal (GI) tract, and identify the major classes of drugs (and their mechanisms of action) used to treat diseases affecting the GI tract.

8. Implement a series of Learning Bridge assignments at your experiential sites to bridge didactic knowledge with experiential experiences.

KEY TERMS AND DEFINITIONS

1. **Acetylcholine receptors:** muscarinic and nicotinic receptors that are activated by acetylcholine and other cholinomimetics.

2. **Adrenergic antagonists:** agents that inhibit the interaction of norepinephrine, epinephrine, and other sympathomimetic drugs with their receptors.

3. **Adrenergic receptors:** receptors that are activated by epinephrine and norepinephrine.

4. **Autonomic nervous system (ANS):** the involuntary and unconscious portion of the nervous system, which, together with the endocrine system, coordinates the integration of daily bodily functions.

5. **Catecholamines:** catechol-containing biogenic amines.

6. **Cholinergic agents:** drugs that stimulate acetylcholine receptors.

7. **Cholinergic antagonists:** agents that block the binding of acetylcholine to its receptors.

8. **Indirect-acting cholinergic agents:** agents that inhibit acetylcholinesterase.

(continues)

9. **Inflammatory bowel disease (IBD):** a chronic inflammatory intestinal disease, divided into ulcerative colitis (UC) and Crohn's disease (CD).

10. **Irritable bowel syndrome (IBS):** a syndrome characterized by relapsing episodes of abdominal discomfort and altered bowel habits (constipation, diarrhea, or both).

11. **JNC 7:** Joint National Committee on the Detection, Evaluation, and Treatment of High Blood Pressure; an organization that provides clinical guidelines to manage elevated blood pressure in the United States.

12. **Monoamine oxidase A (MAO-A):** an enzyme that metabolizes norepinephrine and serotonin.

13. **Monoamine oxidase B (MAO-B):** an enzyme that metabolizes phenylethylamine.

14. **Muscarinic receptors:** receptors that respond to muscarine (a toxic alkaloid from wild mushrooms) and acetylcholine.

15. **Nervous system:** a system of the body consisting of the peripheral nervous system and the central nervous system (CNS).

16. **Neurodegenerative diseases:** diseases that are progressive and involve an irreversible loss of neurons. Examples include Parkinson's disease (PD), Alzheimer's disease (AD), and multiple sclerosis (MS).

17. **Neurotransmitters:** molecules that transmit signals among neuronal cells.

18. **Nicotinic receptors:** ligand-gated ion channels, composed of multiple subunits (two α subunits, one β subunit, one γ subunit, and one δ subunit) that open in response to binding of acetylcholine.

19. **Opiate:** compounds that are structurally related to the compounds found in opium.

20. **Opioid receptors:** δ (delta), μ (mu), and κ (kappa) receptors that are widely distributed in the brain and spinal cord as well as in many peripheral tissues, including vascular, cardiac, lung, and GI tract tissues. Following ligand mediated-activation, these receptors produce diverse effects.

21. **Parasympathetic nervous system:** a major division within the autonomic nervous system that upon stimulation produces diarrhea, sweating, salivation, and lacrimation.

22. **Peptic ulcer disease (PUD):** erosion in the mucous lining of the GI tract (esophagus, stomach, and duodenum).

23. **Positive chronotropic effect:** an effect that increases the rate of heart contraction.

24. **Positive inotropic effect:** an effect that strengthens the contractility of the myocardium.

25. **Postganglionic nerve:** a nonmyelinated nerve fiber that originates in the ganglion but terminates on effector organs.

26. **Preganglionic nerve cell:** a nerve cell that emerges from the CNS and makes a synaptic connection in the ganglia.

27. **RAAS:** renin–angiotensin–aldosterone system.

28. **Sympathetic nervous system:** a major division within the autonomic nervous system that upon stimulation increases the rate and contractility of the heart; relaxes the uterus and detrusor muscle, dilates blood vessels in the skeletal muscles; dilates the trachea, bronchioles, and pupils; regulates body temperature, and stimulates ejaculation.

29. **Sympathomimetics:** agents that are structurally similar to norepinephrine and epinephrine and are able to interact with adrenergic α and β receptor types to produce sympathetic effects.

Introduction

Pharmacology is the study of how a drug interacts with the body to produce a biochemical or physiological effect. Pathophysiology, in contrast, describes how impairment of normal physiological patterns or functions leads to a disease, syndrome, or a disorder. Pharmacology is a science that integrates the sciences of biochemistry, medicinal chemistry, pharmacokinetics, and pharmaceutics to explain how a small molecule such as a drug product interacts with its target to produce a profound and specific therapeutic response.

In this chapter, students are introduced to the sympathetic and parasympathetic nervous systems and therapeutic agents that act through the autonomic nervous system. The pharmacology and pathophysiology associated with depression and neurodegenerative diseases are discussed, and the important therapeutic roles of opioids and other pain medications are addressed. Glucose homeostasis and thyroid functions are discussed to address different classes of therapeutic agents and their mechanisms of action in treating two major disorders of the endocrine system, namely, diabetes mellitus and thyroid disorders. The major drug classes in hypertension, heart failure, and hyperlipidemia are discussed as well, and the therapeutic effects of these classes are emphasized. Pathophysiology that underlies malfunction in the respiratory and gastrointestinal systems is briefly described, and the major classes of therapeutic agents and their mechanisms of action to treat problems associated with these two organ systems are explained. Furthermore, a few commonly used OTC products and their mechanisms of action related to some of these disease states are discussed.

Pharmacology and Related Fields

There are significant differences between pharmacology and other related fields such as biochemistry, medicinal chemistry, pharmacokinetics, pharmaceutics, and pharmacodynamics. A few small overlaps between these fields may, however, confuse students about the exact role of pharmacology in the pharmacy profession.

We will use an example to elucidate the differences between these fields of studies. Suppose Joe Smith is a 20-year-old patient with type 1 diabetes. Joe's pancreas lacks the ability to synthesize the insulin hormone (pathophysiology), so he takes a Humalog insulin shot 15 minutes before each meal. Humalog is provided in a clear aqueous solution dosage form with a neutral pH for subcutaneous injection (pharmaceutics). It consists of two polypeptide chains that are linked together by two disulfide bridges (medicinal chemistry). Upon injection, the insulin is rapidly absorbed (pharmacokinetics) and binds to insulin receptors on myocytes and adipocytes (pharmacodynamics), thereby assisting myocytes in taking up glucose from the blood (pharmacology) so as to reduce hyperglycemia. The absorbed insulin increases the synthesis of glycogen, fatty acids, and proteins (biochemistry).

Before describing the field of pharmacology and its role in therapeutic outcomes any further, it is important to understand two important systems, the autonomic nervous system and the endocrine system, which play major roles in the field of pharmacology.

The Nervous System

The nervous system is divided into two major systems: the peripheral nervous system (PNS) and the central nervous system (CNS). Whereas the CNS consists of the brain and spinal cord

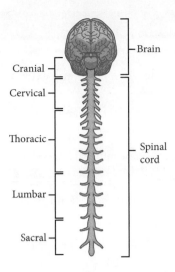

Figure 10.1 The organization of the central nervous system.

(**Figure 10.1**), the peripheral nervous system includes neurons that are found outside the brain and spinal cord but can relay information back and forth with the CNS (**Figure 10.2**). The neurons that directly stem from the brain are called cranial nerves, while the neurons that stem from the spinal cord are called spinal nerves. Humans have 12 cranial nerves. While the first (I) and second (II) cranial nerves originate from the cerebrum, the other 10 cranial nerves (III–XII) originate from the brain stem.

The major pathways of cellular communications in the CNS are neurons—cells with high metabolic and cellular activities in the body. A unique characteristic of neurons is that they synthesize and release only a single type of neurotransmitter at their axonal terminals. Indeed, this phenomenon has assisted scientists in distinguishing different neurons based on the release of their neurotransmitters. For instance, a cholinergic neuron can be differentiated from a dopaminergic neuron based on the differences that exist between acetylcholine and dopamine

The PNS consists of neurons that enter and leave the CNS. While the nervous system as a whole is organized into two major divisions (CNS and PNS), they are not separated from each other and, indeed, function together. Two types of cells are found in the nervous tissue: (1) neurons, which transmit impulses and communicate with other cells, and (2) neuroglia, which are responsible for supporting and nourishing neurons.

The PNS is divided into efferent and afferent nerves. While the efferent nerves carry signals from the brain and spinal cord to the peripheral tissues, the afferent nerves carry signals from the peripheral tissues (skin, skeletal muscles, adipose tissues) to the brain and spinal cord.

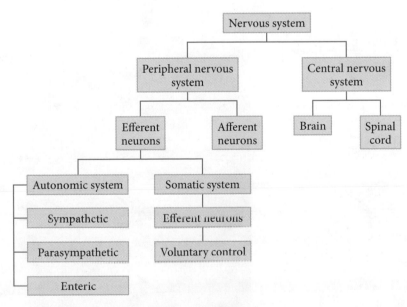

Figure 10.2 The structure and organization of the nervous system.

Adapted from: Clark M, Finkel R, Rey J, Whalen K. *Pharmacology*, 5th ed. Philadelphia: Lippincott Williams & Wilkins; 2012: Chapter 3.

Efferent and Afferent Neurons

Two types of efferent nerve cells are distinguished (**Figure 10.3**):

- Preganglionic nerve cells have their cell body inside the CNS. Such nerves emerge and extend from the CNS to make a synaptic connection in the ganglia.
- Postganglionic nonmyelinated nerve cells have a cell body that originates in the ganglion and ends on effector organs such as cardiac muscles.

In contrast to efferent neurons, afferent neurons transmit signals from the peripheral tissues to the CNS and are important in reflex regulation.

Both efferent and afferent neurons can be long. For instance, afferent neurons that extend from the skin into the spinal cord can be as long as 1 meter.

Autonomic Nervous System

The autonomic nervous system (ANS) is distributed to essentially all organs except for skeletal muscle (skeletal muscle is supplied by the somatomotor nervous system). As the "autonomic" label indicates, the ANS includes the involuntary and unconscious component of the nervous system, which significantly differs from the voluntary nervous system (somatic nervous system). The ANS

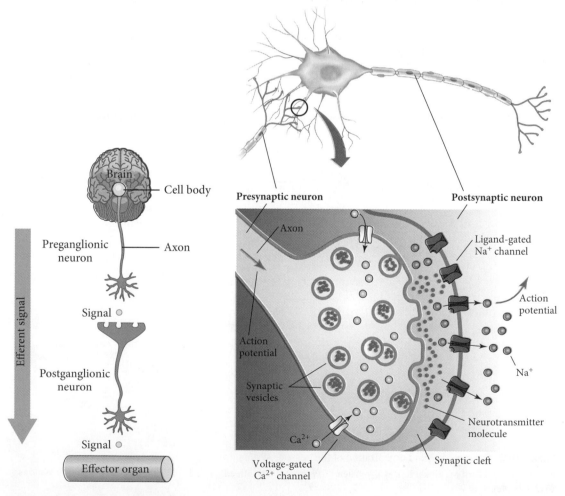

Figure 10.3 Organization of an efferent neuron in the ANS.

Adapted from: Clark M, Finkel R, Rey J, Whalen K. *Pharmacology*, 5th ed. Philadelphia: Lippincott Williams & Wilkins; 2012: Chapter 3.

and the endocrine system collectively coordinate the integration of our daily physiological functions. Many drugs have been developed to affect the ANS or the endocrine system and thereby produce a pharmacologic response to treat a disease state.

The ANS is extended and connected to smooth muscle (e.g., blood vessels, gut wall), cardiac muscle, and glands (e.g., sweat glands, salivary glands). As a result, the ANS controls involuntary functions such as the heartbeat, blood circulation, and secretions from the exocrine glands. In contrast, the somatic system is involved in the voluntary control of skeletal muscle contraction and relaxation for our daily mechanical and functional movements. There are two major divisions within the ANS: the sympathetic and parasympathetic nervous systems.

Sympathetic Nervous System

Sympathetic neurons are part of the efferent ANS. Sympathetic preganglionic neurons originate from the thoracic and lumbar regions of the spinal cord (the first thoracic segment to the third or fourth lumbar segment). Consequently, sympathetic neurons are called the thoracolumbar division of the ANS. The axons of the sympathetic preganglionic neurons leave the spinal cord via the ventral root. From the ventral root, these neurons go through the white rami communicans to reach sympathetic postganglionic neurons. In turn, the axons from sympathetic postganglionic neurons reach the effector organs (target cells) to produce an effect (**Figure 10.4**). A preganglionic sympathetic fiber passes through several ganglia before it ends (synapses) with a postganglionic neuron. In many cases, the sympathetic preganglionic neurons are highly branched and interact with many sympathetic postganglionic neurons. Compared to postganglionic neurons, preganglionic neurons are short.

The sympathetic nervous system is unique in the sense that it adjusts in response to stressful situations such as fear, cold, trauma, and exercise. The effects of sympathetic pharmacological actions are to increase the rate and contractility of the heart; relax the uterus and detrusor muscle; dilate blood vessels in the skeletal muscles; dilate the trachea, bronchioles, and pupils; regulate body temperature when environmental temperature varies; and stimulate ejaculation. The sympathetic nervous system is constantly active, although the degree of activity changes depending on environment factors and organs. This remarkable process assists the human body in adjusting to a constantly changing environment.

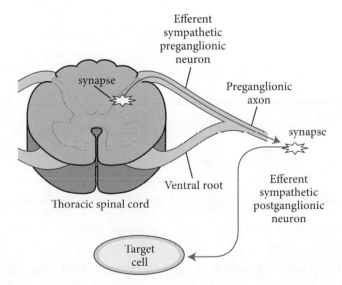

Figure 10.4 The signaling pathway from the thoracic spinal cord to target cells through the sympathetic nervous system.

The aforementioned sympathetic effects occur when the body is in a "fight or flight" situation. When the body is exposed to fear, the best possible reaction to these uncertain situations is to have an increased heart rate and elevated blood pressure, blood flow that shifts from the skin to the skeletal muscles, increased blood glucose to produce energy, and dilation of the bronchioles and pupils to enable a person to breathe and see better. Interestingly, many of these effects are produced by the secretion of catecholamines (particularly epinephrine), which result in the "fight or flight" response.

Parasympathetic Nervous System

As mentioned earlier, humans have 12 cranial nerves. The parasympathetic preganglionic nerves stem from cranial nerves III (oculomotor nerves),VII (facial nerves), IX (glossopharyngeal nerves), and X (vagus nerves in the thorax and upper abdomen). In the parasympathetic system, preganglionic axons are long but the postganglionic axons are short. In contrast, preganglionic axons of the sympathetic nervous system are short and the postganglionic axons are long. Another major difference is that the unique massive branching phenomenon is missing from the parasympathetic neurons, which results in a one-to-one discrete response.

In contrast to the sympathetic nervous system effects, the parasympathetic nervous system seeks to conserve energy to maintain the functions of organs during periods of minimal activity—in other words, to maintain homeostasis. To do so, the parasympathetic nervous system produces many opposite effects to the sympathetic effects: the heart rate is slowed and blood pressure is reduced; GI movements and secretions are stimulated; the absorption of food is stimulated; the retinas of the eyes are protected from excessive light; the urinary bladder and rectum are emptied; and penile erection is stimulated.

Table 10.1 summarizes the effects of the sympathetic and parasympathetic nervous systems.

Table 10.1 Sympathetic and Parasympathetic Effects

Sympathetic Effect	Parasympathetic Effect
Pupil dilation (mydriasis)	Pupil contraction (miosis)
Nasal and lacrimal vasoconstriction	—
Bronchial dilation	Bronchial constriction
Viscous salivary secretion	Increased salivary secretion
Secretion of epinephrine and norepinephrine	—
Increased heart rate and contractility	Decreased heart rate and contractility
Increased arterial blood pressure	Decreased arterial blood pressure
Glycogenolysis and potassium depletion	—
Decreased GI motility (constipation)	Increased GI motility (diarrhea)
Secretion of renin hormone in kidneys	—
Blood vessel dilation to the skeletal muscles	—
Relaxation of detrusor muscle but contraction of trigone and sphincter (urination retention)	Constriction of detrusor muscle but relaxation of trigone and sphincter (urinary urgency)
Stimulation of ejaculation	Relaxation of uterus; stimulation of erection

Data from: Clark M, Finkel R, Rey J, Whalen K. *Pharmacology*, 5th ed. Philadelphia: Lippincott Williams & Wilkins; 2012: Chapter 3.

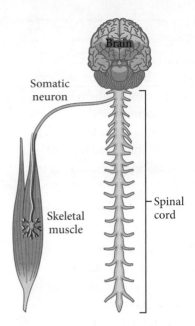

Figure 10.5 The signaling pathway from the somatic nervous system. There is no involvement of ganglia in this pathway.

Somatic Nervous System

The somatic nervous system (SNS) does not contain peripheral ganglia (a peripheral ganglion is a mass cluster of neurons found in the PNS). As a result, the efferent SNS differs from the ANS in that a single myelinated motor neuron that originates in the CNS reaches the effector organ (skeletal muscle) without any involvement of peripheral ganglia. Another difference is that responses in the SNS are much faster than responses in the ANS. The SNS sends sensory information both to and from the CNS. It is responsible for many voluntary muscle movements and includes nerve fibers that are connected to the skin, sensory organs, and skeletal muscles (**Figure 10.5**).

Signaling Between Cells and Organs

Many important pharmacological functions are accomplished by receiving and communicating chemical messages between cells and organs. For instance, hormones that arrive via the bloodstream and neurotransmitters that are released by neurons must reach a cell or an organ to produce an action.

It is important to explain the roles of hormones, neurotransmitters, neuropeptides, and signal transduction before explaining the pharmacological actions of drugs on different organ systems. The significance of signal transduction is described in the *Introduction to Pharmacodynamics* chapter and will not be discussed in detail in this chapter.

Hormones

Hormones have many distinct functions, which may be categorized as follows: (1) growth and differentiation, (2) maintenance of homeostasis, and (3) reproduction. While hormones are the "first messengers," the "second messengers" are just as vital and as potent as hormones. Glucagon and insulin are two examples of hormones that will be discussed elsewhere in this chapter. Examples of "second messengers" include calcium (Ca^{2+}), cyclic adenosine monophosphate (cAMP), inositol triphosphate (IP_3), diacylglycerol, and cyclic guanosine monophosphate (cGMP) (see also the *Introduction to Pharmacodynamics* chapter). A second messenger stimulates or inhibits processes in the cytoplasm or nucleus. For instance, cAMP stimulates cAMP-dependent protein kinase A or PKA. In turn, PKA activates phosphorylase *b*, which in turn converts glycogen phosphorylase *b* to glycogen phosphorylase *a*. The latter enzyme rapidly mobilizes glucose from glycogen (stimulating glycogen breakdown). The overall goal is to increase blood glucose levels.

Growth and Differentiation

Hormones are involved in the growth of an organism and the differentiation of cells. For instance, growth hormone (GH) is important for normal body growth; a deficiency of this hormone results in short stature. The GH protein is synthesized and secreted by somatotrophs in the anterior pituitary of the brain. Another hormone, vitamin D, enhances differentiation of many cells, such as osteoclast precursors, enterocytes, and keratinocytes.

Maintenance of Homeostasis

Almost all hormones affect homeostasis. For example, thyroid hormone controls about 25% of the basal metabolism in most tissues, insulin regulates the blood glucose level by acting on myocytes and adipocytes, and parathyroid hormone (PTH) regulates calcium by promoting the release of calcium from bones and thereby increasing the concentration of calcium in the blood. Sometimes different hormones need each other to maintain homeostasis. For instance, vitamin D and PTH function to control calcium metabolism: PTH stimulates renal synthesis of the active form of vitamin D (1,25-dihydroxyvitamin D), which in turn increases calcium absorption in the GI tract (see also the *Introduction to Nutrients* chapter).

Reproduction

A series of hormones affect reproduction by influencing sex determination during the development of the fetus, sexual maturation during puberty, pregnancy, and lactation. For example, follicle-stimulating hormone (FSH) promotes the development of follicles (as the name of the hormone indicates) in the ovary to release estrogen. Luteinizing hormone (LH) promotes the development of the corpus luteum to release progesterone. Indeed, the combination of estrogen and progesterone in many oral contraceptive drugs blocks the release of both FSH and LH. This inhibitory effect the development of follicles into eggs; consequently, no embryo is formed. The production of prolactin hormone during pregnancy prepares the breasts for lactation.

Neurotransmitters

Neurons communicate with each other through chemical signaling molecules called neurotransmitters. Neurotransmitters are synthesized in the presynaptic region of the nerve terminal. They are stored in vesicles and, when needed by the body, are released into the synaptic cleft (see also Figure 10.3). At that point, they can either bind to receptors on the postsynaptic cell or reenter the presynaptic region through a reuptake mechanism. Some of the released neurotransmitters diffuse away, are degraded, or become inactivated before they reach their receptors on the postsynaptic region.

Two major receptor types are found on the postsynaptic cells.

- Ionotropic receptors have multiple-subunit structures. As the name indicates, they are ion channels. These channels open in response to the binding of neurotransmitters to their receptors. The response to the neurotransmitter is very fast (less than 1 millisecond). A typical neurotransmitter that acts on an ionotropic receptor is acetylcholine (Ach).
- Metabotropic receptors have single-subunit structures. They interact with G proteins, which in turn stimulate production of second messengers to activate protein kinases. The metabotropic response is not as fast as the ionotropic response because activation of a number of molecules takes a longer time. A typical example of a neurotransmitter that acts on a metabotropic receptor is epinephrine.

Neuropeptides

Neuropeptides are identified as definite or probable neurotransmitters. In contrast to neurotransmitters, they are not synthesized in the nerve terminal but rather in the cell body and may co-localize with classic neurotransmitters in neurons. Examples include substance P, endorphin, histamine, cholecystokinin, and somatostatin. For instance, substance P is found in the intestine, peripheral nerves, and the CNS. Substance P is found in large concentrations in the endings of afferent neurons in the spinal cord and may function as a mediator for pain transmission in the dorsal horn.

Drugs Acting on the Autonomic Nervous System

Drugs that act on the ANS are divided into two major classes: cholinergic and adrenergic agents. Important mediators that play important roles in the pharmacology of cholinergic systems are discussed here.

Acetylcholine

Both the sympathetic and parasympathetic nervous systems can use the acetylcholine neurotransmitter to produce an effect (**Figure 10.6**). A preganglionic sympathetic neuron releases acetylcholine, which then acts on the nicotinic receptor on a ganglionic neuron to release norepinephrine in the postganglionic sympathetic nerves. Similarly, the preganglionic parasympathetic neuron releases acetylcholine, which then acts on the nicotinic receptor in the ganglion to release acetylcholine in the postsynaptic cholinergic neurons (**Figure 10.7**).

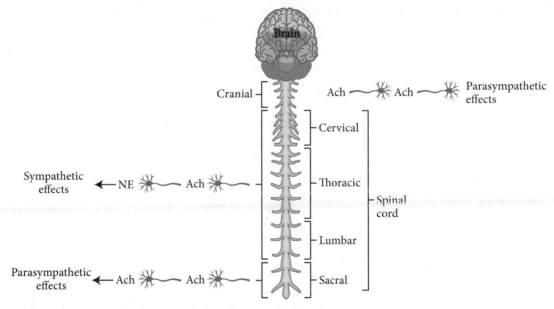

Figure 10.6 The roles of acetylcholine in the CNS.

Adapted from: Nelson LS, et al. *Goldfrank's toxicologic emergencies*, 9th ed. New York: McGraw-Hill; 2010. Available at: http://www.accesspharmacy.com/content.aspx?aID=6504366.

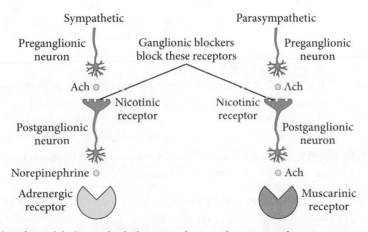

Figure 10.7 The roles of acetylcholine in both the sympathetic and parasympathetic nervous systems.

Adapted from: Clark M, Finkel R, Rey J, Whalen K. *Pharmacology*, 5th ed. Philadelphia: Lippincott Williams & Wilkins; 2012: Chapter 3.

In addition, somatic neurons release acetylcholine that directly acts on nicotinic receptors on skeletal muscles. The nicotinic receptors of autonomic ganglia and skeletal muscle differ, however, and they respond differently to cholinergic agents (see cholinergic agents in this chapter) (**Figure 10.8**).

Acetylcholine is a fairly versatile neurotransmitter that is found in both the central (brain and spinal cord) and peripheral (autonomic nervous system and somatic motor fibers) nervous systems. As Figures 10.6, 10.7, and 10.8 indicate, acetylcholine is a unique neurotransmitter that acts on autonomic effector sites innervated by postganglionic parasympathetic nerves and on skeletal muscle innervated by somatic motor nerves. Acetylcholine receptors account for 5% of all brain neurons, and it has been suggested that acetylcholine in the brain may play an important role in the regulation of sleep–wake states, learning, and memory.

Choline acetyltransferase catalyzes binding of choline molecule to acetate to produce acetylcholine in the synaptic vesicles of cholinergic neurons. This enzyme is abundantly present in the cytoplasm of cholinergic nerve endings. Choline molecules actively enter cholinergic neurons via a transporter mechanism. Acetate inside the neuron then combines with a coenzyme A molecule to form acetyl-CoA. The acetate group is transferred from acetyl-CoA to choline to synthesize acetylcholine. As soon as acetylcholine is synthesized in the cholinergic neurons, it is taken up into synaptic vesicles by a vesicular transporter molecule known as vesicular acetylcholine transfer protein (VAChT). The synaptic vesicles protect acetylcholine from degradation. Following stimulation, Ca^{2+} influx in the cholinergic nerve terminals is a necessary step to release acetylcholine molecules from the synaptic vesicles.

A few molecules, either directly or indirectly, stimulate the release of acetylcholine from nerve endings. Examples include guanidine, aminopyridines, and black widow spider venom. Aminopyridines indirectly stimulate acetylcholine release by blocking K^+ efflux, which results in a delayed repolarization and prolonged Ca^{2+} channel activation. The latter effect results in an increase of Ca^{2+} influx and thereby the release of acetylcholine. Black widow spider venom directly causes acetylcholine to be released; this release explains the severe muscle cramps and diaphoresis caused by this venom.

Acetylcholine binds to its muscarinic receptors and produces central and peripheral parasympathetic effects such as agitation, confusion, seizure, miosis, lacrimation, bronchospasm, and salivation. It can also bind to other types of muscarinic receptors and produce GI motility and constriction of the detrusor muscle (**Figure 10.9**).

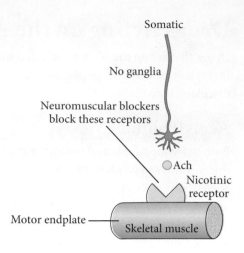

Figure 10.8 The role of acetylcholine in the somatic nervous system.

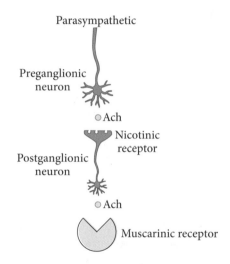

Figure 10.9 The parasympathetic effects of acetylcholine on the muscarinic receptors in cholinergic neurons. Binding of Ach to the muscarinic receptor in the cholinergic cranial neurons results in agitation, confusion, seizure, miosis, lacrimation, bronchospasm, and salivation.

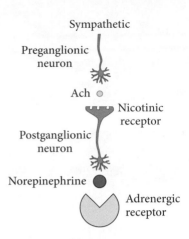

Figure 10.10 The effects of acetylcholine on adrenergic neurons. Binding of Ach to the nicotinic receptor causes the release of norepinephrine. NE binds to its adrenergic neurons and results in nasal vasoconstriction, bronchial dilation, mydriasis, relaxation of the detrusor muscle, tachycardia, and viscous salivation.

Acetylcholine can produce different effects when it binds to the postganglionic nicotinic receptors in autonomic ganglia. It stimulates the release of norepinephrine (NE), which in turn acts on α- and β-adrenergic receptors to produce sympathetic effects such as nasal vasoconstriction, mydriasis, and relaxation of the detrusor muscle (by binding to α receptors) as well as bronchial dilation, tachycardia, glycogenolysis, and potassium depletion (by binding to β receptors). Many of these effects are opposite to what acetylcholine produces in the parasympathetic cholinergic neurons (**Figure 10.10**).

Acetylcholinesterase

Acetylcholine is rapidly hydrolyzed to choline and acetate by the enzyme acetylcholinesterase (AchE). The catalytic activity of AchE is extremely rapid and requires less than 1 millisecond.

Interestingly, some nonspecific esterases can also hydrolyze acetylcholine. For instance, in the plasma, pseudocholinesterase or nonspecific cholinesterase hydrolyzes Ach. The plasma esterases are partly regulated by the endocrine system and are affected by variations in liver function.

Because AchE inactivates acetylcholine, any agent that inhibits AchE will enhance the amount of endogenous acetylcholine. The result of this inhibition will be a high concentration of acetylcholine at the neuromuscular junction and postganglionic neurons

Acetylcholine Receptors

Two types of acetylcholine receptors exist: muscarinic and nicotinic receptors.

Muscarinic Receptors

Muscarinic receptors in the PNS are innervated by postganglionic parasympathetic neurons (see Figure 10.9). The muscarinic cholinergic receptors owe their name to muscarine, a toxic alkaloid found in wild mushrooms. Muscarine has virtually no effect on the nicotinic receptors in the autonomic ganglia, but its stimulatory effect is similar to that of acetylcholine on the smooth muscle. Muscarinic neurons are distributed in all peripheral exocrine glands and organs, but are found in high density in the hippocampus, cortex, and thalamus of the CNS. Several subtypes of muscarinic receptors exist; these receptors are cell-surface receptors and are coupled to G proteins.

Nicotinic Receptors

Nicotinic receptors are ligand-gated ion channels (see the *Introduction to Pharmacodynamics* chapter) that are composed of multiple subunits (two α subunits, one β subunit, one γ subunit, and one δ subunit). They open in response to the binding of acetylcholine to permit the influx of sodium ions. Influx of extracellular sodium ions is necessary for initiation of action potentials in the neurons. Nicotinic receptors are found in the CNS, particularly in the spinal cord; in the autonomic ganglia; and at the skeletal neuromuscular junctions (Figures 10.7 and 10.8).

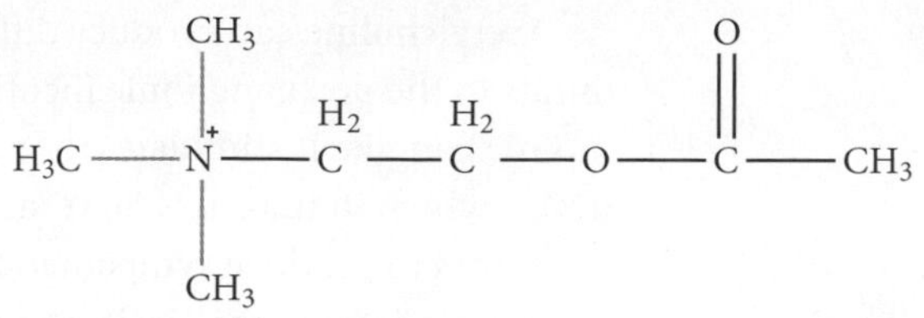

Figure 10.11 Structure of acetylcholine. The nitrogen atom and its attached three methyl groups are necessary to produce the full cholinergic agonistic effect.

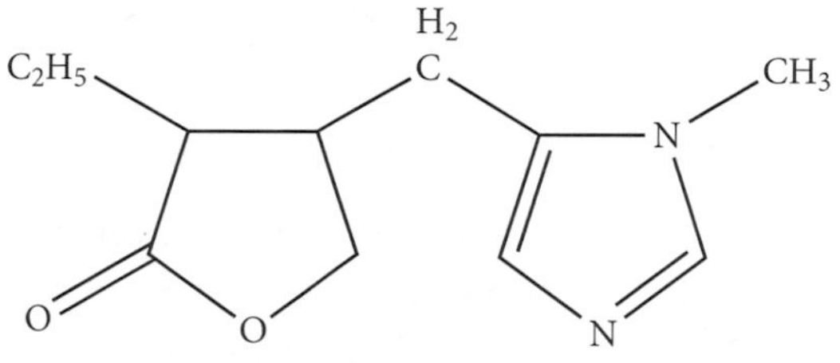

Figure 10.12 Structure of pilocarpine. The tertiary nitrogen atoms (blue) allow this drug to cross the blood–brain barrier and be resistant to the hydrolysis effect of AchE.

Exogenous acetylcholine has no therapeutic application because it undergoes rapid hydrolysis by AchE or by the acidic environment of the stomach. However, some exogenous muscarinic agonists mimic the effects of acetylcholine at muscarinic receptors. **Figure 10.11** shows the structure of acetylcholine. The nitrogen and its attached three methyl groups are the pharmacophore of acetylcholine that produces cholinergic effects.

Cholinergic Agents

Direct-Acting Cholinergic Agonists

Drugs that stimulate acetylcholine receptors are called cholinergic agonists. Important drugs in this class are discussed in the following section.

Pilocarpine

Pilocarpine was originally extracted from the leaflets of South American shrubs of *Pilocarpus* spp. Pilocarpine (Salagen for systemic use or Isopto Carpine as an ophthalmic solution) is stable to hydrolysis by AchE. Being a tertiary amine, pilocarpine does not carry an ionic charge; as a result, it is readily absorbed from the GI tract and is able to cross the blood–brain barrier (**Figure 10.12**).

Pilocarpine, when applied topically to eyes, facilitates drainage of excessive buildup of the aqueous humor resulting from a serious ophthalmic condition, glaucoma. In addition, it causes constriction of the pupils (miosis) and focuses the vision to near objects. Systemically, pilocarpine is used in Sjögren's syndrome (an autoimmune disorder characterized by compromised salivary and lacrimal secretions) and xerostomia (dry mouth resulting from low or absence of saliva secretion). The gel formulation of pilocarpine is susceptible to hydrolysis and should not be stored in the refrigerator for longer than 2 weeks.

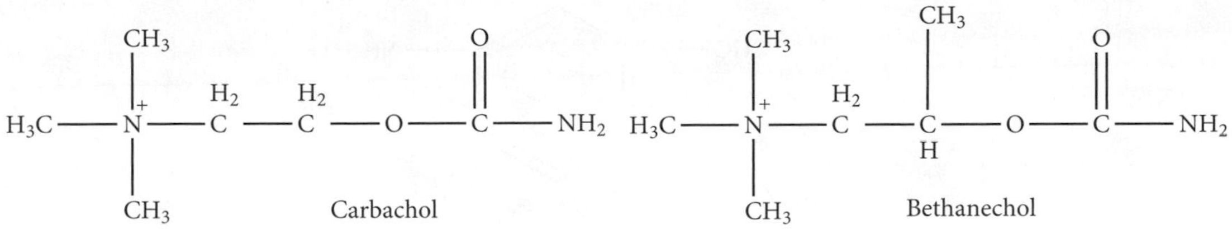

Figure 10.13 Structures of carbachol and bethanechol. The only difference between these structures is the extra methyl group in bethanechol. Due to the lack of the methyl group, bethanechol does not bind to nicotinic receptors.

Due to the effects of pilocarpine, a few other similar agents were synthesized in the 1930s. Two typical examples are carbachol and bethanechol (**Figure 10.13**).

Carbachol

Carbachol (Isopto Carbachol) has both muscarinic and nicotinic effects. It also has a longer duration of action (10 hours) than pilocarpine (6 hours) because it is more resistant to the hydrolysis by AchE (due to the presence of an amide group, compare its structure with that of Ach). Carbachol is used in patients with glaucoma who do not respond or are intolerant to pilocarpine because of ocular irritation or allergic reactions. However, due to its profound cardiovascular (arrhythmia and hypotension) and GI (e.g., abdominal cramps and diarrhea) effects and its long duration of action, therapeutically carbachol is not as useful as pilocarpine. Interestingly, carbachol increases release of epinephrine by stimulating the ganglionic nicotinic receptors.

Bethanechol

Bethanechol (Urecholine) is resistant to hydrolysis by AchE because of its structural features (due to the presence of an amide group, Figure 10.13). Bethanechol's structure is similar to that of carbachol but it contains an additional methyl group on the second carbon. The additional methyl group excludes bethanechol's activity at nicotinic receptors.

Bethanechol is used to treat postoperative and postpartum urinary retention. It has a short duration of action (1 hour) and can be taken on an empty stomach to avoid the cholinergic side effects of nausea and vomiting.

Indirect-Acting Cholinergic Agonists

Indirect-acting cholinergic agents are inhibitors of AchE, responsible for inactivation of the acetylcholine neurotransmitter. Examples of cholinesterase inhibitors include edrophonium, neostigmine, and physostigmine.

Edrophonium

Edrophonium (Enlon; **Figure 10.14**) is a short-acting agent that binds to the enzyme noncovalently. Because it has a quaternary ammonium group, its actions are limited to the periphery. While edrophonium continues to be used for diagnosis of myasthenia gravis, it has largely fallen out of favor due to the availability of better cholinergic agents. Myasthenia gravis, an autoimmune disorder in which the function of skeletal muscles becomes compromised, results from the development of antibody against nicotinic receptors.

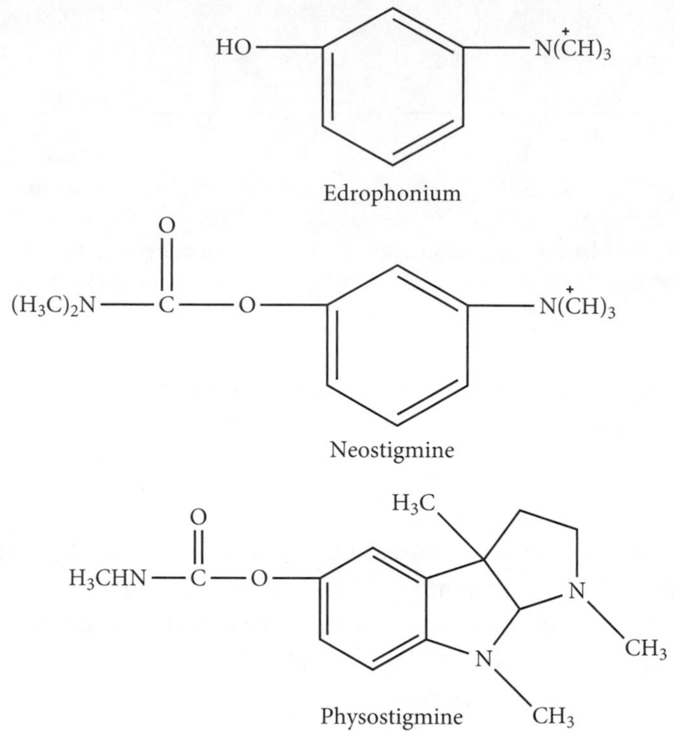

Figure 10.14 Structures of indirect-acting cholinergic agonists. Due to the quaternary amine groups in edrophonium and neostigmine, they have poor GI absorption and minimal penetration through the blood–brain barrier.

Neostigmine and Pyridostigmine

Neostigmine (Prostigmin) and pyridostigmine are reversible inhibitors of AchE that are used in the symptomatic treatment of myasthenia gravis because they can preserve endogenous acetylcholine and consequently expose the motor endplate to adequate concentrations of this neurotransmitter (see Figure 10.8). An oral daily dose of 30 mg pyridostigmine (or 10 mg neostigmine) is usually administered to a patient with myasthenia gravis. Often, incremental doses are given until an optimal response is obtained. Similar to edrophonium, neostigmine is positively charged and has a poor GI absorption and minimal blood–brain barrier penetration. For instance, the effective parenteral dose of neostigmine is 0.5–2 mg but the effective oral dose is much larger (around 20 mg or more). Neostigmine's duration of action is short (usually 1–2 hours). The drug can be used to stimulate the tone of the intestine and urinary bladder.

Physostigmine

Physostigmine has a tertiary amine group (Figure 10.14) which helps this drug to be absorbed readily from the GI tract, subcutaneous tissues, and mucous membranes. It is also used to treat glaucoma because it lowers the intraocular pressure. Because physostigmine is a less polar compound, it can stimulate muscarinic and nicotinic receptors of the ANS and the nicotinic receptors at the neuromuscular junction. Due to the hydrolytic effect of esterases in the plasma, injected physostigmine is broken down into inactive compounds within 2–3 hours. Physostigmine is also an antidote for poisoning from anticholinergic drugs and plants (i.e., tricyclic antidepressants, antihistamines, and plants with an anticholinergic effect).

New indirect-acting cholinergic agents such as donepezil, rivastigmine, and galantamine are used to prevent progression of Alzheimer's disease, which is characterized by loss of cholinergic neurons in the central nervous system. These agents are discussed in a separate section of this chapter ("Neurodegenerative Diseases").

Cholinergic Antagonists

These agents block the binding of acetylcholine to its receptors. Consequently, the sympathetic stimulation remains intact. Neuromuscular blockers, a separate class of anticholinergic drugs, are therapeutically useful to block neurotransmission to skeletal muscles.

Antimuscarinic Agents

Atropine

Atropine (AtroPen; Atropine Care; Isopto Atropine) is a nonselective and competitive muscarinic antagonist. This lipid-soluble tertiary amine readily crosses membrane barriers, particularly the blood–brain barrier, and is well distributed into the CNS (**Figure 10.15**). It has a long duration of action (4–8 hours) and lasts even longer in the eye (at least 3 days). Atropine has both central and peripheral effects. While the CNS effects, such as restlessness, confusion, and excitement, are observed with toxic concentrations, the peripheral antimuscarinic effects in the ocular, gastrointestinal, and genitourinary systems are predictable.

Therapeutically important functions of atropine are restoration of the heart rate following myocardial infarction (MI), reduction of airway secretion during anesthesia, and dilation of the pupil of the eye. Following an MI, vagal stimulation of the heart is increased; atropine administration reduces this vagal stimulation and helps to maintain the hemodynamic state of the patient. Atropine causes the iris sphincter to be relaxed, resulting in dilation of the pupil, which is critically important for ophthalmologic examination. In addition, atropine is used as an antidote to AchE inhibitor poisoning. Atropine is available in different dosage forms (IV, IM, ophthalmic solution, and ophthalmic ointment).

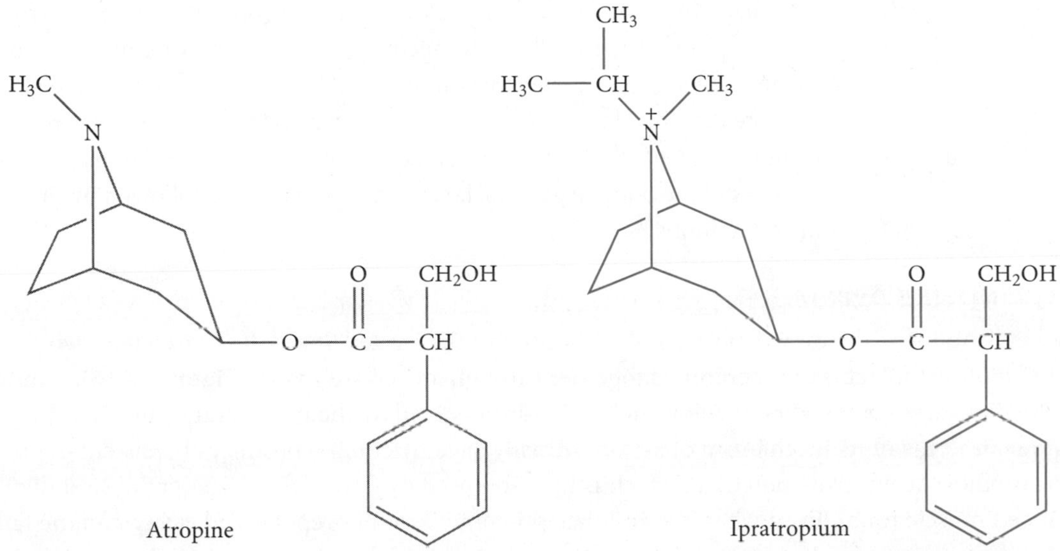

Figure 10.15 Structures of atropine and ipratropium. Atropine, as a tertiary amine and lipophilic compound, readily penetrates the blood–brain barrier. Ipratropium contains a quaternary ammonium group, so its effect is confined to the airways.

Scopolamine

Scopolamine (Transderm Scop for systemic use) is provided as a transdermal patch and is the most effective agent available to treat motion sickness prophylactically. It is also available as an ophthalmic solution (Isopto Hyoscine). Because scopolamine has extensive permeation of the blood–brain barrier (even at low doses), its centrally acting effects are prominent, including drowsiness, amnesia, fatigue, dreamless sleep, and euphoria.

Ipratropium and Tiotropium

Ipratropium (Atrovent HFA) and tiotropium (Spiriva) are used to treat chronic obstructive pulmonary disease (COPD), a disease of the elderly seen in chronic smokers. Both agents are quaternary ammonium compounds and are used in inhalers for their effects on the pulmonary airways. Dry mouth is often reported as an adverse effect.

Benztropine and Trihexyphenidyl

Due to their anticholinergic effect, benztropine (Cogentin) and trihexyphenidyl have been used to treat Parkinson's disease; they reduce the tremor and rigidity associated with this disease. They may be useful in geriatric patient populations who cannot tolerate anti-Parkinsonian agents. Adverse effects associated with their use include sedation, mydriasis, urinary retention, and dry mouth.

Neuromuscular Blockers

Neuromuscular blockers interrupt activation of nicotinic receptors in skeletal muscles. These agents are used as adjuncts to anesthetics in major surgical procedures to relax skeletal muscles. While neuromuscular blockers are used to supplement anesthetic agents, they should not replace general anesthesia. Neuromuscular blockers can be categorized into nondepolarizing blockers and depolarizing blockers.

Nondepolarizing Blockers

Nondepolarizing blocker agents are competitive antagonists of the nicotinic receptors on the skeletal muscles. Examples include atracurium (Atracurium Besylate Injection, from Canada), mivacurium, pancuronium (Pancuronium Bromide, from Canada), vecuronium (Norcuron, from Canada), and rocuronium (Zemuron). Chemically, these agents are quaternary compounds with minimal CNS penetration and, consequently, they are administered by the intravenous route. Nondepolarizing blockers were developed from D-tubocurarine, a natural poison used in arrowheads for hunting in ancient times. Not all muscles are equally sensitive to nonpolarizing agents, however, small skeletal muscles of the body (e.g., jaws, larynx) are relaxed first, followed by the larger muscles of the thorax and limbs.

Depolarizing Agents

Succinylcholine is the only depolarizing agent used in the United States. It forms when two acetylcholine molecules are combined together through an acetate group (**Figure 10.16**). Similar to the depolarizing blockers, succinylcholine is administered by the parenteral route. The drug is unique in terms of its mechanism of action: Initially succinylcholine produces persistent depolarization of the endplate potential, which is then followed by flaccid paralysis (paralysis and reduced muscle tone). Even when the endplate potential becomes repolarized, acetylcholine fails to produce a response due to desensitization of receptor. Initial persistent depolarization is a result of the drug being resistant to the action of acetylcholinesterase. It has a very short duration of action (less than 10 minutes) and undergoes rapid hydrolysis by pseudocholinesterase of the liver and plasma.

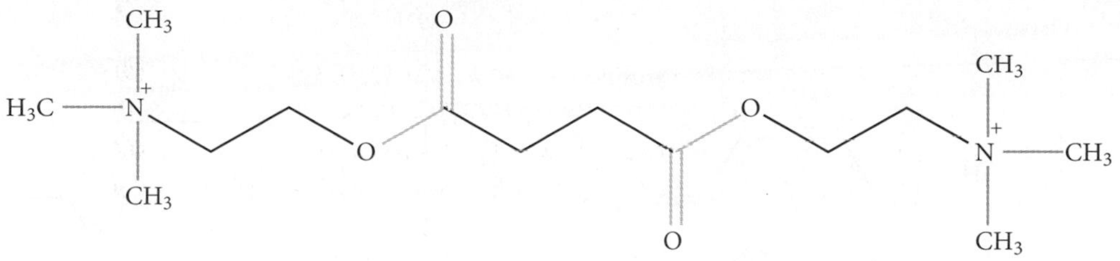

Figure 10.16 Structure of succinylcholine, which has two unique quaternary amino groups and two ester groups. This agent is highly prone to hydrolysis because of the presence of ester groups.

Pharmacogenomics (see also the *Introduction to Pharmacogenomics* chapter) plays an important role here because patients with a genetic variant of plasma pseudocholinesterase hydrolyze succinylcholine slowly, and suffer from prolonged apnea (cessation of breathing for a few seconds during sleep) due to paralysis of the diaphragm. Due to its rapid and short duration of action, succinylcholine is most often used when rapid endotracheal intubation is necessary during the induction of anesthesia.

Adrenergic Agonists

This section describes a few important molecules related to the adrenergic system.

Tyrosine

The amino acid tyrosine serves as the precursor for the synthesis of catecholamine. **Figure 10.17** indicates the enzymes and substrates involved in the synthesis of norepinephrine. For catecholamine biosynthesis, tyrosine is transported to the adrenergic neuron. The enzyme tyrosine hydroxylase is the first (and a rate-limiting) enzyme in the biosynthesis of norepinephrine. While tyrosine hydroxylase is exclusively found in tissues that produce catecholamines, the aromatic amino acid decarboxylase enzyme is present in all tissues.

Catecholamines

A few neurotransmitters have the unique structure of catechol (**Figure 10.18**) and, as a result, are classified as catecholamines. In the adrenal medulla, norepinephrine is converted to epinephrine. While 80% of the catecholamine production of the adrenal medulla consists of epinephrine, 20% is norepinephrine, and both catecholamines are released into the circulation upon stimulation of the adrenal medulla. The release of catecholamines is low in the basal state and during sleep. However, in emergency situations, as in the "fight or flight" response, increased adrenal catecholamine are released in the circulation. In addition, psychological or physical stress or metabolic stress (hypoglycemia and exercise) can increase the release of catecholamines.

The release of norepinephrine is stimulated by an action potential that results in an influx of Ca^{2+} into the presynaptic terminals. Increased Ca^{2+} concentration leads to fusion of norepinephrine-containing vesicles to the presynaptic membrane. Guanethidine is known to block this step, thereby reducing the amount of norepinephrine in the synaptic cleft—an effect referred to as sympathoplegia (a decreased adrenergic outflow). Guanethidine is no longer available in the United States.

Agents that are structurally similar to norepinephrine and epinephrine are able to interact with adrenergic α and β receptors to produce sympathetic effects. These agents are called sympathomimetics. The greatest sympathomimetic activity appears to occur when the benzene ring is separated from the amino group by two carbon atoms (Figure 10.17; see also the *Introduction to Medicinal Chemistry* chapter). While many sympathomimetics act on both adrenergic α and

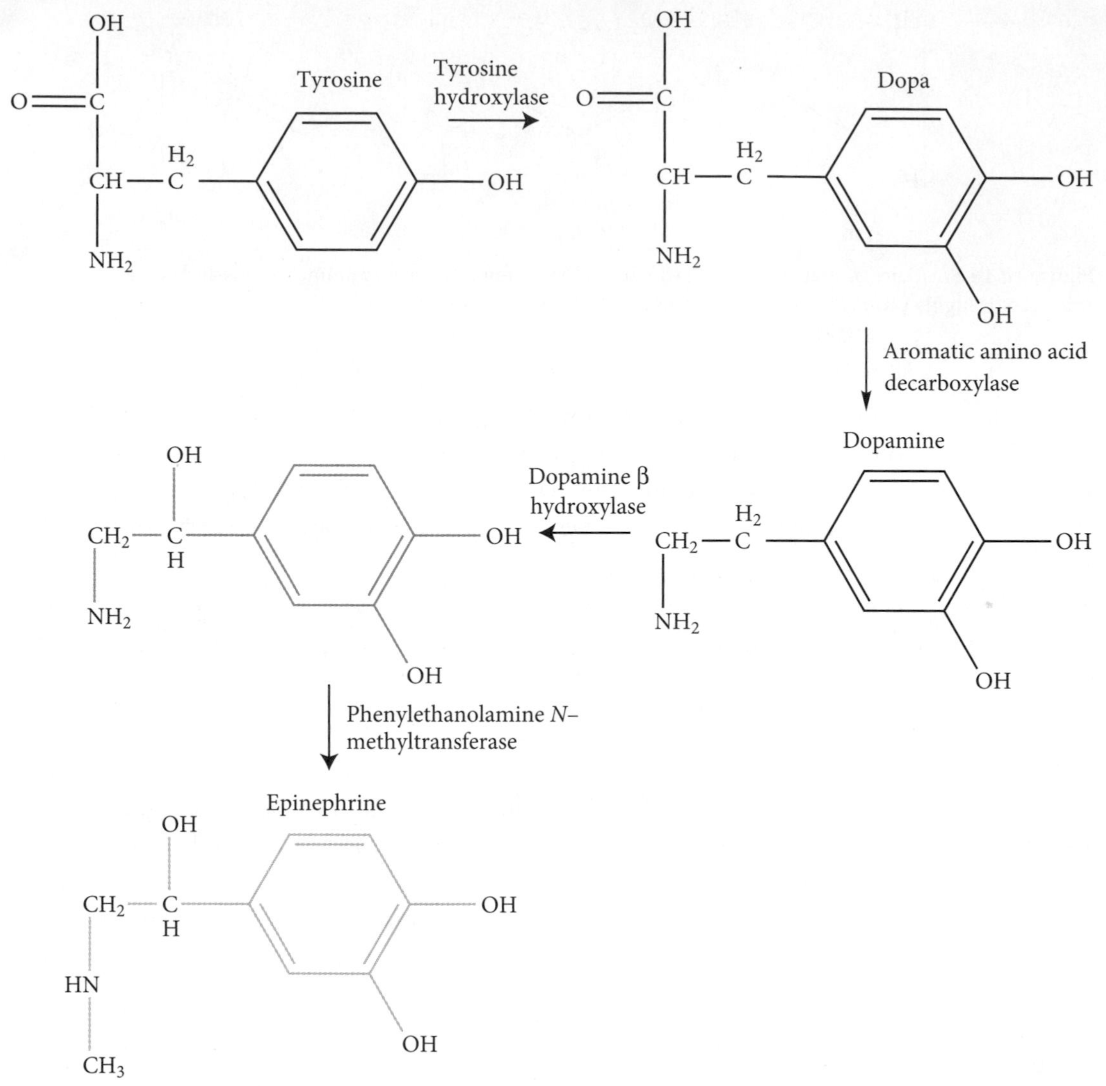

Figure 10.17 Synthesis of norepinephrine and epinephrine from the aromatic amino acid tyrosine.

β receptors (nonselective), a few act selectively (on only one receptor type). For instance, phenylephrine (Sudafed PE Nasal Decongestant) is a selective α_1 receptor agonist and clonidine (Catapres) is a selective α_2 agonist. Isoproterenol (Isuprel), in contrast, acts at both β_1 and β_2 receptors.

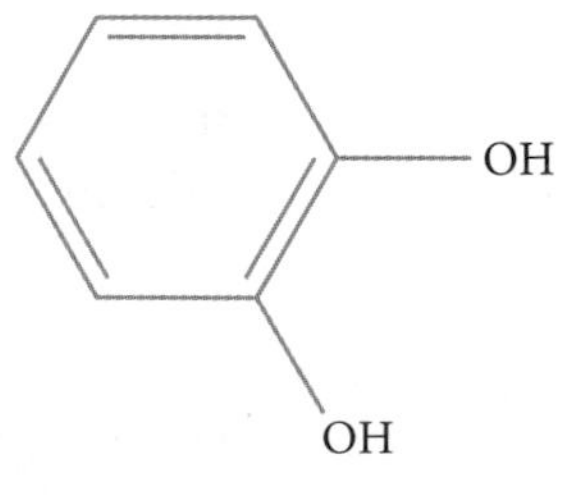

Adrenergic neurons release norepinephrine as the main neurotransmitter. The neurotransmission in the adrenergic neurons mimics the neurotransmission in the cholinergic neurons.

Alpha receptors are subdivided into α_1 and α_2 receptors and β receptors into β_1, β_2, and β_3 receptors. While α receptors stimulate smooth muscle contraction in the blood vessels and genitourinary (GU) tract as well as an increase in the breakdown of glycogen (glycogenolysis), α_2 receptors cause smooth muscle relaxation in the GI tract. Peripheral α_2 receptors also stimulate vasoconstriction of some blood vessels. In addition, α_2 receptors decrease insulin release.

Figure 10.18 A benzene ring with two *adjacent* hydroxyl groups is referred to as "catechol."

Table 10.2 Alpha and Beta Receptor Types and Their Mediated Actions

Receptor Type	α_1	α_2	β_1	β_2
Mediated actions	Increased sweating	Decreased NE, acetylcholine, and insulin release	Tachycardia	Decreased motility
	Vasoconstriction of vascular smooth muscle and hypertension	Vasoconstriction of vascular smooth muscle and hypertension	Increased lipolysis and renin release	Vasodilation
	Increased glucagon release	Platelet aggregation	Increased myocardial contractility	Bronchodilation
	Chronotropic		Both chronotropic and inotropic	Increased glucagon release
	Increased closure of sphincter of the bladder		Increased AV nodal conduction velocity	Increased muscle and liver glycogenolysis
	Mydriasis			Release of potassium

Adapted from Clark M, Finkel R, Rey J, Whalen K. *Pharmacology*, 5th ed. Philadelphia: Lippincott Williams & Wilkins; 2012.

The β_1 receptors mediate lipolysis and renin release and increase the rate and force of myocardial contraction. The β_2 receptors mediate smooth muscle relaxation in the bronchi, blood vessels, and GU and GI tracts; synthesis of glucose (gluconeogenesis) and glycogenolysis in the liver and muscles, and the release of two opposing hormones, insulin and glucagon. In most tissues, β_3 receptors mediate increases in the metabolic rate.

Dopamine is another catecholamine and can stimulate both α_1 and β_1 receptors. Thus it is included among adrenergic agents as well. **Table 10.2** identifies α and β receptors and their mediated actions.

Adrenergic agonists are classified into three sympathomimetic groups: direct acting, indirect acting, and mixed acting.

Direct-Acting Agonists

As their name indicates, these agents directly act on α and β receptors to produce pharmacological effects. They can exhibit selectivity for a specific receptor or nonselectivity for more than one receptor. A few important agents in this category are described next.

Epinephrine

Epinephrine (EpiPen) is a nonselective α- and β-adrenergic agonist that acts on all receptor subtypes (α_1, α_2, β_1, β_2, and β_3 receptors). Epinephrine, at low doses (0.1–0.5 µg/kg/min), increases cardiac output; at higher doses, it produces vasoconstriction. It is used only when patients fail to respond to other traditional therapies for elevating or maintaining normal blood pressure. Epinephrine is used to treat bronchospasm and bronchial asthma, nasal congestion, anaphylactic reactions, and cardiac arrest. In addition, it is included in local anesthetic formulations to reduce systemic absorption and increase duration of action of local anesthetics. Epinephrine is synthesized in the adrenal medulla and constitutes 80% of the catecholamines synthesized in this gland (i.e., it is not produced in extramedullary tissues). This hormone is released directly into the bloodstream.

Epinephrine's major effect is to strengthen the contractility of the myocardium (positive inotropic) and to increase the rate of heart contraction (positive chronotropic). Both effects are mediated by the β_1 receptor. As a result, cardiac output increases. However, epinephrine also increases the oxygen demands on the myocardium. In addition, it stimulates the release of the vasoconstrictive enzyme renin from the kidneys, which increases the production of angiotensin II, a potent vasoconstrictor. The most important role of epinephrine is to stimulate β_2 receptors to treat anaphylactic shock (commonly caused by type I hypersensitivity to allergens; see also the *Introduction to Immunology* chapter). Within a few minutes after a subcutaneous injection of epinephrine, the patient recovers from the anaphylactic shock. A major side effect of epinephrine is cerebral hemorrhage caused by increased blood pressure.

Norepinephrine

Norepinephrine (Levophed) is a potent α_1 and α_2 agonist, has relatively little action on β_2 receptors, and is a major chemical mediator that is released by postganglionic sympathetic nerves. Unlike epinephrine, norepinephrine lacks a methyl group (Figure 10.17); it is also less potent than epinephrine on α receptors of most organs. In contrast to epinephrine, small doses of norepinephrine do not cause vasodilation or lower the blood pressure. The latter effect reflects the fact that norepinephrine constricts the blood vessels of skeletal muscle. Similar to epinephrine, norepinephrine causes hyperglycemia when given in large doses. Both norepinephrine and epinephrine are ineffective when given orally. Norepinephrine is rapidly inactivated by monoamine oxidase (MAO) and catechol-*O*-methyltransferase (COMT). It is never used in the treatment of asthma, nor is it used in combination with local anesthetics.

Isoproterenol

Isoproterenol (Isuprel) has a potent effect on all β receptors and almost no effect on α receptors. It is a powerful vasodilator. Intravenous infusion of isoproterenol lowers peripheral vascular resistance, particularly in skeletal muscle and renal vasculature, which results in increased cardiac output because of positive inotropic and chronotropic effects. While the diastolic pressure falls, the systolic blood pressure often remains unchanged. Isoproterenol is used to stimulate the heart in emergency situations.

Dopamine

Dopamine is often used as a vasopressor in patients with septic shock. At low doses (2 µg/kg/min), dopamine induces D_1-receptor–mediated, cyclic AMP–dependent vascular smooth muscle vasodilation. For this reason, a low-dose dopamine infusion is often used in patients with severe congestive heart failure (CHF). At doses of 1–5 µg/kg/min, dopamine increases renal blood flow and urine output. At higher doses (5–10 µg/kg/min), it improves mean arterial pressure (MAP) as well as heart contractility and rate, mainly by stimulating β_1 receptors. At much higher doses (greater than 15 µg/kg/min), this agent binds to α receptors and produces vasoconstriction, causing the blood pressure to rise.

Similar to norepinephrine, dopamine is a substrate for both MAO and COMT. As a result, it is ineffective when administered orally. In addition, dopamine stimulates the release of norepinephrine from nerve terminals, which subsequently contributes to dopamine's effects on the heart. Dopamine does not cross the blood–brain barrier (due to the presence of hydroxyl groups in the structure, see Figure 10.17), so injecting dopamine usually has no central effects. Due to its adrenergic effect and the stimulation of norepinephrine release, dopamine is used as an antidote in patients with beta-blocker overdose.

Dobutamine

Dobutamine (Dobutrex, from Canada) is a synthetic racemic catecholamine. It acts selectively on β_1 receptors and to some extent on β_2 receptors and vascular α_1 receptors. Its cardiac α_1 and β_1 actions significantly contribute to the positive inotropic activity of dobutamine without producing any changes in peripheral resistance. The positive inotropic effect is beneficial after cardiac surgery. Patients with cardiac decompensation can benefit from use of dobutamine as a short-term treatment. Because this agent has a rapid onset of action and a short half-time (2 minutes), the steady-state plasma dobutamine concentration (C_{pss}) is achieved in approximately 10 minutes once an infusion is started. As a result, dobutamine infusion does not require a loading dose (see the *Introduction to Pharmacokinetics* chapter for more information about the role of loading doses in C_{pss}).

Oxymetazoline

Oxymetazoline (Afrin) acts on α_1 and α_2 receptors and is used as a topical decongestant because of its ability to promote constriction of the nasal mucosa. In addition, it is used in ophthalmic drops (Visine) to relieve eye redness caused by swimming, cold, or contact lenses. Regardless of the route of drug administration, oxymetazoline can be absorbed into the systemic circulation and causes headache, nervousness, and insomnia.

Clonidine

Clonidine (Catapres) acts on central α_2 receptors and reduces blood pressure. Interestingly, when this drug is given orally, it is used for hypertension; when given as an infusion, however, it is helpful for hypotension. The intravenous infusion causes activation of postsynaptic α_2 receptors in vascular smooth muscle. The antihypertensive effect appears to result from activation of α_2 receptors in the lower brain stem region, which then decrease sympathetic outflow from the CNS. Clonidine is effective for smoking cessation, heroin withdrawal, ethanol dependency, prophylaxis of migraines, and attention-deficit/hyperactivity disorder (ADHD) in children, although its official indication is for hypertension. An abrupt discontinuation of clonidine can result in agitation, headache, nervousness, and tremor. Immediate-release clonidine is not equivalent to extended-release clonidine on a dose:dose ratio basis because of the formulations' different pharmacokinetic profiles (the extended-release dosage form requires lower doses).

Phenylephrine

Phenylephrine (Sudafed PE Nasal Decongestant) is a selective α_1 receptor agonist (with no β activity). It has a rapid onset and short duration of action. Because it does not produce tachycardia, it is a useful clinical agent when tachycardia limits the use of other vasopressors. Phenylephrine is not a catecholamine, therefore it is not a target for COMT enzyme (**Figure 10.19**). Because it produces vasoconstriction, it is useful as a nasal decongestant. Large doses of phenylephrine activate β receptors and can cause headache and cardiac irregularities. Although phenylephrine can be found in many OTC products, in some U.S. states (such as Oregon), it is classified as a controlled substance (class IV).

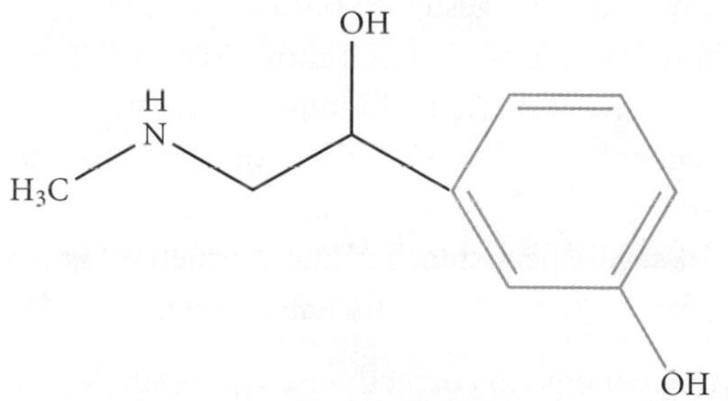

Figure 10.19 Structure of phenylephrine. Because of a lack of a second hydroxyl next to the hydroxyl group, phenylephrine is not considered a catecholamine.

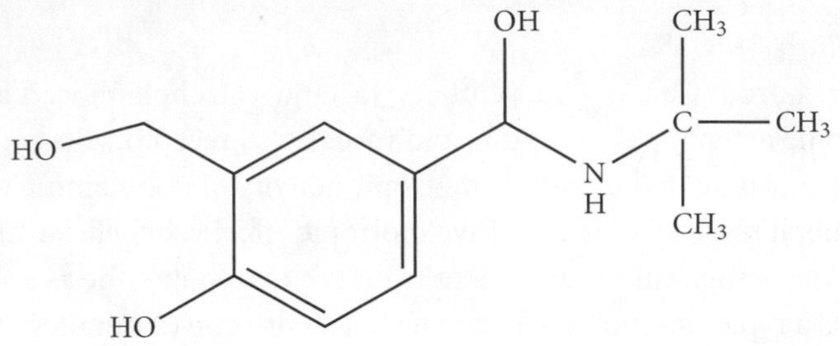

Figure 10.20 Structure of (*R*)-albuterol. Albuterol is a racemic mixture. While (*R*)-albuterol causes bronchodilation, (*S*)-albuterol has no therapeutic effect.

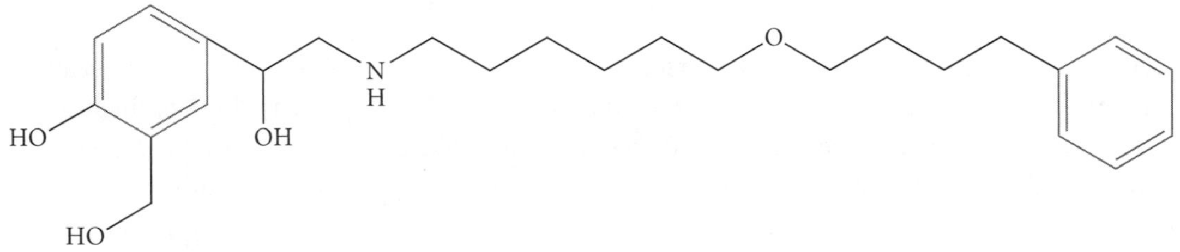

Figure 10.21 Structure of salmeterol. Salmeterol is highly lipophilic due to its long hydrocarbon chain attached to aromatic rings.

Albuterol

Albuterol (Proventil HFA) is a short-acting β_2 agonist (its duration of action is 4–6 hours). In patients with asthma, this agent may be used in a metered-dose inhaler (MDI), with a recommended dose of 2 puffs every 4–6 hours as needed. Albuterol is available as both oral and inhaled formulations. It is a racemic mixture. While (*R*)-albuterol causes bronchodilation, (*S*)-albuterol has no therapeutic effect (**Figure 10.20**). In contrast, levalbuterol is not a racemic mixture and contains only (*R*)-albuterol (see also the *Introduction to Medicinal Chemistry* chapter). One of the major side effects for albuterol is tremor; however, often patients develop tolerance to this side effect.

Salmeterol

Salmeterol (Serevent) is a selective and long-acting β_2 receptor agonist. It is dosed every 12 hours (ideally in the morning and the evening and, in contrast to albuterol, definitely not on an "as needed" basis), should not be used more than twice daily, and provides sustained bronchodilation. Salmeterol is highly lipophilic (**Figure 10.21**) and has been suggested to bind firmly to β_2 receptors, which could explain its long duration of action. It is as effective as ipratropium and is known to be much more selective (at least 50 times) for β_2 receptors than albuterol. In contrast to albuterol, salmeterol's onset of action is slow; thus this agent is not recommended for acute relief of asthmatic symptoms. A combination (Advair Diskus) of salmeterol and an inhaled corticosteroid (fluticasone) has helped many patients with moderate or severe persistent asthma. Salmeterol is useful for patients with frequent and persistent symptoms, particularly nocturnal asthma.

With both albuterol and salmeterol inhalers, educating patients to correctly use those inhalers is critical to achieve the maximum benefit. In particular, patients should know when they should use the quick-acting formulation (albuterol) versus the long-acting formulation (salmeterol).

Indirect-Acting Agonists

Indirect-acting agonists increase the available amount of epinephrine or norepinephrine to stimulate adrenergic receptors. Consequently, two mechanisms of action may be involved:

- Releasing or displacing stored norepinephrine from sympathetic neurons (examples include amphetamine and tyramine, although tyramine is not a clinically useful agent)
- Blocking the reuptake of norepinephrine into sympathetic neurons through blockage of Na^+/K^+-activated ATPase (e.g., cocaine)

Mixed-Action Adrenergic Agonists

The role of these agents is to increase the release of norepinephrine from the presynaptic terminals and to activate adrenergic receptors.

Ephedrine

Ephedrine is a potent CNS stimulant, acts as an agonist at both α and β receptors, as well as stimulates the release of norepinephrine from presynaptic terminals. Despite extensive similarity between epinephrine and ephedrine, ephedrine is not a catechol (**Figure 10.22**). Therefore, ephedrine is not subject to COMT metabolism and can be taken orally. Ephedrine stimulates heart rate and cardiac output and increases peripheral resistance; the latter effect leads to an increase in blood pressure. This agent stimulates the receptors of smooth muscle cells in the bladder, which increases the resistance of the urine outflow (i.e., it causes obstruction in urination). It also stimulates receptors in the lungs and promotes bronchodilation. Ephedrine is used for nasal congestion and to increase the lowered blood pressure caused by anesthesia (anesthesia-induced hypotension).

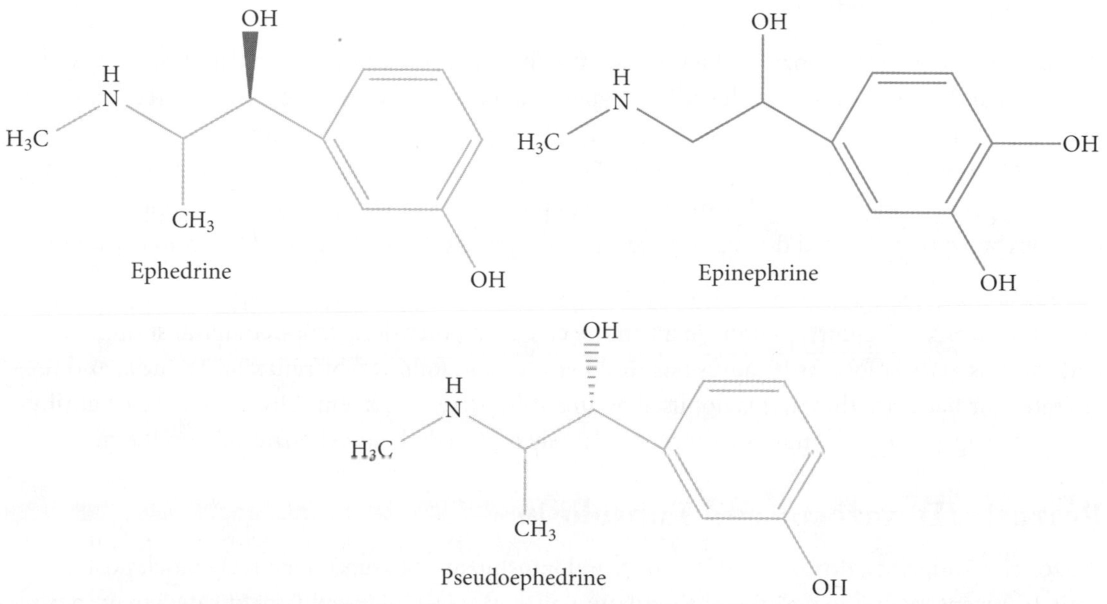

Figure 10.22 Structures of ephedrine, pseudoephedrine, and epinephrine. While epinephrine is a catecholamine, ephedrine and pseudoephedrine are not.

Pseudoephedrine

Pseudoephedrine (SudoGest and Sudafed) is the D-isomer of ephedrine and produces 25% of the effect exerted by ephedrine. It is clinically used to treat nasal decongestion. Pseudoephedrine can be chemically converted to methamphetamine; for this reason, the drug must be sold behind the counter, and in some states (e.g., Oregon) it is a class IV controlled substance drug that requires a prescription to be dispensed. Prior to the implementation of such restrictive policies, pseudo-ephedrine was the most frequently used systemic decongestant. It is a safe nasal decongestant. Doses as high as 180 mg have not been shown to produce any measurable changes in blood pressure or heart rate.

Adrenergic Antagonists

Adrenergic antagonists inhibit the interactions of norepinephrine, epinephrine, and other sympathomimetic drugs with their receptors. Except for phenoxybenzamine (Dibenzyline; see also the *Introduction to Pharmacodynamics* chapter), which is an irreversible antagonist, all of these agents are competitive antagonists. Recognition of the role of adrenergic receptors in the cardiovascular system has encouraged many pharmaceutical companies to synthesize compounds that produce profound effects on the sympathetically innervated organs. Due to the structural differences among the various adrenergic antagonists, they have different affinities and selectivity for the adrenergic receptors. For instance, while a selective β_1 blocker blocks most actions of epinephrine and norepinephrine on the heart, it does not produce an effect on β_2 receptors, which are mainly found in the bronchial smooth muscle.

Alpha-Adrenergic Antagonists

The therapeutic agents in this category reduce elevated blood pressure. As stated earlier, α_1 receptors mediate contraction of arterial, venous, and visceral smooth muscle, whereas α_2 receptors mediate sympathetic output, platelet aggregation, and contraction of some arteries and veins.

Phenoxybenzamine

Phenoxybenzamine (Dibenzyline) is a noncompetitive (irreversible) antagonist of both α_1 and α_2 receptors and is used to reduce the risk of hypertension from excessive release of catecholamines from the adrenal tumor (pheochromocytoma). Pheochromocytoma is a tumor of the adrenal medulla that releases a high concentration of catecholamines into the circulation. Consequently, severe hypertension occurs. While in most cases pheochromocytoma is treated surgically, phenoxybenzamine is used during the presurgical period (10 mg, twice daily, 1–3 weeks before surgery).

By blocking α receptors, phenoxybenzamine causes hypotension, produces nasal stuffiness, and inhibits ejaculation. As it causes postural hypotension followed by reflex tachycardia and precipitates cardiac arrhythmia, it is not used as an antihypertensive agent. More-selective α_1 antihypertensive agents (see the next section) have largely replaced phenoxybenzamine on the market.

Prazosin, Doxazosin, and Tamsulosin

Prazosin (Minipress), doxazosin (Cardura), and tamsulosin (Flomax) selectively block postsynaptic α_1 receptors. In the peripheral vasculature, they also inhibit the uptake of catecholamines in smooth muscle cells, which causes vasodilation and reduces blood pressure. Of note, tamsulosin has the least antihypertensive effect. Because sympathetic neurons stimulate the contraction of trigone and the sphincter, these agents (particularly tamsulosin) are useful in the treatment of obstructive bladder. They block postsynaptic α_1 receptors, thereby relaxing the smooth muscle of the bladder and decreasing the resistance to urinary outflow. The α_1 receptor blockers are often used in addition to other first-line antihypertensive agents.

A serious adverse effect of α_1 blockers is the "first dose" effect, which may consist of transient faintness, palpitations, orthostatic hypotension, and syncope shortly (1–3 hours) after the patient takes the first dose. However, if the patient takes a dose as low as one-third of the normal dose at bedtime, the most serious adverse effect, syncope, can be significantly reduced. There is a risk of fall when these agents are used on a chronic basis. Moreover, these agents cross the blood–brain barrier, and cause depression.

Beta-Adrenergic Antagonists

Beta blockers are not first-line agents for reducing blood pressure; rather, they are often added to thiazide-type diuretics to lower the blood pressure. Indeed, in patients with hypertension but without any compelling indications, thiazide-type diuretics, angiotensin-converting enzyme (ACE) inhibitors, angiotensin-receptor blockers (ARBs), and calcium-channel blockers (CCBs) are used as the initial first-line agents. However, in post-MI patients and patients with coronary artery disease, beta blockers are the first-line agents. While the various beta blockers have different pharmacodynamic properties, they all provide a similar degree of blood pressure lowering effect. The names of all beta blockers, except labetalol and carvedilol, end with -*olol*. Unlike α-receptor blockers, beta blockers usually do not cause sexual dysfunction.

Nonselective Beta Blockers

Propranolol

Propranolol (Inderal LA) is a hydrophobic molecule that is completely absorbed after oral administration. However, because of its high hepatic metabolism during its first passage through the liver, only approximately 25% of an oral dose reaches the systemic circulation. Doses of 40–80 mg/day are used for the treatment of hypertension and angina, although the full antihypertensive effect may not be achieved for several weeks. In addition, propranolol is used for supraventricular arrhythmias/tachycardias and ventricular arrhythmias/tachycardias, myocardial infarction, pheochromocytoma, prophylaxis for migraine, and tremor. It is also used on an "off-label" basis to treat anxiety. Patients with asthma or COPD may develop respiratory crisis if they use propranolol because of its nonselective β_2 receptor blocking activity. Propranolol is also administered intravenously (1–3 mg) to treat life-threatening arrhythmias, albeit with careful monitoring of blood pressure and cardiac function.

In hyperthyroidism, propranolol is useful to protect patients from cardiac arrhythmias. It is not clearly understood why patients with hyperthyroidism are sensitive to adrenergic agents, but one hypothesis is that these patients have more adrenergic receptors than healthy individuals. As a result, propranolol is often given to patients with hyperthyroidism even during pregnancy (its pregnancy risk factor is Category C).

Timolol and Nadolol

Oral timolol (Apo-Timol, from Canada) is well absorbed from the GI tract, but it undergoes extensive first-pass metabolism in the liver. Timolol is used to reduce blood pressure, CHF, and for migraine prophylaxis. In ophthalmology, timolol reduces aqueous humor production in the eyes.

Nadolol (Corgard) is a long-acting beta blocker that is used to treat hypertension and angina pectoris. In unlabeled indications, it is used for migraine prophylaxis and to treat tremors in Parkinson's disease.

Selective Beta Blockers

Atenolol, Metoprolol, and Esmolol

Atenolol (Tenormin), metoprolol (Lopressor), and esmolol (Brevibloc) are β_1-selective blockers; they are also called cardioselective blockers because they do not block β_2 receptors, do not provoke bronchospasm, and do not decrease glycogenolysis. For all these reasons, β_1-selective blockers are

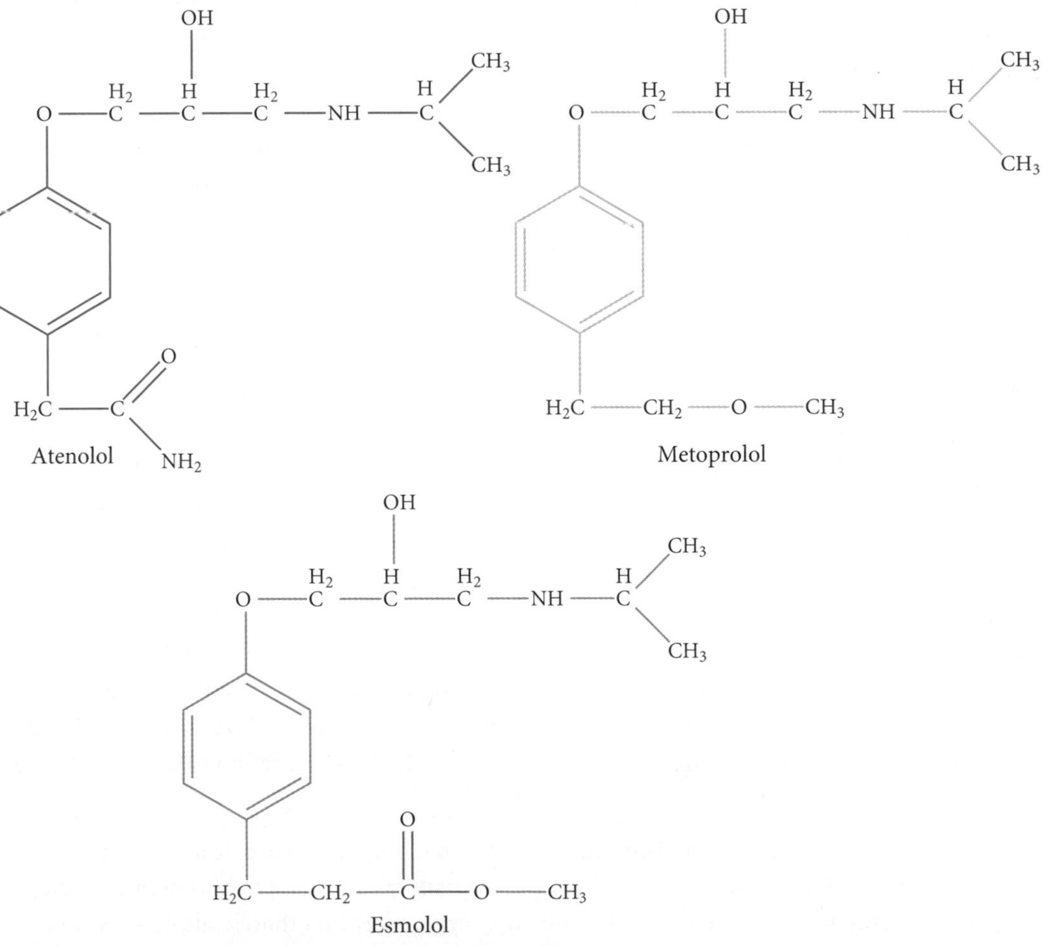

Figure 10.23 Structures of atenolol, metoprolol, and esmolol. Atenolol is the least hydrophobic compound and cannot readily cross the blood–brain barrier. Esmolol, due to presence of an ester group, is prone to hydrolysis.

safer options than nonselective agents to treat patients with asthma or diabetes. However, they may exacerbate asthma when their selectivity is lost (which occurs at high doses).

Atenolol is the least hydrophobic member of this class. The dose of atenolol may need to be adjusted (reduced) in patients with chronic kidney disease. However, atenolol is more hydrophilic than other beta blockers, and does not readily cross the blood–brain barrier. Due to its hydrophilic nature, side effects such as dizziness or drowsiness, which are often seen with other beta blockers, are not observed with atenolol (**Figure 10.23**).

Metoprolol undergoes extensive first-pass metabolism. This agent is often used to treat essential hypertension, angina pectoris, tachycardia, and heart failure, and for migraine prophylaxis. While oral metoprolol has almost full absorption, due to its high first-pass effect (particularly in conjunction with hepatic CYP2D6), its bioavailability is low (approximately 40%). Pharmacogenomics may play an important role in the metabolism of metoprolol. Patients who are poor CYP2D6 metabolizers appear to be at a higher risk (as high as 5 times higher) to experience metoprolol's adverse effects compared with patients who have a normal metabolic profile. Metoprolol tartrate (Lopressor) is an immediate-release dosage form (short acting; its half-life is approximately 6 hours depending on CYP2D6 metabolism) that can be given 2–4 times daily for the treatment of hypertension; metoprolol succinate (Toprol-XL) is an extended-release form (long acting) that is dosed only once per day for the treatment of both hypertension and heart failure.

Esmolol, because of its inclusion of an ester group, is prone to hydrolysis and, therefore, has a short duration of action (Figure 10.23). This agent is used intravenously and often during surgery.

Because these drugs have less effect on β_2 receptors in peripheral vascular tissues, another common side effect of beta blockers, like the coldness of extremities, is rarely seen with β_1-selective blockers.

Nonselective α and β Receptor Blockers

Labetalol and Carvedilol

Labetalol (Trandate) is a racemic mixture that has the potential to block both α and β receptors. Both oral and parenteral dosage forms (the full effect is seen within 2–5 minutes after injection) are available to treat chronic hypertension and hypertensive emergency, respectively. Because labetalol is a hydrophilic drug, it can be used in a pregnancy-induced hypertensive crisis—it has minimal placental transfer (recall from the *Introduction to Pharmacokinetics* chapter that hydrophobic drugs readily cross the placenta, so that ionized or water-soluble drugs are preferred for pregnant women).

Similar to labetalol, carvedilol (Coreg) blocks α_1 and β receptors. In addition, carvedilol has antioxidant and anti-inflammatory effects. The antioxidant effect is due to its ability to bind reactive oxygen species (ROS) and/or reduce the biosynthesis of ROS. Carvedilol is often used for hypertension, CHF, and left ventricular dysfunction following an MI. In contrast to labetalol, it is a very hydrophobic agent and, as a result, it is able to protect cell membranes from lipid peroxidation. Interestingly, carvedilol, when given at high doses, acts similar to calcium-channel blockers. Carvedilol has been effective in reducing mortality and morbidity in patients with mild to severe CHF.

Table 10.3 summarizes the selective and nonselective β-adrenergic blockers.

Table 10.3 A Summary of Selective and Nonselective β-Adrenergic Blockers

Beta Blocker	Blocked Receptor	Pharmacological Effect
Propranolol	β_1 and β_2	↓Blood pressure (BP) ↓Migraine ↓Angina pectoris ↓Symptoms of hyperthyroidism ↓MI ↓Tremors ↑Bronchospasm ↓Glycogenolysis
Timolol	β_1 and β_2	↓BP ↓Glaucoma ↓Migraine ↓CHF ↑Bronchospasm
Nadolol	β_1 and β_2	↓BP ↓Angina pectoris ↓Tremors ↑Bronchospasm
Atenolol, metoprolol, and esmolol	β_1	↓BP
Labetalol	α_1, β_1, and β_2	↓BP ↓CHF
Carvedilol	α_1, β_1, and β_2	↓BP ↓CHF ↓ROS ↓Inflammation

Neurodegenerative Diseases

Two unique characteristics of neurodegenerative diseases are continuous progression and irreversible loss of neurons. Widely prevalent neurodegenerative disorders include Parkinson's disease (PD), Alzheimer's disease (AD), and multiple sclerosis (MS). Of these disease states, the first two conditions are common in the geriatric population. While PD is observed in approximately 1% of patients more than 65 years old, AD has much higher prevalence (10%). The available medications for both PD and AD reduce disease symptoms but are ineffective in producing a permanent and reversible cure. In this section, enzymes and receptors of PD and AD targeted by drugs are briefly discussed.

- Amino acid decarboxylase is present in all tissues. This soluble enzyme requires pyridoxal phosphate (PLP) as a cofactor to catalyze the removal of a carboxylic group from aromatic amino acids (see also the *Introduction to Nutrients* chapter). It catalyzes the conversion of L-dopa to dopamine and 5-hydroxytryptophan to serotonin.

- Monoamine oxidase A (MAO-A) metabolizes norepinephrine and serotonin into inactive compounds. It is present in low concentrations in the brain and in high concentrations in the placenta, intestine, and liver.

- Monoamine oxidase B (MAO-B) metabolizes phenylethylamine (a biogenic amine that is deficient or minimally present in patients with attention-deficit/hyperactivity disorder). This enzyme is present in high concentrations in the basal ganglia and platelets, in low concentrations in the intestine, and in trace amount amount in the placenta.

- Both MAO-A and MAO-B isoforms metabolize, albeit to different extents, monoamine neurotransmitters (dopamine, epinephrine, norepinephrine, serotonin, and tyramine). In neuronal cells, both isoforms are tightly bound to the outer membrane of the mitochondria. MAOs are not present in erythrocytes because these cells lack mitochondria. Concurrent use of MAO inhibitors (MAOIs) such as levodopa, amphetamines, cocaine, and CNS antidepressants can result in serious adverse effects.

- The catechol-*O*-methyltransferase (COMT) enzyme is expressed in the liver but its main function is in the CNS. COMT metabolizes catecholamines by transferring a methyl group to a hydroxyl group of the catecholamine. For example, metabolism of L-dopa to the inactive compound 3-*O*-methyldopa is catalyzed by COMT.

- Glutamate is a major excitatory amino acid in the CNS. It has been suggested that overstimulation of various glutamate receptors causes neuronal cell death. Glutamate has also been suggested to play a role in the pathogenesis of Alzheimer's disease. Magnesium is important for the release of acetylcholine (see the *Introduction to Nutrients* chapter), and overstimulation of glutamate receptors prevents magnesium from entering the cholinergic neurons.

Parkinson's Disease

Parkinson's disease is characterized by the presence of tremor at rest, rigidity, bradykinesia (slowness of movement), and impaired postural stability (instability of balance). As many as 1 million individuals in the United States have PD. The approximate prevalence of PD is 10 per 100,000 persons who are 50–59 years of age and 120 per 100,000 persons who are 80–89 years of age. There is a 2:1 ratio of male-to-female patients who develop PD.

Although the cause of PD is not fully understood, there is a strong connection between degeneration of dopaminergic neurons in the substantia nigra and this disease. In addition, degenerative changes occur in the autonomic ganglia, basal ganglia, spinal cord, and neocortex, involving a variety of neurotransmitters and neuromodulators. Neurotransmitters and neuromodulators affected include acetylcholine, adenosine (which binds to its receptors to change the intercellular levels of second messengers such as cAMP and diacylglycerol), enkephalins (morphine-like endogenous pentapeptides found in the CNS that reduce pain impulses), GABA (an inhibitory neurotransmitter), glutamate, serotonin, and substance P.

Both genetic and environmental factors play roles in the development of PD. For instance, more than 10 genetic mutations are associated with PD. Chronic exposure to pesticides, carbon disulfide, carbon monoxide, and heavy metals (iron and manganese) as well as repeated head trauma can contribute to PD. In addition, drugs such as metoclopramide (Reglan), reserpine, and tetrabenazine (Xenazine) can cause Parkinson-like symptoms. However, upon discontinuation of the triggering medications, these symptoms resolve.

Therapeutic agents used to treat PD can help improve motor (physical movement) and nonmotor (cognitive impairment, depression, fatigue, and sleep disorders) symptoms of patients and help them maintain their day-to-day physical activities. Both pharmacological and nonpharmacological (walking devices, education, exercise, nutrition) treatments are important to consider when treating a patient with PD. The following agents are used in the treatment of PD.

Levodopa plus Carbidopa

In the neurons, levodopa (also known as L-dopa) is synthesized from tyrosine and is subsequently converted to dopamine (recall from Figure 10.17). Levodopa in combination with carbidopa, a peripherally acting agent that inhibits amino acid decarboxylase, work effectively to provide dopamine in the treatment of PD (**Figure 10.24**). The effects of levodopa can be prolonged when added to a COMT or an MAO-B inhibitor. While levodopa crosses the blood–brain barrier, carbidopa does not. The combination of levodopa with carbidopa prevents peripheral levodopa from being converted to dopamine and allows levodopa to be transported into the brain. The combination of these two drugs (which is known as Sinemet)

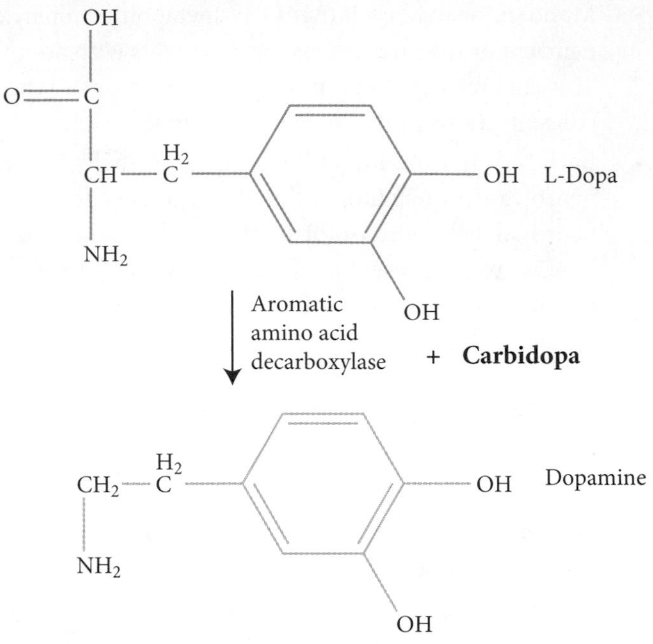

Figure 10.24 The role of carbidopa is to block the peripheral metabolism of levodopa to dopamine by inhibiting an enzyme, the amino acid decarboxylase.

reduces levodopa's peripheral side effects, such as nausea. The newly synthesized dopamine is stored in the presynaptic neurons until it is released to bind to postsynaptic D_1 and D_2 receptors. The dopamine activity is terminated in the neuron via a reuptake by a dopamine transporter. MAO and COMT enzymes are known to metabolize dopamine as well.

In patients with PD, an initial dose of 300 mg/day L-dopa and a dose of 75 mg/day carbidopa are required to provide adequate dopamine in the CNS and inhibit the peripheral activity of L-amino acid decarboxylase, respectively. A complication associated with the chronic use of levodopa is "wearing off" (motor fluctuations) and dyskinesias (involuntary movements of the face, neck, trunk, and extremities); these symptoms can arise as early as 5 to 6 months after starting levodopa therapy. If a patient presents with complaints of "shakiness," it is important to identify whether this effect is caused by a disease-associated tremor or by drug-associated dyskinesia. Levodopa-induced "wearing off" is caused by the increasing loss of neuronal storage of dopamine and the short half-life of levodopa. Another complication of levodopa is "freezing," characterized by a sudden and episodic inhibition of lower-extremity motor function and an increased risk of falls. Patients often complain of having difficulty initiating steps (a feeling of having their feet stuck to the floor). Physical therapy, along with supporting walking devices, are helpful for these patients.

Selegiline

Selegiline (Eldepryl) is a selective MAO-B inhibitor and a weak MAO-A inhibitor. Selegiline extends levodopa's effects; its oral dose is 5 mg, twice daily. Selegiline undergoes first-pass hepatic metabolism and produces L-methamphetamine and L-amphetamine as metabolites. As a result, side effects such as hypertension, tachycardia, diarrhea, insomnia, hallucinations, and jitteriness are common with the use of this medication. To avoid the first-pass metabolism, an orally disintegrating tablet formulation is available that relies on transmucosal absorption. Selegiline is also available as a transdermal dosage form (Emsam), although this version is not indicated for PD, but rather is used for the treatment of major depressive disorder in adults.

Rasagiline (Azilect) is another MAO-B selective inhibitor that is used to treat Parkinson's disease. This drug is not metabolized to amphetamine by-products.

Withdrawal symptoms of selegiline, which occur 24–72 hours after discontinuation, can be severe. Typical withdrawal symptoms include nausea, vomiting, agitation, psychosis, and convulsions. Treatment of withdrawal is usually supportive and may involve a benzodiazepine such as diazepam (Diastat).

Learning Bridge 10.1

AK is a 60-year-old male who was recently diagnosed with an early-stage Parkinson's disease. He has no previous drug allergies. He occasionally uses OTC products for nasal decongestion and sinus problems. For his Parkinson's problem, the neurologist has prescribed selegiline, 5 mg BID.

A. Based on your knowledge of drug interactions of MAOIs, which drugs and food items should you counsel AK about?

B. When should AK take the last dose of selegiline every day?

Entacapone

The COMT enzyme inactivates levodopa in the peripheral tissues. Entacapone (Comtan) selectively inhibits COMT in the periphery, which increases the half-life of levodopa (**Figure 10.25**). The increased concentration of levodopa moves across the blood–brain barrier and reaches the brain. In the brain, levodopa is converted to dopamine. A dose of 200 mg entacapone needs to be given with each dose of carbidopa/levodopa. There is risk of dopaminergic adverse effects, although these effects may be managed by reducing the carbidopa/levodopa dosage. Use of entacapone can cause brownish-orange salivary and urinary discoloration (because a large amount of

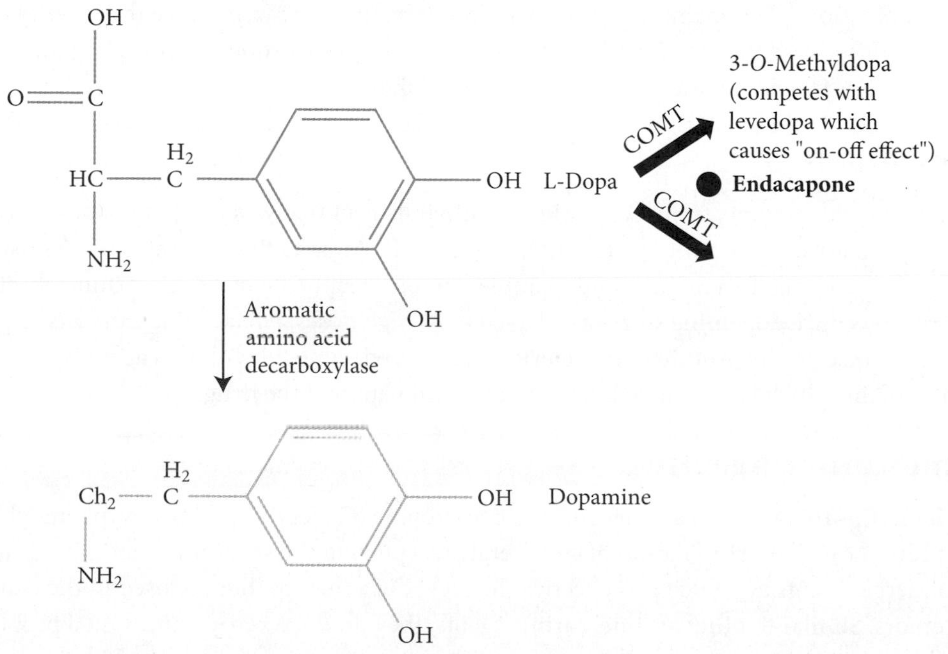

Figure 10.25 Entacapone blocks the metabolism of levodopa so as to increase the concentration of levodopa.

levodopa is converted to melanin, a pigment molecule), so it is important to counsel patients about this harmless effect to increase medication compliance.

A combination of carbidopa–levodopa–entacapone (1:4 carbidopa:levodopa and 200 mg entacapone, collectively known as Stalevo) is available for the treatment of PD. Currently, the FDA is investigating a possible increased risk of cardiovascular events and prostate cancer associated with the use of Stalevo.

Dopamine Agonists

There are two categories of dopamine agonists: ergot-derived and nonergot agonists.

Ergot-Derived Agonists

Bromocriptine (Cycloset) is a typical ergot derivative that activates dopaminergic receptors. Dyskinesia is observed less often with this agent, but the drug produces other severe adverse effects (hallucination, nausea, confusion, lower-extremity edema). Its use is contraindicated in patients with psychiatric illnesses.

Nonergot Agonists

Pramipexole (Mirapex) and ropinirole (Requip) are FDA-approved nonergot dopamine agonists. The nonergot agonists produce fewer adverse effects than the ergot-derived agonists. They can also be used as adjuncts to levodopa therapy in patients with motor fluctuations. Because the risk that younger patients with PD will develop motor complications is high, dopamine agonists are preferred over levodopa. In contrast, because older patients who take dopamine agonists are more likely to develop hallucinations, confusion, and orthostatic hypotension, these patients tend to benefit more from carbidopa/levodopa therapy.

Other nonergot agonists include apomorphine (Apokyn, available only as an injection) and a new agent, rotigotine (Neupro, available as a transdermal patch). Apomorphine is a potent emetic, so an antiemetic should be prescribed whenever this drug is used.

The combination of a dopamine agonist with levodopa therapy can increase the severity of levodopa-induced dyskinesias. Therefore, patients should receive properly counseling on this risk, this is important for those patients with preexisting dyskinesias.

Amantadine

Amantadine (Endantadine, from Canada) is an antiviral agent that was used in the past to treat influenza infections. It has remarkable activity against PD. Amantadine increases the release of dopamine by blocking the reuptake of dopamine into presynaptic neurons. Unfortunately, it loses its effectiveness once dopamine stores are depleted. At high doses, amantadine can cause significant CNS adverse effects. Another characteristic adverse effect noted with this agent is bluish mottling in the skin, which is reversible following discontinuation of the drug.

Antimuscarinic Agents

Examples in this therapeutic category include benztropine (Cogentin) and trihexyphenidyl. These agents prevent excessive stimulation of cholinergic receptors in the striatum. Centrally acting anticholinergic agents are much less effective than levodopa therapy, but are used in the control of mild tremors. Similar to other antimuscarinic agents, they produce xerostomia, visual problems, mood changes, and confusion as adverse effects. These agents are contraindicated in patients with glaucoma, GI obstruction, and benign prostatic hyperplasia (BPH).

Alzheimer's Disease

Alzheimer's disease is the most prevalent type of neurodegenerative disease in patients who are 65 years or older. Patients with AD exhibit the cardinal symptom of difficulty in remembering recent events. As the disease progresses, patients experience confusion, irritability, trouble with speaking, and long-term memory loss and ultimately death. While the disease's cause is not fully understood, it is believed that AD is associated with formation of β-amyloid senile plaques and neurofibrillary tangles in the brain as well as degeneration of cholinergic neurons of the CNS.

The therapy for AD is to moderately assist patients with their daily life activities, as none of the agents available can restore their memory loss. The loss of their memory often causes significant social, psychological, and physical burdens, and may create economic challenges for family members or the patient's caregivers. The primary goal is to treat cognitive difficulties and then to treat psychiatric consequences. As mentioned earlier, none of the therapeutic agents available on the market can prolong life or cure AD. Two major classes of drugs can help AD patients to a moderate extent.

AchE Inhibitors

AchE inhibitors improve cholinergic transmission in AD patients. These agents include donepezil (Aricept), galantamine (Razadyne), and rivastigmine (Exelon). While donepezil and galantamine are competitive inhibitors of AchE, rivastigmine inhibits both AchE and plasma cholinesterase. Rivastigmine use is not associated with any drug interaction, as this agent is not a substrate or inhibitor of CYP-450 enzymes; however, the other two agents mentioned are substrates for these enzymes. Adverse effects associated with all three AchE inhibitors include nausea, vomiting, and diarrhea; these effects are more significant with rivastigmine.

NMDA-Receptor Antagonists

N-methyl-D-aspartate (NMDA) is an ionotropic receptor of glutamate, an amino acid neurotransmitter. Memantine (Namenda) is an antagonist of NMDA receptors in the brain, thereby blocking glutamatergic neurotransmission. Glutamate is an excitatory neurotransmitter that, in excess, affects cognitive function of learning and memory. By blocking NMDA receptors of the brain, excitatory neurotoxicity can be reduced, along with providing neuronal protection.

Memantine is indicated for use in patients with moderate to severe AD. There is no concrete evidence that use of memantine, in combination with AchE inhibitors, provides any additional therapeutic benefit. Favorable pharmacokinetic properties of this drug include 100% oral bioavailability regardless of administration with or without food, low protein binding, and minimal metabolism.

Because depression is quite common in patients with AD (affecting 50% of these individuals), treatment with selective serotonin reuptake inhibitors (SSRIs) may be necessary. Sertraline (Zoloft) and citalopram (Celexa) are often used to treat depression in AD patients.

Multiple Sclerosis

Multiple sclerosis is characterized by demyelination and axonal damage. The condition is inflammatory and autoimmune in nature. MS depletes the myelin sheath (**Figure 10.26**) surrounding CNS axons (i.e., a lipoidal multilayered sheath that wraps around the axon)—an effect that is often caused by penetration of T and B lymphocytes, macrophages, reactive oxygen species, antibodies, and the complement system. Demyelination renders axons susceptible to irreversible damage. MS occurs more frequently in females (1 in 200 women) than in males in the United States and usually is diagnosed in persons between 15 and 45 years of age. The cause of MS is not understood yet, and currently there is no cure for this disease.

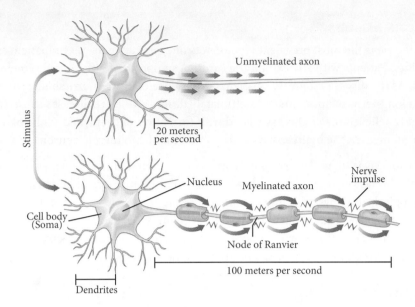

Figure 10.26 The architecture of a neuron. The role of the myelin sheath is to protect the axon and allows faster conduction of action potentials between naked axons.

Treatments for MS are organized into two categories:

- *Symptomatic Therapy:* This treatment is very important to maintain the patient's quality of life. In the case of acute attacks, the standard therapy is an intravenous injection of corticosteroids, particularly high doses of methylprednisolone (Medrol); if methylprednisolone is not available, dexamethasone (Baycadro) can be administered. In addition, high oral doses of methylprednisolone have been shown to be effective in treating acute attacks. Because steroids increase glycogenolysis (see also the *Introduction to Biochemistry* chapter), patients with diabetes mellitus may develop hyperglycemia as a result of such therapy and may require insulin injections to overcome this metabolic adverse effect.

- Disease-Modifying Therapies (DMTs): This treatment is important to reduce the progressive disability experienced by MS patients over time. Interferon IFN-β_{1b} is an effective DMT agent. While its full mechanism of action has not yet been elucidated, it is believed that IFN-β_{1b} has immunomodulating properties that result from reducing IFN-γ secretion by activated lymphocytes or from suppressing T cells. IFN-β_{1a} is given intramuscularly at a dose of 30 µg , once a week. Fingolimod (Gilenya) is the first FDA-approved oral DMT for MS and has been shown to be effective for MS relapses. This sphingosine 1-phosphate receptor agonist sequesters circulating lymphocytes within secondary lymphoid organs and decreases the infiltration of T lymphocytes and macrophages into the CNS. Fingolimod is given daily at a dose of 0.5 mg. The FDA requires that a patient medication guide be provided to patients receiving fingolimod, because this agent's use is associated with bradycardia, increased risk of infections, and optic neuritis.

Anxiety Disorders, Hypnotics, and Depression

The two most frequently occurring mental disorders in clinical practices are depression and anxiety disorders, each of which affects approximately 10% of the adult U.S. population. While some agents are exclusively used to treat one set of disorders, others treat both. This may indicate that the biological principles behind both disorders are similar.

Anxiety Disorders

Anxiety is an adaptive response to stressful situations and is a transient process. It is often triggered by feelings related to either a real concern or a perceived threat that endangers the security of an individual. As an adaptive response, it allows the individual to react to environmental changes. If the anxiety becomes persistent, overwhelming, and affects daily functions, then it is termed anxiety disorders. Unfortunately, because healthcare providers often miss the diagnosis of anxiety disorder, only about one-fourth of patients with such disorders receive appropriate and adequate attention and treatment. Such clinical failure results in increased morbidity and mortality, as these patients may develop other complications such as cardiovascular, cerebrovascular, gastrointestinal, and respiratory disorders.

For healthcare providers, it is important to differentiate between short-term symptoms of anxiety and anxiety disorders. The former are characterized by temporary feelings of fear and can be alleviated by an anxiolytic agent such as a benzodiazepine for 2–3 weeks. By comparison, anxiety disorders need much more attention and treatment because they are linked to far more complex symptoms, such as generalized anxiety disorder, obsessive–compulsive disorder, panic disorder, post-traumatic stress disorder, separation anxiety disorder, social phobia, specific phobias, and acute stress.

This section summarizes the therapeutic agents used to treat anxiety disorders.

Benzodiazepines

Benzodiazepines are the most effective anxiolytic agents in terms of producing rapid relief of acute anxiety symptoms, and all agents in this category are equally effective. Because benzodiazepines are safe and effective, they have replaced earlier-generation anxiolytic agents such as barbiturates. Benzodiazepine therapy does not produce physical dependency during short-term use, so these drugs are safe to use in short-term anxiety disorders.

Benzodiazepines interact with receptors that are directly activated by a major inhibitory neurotransmitter, gamma-aminobutyric acid (GABA). The $GABA_A$ receptors are part of the ligand-gated ion channel signal transduction pathway (see also the *Introduction to Pharmacodynamics* chapter) and have five subunits (two α, two β, and one γ) that form an integral chloride channel. The binding of GABA results in an influx of Cl^- ions, which in turn leads to hyperpolarization of the neuronal cell. This condition makes it more difficult for the cell to depolarize, and subsequently reduces neural excitability. Benzodiazepines enhance the inhibitory effect of GABA by increasing the frequency of Cl^- ion influx into neuronal cells through the $GABA_A$ receptors. The benzodiazepines serve as positive modulators of $GABA_A$ receptors by binding directly to a specific site on the $GABA_A$ receptor distant from the binding site of GABA.

Benzodiazepines are highly hydrophobic drugs (albeit to varying extents), and all of these agents, except clorazepate (Tranxene), are absorbed completely by the oral route. Benzodiazepines are effective in reducing anxiety (social anxiety, performance anxiety, post-traumatic stress, obsessive–compulsive disorder, and phobias), and they produce hypnotic, anticonvulsive, and muscle-relaxing effects. When administered alone, these drugs, even at high doses, do not produce surgical anesthesia, coma, or death.

Benzodiazepines are metabolized extensively by CYP3A4 and CYP2C19. As a result, metabolism of these agents is affected by inhibitors of CYP3A4 (e.g., erythromycin, clarithromycin, ritonavir, itraconazole, ketoconazole). However, oxazepam (Oxpam, from Canada) and lorazepam (Ativan) are conjugated directly and not dependent on CYP3A4 and CYP2C19. Benzodiazepines are classified as controlled substances (Schedule IV).

Benzodiazepines are divided into three categories based on their elimination half-life:

- Short-acting agents ($t_{1/2} < 3$–8 hours) include oxazepam and triazolam (Halcion).
- Intermediate-acting agents ($t_{1/2} = 10$–20 hours) include alprazolam (Xanax), estazolam, lorazepam (Ativan), and temazepam (Restoril).
- Long-acting agents ($t_{1/2} > 24$ hours) include clorazepate (Tranxene), flurazepam (Apo-Flurazepam, from Canada), diazepam (Valium), and quazepam (Doral). These agents should be used only with caution in geriatric patients, as their prolonged effect can cause falls, leading to hip fracture.

Due to their wide range of lipid solubilities, benzodiazepines have different rates of plasma albumin binding, ranging from approximately 70% for alprazolam (less hydrophobic) to nearly 99% for diazepam (hydrophobic). Because of diazepam's high lipid solubility (which also explains why it has such a long $t_{1/2}$), this drug undergoes rapid absorption and distribution (30 minutes) into the CNS.

Buspirone

Buspirone (BuSpar, from Canada) is a mild anxiolytic and is not as effective as benzodiazepines for acute or short-term therapy. However, unlike benzodiazepines, it is devoid of anticonvulsant, muscle relaxant, hypnotic, and dependence properties (it does not bind to the $GABA_A$ receptor to any significant extent). Buspirone does not produce any motor or cognitive impairment, nor does it potentiate the CNS depression effect of alcohol.

Buspirone acts as a partial agonist at 5-HT_{1A} serotonin receptors. It is used as a second-line agent for anxiety disorder because of its delayed onset of effect (more than 1 week). Therefore, it is important to counsel patients who are prescribed buspirone about when to expect the desired effects to occur. Buspirone is absorbed rapidly and completely, but it undergoes extensive first-pass metabolism (the elimination half-life is 2.5 hours); as a result, it must be given 2 to 3 times daily. Its adverse effects include dizziness, fatigue, skin rash, tachycardia, and headaches.

Barbiturates

In the past, barbiturates were used extensively as sedative agents, but they have now been largely replaced by benzodiazepines. They interact with $GABA_A$ receptors by binding at a distinct barbiturate binding site and potentiate GABA-mediated responses. Barbiturates prolong the duration of opening of Cl^- channels, which results in more influx of Cl^- ions into neuronal cells. Conversely, the anesthetic effect of barbiturates results from blocking of Na^+ channels. Compared with benzodiazepines, barbiturates can cause physical dependency and produce severe withdrawal symptoms.

Thiopental (Pentothal), an ultra-short-acting anesthetic, has high lipid solubility and enters the CNS instantaneously. However, its CNS effects are rapidly terminated as it is redistributed from the brain to skeletal muscle. Owing to this profile, thiopental is used to induce anesthesia.

Barbiturates may increase the metabolism of acetaminophen, which reduces the pharmacological effect of acetaminophen.

Hypnotics

All of the hypnotic agents produce dose-dependent CNS depressant effects. Benzodiazepines are the major class of drugs included in this category. However, other agents such as barbiturates and newer drugs such as buspirone, zolpidem (Ambien), zaleplon (Sonata), eszopiclone (Lunesta), and ramelteon (Rozerem) are used to treat sleep disorder. Most hypnotic agents are lipid soluble; thus

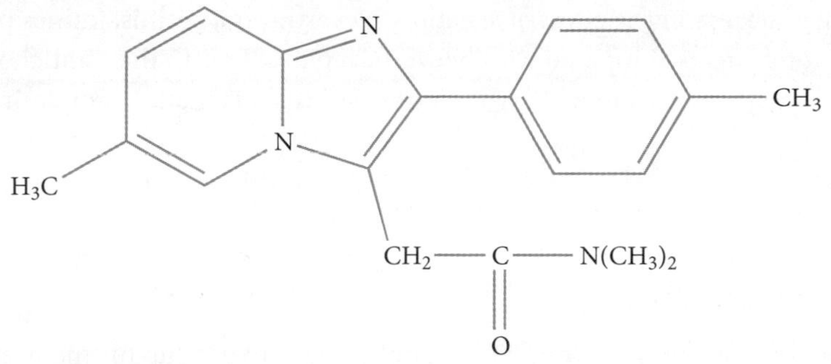

Figure 10.27 Structure of zolpidem.

they are absorbed well from the GI tract and move easily across the blood–brain barrier to become distributed in the brain. In addition, eszopiclone, zaleplon, and zolpidem have a rapid onset of CNS action.

Zolpidem

Zolpidem is structurally dissimilar to benzodiazepines (**Figure 10.27**), but it enhances the activity of GABA by selectively activating the benzodiazepine-1 (BZ$_1$) receptor, a benzodiazepine receptor subtype. This leads to increased chloride conductance and thereby neuronal hyperpolarization, producing sedative and hypnotic effects in less than 1 hour. Because zolpidem acts selectively in binding to BZ$_1$ receptors, but not to BZ$_2$ receptors, it does not produce any effective anxiolytic, muscle relaxant, and anticonvulsant effects.

In January 2013, the FDA recommended a lower starting dose of zolpidem for women. This recommendation was made because the plasma level of zolpidem has been shown to be high in women the morning after the drug administration, which may impair driving or operation of machinery during normal working hours.

Zaleplon

Zaleplon has a rapid onset of action and a relatively short half-life of 1 hour. As a result, it does not produce any psychomotor effect the day after drug administration. This agent is particularly useful for decreasing time for the onset of sleep but not for increasing total sleep time. The most common side effects with its use are dizziness, headache, and somnolence.

Ramelteon

Ramelteon activates melatonin receptors in the CNS. In contrast to zolpidem and the benzodiazepines, ramelteon has no direct effects on GABA receptors. An advantage of this drug is its minimal abuse potential; hence it is not classified as a controlled substance. Ramelteon's adverse effects include dizziness, fatigue, and decreased testosterone and increased prolactin hormone secretion.

Antihistamines

Antihistamines can produce safe hypnotic effects and are found in many OTC products. These agents are effective in treating mild insomnia, especially the first-generation H$_1$ antihistamines such as diphenhydramine (Benadryl), hydroxyzine (Vistaril), and chlorpheniramine (Allerchlor). These agents readily cross the blood–brain barrier and cause sedation. They also compete with histamine in binding to H$_1$ receptors in the GI tract, blood vessels, and respiratory tract and have anticholinergic effects. Their hypnotic effects do not follow a linear dose–response pattern, suggesting a plateau occurs in the effect of sedation. Nevertheless, antihistamines produce less pronounced hypnotic effects compared with benzodiazepines. Due to their anticholinergic effect, patients experience dry mouth and urinary retention, side effects that are not desirable in geriatric patients.

Learning Bridge 10.2

Joe, a recent law school graduate, comes to your pharmacy to pick up his medications. He tells you that he has become extremely anxious about the bar examination, which is scheduled to take place in 5 days. Joe's primary care physician has prescribed buspirone 15 mg BID to help Joe manage his anxiety. A drug utilization review of his patient profile indicates that Joe has also been using rifampin for the last 2 months.

A. Identify three areas you will counsel the patient using buspirone.
B. Will buspirone help Joe in reducing his anxiety during the bar examination? Why?
C. What is your suggestion to Joe?

Depression

Depressive disorders are classified into two main groups: major depression (unipolar depression) and bipolar depression (manic-depressive illness). The lifetime occurrence of major depression is about 15%, and females are at higher risk (2 times higher) for developing this disorder compared to males. Depression is characterized by recurring episodes of the following symptoms for at least 2 weeks: sadness, lack of interest in normal daily activities, poor concentration, insomnia or increased sleep, altered eating habits leading to either weight loss or weight gain, feelings of guilt and worthlessness, decreased energy and libido, and suicidal thoughts. The last symptom is of particular concern, as 10–15% of patients with severe depression attempt suicide. Depressive symptoms can also occur secondary to other disorders such as PD, AD, hypothyroidism, and inflammatory conditions.

Major Depressive Disorder

The highest rates of major depression in adults occur in individuals between 18 and 29 years of age. Approximately 10–20% of these patients have a family member with a history of depression. A major depressive disorder is characterized by experiencing five or more depressive behaviors on a daily basis, such as depressed mood for most of the day, a lack of interest or pleasure in daily activities, significant weight loss or weight gain, insomnia or increased sleep, fatigue, feelings of worthlessness or guilt, difficulty concentrating, and recurrent suicidal ideation without a specific plan.

The underlying cause of the symptoms associated with major depression reflects changes in levels of the neurotransmitters norepinephrine, serotonin (5-HT), and dopamine. Thus, most antidepressant agents potentiate the actions of norepinephrine, serotonin, or dopamine neurotransmitters. The overall goals of treatment are to reduce the symptoms and prevent more episodes of depression. Pharmacists can play important roles by educating patients and their family and friends about two major issues with antidepressants: the delay in achieving the full effect and the importance of adherence.

Antidepressants

Antidepressants are classified by their chemical structures as well as by their mechanisms of action. Factors that influence the selection of one specific antidepressant over others include the patient's history of drug response, pharmacogenetics, past and current medical records, compliance, symptoms, drug interactions, adverse effects, patient preference, and drug cost.

Selective Serotonin Reuptake Inhibitors

Selective serotonin reuptake inhibitors (SSRIs) enhance serotonergic functioning in the brain and are often selected as first-line antidepressants due to their safety (little overdose risk) and improved tolerability. The efficacy of SSRIs in treating patients with major depression is superior to that of other classes of antidepressants. Numerous SSRIs are available, and selecting which drug would best help the patient depends on differences in drug interaction profiles, pharmacokinetic parameters, or cost considerations. All SSRIs are effective in panic disorder. One of the major drawbacks with SSRIs is their delayed response: It takes at least 4 weeks before the full effect is seen (for some patients, it may take as long as 8–12 weeks).

SSRIs' mechanism of action is to block the reuptake of serotonin into neuronal presynaptic end terminals, thereby increasing the availability of serotonin at the synaptic cleft and serotonin receptors. These drugs are well absorbed after oral administration and, except for sertraline (Zoloft), are not affected by food; absorption of setraline is increased with food. All of the SSRIs are metabolized either by CYP-450 or by conjugation reactions. Typical side effects of SSRIs include insomnia, jitteriness, restlessness, agitation, and sexual dysfunction. It has also been suggested that SSRI therapy can cause neurotoxicity such as muscle twitches and tardive dyskinesia. If the drug is abruptly discontinued, it leads to a withdrawal syndrome. Drugs with longer $t_{1/2}$ values are less likely to produce a withdrawal syndrome. To avoid some of the side effects, low initial doses are recommended and should be maintained for the first week of therapy.

Commonly used SSRIs include fluoxetine (Prozac), citalopram (Celexa), sertraline (Zoloft), paroxetine (Paxil), escitalopram (Lexapro), and fluvoxamine (Luvox). As these agents are selective in their action, they have a low affinity for histaminic, adrenergic, and muscarinic receptors and, as a result, they produce fewer anticholinergic and cardiovascular adverse effects than other agents such as tricyclic antidepressants (TCAs). In addition, they do not cause any significant weight gain. Fluoxetine is a unique SSRI; it has a long half-time (50 hours) and is available in a sustained-released dosage form that allows dosing once per week (which increases adherence—a major problem for patients with major depression), and its metabolites are as effective as the parent agent.

Mixed Serotonin and Norepinephrine Reuptake Inhibitors

Mixed serotonin and norepinephrine reuptake inhibitors (SNRIs) bind to transporters for both serotonin and norepinephrine reuptake and increase the actions of both neurotransmitters. These agents are also called second-generation antidepressants. An important feature of SNRIs is that they differ from the TCAs in lacking high affinity for peripheral receptors, including histamine H_1, muscarinic, and α-adrenergic receptors. Three important agents in this class are venlafaxine (Effexor), desvenlafaxine (Pristiq), and duloxetine (Cymbalta).

At low doses, venlafaxine inhibits 5-HT reuptake; at high doses, it inhibits norepinephrine reuptake. Interestingly, the active metabolite of venlafaxine, desvenlafaxine, is also an SNRI. Extended-release venlafaxine has been found to produce better effects in improving social interaction, performance, and some fear factors and to be effective in patients who do not respond well to SSRI therapy. It is important to taper the dose of venlafaxine slowly to reduce the risk of relapse during discontinuation of this drug, because it has a short half-life. Withdrawal symptoms include agitation, dizziness, sweating, and tremor. Sexual adverse effects are a serious problem with venlafaxine use. The drug can also increase blood pressure, so monitoring is necessary.

Duloxetine, another SNRI, is also a weak inhibitor of dopamine reuptake. It has a low affinity for muscarinic cholinergic, H_1-histaminergic, and α_2-adrenergic receptors and is extensively metabolized to inactive metabolites by CYP2D6 and CYP1A2. This agent is well absorbed in the GI tract, but the presence of food decreases the extent of absorption by almost 10%. Postmarketing (Phase IV clinical study; see also the *Introduction to Pharmaceutics* chapter) data have suggested that duloxetine can cause liver toxicity.

Atypical Antidepressants

Bupropion (Wellbutrin) weakly inhibits reuptake of norepinephrine and dopamine, but does not inhibit monoamine oxidase or reuptake of serotonin. This agent has a short half-life, so it requires more frequent dosing. It is also used in smoking cessation, although its exact mechanism of action in this indication is not fully understood (which indicates that increases in dopamine or norepinephrine may have a role in smoking cessation). The use of bupropion is contraindicated in patients who have seizure disorders or have used a monoamine oxidase inhibitor during the past 14 days. Since 2009, the FDA has required the label of bupropion to include a "black box" warning due to the risk of serious neuropsychiatric symptoms (depressed mood, agitation, anxiety, hostility, changes in behavior, suicidal thoughts and behavior, and attempted suicide).

Mirtazapine (Remeron) acts as an antagonist of central presynaptic α_2-adrenergic receptors; it increases noradrenergic and serotonergic activity. This agent also antagonizes 5-HT_2 and 5-HT_3 receptors to reduce anxiety. In addition, it antagonizes histamine receptors, which explains mirtazapine's sedative effect. The most common adverse effects noted with the use of mirtazapine are somnolence, increased appetite, weight gain, xerostomia, and constipation. One of the benefits associated with mirtazapine is its lack of sexual adverse effects (in contrast to SSRIs).

Both *nefazodone* and *trazodone* (Oleptro) act as 5-HT_2 antagonists and mild 5-HT reuptake inhibitors. Since trazodone blocks α_1-adrenergic and histaminergic receptors, it causes dizziness and sedation. Nefazodone's use is limited due to its hepatic toxicity; its label carries a "black box" warning related to its hepatotoxicity.

Tricyclic Antidepressants

Tricyclic antidepressants are well absorbed from the GI tract and, due to their hydrophobic nature, readily cross the blood–brain barrier. They have largely fallen out of favor due to the availability of other antidepressants (particularly SSRIs) that are safer and better tolerated. All TCAs, to varying extents, inhibit the reuptake of norepinephrine and serotonin neurotransmitters. One of the major drawbacks of TCAs is their effect on the cholinergic, adrenergic, and histaminergic systems. Imipramine (Tofranil), desipramine (Norpramin), amitriptyline (Elavil, from Canada), and nortriptyline (Pamelor) are all effective TCAs.

Imipramine is also effective in the cessation of bed-wetting (enuresis); most children who take the drug for this indication respond well within the first week, although the exact mechanism of action is not fully understood. This TCA, however, is recommended only when all other therapies have failed.

TCA poisoning can have severe consequences such as arrhythmias, hypotension, coma, and seizures. Because amitriptyline (**Figure 10.28**) may alter blood glucose levels, it is important to counsel diabetic patients taking this drug to monitor their blood glucose. In addition, be aware that amitriptyline is not approved by the FDA for treating children younger than 12 years of age.

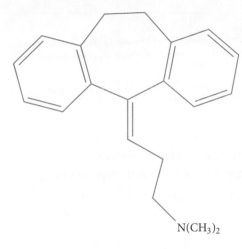

Figure 10.28 Structure of amitriptyline. Pay attention to the tricyclic structure.

$N(CH_3)_2$

Monoamine Oxidase Inhibitors

Monoamine oxidase inhibitors, as their name indicates, inhibit the catalytic activity of MAO, thereby increasing the concentration of norepinephrine, serotonin, and dopamine within the neuronal synapse. Similarly to TCAs, chronic therapy with MAOIs down-regulate both α- and β-adrenergic and serotonergic receptors. As mentioned previously, there are at least two major MAO enzymes: MAO-A and MAO-B. Both MAOIs, phenelzine (Nardil) and tranylcypromine (Parnate), nonselectively inhibit these enzymes. The side effects most frequently observed with MAOIs include postural hypotension, weight gain, anticholinergic effects, and sexual dysfunction. Use of MAOIs is also associated with hypertensive crisis and serotonin syndrome. These agents are not routinely used to treat depression.

Selegiline is available in a transdermal dosage form and is approved by the FDA to treat major depressive disorder. This drug inhibits MAO-A and MAO-B in the brain but has a reduced effect on MAO-A in the GI tract. At least 2 weeks should elapse between the discontinuation of SNRIs or SSRIs and the initiation of MAOIs, so as to avoid serotonergic overstimulation.

A serious drug interaction concern is serotonin syndrome. For instance, concomitant use of a MAO-B inhibitor with antidepressant SNRIs or SSRIs can cause serotonin syndrome, which is characterized by hyperthermia, rigidity, myoclonus, autonomic instability, delirium, and coma. Therefore, the concurrent use of MAO inhibitors and drugs that enhance the amount of norepinephrine, dopamine, serotonin, and tyramine is contraindicated. MAO-B inhibitors are also contraindicated with the opioid agent, meperidine (Demerol).

St. John's Wort

St. John's wort has long been used as an alternative medicine for treating depression. Its mechanism of action has been postulated to involve inhibition of cortisol secretion, increased concentrations of serotonin, and mild MAO inhibition. However, the efficacy of the active ingredient in St. John's wort, hypericum, has long been questioned. St. John's wort is a strong inducer of CYP3A4, so concomitant administration of this drug may affect the concentrations of antidepressants taken by patients with depression.

Learning Bridge 10.3

JJ is a 35-year-old male who was diagnosed with depression about 5 months ago. He has been evaluated by a psychiatrist and is currently on paroxetine 50 mg/day. His depressive symptoms have drastically improved since he started taking the current dosage of paroxetine. JJ, however, has been experiencing sexual dysfunction and has been distressed by this problem. He came to seek your advice on how to overcome this problem.

A. As a healthcare provider, how will you help JJ? Justify your answer.

B. JJ has recently been diagnosed with atypical migraine and has been prescribed sumatriptan tablets to reduce his migraine headaches. Should he take sumatriptan?

Mania and Bipolar Depression

Three types of bipolar depression are distinguished:

- Bipolar I: Characterized by recurrent manic episodes (e.g., increased energy, grandiosity, irritability, euphoria, decreased sleep requirements, psychotic features) and major depressive episodes.
- Bipolar II: Characterized by hypomanic episodes as well as major depressive episodes. Hypomania is elevated or irritable mood that lasts for at least 4 days, but does not cause any significant impairment in functioning. Hypomania can be associated with depression.
- Cyclothymia: Frequent episodes of hypomania and depressive episodes that are not major depressive episodes. The diagnosis of this condition requires episodes to occur over at least a 2-year period.

Mood-stabilizing agents used to treat mania and bipolar depression include lithium, carbamazepine, valproic acid, lamotrigine, and second-generation antipsychotics. These drugs represent the first-line treatment options for bipolar diseases.

Lithium

Lithium (Lithobid) is a monovalent cation that is approved for acute mania and maintenance therapy. It is a first-line agent prescribed for acute mania, acute bipolar depression, and maintenance treatment of bipolar I and II disorders. Lithium produces a prophylactic response in almost 70% of patients and reduces suicide ideation. An abrupt discontinuation or noncompliance can increase the risk of relapse.

Although lithium's full mechanism of action is not known, it has been suggested that chronic lithium administration may change gene expression and has a neuroprotective effect. This drug also inhibits recycling of the inositol substrates needed to generate IP_3 and DAG second messenger system (see also the *Introduction to Pharmacodynamics* chapter) in the cell. Lithium has unique properties that include rapid absorption, wide distribution, minimal protein binding, and unchanged excretion in the urine. To minimize adverse effects, patients taking lithium must undergo periodic thyroid and kidney function tests as well as measurement of the drug concentration in the blood.

In addition, lithium, at a dose of 600 to 1,200 mg/day, is effective against chronic cluster headache attacks (headache with extreme intensity).

The initial side effects of lithium are dose related and occur at peak serum concentrations. To minimize these effects, the drug should be taken in divided doses along with food. Alternatively, extended-release formulations may be used. While transient muscle weakness and lethargy are seen in approximately one-third of patients, polyuria and nocturia can occur in as many as 70% of patients; the latter symptoms may be managed through once-daily bedtime dosing. Similar to digoxin, lithium has a narrow therapeutic window. Moreover, because it is excreted solely by the kidney, the drug will accumulate and cause toxic reactions if used in patients with renal impairment. The therapeutic range of lithium is 0.6–1.2 mEq/L and the toxic plasma concentration level is more than 1.5 mEq/L. Caffeine and theophylline are known to enhance renal elimination of lithium; conversely, thiazide diuretics and NSAIDs increase the serum level of lithium.

Valproic Acid

Valproic acid (Depakote) is used to treat acute manic episodes. It increases the availability or action of GABA. It also mimics the action of GABA at postsynaptic receptor sites. "Black box" warnings associated with valproic acid use are related to hepatic dysfunction and pregnancy (the drug can cause neural tube defects). Valproic acid is significantly protein bound and can displace other agents from protein-binding sites. It can cause blood dyscrasias, an adverse effect that requires monitoring. Liver function tests (LFTs) should be performed prior to and during valproic acid therapy. As mentioned in the *Introduction to Biochemistry* chapter, valproic acid negatively affects the urea cycle in the liver, so it should not be used in patients with hyperammonemia.

Carbamazepine

Carbamazepine (Carbatrol) is a second-line agent for prophylaxis and treatment of bipolar disorders and is generally reserved for lithium-refractory patients. This agent can be used alone but is often prescribed in combination with lithium or valproic acid. Its use is contraindicated in patients with bone marrow depression. Carbamazepine can cause CNS-related adverse effects and fetal harm in pregnancy. The FDA requires a "black box" warning on the drug's label indicating its ability to cause serious reactions (Stevens-Johnson syndrome, pruritus, and rash), particularly in patients of Asian ancestry.

Lamotrigine

Lamotrigine (Lamictal) is approved for bipolar I disorder. It blocks voltage-sensitive Na^+ channels and decreases release of two amino acid neurotransmitters, glutamate and aspartate. Its effect against bipolar depression is enhanced when lamotrigine is combined with valproic acid because the latter agent decreases the clearance of lamotrigine. Similar to carbamazepine, lamotrigine use is associated with life-threatening rash, particularly in pediatric patients ("black box" warning).

Other Agents for Mania and Bipolar Depression

- *Olanzapine/Fluoxetine:* This combination (Symbyax) has most recently been approved by the FDA to treat acute bipolar depression.
- *Quetiapine (Seroquel):* This drug has been approved as a monotherapy to treat acute bipolar depression.
- *Gabapentin (Neurontin):* This agent can be used as an adjunctive therapy for bipolar disorders.
- *Topiramate (Topamax):* This drug can be used for bipolar disorders, although no evidence supporting its effectiveness in these indications has been published. The doses for bipolar disorders are lower than those for the treatment of seizures, and topiramate may cause weight loss.

A few drugs are approved as maintenance therapies in bipolar disorders. For instance, olanzapine (Zyprexa) is used as monotherapy or in combination with other mood-stabilizing drugs. In addition, an atypical antipsychotic drug, aripiprazole (Abilify), is used for maintenance treatment for 6 weeks. Quetiapine, in combination with lithium or valproic acid, is also approved for maintenance therapy of bipolar disorders. However, there is a need to evaluate the safety of antipsychotics as monotherapy or as adjunctive therapy for maintenance treatment.

Learning Bridge 10.4

BC, a graduate student in business school, is started on lithium 300 mg TID for his bipolar disorder.

A. Which laboratory tests are required before initiating lithium therapy?

B. After starting BC on lithium, do you think his plasma level of lithium should be monitored?

C. According to his sister, BC has been urinating frequently and drinking a lot of fluids ever since he started on lithium therapy. What will you tell her to solve BC's problem?

D. His sister also tells you that BC takes prescription-strength ibuprofen for his back pain. What will be your advice?

Antipsychotic Agents

The exact mechanism of action of antipsychotics (which are also called neuroleptics or major tranquilizers) is not known. Both dopamine and serotonin receptor subtypes serve as molecular targets for antipsychotics. The multiple actions of 5-hydroxytryptophan (5-HT; **Figure 10.29**) involve interactions with different 5-HT receptor subtypes. Indeed, multiple 5-HT receptor subtypes are the largest known neurotransmitter-receptor family. These receptor subtypes are G-protein–coupled receptors (see also the *Introduction to Pharmacodynamics* chapter). Most 5-HT receptors (particularly the 5-HT_{2C} receptor) are capable of activating G-proteins independently of an agonist.

There are three subtypes of 5-HT_2 receptors: 5-HT_{2A}, 5-HT_{2B}, and 5-HT_{2C}. The 5-HT_{2A} receptors are widely distributed in the CNS, primarily in serotonergic terminal areas. They are also found in blood platelets, smooth muscle cells, and the GI tract. The 5-HT_{2B} receptors are not located in the brain, but rather are found in the stomach fundus. The 5-HT_{2C} receptors are found in the choroid plexus; the choroid plexus, which is composed of epithelial tissue, is responsible for the production of cerebrospinal fluid (CSF). The 5-HT_{2C} receptors are involved in the control of CSF production, in feeding behavior, and in mood.

Based on antagonism of dopamine and serotonin receptors, antipsychotics are classified into two major categories:

- Typical antipsychotics (also known as first-generation or traditional antipsychotics): These agents are potent antagonists at dopaminergic D_2 receptors.
- Atypical antipsychotics: These agents are potent antagonists at serotonin 5-HT_{2A} receptors; they also antagonize D_2 receptors.

Antipsychotics' labels carry FDA-issued "black box" warnings of a high risk of mortality in patients with dementia-associated psychosis. Antipsychotics are utilized to treat patients suffering from schizophrenia, a complex psychiatric disorder. Schizophrenia is characterized by delusions, hallucinations, disorganized thoughts and speech, and impaired psychosocial functioning. Medication therapy is a must for treating schizophrenia, but nonpharmacological therapies also play important roles in helping patients—for example, patient education, targeted cognitive therapy, social skills, supported housing, and financial support. Indeed, nonpharmacological therapy that involves the family responsible for the care of the patient has improved social functioning and decreased rehospitalization among such patients.

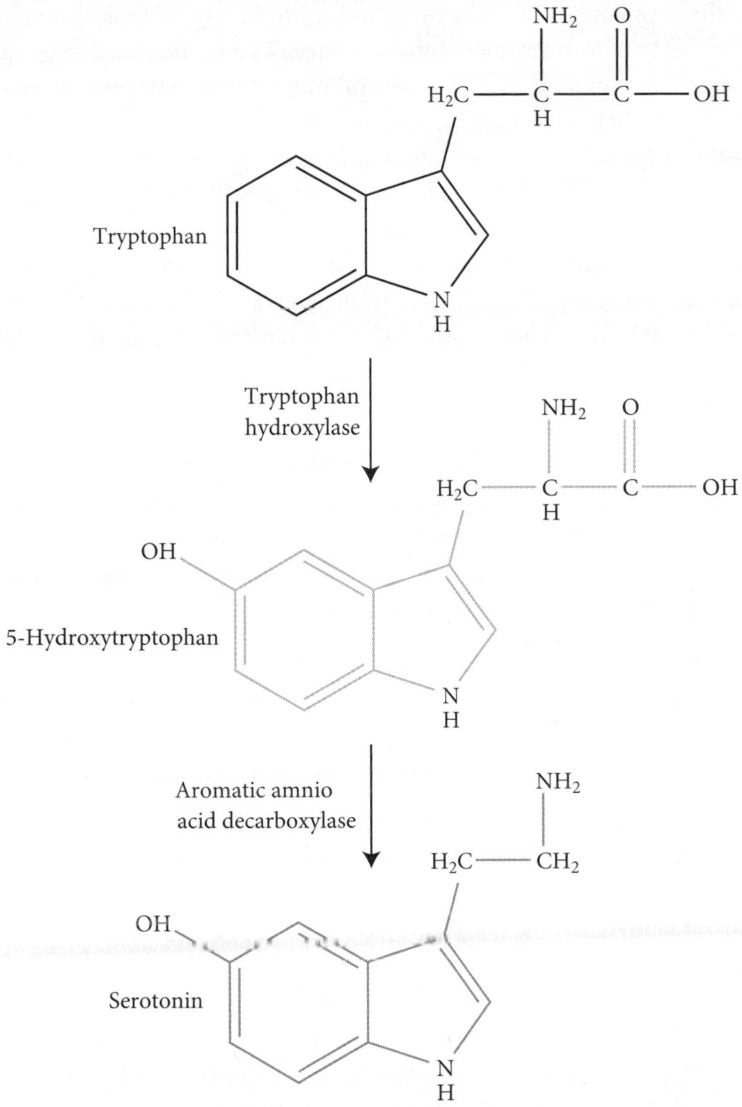

Figure 10.29 Synthesis of 5-hydroxytryptophan (5-HT) and serotonin from the aromatic amino acid tryptophan.

Schizophrenia symptoms are often divided into positive and negative symptoms. Positive symptoms include delusions, disorganized thoughts and speech, hallucinations, and suspiciousness. Negative symptoms include abnormal emotional responses such as inability to experience pleasure or lack of desire to form relationships, lack of motivation, and decreased level of hygiene. The prevalence of schizophrenia is similar among most cultures, and the condition rarely occurs before adolescence or after the age of 40 years. In the United States, the prevalence of this disease is about 1%. While prevalence is equally split between males and females, male patients tend to have their first episode during their early 20s, whereas female patients tend to have their first episode in their early 30s. Schizophrenia is likely caused by multiple physiological and biochemical abnormalities, but its exact cause remains unknown.

Typical Antipsychotics

Typical antipsychotics, also referred to as first-generation antipsychotics, are effective in schizophrenia and other psychotic disorders and are competitive antagonists of D_2 receptors. However, they are more likely to produce orthostatic hypotension and extrapyramidal symptoms (EPS). The extrapyramidal system comprises the neural network in the brain and is affected by the typical antipsychotics (and to a much lesser extent by the atypical antipsychotics). EPS encompass a heterogeneous group of disorders that affect coordination of movement and muscular activity. Interestingly, research into antipsychotic receptor binding in humans has shown that at least 60% D_2 receptor blocking is necessary to reduce positive psychotic symptoms, and blocking of 75% or more of D_2 receptors is associated with EPS. The typical antipsychotics are the major cause of EPS (haloperidol causes the more severe symptoms and chlorpromazine causes the mildest EPS). While typical antipsychotics improve the positive symptoms of schizophrenia, they are not effective in the treatment of negative symptoms. Other agents in this category include chlorpromazine (Largactil, from Canada), fluphenazine (Apo-Fluphenazine, from Canada), haloperidol (Haldol), pimozide (Orap), and thiothixene (Navane).

Atypical Antipsychotics

Atypical antipsychotics (also referred to as second-generation antipsychotics [SGAs]) are linked to a lower incidence of EPS. It has been suggested that the atypical antipsychotics dissociate more rapidly from the D_2 receptor. Except aripiprazole, all other available SGAs have a greater affinity for 5-HT_{2A} receptors than D_2 receptors. In addition to their antipsychotic role, these agents are used in the management of neuropsychotic symptoms of AD.

Currently available atypical antipsychotics include the following drugs: risperidone (Risperdal), quetiapine, olanzapine, aripiprazole, clozapine (Clozaril), and ziprasidone (Geodon). Metabolic complications for atypical antipsychotics can be troublesome. Overall, assessment of patient risk and benefit is warranted, and monitoring during treatment should be considered, when treating patients with atypical antipsychotics.

All atypical antipsychotics antagonize dopamine receptors in the brain and in the periphery. As a result, drugs that increase the amount of dopamine (such as levodopa or amphetamine) will counteract the role of antipsychotics. Two SSRIs used to treat depression, fluoxetine and paroxetine, are known to enhance the plasma concentration of risperidone significantly (approximately 4-fold). In addition to blocking dopamine receptors, atypical antipsychotics block serotonin receptors, particularly 5-HT_{2A} receptors. Their ability to improve negative symptoms and lower the incidence of EPS is suspected to be due to the agents' binding to the 5-HT_{2A} receptors. However, compared with typical antipsychotics, atypical antipsychotics bind to dopamine D_2 receptors with less affinity. For example, the binding affinity of risperidone to the D_2 receptor is 20 times lower than its binding affinity to the 5-HT_{2A} receptor.

Both palperidone and ziprasidone are known to prolong the QT interval—that is, the time from the start of the Q wave to the end of the T wave in the heart's electrical cycle as measured by an electrocardiograph. The QT interval represents depolarization and repolarization of the left and right ventricles (the QT duration is shorter when the heart rate is rapid and is prolonged with a slower heart rate). A prolonged QT interval is indicative of ventricular tachyarrhythmia, which can lead to sudden death.

When patients respond inadequately (or are therapeutically resistant) to multiple antipsychotics, they are said to have a "treatment-resistant" condition, as evidenced by a lack of improvement in positive symptoms and poor improvement in negative symptoms. To date, only clozapine has been shown to be more effective than the other antipsychotics in the management of treatment-resistant schizophrenia. However, any improvement with clozapine in treatment-resistant patients occurs slowly, with the therapeutic response sometimes taking 6 months or longer to appear. In addition, clozapine is known to cause seizures, particularly when it is given in high doses; thus practitioners must be careful when prescribing this drug in patients who have a past or current history of seizure. The drug is also known to cause agranulocytosis and requires regular monitoring.

Table 10.4 Blocking of Different Receptors by Antipsychotic Agents

Drug	Cholinergic (Muscarinic) Receptors	α-Adrenergic Receptors	Serotonin Receptors	Dopamine Receptors	Histamine Receptors (H_1)
Chlorpromazine	+++	+++	+	++	+++
Clozapine			+++	+	++
Fluphenazine	+	+	+	++	+
Haloperidol	+	+	+	+++	+
Risperidone	+	+	+++	+++	+
Thiothixene	+	+	+	+++	+
All antipsychotics				+	

Adapted from: Clark M, Finkel R, Rey J, Whalen K. *Pharmacology*, 5th ed. Philadelphia: Lippincott Williams & Wilkins; 2012: Chapter 13.

Table 10.4 identifies the antagonistic roles of antipsychotics to a series of receptors. Indeed, this table indicates why, for instance, chlorpromazine produces severe anticholinergic side effects (e.g., dry mouth, blurred vision, constipation, nasal stuffiness).

Learning Bridge 10.5

A 50-year-old male diagnosed with schizophrenia was prescribed 10 mg haloperidol daily. Two weeks later, he returned to the doctor with tremor and rigidity. Physical examinations concluded he had cogwheel rigidity.

A. Based on your knowledge of the pathophysiology of Parkinson's disease, blocking which neurotransmitter in the brain can balance the neural circuit of movement?

B. Suggest a therapeutic agent to support your answer.

C. How is quetiapine different from haloperidol in its therapeutic actions and side-effect profile?

Pain Management and Opioids

Pain is one of the major reasons why patients seek medical help, and its emergence often leads to the diagnosis of one or more diseases or disorders. Pain may involve more than one specific area or organ in the body and hence, pain management may be more effective when a multidisciplinary approach is undertaken. In the treatment of pain caused by medical and surgical conditions, medications belonging to different therapeutic classes are used, including oral and parenteral opioids, epidural and local anesthesia, peripheral nerve blockade, NSAIDs, and nonopioid adjuvant drug products.

It is imperative to recognize and treat pain in pediatric patients as well. The basic mechanisms of pain in children and infants are similar to those in adults, with the exception that infants (particularly neonates) may perceive pain more intensely than adults. In neonates, the pain impulse is transmitted along slow-conducting, nonmyelinated C fibers rather than the myelinated Aδ (delta) fibers that transmit pain with a higher conduction velocity. It is not clear how the spinal cord transmits pain signals in this category of patients. Many agents that are used for analgesia in pediatric patients are not available in certain dosage forms; thus their preparation may require compounding the drugs extemporaneously or making dilutions of drugs that are intended for adult patients.

It is important to appreciate that both geriatric and pediatric patient populations might not receive adequate pain control due to their inability to communicate with their care providers. Therefore, the parent or caregiver may play an important role in the overall pain management process.

Opioid Receptors

There are three opioid receptors: δ (delta), μ (mu), and κ (kappa). These receptors have a high sequence homology in the intracellular domains (approximately 60%), but the extracellular loops are quite diverse. Opioid receptors are widely distributed in the brain and spinal cord and in many peripheral tissues, including vascular, cardiac, lung, and GI tract. The functions of these receptors have emerged through research aimed at elucidating the structure–activity relationships of different agonist and antagonist compounds. All opioid receptors consist of an extracellular N-terminus and an intracellular C-terminus, seven transmembrane helices, and a few intracellular loops (recall the serpentine receptors from the *Introduction to Pharmacodynamics* chapter).

Because opioid receptors are coupled to G proteins, the GTP/GDP (guanosine triphosphate/guanosine diphosphate) ratio plays an important role in their functionality. Upon receptor activation, a series of events occurs that includes (1) activation of G proteins, resulting in the inhibition of adenylyl cyclase required for cAMP production; (2) reduction of the opening of voltage-gated Ca^{2+} channels, followed by a decrease in the release of neurotransmitters or an efflux of potassium ion, resulting in hyperpolarization of the cell and reduced neuronal excitability; and (3) activation of protein kinase C (PKC) and phospholipase C (PLC) (see also the *Introduction to Pharmacodynamics* chapter).

Opioids, particularly morphine, are administered by spinal delivery to produce analgesia in some cases. Absorption of most opioids from the GI tract is erratic. However, the absorption through the rectal mucosa is better; thus a few opioids are available as suppositories (morphine and hydromorphone). For some opioids, the transdermal route of administration is employed. In the following sections, various agonists to opioid receptors are discussed.

Morphine

Morphine is the prototype agonist of the μ receptors. Because it is difficult to synthesize morphine, this drug is extracted from poppy seed. The chemical structure of morphine is well known, so many new synthetic agonists have been produced that structurally mimic morphine (**Figure 10.30**). In turn, the effectiveness of morphine is used as a standard to compare the effectiveness of the new analgesics. Morphine exerts its analgesic effect by activating opioid receptors of the CNS, GI tract, and urinary bladder.

As is indicated in Figure 10.30, codeine is methylated morphine and heroin is acetylated morphine. Hydromorphone and hydrocodone are also synthesized by modifying the structure of morphine (**Figure 10.31**). The only difference between hydromorphone and hydrocodone is that the hydroxyl group on hydromorphone is replaced by a methoxy group in the latter, which increases the hydrophobicity of hydrocodone.

Morphine is poorly absorbed in oral dosage forms due to an extensive first-pass effect. In the liver, this drug is mainly metabolized to morphine-3-glucuronide (M3G). To a lesser degree, morphine is metabolized to morphine-6-glucuronide (M6G). Both M3G and M6G are produced by the glucuronyl transferase enzyme in the liver, and both are eliminated by kidneys. While M3G does not have any pharmacological activity, M6G has μ-agonistic effects in the CNS.

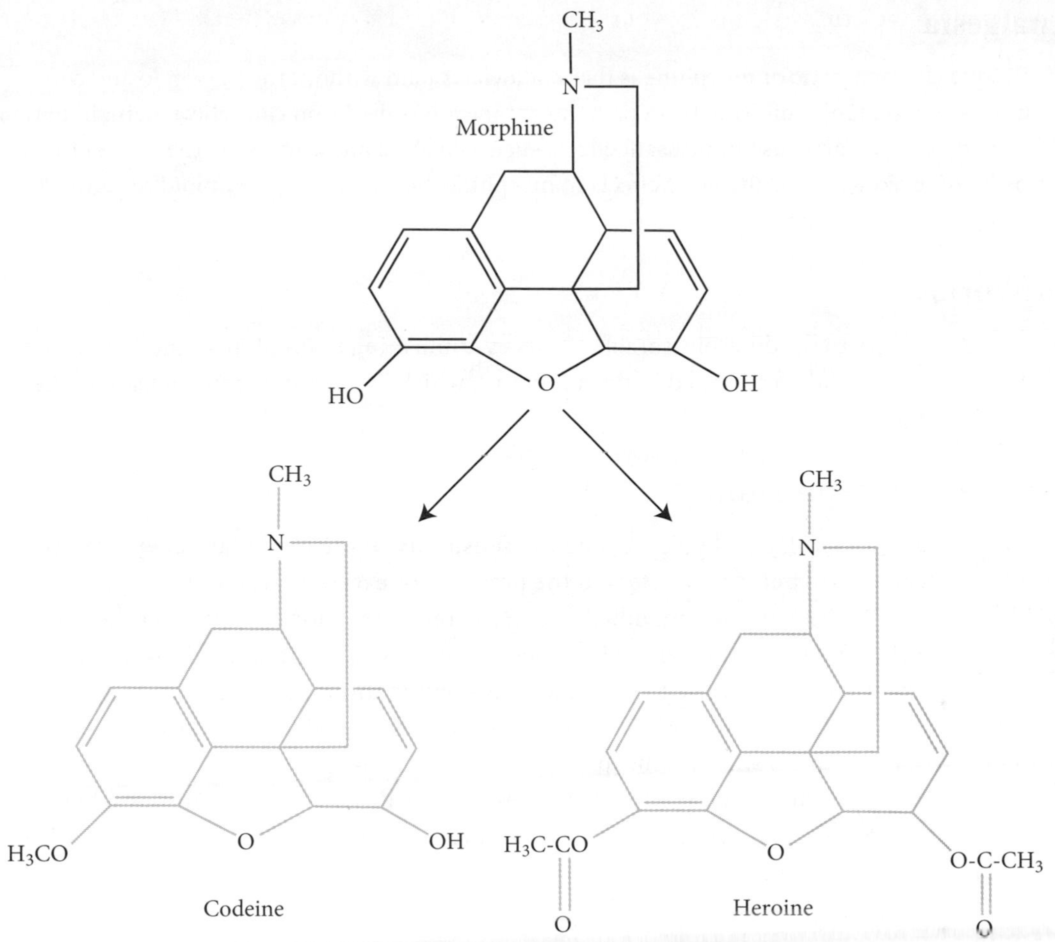

Figure 10.30 Morphine, codeine, and heroin have similar structural and pharmacological properties. While morphine is extracted from the poppy plant, codeine and heroin can be synthesized chemically from morphine.

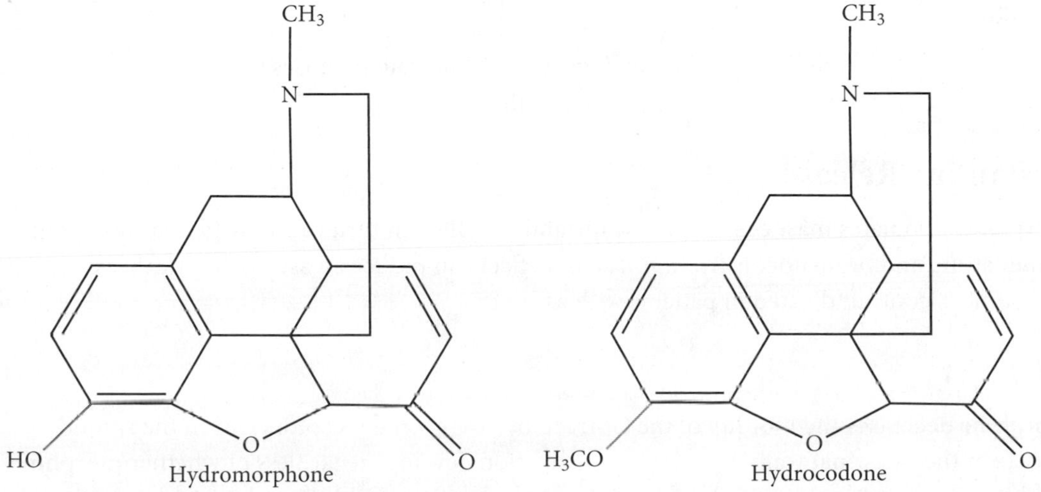

Figure 10.31 Hydromorphone and hydrocodone are synthesized chemically from morphine. Due to its methoxy group, hydrocodone is more hydrophobic than hydromorphone.

Analgesia

The unique characteristic of morphine is that it alleviates pain without the person losing consciousness. For patients suffering from pain, morphine administration can relieve pain; in patients without any pain it can cause unpleasant effects such as nausea and vomiting. The μ receptor is mostly involved with the analgesic effects of morphine, but the other two opioid receptors (δ and κ) contribute in producing analgesia.

Euphoria

Morphine is known to produce pleasurable effects by stimulating μ receptors in the ventral tegmental area (a neuronal area located in the midbrain), which leads to dopamine release in the mesolimbic region.

Respiratory Depression

Morphine reduces ventilation by depressing the sensitivity of the medullary chemoreceptors to hypercapnea (hypercapnea refers to the presence of excessive amounts of CO_2 in the blood), which results in the individual losing the reflex reaction that would otherwise increase breathing to ensure the person has adequate access to oxygen. In addition, morphine depresses the ventilatory response to hypoxia. This combination results in almost no stimulus to breathe and results in seizure. It is the most common cause of death in morphine overdose, particularly in individuals who use morphine with recreational goals in mind. However, with adequate dosing, patients develop tolerance to respiratory depression. Barbiturates, benzodiazepines, and alcohol potentiate the sedation and respiratory depression associated with morphine and other opioids.

Miosis

Stimulation of μ and κ receptors enhances parasympathetic stimulation of the eyes, which causes the pupils to constrict (miosis). Because patients do not develop tolerance to this effect, a pinpoint pupil is a good indication of morphine abuse.

Emesis

Morphine stimulates the chemoreceptor trigger zone, and causes causes vomiting. This is particularly unpleasant when treating patients with cancer.

Histamine Release

Morphine stimulates mast cells to release histamine, which in turn causes urticaria, sweating, vasodilation, and bronchoconstriction. The last effect can induce an asthmatic attack; as a result, morphine is contraindicated in patients with asthma.

GI Tract

Morphine decreases the motility of the GI tract, by acting on μ receptors within the smooth muscle of the intestinal wall. As a result, constipation develops regardless of whether morphine is taken on an acute or chronic basis. Patients treated with morphine can benefit from use of a stimulant laxative such as senna (Senokot). While nausea, vomiting, sedation, pruritus, and other adverse effects of opioids eventually subside within a few days, patients do not develop tolerance to constipation.

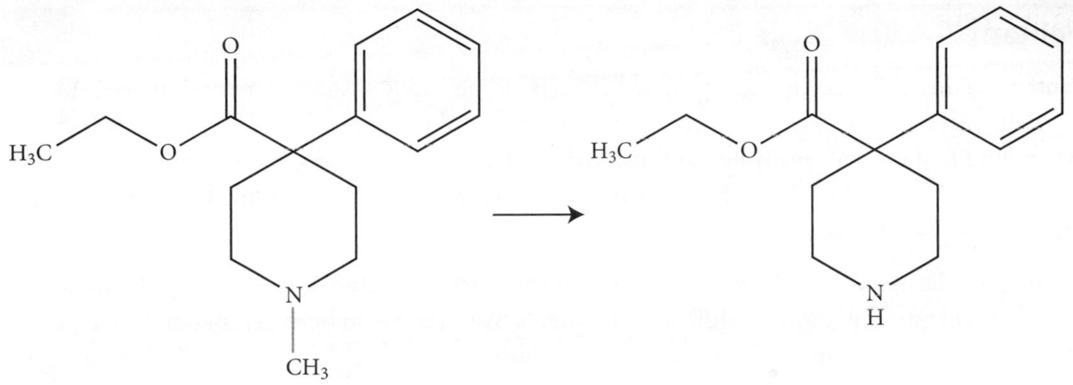

Figure 10.32 Metabolism (*N*-demethylation) of meperidine produces normeperidine, which causes serious adverse effects including anxiety, tremors, and generalized seizure.

Cough-Suppressant Activity

Morphine can produce an antitussive effect. This cough suppression occurs via an agonistic effect on the μ and κ receptors. Interestingly, before the side effects of heroin were discovered in the early 1900s, heroin was used to treat coughs.

Cardiovascular Effects

At large doses, morphine reduces heart rate and causes bradycardia. In addition, high doses of morphine result in arteriolar and venous dilation, which ultimately leads to hypotension. This hypotension appears to be mediated by degranulation of histamine-containing vesicles, which results in the release of histamine.

Meperidine

Meperidine (Demerol) produces a strong analgesic response, is able to inhibit the ascending pain pathways, alters the perception of and response to pain, and causes CNS depression. These effects are produced when meperidine binds to μ and κ receptors. Meperidine is used to treat moderate-to-severe pain and is often administered as an adjunct to anesthesia and preoperative sedation. However, it can cause hypotension when administered postoperatively.

All opioids except meperidine reduce the strength, duration, and frequency of uterine contractions, causing delay in labor when they are administered to women in active labor. Accordingly, it is safe to give meperidine during labor; indeed, it has been suggested that the duration and frequency of uterine contractions may be increased by meperidine.

Meperidine is either hydrolyzed to an inactive metabolite, meperidinic acid, or else undergoes *N*-demethylation to normeperidine (**Figure 10.32**). The latter metabolite produces anxiety, tremors, and generalized seizure (particularly in patients with renal impairment, a condition that causes accumulation of the metabolite to toxic levels). Meperidine metabolites are excreted in the urine.

Naloxone, an opioid antagonist, does not reverse all effects of meperidine; as a result, meperidine should not be given in doses higher than 600 mg/day. Meperidine is also contraindicated in combination with MAOIs or within 14 days of taking MAOIs or SSRIs because of the risk of CNS adverse effects (seizures and confusion).

Fentanyl

Fentanyl (Duragesic) is chemically related to meperidine and is a very potent opioid, in fact, its analgesic effect is 100 times more potent than that of morphine. Because it is a hydrophobic compound fentanyl can easily be administered via the parenteral, transmucosal, and transdermal routes. It accumulates in skeletal muscle and fat and is released slowly into the blood, where it is metabolized by CYP3A4.

The transdermal dosage form of fentanyl is particularly important when patients are noncompliant or oral administration is difficult for patients. An increase in body temperature releases more (30%) active compound through the skin. The onset of action for the transdermal dosage form is 5–10 minutes; thus this dosage form is used for the management of moderate-to-severe chronic pain. Because of the slow release, the analgesic effect is still seen 8–16 hours after patch application a factor that must be taken into consideration when treating a patient overdosed with a fentanyl patch.

Methadone

Methadone (Dolophine) is the only long-acting, liquid opioid agonist currently available. It has a long half-life, so dosing intervals of 8 to 12 hours are permitted. Methadone produces less of a euphoric effect compared to morphine. Its action is mediated by binding to μ receptors. It also acts as an antagonist to the NMDA receptor. Methadone is used in controlling the withdrawal symptoms of opioid-dependent patients. Because it has oral efficacy, a longer duration of action, and a low cost, it is a popular narcotic analgesic.

Oxycodone

Oxycodone (OxyContin) is an oral μ opioid with an analgesic effect that is used for moderate-to-severe pain; it may also be used in combination with nonopioid analgesics. Oxycodone has been used as an alternative analgesic to morphine, but its side effects are similar to those of morphine. Because it is available in both immediate-release and controlled-release oral dosage forms, it is very useful in treating both persistent and acute pain. Unfortunately, the drug is frequently abused, with illicit users often presenting false prescriptions to pharmacies.

Codeine

Codeine (Codeine Contin, from Canada) is prescribed in the treatment of moderate pain, and is often combined with acetaminophen. Its side effects are very similar to those produced by morphine (i.e., euphoria, sedation, constipation). Codeine is particularly useful as an oral antitussive. However, due to its side-effect profile, codeine has been replaced by dextromethorphan (Delsym) as an OTC product (**Figure 10.33**). Dextromethorphan also acts as an NMDA receptor antagonist. However, because large doses of dextromethorphan can cause hallucinations, confusion, excitation, seizures, and respiratory suppression, the FDA has issued warnings regarding dextromethorphan's potential for abuse.

Hydrocodone

Hydrocodone is used for pain in combination with other analgesic agents (acetaminophen and ibuprofen). Vicodin (hydrocodone/acetaminophen) is available in strengths of 5/500, 7.5/750, and 10/660 (hydrocodone mg/acetaminophen mg). Vicoprofen (hydrocodone/ibuprofen) is available in one strength: 7.5 mg hydrocodone/200 mg ibuprofen. Its pharmacologic properties are similar to those of morphine.

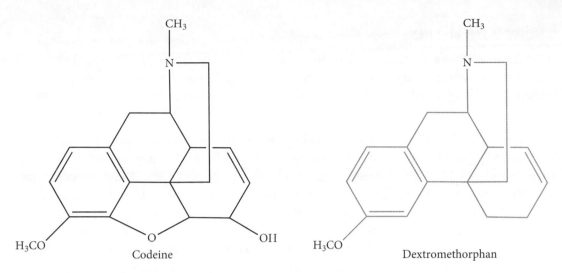

Figure 10.33 Methadone and dextromethorphan are structurally and pharmacologically similar, but are used for different indications. Dextromethorphan has relatively few adverse effects compared to codeine.

Opioid Agonist–Antagonist Derivatives

Opioid agonist–antagonist derivatives have a lower risk of abuse, as they have a ceiling analgesic effect. They are agonists at the κ receptors, but also bind to μ receptors as weak antagonists. The result is more dysphoria (depression and anxiety at high doses such as 60–90 mg) and a lower risk of respiratory depression.

Pentazocine (Talwin) is the prototype agent in this category. Its CNS effects are similar to those of the morphine-like opioids. Pentazocine's cardiovascular effects differ from those of other opioid agonists, however; at high doses, it increases both blood pressure and heart rate. Pentazocine is used as pain medication as well as a sedative prior to surgery.

Another important agent in this category is buprenorphine (Subutex). Buprenorphine has been approved for opioid withdrawal and is often used at the beginning of withdrawal treatment. Suboxone is a combination product that includes both buprenorphine and the opiate antagonist naloxone. Suboxone is used in the maintenance therapy of individuals who are addicted to opiates.

Naloxone is an antagonist that competitively binds to opioid receptors but does not produce any analgesic or other opioid-like effects. As a result, it is used to remedy the toxicity of agonist and agonist–antagonist opioid derivatives. Naltrexone (ReVia) is also an antagonist agent to opioid receptors, but it has longer duration of action compared to naloxone. For instance, a single dose of naltrexone blocks the effects of heroin for two full days. Acute overdose of heroin is often indicated by respiratory depression, coma, skeletal muscle floppiness, cold and clammy (sweaty) skin, miosis, pulmonary edema, bradycardia, hypotension, and death. Opioid antagonists are very useful not only for mitigating these overdose effects but also for treating withdrawal from opioid addiction.

Learning Bridge 10.6

A patient with shoulder dislocation was released from the emergency room with a prescription for Ultracet starting at 50 mg po BID. The on-call resident overlooked the fact that the patient is taking fluoxetine for obsessive–compulsive disorder (OCD) as well. Identify the problems that the patient will face with the new prescription.

Heart Failure

Heart failure (HF) is a medical condition in which the heart is unable to provide adequate cardiac output to meet the metabolic needs of the body. Approximately 6 million Americans have heart failure. Each year 600,000 patients are newly diagnosed with HF, and approximately 10% of patients are more than 75 years old.

Abnormalities that reduce ventricular filling (diastolic dysfunction) or myocardial contractility (systolic dysfunction) can lead to HF. The two major risk factors for heart failure are coronary artery disease (CAD) and hypertension. Heart failure is a gradually progressing disorder that may be initiated by myocardial injury, which is then followed by a series of compensatory responses as the body attempts to maintain adequate cardiac output. These compensatory responses include release of several mediators (angiotensin II, norepinephrine, aldosterone, pro-inflammatory cytokines, and vasopressin), as well as activation of the sympathetic nervous system and the renin–angiotensin–aldosterone system (RAAS), resulting in hypertension and sodium and water retention. These compensatory mechanisms produce the symptoms of heart failure.

Cardiac output is the volume of blood pumped by the heart in 1 minute (mL blood/min). Accordingly, it is a function of the heart rate and stroke volume and can be measured by the following equation:

Cardiac output (mL/min) = heart rate (beats/min) × stroke volume (mL/beat)

The heart rate is simply the number of heart beats per minute, and the stroke volume is the volume of blood (mL) that is pumped out of the heart per each beat. As an example, the cardiac output for an average healthy individual with a resting heart rate of 70 beats/minute and a resting stroke volume of 70 mL/minute is calculated as follows:

Cardiac output = 70 (beats/min) × 70 (mL/beat) = 4,900 mL/min

As this equation indicates, cardiac output can be increased by an increase in either the heart rate or the stroke volume. The total volume of blood of an average person is approximately 5 liters, so the entire volume of blood is pumped by the heart during each minute when the body is at rest.

Patients with symptomatic heart failure are treated with an ACE inhibitor, a selective beta blocker (carvedilol, metoprolol succinate, or bisoprolol), and a diuretic. If the ACE inhibitor is not tolerated, contraindicated, or is not effective (as in many African American patients), an angiotensin II receptor blocker is substituted. In addition, treatment with digoxin is known to improve HF symptoms and reduce hospitalizations.

When beta blockers are prescribed in heart failure, it is important to gradually increase the dose until the target therapeutic dose is achieved. However, if the reduction in heart rate becomes a concern, the target dose may not be attained. As such, the optimal dose of the agent and adequate heart rate should be considered seriously.

In acute HF, a loop diuretic is used; in chronic HF, the combination of a loop diuretic, a spironolactone diuretic, and an ACE inhibitor is used. In addition to sodium restriction, diuretics should be prescribed to patients with signs of peripheral edema or pulmonary congestion.

ACE Inhibitors

ACE inhibitors are known to increase survival of patients with CHF. This class of agents reduces disease progression and frequency of hospitalization from complications of HF. In addition, patients with asymptomatic left ventricular dysfunction and those who have experienced a myocardial infarction in the past should receive ACE inhibitors. ACE inhibitors are able to decrease left ventricular (LV) volume and prevent fibrosis. These agents can reduce both preload and afterload, increase cardiac output, and reduce the levels of two mediators, epinephrine and aldosterone, by virtue of decreased angiotensin II formation.

ACE inhibitors inhibit the conversion of angiotensin I (AngI) to the active angiotensin II (AngII). As a result, the active circulation of AngII is reduced, which in turn lowers blood pressure and enhances natriuresis (excretion of sodium in the urine).

As a result of a decreased level of active AngII, ACE inhibitors cause the following effects: (1) a reduction in the output of the sympathetic nervous system (reduced release of norepinephrine and epinephrine); (2) increased vasodilation of the vascular smooth muscle; (3) a reduced level of sodium retention and water; (4) an increased level of bradykinin; (5) an increased level of prostaglandins; and (6) an increased level of renin. Renin is important for the synthesis of AngI from angiotensinogen in the blood. AngI is converted to AngII by the angiotensin-converting enzyme (ACE).

Four problems observed with ACE inhibitors are angioedema (when the face and lips are swollen), hyperkalemia, and persistent cough. In addition, these agents are contraindicated during pregnancy.

ACE inhibitors are classified into three groups based on their chemical structures:

- Sulfhydryl group-containing ACE inhibitors: captopril (Apo-Capto, from Canada)
- Dicarboxylate-containing ACE inhibitors: lisinopril (Prinivil), benazepril (Lotensin), enalapril (Vasotec), quinapril (Accupril), moexipril (Univasc), ramipril (Altace)
- Phosphate-containing ACE inhibitors: fosinopril (Apo-Fosinopril, from Canada)

There are currently 11 ACE inhibitors marketed in the United States, which exhibit different potencies. Except for lisinopril and enalapril, the presence of food in the GI tract slows or reduces the absorption of ACE inhibitors.

Some of the ACE inhibitors, such as enalapril, have shown promise in reducing the incidence of MI, stroke, and death from arrhythmia. Both captopril and lisinopril produce renoprotection (indicated by changes in albumin excretion), particularly in patients with diabetes mellitus (DM) and renal failure. In addition, ACE inhibitors are known to reduce progression of retinopathy in DM type 1.

The renoprotective roles of ACE inhibitors result from several mechanisms. First, ACE inhibitors reduce glomerular capillary pressure by decreasing the arterial blood pressure and dilating the efferent arterioles of the kidneys, thereby reducing the risk of glomerular injury. Second, ACE inhibitors increase the selective permeability of glomerular filtration; that is, they significantly reduce the loss of renal protein into Bowman's capsule. Increased selective permeability, in turn, reduces exposure of the mesangium to proteinaceous factors that often promote mesangial cell growth. Stimulation and expansion of the mesangial growth lead to nephropathy (mesangial cells create a layer surrounding the glomerular capillaries). Third, because AngII is a growth factor, reducing the amount of AngII reduces the rate of mesangial cell growth (**Figure 10.34**).

Nonsteroidal anti-inflammatory drugs (NSAIDs) can worsen HF: Prostaglandins are responsible for vasodilation of afferent arterioles, and NSAIDs inhibit the synthesis of prostaglandins. The inhibition of prostaglandins results in a higher glomerular filtration rate (GFR) pressure along with a higher blood flow. Other drugs that should be avoided in patients with HF are two calcium-channel blockers, verapamil and diltiazem.

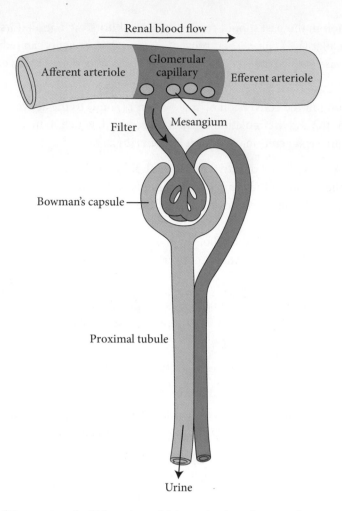

Figure 10.34 ACE inhibitors protect the kidneys by multiple mechanisms, but most importantly by inhibiting the expansion of mesangial cell growth.

Angiotensin-Receptor Blockers

Angiotensin-receptor blockers are known to reduce both LV pressure and volume. They are used for the treatment of hypertension because they block angiotensin type 1 (AT_1) receptors that are expressed in vascular smooth muscle, proximal tubule of the nephron, and adrenal medullary cells. This blockage of AT_1 receptors relaxes smooth muscle and leads to vasodilation, increasing renal salt and water excretion, reducing plasma volume, and decreasing cellular hypertrophy. Interestingly, because the AT_1 receptors have a feedback inhibitory mechanism that reduces the release of renin, blockage of AT_1 receptors results in an increase in renin and AngII levels. In contrast to ACE inhibitors, ARBs do not increase bradykinin levels and, as a result, are less likely to cause persistent cough. Well-known ARBs include candesartan (Atacand), losartan (Cozaar), telmisartan (Micardis), valsartan (Diovan), olmesartan (Benicar), and eprosartan (Teveten). Similar to ACE inhibitors, ARBs cause hypotension, hyperkalemia, and reduced renal function. It is not recommended to combine an ACE inhibitor with an ARB to treat hypertension.

Beta Blockers

A well-documented body of evidence indicates that beta blockers reduce morbidity and mortality in patients with HF. Therefore, HF patients are likely to receive beta blocker treatment even if their symptoms are well controlled with an ACE inhibitor or a vasodilator, and even if they do not suffer from edema. Beta blockers are also recommended for asymptomatic patients with a reduced LV ejection fraction (LVEF) to reduce the risk of progression to HF.

Beta blockers antagonize the sympathetic neurons, so they are useful in reducing the progress of HF by terminating or reversing ventricular remodeling, reducing myocyte death from catecholamine-induced necrosis or apoptosis, improving LV systolic function, reducing heart rate, reducing myocardial oxygen demand, and inhibiting renin release. Due to the negative inotropic effect caused by beta blockers, initiation of a beta blocker at normal doses in patients with HF can lead to symptomatic worsening or acute decompensation. To reduce the risk of acute decompensation, such therapy should be initiated at a low dose, followed by incremental increases of the dose. The most commonly used beta blockers include carvedilol (also exerts α-blocking properties; initial dose of 3.125 mg twice daily), carvedilol CR (initial dose of 10 mg once daily), metoprolol succinate (initial dose of 12.5 mg once daily), and bisoprolol (Zebeta; initial dose as low as 1.25 mg once daily).

Diuretics

Diuretics are used to reduce venous pressure, inhibit reabsorption of Na^+ and Cl^- ions from the renal tubules, decrease plasma volume, and decrease venous return to the heart (i.e., reduce ventricular preload). As a result, salt and water retention, edema, and pulmonary congestion are reduced and cardiac overwork and oxygen demand are decreased. While diuretics have no direct effect on cardiac contractility, a decrease in the cardiac size leads to improved pump efficiency, a critical benefit in improving systolic failure.

While furosemide (Lasix), torsemide (Demadex), and bumetanide (Burinex, from Canada) are effective diuretics at the loop of Henle, thiazides and potassium-sparing diuretics are effective at the distal portion of the renal tubule. Intravenous loop diuretics—especially furosemide—are used in the treatment of decompensated heart failure; furosemide, for example, reduces preload within 10 minutes. Torsemide has a better oral absorption and a longer duration of action compared to furosemide.

Patients who use a combination of thiazides and a loop diuretic may potentially develop dehydration, hyponatremia, or hypokalaemia. Consequently, electrolyte and renal function should be monitored every 2–3 days when combination therapy is prescribed (close monitoring of patients' electrolyte abnormalities, renal dysfunction, and symptomatic hypotension is required). More detailed information about diuretics is provided in the "Diuretics" section later in this chapter.

Vasodilators

Vasodilators are effective in reducing cardiac size, adjusting venous return (preload), and decreasing the resistance to ventricular ejection (i.e., afterload—increased afterload is a major factor in HF). Nitroglycerin is often used to treat severely acute HF. Oral vasodilators such as hydralazine (Apo-Hydralazine, from Canada) and isosorbide dinitrate (Isordil), when given in combination, have proved effective in reducing mortality in African Americans. The mechanism of action for isosorbide dinitrate is enhanced synthesis of cyclic guanosine monophosphate (cGMP), which in turn stimulates relaxation of the vascular smooth muscle.

Inotropic Drugs

A positive inotropic effect increases cardiac contractility, which in turn leads to increased cardiac output. The inotropic drugs that are often used for this purpose are β_1-receptor agonists such as dopamine and dobutamine and type III phosphodiesterase inhibitor, milrinone (Primacor, from Canada) for short-term IV therapy. Because all inotropic drugs increase intracellular calcium,

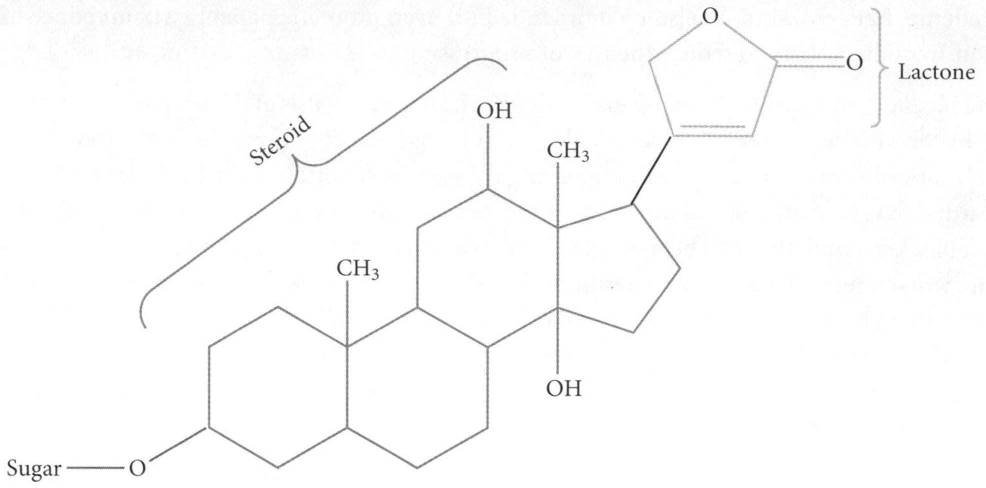

Figure 10.35 A typical digitalis structure and its constituents.

they enhance cardiac contractility. However, the use of inotropic drugs should be reserved for patients with acute decompensated heart failure (ADHF) who are unresponsive to vasodilators and diuretics.

When selecting an inotropic agent, it is important to take into consideration whether a patient is being treated with a beta blocker—being on a beta blocker reduces the response to the typical doses of the β_1-receptor agonists. Patients taking beta blockers should instead be treated with type III phosphodiesterase inhibitors because these drugs' mechanism of action is independent of β receptors.

Digitalis

Digitalis comprises a family of plants that serve as a source of cardiac glycosides of medicinal importance. The structure of digitalis is shown in **Figure 10.35**. All of the cardiac glycosides have a steroid nucleus and a series of sugars at carbon 3. Cardiac glycosides lack an ionizable group and, as a result, their solubility is not pH dependent.

The only cardiac glycoside that is available in the United States is digoxin, which is the prototype for cardiac glycosides. Oral digoxin has a good absorption profile (80% absorbed after oral administration). Digoxin is distributed in different tissues including the CNS. Approximately 70% of the parent drug is excreted unchanged by the kidneys. Consequently, renal disorders can affect the digoxin levels in the body.

Cardiac glycosides increase the Ca^{2+} concentration in the surrounding area of the contractile proteins during systole. Digoxin inhibits the cardiac Na^+/K^+-ATPase pump, leading to a resultant increase in intracellular sodium concentration. The Na^+/K^+-ATPase pump is responsible for removal of intracellular sodium through an exchange with potassium influx. When the pump is blocked, the increased intracellular Na^+ reduces the driving force for Na^+/Ca^{2+} exchange, which results in a higher intracellular Ca^{2+} concentration in cardiac myocytes. The increased Ca^{2+} level causes an increase in cardiac contraction as well as cardiac output. Digoxin can be used to treat severe LV systolic dysfunction following diuretics and ACE inhibitor treatment.

Digoxin has several notable side effects, including anorexia, nausea, and vomiting. Patients who take chronic digitalis are prone to toxicity due to an excessive calcium accumulation in cardiac cells (i.e., calcium overload), which may result in arrhythmias. In addition, acute intoxication is often caused by suicidal or accidental overdose with digitalis—a condition that has severe medical consequences such as cardiac depression and cardiac arrest. A decrease in the serum potassium level can potentiate the cardiotoxicity of digoxin (which explains the drug–drug interactions of digoxin with thiazide and loop diuretics). However, the serum potassium level should not rise above 5 mEq/L. A serum concentration of digoxin exceeding 2.4 ng/mL is toxic. Digoxin immune Fab (DigiFab) is an antidote agent to treat digoxin toxicity. It binds to digoxin, and the drug-antibody complex is excreted by the kidneys.

Aldosterone Antagonists

Aldosterone antagonists block the mineralocorticoid receptors in nephrons of the kidney. Two such agents available in the U.S. market are spironolactone (Aldactone) and eplerenone (Inspra). These agents inhibit sodium reabsorption and potassium excretion by the kidney. In the heart, aldosterone antagonists are useful agents that inhibit the cardiac extracellular matrix and collagen deposition, thereby preventing the cardiac fibrosis and ventricular remodeling that might otherwise occur after a myocardial infarction. While spironolactone has a high affinity for androgen and progesterone receptors, eplerenone has a low affinity for these receptors. Spironolactone may produce gynecomastia and other sexual adverse effects. Eplerenone is contraindicated in patients with creatinine clearance (CrCl) of 30 mL/min or less and serum K^+ greater than 5.5 mEq/L. Recently, it was shown that aldosterone antagonists prevent the systemic pro-inflammatory state and oxidative stress, both of which are caused by aldosterone.

Because aldosterone antagonists spare K^+ excretion, monitoring of the K^+ level is important to avoid hyperkalemia. As a result, it is important for pharmacists to counsel patients not to take supplemental potassium when starting aldosterone antagonists.

Learning Bridge 10.7

BB, a patient with CHF, was stabilized for the past four years with furosemide, ramipril, and carvedilol. In addition, BB claims to be on a salt-restricted diet. Ten days ago, BB came to the clinic with the complications of serious edema and weight gain.

A. What will be your suggestions to treat BB's edema?
B. Do you need to monitor any electrolytes following the suggested intervention(s)?

Hypertension

Hypertension is the medical condition of having a persistently elevated arterial blood pressure. It is one of the major risk factors for cardiovascular (CV) disease in the United States. Indeed, hypertension is called the (silent killer) because it does not necessarily produce any symptoms to warn patients of their elevated blood pressure. It is very important to diagnose hypertension to reduce CV morbidity and mortality. In fact, there is a clear correlation between blood pressure and CV morbidity and mortality. The seventh report of the Joint National Committee on the Detection, Evaluation, and Treatment of High Blood Pressure (JNC 7) provides effective treatment guidelines to manage hypertension in the United States.

There are two types of hypertension:

- *Essential hypertension:* This form of hypertension is caused by an unknown pathophysiology. etiology. Although incurable, this most prevalent form of the disease (accounting for more than 90% of all cases) can be successfully managed by therapeutic agents.

- *Secondary hypertension:* This form of hypertension is caused by various medical conditions affecting the kidneys, arteries, heart, or endocrine glands or is induced by specific drug therapy. The most common cause of secondary hypertension is severe chronic kidney disease. In contrast to essential hypertension, secondary hypertension occurs in only a small percentage of the population (fewer than 10% of all cases).

While awareness of hypertension seems to be high, treatment and management of this blood pressure condition seem to fall short in the United States. For instance, data collected from 2003 to 2006 by the National Health and Nutrition Examination Survey and the National Center for Health Statistics indicated that 77.6% of all persons with hypertension in the United States were aware of their disease. The same study found that only 67.9% of patients were receiving some form of antihypertensive treatment and only 44.1% of all patients had a controlled blood pressure.

Approximately one-third of the U.S population (men and women) has a blood pressure that is higher or equal to 140/90 mm Hg. Different ethnic groups have different prevalence rates. For instance, the highest prevalence is found among non-Hispanic blacks (45% in women, 44% in men) and non-Hispanic whites (31% in women, 34% in men). The prevalence rates among Mexican Americans are 32% in women and 26% in men; the rates for American Indians/Alaska Natives are 25% in both women and men.

To diagnose hypertension, more than one blood pressure reading is required. Often the clinician will measure the blood pressure a few times during two or more clinical visits before a patient is finally diagnosed with hypertension. Indeed, JNC 7 recommends blood pressure assessment in adults (age greater than or equal to 18 years) to be based on the average of two or more blood pressure values from two or more clinical visits.

The major goal in treating hypertension is to reduce hypertension-associated complications, particularly progression to any CV risk. The normal blood pressure is less than 120/80 mm Hg (systolic/diastolic). Achieving different systolic/diastolic pressures is associated with different levels of hypertension. For instance, while a blood pressure less than 140/90 mm Hg is the goal to reduce CV risk, a blood pressure of less than 130/80 mm Hg is the goal for patients with diabetes and patients with significant chronic kidney disease. In addition, the American Heart Association recommends a blood pressure less than 130/80 mm Hg for patients with known coronary artery disease (MI, stable angina, and unstable angina) or atherosclerotic vascular disease (ischemic stroke, transient ischemic attack, peripheral arterial disease, and abdominal aortic aneurysm).

Many factors contribute to elevated blood pressure, including defects in the renin–angiotensin–aldosterone system (RAAS), disorders in natriuretic hormone and electrolytes (sodium and calcium), abnormal neuronal mechanisms, hyperinsulinemia, and use of drugs such as steroids, contraceptives, alcohol, cyclosporine, sympathomimetics, MAO inhibitors, TCAs, and NSAIDs. A variety of physiological conditions can result in elevated blood pressure as well. For instance, some specific electrolyte disorders can lead to hypertension. Hypocalcemia (or calcium deficiency; see also the *Introduction to Nutrients* chapter) can disturb the balance between intracellular and extracellular calcium concentrations. An increased intracellular calcium concentration will, in turn, increase peripheral vascular resistance. As a result, dietary calcium supplementation may reduce blood pressure. In another physiological condition leading to hypertension, both α and β presynaptic receptors may provide negative and positive feedback to the norepinephrine-containing vesicles of the neurons. While stimulation of presynaptic α-receptors inhibits norepinephrine release, stimulation of presynaptic β-receptors will increase norepinephrine release.

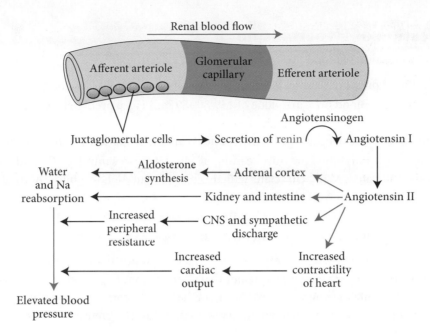

Figure 10.36 Renin has a profound effect on blood pressure by affecting a cascade of physiological events.

Increased insulin secretion from the pancreas cells is known to increase blood pressure by different mechanisms. For instance, an increase in insulin concentration can lead to greater retention of renal Na^+, which in turn will enhance sympathetic nervous system activity. Because insulin can have growth hormone–like actions, it can cause hypertrophy of vascular smooth muscle cells. In addition, insulin can increase intracellular calcium, leading to increased vascular resistance.

The RAAS is involved with most regulatory components of blood pressure and makes significant contributions to the homeostatic regulation of blood pressure. The kidney regulates RAAS activation and regulation. Because the RAAS regulates sodium, potassium, and blood volume, it strongly influences vascular tone and the sympathetic nervous system. The juxtaglomerular cells of the kidney play a major role in the development of blood pressure; they function as baroreceptor sensors. This function arises because decreased renal artery pressure, decreased kidney blood flow, or decreased delivery of sodium and chloride to the distal tubule stimulates the juxtaglomerular cells to secrete renin. **Figure 10.36** describes the effects of renin on multiple pathways that affect blood pressure. Because β-receptors are also found on the surface membranes of juxtaglomerular cells, a beta blocker can inhibit the release of renin as well.

Blood pressure is diagnosed by measuring the pressure in the arterial wall and is given in the unit "millimeters of mercury" (mm Hg). Both systolic and diastolic pressures are measured. Systolic pressure represents the peak value, which is achieved during cardiac contraction; diastolic pressure represents the pressure when the cardiac chambers are filled following contraction. Approximately 65% of the cardiac cycle is spent in diastole and 35% in systole. The difference between systolic and diastolic pressures, called the pulse pressure, represents arterial wall tension. In patients who are 50 years or older, systolic pressure is a stronger predictor of a CV disease than diastolic pressure.

The blood pressure is lowest during sleep, but increases sharply a few hours prior to awakening, with the highest blood pressure occurring in the midmorning. During physical activity or emotional stress, blood pressure readings may increase as well.

Classification of Hypertension

The JNC 7 classification of blood pressure includes four categories:

- *Normal:* Blood pressure reading less than 120/80 mm Hg (systolic/diastolic).
- *Prehypertension:* Blood pressure value of 139/80–89 mm Hg; a prehypertensive state for which no medication is necessary. However, in compelling cases, diuretics may be used. Blood pressure values of prehypertensive patients are likely to increase in the future.
- *Stage 1 hypertension:* Blood pressure reading of 140–159/90–99 mm Hg. Thiazide diuretics are usually indicated. Many clinicians will also consider an ACE inhibitor, ARB blocker, beta blocker, or calcium-channel blocker.
- *Stage 2 hypertension:* Blood pressure reading greater than 160/100 mm Hg. A combination of a thiazide-type diuretic with other antihypertensive agents is used.

In addition to these categories, hypertensive emergency and urgency are conditions in which the blood pressure values are very high (greater than 180/120 mm Hg). Hypertensive emergency is characterized by acute or progressing target-organ damage. In contrast, a high blood pressure without acute or progressing target-organ injury is classified as hypertensive urgency.

Treatment of Hypertension

The overall goal in treating and managing hypertension is to decrease CV morbidity and mortality. Medications play an important role in providing significant clinical benefits, because the increased risks of CV disease and death associated with elevated blood pressure are significantly reduced by antihypertensive therapy. Nevertheless, medical therapy of hypertension is a complex process, as the disease is rarely symptomatic. While monotherapy is often used for the treatment of mild and moderate hypertension, multiple drugs are used, in a stepwise fashion, to reach an adequate blood pressure control for complicated conditions.

The most commonly used antihypertensive drugs are ACE inhibitors, angiotensin II receptor blockers, beta blockers, calcium-channel blockers, diuretics, aldosterone antagonists, and direct renin inhibitors. In addition, nonpharmacologic approaches, such as salt restriction and weight reduction, are considered along with the medical therapy. For instance, a reasonable dietary goal is to have 70–100 mEq of sodium per day, which can be achieved by avoiding salting food during or after cooking. Changing eating habits can also be beneficial. For instance, eating more fruits and vegetables and less fat and reducing alcohol consumption (i.e., drinking two or fewer drinks per day) can lower blood pressure.

Age and ethnicity are other factors that one should take into consideration when treating patients with hypertension. For instance, elderly patients of almost all ethnicities respond better to diuretics and beta blockers compared to ACE inhibitors. African Americans of all ages do not respond well to ACE inhibitors but respond better to diuretics and calcium-channel blockers.

Reducing weight can help reduce blood pressure in 75% of overweight patients with mild to moderate hypertension. Regular exercise has been shown to normalize blood pressure.

Diuretics

Diuretics increase the rate of urine flow as well as the rate of Na^+ and Cl^- excretion. Sodium chloride is the major determinant of the volume of the extracellular fluid and, consequently, is a good target for diuretics to reduce extracellular fluid volume by decreasing total body NaCl. Therefore, a drug that blocks the proximal tubular reabsorption of NaCl is a powerful and useful diuretic.

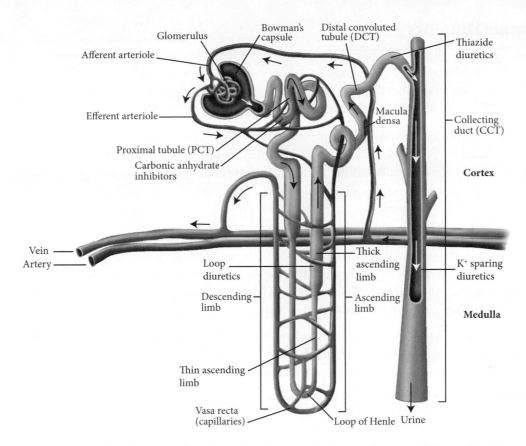

Figure 10.37 A simple architecture of a nephron that demonstrates the site of action of different diuretics.

A nephron contains four segments: the proximal convoluted tubule (PCT), the thick ascending limb of the loop of Henle (TAL), the distal convoluted tubule (DCT), and the cortical collecting tubule (CCT). Each of these sections has a different mechanism for reabsorbing sodium and other electrolytes. (**Figure 10.37**).

Depending on the mode of action, diuretics are classified as carbonic anhydrate inhibitors, loop diuretics, thiazide diuretics, thiazide-like diuretics (similar in action but do not have the structure of thiazides), or potassium-sparing diuretics. Keep in mind that diuretics not only increase the excretion of Na and Cl ions, but may also increase the excretion of other cations such as K^+, H^+, Ca^{2+}, and Mg^{2+}; anions such as HCO_3^- and $H_2PO_4^-$; and uric acid.

While HCO_3^-, NaCl, glucose, and amino acids are reabsorbed via specific transport systems in the early part of the PCT, potassium ions are reabsorbed via the paracellular pathway. In contrast, water is passively reabsorbed to maintain the osmolality of the proximal tubular fluid. As the tubule fluid proceeds along the length of the proximal tubule, the luminal concentrations of these ions/molecules decrease. A significant portion of filtered sodium and potassium ions (65%), 85% of the HCO_3^-, and 60% of the water are reabsorbed in the proximal tubule. In addition, all of the filtered glucose and amino acids are reabsorbed in the proximal tubule.

Despite the fact that the cortical collecting tubule reabsorbs only 2–5% of NaCl, it plays an important role in the diuretic action. The CCT is the final site of NaCl reabsorption and, as a result, is responsible for the regulation of body fluid volume and for determining the final sodium concentration of the urine. In addition, the CCT is the most important site of potassium secretion.

Thiazide Diuretics

For most patients with hypertension, thiazide diuretics are the first-line therapy. However, for patients without compelling indications, ACE inhibitors, ARBs, or CCBs may be used as first-line therapy. Extensive studies have shown that thiazide diuretics can significantly reduce the risk of stroke, MI, CV disease, and CV-related mortality.

Thiazide agents block the Na/Cl transporter (inhibit NaCl reabsorption) from the luminal side of epithelial cells in the distal convoluted tubule. These drugs can decrease Na^+ and water retention, blood volume, cardiac output, and peripheral resistance—all effects that lead to lower blood pressure. In contrast to loop diuretics, thiazides enhance Ca^{2+} reabsorption. As a result, these agents can mask hypocalcemia caused by hyperparathyroidism, carcinoma, and sarcoidosis (growth of inflammatory cells in the lungs, eyes, and skin).

All thiazides can be administered orally. The mainstay thiazide therapy is hydrochlorothiazide (Microzide). Chlorothiazide (Diuril) is the only thiazide that, in addition to oral tablets and suspension formulations, is available for parenteral administration. Chlorthalidone (Thalitone) is slowly absorbed and has a longer duration of action.

Thiazides are secreted in the proximal tubule by the active tubular secretion system (see also the *Introduction to Pharmacokinetics* chapter); as a result, their release competes with the secretion of uric acid. This competition blocks uric acid secretion and consequently elevates the serum uric acid level, which can cause problems for patients with gout. Chlorthalidone is almost twice as potent as hydrochlorothiazide in lowering blood pressure.

Loop Diuretics

Loop diuretics specifically block NaCl reabsorption in the thick ascending limb (Figure 10.37) and inhibit the cotransport of sodium, potassium, and chloride. Because of the large NaCl absorptive capacity of the thick ascending limb, loop diuretics are the most effective diuretic agents available on the market. Furosemide is the mainstay drug in this category. While furosemide, bumetanide, and torsemide are sulfonamide derivatives, ethacrynic acid is not. Thus this agent is a good choice for patients who are allergic to sulfonamide.

All of the loop diuretics act via the same mechanism. These agents are very effective in patients with severe chronic kidney disease (i.e., when the GFR is less than 30 mL/min; see also the *Introduction to Nutrients* chapter) or severe edema. The loop diuretics are short-acting agents, with diuresis occurring over a 4-hour period following a dose. Note that when loop diuretics are used in tandem with aminoglycosides (e.g., gentamicin, neomycin, kanamycin), there is a risk that the patient may develop ototoxicity.

Loop diuretics are not first-line therapies for hypertension, but rather are usually reserved for situations in which the patient does not respond to a thiazide agent or the response is inadequate. Because thiazides cause excretion of K^+ and Na^+, but not Ca^{2+}, use of these agents in patients with hypercalcemia can be problematic. Notably, furosemide is usually a better choice than thiazides for the treatment of patients with hypercalcemia.

As mentioned earlier in this chapter, prostaglandins play an important role in maintaining glomerular filtration by causing vasodilation of the afferent arteriole. NSAIDs are known to inhibit the synthesis of prostaglandins. If NSAIDs are used together with loop diuretics, the efficacy of loop diuretics is decreased.

Potassium-Sparing Diuretics

Because they cause Na$^+$ excretion but decrease potassium and hydrogen ion excretion, agents in this category are called potassium-sparing diuretics. Spironolactone and eplerenone are two steroid derivatives that act as antagonists of aldosterone receptors in the collecting tubules of the nephron. Aldosterone is a mineralocorticoid hormone secreted by the adrenal cortex of the body. Both potassium-sparing agents reduce the expression of genes controlling the synthesis of epithelial sodium ion channels and Na$^+$/K$^+$-ATPase pumps and have a long duration of action (24–72 hours). In addition, both agents have long-term benefits in heart failure. Amiloride (Midamor, from Canada) and triamterene (Dyrenium) are also classified as potassium-sparing agents and block the epithelial sodium channels in the DCT and CCT of the nephron. However, these two agents have a shorter duration of action (12–24 hours) than spironolactone and eplerenone.

Potassium-sparing agents cause hyperkalemia, so they should not be given with potassium supplements. In addition, one has to be careful if they are prescribed with ACE inhibitors and angiotensin receptor blockers, as the risk of hyperkalemia is even greater.

Beta Blockers

In hypertensive patients with no compelling indications, treatment should be initiated with other agents (thiazides, ACE inhibitors, ARBs, and CCBs) before a beta blocker is used. Beta blockers are considered first-line agents to treat specific compelling indications (i.e., post-MI and coronary artery disease). While a few mechanisms of action have been suggested for beta blockers, none of those mechanisms alone can consistently explain the reduction of blood pressure. As mentioned elsewhere in this chapter, beta blockers produce negative chronotropic and inotropic effects and, consequently, can reduce the cardiac output, an ability that makes them useful as antihypertensive agents.

Because β-receptors are present on the membranes of juxtaglomerular cells, a beta blocker can inhibit the release of renin. To some degree there is a link between plasma renin concentration and the antihypertensive efficacy of a beta blocker. Research has suggested that hypertensive patients with low plasma renin concentrations respond well to beta blockers; thus some additional mechanism must account for the antihypertensive effect of a beta blocker. While pharmacodynamic and pharmacokinetic differences (e.g., first-pass metabolism, route of elimination, degree of hydrophilicity or hydrophobicity, and serum half-life) are observed among beta blockers, all of these agents provide a similar degree of blood pressure lowering effects. Surprisingly, beta blockers are more effective in hypertensive patients who are white and young compared to black and elderly patients.

When considering beta-blocker therapy, it is important to remember the sites of β receptors. While β_1 receptors are found in the heart and kidney, β_2 receptors are found in the lungs, liver, pancreas, and arteriolar smooth muscle. Stimulation of β_1 receptors increases heart rate, contractility, lipolysis, and renin release, whereas β_2 receptor stimulation results in bronchodilation and vasodilation (see also Table 10.2). Accordingly, cardioselective beta blockers will not cause bronchospasm or vasoconstriction. Blocking β_1 receptors may, however, mask, a warning sign of hypoglycemia. As such, patient education is critical when counseling patients with diabetes who use antidiabetic agents and are also prescribed beta blockers.

Cardioselective beta blockers such as atenolol, metoprolol, and nebivolol (Bystolic) are preferred when using a beta blocker as an antihypertensive agent. This is particularly true when treating hypertensive patients who also suffer from asthma or diabetes. The cardioselectivity of beta blockers, however, is dose dependent. At higher doses, a cardioselective agent acts on both β_1 and β_2 receptors. The exact dose that leads to the loss of the cardioselectivity varies from patient to patient. Propranolol and atenolol are the most and least lipophilic drugs, respectively. The lipophilic nature of propranolol explains why a higher concentration of this agent reaches the brain compared to atenolol at equivalent doses.

Because beta blockers antagonize β receptors in the myocardium, they can cause bradycardia and atrioventricular conduction abnormalities and increase the risk of developing acute heart failure. However, a decrease in the heart rate may be helpful for patients with atrial arrhythmias (atrial fibrillation and atrial flutter).

It is important to advise patients not to discontinue therapy abruptly because of the risk of cardiac events such as unstable angina, MI, or even death in patients with coronary disease. Up-regulation of β receptors is associated with these events. In addition, abrupt cessation can lead to rebound hypertension. Therefore, discontinuation of beta blockers should always be gradual, with a dose reduction occurring over 1 to 2 weeks.

ACE Inhibitors

Most clinicians prefer to prescribe ACE inhibitors as first-line therapy to treat hypertension. However, if an ACE inhibitor is not used as the first-line therapy, it can be considered as a second-line agent for this indication. Similar to beta blockers, ACE inhibitors are most effective in young white patients. For patients with diabetes and hypertension and those with heart failure and diabetes, ACE inhibitors are first-line agents.

As described earlier, angiotensin II is a major player in the regulation of the arterial blood pressure; ACE inhibitors block the conversion of angiotensin I to angiotensin II. Angiotensin II is an effective vasoconstrictor that promotes aldosterone release. The release of aldosterone increases sodium and water reabsorption, with accompanying potassium loss. While ACE is widely distributed in many tissues and different cell types, it is predominantly present in endothelial cells lining the blood vessels. Hence, the major site for the production of angiotensin II is the blood vessels.

ACE inhibitors have some other antihypertensive roles as well. These agents block degradation of bradykinin and promote the synthesis of vasodilating molecules such as prostaglandin E_2 and prostacyclin. Indeed, an increased amount of bradykinin enhances the antihypertensive effects of ACE inhibitors, albeit at the cost of persistent dry cough production (in 10–20% of patients). This dry cough does not cause respiratory illness, but rather is troublesome to patients and can lead to noncompliance issues.

Another major side effect of ACE inhibitors is elevation of the serum potassium level. Consequently, patients with chronic kidney disease or those who use potassium supplements, potassium-sparing diuretics, ARBs, or direct renin inhibitors are at risk of developing hyperkalemia when they concurrently take ACE inhibitors. Monitoring serum potassium and creatinine levels within the first month of initiating or increasing the dose of an ACE inhibitor is helpful as a means to prevent hyperkalemia. Although ACE inhibitors protect the diabetic kidney, perhaps the most severe adverse effect associated with these agents is development of acute kidney failure (occurs in fewer than 1% of patients).

A less frequently observed side effect is angioedema (lip and tongue swelling and possibly difficulty breathing). This side effect occurs in fewer than 1% of users, though it is often seen in African Americans and smokers. One has to anticipate a small decrease in the GFR and an increase in the serum creatinine when an ACE inhibitor is used. These effects result from inhibition of angiotensin II–mediated vasoconstriction of the efferent arteriole of the glomerulus in the kidney.

Most ACE inhibitors are given once daily, but when higher doses are required, these agents are given twice daily to maintain 24-hour effects, particularly with enalapril, benazepril, quinapril, and ramipril. ACE inhibitors are contraindicated in patients on lithium therapy (ACE inhibitors can increase lithium serum concentrations) and during pregnancy (they cause renal damage to the fetus).

Learning Bridge 10.8

In his physician's office, a 32-year-old male state government official was diagnosed with type 2 diabetes and hypertension. He was started on metformin and a sulfonylurea agent for diabetes. For his blood pressure management, you as an ambulatory care pharmacist were asked to recommend an agent from the therapeutic categories of beta blockers or ACE inhibitors.

A. What will your recommendation be? Justify your answer by citing the advantages and disadvantages of your choice.

B. The patient was prescribed lisinopril 5 mg po, once daily. His systolic and diastolic pressure readings returned to normal, but he complained of persistent cough. What will your recommendation be?

Angiotensin II Receptor Blockers

While an ACE inhibitor inhibits formation of angiotensin II, an ARB blocks the binding of angiotensin II to its type 1 (AT_1) receptor. Binding of angiotensin II to the AT_1 receptor triggers a series of events that includes vasoconstriction, aldosterone release, sympathetic activation, antidiuretic hormone release, and constriction of the efferent arterioles of the glomerulus in the kidney. Therefore, blocking the AT_1 receptors can reduce an elevated blood pressure.

ARBs are selective blockers of the AT_1 receptors, but do not have any effect on AT_2 receptors (stimulation of the AT_2 receptor opens K^+ channels, inhibits cell growth, and increases synthesis of nitric oxide, which is followed by increased intracellular concentration of cGMP). Compared to ACE inhibitors, ARBs do not block the breakdown of bradykinin; this characteristic is of particular interest, because bradykinin has a vasodilating effect. Since ARBs do not impede the metabolism of bradykinin, they do not produce any significant dry cough. Therefore, ARBs are good alternatives for patients who require ACE inhibitors but who experience an annoying and persistent dry cough with those medications.

Extensive research has indicated that the ARBs' benefits in reducing CV disease are similar to those of ACE inhibitor therapy in hypertension. In addition, a combination of an ACE inhibitor with an ARB did not show additional CV benefits, suggesting that concurrent use of an ACE inhibitor and an ARB for the management of hypertension is not necessary.

ARBs are more beneficial for patients with type 2 diabetes and nephropathy, which suggests that their effects on the efferent arteriole may be different from the effects of ACE inhibitors. Consequently, ARBs do not lead to renal failure for patients with renal artery stenosis. In contrast to ACE inhibitors, most ARBs have long half-lives and require once-daily dosing. A few ARBs such as candesartan, eprosartan, losartan, and valsartan have short half-lives and may require twice-daily dosing. Addition of low doses of a thiazide-type diuretic to an ARB regimen can increase the antihypertensive effect of the ARB agent. Similar to the case for ACE inhibitors, use of ARBs is contraindicated during pregnancy.

Renin Inhibitors

Inhibition of renin action can reduce the formation of angiotensin I and angiotensin II and, as a result, lowers blood pressure (Figure 10.36). A recently approved selective renin inhibitor, aliskiren (Tekturna), is used in the treatment of hypertension. It has a long half-life (24 hours; given once daily) and is eliminated unchanged through biliary excretion. Aliskiren reduces blood pressure similar to an ACE inhibitor or ARB. Although this agent does not produce a dry cough, researchers have not determined whether it has the other side effects associated with angiotensin antagonists/ACE inhibitors. Aliskiren can be combined with ACE inhibitors or ARBs if necessary. Similar to ACE inhibitors and ARBs. it is contraindicated in pregnancy because of fetal toxicity. In addition, renin inhibitors can cause potassium retention. In 2012, the FDA announced a new contraindication regarding the concurrent use of aliskiren and ACE inhibitors or ARBs in patients with diabetes or renal impairment.

As this discussion suggests, renin inhibitors, ACE inhibitors, and ARBs have, to some extent, similar mechanisms of action. **Table 10.5** summarizes the differences and similarities among these three classes of antihypertensive agents.

Table 10.5 Characteristics of Three Classes of Antihypertensive Agents

Characteristic	Angiotensin-Converting Enzyme Inhibitors	Angiotensin II Receptor Blockers	Renin Inhibitors
Mechanism of action	Inhibit the formation of angiotensin II from angiotensin I	Block the binding of angiotensin II to its type 1 (AT_1) receptor	Reduce the formation of angiotensin I and angiotensin II
Use	First-line therapy to treat hypertension, particularly in patients with both diabetes and hypertension	If an ACE inhibitor is not effective in reducing blood pressure or cannot be tolerated, ARBs can be used	To reduce blood pressure
Maximum antihypertensive effect	In less than 1 day (for many patients, after 6–8 hours)	In less than 1 day (for many patients, after 6–8 hours)	Within 2 weeks
Gender and age	Most effective in young white patients	Effective in African American patients	Unknown
Degradation of bradykinin	No	Yes	Unknown
Cough	High prevalence (10–20% of patients)	Small prevalence (fewer than 3% of patients)	Small prevalence (fewer than 1% of patients)
Risk of angioedema	Increases	None	Unknown
Serum potassium level	Increases	Increases	Increases
Contraindications	Patients on lithium therapy; during pregnancy	During pregnancy (due to injury and death of the developing fetus)	During pregnancy (due to injury and death of the developing fetus); in combination with an ACEI or an ARB in patients with renal impairment (due to nephrotoxic effect)

Calcium-Channel Blockers

Calcium-channel blockers (CCBs) are used as a first-line therapy to treat hypertension. In addition, they are used in coronary artery disease and in patients who have both diabetes and hypertension. They are also used in combination with other antihypertensive agents.

CCBs' mechanism of action is to block Ca^{2+} channels and thereby reduce the influx of calcium across the cell membrane of cardiac and smooth muscle cells. In the absence of CCBs, when vascular smooth muscle cell is stimulated, the voltage-sensitive calcium channels in the cell membrane open to promote calcium influx. This influx, in turn, releases stored calcium from the sarcoplasmic reticulum (SR; the network of tubules that surrounds the myofibrils). The increased intracellular free calcium binds to calmodulin, a step that is followed by activation of myosin light-chain kinase. The latter enzyme enables myosin to be phosphorylated and interact with actin to produce contraction.

There are two types of calcium channels: a high-voltage channel (L-type) and a low-voltage channel (T-type). The CCBs currently available in the U.S. market are L-type channel blockers.

Except for amlodipine (Norvasc) and felodipine (Plendil, from Canada), all CCBs have negative inotropic effects. Structurally, two subclasses of CCBs are distinguished: non-dihydropyridines such as verapamil (Calan) and diltiazem (Cardizem), and dihydropyridines (all other CCBs) (**Figure 10.38**). From a pharmacodynamic point of view, agents belonging to one class differ from those in other classes, but all CCBs have similar antihypertensive effectiveness.

Non-dihydropyridines decrease heart rate and slow atrioventricular nodal conduction. Verapamil produces negative inotropic and chronotropic effects, which can cause systolic heart failure in high-risk patients; diltiazem produces these effects to a lesser extent.

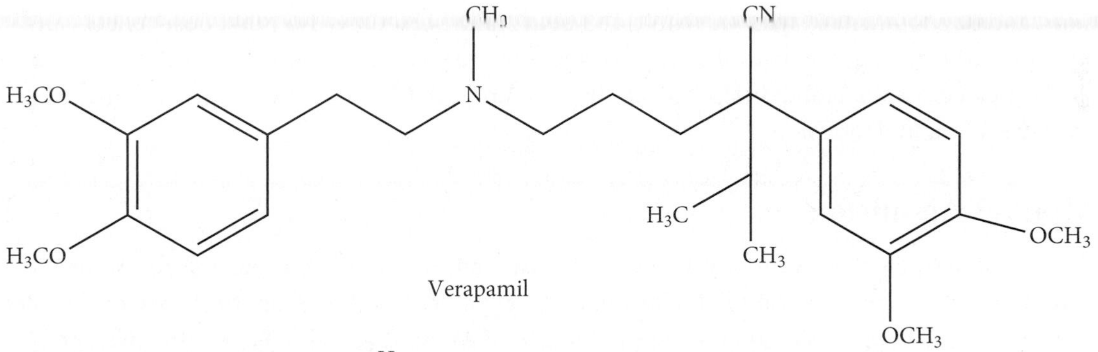

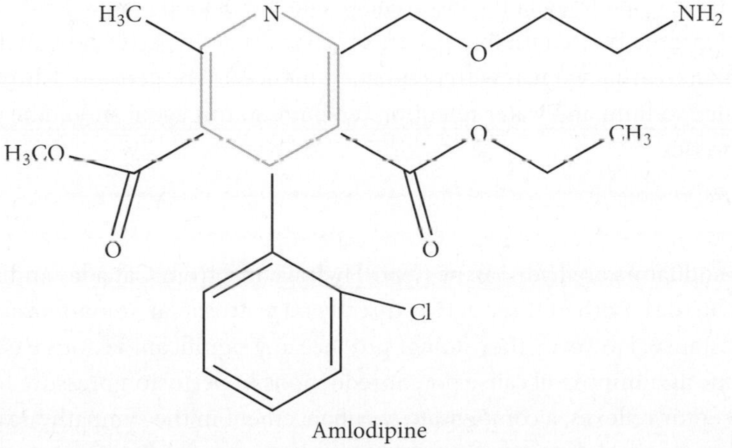

Figure 10.38 Structure of a non-dihydropyridine calcium-channel blocker, verapamil, and a dihydropyridine, amlodipine. Notice the pyridine ring in the structure of amlodipine.

In contrast, because of dihydropyridines' peripheral vasodilating effect, these agents can cause a baroreceptor-mediated reflex increase in heart rate. Dihydropyridines do not change the conduction rate through the atrioventricular node, so they do not produce supraventricular tachyarrhythmias. Of note, Amlodipine has shown to be more effective than lisinopril in treating African American patients with hypertension.

Verapamil causes significant drug interactions because it is capable of inhibiting CYP3A4. In addition, because of the increased risk of heart block with non-dihydropyridines, a healthcare practitioner has to be careful when prescribing verapamil and diltiazem in combination with a beta blocker. A dihydropyridine derivative agent should be given if a CCB is needed in combination with a beta blocker to treat hypertension.

Alpha Receptor Blockers

Alpha-1 receptor blockers act as competitive antagonists of the α_1 receptors in the peripheral vasculature and block the uptake of catecholamines in smooth muscle cells. The most frequently used agents in this category include prazosin (Minipress), terazosin (Apo-Terazosin, from Canada), and doxazosin (Cardura). Evidence-based studies have indicated that thiazide-type diuretics, when compared to α_1 blockers, are more effective in preventing CV disease in patients with hypertension. Alpha-1 receptor blockers are typically used in combination with first-line antihypertensive agents.

In addition to their role as antihypertensive agents, the α_1 blockers can provide benefits in men with BPH. These drugs antagonize postsynaptic α_1 receptors that are located on the prostate capsule, thereby reducing the resistance to urinary outflow.

One serious side effect of α_1 blockers is the "first dose" effect that is produced either by the first initial dose or during dose escalation. This effect is characterized by transient dizziness, palpitations, and development of syncope within 1–3 hours of the first dose. The "first dose" effect can be improved by taking the first initial dose or the subsequent increased dose at bedtime. Since α_1 blockers can cross the blood–brain barrier, they can produce CNS side effects such as lethargy, vivid dreams, and depression.

Alpha-2 Agonists

In contrast to α_1 blockers, centrally acting α_2 agonists can stimulate α_2 receptors in the brain and lower blood pressure. This stimulation can reduce sympathetic outflow from the vasomotor center in the brain and decreases blood pressure. A few agents in this category are clonidine (Catapres), guanabenz (Wytensin, from Canada), guanfacine (Tenex), and methyldopa (Apo-Methyldopa, from Canada). While clonidine is often used in patients with resistant hypertension, methyldopa is the drug of choice when treating women with pregnancy-induced hypertension. Chronic use of methyldopa can induce sodium and water retention (edema), so this agent should be given in combination with a diuretic.

Vasodilators

Two frequently used vasodilators are hydralazine (Apo-Hydralazine, from Canada) and minoxidil (Loniten, from Canada). Both of these agents directly relax arteriolar smooth muscle and decrease peripheral resistance. However, they do not produce any significant venous vasodilation. Because both hydralazine and minoxidil cause potent reductions in perfusion pressure followed by activation of baroreceptor reflexes, a compensatory enhancement in the sympathetic outflow is produced. This effect increases heart rate, cardiac output, and release of renin. The compensatory mechanism is worse with minoxidil compared with hydralazine. However, the compensatory baro-receptor response can be alleviated by combining vasodilators with a beta blocker.

Because hydralazine can cause a dose-dependent lupus-like syndrome (see also the *Introduction to Immunology* chapter), it has limited clinical use for chronic management of hypertension. Minoxidil can cause hirsutism (increased hair growth on the face, arms, back, and chest), so it has also been used (topically in Rogaine) to stimulate hair growth. Minoxidil is reserved for treating resistant hypertension and for patients who require hydralazine but experience serious drug-induced lupus-like side effects with the agent.

Hyperlipidemia

In the United States, deaths caused by atherosclerosis outnumber deaths caused by cancer, accidents, chronic lung disease, and diabetes combined. Atherosclerosis, a condition in which blood vessels become narrowed by plaque formation, is caused by abnormalities in plasma lipoproteins, and is a significant factor contributing to coronary heart disease (CHD). CHD can be caused by atherosclerosis of small blood vessels of the heart. Hyperlipidemia occurs in approximately 16% of adults in the United States. Premature coronary atherosclerosis results in ischemic heart disease and is the most common consequence of dyslipidemia.

It is important to understand the differences between dyslipidemia, hyperlipidemia, and hyper-lipoproteinemia. Dyslipidemia is defined as any abnormality in the function of lipids: total cholesterol, low-density lipoprotein cholesterol (LDL-C), triacylglycerols, and high-density lipoprotein cholesterol (HDL-C), or a combination of these abnormalities. Hyperlipidemia is defined as a high plasma concentration of these lipids, and hyperlipoproteinemia is defined as having an increased serum concentration of the lipoprotein macromolecules.

The major risk factors for CHD are elevated LDL, decreased HDL, cigarette smoking, hypertension, type 2 diabetes, advancing age, and family history of CHD events. Interestingly, when total cholesterol levels are lower than 160 mg/dL, the risk of CHD is significantly reduced, even in the presence of other risk factors. LDL cholesterol plays an important role in CHD: For every 1 mg/dL change in LDL-C, the relative risk for CHD is proportionally changed by approximately 1%. However, this correlation is weaker in women and elderly patients. By comparison, for every 1 mg/dL increase in HDL-C, the risk of future cardiovascular disease is reduced by 2%. An inverse correlation exists between HDL-C and CHD, because HDL-C is involved in reversing cholesterol transport by delivering cholesterol from the cell wall to the liver for cholesterol clearance. In addition, HDL-C can prevent LDL-C oxidation and may inhibit platelet aggregation and activation.

Factors such as elevated plasma cholesterol levels and consumption of foods rich in saturated (animal) fats are associated with development of CHD. There is a correlation between consumption of excess saturated fat and elevated cholesterol levels. Therefore, it is important to reduce the intake of saturated fat when treating hypercholesterolemia. Fasting lipoprotein levels should be tested once every 5 years in adults 20 years or older. A follow-up lipoprotein profile screening is required if total cholesterol is 200 mg/dL or HDL-C is less than 40 mg/dL. Patients with diabetes should have a fasting lipid profile tested more often (once per year). For nonfasting screening, the measurement of HDL-C and total cholesterol (TC) is necessary.

The Adult Treatment Panel III (ATP III) of the National Cholesterol Education Program has established a series of ranges to help clinicians with their diagnosis of lipid disorders. **Table 10.6** indicates the values assigned for triacylglycerols (TG), LDL-C, and HDL-C.

Table 10.6 Ranges for Lipid Levels Based on the Adult Treatment Panel III Guidelines

Lipid	Normal (mg/dL)	Borderline (mg/dL)	High (mg/dL)	Very High (mg/dL
Total cholesterol	< 200	200–239	240	≥240
Triacylglycerols	<150	150–199	200–499	≥500
LDL-C	<100	100–129	130–189	≥190
HDL-C	40	—	>60	—

Cholesterol

Cholesterol, triacylglycerols, and phospholipids are the major lipids in the body. Cholesterol, an important biological lipid, not only is essential to maintain the integrity of the cell membrane, but also serves as a precursor for the synthesis of the steroid hormones, vitamin D, and bile acids. Cholesterol, either derived from food or as endogenously secreted molecule, is transported through the circulation by lipoprotein molecules. The majority of endogenous cholesterol synthesis occurs in the liver, where a small fraction of the cholesterol production is incorporated into the membrane of hepatocytes and the rest is in the form of free cholesterol, bile acids, and cholesteryl esters.

Cholesterol synthesis occurs in the cytoplasm from acetyl CoA. Approximately 50% of the total cholesterol pool in the body is derived from *de novo* biosynthesis. Total cholesterol and LDL-C increase throughout the life span in both men and women—a trend caused not by synthesis of more cholesterol, but rather by consumption of cholesterol-enriched food. The acetyl-CoA that is used in cholesterol biosynthesis is derived from β-oxidation of fatty acids or the end product of glycolysis, pyruvate. All of the reduction reactions of cholesterol biosynthesis use NADPH as the reducing agent. Recall that the pentose phosphate pathway is important for the production of NADPH (see also the *Introduction to Biochemistry* chapter).

Human cells synthesize 1 g of cholesterol each day, mainly in the liver. In the first stage of cholesterol synthesis, two acetyl-CoA condense to form acetoacetyl-CoA, in a reaction catalyzed by a thiolase. Acetoacetyl-CoA, in turn, is converted to β-hydroxy-β-methylglutaryl-CoA (HMG-CoA). HMG-CoA reductase is the major regulatory enzyme in cholesterol biosynthesis as well as a key enzyme in the conversion of HMG-CoA to mevalonate. Insulin (by having a stimulatory effect) and glucagon (by having an inhibitory effect) control the activity of HMG-CoA reductase. In addition, cholesterol is subject to feedback inhibition, through regulation of transcription and translation of the HMG-CoA reductase enzyme (**Figure 10.39**).

Plasma Lipoproteins

Plasma lipoproteins are composed of phospholipid, cholesterol, and protein, and the cores of these molecules comprise packages of triacylglycerol and cholesterol ester. The lipid/protein ratio, and therefore the density, of plasma lipoproteins varies. Thus these particles may be separated by ultracentrifugation into fractions classified as chylomicrons, high-density lipoprotein (HDL), low-density lipoprotein (LDL), and very-low-density lipoprotein (VLDL).

Due to the water insolubility of lipids, they cannot travel freely from the tissue of origin to other tissues to be stored or consumed. Circulating plasma lipoproteins, therefore, facilitate movement of lipids in the blood.

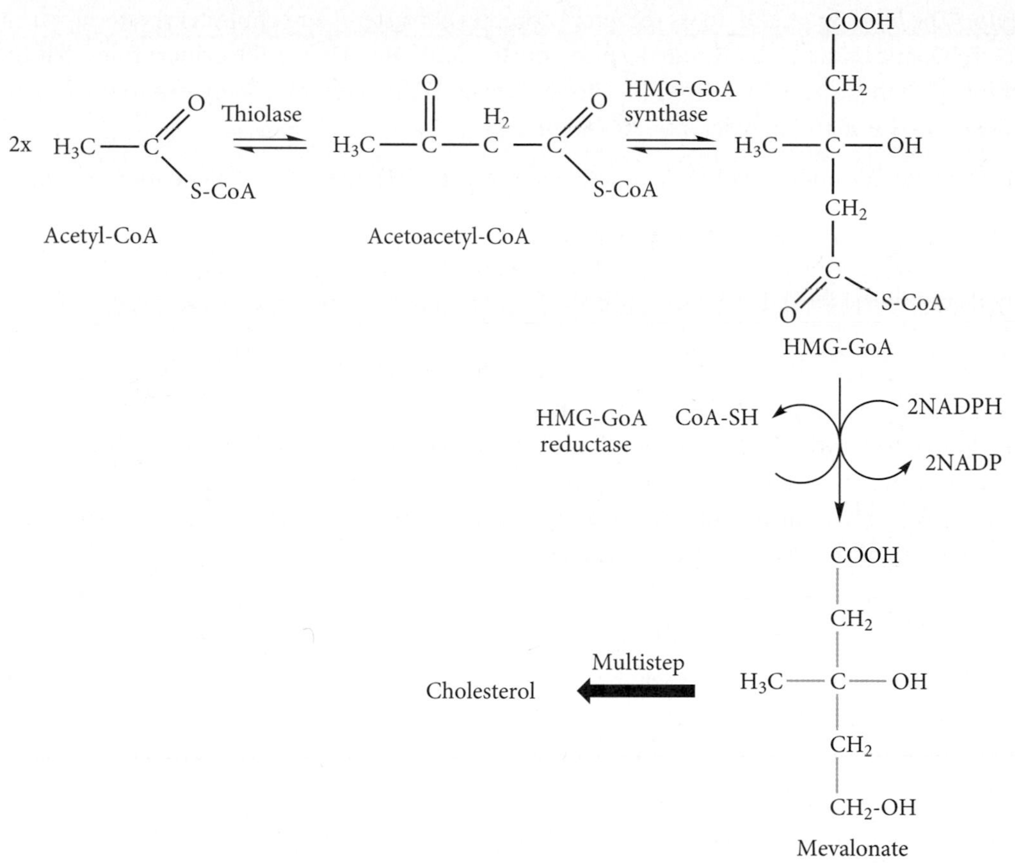

Figure 10.39 Synthesis of cholesterol from acetyl-CoA. The HMG-CoA reductase enzyme catalyzes the rate-limiting step in the biosynthesis of cholesterol. For this reason, it represents an excellent target for drug development to reduce the synthesis of cholesterol.

Chylomicrons

Chylomicrons carry fatty acids, which are obtained from the diet, to tissues for use or storage. Amongst the lipoproteins, chylomicrons are largest in size but least in density. These particles contain the highest concentration of TAG. Chylomicrons include apolipoproteins B-48, B-100, and E and are catabolized by lipoprotein lipase (LPL). Fasting affects the plasma concentration level of chylomicrons (after a fast of 12–14 hours, there are almost no chylomicrons in the plasma).

Low-Density Lipoprotein

Excess fatty acids from the diet or excess carbohydrates are converted to triacylglycerols in the liver; these molecules, in turn, are packaged with specific apolipoproteins to form the lipoprotein known as VLDL. From the liver, VLDL molecules enter the capillaries and are transported to the myocytes and adipocytes. In these tissues, one of the apolipoproteins, apoC-II, activates lipoprotein lipase to release fatty acids from the triacylglycerol component of VLDL. These new lipoproteins are no longer VLDLs, but rather become LDLs that deliver cholesterol to extrahepatic tissues (including coronary arteries). Thus VLDL is a precursor for almost all LDL molecules found in the circulation.

The LDL receptors play an essential role in clearing circulating LDL from the plasma. LDL is rich in both cholesterol and cholesteryl esters, which together make up almost 50% of LDL. After the conversion of VLDL to LDL, the only apolipoprotein that remains in the plasma is apoB-100 (Apo B makes up almost all of the LDL at this point), which facilitates binding of LDL to its receptor. The binding of LDL to its receptor promotes cholesterol and cholesteryl ester uptake into the extrahepatic tissues, which contain receptors for apoB-100. Due to the critical roles that LDL receptors play in clearing LDL from the blood, defects in these receptors can lead to the genetic disease known as familial hypercholesterolemia.

To calculate the amount of LDL and total cholesterol (CH), the following equations are used:

$$LDL = Total\ cholesterol - (HDL + TG/5)$$

$$Total\ cholesterol = (LDL + HDL + TG/5)$$

When LDL permeability increases because of a dysfunction of vascular endothelial cells, LDL becomes oxidized within arterial lesions, which in turn recruit monocytes. Monocytes are converted to macrophages capable of engulfing oxidized LDL. These macrophages, filled with oxidized LDL, become foam cells that accelerate formation of plaque. Rupture of the formed plaques results in thrombosis. When the plaque becomes large, it blocks the arteries leading to a reduction of blood flow and oxygen to the heart or brain.

High-Density Lipoprotein

HDLs are lipoprotein complexes that are smaller and denser than LDL. They are called "good cholesterol" because they transport cholesterol from extrahepatic tissues back to the liver, thereby lowering total serum cholesterol. In the liver, some of this cholesterol is converted to bile salts (see also the *Introduction to Nutrients* chapter).

The major apolipoprotein in HDL is apoA-I, which is important for the production of this lipoprotein. A low plasma concentration of apoA-I increases the risk of CHD.

HDL molecules bind to their cell membrane receptors in the liver and adrenal glands and deposit cholesterol and other lipids that enter the bloodstream. Later, the cholesterol-depleted HDL dissociates from the plasma membrane receptors and recirculates in the blood, once again extracting lipids from chylomicron and VLDL particles.

Therapeutic Agents in the Treatment of Hyperlipidemia

The initial therapies for hyperlipidemia consist of lifestyle changes, regular exercise, and a minimal intake of saturated fat and cholesterol. In addition, many pharmacological agents are available to treat this condition. While some agents reduce the absorption of cholesterol or decrease the synthesis of VLDL, LDL, and TG, others increase VLDL clearance, enhance LDL catabolism, or increase HDL. All of these agents, except resins, are contraindicated in patients with chronic liver diseases. Among these agents, niacin is most effective in increasing HDL, statins are most effective in reducing LDL, and fibric acids are the most effective in lowering triacylglycerol levels.

HMG-CoA Reductase Inhibitors

Statins structurally mimic mevalonate; thus they competitively inhibit the rate-limiting and regulatory enzyme of cholesterol biosynthesis, HMG-CoA reductase (Figure 10.39). Statins are the first-line agents for treating hyperlipidemia. In addition to inhibiting cholesterol synthesis, higher doses of the more potent statins—atorvastatin (Lipitor), simvastatin (Zocor), and rosuvastatin (Crestor) reduce triacylglycerol levels and increase HDL-C. Research data support the contention that simvastatin, pravastatin (Pravachol), lovastatin (Mevacor), atorvastatin, and rosuvastatin can reduce fatal and nonfatal CHD events, strokes, and total mortality. In November 2013, the American Heart Association and the American College of Cardiology developed a series of new guidelines for patients to receive statins. Four groups of patient populations have been identified in these new guidelines which include: 1) diabetic patients who are 40–75 years of age, 2) patients with cardio-vascular disease, 3) patients with a high LDL level (≥190 mg/dL), and patients who are 40–75 years of age with an estimated 10–year risk of cardiovascular disease of ≥ %7.5.

Statins reduce serum cholesterol levels and increase the expression of the LDL receptor gene. Having a larger number of LDL receptors on the surface of hepatocytes promotes removal of LDL from the blood and, as a result, lowers LDL-C levels (by 20–55%, depending on the dose of the statin drug). Some studies have even shown that statins can facilitate the removal of LDL precursors (VLDL and intermediate-density lipoprotein [IDL]) by decreasing hepatic VLDL production. In addition, statins reduce triacylglycerol levels that are higher than 250 mg/dL; as a consequence, patients who suffer from hypertriglyceridemia experience a 35–45% reduction in their TG levels. Interestingly, statin therapy increases endothelial production of the vasodilator nitric oxide, thereby improving the endothelial function as well.

It is important to counsel patients to take their statins in the evening because cholesterol is predominantly synthesized by the liver during the night. Absorption of lovastatin is better when the drug is taken with food in the evening. Advicor (lovastatin + niacin) should be taken at bedtime with snacks. Because atorvastatin has a long half-time, it can be taken at any time of the day. Rosuvastatin dosages need to be adjusted in patients with severe renal failure (CrCl less than 30 min/mL/1.73 m^2). In addition, antacids are known to reduce the serum level of rosuvastatin.

The statins, except simvastatin and lovastatin, are administered in an active form, the β-hydroxy acid form. Simvastatin and lovastatin are prodrugs that are administered as inactive lactones; they become active upon their biotransformation in the liver to their respective β-hydroxy acids. All statins are subject to an extensive hepatic first-pass effect. As a result, their bioavailability varies between 5% and 30% of the administered doses. Except for atorvastatin and rosuvastatin (which have a 20-hour half-life), statins have a short half-life (1–4 hours). Simvastatin has a half-life of 12 hours. Protein binding of statin agents is high; more than 95% of statins and their metabolites can bind to plasma proteins (the only exception is pravastatin and its metabolites, which have only 50% protein binding ability).

Two major side effects observed with statins are myopathy and rhabdomyolysis (between 1987 and 2001, the FDA recorded 42 deaths from rhabdomyolysis induced by statins). Both of these side effects are related to the dose and plasma concentration of the statin. As a result, any factor that inhibits statin metabolism can lead to myopathy; such factors include age (especially age greater than 80 years), hepatic or renal failure, diabetes mellitus, small body size, and untreated hypothyroidism. In addition, concomitant use of drugs (or food) that reduce statins' metabolism can lead to myopathy and rhabdomyolysis. The most common drug interactions have been noted with agents such as digoxin, warfarin, macrolide antibiotics, and azole antifungals. In addition, HIV protease inhibitors cause a reduction of statin metabolism. It has been shown that grapefruit juice inhibits CYP3A4 and, as a result, metabolism of statin that are metabolized by CYP3A4 are affected (however, eight ounces or less of grapefruit juice/day will not cause muscle injury to any significant extent).

Lovastatin, atorvastatin, and simvastatin (LAS) are primarily metabolized by CYP3A4 and 3A5. Fluvastatin is metabolized (50–80%) by CYP2C9. Pravastatin is not metabolized to any significant extent by the CYP system, but rather is excreted unchanged in the urine.

Pregnant or nursing women should not take statins.

Resins

Bile-acid sequestrants are also called resins. Cholestyramine (Questran) and colestipol (Colestid) are anion exchangers and were the first lipid-lowering agents to reach the market. As they are not absorbed from the intestine, they are the safest lipid-lowering agents. These agents are often prescribed for patients 11–20 years of age. In addition, they are used as second-line agents if statin therapy does not adequately lower LDL-C levels. Maximal doses of resins are effective in reducing LDL-C levels by as much as 25%; however, these agents cause bloating and constipation, which may lead to noncompliance issues. A newer agent, colesevelam (Welchol), is available in tablet and powder formulations (the powder must be mixed with water). However, the safety and efficacy of colesevelam in pregnant women and pediatric patients have not been studied yet.

Resins (Questran 4–6 g powder/daily) may be taken with food and nonfat yogurt. The mixture can be chilled overnight to improve the taste. The effectiveness of resins needs to be assessed after 6 weeks of therapy as part of monitoring their GI side effects. Patients should take a given dose with the largest meal.

As mentioned earlier, resins are anion exchangers that exchange Cl⁻ ions for the highly positively charged bile acids. Because of the large size of the complex formed with the bile acids, these agents are excreted in the stool. The interruption of enterohepatic recycling (reabsorption) of bile acids promotes the oxidation of cholesterol to bile acid. This process reduces the hepatic cholesterol content and stimulates the production of LDL receptors in the liver.

Due to their ion exchange ability, resins bind many organic salts, including warfarin and levothyroxine, thiazides, furosemide, and propranolol. Therefore, patients should take these medications 1 hour before or 4 hours after a resin administration.

Statins, when given in combination with cholestyramine and colestipol, can produce 20–30% better reductions in LDL-C than a statin given alone.

Nicotinic Acid

Niacin (Niaspan) is also one of the oldest lipid-lowering agents that affects virtually all lipid parameters. Most notably, it increases HDL levels by 30–40% and decreases TG levels by 35–45% (with TG, the maximal effect is seen within 4–7 days). Niacin is also a water-soluble vitamin (vitamin B_3) that functions as a vitamin following its conversion to one of the electron carrier coenzymes, NAD or NADP. To realize the lipid-lowering effect, much larger doses of niacin are needed than those required as a vitamin (see also the *Introduction to Nutrients* chapter).

The role of niacin in adipocytes is to inhibit hormone-sensitive lipase and thereby inhibit the lipolysis of TG, which in turn reduces the transport of free fatty acids to the liver and decreases hepatic TG synthesis. It has been suggested that niacin may inhibit diacylglycerol acyltransferase-2, which functions as a rate-limiting enzyme in TG synthesis. A reduction of TG synthesis reduces hepatic VLDL production, which explains the concomitant reduction of LDL levels. Niacin increases HDL-C levels not by increasing HDL-C synthesis, but rather by decreasing clearance of apoA-I.

Niacin's half-life is approximately 1 hour, which explains why it must be taken two or three times per day. At lower doses, only the major metabolite, nicotinuric acid, is found in the urine. At higher doses, a larger amount of unchanged nicotinic acid is excreted in the urine.

Three major side effects of niacin are flushing, pruritus (face, upper trunk, and skin rashes), and dyspepsia. Flushing and pruritus are prostaglandin mediated; NSAIDs (such as acetyl salicylic acid) 325 mg or ibuprofen 200 mg taken 30 minutes before niacin administration) can, therefore, help to alleviate these side effects. The flushing side effect is more likely to occur when a patient begins the niacin therapy, when the drug is consumed with hot beverages (e.g., coffee, tea) or alcohol, or when an established dose is increased. If the patient experiences dry skin as a result of niacin use, skin moisturizers are advised. If the drug is taken with food, other side effects such as dyspepsia, nausea, vomiting, and diarrhea are less likely to occur. It is important to avoid niacin in patients with any history of peptic ulcer because niacin can promote recurrence of ulcer disease.

The most severe side effect of niacin is hepatotoxicity, a condition indicated by high serum transaminases. Dosage forms of niacin include immediate release (Niacor), extended release (Niaspan), and controlled/slow release (Slo-Niacin). Both regular niacin (Niacor) and controlled-release niacin (Slo-Niacin) have been reported to cause severe liver toxicity. By comparison, extended-release niacin is less likely to cause severe hepatotoxicity due to its less frequent dosing. However, this formulation can also cause flushing and pruritus like the regular niacin. The likelihood of developing severe hepatotoxicity is high among patients who ingest more than 2 g niacin without a clinician's supervision. Interestingly, when an LDL-C reduction of 50% or more is achieved, there is a greater risk of niacin toxicity. Niaspan is the only FDA-approved niacin formulation indicated for treating dyslipidemia.

To avoid hepatotoxicity, a series of precautions needs to be taken when patients are prescribed niacin. For instance, baseline (before a therapy is initiated) liver function tests (LFTs) should be performed. Niacin causes hyperglycemia because it increases insulin resistance; thus blood glucose levels should be monitored at least weekly until the values become stable. In addition, sustained-release niacin (Slo-Niacin 1–2 g/day) requires monthly LFTs, followed by LFTs after 12 weeks and annually. Diabetic patients should be subjected to a routine fasting glucose (FG) test. Because niacin can increase serum uric acid levels, precautions should be taken with patients suffering from gout. Thus, in patients with a history of gout who are taking niacin, it is necessary to check their uric acid levels.

If patients switch from niacin to Advicor (lovastatin + niacin), the amount of niacin in the combination therapy should be less than the dose in niacin therapy only. In other words, Advicor should not be substituted for equivalent doses of immediate-release niacin.

It is important to increase the immediate-release niacin dose gradually. Patients can take 100 mg three times daily during the first week, 200 mg three times daily during the second week, 350 mg three times daily during the third week, and 500 mg three times daily during the fourth week. After establishing a stable dose, transaminases, serum albumin, fasting glucose, and uric acid levels should be measured. The maximum dose of Niaspan given per day is 2,000 mg (for instance, 1,000 mg twice daily).

Niacin should not be taken concomitantly with resins; a gap of 4 hours is permissible to avoid drug interaction. Myopathy can arise when this drug is used simultaneously with statins or gemfibrozil. In addition, niacin can increase bleeding risk, so caution is advised when patients are candidates for surgery.

Fibric Acids

Gemfibrozil (Lopid) and fenofibrate (TriCor) are the two most frequently prescribed fibric acids. Fibric acids are best known for reducing TG, but their exact mechanism of action is not fully understood. It is believed that fibrates activate peroxisome-proliferator activated receptor-alpha, a hepatocyte-specific transcription factor that promotes gene expression of specific enzymes involved in fatty acid β-oxidation in mitochondria and peroxisomes, decreases fatty acid and TG synthesis, reduces production of VLDL, increases lipoprotein lipase (LPL) synthesis, and reduces expression of apoC-III. A reduction in hepatic production of apoC-III can enhance the removal of VLDL. Fenofibrate is more effective than gemfibrozil at increasing HDL levels.

While gemfibrozil should be taken 30 minutes before a meal, fenofibrate can be taken either with or without food. It is also important to screen the patient with a total fasting lipid panel (HDL, LDL, total cholesterol, TG) and to assess fibrates' therapeutic effectiveness after 6 weeks.

Side effects associated with fibrates include dizziness, dyspepsia, and gallstones. The risk of myopathy increases when these agents are combined with statins. To reduce the risk of myopathy, statin doses should be reduced when a statin is combined with a fibrate. Fibrates are contraindicated in patients with chronic liver disease. These drugs increase warfarin's effectiveness and are metabolized by CYP3A4.

In patients with TG levels less than 400 mg/dL, fibrates reduce TG levels by almost 50% and increase HDL-C concentrations by about 15%. However, not all fibrates can reduce LDL-C levels. Second-generation agents, such as fenofibrate and bezafibrate (Bezalip SR, from Canada), can lower LDL levels (by 15-20%) along with a decrease of VLDL levels. Fibrates have a high protein binding profile (more than 95%), and their half-life varies significantly, with gemfibrozil having the shortest half-life (1.1 hours) and fenofibrate having the longest half-life (20 hours).

Inhibition of Dietary Cholesterol Uptake

This class of lipid-lowering drugs inhibits cholesterol absorption by enterocytes in the small intestine. Such agents are often used in combination with statins. Ezetimibe (Zetia) was the first compound approved in this class; it is available as a 10 mg tablet. However, ezetimibe does not affect intestinal triglyceride absorption. Similar to other lipid-lowering agents, ezetimibe is contraindicated in patients with moderate to severe liver disease.

Ezetimibe is highly water insoluble. After its administration, it undergoes glucuronidation in the intestinal epithelium and enters the enterohepatic recirculation. Because resins can inhibit absorption of ezetimibe, ezetimibe and resins should not be administered together. Otherwise, there are no other significant drug interactions for ezetimibe.

Some drug therapy combinations include both statins and other lipid-lowering agents. Examples are ezetimibe/simvastatin (Vytorin, 10 mg/10 mg to 10 mg/80 mg), lovastatin/niacin (Advicor, 20 mg/500 mg to 20 mg/1,000 mg), and amlodipine/atorvastatin (Caduet, 10 mg/20 mg).

Omega-3 ethylester (Lovaza, 1 g capsule) is the first FDA-approved omega-3 fatty acid; it seems to be effective for patients with TG levels greater than 500 mg/dL. While the mechanism of action for omega-3 is not yet fully understood, researchers have suggested that this agent increases hepatic β-oxidation of fatty acids and reduces hepatic synthesis of triacylglycerols (see also the *Introduction to Nutrients* chapter).

Learning Bridge 10.9

AA, a patient with hyperlipidemia, has been taking atorvastatin 40 mg daily for the past 1.5 years. On a recent visit, the doctor prescribed him a niacin tablet, 500 mg/day, for the first month and told him to increase the dose to 1,000 mg/day after this point.

As an intern pharmacist, what will be your advice to AA on the dermatological adverse effects of niacin?

Drugs That Modulate the Endocrine System

Thyroid Disorders

Thyroid hormones include thyroxine (T_4), tri-iodothyronine (T_3), and calcitonin. While thyroxine and tri-iodothyronine are involved in metabolism and growth, calcitonin serves as an important regulator of calcium homeostasis. In this section, only thyroxine and tri-iodothyronine will be discussed (calcitonin is described in the *Introduction to Nutrients* chapter). Thyroxine (T_4) and tri-iodothyronine (T_3) are amino acid derivatives and contain four and three iodine residues, respectively (**Figure 10.40**).

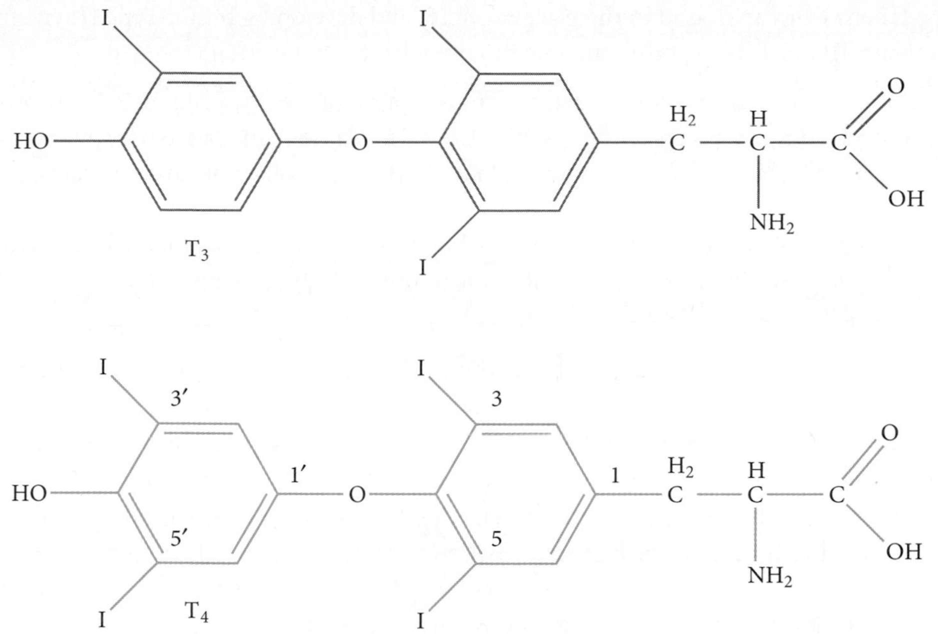

Figure 10.40 The structures of tri-iodothyronine (T$_3$) and thyroxine (T$_4$).

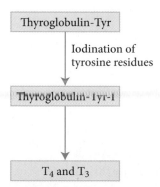

Figure 10.41 Synthetic pathway for the production of T$_3$ and T$_4$ from thyroglobulin.

The thyroid gland synthesizes, stores, and secretes T$_3$ and T$_4$. Tri-iodothyronine has a binding affinity that is 10–15 times higher than that of T$_4$ for thyroid hormone receptors. All cell types within the body require a constant amount of thyroid hormones for proper functioning. These hormones are synthesized by mono- and di-iodination of tyrosine residues (MIT and DIT, respectively), followed by coupling of two tyrosine (Tyr) residues through an ether linkage to produce T$_3$ (MIT and DIT) and T$_4$ (DIT + DIT). Tyrosine residues are derived from a protein called thyroglobulin (Tg). When needed, stored T$_4$ and T$_3$ are released from the Tg by proteolysis (**Figure 10.41**).

Once dietary iodides (I$^-$) are taken up by the thyroid gland, they become oxidized to iodine by thyroid peroxidase. This step is crucial to make the iodides more reactive so that they can covalently bind to the tyrosine molecules on thyroglobulin. Thyroid peroxidase is a heme-containing, membrane-bound enzyme, found at the apical membrane of the thyroid cells. Antithyroid drugs such as propylthiouracil (Propyl-Thyracil, from Canada) and methimazole (Tapazole) inhibit thyroid peroxidase, so they are good choices for treating hyperthyroidism. Inorganic ions, including bromine, fluorine, and lithium, are known to inhibit iodide transport into the thyroid gland.

Thyroxine (T$_4$) is synthesized and released from the thyroid gland in high concentrations into the plasma. The deiodination process predominantly occurs in the target tissues and plays a crucial role in the thyroid hormones' overall activity. Most cells are capable of deiodinating T$_4$ to T$_3$, and tissues such as kidney and liver cells have high expression of deiodinase. The deiodination process is catalyzed by three types of deiodinase enzymes:

- Type I enzymes are widely distributed in peripheral tissues, including the liver and the kidney.
- Type II enzymes are found in the CNS, pituitary, and thyroid gland.

- Type III enzymes are found in the placenta, skin, and developing brain. Type III enzymes inactivate T_4 and T_3 by deiodinating the inner ring at the 5' position.

Tri-iodothyronine is the master regulator of transcription of specific genes in cellular processes (i.e., genes involved in energy metabolism, the citric acid cycle, and oxidative phosphorylation). Therefore, thyroid hormones play an important role in the metabolism of carbohydrates, proteins, and lipids in different tissues. Because T_4 and T_3 are water insoluble, in order to circulate into the blood and reach their site of action, they must be bound to transport proteins such as thyroxine-binding globulin (TBG), transthyretin (TTR), and albumin. Approximately 99.96% of circulating T_4 and 99.5% of T_3 are bound to these proteins.

Thyroid hormone secretion is regulated by three hormones of the hypothalamic–pituitary–thyroid axis—namely, thyrotropin-releasing hormone (TRH), thyroid-stimulating hormone (TSH), and thyroid hormones (T_4 and T_3). TRH is a short peptide (a tripeptide) that is released by the hypothalamus and stimulates the synthesis and release of TSH, a glycoprotein hormone, from the anterior pituitary. TSH, in turn, signals the thyroid gland to release thyroid hormones. Similar to any other feedback mechanism, the production and release of TRH and TSH are regulated by feedback from the circulating free thyroid hormones. The thyroid gland's production of sufficient levels of hormones sends signals to suppress the production and release of TRH and TSH, and vice versa.

Today, with improved technology, very sensitive and accurate TSH assays can detect low concentrations of TSH to diagnose whether TSH secretion is subnormal. The normal serum levels of TSH, T_3, and T_4 are 0.4–4 mIU/L, 60–180 ng/dL, and 4–11 μg/L, respectively. In clinical settings, measurement of TSH alone is often used as the first-line thyroid function test.

Two major disorders are associated with thyroid hormone secretion: hypothyroidism and hyperthyroidism.

Hypothyroidism

Hypothyroidism is a thyroid disorder that results from decreased thyroid hormone production. Because hypothyroidism develops slowly, it is somewhat difficult to diagnose this disease. Hypothyroidism is a major endocrine problem. Primary hypothyroidism is caused by a nonfunctional thyroid gland. In contrast, secondary hypothyroidism, which is less common, is a result of pituitary failure to secrete TSH. Owing to their catabolic and metabolic effects, thyroid hormones are essential for growth and development during embryonic life. If thyroid deficiency in a pregnant mother is not corrected, then it may result in fetal and neonatal mental retardation and/or cretinism.

An elevated plasma concentration of TSH is the first evidence of primary hypothyroidism. Initially, many patients have a normal range of the free (unbound) T_4 (compensated hypothyroidism) and a few, if any, symptoms of hypothyroidism. However, as the disease progresses, the plasma concentration of free T_4 falls below the normal range. Interestingly, thyroid hormone production will shift toward T_3, which will often be maintained in the normal range despite the low T_4 level.

A significant percentage (more than 90%) of hypothyroidism cases occur as a consequence of (1) destruction of the thyroid gland by antibodies produced against the gland (autoimmune destruction), also known as Hashimoto's disease; and (2) radioiodine or surgical treatment of hyperthyroidism. In addition, certain drug therapy, TSH deficiency, abnormal synthesis of T_4 T4/T3 T_3, and severe iodine deficiency may result in a hypothyroid state. Clinical symptoms of hypothyroidism include lethargy, cold intolerance, weight gain, constipation, dryness of skin and hair, muscle cramps, myalgia, and bradycardia. In addition, women may experience menorrhagia and infertility.

In adults, the most common cause of spontaneous hypothyroidism is Hashimoto's disease. Patients with Hashimoto's disease produce antibodies that attack thyroid peroxidase. In contrast, iatrogenic hypothyroidism is caused by exposure to excessive radiation or surgical procedure in the neck. However, there is a delay in the development of hypothyroidism following radioiodine therapy, with the condition occurring within 3 months to a year after ^{131}I therapy.

Hypothyroidism is managed by thyroxine replacement, starting with low doses, and periodic monitoring of TSH in the serum. The dose of thyroxine should be gradually increased over several months until a euthyroid state is achieved.

It is critical to recognize any thyroid hormone deficiency and correct hypothyroidism, particularly to maintain infants' normal growth and mental development. While hypothyroidism is rarely caused by iodine deficiency, in patients with autoimmune thyroiditis, the synthesis of thyroid hormones is blocked. This condition results in increased secretion of TSH and thyroid enlargement.

The major goal in treating hypothyroidism is to increase the amount of thyroid hormone so as to maintain normal growth and metabolism. In children, thyroid hormone replacement is necessary for neurological development and to reverse the biochemical abnormalities associated with hypothyroidism. Drug therapy with T_4 is preferred, as T_4 is readily available as levothyroxine sodium (Levothyroid). Monitoring TSH concentrations is important to gauge the adequacy of treatment.

Treatment of Hypothyroidism

The goals of hypothyroidism treatment are to provide adequate thyroid hormone and maintain the patient's TSH within the normal range. Levothyroxine (T_4) is the first-line therapy for treatment of hypothyroidism. A series of synthetic preparations are available in the market, including levothyroxine, liothyronine (Cytomel), and liotrix (Thyrolar). Levothyroxine is relatively inexpensive and has been shown to produce effective results. Synthetic T_3 is more active than T_4, but administration of T_4 results in its conversion to T_3. In other words, levothyroxine serves as a precursor for T_3.

Levothyroxine has good oral bioavailability (80%) and a half-life of approximately 7 days. The maximal absorption of levothyroxine is achieved when it is taken on an empty stomach. The required dose of levothyroxine depends on factors such as age, the presence of absorption disorders, and the severity and duration of hypothyroidism. Pregnant women require a higher dose of the hormone because of increased inactivation of the hormone by the placental deiodinase, and because of the need to transfer T_4 to the fetus. Initial doses of 50 μg and 25 μg are adequate for young and elderly patients, respectively. However, for most patients, after reaching a steady-state level, a daily dose of 125 μg levothyroxine based on a ratio of 1.7 μg/kg/day is adequate.

To monitor the adequacy of thyroid hormone replacement, TSH concentration should be measured. An elevated TSH concentration indicates insufficient hormone replacement. Both TSH and T_4 concentrations should be monitored every 6 weeks until a euthyroid state is achieved. Clinical studies have shown that aggressive therapy with levothyroxine is critical for children with hypothyroidism to ensure their normal development. In addition, thyroid hormone supplementation is necessary for fetal growth during pregnancy; levothyroxine is considered the drug of choice for this indication (it is one of the few agents belonging to pregnancy category A).

The relationship between T_4 concentration and TSH is not linear; as a result, even a very small change in T_4 concentration can result in a significant change in TSH level. Numerous foods and drugs can reduce the absorption of levothyroxine. For instance, foods such as soybean formula, dietary fiber supplements, and coffee, along with drugs such as cholestyramine, calcium carbonate, sucralfate, aluminum hydroxide, and ferrous sulfate, can reduce the absorption of levothyroxine. In addition, ranitidine (Zanta) and proton pump inhibitors may reduce the absorption of levothyroxine.

Unfortunately, T_3 is not a good option to treat hypothyroidism because it has been shown to increase the incidence of cardiac adverse effects, has a higher cost, and is difficult to monitor with conventional laboratory tests. A combination of T_3 and T_4 (liotrix) in a 4:1 ratio is available on the market. This drug is expensive, and clinical studies have shown that a combination of T_4 and T_3 is not superior to T_4 alone.

Thyroid hormone therapy does not have any significant side effects. The only side effects of thyroxine are noted when high doses of thyroid hormone are administered and may consist of heart failure, angina pectoris, and myocardial infarction. An allergic reaction may occur as well. Synthroid tablets do not produce any allergic reaction, as the formulation is devoid of any dye substance and allergenic excipients.

Learning Bridge 10.10

JB, a 40-year-old male, has been taking levothyroxine tablets, 25 µg, once daily, for his hypothyroidism for about a month. Although JB feels better than before he was prescribed the medication, he still complains of being extremely lethargic in the morning and constipated. Other than this medication, JB is not taking any prescription drug. As a pharmacy intern, you asked him whether he is taking any OTC product. JB admitted taking Prevacid regularly to get relief from indigestion caused by the stress of the managerial position in which he is employed.

A. Indicate why JB is not getting total relief from his levothyroxine treatment.
B. How will you counsel JB?

Hyperthyroidism

Hyperthyroidism refers to an overactive thyroid gland. This term also refers to thyrotoxicosis, in which cells become exposed to high levels of the thyroid hormones; in other words, thyrotoxicosis can occur from elevated T_4 levels. Hyperthyroidism can occur as the result of (1) ingestion of iodine; (2) Graves's disease (the most common cause); (3) thyroiditis (often caused by viral infection); and (4) excessive ingestion of thyroid hormones.

Graves's disease is the most common cause of hyperthyroidism. It arises when thyroid-stimulating antibodies act as agonists to TSH receptors, which results in hypersecretion of T_4. Similar to the action of TSH, when these antibody molecules bind to the TSH receptor, they activate G-protein and the adenylate cyclase enzyme (see also *Introduction to Pharmacodynamics* chapter). Patients suffering from Graves's disease lack the regulatory mechanism that governs secretion and synthesis of T_4. Graves's disease is approximately eight times more common in women than in men.

Many of the clinical symptoms of hyperthyroidism are the opposite of the symptoms seen with hypothyroidism. These symptoms include weight loss despite normal appetite, sweating, heat intolerance, fatigue, palpitation, agitation and tremor, muscle weakness, angina and heart failure, diarrhea, and exophthalmos (protrusion of the eyeballs).

Treatment of Graves's disease can consist of antithyroid drug therapy, radioiodine treatment, or thyroidectomy. The overall therapeutic goals for patients with hyperthyroidism are to inhibit secretion of excessive thyroid hormones and reduce the symptoms associated with this endocrine imbalance.

Treatment of Hyperthyroidism

Thioamides

Propylthiouracil (PTU, from Canada, as 50 mg tablet) and methimazole (Tapazole or MMI as 5 and 10 mg tablets) are available in the United States as treatments for hyperthyroidism. Both agents inhibit the biosynthesis of the thyroid hormone by serving as false substrates for the thyroid peroxidase enzyme. As a result, thyroid peroxidase cannot oxidize iodide to iodine, which in turn inhibits MIT and DIT formation. In addition, PTU inhibits the peripheral conversion of T_4 to T_3 within a few hours of administration.

Both PTU and MMI are absorbed from the GI tract quite well (80–95%). The half-life of PTU is 1–2.5 hours; that of MMI is 6–9 hours. While the extent to which PTU binds to plasma albumin varies, MMI does not become bound to plasma protein at all. MMI is able to cross the placenta and is found in breast milk. Placental transfer of MMI results in elevated TSH and low T_4 levels in fetuses. Both PTU and MMI have a slow onset of action, and the full therapeutic effect takes from 4 to 8 weeks to be realized after therapy begins.

Most adverse effects associated with thioamide use are minor and do not require discontinuation of therapy. Reversible agranulocytosis, however, is an important adverse effect of thioamides. This condition is characterized by fever, malaise, oropharyngeal infections, and decreased granulocyte count. The American Thyroid Association and the FDA recommend that PTU should not be considered as a first-line therapy in either adults or children due to the risk of hepatoxicity. However, during the first trimester of pregnancy when there is a risk of MMI-induced thyroid toxicity to the fetus, PTU is prescribed despite this recommendation.

Iodides (Saturated Solution of Potassium Iodide and Lugol's Solution)

Iodide inhibits the release of thyroid hormones from proteolysis of Tg. It can be used as a presurgical medication prior to thyroid surgery. Saturated solution of potassium iodide (SSKI) should not be used 3–7 days following radioactive iodine treatment so as to concentrate the radioactive iodide in the thyroid. Commonly occurring adverse effects with iodide therapy include hypersensitivity reactions such as rashes, drug fever, rhinitis, and conjunctivitis. In addition, salivary gland swelling and gynecomastia may occur.

Adrenergic Blockers

Adrenergic blockers are useful to reduce the symptoms associated with hyperthyroidism. For instance, symptoms such as palpitations, anxiety, and tremor can be alleviated by propranolol (20–40 mg, four times daily). Beta blockers are used as adjunctive agents, along with antithyroid drugs, radioactive iodine (RAI), or iodides. However, nonselective agents should not be used in patients with asthma and COPD, sinus bradycardia, and spontaneous hypoglycemia. Also, beta blockers should not be used in patients taking monoamine oxidase inhibitors or tricyclic antidepressants. Calcium-channel blockers may be substituted for beta blockers in patients with these conditions.

Radioactive Iodine

Sodium iodide-131 (^{131}I) is used to treat Graves's disease; it becomes well concentrated in the thyroid gland. Sodium iodide-131 emits beta particles with a half-life of 8 days. While other organs can also take up ^{131}I, organification of the absorbed iodine can take place only in the thyroid gland. Like other radioactive drugs, sodium iodide-131 is contraindicated during pregnancy.

When treatment for hyperthyroidism is initiated, patients need to be evaluated on a monthly basis until they reach a euthyroid condition. During the evaluation process, indications such as tachycardia, weight loss, and heat intolerance should be carefully investigated.

Diabetes

Diabetes mellitus (DM) is a metabolic disease. According to the American Diabetes Association, approximately 25.8 million people in the United States had diabetes in 2011 (8.3% of the population). In addition, 79 million people were prediabetic. Diabetes mellitus is a progressive disease and, if untreated, will gradually affect many organ systems.

Diabetes mellitus is associated with deficiencies in carbohydrate, fat, and protein metabolism and progressively results in chronic and severe complications. According to the American Diabetes Association, the cost of DM totaled approximately $174 billion in 2007. In addition, DM has many complications and is the leading cause of blindness in adults between 20 and 74 years old. This disease is also a leading cause of kidney failure and accounts for 60% of lower-extremity nontraumatic amputations in the United States.

There are two major types of diabetes, designated as types 1 and 2. In type 1 diabetes, the pancreas does not produce insulin. In type 2 diabetes, cells fail to respond to insulin, there is decreased muscular uptake of glucose, or the secretion of insulin is inadequate. In addition, gestational diabetes may occur in pregnant women.

The clinical presentations of type 1 and type 2 diabetes differ in important ways. Although type 1 diabetes can occur at any age, approximately 75% of cases appear before 20 years of age and the remaining 25% develop during adulthood. Patients with type 1 diabetes are often thin, whereas patients with type 2 diabetes are often obese. Untreated patients with type 1 diabetes may develop life-threatening ketoacidosis (KDA). Indeed, 20–40% of patients with type 1 disease present with diabetic KDA following several days of polyuria, polydipsia, polyphagia, and weight loss. While insulin resistance is common in type 2 disease, it is absent in type 1 diabetes. Furthermore, some rare types of diabetes are caused by infections, drugs, and pancreatic destruction.

Diabetes mellitus is diagnosed based on the blood glucose concentration:

- 200 mg/dL or greater (at any given time)
- 200 mg/dL or greater after 2 hours of an oral load (75 g glucose) and after 8 hours of an overnight fast
- 126 mg/dL or greater after 8 hours of an overnight fast

Insulin is a 5.8-kDa hormone that is synthesized as an inactive polypeptide, preproinsulin, in the β cells of the pancreas. The cleavage of the pre (signal peptide), and then the pro sequence C-Peptide, by a proteolytic enzyme produces active insulin. The active insulin has two polypeptide chains, A and B. The C-peptide can be used as a marker for endogenous insulin formation.

Diabetes and Metabolic Complications

Insulin is an anabolic hormone whose blood concentration in fasting healthy adults is approximately 10 mU/L. However, this value rises immediately following a meal to 60 mU/L, then returns to the basal level after 1–4 hours. Almost all tissues in mammalians express insulin receptors, but such receptors are found in especially high concentrations in cells of energy-storing tissues such as liver, muscle, and fat. For instance, an erythrocyte may have only 30 insulin receptors, while a myocyte may contain 300,000 insulin receptors. Hepatocytes, myocytes, and adipocytes are the main targets for insulin.

Although insulin does not affect the uptake of glucose by hepatocytes, it affects the liver through other metabolic pathways. Hepatic glucose uptake is not affected by insulin due to the presence of the glucose transport system (glucose transporter 2 [GLUT2]) in the cell membrane

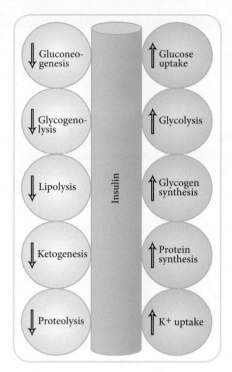

Figure 10.42 Insulin has both stimulatory and inhibitory effects on many biochemical pathways.

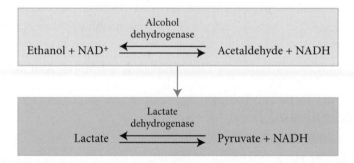

Figure 10.43 Alcohol inhibits gluconeogenesis by promoting removal of pyruvate, the substrate for gluconeogenesis.

of hepatocytes. Because of the active role that GLUT2 plays in the hepatocytes, the concentrations of glucose in the liver and in the blood are almost identical (5 mM).

When insulin is released from the pancreas in healthy individuals, a high blood glucose level becomes apparent. Under these circumstances, the body should not synthesize glucose (i.e., it should inhibit gluconeogenesis). Gluconeogenesis and glycolysis have counterbalancing regulatory mechanisms; thus, when one is inhibited, the other is often stimulated. In other words, when gluconeogenesis is inhibited, glycolysis is stimulated and vice versa. Insulin, however, stimulates the glycogen synthase enzyme in the liver and muscle to promote glycogen synthesis. Insulin is released as a result of a high blood glucose level, and one way to handle the excess glucose is to store it in a form of glycogen in both liver and muscle. By the same token, the degradation of glycogen should be inhibited when the blood glucose level is high. As a result, insulin inhibits glycogenolysis. **Figure 10.42** summarizes the metabolic pathways that are affected by insulin.

It is important to counsel diabetic patients to avoid excessive use of alcohol. Alcohol, similar to insulin, inhibits gluconeogenesis and causes hypoglycemia. In addition, alcohol slows the citric acid cycle by depleting NAD^+ and increasing NADH (**Figure 10.43**).

Insulin stimulates amino acid uptake into muscle tissue as well as transcription of ribosomal RNA and a few initiation factors for protein synthesis. Overall, the synthesis of proteins is stimulated by insulin. Conversely, insulin inhibits proteolysis to reduce the amount of free amino acids in the circulation (recall the discussion of glucogenic amino acids from the *Introduction to Biochemistry* chapter).

Insulin promotes the formation of acetyl-CoA, a precursor for fatty acid synthesis. The activity of the pyruvate dehydrogenase complex located inside mitochondria is stimulated by insulin as well. Stimulation of pyruvate dehydrogenase leads to depletion of the pyruvate needed for gluconeogenesis. Because acetyl-CoA serves as the precursor for fatty acids, the synthesis of fatty acids is also promoted. Most importantly, insulin stimulates the acetyl-CoA carboxylase enzyme, which uses acetyl-CoA molecules to initiate fatty acid synthesis. Fatty acids, in turn, are used to synthesize triacylglycerols. The regulatory enzyme, HMG-CoA reductase, which functions essentially to synthesize cholesterol, is stimulated by insulin as well. The increased concentration of acetyl-CoA molecules and induction of HMG-CoA reductase play important roles in the synthesis of cholesterol.

During the lipolysis process, triacylglycerols within adipocytes become degraded into glycerol and fatty acids by a hormone-sensitive lipase enzyme. While the fatty acids serve as an energy source, the glycerol component acts as a precursor for the synthesis of glucose (via gluconeogenesis). In conditions of elevated blood glucose, insulin inactivates hormone-sensitive lipase by a dephosphorylation mechanism, resulting in inhibition of lipolysis.

Marathon runners should not eat large amounts of carbohydrate-rich foods immediately before their race because ingestion of carbohydrates will promote insulin secretion, putting the body in an anabolic state rather than a catabolic state. As a result, glycogen degradation, lipolysis, and proteolysis and energy production will be inhibited. In addition, this condition will trigger hypoglycemic symptoms.

Glucagon Hormone and Blood Glucose

Glucagon is a hormone that is released from α cells of the pancreas and is known to influence many metabolic reactions. Of particular interest here is its role in providing adequate supplies of glucose to the blood. When the blood has a low glucose level, it is better to slow down glycolysis. In this situation, glucagon suppresses synthesis of pyruvate kinase (the last enzyme involved in the 10th—and last—step of glycolysis). In effect, this condition favors gluconeogenesis over glycolysis. Because pyruvate synthesis is the last step as well as a rate-limiting step in the glycolysis pathway, it is an appropriate step for regulation.

Glycogen phosphorylase *a* enzyme degrades glycogen into glucose monomers. Glucagon increases the amount of glycogen phosphorylase *a*, thereby triggering glycogen degradation in the liver. As a result, the liver sends glucose to the blood in an attempt to maintain the normal concentration of glucose (5 mM). Glucagon injection is used to treat severe hypoglycemia in diabetic patients and when intravenous glucose is not available.

Glucagon also stimulates the release of catecholamines. It may be used to treat a patient who has overdosed on a beta blocker and is experiencing severe bradycardia and profound hypotension. An intravenous injection of glucagon (3–10 mg) followed by a continuous IV infusion is required to increase the secretion of epinephrine and norepinephrine to compete with the beta blocker. However, the dose used here is higher (3–10 mg) than the dose used in a hypoglycemic condition (0.5–2 mg).

Because glucagon is degraded extensively in the liver and kidneys ($t_{1/2}$ is 5 minutes), commercially available glucagon hormone (GlucaGen, 1 mg) is administered either intravenously, intramuscularly, or subcutaneously. Although the blood glucose level is restored within 10 minutes, the patient should still have enough liver glycogen for glucose supply.

It is important to counsel diabetic patients to limit the amount of coffee and tea they consume. Caffeine and tea contain xanthine and theophylline, respectively. Both substances stimulate cAMP production, which activates glycogen phosphorylase *a*; this enzyme increases glycogenolysis, resulting in hyperglycemia.

Analysis of the gene that expresses glucagon revealed that it expresses two other products: glucagon-like peptide 1 (GLP-1; physiologically acts as an incretin) and glucagon-like peptide 2 (GLP-2). The glucagon gene expresses proglucagon in the pancreas, GI tract, and the brain. In pancreatic cells, proglucagon is converted into glucagon; in the GI tract and brain cells, proglucagon is converted into GLP-1 and GLP-2. Interestingly, GLP-1 has an opposite effect to glucagon. GLP-1 lowers the blood glucose level by three mechanisms: (1) stimulating the secretion of insulin and inhibiting the release of glucagon; (2) inhibiting gastric secretions, which decreases the absorption of glucose following meals; and (3) reducing appetite. Recognition of these metabolic effects has prompted researchers to synthesize GLP-1–like drugs to treat type 2 diabetes, for which the therapeutic goal is to increase insulin secretion from the pancreas. For example, exenatide (Byetta), an analog of GLP-1, is used to treat type 2 diabetes. Exenatide is administered as a subcutaneous injection 30–60 minutes prior to meals. GLP-1 (incretin) release from the intestine is stimulated by the meal, but this peptide is rapidly inactivated by the dipeptidyl peptidase IV (DPP-IV) enzyme.

Amylin is another peptide hormone that is produced in pancreatic β cells (for every 10 insulin molecules, one amylin molecule is produced). Amylin is co-secreted with insulin and interacts with amylin receptors on the plasma membrane (mostly in the CNS) to inhibit glucagon and gastric acid secretion. It also delays gastric emptying, thereby suppressing appetite. The drug pramlintide (Symlin) mimics amylin and is used to treat diabetes, particularly in patients with type 1 disease that is not adequately controlled with insulin therapy.

Table 10.7 summarizes the effect of insulin, glucagon, GLP-1, and amylin hormones.

Blood Glucose Level

Nonenzymic binding of glucose to hemoglobin (Hb) results in the formation of hemoglobin A1c (HbA_{1c}). A 6% HbA_{1c} measurement corresponds to an estimated average of 126 mg hemoglobin per deciliter blood over the preceding 3 months. Such an HbA_{1c} value may be obtained to determine how well a treatment has normalized the blood glucose levels in a person with diabetes over the past 3 months. If serum glucose is high, more Hb molecules are glycated (HbA_{1c}). Because the

Table 10.7 Physiological Effects of Insulin, Glucagon, GLP-1, and GLP-2 Hormones

Effect	Insulin	Glucagon	GLP-1	Amylin
Blood glucose level	↓	↑	↓	↓
Gastric acid secretion	↓	↑	↓	↓
Gastric emptying	↓	↑	↓	↓
Serum potassium level	↓	↑	Unknown	Unknown

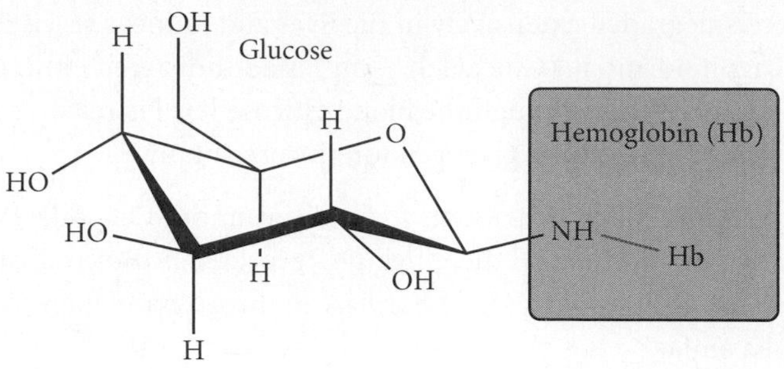

Figure 10.44 Nonenzymic binding of glucose to hemoglobin A (glycation) results in the formation of hemoglobin A1c (HbA_{1c}).

glucose molecule covalently attaches to the Hb, the hemoglobin molecule remains glycated throughout its life span (at least 90 days) (**Figure 10.44**).

At blood glucose levels greater than 97 mg/dL, each 1% of HbA_{1c} corresponds to approximately 30 mg/dL of glucose: 5% = 97 mg/dL; 6% = 126 mg/dL; 7% = 154 mg/dL; 8% = 183 mg/dL; and 9% = 212 mg/dL. Good glycemic control for a patient with diabetes is defined as less than 7% HbA_{1c}. HbA_{1c} should be measured 2–4 times per year.

Glycemic Control

For a nondiabetic individual or a prediabetic patient (with HbA_{1c} = 5.7–6%), the Hb_{A1c} goal is less than 5.7%. For a recently diagnosed diabetic patient with HbA_{1c} greater than 8%, the Hb_{A1c} goal is less than 7%. For a diabetic patient who has been diagnosed for many years and still has Hb_{A1c} greater than 8%, the goal is 7–8%.

Type 1 Diabetes

In type 1 diabetes, pancreatic β cells are destroyed by the immune system (autoimmune destruction), thereby preventing any production of insulin. Destruction of pancreatic β cells leads to a lack of both insulin and amylin. β-cell destruction begins during infancy and progressively continues over years; by the time a patient is diagnosed with type 1 diabetes, approximately 80% of the β cells are destroyed. Many scientists believe that this condition is brought on by exposure to viruses that cause antibodies or cytotoxic T cells (CTL) to destroy pancreatic islets. However, it is unknown whether other environmental factors might initiate the autoimmune process.

Diabetic Ketoacidosis

Diabetic ketoacidosis (DKA) is serious form of ketosis that, if not treated, is fatal. A few parameters are indicative of DKA, such as blood glucose concentration greater than 300 mg/dL, blood pH less than 7.2, and concentration of ketone bodies greater than 90 mg/dL (normal ketone body concentration is less than 3 mg/dL). Due to a lack of insulin, a person with untreated type 1 diabetes is also likely to develop hyperkalemia (see Table 10.7), which may precipitate cardiac arrest. The most important treatment for DKA is intravenous administration of regular insulin (10 units/h). Given that insulin promotes entry of K^+ into the cells, insulin therapy may cause hypokalemia, thus one must measure plasma K^+ levels every hour until the DKA is alleviated.

When insulin hormone is lacking in the body, the cells (particularly hepatocytes) use oxaloacetate for gluconeogenesis to synthesize glucose (recall that insulin inhibits gluconeogenesis and a lack of insulin stimulates gluconeogenesis). The depletion of oxaloacetate slows down the citric

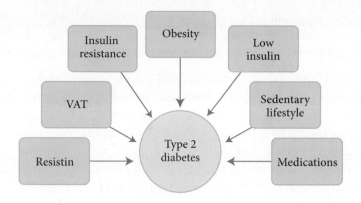

Figure 10.45 Many factors are involved with the development of type 2 diabetes.

acid cycle. As a result, the acetyl-CoA that is produced by β-oxidation of fatty acids, rather than being used in the citric acid cycle, accumulates in the cells. Because little coenzyme A is present in the cell, acetyl-CoA is broken down to release coenzyme A—a process that also favors the synthesis of ketone bodies (acetoacetate, β-hydroxybutyrate, and acetone). These acidic ketones are released into the blood and reduce the pH of the blood, causing a life-threatening condition.

Type 2 Diabetes

Type 2 diabetes may occur in any age group, but most often arises in patients with a sedentary lifestyle. Approximately 80% of all patients with type 2 diabetes are obese. In type 2 diabetes, the pancreas can produce insulin but myocytes and adipocytes do not respond adequately to the insulin hormone (referred to as "insulin resistance"). Type 2 diabetes is more prevalent than type 1 disease, and 90% of all patients with diabetes have this form of the disease.

Many risk factors contribute to the development of type 2 diabetes, including family history (i.e., diagnosed parents or siblings), obesity, sedentary lifestyle, race or ethnicity (Native Americans, African Americans, Hispanic Americans, and Asians/South Pacific Islanders), hypertension (usually 140/90 mm Hg in adults), dyslipidemia (high TG and low HDL), polycystic ovary syndrome, and a history of gestational DM. **Figure 10.43** highlights some of the factors that predispose individuals to develop type 2 diabetes.

As part of the management of type 2 diabetes, it is important to encourage patients to undertake dietary and exercise modifications and to educate them to implement self-monitoring of blood glucose (SMBG). Regular exercise and knowledge of their blood glucose levels can prevent worsening of type 2 diabetes symptoms or complications. In other words, type 2 disease is not as severe as type 1 disease, and it is possible to control this form with exercise and a healthy diet. However, if these efforts fail, oral drug therapy is initiated to stimulate the pancreas to produce more insulin or to reduce insulin resistance. Persons with type 2 diabetes who have a glucose level greater than 250 mg/dL or HbA_{1c} greater than 10% may also require insulin injections (0.1–0.2 U/kg/day). Depending on medication adherence, most individuals with type 2 diabetes and HbA_{1c} greater than 9% are likely to use two or more antidiabetic agents (combination therapy) to reach the optimal goal. For instance, combination oral agents consisting of metformin and glyburide (Glucovance) or metformin and glipizide (Metaglip) can effectively reduce a high HbA_{1c}.

Following consumption of a carbohydrate-rich food, insulin is secreted by the pancreas, enters the portal vein, and is transported to the liver. Insulin also suppresses glucagon secretion, and in the liver it reduces gluconeogenesis. However, patients with type 2 diabetes fail to suppress glucagon release, which results in hyperglucagonemia and continued gluconeogenesis. As a result, these patients have two sources of glucose in the postprandial state (following a meal): the carbohydrate in the food and the continued gluconeogenesis occurring in the liver.

While a person is in a fasting state, 75% of the body's glucose supply may be utilized by non–insulin-dependent tissues (brain, liver, and GI tissues), and 25% is used by muscle that is dependent on insulin. Due to the unique ability of glucose to provide ATP, the brain's glucose uptake occurs at the same rate during both fed and fasting periods. Approximately 80% of the glucose that is taken up by peripheral tissues is used by the skeletal muscle; only a small percentage (5%) is used by adipocytes. Nevertheless, adipocytes play an important role in maintaining glucose homeostasis. For instance, small increments in the plasma insulin concentration result in a marked reduction in the plasma fatty acid level, and this reduction increases the uptake of glucose by muscle and decreases gluconeogenesis in the liver. As a result, the risk of hyperglycemia is reduced.

Weight gain has been associated with the development of type 2 diabetes. The relative amounts of two adipose hormones, resistin and adiponectin, in the body are altered in type 2 diabetes. Adiponectin is a peptide hormone that inhibits hepatic gluconeogenesis and increases glucose transport and fatty acid oxidation in myocytes; the level of adiponectin is reduced in obesity. Resistin is a polypeptide hormone that blocks the action of insulin; the level of resistin is elevated in obesity.

Another factor associated with obesity and development of type 2 diabetes is visceral adipose tissue (VAT), which refers to fat cells located within the abdominal cavity. VAT explains the variation in insulin resistance seen in African Americans patients. Such tissue has a higher rate of lipolysis than subcutaneous fat, resulting in an increased level of plasma fatty acid. These fatty acids decrease glucose uptake by skeletal muscle.

Gestational Diabetes

During late pregnancy, plasma fatty acids levels become elevated. This increased level of free fatty acids may block the uptake of glucose by myocytes and stimulate hepatic gluconeogenesis, which in turn precipitates insulin resistance. Gestational diabetes is one of the most common complications of pregnancy, affecting approximately 7% of all pregnant women in the United States. Often, gestational diabetes is treated by diet and exercise and the condition is resolved following delivery.

Diabetic Complications

It is very important to reduce any risk of microvascular complications (retinopathy, nephropathy, neuropathy) and macrovascular complications (stroke and CVD) in both type 1 and type 2 diabetes. Current American Diabetes Association guidelines state that the target HbA_{1c} goal to prevent microvascular or macrovascular complications is less than 7%.

Metabolic Syndrome

Metabolic syndrome, also referred to as insulin resistance, is associated with CV risk factors including hyperinsulinemia, hypertension, abdominal obesity, dyslipidemia, and coagulation disorders. While metabolic syndrome is a risk indicator, it does not represent an absolute risk because it does not include other risk factors, such as age and sex. Nevertheless, patients with metabolic syndrome are at increased risk for CV disease and type 2 diabetes.

Central obesity is recognized as a key factor in the development of metabolic syndrome and can be assessed by using waist circumference, which is a good marker for VAT. An individual with three or more of the following risk factors is considered to have a metabolic syndrome:

- Abdominal obesity with a waist circumference greater than 102 cm for men or greater than 88 cm for women
- Triacylglycerol level equal to or greater than 150 mg/dL
- HDL level less than 40 mg/dL for men or less than 50 mg/dL for women
- Blood pressure equal to or greater than 130/80 mm Hg
- Fasting glucose equal to or greater than 110 mg/dL

The American Diabetes Association recommends overweight (BMI = 25 kg/m²) individuals (at any age) who have at least one other risk factor be screened for type 2 diabetes. The screening test is either fasting plasma glucose, HbA_{1c}, or a 2-hour oral glucose load test.

Blurred Vision

Concentration of glucose in the aqueous humor of the eye is at least 5 times higher than that in the lens. This leads to diffusion of glucose from the aqueous humor to the lens. The enzyme known as aldose reductase catalyzes conversion of glucose to sorbitol (a sugar). Sorbitol molecules do not diffuse through cell membranes and, as a result, accumulate in the lens. There, they precipitate lens proteins, which in turn cause an osmotic imbalance in the lens. This eventually leads to blurred vision and then cataract. It remains to be seen whether an experimental aldose reductase inhibitor can be used clinically to prevent cataracts or optic neuropathy.

Hyperglycemia

The symptoms of hyperglycemia are indicated by the mnemonic UFAT: Urination, Fatigue, Agitation, and Thirst. The high blood glucose level associated with this condition exceeds the kidneys' reabsorption capacity for glucose, which allows glucose to spill into urine (glucosuria). This causes osmotic diuresis and excessive urination (polyuria) as well as dehydration (polydipsia). The polyuria also causes a urinary loss of Na^+ and K^+. In healthy individuals, all of the filtered glucose molecules are reabsorbed in the proximal tubule.

The excess of glucose in hyperglycemia binds to many tissue proteins in a nonenzymatic manner. The resulting glycated proteins are called advanced glycosylation end products (AGEs). Macrophage receptors, upon binding to AGEs, release cytokines such as interleukin 1 (IL-1) and tumor necrosis factor (TNF) (see also the *Introduction to Immunology* chapter). The release of these cytokines increases the proliferation of endothelial cells and degrades mesenchymal cells (cells that differentiate into osteoblasts, adipocytes, myoblasts, and chondroblasts).

The normal blood glucose level is 5 mM (approximately 90 mg/dL). Even under the condition of starvation, this concentration should not be lower than 2.5 mM. An adequate concentration of glucose in the blood is necessary to supply enough glucose to both the brain and erythrocytes: Nerve cells (which use many ATP molecules) and erythrocytes (which lack mitochondria that might otherwise produce enough ATP molecules) need a constant supply of glucose.

Retinopathy

Diabetes is the leading cause of nontraumatic blindness. The blood vessels of the eyes in persons with diabetes are prone to microaneurysms, fragile vessels, leakage, and hemorrhage. These pathologic complications are collectively referred to as diabetic retinopathy. Because early-stage retinopathy can be reversed with improved glycemic control, it is imperative that patients with established retinopathy see an ophthalmologist or an optometrist. Unfortunately, more advanced retinopathy cannot be reversed through improved glycemic control.

Nephropathy

Nephropathy results in the development of end-stage renal disease. When a patient is newly diagnosed with type 2 diabetes, it is important to carry out a urinary analysis for albumin (i.e., measure the risk of microalbuminuria). Microalbuminuria may be an early indication of diabetic nephropathy. While macroalbuminuria (or simply albuminuria) is characterized by a high concentration of albumin (more than 300 mg/24 hours) in the urine and is indicative of glomerular damage, microalbuminuria is defined by identification of 30–300 mg albumin/24 hours in the urine. Microalbuminuria rarely occurs in patients with type 1 diabetes.

Because many factors can affect the amount of albumin in the urine, microalbuminuria should be assessed on two separate occasions over a period of 3–6 months. In addition, factors that affect the amount of albumin in the urine should be taken into consideration (i.e., conditions that may cause temporary elevations in the urinary albumin excretion such as exercise, urinary tract infections, hypertension, short-term hyperglycemia, and heart failure). ACE inhibitors and ARBs, due to their effectiveness in reducing intraglomerular pressure, are the first-line agents prescribed to prevent the progression of renal disease in patients with type 2 diabetes.

Peripheral Neuropathy

Neuropathy describes the inability of neurons to transmit information back and forth from the brain and spinal cord to the rest of the body. As a result of peripheral neuropathy, patients with diabetes may experience muscle weakness, pain in the extremities, urinary incontinence, numbness or loss of sensation in the feet, and sexual impotence. Claudication and nonhealing foot ulcers are common complications in patients with type 2 diabetes. Therefore, it is important to advise patients to cease smoking and correct lipid abnormalities, along with initiating antiplatelet therapy. Paresthesias, numbness, and pain in the feet are often the predominant symptoms of peripheral neuropathy. When neuropathy is painful, patients can use low-dose tricyclic antidepressants, anticonvulsants (gabapentin, pregabalin, carbamazepine), duloxetine, and venlafaxine to obtain relief. Interestingly, topiramate (Topamax) is also effective in this indication; it reduces peripheral neuropathy symptoms and can stimulate weight loss in patients with diabetes.

Peripheral neuropathy can affect the cell body (neuronopathy or ganglionopathy), myelin (myelinopathy), and the axon (axonopathy) of nerve cells. These conditions present with distinct clinical manifestations.

Learning Bridge 10.11

Joe is a 45-year-old, obese male who was diagnosed with type 2 diabetes 5 months ago. Despite being advised by his primary physician to become more active, he maintains a sedentary lifestyle. He is currently taking metformin 1,000 mg twice a day. His HbA_{1c} was 8.5% at his last doctor's visit. When he came to refill his medication, Joe complained about burning and tingling sensations in his feet. You suspected peripheral neuropathy and advised him to see a physician immediately.

A. What are the treatment options to treat diabetic neuropathy?
B. Can you delay the occurrence of diabetic neuropathy?
C. How will you counsel Joe on lifestyle modifications?

Diabetes Management

The main goals of diabetes management are to educate patients about symptoms (particularly hypoglycemia) and awareness of their daily blood glucose level, to decrease the risk for complications (both microvascular and macrovascular complications), to improve symptoms, and to improve the quality of life. While achieving glycemic control that leads to less than 7% HbA_{1c} is desirable to reduce the risk for development of microvascular complications, smoking cessation and treatment of dyslipidemia and hypertension are required for the management of macrovascular complications. Hyperglycemia increases the risk for microvascular disease and causes poor wound healing. As mentioned previously, DKA is the most severe consequence of type 1 diabetes; to treat this condition, hospitalization and intravenous insulin injection are required. Simply put, blood glucose control alone is not sufficient to reduce the risk of macrovascular complications.

Hypoglycemia

The most common adverse reaction to insulin and oral antidiabetic drugs is hypoglycemia. It can cause serious complications and if prolonged can be fatal. Hypoglycemia symptoms include the following:

- Neurogenic symptoms appear at a blood glucose level of 40–60 mg/dL and include sweating, hunger, paresthesias, palpitations, tremor, and anxiety.
- Neuroglycopenic symptoms appear at a blood glucose level less than 40 mg/dL and consist of confusion, convulsions, drowsiness, blurred vision, and coma. A blood glucose level less than 10 mg/dL leads to permanent brain damage and death.

Hypoglycemic symptoms that occur during the day are manageable. For instance, giving fruit juice or a few sugar cubes will immediately alleviate the symptoms. Hypoglycemia that occurs during night (sleep) is difficult to detect; morning signs indicative of nocturnal hypoglycemia include morning headaches, night sweats, and symptoms of hypothermia.

All of the following conditions may cause hypoglycemia:

- Certain drugs: insulin, oral antidiabetic drugs (particularly sulfonylureas), ethanol, and quinine (an antimalarial agent)
- Critical illnesses of hepatic, renal, and cardiac origin and sepsis
- Deficiencies of cortisol, glucagon, norepinephrine, and epinephrine
- Insulinoma

Insulinoma is the excessive production and release of insulin by β cells. The excessive amount of insulin carries a large amount of glucose into the cells, which results in hypoglycemia. The lack of glucose means fewer ATP molecules are available in the brain—a condition that, if not treated, leads to brain damage. For conditions where the insulin level should be low (such as during fasting or exercise), the high insulin concentration results in hypoglycemia. In a healthy person in a fasting or exercise state, insulin level would decrease to promote gluconeogenesis and thereby maintain normal levels of blood glucose. In addition, the low insulin level promotes lipolysis to release fatty acids and thereby provide energy during exercise or fast.

Insulin also promotes cellular uptake of potassium. In patients with a deficiency of insulin (diabetes), potassium does not move into the cells efficiently, which results in hyperkalemia. Patients with insulinoma, however, develop hypokalemia. For this reason, these individuals should avoid drugs that cause potassium depletion, such as corticosteroids, diuretics, aldosterone antagonists, and amphotericin B (Fungizone, from Canada). A plasma C-peptide level of 2 nmol/L or greater is indicative of insulinoma.

For patients with type 1 diabetes, in addition to insulin administration, consumption of a balanced and healthy diet is important to maintain a healthy body weight. Careful monitoring of the amounts of carbohydrate and fat in the diet is imperative. In contrast, for patients with type 2 diabetes, weight loss is an important factor in maintaining glycemic control. Exercise is also important to improve the sensitivity of tissue cells to insulin and to reduce CV risk factors. It is important to advise patients to select an exercise regimen that they are likely to adhere to or to begin with slow-paced exercise if they have a sedentary lifestyle.

In addition to different insulin injection formulations (for both type 1 and 2 diabetes), eight classes of oral antidiabetic agents (only for type 2 diabetes) are available in the United States.

Insulin Injections

Lipohypertrophy, which is indicated by an enlargement of subcutaneous fat depots, occurs frequently with insulin injections when patients administer insulin to the same anatomic site of their body. Lipohypertrophy may also cause tissue damage and irregular absorption of insulin. Counsel your patients to rotate the sites of injection within one anatomic region (for instance, in the abdominal area) rather than injecting insulin in a different anatomic region. If burning, itching, or swelling occurs at the sites of injections, counsel your patients to contact their providers.

Several different synthetic preparations of insulin injections are available, which have different characteristics such as strength, onset, and duration of action. To establish these characteristics, insulin hormones are manipulated (analogs) to produce physiochemical and pharmacokinetic advantages by changing one or more amino acids along the insulin's polypeptide chains. Today, two strengths of insulin injections are available in the United States: 100 units/mL (which corresponds to 3.6 mg/mL) and 500 units/mL. The 500 units/mL regular insulin is available for patients who need a higher strength. All other insulin injections are provided as 100 units/mL, so one has to be careful with the 500 units/mL strength to avoid a serious dispensing error. If a patient needs lower doses of insulin, dilution of 100 units/mL insulin can be achieved by using diluents and empty bottles that can be obtained from the manufacturers of the insulin injection.

In the past, the insulin injections were prepared from either beef or pork sources. For instance, bovine insulin (which differs from human insulin by only three amino acids) was used for type 1 diabetes. Because of concerns about mad cow disease, it is no longer available in the United States; instead, recombinant DNA is used to manufacture insulin. For instance, Eli Lilly and Sanofi-Aventis use *Escherichia coli* and Novo Nordisk uses *Saccharomyces cerevisiae* (yeast organism) for the synthesis and production of injectable insulin (see also the *Introduction to Cell Biology* chapter).

For an insulin molecule to be absorbed in an active form through blood capillaries, it must attain a monomer structure. Six insulin molecules can naturally self-associate into a hexamere upon subcutaneous injection. To dissociate the hexameric structure prior to absorption, one can add additives such as protamine and zinc or substitute one or more amino acids along the insulin chains.

Lispro (Humalog), aspart (Novolog), and glulisine (Apidra) insulin dissociate rapidly to monomers because of amino acid changes. In insulin lispro, lysine and proline in the B chain are reversed (hence the name lispro). This structural change results in the fast onset of short-acting insulin (less than 15 minutes). In insulin aspart, proline is changed to aspartic acid. These structural changes do not allow insulin to self-associate, which results in a short-acting insulin. Insulin glulisine has two amino acid exchanges: Lysine is replaced by glutamic acid and asparagine is replaced by lysine. Again, these structural changes result in a short-acting, fast-onset preparation. All three rapid-acting insulin formulations (lispro, aspart, and glulisine) have less tendency to cause hypoglycemia (a major concern for many antidiabetic agents). Therefore, patients with diabetes who use these drugs do not need to eat snacks between meals.

Glargine (Lantus) insulin is synthesized by changing four amino acids. It reaches its isoelectric point (6.8) at the site of injection and becomes insoluble. This insolubility prolongs glargine's absorption. In other words, while glargine is buffered to a pH of 4, at the site of injection with a neutral pH of the body, it rapidly builds the insoluble hexameric form and slowly dissolves into monomers and dimers. Because of the important role that the pH plays in its action, glargine should not be mixed with other insulin preparations. Glargine is a long-acting insulin injection (24-hour duration).

Another long-acting insulin, detemir (Levemir), has a different composition. In detemir, a 14-carbon fatty acid is attached at amino acid 29 in the B chain of the insulin molecule. The attached fatty acid facilitates the insulin chains' attachment to interstitial albumin at the subcutaneous injection site. The prolonged action of detemir is produced as the drug slowly dissociates from the interstitial albumin to enter the capillaries.

NPH stands for "neutral protamine Hagedorn." Protamine, as the name indicates, is a protein isolated from fish. This protein, together with zinc, facilitates aggregation of insulin molecules, which in turn prolongs the duration of action of insulin (18–24 hours).

A few factors play important roles in the absorption of insulin from a subcutaneous depot—for instance, the concentration of the insulin, additives to the insulin preparations, buffering of the solution, inconsistent suspension (gently rolling the vial back and forth can alleviate this problem), blood flow to the injection area (rub the injection area to increase skin temperature), and the injection site. Abdominal fat, the posterior upper arms, the lateral thigh area, and the superior buttocks are the best sites for injection of regular or NPH insulin preparation; all other insulin preparations retain their absorption profile at all sites of injection.

Regular insulin is the only insulin solution that can be given intravenously; it is a clear solution and can be mixed with all other insulin solutions except insulin glargine and insulin detemir. When mixing regular insulin with other insulin injections, regular insulin should be drawn first.

Insulin is metabolized in the liver, muscle, and kidney. While the liver accounts for 20% to 50% of insulin's metabolism in a single pass, 15% to 20% of insulin metabolism takes place in the kidney. The latter process may explain why a lower insulin dose is required in patients with end-stage renal disease.

Researchers have explored a variety routes of administration for insulin in an effort to increase compliance with therapy and reduce the cost for patients. The pulmonary route of insulin administration is especially attractive because of the lungs' large alveolar-capillary network for drug absorption. The first inhalation insulin was approved in early 2003 (Exubera), but was eventually discontinued due to its potential for causing lung cancer. Another inhaled insulin preparation (Afrezza) is currently undergoing clinical trials for efficacy and safety.

Most of the insulin preparations are neutral in terms of pH, a characteristic that improves their stability. The major exception is the long-acting insulin known as glargine, which is provided in an acidic solution.

The primary route of insulin administration is subcutaneous. While intermediate-acting insulin preparations (which are suspensions) are cloudy solutions, rapid-, short-, and long-acting insulin preparations are "clear" solutions. Pharmacists should avoid using this "clear" designation as an indicator of the kind of insulin injection or preparation, because such clarity is not unique to any particular preparation and can cause errors in dispensing and administration of insulin preparations.

Table 10.8 Insulin Preparations

Generic	Brand	Onset	Duration	Comments
Rapid-Acting Insulin				
Lispro	Humalog	<15 min	3 hr	Usually administered in association with meals.
Aspart	Novolog	<15 min		
Glulysine	Apidra	<15 min		
Short-Acting Insulin				
Regular insulin	Novolin R, Humulin R	0.5–1 hr	3–6 hr	Inject 30 minutes before a meal; it is the only formulation that can be administered intravenously.
Intermediate-Acting Insulin				
Insulin zinc	Insulin Lente	3–4 hr	12–18 hr	Should not be used for emergency situations; available in suspension forms; often administered at bedtime (i.e., after a few daytime injections of rapid- or short-acting insulin).
Human NPH	Novolin N, Humulin N	1–3 hr		
Long-Acting Insulin				
Glargine	Lantus	3–4 hr	24 hr	Should not be diluted or mixed with any other insulin or solution; should be administered once daily, at any time of day but at the same time of each day; has an acidic pH.
Detemir	Levemir	3–4 hr	18–24 hr	Should not be diluted or mixed with any other insulin or solution; duration is dose dependent; has a fatty acid attachment. • 0.1–0.2 unit/kg: 6–12 hr • 0.6 unit/kg: 20 hr • > 0.6 unit/kg: 22 hr
Ultralente	—	6–10 hr	18–20 hr	Rarely prescribed.
Premixed Insulin				
Insulin NPH/insulin regular	Novolin 70/30; Humulin 50/50	0.5–1 hr	18–24 hr	Administered once or twice daily (before breakfast and dinner); the pen in use should not be refrigerated and the insulin should not be mixed or diluted with other insulin.
Insulin aspart protamine/insulin aspart	Novolog 70/30	<15min	18–24 hr	Intermediate-acting characteristics; store unopened vials in refrigerator; vials (in use) may be stored at room temperature for up to 28 days. Do not use if it is frozen; administer within 15 minutes before a meal; the pen in use should not be refrigerated and should be discarded after 14 days.

Data from: *Pharmacotherapy: A Pathophysiologic Approach*, 7th ed.; *Remington: The Science and Practice of Pharmacy*, 21st ed.; *Drug Information Handbook*, 18th ed.; and *Comprehensive Pharmacy Review*, 7th ed.

The insulin solution should not be shaken because insulin is a polypeptide that upon shaking will be denatured, thereby rendering the insulin inactive. Gently rolling the vials in the hands (10 times) should be advised.

The four major insulin preparations are classified as rapid acting, short acting, intermediate acting, and long acting, based on their onset and duration of action. Premixed insulin preparations are also available. **Table 10.8** identifies the various insulin preparations.

Oral Antidiabetic Agents

The classes of oral antidiabetic agents available in the U.S. market include glucosidase inhibitors, biguanides, meglitinides, peroxisome proliferator-activated receptor agonists (thiazolidinediones or glitazones), dipeptidyl peptidase 4 (DPP-4) inhibitors, GLP-1 agonists, dopamine agonists, and sulfonylureas. Two important considerations arise with these antidiabetic agents: (1) none of them are of any use for type 1 diabetes and (2) all of them are contraindicated in patients with ketoacidosis. A patient with type 2 diabetes with a glucose level greater than 250 mg/dL or HbA$_{1c}$ greater than 10% is prescribed injectable insulin (0.1–0.2 U/kg/day). While biguanides and thiazolidinediones are able to reduce insulin resistance and, therefore, are often categorized as insulin sensitizers, sulfonylureas and meglitinides are categorized as insulin secretagogues due to their ability to enhance the release of insulin from pancreas.

Sulfonylureas

As their names indicate, sulfonylureas have sulfonamide and urea functional groups (**Figure 10.46**). All drugs in this class are highly protein bound and block the ATP-gated K$^+$ channels in the plasma membrane of β cells to stimulate the secretion of endogenous insulin. These drugs may cause a weight gain of 1–2 kg. Normally, the uptake of glucose through GLUT2 on the β cells stimulates the release of insulin. Inside the β cells, just as in any other cells, glucose undergoes glycolysis, which leads to an increased number of ATP molecules. These ATP molecules close the ATP-gated K$^+$ channels in the plasma membrane, which results in depolarization of the membrane. This depolarization process, in turn, opens Ca^{2+} channels in the membrane and is followed by calcium influx and insulin release.

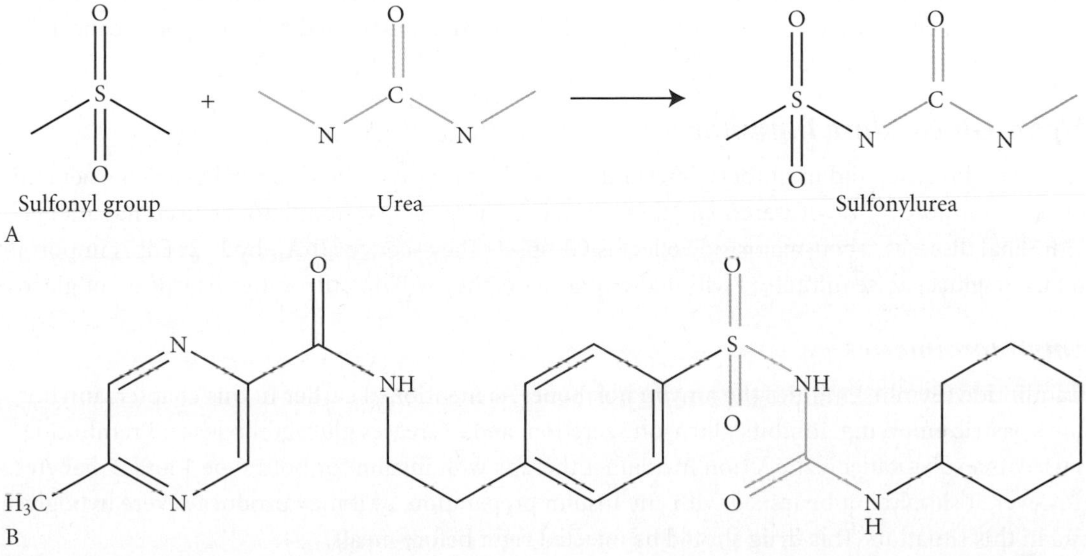

Figure 10.46 (A) Sulfonylurea has both sulfonamide and urea functional groups. (B) Structure of glipizide.

First-generation sulfonylureas include tolbutamide (Apo-Tolbutamide, from Canada), which has a relatively short duration of action ($t_{1/2} \approx 10$ hours), and chlorpropamide (Apo-Chlorpropamide, from Canada Diabinese), which has a longer duration of action ($t_{1/2} = 36$ hours). Second-generation sulfonylureas include glipizide (Glucotrol), glyburide (DiaBeta), and glimepiride (Amaryl). They have a long duration of action (approximately 24 hours), and their plasma levels are increased when they are combined with salicylate, sulfonamide, MAOIs, and choramphenicol. Glyburide does not effectively cross the placenta, which makes it a safe drug for use in pregnancy. All of the second-generation agents reduce HbA_{1c} by 1–2%.

Meglitinides

Agents in this class are repaglinide (Prandin) and nateglinide (Starlix). They have a similar mechanism of action to sulfonylureas, but provide a shorter duration of action than the second-generation sulfonylureas (2 hours versus 24 hours). Meglitinides may be used with other antidiabetic agents (except sulfonylureas) and reduce HbA_{1c} by 1–2%. They are particularly useful if a patient is allergic to sulfonylurea.

Biguanides

Metformin (Glucophage) is the drug of choice in initiating antidiabetic treatment. It inhibits gluconeogenesis and reduces triacylglycerol synthesis. However, it is the only agent among the oral antidiabetic agents that can cause lactic acidosis. Because of this side effect, patients should avoid drinking alcohol, as alcohol potentiates lactic acid formation. Metformin should not be used in patients with renal or hepatic diseases. To reduce stomach upset, it should be taken with food (the therapeutic dose is more than 1 g/day). Metformin reduces HbA_{1C} by 1–2%.

Thiazolidinediones

The two agents of the thiazolidinedione (TZD) class are rosiglitazone (Avandia) and pioglitazone (Actos). They activate PPARγ, a nuclear hormone receptor associated with glucose metabolism and adipocyte differentiation. These agents reduce the level of circulating fatty acids in the blood by stimulating glyceroneogenesis (synthesis of triacylglycerols; see also the *Introduction to Biochemistry* chapter). These "long-acting" (more than 24 hours) oral agents are known to cause weight gain and edema. The FDA requires a "black box" warning on rosiglitazone's label because this drug can cause or exacerbate CHF. In addition, the FDA requires a "black box" warning on pioglitazone's label because of the risk of heart failure and the increased risk of bladder cancer. Thiazolidinediones reduce HbA_{1c} by 1–2%.

Alpha-Glucosidase Inhibitors

Acarbose (Precose) and miglitol (Glyset) inhibit α-glucosidase in the intestinal brush border and decrease the absorption of starch and disaccharides. These agents should not be used in patients with renal diseases. Their major side effect is GI upset. They reduce HbA_{1c} by 1–2%. It is important to take α-glucosidase inhibitors with food; otherwise, they will not affect the absorption of glucose.

Amylinomimetics

Pramlintide (Symlin) mimics the amylin hormone. As mentioned earlier in this chapter, amylin slows gastric emptying, inhibits glucagon secretion, and decreases glucagon release. Pramlintide is used as a subcutaneous injection in adjunct therapy with insulin for both type 1 and 2 diabetes. However, it should not be mixed with any insulin preparation, as it may produce severe hypoglycemia in this situation. This drug should be injected right before meals.

Dipeptidyl Peptidase 4 Inhibitors

The incretin hormone stimulates β cells to release insulin; it also inhibits the release of glucagon. Dipeptidyl peptidase 4 (DPP-IV), in turn, inhibits incretin. Sitagliptin (Januvia) and saxagliptin (Onglyza) are inhibitors of DPP-IV that can increase the incretin level. DPP-IV inhibitors are often used in combination with sulfonylureas or biguanide. Sitagliptin is excreted by the kidneys, so precautions should be taken when prescribing it to patients with renal diseases. Sitagliptin is known to reduce HbA_{1C} by 0.6–1.2%.

Incretin Mimics

Exenatide (Byetta) is a subcutaneous injection that mimics incretin. As a result, it stimulates β cells to release insulin and inhibits the release of glucagon. In addition, it slows gastric emptying to slow glucose absorption into blood (this agent should not be given after ingestion of food). Exenatide should not be given with drugs that require rapid GI absorption. It is known to cause weight loss and reduces HbA_{1c} by 0.5–1%. Nausea is often an initial adverse effect with exenatide, and patients should be counseled to drink plenty of fluids.

Sodium Glucose Transporter 2 Inhibitors

Sodium glucose transporter 2 (SGL-2) inhibitors block the active reabsorption of glucose in the proximal tubule of the kidney. SGL-2 is a potential target for the development of other classes of antidiabetic agents. In March 2013, canagliflozin, an SGL-2 inhibitor drug, was approved by the FDA for treating patients with type 2 diabetes. Canagliflozin is the first SGLT-2 inhibitor to enter the U.S. market.

Respiratory System

As explained in the *Introduction to Biochemistry* chapter, during oxidative phosphorylation, most of the body's tissues depend on oxygen to produce ATP. We constantly need to breathe in oxygen so that oxygen can be distributed to the various tissues. In turn, the by-product of oxygen consumption, CO_2, needs to be exhaled. Simply put, the major role of the respiratory system is to take in oxygen through inhalation, distribute that oxygen to the body's tissues, and remove accumulated CO_2 from the tissues by exhalation. The respiratory system consists of the lungs (a gas-exchanging organ) and the chest wall. It also includes respiratory muscles and nerves that connect these muscles to the brain.

At rest, we breathe 12–15 times per minute, and with each breath we inspire and expire approximately 500 mL of air. As part of the oxygen–carbon dioxide exchange process, 250 mL of O_2 enters the body per minute and 200 mL of CO_2 is excreted. Other gases are also found in expired air including methane (from the intestines), alcohol, and acetone (produced in different biochemical pathways). Interestingly, more than 250 different volatile substances have been identified in human breath.

The air we breathe goes through the nose or mouth, the pharynx, the larynx (the upper airways), and then passes down the trachea and enters the alveoli through the respiratory bronchioles and alveolar ducts. In the alveoli, oxygen comes in contact with the venous blood in the pulmonary capillaries. Between the trachea and the alveolar sacs, the airways divide approximately 23 times. These multiple divisions dramatically enhance the total cross-sectional area of the airways, from 2.5 cm² in the trachea to 11,800 cm² in the alveoli.

Two types of epithelial cells line the alveoli. Type I cells cover approximately 95% of the alveolar epithelial surface area. Type II cells are thicker and make up 5% of the surface area; they secrete surfactant and participate in alveolar repair. In addition to these two cell types, the alveoli contain other specialized cells including macrophages, lymphocytes, plasma cells, neuroendocrine cells, and mast cells. The mast cells secrete heparin, lipids, histamine, and a series of proteases that contribute to allergic reactions. Surfactant, a lipid-containing protein, is produced in the lungs and found in the fluid lining the alveolar epithelium. Surfactant reduces surface tension in the lungs, thereby allowing the expansion of alveoli.

The autonomic nervous system innervates the walls of the bronchi and bronchioles with (1) efferent parasympathetic fibers that cause bronchoconstriction, pulmonary vasodilation, and bronchial secretion and (2) sympathetic fibers that cause bronchial smooth muscle relaxation, pulmonary vasoconstriction, and inhibition of bronchial secretion. For instance, the bronchial epithelium and smooth muscle contain β_2-adrenergic receptors. While stimulation of β_2 receptors increases bronchial secretion and mediates bronchodilation, stimulation of α_1-adrenergic receptors inhibits bronchial secretion.

Abnormalities in the airway's functions may lead to chronic obstructive pulmonary disease (COPD), exemplified by chronic bronchitis and emphysema. From a clinical standpoint, it is important to distinguish between asthma and COPD. **Table 10.9** identifies the differences between these two diseases.

Asthma

Asthma is caused by bronchoconstriction and is characterized by chronic wheezing, cough, and a feeling of tightness in the chest. Three underlying characteristics of asthma are

- *Airway obstruction.* Leukotrienes that are released from eosinophils and mast cells can cause bronchoconstriction.

Table 10.9 Differences between Asthma and COPD

Asthma	COPD
Asthma is a chronic inflammatory disease of the airways of the lung. Its onset typically occurs during childhood or adolescence, and is a result of genetic predisposition and environmental exposures.	COPD is caused by chronic bronchitis or emphysema. Most commonly, it occurs in smokers (85% of diagnosed cases). In addition, risk factors such as genetic predisposition, environmental exposures (dusts and chemicals), and air pollution contribute to COPD.
Exacerbations are caused by chronic wheezing, cough, shortness of breath, and a feeling of tightness in the chest. Cold air, exposure to chemicals, or exercise may trigger these exacerbations.	Exacerbations are often caused by respiratory tract infections. For this reason, antimicrobial therapy is used during acute exacerbations of COPD.
Patients with asthma who receive appropriate treatment have near-normal lung function and are symptom free between exacerbations.	Patients with COPD rarely experience a day without symptoms.
The inflammatory process in asthma is treated most effectively with corticosteroids, and bronchial constriction is prevented/treated with inhaled β_2-adrenergic receptor agonists.	Bronchodilators represent the mainstay of drug therapy (long-acting bronchodilators). Smoking cessation slows the progression of COPD. Corticosteroids do not have any significant anti-inflammatory effect in COPD and, as a result, the use of corticosteroids is controversial.

- *Airway inflammation.* In inflammatory reactions, proteins released from eosinophils can damage the airway epithelium and contribute to the hyperresponsiveness. In addition, other mediators (amines, neuropeptides, chemokines, and interleukins) produce inflammation in the lungs.
- *Airway hyperresponsiveness.* An immune reaction has been linked to asthma, indicated by high plasma IgE levels. Allergens, particles that stimulate IgE production and release, include proteins (e.g., house mite dust, cockroach feces, animal danders, molds, pollens). The IgE antibodies bind to mast cells in the airway mucosa. Upon reexposure to the allergen, the antigen–antibody interaction on the surface of the mast cells initiates the synthesis and secretion of histamine, tryptase, leukotrienes C_4 and D_4, and prostaglandin D_2. These mediators cause muscle contraction and vascular leakage, which ultimately lead to acute bronchoconstriction. Bronchoconstriction is not always caused by allergens, instead, it may result from viral respiratory infections. In addition, bronchoconstriction can be caused by exercise, and inhalation of cold air and sulfur dioxide (so-called nonspecific bronchial hyperreactivity).

Asthma is also characterized by alteration of the bronchial mucosa—namely, thickening of the lamina reticularis that lies under the airway epithelium. This thickening process also causes hyperplasia of the cells of the airway wall vessels, smooth muscle, secretory glands, and goblet cells.

Two forms of asthma are distinguished: mild and severe. In the mild form of the disease, symptoms occur only occasionally and are often caused by exposure to allergens, exercise, or viral upper respiratory infection. In contrast, severe asthma is associated with frequent attacks of wheezing dyspnea, particularly at night. Because both short-term and long-term treatments are available, these clinical symptoms are manageable.

When patients experience symptoms, reversing the contraction of smooth muscle is the easiest and fastest way to treat them. Short-term relief can be achieved by administering β-receptor agonists. Long-term control is achieved with inhaled corticosteroids, leukotriene pathway antagonists, or inhibitors of mast cell degranulation. Severe asthma has also been treated with a monoclonal antibody, omalizumab, which reduces IgE and thereby mitigates allergic sensitization.

β_2 agonists bind to the β_2 receptors present on the lungs to cause bronchodilation, which can relieve mild to moderate asthma attacks. Other drugs, such as steroids, are used to reduce inflammation. Inhibitors of leukotriene synthesis or leukotriene receptor antagonists have also shown to produce desirable outcomes in patients with asthma. The following subsections profile the drugs used in the treatment of asthma.

Inhaled Corticosteroids

Inhaled corticosteroids (ICS) are the first-line therapy for patients with persistent asthma. Although the optimal dose and schedule of ICS are unknown, these agents are often administered twice daily. Corticosteroids have anti-inflammatory effects and inhibit the infiltration of asthmatic airways with lymphocytes, eosinophils, and mast cells.

Inhaled corticosteroids are equally effective in both children and adults. Doses of less than 400 µg beclomethasone (QVAR) or equivalent are effective, although some patients—particularly those who are resistant to corticosteroids—may need higher doses (up to 2000 µg/day). Inhaled corticosteroids are considered long-term "controllers," whereas beta agonists are referred to as short-term "relievers." An ICS can be added to a long-acting β-receptor agonist, such as salmeterol or formoterol, to improve asthma control.

Because steroids produce many side effects, patients should receive the minimal dose required to control asthma, and thereafter the dose should be slowly reduced. To reduce the side effects, corticosteroids are administered as inhaled medications rather than as oral or parenteral formulations. The latter two dosage forms are used only if patients have an urgent need for relief, do not respond well to other bronchodilators, or experience worsening symptoms with other bronchodilators.

It has been suggested that once-daily dosing of budesonide (Pulmicort), mometasone (Asmanex), and ciclesonide (Alvesco) is effective when the dose is 400 µg. If the daily dose requirement is more than 800 µg, a metered-dose inhaler (MDI) should be used. To reduce the risk of oropharyngeal side effects, a spacer device should be employed. Most ICS are administered as a daily dose of 4 puffs (2 puffs every 12 hours). Of note, MDIs do not work properly in cold temperatures.

Because inhaled steroids increase the risk of oropharyngeal candidiasis, patients need to rinse their mouth (gargle water and spit it out) after the administration of an ICS. The use of ICS is often continued for 10–12 weeks before making a decision to withdraw or continue with the therapy. Chronic use of ICS productively reduces symptoms, diminishes bronchial reactivity, and improves pulmonary function in patients with mild asthma. Because proper inhalation technique is important in improving the symptoms, pharmacists should counsel and teach patients to use the inhaler accurately.

Sympathomimetic Agents

The adrenoceptor agonists elicit the following antiasthmatic effects: airway smooth muscle relaxation, inhibition of the release of inflammatory mediators, prevention of microvascular leakage (which often leads to inflammation), and increased mucociliary transport. Adrenergic agonists activate adenylyl cyclase (AC) via coupling to stimulatory G-protein (Gs); AC activation is followed by increased production of intracellular cAMP (see also the *Introduction to Pharmacodynamics* chapter). However, sympathomimetic agents can cause tachycardia, arrhythmias, worsening of angina pectoris, and skeletal muscle tremor as side effects.

The most compelling effect of β adrenoceptor agonists in the airway is to relax the airway smooth muscle. The members of this drug class that have been used in the treatment of asthma include epinephrine, ephedrine, isoproterenol (Isuprel), and albuterol (ProAir or Proventil). Of note, both epinephrine and isoproterenol enhance the rate and force of cardiac contraction and, as a result, are reserved for special situations.

When epinephrine is injected subcutaneously (or inhaled), it produces rapid bronchodilation. The maximal bronchodilation effect is seen approximately 15 minutes after inhalation and lasts 60–90 minutes. Epinephrine is very effective in treating acute vasodilation, shock, and bronchospasm associated with anaphylaxis in an emergency situation. However, it has largely been replaced by more selective β_2 agonists in treating asthma.

Adrenoceptor agonists are administered by inhalation to reduce any systemic effects and produce significant localized effects on airway smooth muscle. The effectiveness of the inhalers depends on drug particle size and the pattern of breathing. For instance, bronchodilation is increased by slowly inhaling the drug and then holding the breath for 5–10 seconds. β_2 adrenoceptor agonists, when taken on an "as needed" basis, are considered safe bronchodilators to treat asthma.

Albuterol is the sympathomimetic agent most commonly used for treatment of the bronchoconstriction of asthma. Other β_2-selective agonists have also been used to treat asthma, including terbutaline (Bicanyl, from Canada), metaproterenol (Apo-Orciprenaline, from Canada), and pirbuterol (Maxair) in an MDI (terbutaline is the only one of these medications available in a subcutaneous injection dosage form). Compared to epinephrine, the structures of these drugs have larger substitutions on the amino group and the hydroxyl groups of the aromatic ring. These agents are effective both as inhalation medications and oral formulations. Because larger particles are used in nebulizers (much larger than those from an MDI), higher dose is necessary for its dosing (i.e., 2.5–5.0 mg versus 100–400 µg). Nebulizers are not superior to inhalers, but rather are used by patients who cannot coordinate inhalation from an MDI or simply cannot use an MDI.

Most β_2-selective agonists are racemic mixtures, in which only the R isomer activates the β_2 receptor (see also the *Introduction to Medicinal Chemistry* chapter). Levalbuterol (Xopenex) is a purified preparation of the R isomer of albuterol, although whether levalbuterol is better than albuterol remains controversial. In addition to being available as inhalers, albuterol (and terbutaline) is available in tablet form; doses are typically 1–3 tablets daily. Because tablets do not produce a better effect than inhalers, they are rarely prescribed.

Two long-acting (for at least 12 hours) β_2-selective agonists are available in the United States: salmeterol (Serevent) and formoterol (Foradil). Their longer duration of action results from their high lipid solubility. Figures 10.20 and 10.21 show the structures of albuterol and salmeterol, respectively.

For two obvious reasons, long-acting β_2-selective agonists are not better than albuterol. First, they do not have an anti-inflammatory effect and, as a result, they are not recommended as monotherapy for asthma. Second, due to their long-lasting effect, they should not be used in acute bronchospasm. However, because these agents do not interact with inhaled corticosteroids, they can be used together with steroids, as in the combination of fluticasone + salmeterol (Advair Diskus 100/50). Diskus is a dry-powder inhaler that patients need to breathe rapidly. In contrast, an MDI inhaler (e.g., albuterol) requires slow inhalation. Long-acting β_2-selective agonists are not the first-line treatment of asthma; indeed, their label carries a "black box" warning about the risk of asthma-related deaths.

Methylxanthine Agents

Use of theophylline (Theo-24; also found in tea) has significantly declined over the years, yet its very low cost is an important advantage for patients who live in societies with limited healthcare resources. Methylxanthine agents inhibit several members of the phosphodiesterase (PDE) family, including phosphodiesterase 4 (PDE4). Because PDE4 inactivates (hydrolyzes) cAMP, the PDE4 inhibition results in higher concentrations of intracellular cAMP, which (among other mechanisms) leads to increased relaxation of airway smooth muscle. In addition, the inhibition of PDE4 in inflammatory cells diminishes the secretion of cytokines and chemokines. The latter effect decreases immune cell migration and activation.

A second mechanism of action for methylxanthine agents has been suggested to be inhibition of cell-surface receptors for adenosine. Adenosine is known to promote contraction of airway smooth muscle. At low concentrations, methylxanthines inhibit presynaptic adenosine receptors in sympathetic nerves, resulting in increased catecholamine release from nerve endings. This finding may explain the positive chronotropic and inotropic effects of methylxanthine agents.

Theophylline has a narrow therapeutic window. Its toxic reactions correlate well with the plasma level of the agent. While theophylline is effective at plasma concentrations of 5–20 µg/mL, at higher doses (e.g., plasma concentrations of 15 µg/mL) it leads to anorexia, nausea, vomiting, abdominal discomfort, headache, and anxiety. In even higher doses, such as plasma levels greater than 40 µg/mL, its toxicity extends to seizures and arrhythmias.

Antimuscarinic Agents

Atropine works as a bronchodilator by inhibiting binding of acetylcholine at postganglionic muscarinic receptors. Antimuscarinic agents are useful for patients who cannot tolerate β_2 agonists. When atropine is given intravenously, it causes bronchodilation at a lower dose than the dose that causes an increase in the heart rate. Giving atropine as an inhaler drug can reduce its systemic effects on the heart.

A more selective quaternary ammonium derivative, ipratropium bromide (Atrovent HFA), can reduce the cardiac side effect due to its poor systemic absorption.

Tiotropium (Spiriva) is a long-acting (24-hour duration of action), selective antimuscarinic agent that is used as an inhaler medication for the treatment of COPD.

Cromolyn

Cromolyn (Gastrocrom) inhibits the early response of mast cells following exposure to an antigen. Notably, the inflammatory response of eosinophils to allergens is inhibited by this drug. Cromolyn can effectively prevent asthma attacks induced by antigen exposure and exercise. A consistent and regular dosing, such as four times daily, slightly reduces the level of bronchial hyperreactivity. Because cromolyn has a low bioavailability, it is used only in aerosol form (delivered by nebulizer or MDI). As a result, any systemic side effect is reduced and the drug remains confined to the sites of administration. Side effects include throat irritation, cough, and mouth dryness. Cromolyn cannot act on airway smooth muscle, so it is used only in asthma prophylaxis. Solutions of cromolyn are taken as nasal sprays or eye drops to reduce symptoms of allergic rhinoconjunctivitis.

Leukotriene Pathway Inhibitors

Leukotrienes are involved in many inflammatory diseases and, in turn, inhibition of their synthesis can help reduce airway inflammation. The enzyme 5-lipoxygenase catalyzes the synthesis of leukotrienes from arachidonic acid, when the former are produced by the inflammatory cells of the airways such as eosinophils, mast cells, macrophages, and basophils. Leukotrienes (LTD_4) cause bronchoconstriction, enhance bronchial reactivity, produce mucosal edema, and stimulate mucus hypersecretion.

Two mechanisms are exploited to counteract the role that leukotrienes play in asthma. First, the 5-lipoxygenase enzyme is inhibited to decrease the synthesis of leukotrienes. Second, direct inhibition of the binding of LTD_4 to its receptor on target tissues can prevent inflammatory actions. Zileuton (Zyflo) is a 5-lipoxygenase inhibitor, and zafirlukast (Accolate) and montelukast (Singulair) are inhibitors of the LTD_4 receptor. Both inhibitory mechanisms have been shown to produce effective responses in treating asthma. These leukotriene pathway inhibitors are administered orally, and they are useful in patients who struggle with inhalers (particularly montelukast, which is approved for use in children 6 years or younger).

Anti-IgE Monoclonal Antibodies

This category of drugs represents a new approach to treat asthma, but due to its cost, it is not widely used. Antibody against immunoglobulin E (IgE) inhibits the binding of IgE to mast and other inflammatory cells. However, the drug does not inhibit IgE that is already bound to the mast cells.

Administration of omalizumab (Xolair) for a 10-week trial has been found to significantly lower plasma IgE level; it also significantly reduces the level of the early and late bronchospastic responses to antigens. The most important effect of omalizumab is to reduce the frequency and severity of asthma exacerbations. This drug can significantly (88%) reduce exacerbations that might otherwise require hospitalization. As a result, monoclonal antibody is an effective treatment option for selected individuals with severe asthma characterized by frequent exacerbations.

Chronic Obstructive Pulmonary Disease

COPD is characterized by an airflow abnormality that is not fully reversible. This chronic and progressive lung disease has been associated with increased prevalence and mortality during the past two decades. It is the fourth leading cause of death in the United States. Most patients with COPD exhibit chronic bronchitis and emphysema caused by chronic smoking. This pulmonary disease occurs mostly in older patients, triggers neutrophilic inflammation (not eosinophilic inflammation as in asthma), and does not respond well to ICS. With continued cigarette smoking, a progressive loss of pulmonary function takes place over time.

Emphysema

Emphysema is a severe pulmonary disease that can result in the replacement of alveoli with large air sacs. In addition, patients may experience a loss of elastic tissues and inefficient gas exchange in the lung. Alternatively, emphysema may cause airway obstruction during breathing.

Heavy cigarette smoking is the most common cause of emphysema. The smoke increases the number of pulmonary alveolar macrophages; these macrophages, in turn, release neutrophil chemotactic factors that recruit neutrophils. The neutrophils releases elastase, proteinases, and metalloproteinases to promote elastolysis and emphysema. Alpha$_1$ antitrypsin is a plasma protein that inactivates elastase and other proteases, and nicotine is known to inhibit α_1 antitrypsin. The end result is an increased destruction of lung tissue.

Treatment of COPD

Approaches to treat COPD are quite similar to the treatment of asthma. However, the expected benefits are less for COPD than for asthma. While currently there is no cure for this disease, rather than managing symptoms, healthcare efforts focus on preventing COPD. Because this respiratory disease is caused by cigarette smoking or air pollution, smoking cessation and avoidance of exposure of air pollution are the most effective means of reducing the progression of COPD.

Because exacerbations in COPD are often caused by bacterial infection of the lower airways, routine antibiotic therapy is also employed to treat COPD. In addition, patients with COPD should receive the annual influenza vaccine. In the treatment of COPD, a series of agents are used: short-acting β_2 agonists for relief of acute symptoms (indeed, bronchodilators are the major treatment), anticholinergic drugs (ipratropium bromide), or a combination of both β_2 agonists and anticholinergic drugs. In addition, theophylline is used in COPD because it can improve the contractile function of the diaphragm, thereby enhancing ventilatory capacity.

In addition to the single ingredient inhaler mentioned previously, some inhaler formulations contain two medications. For instance, inhalers containing fluticasone and salmeterol (Advair Diskus), or budesonide and formoterol (Symbicort), are used to treat both and COPD. The combination therapy has several benefits over other single-agent inhalers—namely, synergistic actions between both medications, delivery of both drugs to the same cells in the airways, and greater effectiveness than single long-acting beta agonists or steroids.

Antioxidants such as vitamins C and E and *N*-acetyl-cysteine have also been shown to be effective in the treatment of COPD, as oxidative stress plays an important role in pathogenesis of COPD. In contrast, leukotriene modifiers and mast cell stabilizers have not been studied extensively for this indication and currently are not recommended for routine use in the treatment of COPD.

Gastrointestinal Drugs

The gastrointestinal system includes several organs, each with a distinct function. Specifically, the GI system includes the stomach, liver, pancreas, small intestine (which includes the duodenum, jejunum, and ileum), and large intestine. The GI tract ends in the rectum. All of these organs have different pH, surface area, and secretions and, therefore, differently influence drug absorption. The GI system interacts with other organ systems to ensure effective homeostasis of the body. The GIT is highly vascularized and contains lymphatic channels responsible for immune responses. Enteric neurons control bowel movement, regulate luminal fluids, and perform involuntary functions.

The absorption of drugs in the GI tract occurs through the epithelial cells, with drugs entering into the blood capillaries of the lamina propria and then traveling through capillaries to the rest of the body. The main functions of the GI tract are to facilitate nutrient intake, digestion, and elimination of wastes. While the mouth processes the food and mixes it with salivary amylase, the esophagus moves the food downward into the stomach. The lower esophageal sphincter plays an important role in preventing reflux of the gastric contents.

Food in the stomach is mixed with pepsin and hydrochloric acid (HCl); HCl sterilizes the upper gut. In addition, the stomach secretes intrinsic factor, which is important for vitamin B_{12} absorption (see also the *Introduction to Nutrients* chapter). The food in the stomach mixes further with pancreatic juice and bile in the duodenum to facilitate digestion. A series of digestive zymogens are released from the pancreas to facilitate digestion of macromolecules such as carbohydrate, protein, and fat. In addition, the pancreas releases bicarbonate to optimize the pH for activation of these zymogens. The bile acid that is secreted from the gallbladder plays a crucial role in the digestion of fats as well (see also the *Introduction to Nutrients* chapter).

The pH of the small intestine is higher than the pH of the stomach due to secretion of bicarbonate from the pancreas, which enters the small intestine. The transit time of food and drugs in the small intestine is in the range of minutes to a few hours.

Because the GI tract plays an important role in the digestion, absorption, and elimination of food and drugs, a malfunction in this area may lead to diseases of the stomach, intestine, biliary tree, and pancreas. For instance, a simple lack of lactase enzyme (lactase deficiency) results in the production of gas and diarrhea. Other examples of GI disorders include celiac disease, bacterial infections, Crohn's ileitis, dehydration, electrolyte disorders, and malnutrition (see also the *Introduction to Nutrients* chapter).

Treatment of GI Diseases

GI diseases are often indicated by the following signs and symptoms:

- Abdominal or chest pain (the latter is often confused with heart problems)
- GI disturbances (nausea, vomiting), dysphagia or odynophagia (difficult or painful swallowing, respectively), and anorexia

- Altered bowel movements (diarrhea or constipation)
- GI bleeding

In addition, GI diseases can be complicated by factors such as dehydration, sepsis, and shock. Several agents, including over-the-counter remedies, are available to treat GI diseases.

Gastroesophageal reflux disease (GERD) is a GI disorder that is often caused by ulceration and erosion of the mucous layer lining the upper portion of the GI tract by upward movement of gastric contents into the esophagus. Available treatment for acid-peptic diseases seeks to reduce intragastric acidity by controlling hydrogen acid secretion, improving mucosal defense, and, in some cases, using antibiotics to eradicate *H. pylori* bacteria. In addition, elevating the head during sleep, decreasing fat intake, smoking cessation, avoiding lying down within 3 hours of eating, losing weight, avoiding alcohol, and eating smaller meals can help to manage the symptoms of GERD. Conversely, consumption of spicy food, orange juice, tomato juice, and coffee can irritate the esophageal mucosa.

GERD has a high prevalence in Western countries, and research studies have indicated that obesity is associated with its development. In the United States, approximately 60 million people experience GERD symptoms on a monthly basis. The clinical presentation of GERD is characterized by heartburn (the most common complaint), indicated by a burning sensation and pain behind the breastbone, in the neck and throat (the pain usually occurs after heavy meals, particularly those rich in fats); hypersalivation and belching; and unexplained weight loss. Acid suppression is the mainstay of therapy for GERD.

In healthy individuals, there is a balance between gastric acid secretion and an effective mucosal defense and repair mechanism in the GI tract. However, when the mucous lining of the GI tract (esophagus, stomach, and duodenum) becomes eroded, peptic ulcer disease (PUD) develops.

Antacids

Many agents in this category are classified as OTC products. Their main role is to neutralize stomach acid by reacting with protons in the lumen of the gut. Magnesium hydroxide, $Mg(OH)_2$, and aluminum hydroxide, $Al(OH)_3$, are often used as antacids. These agents have opposite effects on bowel movement: While magnesium hydroxide (Fleet) has a laxative effect, aluminum hydroxide (Dermagran) causes constipation. None of the agents are absorbed from the gut absorbed from the gut, in contrast to other antacids such as calcium carbonate and sodium bicarbonate, which are absorbed well from the gut. As a result, calcium carbonate and sodium bicarbonate have systemic effects and, therefore, are less popular as antacids.

H_2 Receptor Antagonists

Histamine2 (H_2) receptors can be found on many cell types, including cells of the gastric mucosa, heart, lung, CNS, uterus, and immune system. When histamine binds to the H_2 receptor, it stimulates activation of adenyl cyclase, which in turn increases cAMP production, leading to activation of cAMP-dependent protein kinase in smooth muscle and in parietal cells of the stomach. The outcome of the histamine binding is to increase gastric acidity through stimulation of the H^+/K^+-ATPase pump, resulting in the release of protons into the gastric lumen. Cimetidine (Tagamet HB 200), ranitidine (Zantac), famotidine (Pepcid), and nizatidine (Axid) inhibit stomach acid production by inhibiting the binding of histamine to H_2 receptors. These agents are effective in the treatment of GERD, peptic ulcer disease, and non-ulcer dyspepsia. When the oral routes are not

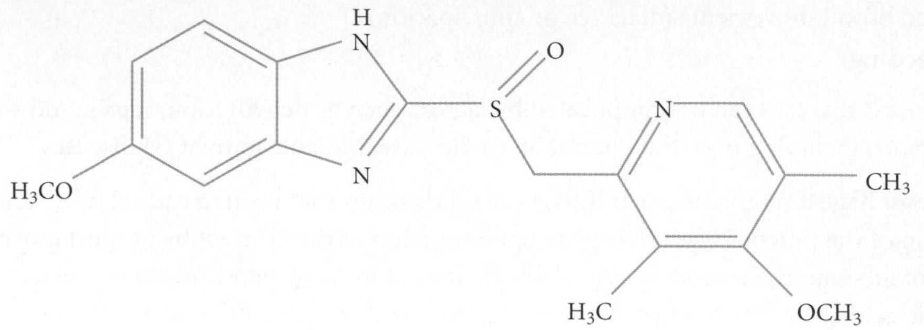

Figure 10.47 Structure of omeprazole.

feasible means of drug delivery, intravenous and intramuscular formulations of cimetidine, raniti-dine, and famotidine can be employed.

The side effects of H_2 receptor antagonists are minor (occurring in fewer than 3% of patients), but often include diarrhea, headache, drowsiness, fatigue, muscular pain, and constipation. The intravenous administration may add minor CNS side effects such as confusion, hallucinations, and slurred speech. Cimetidine is rarely used, as this drug interacts with many other agents.

H_2 receptor antagonists cross the placenta and are secreted in breast milk. Consequently, these agents should be used with caution in women during pregnancy or while breastfeeding.

Proton Pump Inhibitors

Proton pump inhibitors (PPIs) are potent gastric acid suppressors. As their name indicates, they inhibit the gastric H^+/K^+-ATPase pump. The daily production of acid (basal and stimulated) is reduced by as much as 80–95% when PPIs are used. Six proton pump inhibitors are available for clinical use: omeprazole (Prilosec OTC), esomeprazole (Nexium), lansoprazole (Prevacid), dexlan-soprazole (Dexilant), rabeprazole (AcipHex), and pantoprazole (Protonix). These drugs have very similar pharmacologic properties. All of them are lipophilic (**Figure 10.47**), weak bases that easily diffuse into parietal cells and become protonated and concentrated there (more than 1,000-fold).

Proton pump inhibitors are prodrugs that become activated in an acidic environment at the right physiological site. Any activation at an acidic milieu, however, will release the active agent before it reaches the actual site of action (i.e., before it reaches the parietal cells). Consequently, PPI tablets have an enteric coating that protects from unwanted earlier activation in the stomach. These prodrugs are rapidly absorbed into the systemic circulation, diffuse into the parietal cells, and accumulate in the acidic secretory canaliculi. There, PPIs become activated and covalently bound to the sulfhydryl groups of cysteines in the H^+/K^+-ATPase pump. While PPIs are rapidly metabolized in the liver ($t_{1/2} = 1$–2 hours), due to their irreversible inhibition of the proton pump, their pharmacologic effect persists for 24 hours (i.e., until the gene expression allows new synthesis of the H^+/K^+-ATPase pump). Full effects from these agents take 3–4 days to become evident.

Because PPIs block the final step in acid production, they are much more effective than H_2 receptor inhibitors for GERD and peptic ulcer. The major side effects of these agents are diarrhea, abdominal pain, and headache. They are also effective in the treatment of non-ulcer dyspepsia, the prevention of stress-related mucosal bleeding, and the treatment of Zollinger-Ellison syndrome. Zollinger-Ellison syndrome is a progressive and life-threatening syndrome that is caused by ulcer-ation of the upper jejunum, excessive gastric acid secretion, and pancreatic nonbeta-cell tumors.

These acid-suppressing agents will affect drugs that need the normal acidic milieu of the stomach to have the desired effect. For instance, the oral bioavailability of vitamin B_{12}, digoxin, ketoconazole, and iron supplements is affected by PPIs. Among the currently available PPIs, lansoprazole and esomeprazole are also indicated for the treatment and prevention of gastric ulcer caused by NSAIDs.

Sucralfate

Sucralfate (Carafate) is a small but poorly soluble molecule. In an acidic milieu, sucralfate undergoes extensive cross-linking (polymerization). The viscous polymer produces a cytoprotective effect by adhering to injured epithelial cells of the GI tract and provides coating over ulcer beds for as long as 6 hours after a single dose. Sucralfate is able to accelerate the treatment of peptic ulcers and reduces the recurrence rate. Although it must be taken 4 times daily, it does not produce any major side effect due to its insolubility and lack of systemic effects.

Misoprostol

The gastric mucosa's major synthesized prostaglandins are prostaglandin E_2 (PGE_2) and prostacyclin (PGI_2). These prostaglandins bind to the EP3 receptor on parietal cells, thereby reducing the intracellular cAMP concentration and the rate of gastric acid secretion. Another function of PGE_2 is to prevent gastric injury by stimulating mucin production, enhancing bicarbonate secretion, and increasing mucosal blood flow. Nevertheless, gastric acid suppression has been suggested to be the most important effect of misoprostol, though this effect is dose dependent (oral doses of 100–200 µg). The recommended dose for ulcer prophylaxis is 200 µg, taken 4 times daily. Because NSAIDs are known to inhibit cyclooxygenase enzymes and thereby reduce the synthesis of prostaglandins, the synthetic prostaglandin E_2 analog, misoprostol, seems to be effective in mitigating the NSAID-induced mucosal damage. However, misoprostol needs to be taken multiple times during the day, and it is not a first-line therapy for the treatment of NSAID-induced mucosal damage.

Misoprostol is rapidly absorbed after oral administration. The presence of food and antacids in the GI tract decreases its rate of absorption, resulting in delayed and reduced peak plasma concentrations.

The side effects of misoprostol are another reason why this agent is rarely used. They include diarrhea (30%) and exacerbations of inflammatory bowel disease (IBD); hence this medication should be avoided in patients with IBD. In addition, due to misoprostol's increased effect on uterine contractility, it is contraindicated during pregnancy.

Bismuth

Bismuth (Pepto-Bismol) is a unique molecule with many pharmacologic roles in GI diseases. Bismuth can build a protective coat on ulcerated tissue, stimulates mucosal protection, has anti-inflammatory and antibacterial effects, and is capable of sequestrating enterotoxins. Bismuth is effective against *H. pylori*, the causative bacterium in infection-related peptic ulcer disease.

Bismuth reduces stool liquidity in infectious diarrhea, but causes black stools and black staining of the tongue. This agent is used frequently for the treatment of traveler's diarrhea. Upon administration of bismuth, it interacts with the stomach's HCl to form bismuth oxychloride. Some bismuth preparations contain salicylic acid, so one must be careful if patients are allergic to salicylic acid or when salicylic acid is contraindicated (e.g., in children to avoid Reye's syndrome).

Antibiotics

Recurrent non-NSAID-induced peptic ulcers are often associated with chronic infection with *H. pylori* bacteria. In such cases, eradication of the bacteria results in rapid healing of peptic ulcers and reduces the rate of recurrence.

Several different combinations of antibiotics and antacids are used to treat peptic ulcers. Two forms of therapy are employed for a 2-week course of medication:

- *Triple therapy* includes a PPI, clarithromycin (Biaxin), and amoxicillin (Moxatag). Metronidazole (Flagyl) can be used if patients are allergic to penicillin. Clarithromycin is a potent CYP3A4 inhibitor and can cause drug–drug interactions.
- *Quadruple therapy* includes a PPI, metronidazole, tetracycline (Apo-Tetra, from Canada), and bismuth subsalicylate.

Metronidazole interacts with bacterial DNA to disrupt the helical DNA structure. Substitution of the prescribed antibiotic with another option is not recommended, for instance, the clinician should not change clarithromycin to erythromycin. Due to the increased risk of bacterial resistance, these treatment regimens should always include two antibiotics. Much as with other antibiotic therapy, it is important to counsel patients that they should complete the entire course to fully eradicate the *H. pylori* bacteria. Although clarithromycin, amoxicillin, and metronidazole can be taken without food, the presence of food will reduce the stomach upset often experienced with clarithromycin and metronidazole. In contrast, tetracycline should be taken on an empty stomach; in addition, the patient should take this drug at least 2 hours after taking antacids, dairy products, or iron supplements due to the chelating ability of tetracycline.

Drugs Used for Irritable Bowel Syndrome

Irritable bowel syndrome (IBS) is characterized by relapsing episodes of abdominal discomfort, pain, bloating, distension, cramps, and altered bowel habits (constipation, diarrhea, or both). This condition is 3 times more prevalent in women than in men. In approximately 80% of patients, psychological factors play important roles in the pathogenesis of IBS. The therapeutic goals are to treat the diarrhea and abdominal pain as well as to improve the IBS symptoms and patients' quality of life.

Anticholinergic agents such as dicyclomine (Bentyl) and hyoscyamine (Anaspaz) are effective options for treating diarrhea because they decrease GI motility by relaxing smooth muscle in the gut. Hyoscyamine also decreases urgency and urinary leakage. Because psychological factors are often involved in the development of IBS, TCAs can provide additional therapeutic benefit. TCAs (e.g., amitriptyline, desipramine, doxepin) can improve IBS symptoms (abdominal pain and altered bowel habits). In patients with severe IBS, other antidepressants such as SSRIs may be used.

Loperamide (Imodium) is an antidiarrheal OTC agent (available in capsule, solution, and chewable tablet forms) that inhibits the calcium-binding protein calmodulin and, as a result, controls chloride secretion. It has been suggested that the antidiarrheal effect of loperamide is 40–50 times higher than morphine's antidiarrheal effect. In addition, through the opioid receptor, this agent acts on intestinal muscles to inhibit peristalsis. The initial oral adult dose of loperamide is 4 mg, followed by 2 mg administered after each loose stool. Loperamide may cause dizziness and constipation, but with correct dosing these side effects are minimized. The maximum dose of loperamide is 16 mg/day. Because loperamide is an OTC agent, pharmacists can play an important role in correct dosing and effective counseling. For instance, if the patient, in addition to the diarrhea, has a high fever or bloody stool, or if the effect of loperamide is not seen within 48 hours, the patient needs to be referred to a healthcare provider. Similar to bismuth, loperamide is also used to treat traveler's diarrhea.

Drugs Used in Inflammatory Bowel Disease

As the name indicates, IBD is a chronic inflammatory intestinal disease. It significantly affects GI functions and produces consequences such as diarrhea, abdominal pain, bleeding, anemia, and weight loss. Two types of IBD are distinguished: ulcerative colitis (UC) and Crohn's disease (CD). The underlying causes for both UC and CD include infection, genetics, immune deficiency, and environmental factors.

Ulcerative colitis is a mucosal inflammatory condition confined to the rectum and colon. It is more common in men, and usually occurs in persons between 30 and 40 years of age. Symptoms of UC include rectal bleeding, abdominal pain, and diarrhea followed by rectal urgency. With mild UC, the first-line therapy consists of aminosalicylates. If a patient does not respond to amino-salicylates, corticosteroids are prescribed. If corticosteroids fail to produce any therapeutic benefit, immunosuppressants such as azathioprine (Imuran) or 6-mercaptopurine (Purinethol) can be used. Moderate to severe UC can be treated with antibody therapy such as infliximab (Remicade). In severe cases, intravenous steroids are the first-line therapy and are administered in the hospital setting; if the patient does not respond within 7 days, surgery or intravenous cyclosporine is employed.

Crohn's disease is characterized by transmural inflammation of any part of the GI tract (from mouth to anus). It is more common in women, and often occurs in persons between 20 and 30 years of age. Patients experience frequent rectal bleeding. For mild to moderate CD, oral ami-nosalicylates are the initial therapy; the combination of aminosalicylates and antibiotics (met-ronidazole or ciprofloxacin) is also effective. For patients with moderate to severe cases, steroids (prednisone and budesonide) are effective agents (but are not appropriate as maintenance therapy). If a patient does not respond to steroids, azathioprine or 6-mercaptopurine can be prescribed. Indeed, 6-mercaptopurine is the best agent for preventing relapse of CD after surgical intervention. However, if a patient cannot tolerate azathioprine, 6-mercaptopurine will not be effective, either. Azathioprine blocks purine metabolism and, therefore, inhibits synthesis of nucleotides. In addition, it inhibits mitosis during cell proliferation.

Adalimumab (Humira; a TNF blocker) also seems to be effective in controlling CD. Initially, a daily dose of 160 mg is taken for 2 days, followed by a daily dose of 80 mg for 2 weeks (day 15), and then a maintenance dose of 40 mg every other week (i.e., beginning of day 29). As its name indicates, adalimumab is a recombinant monoclonal antibody ("mab" is an abbreviation for "monoclonal antibody"). It binds to TNF-α, which in turn reduces the binding of TNF-α to its receptor; this ultimately slows down cytokine-driven inflammatory processes.

The major goals of IBD management are to control acute exacerbations of the disease and to dampen the generalized inflammatory response on a long-term basis. To date, no medication has been able to achieve both of these goals simultaneously. For example, glucocorticoids are often used for moderate to severe IBD, but due to their side effects, they are inappropriate for long-term use. Conversely, immunosuppressive agents, such as azathioprine, are preferred for long-term management. However, because it takes several weeks for a therapeutic effect to appear, these drugs are not effective in acute cases. In November 2011, the FDA issued a warning about a possible role for azathioprine in development of a rare malignancy, hepatosplenic T-cell lymphoma.

Topical aminosalicylates are the treatment of choice for distal UC that involves only the rectum. Indeed, the topical formulations of these drugs are more effective than the oral formulations. Topical aminosalicylates can be administered as a nightly suppository or enema. In addition, rectally administered steroids may be used in combination with aminosalicylates. However, if a patient cannot tolerate topical drugs, oral steroids or aminosalicylates are useful. While oral ami-nosalicylates are effective for maintenance therapy, topical (or oral) steroids are not.

Among the aminosalicylates, sulfasalazine (Azulfidine; 4–6 g/day) is metabolized by the gut bacteria to the active ingredient, mesalamine. Mesalamine is also known as 5-aminosalicylic acid (5-ASA). It is not clear how 5-ASA works, but it probably inhibits the synthesis of prostaglandins (by inhibiting COX enzymes) and inflammatory leukotrienes. Other agents in this category are mesalamine (Asacol; 2.3–4.8 g/day) and balsalazide (Colazal; 6.75 g/day). Oral corticosteroids are reserved for patients who fail to respond to oral aminosalicylates. The corticosteroids that are often used for IBD are prednisone (40–60 mg/day), methylprednisolone (Solu-Medrol; 16 mg, three times daily), and budesonide (Enocort; 9 mg/day).

Two antibiotics are used in the treatment of IBD (only for CD): metronidazole (Flagyl) and ciprofloxacin (Cipro). Ciprofloxacin causes diarrhea as well as tendonitis and cartilage deterioration (see also the *Introduction to Microbiology* chapter).

Glucocorticoids are sometimes used to treat chronic UC and Crohn's disease, particularly in acute exacerbations and in patients who do not respond well to rest, diet, and sulfasalazine therapy. For instance, hydrocortisone (Cortef) and oral prednisone is used for mild and severe UC, respectively. The dose of prednisone can be increased for patients with severe UC with fever, anorexia, and anemia.

Live vaccines should not be administered in patients who are taking infliximab, cyclosporine, and methotrexate (Rheumatrex). Methotrexate inhibits dihydrofolate reductase and purine synthesis; tetrahydrofolate is the product of the dihyrofolate reductase enzyme and is important for the synthesis of thymine in DNA (see also the *Introduction to Nutrients* chapter). Methotrexate also reduces IL-1 and IL-2 and induces T-cell apoptosis. However, it can cause leukopenia (low number of white blood cells). In addition, a strong drug interaction occurs between methotrexate and an NSAID, which can be fatal (NSAIDs can reduce the excretion of methotrexate). Methotrexate is also an antineoplastic agent and can depress bone marrow when taken in high doses.

A series of OTC products is also available in the United States for the treatment of GI diseases. For instance, antacids such as aluminum hydroxide and magnesium hydroxide; calcium carbonate; and histamine H_2 antagonists such as ranitidine and famotidine are available to reduce symptoms in gastroesophageal reflux and dyspepsia. Other OTC products such as simethicone (Ovol, from Canada) are used as antiflatulents to alleviate the symptoms of gas. Finally, some PPIs are available as OTC products (omeprazole).

Laxatives

To get relief from constipation, patients may use fiber supplements, stool softeners, enemas, and laxatives. Laxatives work by various mechanisms to increase bowel movements: stimulation of the bowel wall; bulk formation of the stool, which induces reflex contraction of the bowel; softening of hard stool; and lubricative action that eases passage of stool through the rectum. In addition, osmotic laxatives are used, albeit only as needed, as they often cause abdominal pain. Other medications should not be taken within 1 hour of taking osmotic laxatives.

Bulk-Forming Laxatives

Bulk-forming laxatives consist of natural or synthetic hydrophilic polysaccharide derivatives that absorb water and thereby increase stool bulk to facilitate peristalsis. This effect is achieved after taking the medication for 2–3 days. Although they are quite safe, it is important to recognize that these products are cable of binding to digoxin, warfarin, calcium complexes, and tetracycline; thus the laxatives' administration should be separated from the administration of these drugs to avoid any effect on the drugs' actions. Pharmacists should advise patients taking a bulk-forming laxative to drink plenty of water. Examples of bulk-forming laxatives include psyllium (Metamucil), methylcellulose (Citrucel), and calcium polycarbophil.

Emollient Laxatives (Stool Softeners)

These laxatives serve as surfactants by absorbing water and fat into stool. It takes 2–3 days to achieve the full effect, and the product may cause systemic absorption. An example is docusate (Doc-Q-Lace). Due to their delayed action, emollient laxatives are not good choices to treat acute constipation.

Stimulant Laxatives

As their name indicates, these laxatives stimulate bowel motility and increase secretion of liquid into the bowel. An example is Fleet Bisacodyl, which is often used for bowel evacuation prior to an examination. Senna (Senokot) is a good choice for this indication, provided patients who are using opioids receive proper counseling beforehand.

Saline and Osmotic Laxatives

These agents create an osmotic gradient that draws water into the intestine. Rectal administration has a faster effect (less than 30 minutes) compared with oral administration (1–4 hours). Saline and osmotic laxative agents contain magnesium, so caution should be used when they are taken by patients with impaired renal function. Examples include magnesium hydroxide (Milk of Magnesia), magnesium citrate, and magnesium sulfate. In addition, glycerin acts as a hyperosmotic laxative, having an onset of action of 30 minutes. Glycerin suppositories are safe for use in infants.

Lubricant Laxatives

Lubricant laxatives emulsify the intestine, with the onset of action occurring in 6 hours. These products can reduce the absorption of fat–soluble vitamins. Examples include mineral oil and olive oil.

Chloride-Channel Activators

The only available agent in this class is lubiprostone (Amitiza), which facilitates the passage of stool by activating Cl⁻ channels to increase fluid secretion in the intestinal lumen. This product is often used for idiopathic chronic constipation and IBS with constipation in women. Only bulk-forming laxatives or stool softeners should be prescribed to pregnant women.

Learning Bridge 10.12

After he was diagnosed with *Helicobacter pylori* infection, JJ was prescribed a regimen of a proton pump inhibitor (PPI), amoxicillin, and clarithromycin. When he came to the pharmacy to fill his prescriptions, he realized that he had forgotten to tell the doctor that he developed a rash and hives when he took Augmentin for a serious bronchial infection.

A. How will you help JJ?
B. Discuss a noninvasive test to detect *H. pylori* infection.

Golden Keys for Pharmacy Students

1. The CNS is composed of the brain and spinal cord, and the peripheral nervous system consists of neurons that are found outside the brain and spinal cord but are capable of transmitting signals back and forth with the CNS.

2. The peripheral nervous system is divided into efferent and afferent nerves. While the efferent nerves carry signals from the brain and spinal cord to the peripheral tissues, the afferent nerves carry signals from the peripheral tissues (skin, skeletal muscles, adipose tissues) to the brain and spinal cord.

3. In the parasympathetic system, the preganglionic neurons are long but the postganglionic neurons are short. In contrast, in the sympathetic nervous system, the preganglionic neurons are short and the postganglionic neurons are long.

4. Exogenous acetylcholine has no therapeutic application because it undergoes rapid hydrolysis by AchE or by the acidic environment of the stomach.

5. Epinephrine's major effects are to strengthen the contractility of myocardium (positive inotropy) and to increase the rate of contraction (positive chronotropy).

6. Norepinephrine is a potent α_1 and α_2 agonist, but has relatively little action on β_2 receptors. This major chemical mediator is released by postganglionic sympathetic nerves.

7. Albuterol is a short-acting β_2 agonist; its duration of action is 4–6 hours.

8. Salmeterol is a selective and long-acting β_2 receptor agonist. It is dosed every 12 hours.

9. Pseudoephedrine (SudoGest and Sudafed) is the D-isomer of ephedrine and produces 25% of the effect associated with ephedrine. It is clinically used as a nasal decongestant. Because this drug can be converted to methamphetamine, pseudoephedrine must be sold behind the counter.

10. A serious adverse effect of α_1 blockers is a "first dose" effect, which can cause transient faintness, palpitations, orthostatic hypotension, and syncope shortly (1–3 hours) after the first dose.

11. Beta blockers are not first-line agents for reducing blood pressure, but rather are typically added to a thiazide-type diuretic to lower the blood pressure.

12. For hypertensive patients without any compelling indications, thiazides, ACE inhibitors, angiotensin receptor blockers, and calcium-channel blockers are used as the initial first-line agents.

13. In patients with hyperthyroidism, propranolol is useful to prevent cardiac arrhythmias. However, patients with asthma or COPD may develop bronchoconstriction if they take propranolol because of its nonselective β-receptor blocking effect.

14. β_1-selective blockers are also called cardioselective blockers because they do not block β_2 receptors, do not provoke bronchospasm, and do not decrease glycogenolysis. They are safer than nonselective agents for patients with asthma or diabetes.

15. The selective β_1 blocker atenolol is the least hydrophobic member of this drug class. As a result, it cannot readily cross the blood–brain barrier. Moreover, side effects such as dizziness or drowsiness, which are often seen with other beta blockers, do not occur with atenolol.

16. Oral metoprolol undergoes almost full absorption, but due to its high first-pass effect, its bioavailability is relatively low (approximately 40%).

17. Labetalol is a hydrophilic drug. It can be used in pregnancy-induced hypertensive crisis as it has minimal placental penetration.

18. Metoprolol tartrate is an immediate-release dosage form (short-acting; $t_{1/2} \approx 6$ hours) that can be given 2–4 times daily to treat hypertension. In contrast, metoprolol succinate is an extended-release form (long-acting) and is dosed only once per day for the treatment of both hypertension and heart failure.

19. Combination of a dopamine agonist with levodopa can increase the severity of levodopa-induced dyskinesia.

20. Because depression is quite common in patients with Alzheimer's disease, treatment with selective serotonin reuptake inhibitors is often useful in such individuals.

21. Benzodiazepines are highly hydrophobic drugs (although to different extents), and all of these agents, except clorazepate (Tranxene), are absorbed completely from the GI tract. Benzodiazepines are classified as controlled substances (Schedule IV).

22. The exact mechanism of action of antipsychotics is not known. Both dopamine and serotonin and their subtype receptors play important roles in producing effects.

23. Based on their actions on dopamine receptors and 5-HT_{2A} receptors, antipsychotics are classified into two major classes: typical antipsychotics and atypical antipsychotics.

24. There are three opioid receptors—δ (delta), μ (mu), and κ (kappa)—which have highly conserved sequences (approximately 60%). The highest diversity in their structures is found in the extracellular loops of the receptors.

25. The μ receptors are highly involved in producing the analgesic effects of morphine within the brain.

26. Stimulation of μ and κ receptors results in enhanced parasympathetic stimulation of the eyes. As patients do not develop tolerance to this effect, a pinpoint eye is a good indication of morphine use (or abuse).

27. Morphine decreases gastric motility, an effect that is believed to result from its actions on μ receptors within the smooth muscle of the intestinal wall.

28. Barbiturates, benzodiazepines, and alcohol potentiate sedation and respiratory depression of opioids.

29. All opioids, with the exception of meperidine, reduce the strength, duration, and frequency of uterine contractions; hence these medications may delay the onset of labor.

30. Buprenorphine has been approved for treatment of opioid withdrawal; it is often used at the beginning of a detoxification regimen.

31. Captopril and lisinopril provide renoprotection (indicated by changes in albumin excretion), particularly in patients with diabetes mellitus and renal failure. In addition, ACE inhibitors are known to reduce the progression of retinopathy in DM type 1.

32. Digoxin concentrations in the plasma that exceed 2.4 ng/mL are toxic. Digoxin immune Fab (DigiFab) is an antidote agent used to treat digoxin toxicity.

33. Because aldosterone antagonists spare K^+ excretion, monitoring of K^+ level is important to avoid hyperkalemia when such drugs are prescribed. Pharmacists should counsel patients to avoid taking supplemental potassium before starting aldosterone antagonist treatment.

34. Diuretics not only increase the excretion of Na^+ and Cl^- ions, but also may increase the excretion of cations such as K^+, H^+, Ca^{2+}, and Mg^{2+}; anions such as HCO_3^- and $H_2PO_4^-$; and uric acid.

35. Essential hypertension is caused by an unknown pathophysiological etiology. It can be controlled but not cured and is the most prevalent form of hypertension (more than 90% of cases).

36. In contrast to loop diuretics, thiazides enhance Ca^{2+} reabsorption. As a result, these agents can mask hypocalcemia caused by hyperparathyroidism, carcinoma, and sarcoidosis.

37. Chlorothiazide (Diuril) is the only thiazide that is available for parenteral administration (it can be taken orally as tablets or suspensions).

38. While furosemide, bumetanide, and torsemide are sulfonamide derivatives, ethacrynic acid is not. Ethacrynic acid is a good choice for patients with hypertension who are allergic to sulfonamide.

39. Use of ACE inhibitors and ARBs is contraindicated during pregnancy.

40. Inhibition of renin's action can reduce the formation of angiotensin I and angiotensin II and, as a result, lowers blood pressure.

41. Compared to lisinopril, amlodipine has shown to be more effective in African American patients with hypertension.

42. In contrast to α_1 blockers, centrally acting α_2 agonists can stimulate α_2 receptors in the brain and lower blood pressure.

43. Pregnant or nursing women should not take statins.

44. Only lovastatin, atorvastatin, and simvastatin are primarily metabolized by CYP3A4 and CYP3A5.

45. If patients switch from niacin to Advicor (which contains both lovastatin and niacin), the niacin dose in the combination therapy should be less than the dose of the individual niacin therapy.

46. Fenofibrate is more effective than gemfibrozil in increasing HDL levels.

47. The goals of hypothyroidism treatment are to ensure adequate thyroid hormone levels in the body and maintain the patient's TSH within the normal range.

48. Thyroid hormone is necessary for fetal growth during pregnancy. Levothyroxine is considered the drug of choice for treating hypothyroidism in pregnant women, as it is a pregnancy category A drug.

49. Insulin is an anabolic hormone. Its blood concentration in fasting healthy adults is approximately 10 mU/L, but increases immediately to 60 mU/L following a meal and then returns to the basal level 1–4 hours later.

50. Diabetic ketoacidosis (DKA) is an uncontrolled form of ketosis that, if not treated, can be fatal.

51. All three rapid-acting insulin formulations (lispro, aspart, and glulisine) have a lower tendency to cause hypoglycemia (a major concern for many antidiabetic agents).

52. Regular insulin is the only insulin solution that can be administered intravenously. This clear solution can be mixed with most insulin preparations except glargine and detemir.

53. Oral antidiabetic agents are ineffective as treatments for type 1 diabetes and are contraindicated in patients with ketoacidosis.

54. The symptoms of hyperglycemia are identified by the mnemonic UFAT: Urination, Fatigue, Agitation, and Thirst.

55. Bronchial dilation is achieved by slowly inhaling β_2 agonists and then holding the breath for 5–10 seconds.

56. Advair Diskus is a dry-powder inhaler that needs to be inhaled rapidly. An MDI inhaler (albuterol) requires slow inhalation.

57. Zileuton is a 5-lipoxygenase inhibitor, and zafirlukast and montelukast are antagonists of the LT receptor. Both inhibitors are effective in asthma treatment. Montelukast, unlike the other agents, is only approved for children 6 years or younger.

58. While PPIs are rapidly metabolized in the liver ($t_{1/2} = 1–2$ hours), due to their irreversible inhibition of the proton pump, their pharmacologic effect persists for 24 hours (i.e., until the gene expression permits new synthesis of the H^+/K^+-ATPase pump). However, their full effect is achieved only 3–4 days after therapy is begun.

59. To treat constipation during pregnancy, a bulk-forming laxative or a stool softener may be used. Senna may be recommended to treat constipation caused by opioid medications. Glycerin suppositories are safe to treat constipation in infants.

Learning Bridge Answers

10.1 A. Although selegiline selectively inhibits MAO-B, at higher concentrations it can serve as a nonselective MAO inhibitor. MAO inhibitors block the metabolism of catecholamines; hence consumption of tyramine-containing foods such as cheese, herring, chocolate should be avoided when taking MAOIs (because tyramine acts as a catecholamine and MAO inhibitors prevent the inactivation of tyramine). Over-the-counter nasal decongestants contain sympathomimetic amines and can potentially stimulate the adrenergic system. Chances of hypertensive crisis are enhanced when an OTC nasal decongestant is used along with selegiline, so this combination should be avoided.

B. Selegiline is metabolized in the liver to amphetamine and methamphetamine. Amphetamine and methamphetamine are CNS stimulants and can cause insomnia and jitteriness. AK should not take the last dose of selegiline at bedtime; rather, he should be advised to take it in the early evening.

10.2 A. Joe should not stop taking buspirone if he does not get instant relief from anxiety. It can take several weeks before the anxiolytic effects become apparent. The patient should be assured that taking buspirone for an extended period of time is safe, as this drug (unlike benzodiazepines) does not produce dependency. Lastly, the patient should be aware of buspirone's adverse reactions (headache, dizziness).

B. As mentioned in the previous answer, buspirone's full effect usually requires a few weeks to emerge (sometimes it can take as long as 6 weeks). Rifampin significantly reduces (10-fold reduction) the plasma concentration of buspirone because of CYP3A4 induction, so buspirone is not a good choice for this patient.

C. Tell the patient that you would be happy to call his physician and ask him to switch the prescription for buspirone to propranolol 10 mg/daily to manage the patient's anxiety during the bar examination. Keep in mind that rifampin also affects benzodiazepines. Joe should discontinue using propranolol after taking the examination. In addition, make sure that Joe does not have pulmonary problems (asthma or COPD) because propranolol negatively affects these respiratory diseases.

10.3 A. Paroxetine can significantly impair sexual function, which can cause additional distress to a clinically depressed patient. JJ should be advised to talk to his psychiatrist about taking mirtazapine, an atypical antidepressant that does not cause sexual dysfunction. If the doctor agrees to prescribe mirtazapine, the paroxetine dose should be gradually tapered down to avoid withdrawal symptoms. Mirtazapine can cause significant sedation and should be taken at night.

B. Whether JJ is taking paroxetine or mirtazapine, serotonin agonists (including sumatriptan co-administration) can trigger serotonin syndrome. Serotonin syndrome is characterized by symptoms including tremor, rigidity, and myoclonus, along with autonomic instability, nausea, and vomiting. Because triptans are the first-line treatments for migraine, JJ should take sumatriptan—but careful monitoring for serotonin syndrome is warranted during initiation and dose escalation.

10.4 A. Lithium can affect different organs in the body; hence, prior to initiating lithium therapy, baseline values for electrolyte levels, BUN, creatinine, TSH, and thyroxine should be obtained, along with a CBC (complete blood count).

B. Lithium has a narrow therapeutic window and its adverse effects are dose related. Therefore, periodic monitoring of the serum lithium level is required.

C. Lithium can trigger nephrogenic diabetes insipidus, an endocrine disorder characterized by polyuria and polydipsia. This condition results from lithium-mediated inhibition of the action of antidiuretic hormone (ADH) on the kidney in preserving water of the body. Despite his symptoms, BC should continue taking fluid to prevent dehydration.

D. Ibuprofen is classified as an NSAID. Any NSAID can increase lithium concentration in the blood, subsequently leading to toxic reactions. BC's sister should consult his physician and request prescription-strength acetaminophen (which is not an NSAID) for back pain.

10.5 A. The nigrostriatal pathway in the brain is important for normal movement and posture of the body. This pathway is balanced by the action of dopamine and acetylcholine. Haloperidol is a potent antagonist of dopamine receptors in the mesolimbic area of the brain. In addition, it blocks dopaminergic receptors in the nigrostriatal pathway, resulting in excessive activation of cholinergic signaling. As a result, tremor and rigidity occur. The goal should be to counteract the excessive cholinergic stimulation in this pathway.

B. Centrally acting anticholinergics such as benztropine or trihexiphenidyl should be used to counteract excessive cholinergic stimulation.

C. Quetiapine is a second-generation antipsychotic that has the advantage of improving both the positive and negative symptoms of schizophrenia. This drug does not cause any problem with motor function (like that seen in this patient on haloperidol). Haloperidol affects only the positive symptoms of schizophrenia. Quetiapine's important side effects are weight gain and hyperglycemia (an adverse effect associated with the entire drug class), sedation, and cataract formation.

10.6 A. Important considerations include (1) determining whether BB is actually on a salt-restricted diet and (2) determining BB's compliance with the diuretic dose. If you are satisfied with these evaluations, the furosemide dose or frequency can be increased to augment diuresis. Furosemide may be administered by continuous infusion to be more effective and to avoid GI absorption. Co-administration of furosemide with a thiazide diuretic can decrease edema and weight gain.

B. Serum electrolytes need to be checked to make sure electrolytes are normal—particularly the serum K^+ level, which is decreased by both thiazides and loop diuretics.

10.7 Ultracet contains two analgesics, acetaminophen and tramadol. Tramadol, in addition to its opioid properties, can inhibit the reuptake of norepinephrine and 5-HT in the nerve terminals, similar to tricyclic antidepressants. This drug should not be used with an SSRI such as fluoxetine because it potentiates serotonergic function and increases the risk of serotonin syndrome.

10.8 A. Both ACE inhibitors and beta blockers are effective treatment options for managing hypertension. As this patient has diabetes, an ACE inhibitor is preferred over a beta blocker, because ACE inhibitors delay nephropathy and decrease microglobinuria. Beta blockers, in contrast, blunt hypoglycemic responses (tachycardia, skeletal muscle tremors), which can lead to a life-threatening condition.

B. ACE inhibitors can produce cough (at least in 10–20% of cases) because these agents inhibit bradykinin degradation. Bradykinin buildup stimulates the cough center of the brain. Patients who are intolerant to ACE inhibitors because of cough can be switched to an angiotensin receptor blocker, as with the patient in this case.

10.9 Niacin can cause flushing and pruritus in the extremities. This reaction is mediated by prostaglandins that are involved in mediating inflammatory reactions in the body. Taking an OTC NSAID such as aspirin or ibuprofen 30 minutes prior to taking niacin can decrease these symptoms. Aspirin, ibuprofen, and other NSAIDs can inhibit prostaglandin formation in the cells by inhibiting cyclooxygenase (COX-1 and COX-2).

10.10 A. Upon questioning, JB admitted taking Prevacid and levothyroxine just before lunch. Prevacid contains lansoprazole, which can markedly decrease levothyroxine absorption. As a result, all symptoms of hypothyroidism could not be resolved with the current dosage of levothyroxine.

B. JB should be advised to take levothyroxine in the morning and lansoprazole just before meals to enhance the absorption of thyroxine.

10.11 A. Diabetic neuropathic pain can be treated by anticonvulsants such as topiramate, pregabalin, and gabapentin. TCAs (imipramine, nortriptyline) and NSRIs (duloxetine, venlafaxine) can also be used in this condition. Currently, there is no specific drug available on the market that can target the neuropathic pain.

B. Yes, diabetic neuropathy can be delayed by lowering blood glucose levels. Joe's HbA_{1c} is high; it should be less than 7%. Both medications and lifestyle modifications can be used to lower blood glucose levels.

C. Joe needs to exercise regularly for at least 30 minutes, 5 times per week, and remain active to lose 5% to 10% of his body weight. To reduce his obesity, he should be referred to a dietician to counsel him on correct food and calorie intake.

10.12 A. Augmentin contains amoxicillin, an aminopenicllin that is widely used for respiratory tract infections. JJ has a previous history of penicillin allergy (rash, hive, urticaria) and cannot take amoxicillin for *H. pylori* eradication. Metronidazole should be substituted for amoxicillin.

B. In addition to using endoscopy, the presence of *H. pylori* can be detected by a urea breath test. *H. pylori* produces urease, which is responsible for the degradation of urea to carbon dioxide and ammonia. In the urea breath test, radiolabeled urea is ingested, and radiolabeled carbon dioxide produced by the bacteria is then detected in the breath.

Problems and Solutions

Problem 10.1 At the neuromuscular junction, pancuronium:

- **A.** Blocks the action of muscarinic receptors.
- **B.** Blocks the action of nicotinic receptors.
- **C.** Blocks the breakdown of acetylcholine.
- **D.** Depletes the storage sites of acetylcholine.

Solution 10.1 B is correct.

Problem 10.2 Muscarinic receptors are:

- **A.** G-protein coupled proteins.
- **B.** Ligand gated ion channels.

Solution 10.2 A is correct.

Problem 10.3 Action of succinylcholine is terminated by an esterase present in:

- **A.** Plasma.
- **B.** Neuromuscular junctions.
- **C.** Both A and B.

Solution 10.3 A is correct.

Problem 10.4 A patient who has undergone GI surgery is having difficulty with urination. Which of the following agents can be used to treat this postoperative complication?

- **A.** Carbachol
- **B.** Scopolamine
- **C.** Bethanechol
- **D.** Edrophonium

Solution 10.4 C is correct.

Problem 10.5 Indirectly acting sympathomimetics like ephedrine:

- **A.** Stimulate NE release from the nerve terminal.
- **B.** Activate α receptors.
- **C.** Activate β receptors.
- **D.** All of the above.

Solution 10.5 D is correct.

Problem 10.6 Dobutamine increases the contraction of the heart. Although it activates both α and β receptors, its inotropic effect is caused by activation of cardiac:

- **A.** α_1 receptors.
- **B.** β_1 receptors.
- **C.** Both A and B.

Solution 10.6 B is correct.

Problem 10.7 A 45-year-old male has recently been diagnosed with pheochromocytoma. Prior to surgery, he will be treated with:

- **A.** Prazosin.
- **B.** Phentolamine.

C. Phenoxybenzamine.

D. Phenylephrine.

Solution 10.7 C is correct.

Problem 10.8 Which of the following is an adverse effect of fingolimod?

A. Bone marrow depression

B. Hemolytic anemia

C. Vivid dreams

D. Risk of infections

Solution 10.8 D is correct.

Problem 10.9 All of the following statements regarding Alzheimer's disease (AD) are true *except*:

A. AD is characterized by dementia and significant memory loss.

B. AD is characterized by formation of β-amyloid plaques in the brain.

C. AD is characterized by the presence of neurofibrillary tangles.

D. Cholinergic agonists are effective therapeutic agents for AD.

Solution 10.9 D is correct.

Problem 10.10 Which of the following agents stimulates release of dopamine in the substantia nigra?

A. Levodopa

B. Entacapone

C. Selegiline

D. Amantadine

Solution 10.10 D is correct.

Problem 10.11 Which of the following effects is produced by normeperidine, a major metabolite of meperidine?

A. Increases blood pressure

B. Causes convulsions

C. Decreases heart rate

D. Increases dopamine release

Solution 10.11 B is correct.

Problem 10.12 Fentanyl is metabolized by:

A. CYP1A2.

B. CYP3A4.

C. CYP2D6.

D. Plasma esterase.

E. Nitroreductase.

Solution 10.12 B is correct.

Problem 10.13 Which of the following drugs activates kappa (κ) opioid receptors and is a weak antagonist at mu (μ) receptors?

A. Naloxone

B. Oxymorphone

    C. Methadone

    D. Pentazocine

Solution 10.13 D is correct.

Problem 10.14 What is the proposed mechanism of anxiolytic activity for buspirone?

    A. A decrease in GABAergic function in the brain

    B. A partial agonist activity at 5-HT$_{1A}$ receptors

    C. An agonist activity at brain adrenergic receptors

    D. An antagonist activity at brain dopaminergic receptors

Solution 10.14 B is correct.

Problem 10.15 A 79-year-old man with poor liver function was treated with a benzodiazepine for acute anxiety. Which agent was chosen for this indication?

    A. Oxazepam

    B. Diazepam

    C. Clonazepam

    D. Clorazepate

    E. Chlordiazepoxide

Solution 10.15 A is correct.

Problem 10.16 True or false: Zolpidem nonselectively activates benzodiazepine (BZ) receptors.

    A. True

    B. False

Solution 10.16 B is correct.

Problem 10.17 Which of the following agents can cause liver toxicity?

    A. Selegiline

    B. Nortryptiline

    C. Nefazodone

    D. Setraline

Solution 10.17 C is correct.

Problem 10.18 Although used for smoking cessation, bupropion use is associated with increased risk of:

    A. Tachycardia.

    B. Bronchoconstriction.

    C. Hypertension.

    D. Seizure.

Solution 10.18 D is correct.

Problem 10.19 Which of the following agents blocks the reuptake of both norepinephrine and serotonin?

    A. Selegiline

    B. Venlafaxine

   C. Mirtazapine

   D. Trazodone

Solution 10.19 B is correct.

Problem 10.20 Which of the following agents can cause birth defects?

   A. Olanzapine

   B. Lamotrigine

   C. Valproic acid

   D. Quetiapine

Solution 10.20 C is correct.

Problem 10.21 What is the mechanism of action for valproic acid?

   A. Blockade of potassium channels

   B. Blockade of calcium channels

   C. Facilitation of GABA-mediated actions in the CNS

   D. Glutamate receptor antagonism

Solution 10.21 C is correct.

Problem 10.22 Lamotrigine inhibits the release of:

   A. Glutamate.

   B. GABA.

   C. Glycine.

   D. NE.

Solution 10.22 A is correct.

Problem 10.23 All of the following symptoms are "positive symptoms" of schizophrenia *except*:

   A. Delusions.

   B. Hallucinations.

   C. Absence of motivation.

   D. Disorganized speech.

Solution 10.23 C is correct.

Problem 10.24 True or false: Second-generation antipsychotics have the drawback of causing metabolic abnormalities.

   A. True

   B. False

Solution 10.24 A is correct.

Problem 10.25 Which of the following agents produces ECG abnormalities?

   A. Risperidone

   B. Ziprasidone

   C. Olanzapine

   D. Quetiapine

Solution 10.25 B is correct.

Problem 10.26 First-generation antipsychotics exhibit which of the following effects in schizophrenia? (Choose all that apply.)

    A. Create extrapyramidal symptoms

    B. Relieve positive symptoms

    C. Relieve negative symptoms

Solution 10.26 Both A and B are correct.

Problem 10.27 Digoxin increases the intracellular concentration of _____ ions necessary for cardiac contraction.

    A. Na^+

    B. Ca^{2+}

    C. Mg^{2+}

Solution 10.27 B is correct.

Problem 10.28 Beta blockers used in congestive heart failure cause which beneficial effect?

    A. Diuresis

    B. Attenuation of deleterious effects from catecholamine

    C. Blockade of angiotensin II receptors

    D. Increased heart rate

    E. Stimulation of β receptors in the lungs

Solution 10.28 B is correct.

Problem 10.29 Dobutamine in CHF produces:

    A. Bronchodilation.

    B. Depression.

    C. Vasodilation.

    D. Positive inotropy.

Solution 10.29 D is correct.

Problem 10.30 ACE inhibitors, when used in CHF, decrease all of the following *except*:

    A. Plasma aldosterone.

    B. Blood pressure.

    C. Plasma sodium.

    D. Cardiac fibrosis.

    E. Plasma renin.

Solution 10.30 E is correct.

Problem 10.31 Compared to spironolactone, amiloride has a _____ duration of action.

    A. longer

    B. shorter

Solution 10.31 B is correct.

Problem 10.32 Problems with hearing can occur with which class of diuretics?

    A. Osmotic

    B. Loop

   C. Potassium-sparing

   D. Thiazides

Solution 10.32 B is correct.

Problem 10.33 Hydrochlorothiazide acts at the _____ of the nephron and inhibits the _____ transporter.

   A. proximal convoluted tubule; Na/K/Cl

   B. proximal convoluted tubule; Na/K

   C. distal convoluted tubule, Na/Cl

   D. distal convoluted tubule, Na/Ca

Solution 10.33 C is correct.

Problem 10.34 Identify the incorrect statement regarding metoprolol.

   A. It antagonizes the actions of β_1 receptors of the heart

   B. It produces negative inotropic and chronotropic effects

   C. It loses receptor selectivity with increased dose

   D. It increases renin release from the kidney

Solution 10.34 D is correct.

Problem 10.35 Ramipril inhibits:

   A. Conversion of prorenin to renin.

   B. Conversion of angiotensinogen to angiotensin I.

   C. Conversion angiotensin I to angiotensin II.

   D. Angiotensin AT2 receptors.

Solution 10.35 C is correct.

Problem 10.36 Which of the following calcium-channel blockers has maximal depressant effect on the heart?

   A. Diltiazem

   B. Amlodipine

   C. Verapamil

   D. Felodipine

Solution 10.36 C is correct.

Problem 10.37 Atorvastatin, when combined with fenofibrate, increases the risk of:

   A. Abdominal pain.

   B. Renal failure.

   C. Optic neuritis.

   D. Increased serum uric acid concentration.

   E. Myopathy.

Solution 10.37 E is correct.

Problem 10.38 A major toxicity of fenofibrate is the increased risk of:

   A. Bloating and constipation.

   B. Gallstone formation.

C. Hyperuricemia.
D. Seizure.
E. Hypertension.

Solution 10.38 B is correct.

Problem 10.39 Which of the following is (are) true about colesevelam?

A. It increases the conversion of cholesterol to bile acid formation in the gallbladder.
B. It increases hepatic LDL receptors.

Solution 10.39 Both A and B are true.

Problem 10.40 Simvastatin lowers serum cholesterol by:

A. Inhibiting hepatic synthesis of fatty acids.
B. Shunting hepatic cholesterol into bile acid synthesis.
C. Increasing the hepatic expression of LDL receptors.
D. Increasing the expression of lipoprotein lipase.

Solution 10.40 C is correct.

Problem 10.41 Albuterol, a β_2-agonist, increases the intracellular production of cAMP. Which of the following agents can also increase cAMP levels?

A. Cromolyn
B. Zafirlukast
C. Theophylline
D. Budenoside

Solution 10.41 C is correct.

Problem 10.42 A 70-year-old patient with asthma was admitted in the ER with overdose of theophylline. At toxic doses, theophylline can cause:

A. Cerebral hemorrhage.
B. Seizure.
C. Acute renal failure.

Solution 10.42 B is correct.

Problem 10.43 For asthma treatment, why are inhaled glucocorticoids preferred over oral therapy?

A. Reduced cost
B. Lower bioavailability by oral route
C. Minimal adverse effects

Solution 10.43 C is correct.

Problem 10.44 What is the mechanism of action of nizatidine?

A. It facilitates degradation of histamine.
B. It inhibits synthesis of histamine.
C. It depletes storage sites for histamine.
D. It inhibits histamine from binding to its receptors.

Solution 10.44 D is correct.

Problem 10.45 Misoprostol is indicated for the treatment of NSAID-induced ulcers. What is the most common adverse effect associated with its use?

A. Headache
B. Dizziness
C. Diarrhea
D. Constipation

Solution 10.45 C is correct.

Problem 10.46 Which of the following antacids exerts antibacterial effects?

A. Magnesium hydroxide
B. Calcium carbonate
C. Bismuth subsalicylate
D. Aluminum hydroxide

Solution 10.46 C is correct.

Problem 10.47 All of the following statements regarding omeprazole are correct *except*:

A. It is formulated in enteric-coated form to prevent premature activation.
B. It is concentrated in the parietal cell acid secretory canaliculi.
C. It irreversibly inhibits the H^+/K^+-ATPase pump.
D. Its effectiveness in acid suppression is equivalent to that of H_2 antagonists.

Solution 10.47 D is correct.

Problem 10.48 "Coupling" in thyroid hormone biosynthesis involves:

A. Increased iodine uptake in the thyroid gland.
B. Iodination of the precursor amino acid.
C. An ether bridge between mono- and di-iodinated amino acid residues.
D. Storage of newly synthesized thyroid hormone in thyroglobulin residues.

Solution 10.48 C is correct.

Problem 10.49 All of the following describe the symptoms of hypothyroidism *except*:

A. Lethargy.
B. Heat intolerance.
C. Bradycardia.
D. Constipation.

Solution 10.49 B is correct.

Problem 10.50 Which of the following agents/measures inhibits synthesis of the thyroid hormone in hyperthyroidism?

A. Propylthiouracil
B. Propranolol
C. Lugol's solution
D. Decreased intake of dietary iodine

Solution 10.50 A is correct.

Problem 10.51 Which of the following is an adverse effect of propylthiouracil?

 A. Lacrimation
 B. Bradycardia
 C. Agranulocytosis
 D. Lethargy

Solution 10.51 C is correct.

Problem 10.52 What is the most important complication associated with insulin therapy?

 A. Pancreatitis
 B. Hypokalemia
 C. Angina
 D. Hypoglycemia
 E. Respiratory distress

Solution 10.52 D is correct.

Problem 10.53 Mr. SAK has just begun treatment with metformin. He should be monitored for the development of which of the following adverse effects?

 A. Hypercalcemia
 B. Elevated uric acid
 C. Lactic acidosis
 D. Hypertension
 E. Polyuria

Solution 10.53 C is correct.

Problem 10.54 Insulin lispro is generally administered:

 A. 1 hour after breakfast.
 B. 1 hour after dinner.
 C. At bedtime.
 D. Immediately before a meal.

Solution 10.54 D is correct.

Problem 10.55 Which of the following agents inhibits degradation of incretin hormones?

 A. Glimeperide
 B. Sitagliptin
 C. Pioglitazone
 D. Metformin

Solution 10.55 B is correct.

References

1. Am OB, Amit T, Youdim MB. Contrasting neuroprotective and neurotoxic actions of respective metabolites of anti-Parkinson drugs rasagiline and selegiline. *Neurosci Lett.* 2004;355:169–172.

2. American Diabetes Association. Diabetes facts and figures. Available at: http://www.diabetes.org/diabetes-basics/diabetes-statistics/. Accessed November 17, 2012.

3. American Diabetes Association. Diabetic nephropathy. *Diab Care.* 2004;27(suppl 1):S79–S83.

4. Anderson LB, Anderson PB, Anderson BT, Bishop A, & Anderson J. Effects of selective serotonin reuptake inhibitors on motor neuron survival. *International Journal of General Medicine*, 2009:2 109–115.

5. Bainbridge JL, Corboy JR. Multiple sclerosis. In: DiPiro JT, Talbert RL, Yee GC, et al. *Pharmacotherapy: a pathophysiologic approach*, 8th ed. New York, NY: McGraw-Hill; 2011. Available at: http://www.accesspharmacy.com/content.aspx?aID=7984977.

6. Barnes PJ. Pulmonary pharmacology. In: Barnes PJ, ed. *Goodman & Gilman's the pharmacological basis of therapeutics*, 12th ed. New York, NY: McGraw-Hill; 2010. Available at: http://www.access-pharmacy.com/content.aspx?aID=16671685.

7. Barrett KE, Barman SM, Boitano S, Brooks H. The autonomic nervous system. In: Barrett KE, Barman SM, Boitano S, Brooks H: *Ganong's review of medical physiology*, 23rd ed. New York, NY: McGraw-Hill; 2011. Available at: http://www.accesspharmacy.com/content .aspx?aID=5241045, 2009.

8. Barrett KE, Barman SM, Boitano S, Brooks HL. Excitable tissue: nerve. In: Barrett KE, Barman SM, Boitano S, Brooks HL, eds. *Ganong's review of medical physiology*, 24th ed. New York, NY: McGraw-Hill; 2012. Available at: http://www.accesspharmacy.com/content .aspx?aID=56260716.

9. Barrett KE, Barman SM, Boitano S, Brooks H. Neurotransmitters and neuromodulators. In: Barrett KE, Barman SM, Boitano S, Brooks H, eds. *Ganong's review of medical physiology*, 23rd ed. New York, NY: McGraw-Hill; 2011. Available at: http://www.accessmedicine.com/content .aspx?aID=5241648.

10. Barrett KE, Barman SM, Boitano S, Brooks H. Pulmonary function. In: Barrett KE, Barman SM, Boitano S, Brooks H, eds. *Ganong's review of medical physiology*, 23rd ed. New York, NY: McGraw-Hill; 2010. Available at: http://www.accesspharmacy.com/content.aspx?aID=5245931.

11. Baumann TEJ, Strickland JM, Herndon CM. Pain management. In: DiPiro JT, Talbert RL, Yee GC, et al. *Pharmacotherapy: a pathophysiologic approach*, 8th ed. New York, NY: McGraw-Hill; 2011. Available at: http://www.accesspharmacy.com/.

12. Benowitz NL. Antihypertensive agents. In: Katzung BG, Masters SB, Trevor AJ. *Basic & clinical pharmacology*, 11th ed. New York, NY: McGraw-Hill; 2009. Available at: http:// www.accesspharmacy.com/content.aspx?aID=4517715.content.aspx?aID=7986332.

13. Bersot TP. Drug therapy for hypercholesterolemia and dyslipidemia. In: Brunton LL, Chabner BA, Knollmann BC. *Goodman & Gilman's the pharmacological basis of therapeutics*, 12th ed. New York, NY: McGraw-Hill; 2010. Available at: http://www.accesspharmacy.com/content. aspx?aID=16669341.

14. Biaggioni I, Robertson D. Adrenoceptor agonists and sympathomimetic drugs. In: Katzung BG, Masters SB, Trevor AJ. *Basic & clinical pharmacology*, 11th ed. New York, NY: McGraw-Hill; 2009. Available at: http://www.accesspharmacy.com/content.aspx?aID=4520412.

15. Boushey HA. Drugs used in asthma. In: Katzung BG, Masters SB, Trevor AJ, eds. *Basic & clinical pharmacology*, 12th ed. New York, NY: McGraw-Hill; 2012. Available at: http:// www.accessmedicine.com/content.aspx?aID=55823726.

16. Brown JH, Laiken N. Muscarinic receptor agonists and antagonists. In: Brunton LL, Chabner BA, Knollmann BC. *Goodman & Gilman's the pharmacological basis of therapeutics*, 12th ed. New York, NY: McGraw-Hill; 2010. Available at: http://www.accesspharmacy.com/content .aspx?aID=16660596.

17. Chen JJ, Nelson MV, Swope DM. Parkinson's disease. In: DiPiro JT, Talbert RL, Yee GC, et al. *Pharmacotherapy: a pathophysiologic approach*, 8th ed. New York, NY: McGraw-Hill; 2011. Available at: http://www.accesspharmacy.com/content.aspx?aID=7986138.

18. Clark M, Finkel R, Rey J, Whalen, K. *Pharmacology*, 5th ed. Philadelphia, PA: Lippincott Williams & Wilkins; 2012.

19. Crismon L, Argo TR, Buckley PF. Schizophrenia. In: DiPiro JT, Talbert RL, Yee GC, et al. *Pharmacotherapy: a pathophysiologic approach*, 8th ed. New York, NY: McGraw-Hill; 2011. Available at: http://www.accesspharmacy.com/content.aspx?aID=7987911.

20. Curry SC, Mills KC, Ruha A-M, O'Connor AD. Neurotransmitters and neuromodulators. In: Nelson LS, Lewin NA, Howland MA, et al. *Goldfrank's toxicologic emergencies*, 9th ed. New York, NY: McGraw-Hill; 2010. Available at: http://www.accesspharmacy.com/content .aspx?aID=6504366.

21. Drayton SJ. Bipolar disorder. In: DiPiro JT, Talbert RL, Yee GC, et al. *Pharmacotherapy: a pathophysiologic approach*, 8th ed. New York, NY: McGraw-Hill; 2011. Available at: http://www. accesspharmacy.com/content.aspx?aID=7989283.

22. Ebadi M. *Desk reference of clinical pharmacology*, 2nd ed. Boca Raton, FL: CRC Press; 2007.

23. Else T, Hammer GD, McPhee SJ. Disorders of the adrenal medulla. In: McPhee SJ, Hammer GD. *Pathophysiology of disease: an introduction to clinical medicine*, 6th ed. New York: McGraw-Hill; 2009. Available at: http://www.accesspharmacy.com/content.aspx?aID=5368271.

24. Ferrucci L, Studenski S. Clinical problems of aging. In: Fauci AS, Braunwald E, Kasper DL, et al. *Harrison's principles of internal medicine*, 18th ed. New York, NY: McGraw-Hill; 2011. Available at: http://www.accesspharmacy.com/content.aspx?aID=9099513.

25. Fiscella RG, Lesar TS, Edward DP. Glaucoma. In: DiPiro JT, Talbert RL, Yee GC, et al. *Pharmacotherapy: a pathophysiologic approach*, 8th ed. New York, NY: McGraw-Hill; 2011. Available at: http://www.accesspharmacy.com/content.aspx?aID=7998061.

26. Gourley DR, Eoff JC, eds. *The APhA complete review for pharmacy*, 9th ed. Washington DC: APhA; 2012.

27. Handelsman Y, Mechanick JI, Blonde L, et al. American Association of Clinical Endocrinologists medical guidelines for clinical practice for developing a diabetes mellitus comprehensive care plan. *Endocrine Pract.* 2011;17(S2):1–53.

28. Hasler WL, Owyang C. Approach to the patient with gastrointestinal disease. In: Longo DL, Kasper DL, Jameson JL, et al., eds. *Harrison's principles of internal medicine*, 18th ed. New York, NY: McGraw-Hill; 2012. Available at: http://www.accesspharmacy.com/content.aspx.

29. Hauser SL, Beal MF. Biology of neurologic diseases. In: Fauci AS, Braunwald E, Kasper DL, et al. *Harrison's principles of internal medicine*, 18th ed. New York, NY: McGraw-Hill; 2011. Available at: http://www.accesspharmacy.com/content.aspx?aID=9144786.

30. Hilal-Dandan R. Renin and angiotensin. In: Brunton LL, Chabner BA, Knollmann BC. *Goodman & Gilman's the pharmacological basis of therapeutics*, 12th ed. New York, NY: McGraw-Hill; 2010. Available at: http://www.accesspharmacy.com/content.aspx?aID=16667140.

31. Ives HE. Diuretic agents. In: Katzung BG, Masters SB, Trevor AJ. *Basic & clinical pharmacology*, 11th ed. New York, NY: McGraw-Hill; 2009. Available at: http://www.accesspharmacy.com/content .aspx?aID=4509054.

32. Jameson JL. Principles of endocrinology In: Fauci AS, Braunwald E, Kasper DL, et al. *Harrison's principles of internal medicine*, 18th ed. New York, NY: McGraw-Hill; 2011. Available at: http:// www.accesspharmacy.com/content.aspx?aID=9139719.

33. Jonklaas J, Talbert RL. Thyroid disorders. In: DiPiro JT, Talbert RL, Yee GC, et al. *Pharmacotherapy: a pathophysiologic approach*, 8th ed. New York, NY: McGraw-Hill; 2011. Available at: http://www.accesspharmacy.com/content.aspx?aID=7991868.

34. Katzung BG, White PF. Skeletal muscle relaxants. In: Katzung BG, Masters SB, Trevor AJ. *Basic & clinical pharmacology*, 11th ed. New York, NY: McGraw-Hill; 2009. Available at: http://www .accesspharmacy.com/content.aspx?aID=4514997.

35. Katzung BG, Trevor AJ, Masters SB. Drugs used in gastrointestinal disorders. In: Katzung BG, Trevor AJ, Masters SB, eds. *Pharmacology: examination & board review*, 9th ed. New York, NY: McGraw-Hill; 2010. Available at: http://www.accesspharmacy.com/content.aspx?aID=6547642.

36. Kishor S, Jaina KS, Kathiravanb MK, et al. The biology and chemistry of hyperlipidemia. *Bioorgan Med Chem*. 2007;15:4674–4699.

37. Lacy CF, Armstrong LL, Goldman MP, Lance LL. *Drug information handbook*, 18th ed. Hudson, OH: Lexicomp; 2009.

38. Lemke TL, Williams DA, Roche VF, Zito SW. *Foye's principles of medicinal chemistry*, 7th ed. New York: Wolters Kluwer/Lippincott Williams & Wilkins; 2012.

39. Lewis EJ, Hunsicker LG, Clarke WR, et al. Renoprotective effect of the angiotensin-receptor antagonist irbesartan in patients with nephropathy due to type 2 diabetes. *N Engl J Med*. 2001;345:851–860.

40. Maclaren R, Rudis MI, Dasta JF. Use of vasopressors and inotropes in the pharmacotherapy of shock. In: DiPiro JT, Talbert RL, Yee GC, et al. *Pharmacotherapy: a pathophysiologic approach*, 8th ed. New York, NY: McGraw-Hill; 2011. Available at: http://www.accesspharmacy.com /content.aspx?aID=7974733.

41. Mader SS. *Human biology*, 9th ed. New York, NY: McGraw-Hill; 2006.

42. Manini AF. Monoamine oxidase inhibitors. In: Manini AF, ed. *Goldfrank's toxicologic emergencies*, 9th ed. New York, NY: McGraw-Hill; 2011. Available at: http://www.accesspharmacy.com/content .aspx?aID=6519667.

43. May R, Smith PH. Allergic rhinitis. In: DiPiro JT, Talbert RL, Yee GC, et al. *Pharmacotherapy: a pathophysiologic approach*, 8th ed. New York, NY: McGraw-Hill; 2011. Available at: http://www .accesspharmacy.com.

44. Melton ST, Kirkwood CK. Anxiety disorders I: generalized anxiety, panic, and social anxiety disorders. In: DiPiro JT, Talbert RL, Yee GC, et al. *Pharmacotherapy: a pathophysiologic approach*, 8th ed. New York, NY: McGraw-Hill; 2011. Available at: http://www.accesspharmacy .com/content.aspx?aID=7989670.om/content.aspx?aID=7998284.

45. Mihic SJ, Harris RA. Hypnotics and sedatives. In: Brunton LL, Chabner BA, Knollmann BC. *Goodman & Gilman's the pharmacological basis of therapeutics*, 12th ed. New York, NY: McGraw-Hill; 2010. Available at: http://www.accesspharmacy.com/content.aspx?aID =16663643.

46. Mills JC, Stappenbeck TS, Bunnett NW. Gastrointestinal disease. In: Mills JC, Stappenbeck TS, Bunnett NW, eds. *Pathophysiology of disease: an introduction to clinical medicine*, 6th ed. New York, NY: McGraw-Hill; 2010. Available at: http://www.accesspharmacy.com/content.aspx?aID =5369402.

47. Moore TD, Anderson JR. Heart failure. In: DiPiro JT, Talbert RL, Yee GC, et al. *Pharmacotherapy in primary care*. New York, NY: McGraw-Hill; 2008. Available at: http://www.accesspharmacy. com/content.aspx?aID=3600546.

48. Nahata MC, Taketomo C. Pediatrics. In: DiPiro JT, Talbert RL, Yee GC, et al. *Pharmacotherapy: a pathophysiologic approach*, 8th ed. New York, NY: McGraw-Hill; 2011. Available at: http://www. accesspharmacy.com/content.aspx?aID=7967211.

49.   Nelson LS, Olsen D. Opioids. In: Nelson LS, Lewin NA, Howland MA, et al. *Goldfrank's toxicologic emergencies*, 9th ed. New York, NY: McGraw-Hill; 2010. Available at: http://www.accesspharmacy.com/content.aspx?aID=6511222.

50.   O'Donnell JM, Shelton RC. Drug therapy of depression and anxiety disorders. In: Brunton LL, Chabner BA, Knollmann BC. *Goodman & Gilman's the pharmacological basis of therapeutics*, 12th ed. New York, NY: McGraw-Hill; 2010. Available at: http://www.accesspharmacy.com/content.aspx?aID=16663059.

51.   Park SH. Bipolar disorders. In: Sutton SS. *McGraw-Hill's NAPLEX® review guide*. New York, NY: McGraw-Hill; 2010. Available at: http://www.accesspharmacy.com/content.aspx?aID=7254936.

52.   Parker RB, Cavallari LH. Systolic heart failure. In: DiPiro JT, Talbert RL, Yee GC, et al. *Pharmacotherapy: a pathophysiologic approach*, 8th ed. New York, NY: McGraw-Hill; 2011. Available at: http://www.accesspharmacy.com/content.aspx?aID=7970780.

53.   Parmley WW, Katzung BG. Drugs used in heart failure. In: Katzung BG, Masters SB, Trevor AJ. *Basic & clinical pharmacology*, 11th ed. New York: McGraw-Hill 2009. Available at: http://www.accesspharmacy.com/content.aspx?aID=4518357.64636.

54.   Patel PM, Patel HH, Roth DM. General anesthetics and therapeutic gases. In: Brunton LL, Chabner BA, Knollmann BC. *Goodman & Gilman's the pharmacological basis of therapeutics*, 12th ed. New York, NY: McGraw-Hill; 2010. Available at: http://www.accesspharmacy.com/content.aspx?aID=166.

55.   Patrick GL. *An introduction to medicinal chemistry*, 2nd ed. New York, NY: Oxford University Press; 2001.

56.   Prendergast TJ, Seeley EJ, Ruoss SJ. Pulmonary disease. In: Prendergast TJ, Seeley EJ, Ruoss SJ, eds. *Pathophysiology of disease: an introduction to clinical medicine*, 6th ed. New York, NY: McGraw-Hill; 2010. Available at: http://www.accesspharmacy.com/content.aspx?aID=5369033.

57.   Rao RB. Neurologic principles. In: Rao RB, ed. *Goldfrank's toxicologic emergencies*, 9th ed. New York, NY: McGraw-Hill; 2011. Available at: http://www.accesspharmacy.com/content.aspx?aID=6506076.

58.   Remington. *The science and practice of pharmacy*, 21st ed. Philadelphia: Lippincott Williams & Wilkins; 2005.

59.   Sanders-Bush E, Hazelwood L. 5-Hydroxytryptamine (serotonin) and dopamine. In: Brunton LL, Chabner BA, Knollmann BC. *Goodman & Gilman's the pharmacological basis of therapeutics*, 12th ed. New York, NY: McGraw-Hill; 2010. Available at: http://www.accesspharmacy.com/content.aspx?aID=16662305.

60.   Saseen JJ, Maclaughlin EJ. Hypertension. In: DiPiro JT, Talbert RL, Yee GC, et al. *Pharmacotherapy: a pathophysiologic approach*, 8th ed. New York, NY: McGraw-Hill; 2011. Available at: http://www.accesspharmacy.com/content.aspx?aID=7969921.

61.   Schimmer BP, Funder JW. ACTH, adrenal steroids, and pharmacology of the adrenal cortex In: Brunton LL, Chabner BA, Knollmann BC. *Goodman & Gilman's the pharmacological basis of therapeutics*, 12th ed. New York, NY: McGraw-Hill; 2010. Available at: http://www.accesspharmacy.com/content.aspx?aID=16674048.

62.   Senz A, Nunnink L. Review article: inotrope and vasopressor use in the emergency department. *Emerg Med Australas.* 2009;21:342–351.

63.   Sharkey KA, Wallace JL. Treatment of disorders of bowel motility and water flux; anti-emetics; agents used in biliary and pancreatic disease. In: Brunton LL, Chabner BA, Knollmann BC, eds. *Goodman & Gilman's the pharmacological basis of therapeutics*, 12th ed. New York, NY: McGraw-Hill; 2010. Available at: http://www.accessmedicine.com/content.aspx?aID=16675372.

64. Shargel L, Mutnick AH, Souney PF, Swanson LN. *Comprehensive pharmacy review*, 7th ed. Philadelphia, PA: Lippincott Williams & Wilkins; 2010.

65. Slattum PW, Swerdlow RH, Hill AM. Alzheimer's disease. In: DiPiro JT, Talbert RL, Yee GC, et al. *Pharmacotherapy: a pathophysiologic approach*, 8th ed. New York, NY: McGraw-Hill; 2011. Available at: http://www.accesspharmacy.com/content.aspx?aID=7984697.

66. Stone NJ, Robinson J, Lichtenstein AH, Merz NB, et al. Guideline on the Treatment of Blood Cholesterol to Reduce Atherosclerotic Cardiovascular Risk in Adults. Journal of the American College of Cardiology doi: 10.1016/j.jacc.2013.11.002. 2013. Available at: http://content.onlinejacc.org/article.aspx?articleid=1770217

67. Talbert RL. Dyslipidemia. In: DiPiro JT, Talbert RL, Yee GC, et al. *Pharmacotherapy: a pathophysiologic approach*, 8th ed. New York, NY: McGraw-Hill; 2011. Available at: http://www.accesspharmacy.com/content.aspx?aID=7974214.

68. Taylor P. Anticholinesterase agents. In: Brunton LL, Chabner BA, Knollmann BC. *Goodman & Gilman's the pharmacological basis of therapeutics*, 12th ed. New York, NY: McGraw-Hill; 2010. Available at: http://www.accesspharmacy.com/content.aspx?aID=16660859.

69. Teter CJ, Kando JC, Wells BG. Major depressive disorder. In: DiPiro JT, Talbert RL, Yee GC, et al. *Pharmacotherapy: a pathophysiologic approach*, 8th ed. New York, NY: McGraw-Hill; 2011. Available at: http://www.accesspharmacy.com/content.aspx?aID=7988626.

70. Trevor AJ, Katzung BG, Masters SB. Cholinoceptor blockers and cholinesterase regenerators. In: Trevor AJ, Katzung BG, Masters SB. *Pharmacology: examination & board review*, 9th ed. New York, NY: McGraw-Hill; 2010. Available at: http://www.accesspharmacy.com/content.aspx?aID=6543531.

71. Trevor AJ, Katzung BG, Masters SB. Drugs used in hypertension. In: Trevor AJ, Katzung BG, Masters SB. *Pharmacology: examination & board review*, 9th ed. New York, NY: McGraw-Hill 2010. Available at: http://www.accesspharmacy.com/content.aspx?aID=6543753.

72. Trevor AJ, Katzung BG, Masters SB. Sedative-hypnotic drugs. In: Trevor AJ, Katzung BG, Masters SB. *Pharmacology: examination & board review*, 9th ed. New York, NY: McGraw-Hill; 2010. Available at: http://www.accesspharmacy.com/content.aspx?aID=6544555.

73. Triplitt CL, Reasner CA. Diabetes mellitus. In: DiPiro JT, Talbert RL, Yee GC, et al. *Pharmacotherapy: a pathophysiologic approach*, 8th ed. New York, NY: McGraw-Hill; 2011. Available at: http://www.accesspharmacy.com/content.aspx?aID=7990956.

74. UpToDate. Waltham, MA: 2012. Available at: http://www.uptodate.com/online with subscription.

75. Wallace JL, Sharkey KA. Pharmacotherapy of gastric acidity, peptic ulcers, and gastroesophageal reflux disease. In: Wallace JL, Sharkey KA, eds. *Goodman & Gilman's the pharmacological basis of therapeutics*, 12th ed. New York, NY: McGraw-Hill; 2011. Available at: http://www.accesspharmacy.com/content.aspx?aID=16675229.

76. Wallace JL, Sharkey KA. Pharmacotherapy of inflammatory bowel disease. In: Wallace JL, Sharkey KA, eds. *Goodman & Gilman's the pharmacological basis of therapeutics*, 12th ed. New York, NY: McGraw-Hill; 2011. Available at: http://www.accesspharmacy.com/content.aspx?aID=16675684.

77. Waxman SG. Fundamentals of the nervous system. In: Waxman SG, ed. *Clinical neuroanatomy*, 26th ed. New York, NY: McGraw-Hill; 2011.

78. Westfall TC. Neurotransmission: the autonomic and somatic motor nervous systems. In: Brunton LL, Chabner BA, Knollmann BC. *Goodman & Gilman's the pharmacological basis of therapeutics*, 12th ed. New York, NY: McGraw-Hill; 2010. Available at: http://www.accesspharmacy.com/content.aspx?aID=16659803.

79. Westfall TC, Westfall DP. Adrenergic agonists and antagonists. In: Brunton LL, Chabner BA, Knollmann BC. *Goodman & Gilman's the pharmacological basis of therapeutics*, 12th ed. New York, NY: McGraw-Hill; 2010. Available at: http://www.accesspharmacy.com/content.aspx?aID=16661344.

80. Williams DM, Bourdet SV. Chronic obstructive pulmonary disease. In: DiPiro JT, Talbert RL, Yee GC, et al. *Pharmacotherapy: a pathophysiologic approach*, 8th ed. New York, NY: McGraw-Hill; 2011. Available at: http://www.accesspharmacy.com/content.aspx?aID =7975888.

81. Wuttke H, Rau T, Heide R, et al. Increased frequency of cytochrome P450 2D6 poor metabolizers among patients with metoprolol-associated adverse effects. *Clin Pharmacol Ther*. 2002;72:429–437.

82. Wyatt C, Moos PJ, Brown TG. Pulmonary pathology. In: Wyatt C, Moos PJ, Brown TG, eds. *Pathology: the big picture*. New York, NY: McGraw-Hill; 2008. Available at: http://www.accessmedicine.com /content.aspx?aID=57053485.

83. Yaksh TL, Wallace MS. Opioids, analgesia, and pain management. In: Brunton LL, Chabner BA, Knollmann BC. *Goodman & Gilman's the pharmacological basis of therapeutics*, 12th ed. New York, NY: McGraw-Hill; 2010. Available at: http://www.accesspharmacy.com/content.aspx?aID =16663974.

84. Zipitis CS, Akobeng AK. Vitamin D supplementation in early childhood and risk of type 1 diabetes: a systematic review and meta-analysis. *Arch Dis Child*. 2008;93:512–517.

Introduction to Toxicology

Fawzy Elbarbry

OBJECTIVES

1. Understand the scientific and clinical application of toxicology.

2. Use different dose–response curves to assess safety of a drug.

3. Define and understand the clinical use of the therapeutic index and margin of safety.

4. Recognize the different factors that may influence a drug's toxicity.

5. Recognize the different approaches that are used to manage a poisoned patient.

6. Understand the clinical features and treatment of poisoning from commonly used drugs and environmental chemicals.

7. Provide examples of drugs that can cause selective organ toxicity.

8. Implement a series of Learning Bridge assignments at your experiential sites to bridge your didactic learning with your experiential experiences.

KEY TERMS AND DEFINITIONS

1. **Acute toxicity:** The adverse effects of a substance that result either from a single exposure or from multiple exposures in a short space of time (usually less than 24 hours).

2. **Antidote:** A remedy or substance that can neutralize or counteract a form of poisoning.

3. **Chronic toxicity:** The adverse health effects from repeated exposures, often at lower levels, to a substance over a longer time period (months or years).

4. **Decontamination:** The process of cleansing the human body to remove contamination by hazardous materials such as chemicals, radioactive substances, and infectious material.

5. **Dialysis:** A process for removing waste and excess water from the blood, which is used primarily to perform many of the normal duties of the kidneys in people with renal failure.

6. **Genetic polymorphism:** The simultaneous occurrence in the same locality of two or more discontinuous genetic variants of a specific trait in such proportions that the rarest of them cannot be maintained just by recurrent mutation or immigration.

7. **Median effective dose (ED_{50}):** A drug dose that is required to produce a specific effect in 50% of the population.

8. **Median lethal dose (LD_{50}):** A statistically derived single dose of a substance at which 50% of the individuals (usually experimental animals in acute toxicity studies) are expected to die.

9. **Medication error:** Any avoidable event that may cause or lead to inappropriate medication use or harm to the patient.

10. **Therapeutic index:** A statement of how selective a drug is in producing its therapeutic effect versus causing undesirable effects.

Introduction

According to the philosophical definition of poisons offered by the Renaissance physician Paracelsus (1493–1541), every drug or chemical is a potential poison based on its dose. Dosage regimens of drugs, then, should be adjusted based on patients' conditions to keep plasma levels of drugs within their therapeutic ranges. Unfortunately, due to errors made by patients or healthcare providers, drug levels may sometimes exceed their maximum therapeutic concentrations leading to toxicity. It is crucial that pharmacists are aware of the early signs of toxicity to allow for early diagnosis and treatment of affected patients. Recognition of specific antidotes and special detoxification techniques for toxic agents may rescue patients in both hospital and community settings.

This chapter discusses the various factors that may influence drug toxicity. These factors include, but are not limited to, patients' age, gender, concurrent medications, concurrent medical conditions, and genetic predispositions, in addition to outright medication errors. Additionally, this chapter identifies the different approaches that are followed to manage poisoned patients. These approaches include clinical stabilization, decontamination, enhancement of poison elimination, use of antidotes, and prevention of reexposure. Finally, the chapter lists those drugs that are most frequently implicated in select organ toxicity.

What Is Toxicology?

The U.S. Food and Drug Administration (FDA) and pharmaceutical companies spend a significant amount of time and financial resources to make sure that new drugs are both effective and safe. Despite these efforts, no drug can ever be considered entirely safe. In addition to its intended therapeutic effect, a drug may have unintended (and mostly undesirable) effects, called adverse drug reactions or side effects. The nature of these adverse reactions can range in severity from immediate death to subtle changes that may not be recognized until months or years later. Drug toxicity is often classified according to the level of drug-induced pathological effect into four categories: cell death or tissue injury, altered cellular function, immunological or hypersensitivity, and cancer.

Toxicology is often regarded as the science that deals with the harmful effects—poisoning or toxicity—of drugs. Most pharmaceutical agents may be nontoxic and even beneficial in small amounts, but when the dose is increased, adverse effects may arise (**Table 11.1**).

Toxicology is concerned with studying the relationship between exposure level (dose) and its deleterious effects on the living organism, examining the nature of these effects, and predicting

Table 11.1 Dose-Dependent Effects of Selected Drugs/Chemicals

Drug/Chemical	Therapeutic Concentration	Toxic Concentration	Lethal Concentration
Acetaminophen (Tylenol)	10–20 mg/L	400 mg/L	1,500 mg/L
Diazepam (Valium)	0.5–2.5 mg/L	5–20 mg/L	> 50 mg/L
Ethanol (ethyl alcohol)	500 mg/L	1,000 mg/L	5,000 mg/L
Lithium (Lithobid)	4–8 mg/L	13.9 mg/L	> 13.9 mg/L
Meperidine (Demerol)	0.6 mg/L	5 mg/L	30 mg/L
Secobarbital (Seconal)	1.0 mg/L	7.0 mg/L	> 10 mg/L

the probability of their occurrence. The terms "poison," "toxic agent," and "toxicant" will be considered synonymous in this chapter.

The adverse effects (toxicity) manifested by an organism in response to a toxic agent can be acute or chronic. Acute toxicity refers to the effects that result from either a single exposure or from multiple exposures in a short space of time (usually less than 24 hours). To be recognized as acute toxicity, the adverse effects should occur within 14 days of the administration of the substance. For example, inhalation of a high concentration of cyanide may cause immediate injury by inhibiting respiration, with death following in a matter of minutes if not treated immediately (see the *Introduction to Biochemistry* chapter for the lethal mechanism of cyanide). Chronic toxicity describes the adverse health effects that result from repeated exposures, often at lower levels, to a substance over a longer period of time (months or years). For example, chronic exposure to low concentrations of cyanide, such as in individuals whose diet includes significant amounts of cyanogenic plants like cassava, may cause demyelination, lesions of the optic nerve, ataxia, hypertonia, goiters, and depressed thyroid function.

Dose–Response Curves

The dose–response relationship is a correlative relationship that describes the effect of different levels of exposure (doses) on an organism. Understanding the causal relationships between dose and effect is central to toxicology to determine "safe" and "toxic" levels and therapeutic dosages of drugs, as well as potential pollutants to which humans or other organisms are exposed (see the *Introduction to Pharmacodynamics* chapter for more details about the dose–response relationship). Exposure of different individuals to the same dose of a single drug or to similar drugs may result in a wide variation in response. This so-called interindividual variation may be attributed to several causes, such as genetic variations, age, gender, disease condition, and administration of interacting drugs. Generally, the majority of the individuals will show an "average/therapeutic" effect, while a very few will show either a minimal or a toxic effect. In turn, a graph of the magnitude of response versus the number of individuals encountering this response will normally be depicted as a bell-shaped distribution curve (**Figure 11.1**). In this graph, the majority of the

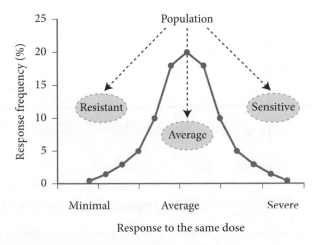

Figure 11.1 Frequency distribution curve. Individuals were exposed to the same dose of a hypothetical chemical, and the curve showing an average effect, lower than average effect (resistant), or higher than average effect (sensitive) was plotted.

responders fall in the middle and experience the average effect from the drug dose. Responders at the far left of the curve are typically resistant or less susceptible, whereas those at the far right are hypersusceptible.

In a normally distributed population, approximately 68% of the population lies within one standard deviation (SD) of the mean; 95% of the population lies within two SD of the mean; and 99.7% of the population lies within three SD of the mean. The SD, calculated using a statistical formula, is widely utilized to estimate the percentage of the test population who tend to deviate most from those who respond with a tendency around the mean. From this estimate of deviation, we can predict what percentage of the population would tend to not respond similarly to the "average" individual (i.e., an individual who has a response tendency around the mean).

This frequency distribution curve works well for quantal data—that is, "all or none" responses, such as death, hypnosis, or tumor production. Such a relationship is called a "quantal dose–response relationship."

Exposure of individuals to escalating doses will normally result in a curve that is characterized by a dose-dependent increase in the severity or magnitude of response. Such dose–response curves are used by toxicologists to derive dose estimates of chemical substances. Median lethal dose (LD_{50}) is a statistically derived single dose of a substance at which 50% of the individuals (usually experimental animals in acute toxicity studies) are expected to die (**Figure 11.2**).

Figure 11.2 also shows an estimation of the drug dose that is required to produce a specific effect—analgesia in this case—in 50% of the population. This dose is called the median effective dose (ED_{50}). Additionally, and as long as the specific end point is indicated, the dose–response curve can be used to derive other dose estimates that may indicate the safety, effectiveness, or toxicity of the substance under investigation. Examples of these dose estimates are shown in **Table 11.2**.

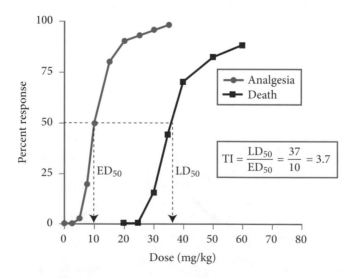

Figure 11.2 Quantal dose–response curve. Animals were injected with an escalating dose of a hypothetical analgesic drug, and their responses (analgesia or mortality) were determined and plotted. The graph shows how LD_{50}, ED_{50}, and TI were determined.

Table 11.2 Examples of Dose Estimates Terms Commonly Used to Indicate the Safety, Effectiveness, or Toxicity of a Chemical

Dose	Indication
ED_0	Dose effective in 0% of the population
ED_{10}	Dose effective in 10% of the population
ED_{50}	Dose effective in 50% of the population
ED_{99}	Dose effective in 99% of the population
TD_0	Dose causes adverse toxic effects in 0% of the population
TD_{10}	Dose causes adverse toxic effects in 10% of the population
TD_{50}	Dose causes adverse toxic effects in 50% of the population
TD_{99}	Dose causes adverse toxic effects in 99% of the population
LD_0	Dose causes mortality (death) in 0% of the population
LD_1	Dose causes mortality (death) in 1% of the population
LD_{50}	Dose causes mortality (death) in 50% of the population

Learning Bridge 11.1

A toxicity study was conducted on a group of male Sprague-Dawley rats to examine the acute toxicity of a new investigational antihypertensive drug, FAE. Based on the dose–response graph shown in **Exhibit 11.1**, what is the LD_{50} of FAE?

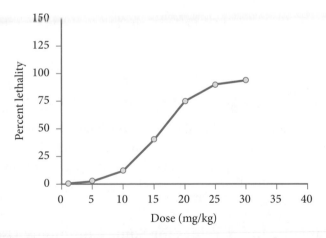

Exhibit 11.1 A dose–response graph of a new investigational antihypertensive drug administered to male Sprague-Dawley rats.

A. 5 mg/kg
B. 17 mg/kg
C. 50 mg/kg
D. There is not enough information to answer this question.

Therapeutic Index and Margin of Safety

The *therapeutic index* (TI), also known as the therapeutic ratio, is a statement of how selectively a drug produces its therapeutic effect versus causing undesirable effects such as death in animal studies and toxicity in human studies. Quantitatively, and as illustrated in Figure 11.2, TI is the ratio of $\left(\frac{LD_{50}}{ED_{50}}\right)$ in animal studies or $\left(\frac{TD_{50}}{ED_{50}}\right)$ in humans. Generally, a drug with a higher therapeutic index (i.e., having a large difference between toxic and therapeutic doses) is preferable to a drug with a lower TI, as patients may need to take a much higher dose of such a drug to achieve toxic/lethal levels compared to therapeutic levels. Conversely, drugs with lower TI (i.e., having small differences between therapeutic and toxic doses) must have their doses titrated carefully, and tight monitoring of their blood level may be required to achieve therapeutic effects while minimizing toxicity. **Table 11.3** illustrates how TI varies among pharmaceutical agents.

As just one data point along the entire range of potential responses, the median dose (i.e., LD_{50} and ED_{50}) does not fully describe the threshold dose level (the point at which toxicity first appears) and the slope (the percentage of the population responding per unit change in dose) of the dose–response curve. Both the slope and the threshold of the curve are important in predicting the therapeutic and toxic effects of a drug at specific dose levels. For example, two drugs might have the same LD_{50}, but clinically have different degrees of health hazards. As an example, in **Figure 11.3**, drug A and drug B have a similar LD_{50} value (20 mg/kg), but different thresholds and slopes. Drug A has a higher initial lethal threshold, but a steeper slope; thus only small additional doses of drug A are needed to reach the 50% lethality level. In contrast, drug B has a lower initial threshold, but a relatively flat slope; thus larger changes in dosage may be required before 50% of the population die.

To overcome the limitations of LD_{50} and ED_{50} values in assessing the safety and toxicity of a drug, the margin of safety (MOS) is often used by toxicologists for risk assessment purposes. Utilization of MOS depends on using ED_{99} for the desired effect and LD_1 for the undesired, or lethal, effect.

$$\text{Margin of Saftey} = \frac{LD_1}{ED_{99}}$$

The margin of safety is more critical than the TI, because it takes into account the possible overlap in dose–response curves for the desired and undesired effects. For example, in Figure 11.2, doses less than ED_{90} do not cause toxicity, whereas effective doses greater than ED_{90} may result into toxicity in addition to their desirable (analgesic) effect.

Table 11.3 Therapeutic Index Values for Some Commonly Used Drugs/Chemicals

Drug	Indication	Therapeutic Index
Digoxin (Lanoxin)	Atrial fibrillation/flutter	2:1
Ethanol	Sedative	10:1
Cocaine	Stimulant/local anesthetic	15:1
Morphine (Kadian)	Analgesic	70:1
Diazepam (Valium)	Sedative/hypnotic	100:1
Nitrous oxide	Anesthetic agent	150:1
Marijuana	Sedative/analgesic	1,000:1

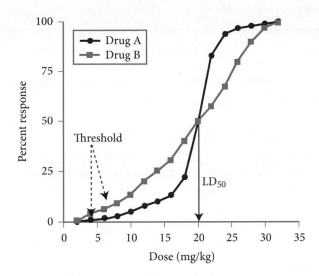

Figure 11.3 Quantal dose–response curves of two drugs that have similar LD_{50} values, but different thresholds and slopes. Different degrees of health hazards would be expected for these drugs.

Factors Influencing Toxicity

Several factors appear to predispose an individual patient to drug toxicity. These factors can be generally attributed to the drug itself (e.g., narrow therapeutic index), the patient (e.g., age), the healthcare provider (e.g., medication errors), or a combination of these factors, as illustrated in **Figure 11.4**. In most of the cases, these factors are associated with altering the pharmacokinetic or pharmacodynamic characteristics of the drug. Recognition of these predisposing factors is important in ultimately preventing—or at least reducing the risk of—toxicity.

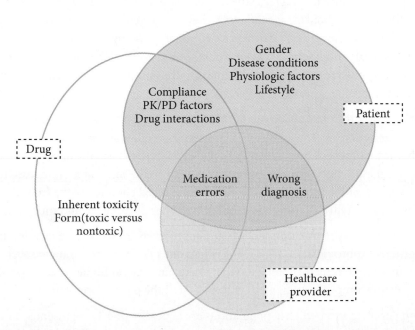

Figure 11.4 Factors that influence the risk of drug toxicity. Drug-induced toxicity is multifactorial in origin. Inherent properties of the drug, the patient's physiological factors, and medication errors by healthcare providers all affect the risk of toxicity.

Age

Risk of toxicity is particularly high in very young and very old patients. During the early neonatal period, the organs responsible for drug metabolism and excretion are not fully developed. Therefore, the rate of drug elimination is usually slower in this age group, and these patients may have a higher risk of toxicity. For example, the elimination half-life of the H_2-receptor antagonist famotidine (Pepcid) was found to be 10.5 ± 5 hours in neonates 5–19 days of age compared to 3 ± 1 hours in adults. This long half-life in neonates occurs secondary to the immaturity of glomerular filtration in such patients and the tubular secretion of famotidine (approximately 78% eliminated as unchanged drug in urine). However, even the use of appropriate doses of specific medications in children has produced unexpected toxicity that often cannot be explained by changes in the drug's pharmacokinetics. Accordingly, increased sensitivity of specific drug receptors in the developing child may account for the observed toxicity in infants compared to adults. For example, the high concentration of dopamine-2 receptors in infants compared to adults may explain why dopamine antagonists such as chlorpromazine (Largactil, from Canada) are more likely to cause acute dystonia in infants than adults.

Aging is associated with several changes in body composition and organ functions that may also predispose elderly patients to drug toxicity. The annual rate of drug-induced toxicity for individuals aged 65 years or older is estimated to be more than twice the rate for those persons younger than 65 years of age.

Aging may have a significant effect on the pharmacokinetics and pharmacodynamics of a drug. Although several organs may contribute to drug elimination from the body, both the liver and the kidneys play major roles in drug elimination through metabolism and excretion, respectively. Age-related decreases in the masses of the liver and kidneys, coupled with decreases in function, play an important role in the reduction of drug elimination in elderly patients, increasing the potential for toxicity if the dose is not adjusted accordingly. For example, the intrinsic activity of cytochrome P450 (CYP) enzymes is significantly reduced in the elderly. With drugs that are highly dependent on this pathway (e.g., long-acting benzodiazepines such as diazepam and chlordiazepoxide), a decrease in hepatic clearance can increase the drug's concentration and lead to toxicity. In addition to altered hepatic metabolism, age influences hepatic perfusion. Aging significantly decreases liver blood flow and, therefore, decreases hepatic elimination of high-extraction-ratio drugs such as propranolol (Inderal) and lidocaine (Xylocaine) (see also the *Introduction to Pharmacokinetics* chapter). **Table 11.4** indicates age-related variations in the elimination half-lives of some commonly used medications.

Aging may also alter the pharmacodynamic behaviors of drugs. These alterations may include changes in the number or binding affinity of target receptors, changes in signal transduction, and alteration in homeostatic mechanisms. For example, older patients usually have higher susceptibility to the anticholinergic effects of medications. Such high risk of anticholinergic toxicity may be attributed to a smaller number of cholinergic neurons, reduced choline uptake from the periphery, a lower rate of choline acetyltransferase, and a smaller number of nicotinic and muscarinic receptors.

Additionally, the elderly population tends to use more medications and have more illnesses than younger age groups. Approximately 15–45% of older adults develop moderate to severe forms of cognitive impairment from medication use, which may put them at higher risk of overdose or cause them to be noncompliant compared with the rest of the patient population.

Finally, both geriatric and pediatric populations are generally poorly represented in clinical trials. Thus risk of toxicity is generally higher in these populations simply because of a lack of knowledge about these risks.

Table 11.4 Age-Related Variations in the Elimination Half-lives of Some Commonly Used Medications

Drug Name	Route of Elimination	Age	Half-life (hours)
Valproic acid (Depakene)	Primarily metabolism by the liver	Neonates[1] Infants[2] Children[3] Adults[4] Geriatrics	17.2 12.5 ± 2.8 11 ± 4 11.9 ± 5.7 15.3 ± 1.7
Gentamicin (Garamycin)	Primarily glomerular filtration by the kidney	Neonates Infants Adults Young geriatrics Old geriatrics	6 ± 2 4 ± 1 2 ± 1 3.5 ± 2 4 ± 1
Vancomycin (Vancocin)	Primarily glomerular filtration by the kidney	Neonates Infants Adults Geriatrics	6.7 5.6 ± 2.1 7 ± 1.5 12.1 ± 0.8
Digoxin	70% glomerular filtration and tubular secretion; 30% biliary excretion and some gut flora elimination	Neonates Children Adults	44 ± 13 37 ± 16 36 ± 8

Notes:
1. Neonates: < 4 weeks.
2. Infants: 4 weeks to < 1 year.
3. Children: 3 years to < 16 years.
4. Adults: 18 years to < 60 years.

Concurrent Diseases

Comorbid conditions such as cardiovascular disease, obesity, or hepatitis can alter the pharmacokinetics or pharmacodynamics of drugs, and increase the risk of toxicity in patients with these conditions relative to comparatively healthy individuals. Congestive heart failure, for example, reduces hepatic blood flow and may reduce the elimination of drugs with a high hepatic extraction ratio when those agents are administered intravenously. Kidney impairment may result in accumulation of drugs or metabolites that are renally excreted to a high extent. This results in a higher-than-normal plasma concentration and exaggerated response, especially for drugs with a narrow therapeutic window. Concurrent diseases may also increase the risk of toxicity by enhancing the pharmacodynamic response to drugs. For example, patients with hypothyroidism usually experience exaggerated responses from the usual doses of digoxin. Factors contributing to this toxicity are the increased receptor sensitivity and decreased renal excretion of digoxin in hypothyroidism.

Concurrent Medications/Diet

Generally, the number and severity of toxic reactions increase disproportionately with the number of drugs and alternative medicines or natural products taken. Alterations in drugs pharmacokinetics, especially bioavailability and elimination, and pharmacodynamics are the main concerns with drug–drug interactions. Oral bioavailability, and therefore plasma level, of drugs can be increased after inhibition of p-glycoprotein, a transporter protein expressed on the luminal surfaces of intestinal epithelial cells. Also, inactivation of gut flora that extensively destroys some drugs, such as digoxin, prior to absorption can result in higher-than-normal bioavailability and higher risk of toxicity. Inhibition of drug-metabolizing enzymes, especially the cytochrome P450

Table 11.5 Examples and Mechanisms of Pharmacokinetics (PK) and Pharmacodynamics (PD) in Drug–Drug Interactions That Result in Toxicity

PK/PD Parameters	Examples and Mechanism of Increased Toxicity
Absorption (bioavailability)	• Tetracycline (Apo-tetra, from Canada) increases the risk of toxicity from digoxin. Tetracycline inactivates gut flora that extensively destroy digoxin and reduce its oral bioavailability. • Quinidine (Apo-Quinidine, from Canada) increases the risk of toxicity from digoxin. Quinidine is a potent inhibitor for the p-glycoprotein transporter that is responsible for preventing digoxin molecules from reaching the systemic circulation and effectively limiting its bioavailability.
Distribution	• Ibuprofen (Advil) increases the risk of bleeding from warfarin (Coumadin). Ibuprofen displaces warfarin (approximately 99% plasma protein bound) from protein-binding sites and increases the unbound drug concentration.
Metabolism	• Erythromycin (E.E.S.) increases the risk of toxicity from verapamil (Calan). Erythromycin inhibits CYP3A4, thereby minimizing the hepatic first-pass extraction and systemic clearance of verapamil. • β–blockers increases the risk of toxicity from lidocaine. β–blockers decrease hepatic blood flow and reduce the clearance of the high-extraction-ratio lidocaine.
Excretion	• NSAIDs increase the risk of toxicity from lithium. NSAIDs decrease renal blood flow and, therefore, the glomerular filtration rate and lithium clearance. • Salicylates increase the risk of toxicity from methotrexate (Rheumatrex). Salicylates compete with methotrexate for the same drug transport protein in the proximal renal tubule, resulting in reduced methotrexate excretion.
PD interactions	• Thiazide diuretics increase toxicity from digoxin. Thiazide diuretics deplete potassium, resulting in sensitization of the heart to digoxin therapy. • St. John's wort (an herbal treatment for depression) increases the toxicity of selective serotonin reuptake inhibitors (SSRIs) such as fluoxetine (Prozac). St. John's wort has both serotonin agonist and serotonin reuptake inhibitory effects, so it creates additive serotonin toxicity.

family, may significantly increase the risk of toxicity with drugs that are extensively metabolized by these enzymes (see also the *Introduction to Medicinal Chemistry* chapter). Drugs that reduce organ perfusion, such as NSAIDs and β–blockers, may reduce the hepatic or renal elimination rate of drugs that are mostly eliminated by hepatic metabolism and renal excretion, respectively.

Pharmacodynamic interactions can also precipitate severe and multiple toxic reactions. These interactions generally result from the concurrent administration of drugs having the same pharmacologic actions or from alteration of the sensitivity or the responsiveness of the tissues to one drug by another drug. A good understanding of the pharmacology of each drug is the key to predicting many of these interactions. **Table 11.5** shows examples of pharmacokinetics and pharmacodynamics in drug–drug interactions that can result in toxicity.

In addition to the modes of interaction presented in Table 11.5, an increased toxicity, when two chemicals are given together, may be attributed to an additive, potentiation, or synergistic effect. An *additive* effect occurs when the toxicity resulting from combining two chemicals is equal to the sum of the response of each chemical given alone. *Potentiation* occurs when the toxicity of one chemical is greatly enhanced by adding another chemical that does not have inherent toxicity by itself (see the *Introduction to Pharmacodynamics* chapter for more examples). A *synergistic* effect occurs when the combined effects of two chemicals are much greater than the sum of the effects of each agent given alone. **Table 11.6** illustrates the quantitative definitions of these interaction types, with specific examples.

Table 11.6 Quantitative Illustration of the Types of Combined Toxicity from Administration of Two Agents, A and B, with Specific Examples

	Toxic Effect of Drug A	Toxic Effect of Drug B	Combined Toxicity	Example
Addition	40	60	100	Co-administration of CNS depressant agents such as alcohol and tranquilizers often causes depression equal to the sum of that caused by each drug alone.
Potentiation	0	80	100	Isopropanol does not have inherent hepato-toxicity, but it greatly enhances the toxicity of carbon tetrachloride when the two chemicals are given together. Such interaction can occur in the industrial workplace.
Synergism	10	50	100	The combination of ethanol and carbon tetra-chloride results in a hepatotoxicity response that is much greater than the sum of hepato-toxicity from each chemical alone.

Genetic Factors

Advances in the field of pharmacogenomics have shown that genetic makeup is an important determinant of drug-induced toxicity. Extensive research into drug-metabolizing enzymes in the last two decades has identified several allelic variants with catalytic activities different from those of wild-type genes. Analyzing these genetic variations and polymorphisms might help in identifying those patients who may show resistance or toxicity reactions. A relatively high incidence of polymorphism has been shown with at least five of the major CYP enzymes (CYP2A6, CYP2C9, CYP2C19, CYP2D6, and CYP3A4) responsible for drug biotransformation (see also the *Introduction to Pharmacogenomics* chapter). For example, the *S*-enantiomers of warfarin are mainly responsible for its anticoagulant effect and are metabolized by CYP2C9. Individuals carrying the variant CYP2C9 alleles *2 and *3 have a significantly reduced rate of warfarin clearance and are more susceptible to bleeding complications. Similarly, several studies have indicated a relationship between the CYP2A6*4 allele and susceptibility for lung cancer from smoking. It has been suggested that individuals carrying the defective CYP2A6*4 allele might require fewer cigarettes to achieve sufficient levels of nicotine in the blood.

Approximately 5–10% of the population carries two decreased-activity alleles for CYP2D6. These "poor CYP2D6 metabolizers" have a higher risk of toxicity from antidepressants that are extensively eliminated via CYP2D6-mediated metabolism. Conversely, "ultrarapid CYP2D6 metabolizers" have a higher toxicity risk from drugs such as codeine (PMS-codeine, in Canada) and tramadol that are metabolized by CYP2D6 to pharmacologically active metabolites. A tragic case was reported in a Canadian newspaper in which a 13-day-old baby died when his mother, later identified as "ultrarapid CYP2D6 metabolizer," was prescribed codeine and acetaminophen. Administration of codeine by this nursing mother, who is an ultra-rapid metabolizer, may have led to abnormally high levels of morphine in her breast milk. Her nursing infant may have been exposed to an overdose of morphine.

Genetic polymorphism in conjugating enzymes also occurs. Among these enzymes, *N*-acetyltransferase (NAT) was one of the first to be found to have a genetic bias. Patients with low NAT activity, known as "slow acetylators," are more likely to exhibit toxicity symptoms from isoniazid (Isotamine, from Canada) and hydralazine (Apo-hydralazine, from Canada) when administered standard doses, compared with "fast acetylators." Similarly, genetic variability in the catalytic activity of glutathione-*S*-transferase (GST) may be linked to individual susceptibility to hepatotoxicity from drugs such as acetaminophen and troglitazone. Individuals with a defective enzyme, thiopurine *S*-methyltransferase, are unable to metabolize thiopurines and have higher susceptibility for toxicity, especially leukopenia, from azathioprine (Imuran) and 6-mercaptopurine (Purinethol)—drugs that are used in the treatment of leukemia and autoimmune diseases, respectively.

Polymorphism in cellular proteins and receptors may also result in variations in the pharmacodynamic response of an individual. Polymorphism in the G-protein–coupled receptor of bradykinin results in a cough when affected individuals take angiotensin-converting enzyme (ACE) inhibitors. Similarly, deficiency of glucose-6-phosphate dehydrogenase leads to hemolysis in patients taking drugs with high redox potential, such as sulfonamides and dapson. Approximately 1–2% of the population may have mutations in the genes encoding for the cardiac ion channels that render them more vulnerable to long-QT syndrome and sudden cardiac death from exposure to certain drugs such as terfenadine and antiarrhythmic agents. Advances in the pharmacogenomics research field are expected to provide the pharmaceutical industry and the clinicians with useful biomarkers to optimize drug therapy and minimize drug toxicity.

Gender

Analysis of data from the FDA Adverse Events Reporting System and other data resources reveals that women have a higher risk of drug-induced toxic reactions than men. Although this gender-related difference in the frequency of experiencing toxic reactions could be due to over-dosing, differences in immunological and hormonal makeup, or women's tendency to take more medications than men, it is more likely that gender-related differences in pharmacokinetic and pharmacodynamic factors play the major role.

Because of women's body size and composition, drugs have generally low clearance and/or volume of distribution in women, which may result in higher drug concentrations even from normal doses. For example, women are more vulnerable to the sedation and drowsiness effects of antihistamines compared to men. This can be explained by the lower activity of CYP2D6, the enzyme responsible for the metabolic elimination of antihistamines, in women compared to men. When adjusted for body surface area, glomerular filtration, tubular secretion, and tubular reabsorption are all lower in women than men and, therefore, renal clearance is generally slower in women. This may explain the fact that hospitalization due to toxic reactions from diuretics, such as torsemide (Demadex), is more prevalent among women.

Gender-related differences in pharmacodynamics have been also extensively studied. For example, women are more sensitive to pain and more susceptible to chronic and postsurgical pain conditions. Similarly, female sex is a risk factor for prolonged QT interval and potentially fetal arrhythmias. Class I and III antiarrhythmic agents show a higher incidence of torsades de pointes tachycardia in women. Additionally, digoxin therapy has been associated with a significantly elevated mortality compared with placebo therapy in women.

Medication Errors

Medication errors include any avoidable event that may cause or lead to inappropriate medication use or harm to the patient. Since 2000, more than 95,000 reports of mediation errors have been sent to the FDA. Given that these reports are voluntary, the exact number of medication errors is believed to be higher. Although not all medication errors result in significant toxicity problems, 7% are serious enough to cause severe harm and death. These medication errors can occur in any stage of the drug therapy process, including the prescribing, dispensing, and administering stages. Given that medication errors usually occur because of multiple and complex factors, reduction and prevention of these errors require a collaborative effort from all parts of the healthcare system—including both healthcare professionals and patients.

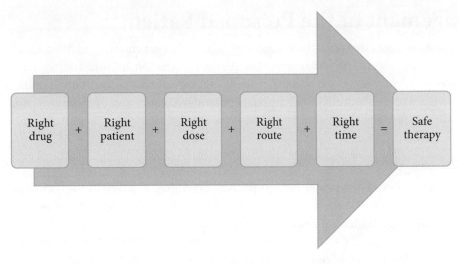

Figure 11.5 The traditional "Five Rights" approach to minimize medication errors in healthcare settings.

Several practical measures have been suggested to reduce medication errors in hospitals and other healthcare settings. Generally these approaches involve inspection of the systems involved in prescribing, documenting, transcribing, dispensing, administering, and monitoring of therapy to make sure the traditional "Five Rights" of safe medication administration have been met (**Figure 11.5**).

Learning Bridge 11.2

During your first day of introductory pharmacy practice experience, your preceptor gives you the following assignment (shown in **Exhibit 11.2**), which was taken from four patient profiles and was organized by another intern at your pharmacy. Examine the pharmacologic effects and pharmacokinetic properties of the following drugs and assess the consequences of their simultaneous use.

Exhibit 11.2 Interactions Between Drugs A and B

Patient Name	Drug A	Drug B	Result of Simultaneous Administration
MR	**Itraconazole** A potent inhibitor for CYP3A4	**Midazolam** Has a low bioavailability due to substantial first-pass metabolism by CYP3A4 in the intestinal epithelium	
PJ	**Nonsteroidal anti-inflammatory drugs** Competes with and displaces drugs from plasma protein-binding sites	**Warfarin** 98–99% plasma protein binding	
SK	**Probenecid** Acts as an active tubular secretion inhibitor	**Methotrexate** Excreted by active secretion by the kidneys	
AR	**Ciprofloxacin** Potent inhibitor of CYP1A2	**Theophylline** Extensively metabolized by CYP1A2 and to a lesser extent by CYP3A4	

Management of the Poisoned Patient

General treatment goals should include clinical stabilization, prevention of further absorption of the poison (decontamination), enhancement of poison elimination, administration of antidote, clinical follow-up, and prevention of reexposure. Specific treatment depends on identification of the poison, its route and amount of exposure, its pharmacokinetics and pharmacodynamics, the duration of exposure, and the past medical history of the patient.

Clinical Stabilization

Assessing and supporting the vital functions (airway, breathing, and circulation—collectively known as the ABCs) must be the initial concern in managing drug toxicity. Additional interventions, such as oxygen administration, continuous cardiac monitoring, and determination of blood glucose, arterial blood gases (ABGs), and electrolyte levels, should be included in patients with concerning histories. Dextrose, oxygen, naloxone, and thiamine—the "coma cocktail"—often are given empirically to patients with depressed mental status. After ensuring that vital signs have been addressed, close physical examination and laboratory findings should be performed to narrow the diagnosis to a particular class of poisons. Results from a basic metabolic panel, ABGs, electrocardiogram (EKG), x-rays, and serum levels may prove useful and may be utilized based on the history or suspicion.

For example, salicylate toxicity is recognized by a pattern of symptoms including nausea, vomiting, tinnitus, diaphoresis, hypoglycemia, hyperthermia, seizures, respiratory alkalosis, metabolic acidosis, and high serum salicylate concentration. Because of their formulation, however, salicylates have the potential for delayed or continual absorption from the gastrointestinal tract. Therefore, decreased salicylate levels do not always indicate resolving toxicity, and serial levels are typically indicated in case of an acute toxicity.

Decontamination

Prevention of further poison absorption during the early stage of toxicity can significantly reduce the amount reaching the patient's systemic circulation, thereby minimizing toxicity. For toxins presented by the ocular or topical route, the main intervention is rapid and thorough irrigation of the exposed areas. A patient who was exposed to toxins through inhalation should be moved from the toxic environment to fresh air.

The four main methods used for gastric decontamination to prevent continued absorption of an oral poison are induction of emesis with ipecac, gastric lavage, single-dose or multiple-dose activated charcoal, and whole-bowel irrigation. Several research articles indicate that there is only limited evidence to support routine use of these gastric decontamination methods. Therefore, the decision about gastric decontamination should be made on an individual case basis after full understanding of the indication, contraindications, benefits, and risks of each technique, as shown in **Table 11.7**.

Enhancement of Poison Elimination

This approach is intended to enhance the elimination of a previously absorbed substance at a rate greater than that provided by the intrinsic elimination pathways. The most commonly used methods employed in this regard include manipulation of urinary pH, multiple-dose activated charcoal, and dialysis.

Table 11.7 Commonly Used Gastric Decontamination Techniques

Gastric Decontaminant	Contraindications	Adverse Reactions	Comments
Syrup of ipecac	1. **Patient's age**: younger than 6 months 2. **Patient's condition**: CNS depression, seizures, comorbid condition that would be compromised by vomiting 3. **Poison**: strong acids, alkali, sharp objects, poison with rapid onset of action, hydrocarbons	Diarrhea, prolonged emesis, lethargy	No longer recommended for general use
Gastric lavage	1. **Patient's condition**: risk of gastric perforation or hemorrhage, absent airway protection reflexes, combative 2. **Poison**: acids, alkali, hydrocarbons, too large to fit into the lumen of the lavage tube	Aspiration (<10%), gastric and esophageal perforation (1%)	Considered for life-threatening toxicity that cannot be treated with other approaches
Activated charcoal	1. **Patient's condition**: absent airway protection reflexes, gastrointestinal perforation 2. **Poison**: corrosives	Constipation, mechanical obstruction of airways, bowel obstruction, may prevent absorption of orally administered medications	Should be given in an amount equal to 10 times the weight of the ingested poison
Whole-bowel irrigation	1. **Patient's condition**: absent airway protection reflexes, nonintact gastrointestinal tract, persistent vomiting, diarrhea 2. **Poison**: corrosives	Electrolyte disturbance, nausea, abdominal cramp	Significant amount of the toxicant can be absorbed before the process clears the gastric lumen from unabsorbed material

Manipulation of Urinary pH and Forced Diuresis

The basic principle of this approach is to change the pH of the urinary filtrate to a level sufficient to ionize the poison and prevent its tubular reabsorption back to plasma. Urinary alkalinization, such as by sodium bicarbonate, is commonly used to enhance the renal excretion of weakly acidic drugs, such as phenobarbital (PMS-Phenobarbital, from Canada) and acetyl salicylic acid (Aspir-low). Rare, but serious complications of this method include metabolic alkalosis, fluid overload, and hypernatremia. Acidification of urine, such as by ammonium chloride, is not commonly used to remove basic poisons, such as amphetamine (Adderall), because of the acute renal failure and electrolyte disturbances associated with acidification.

Multiple-Dose Activated Charcoal

Multiple-dose activated charcoal (MDAC) includes repetitive oral administration of activated charcoal and has been shown to increase the nonrenal clearance of various substances. Charcoal, through its binding to the poison in the gastrointestinal tract, maintains a concentration gradient such that the toxin passes continuously from the blood into the gut lumen, where it is adsorbed to charcoal.

Interruption of the enterohepatic circulation of drugs is another mechanism by which MDAC is thought to produce its beneficial effect. Agents for which MDAC has been shown to be an effective means of enhanced clearance include carbamazepine (Tegretol), dapson, digoxin (Lanoxin), phenobarbital, salicylates, theophylline (Theo-24), and agents that undergo enterohepatic circulation.

Dialysis

This technique removes toxic agents through a semipermeable dialysis membrane. Dialysis techniques are effective in removing drugs that are water soluble, have a low molecular weight (less than 500 daltons), have a small volume of distribution (less than 0.5 L/kg), and are not significantly bound to plasma proteins.

Hemodialysis is more efficient than peritoneal dialysis and has been well studied as a treatment for toxicity. Hemodialysis has been shown to be clinically effective in life-threatening poisoning of alcohols, lithium, metformin (Glucophage), paraldehyde, and theophylline. However, hemodialysis is not effective in managing poisoning of many other drugs, such as amphetamines, antidepressants, benzodiazepines, digoxin, and opioids.

Use of Antidotes

The effects of poisons can be prevented or attenuated by administration of specific antidotes. Appropriate use of antidotes, through correct identification of a specific poison, can significantly reduce mortality and morbidity rates. Available antidotes vary widely in their mechanism of action, as described here:

- *Physical binding of the toxin:* The antidote (e.g., the Fab fragment, which is specific to digoxin) binds physically to the toxin, facilitating its systemic clearance and/or preventing its harmful effects *in vivo.*

- *Pharmacologic antagonism of the toxin:* The antidote (e.g., atropine, which is specific to organophosphate insecticides) interferes with the pharmacologic effect of the toxin at the receptor level.

- *Biochemical antagonism of the toxin:* The antidote interacts chemically with the biological system to minimize the toxicity of the poison. For example, cyanide poisoning can be treated by administration of sodium nitrite, which induces formation of methemoglobin. The latter serves as an alternative binding site for cyanide, thereby increasing the body's detoxification capacity for cyanide.

Table 11.8 summarizes the clinical features and treatment of toxicity for selected substances.

Follow-Up and Prevention of Reexposure

Supportive care and close monitoring of the poisoned patient should continue until clinical and laboratory abnormalities have resolved. Management of poisoning should not rely solely on the blood levels of the poison, however—toxicity does not always correlate with blood level, especially if the metabolites are also responsible for toxicity.

Because poisoning is a preventable illness, prevention is an important part of toxicology. Examples of preventive approaches including the following measures:

- Patients and family members should be educated about the safe use of medication or chemicals based on the labeling instructions. Confused patients should be assisted with administration of their medications.

- Educate the public to notify the appropriate agencies or health departments in case of environmental or workplace exposure.

- Young children and patients at risk for intentional overdose should have a limited or no access to poisons.

- Alcoholic beverages, medications, household products (e.g., automotive, cleaning, fuel, pet-care, and toiletry products), and vitamins should be kept in locked or child-proof cabinets to prevent children from accessing them.

- Depressed and psychotic patients should receive psychiatric assessment, disposition, and follow-up. They should be given prescriptions for a limited supply of drugs and with a limited number of refills and be monitored for compliance and response to therapy.

Table 11.8 Clinical Features and Treatment of Specific Toxic Syndromes and Poisonings from Commonly Used Drugs and Industrial Solvents

Drug/Toxicant	Available Forms	Clinical Toxicity Features (Lab Findings)	Treatment
Acetaminophen	Example: Tylenol Tablets, syrup, drops	Nausea, vomiting, diaphoresis, abdominal pain, hepatic failure (High serum acetaminophen level)	GI decontamination: activated charcoal Antidote: *N*-acetyl-L-cysteine (Acetadote)
Benzodiazepines	Examples: diazepam (Valium), lorazepam (Ativan)	Drowsiness, ataxia, confusion	GI decontamination: activated charcoal, cathartic, gastric emptying Antidote: flumazenil (Romazicon)
β–Adrenergic blockers	Examples: propranolol (Inderal), atenolol (Tenormin)	Hypotension, bradycardia, bronchospasm (Blood glucose; hypoglycemia)	GI decontamination: activated charcoal, gastric lavage Antidote: glucagon
Calcium-channel blockers	Example: verapamil (Calan)	Hypotension, bradycardia, pulmonary edema	GI decontamination: activated charcoal, gastric lavage, whole-bowel irrigation Antidote: glucagon, calcium chloride
Cyanide	Industrial chemicals, nail-polish removers	Headache, dyspnea, ataxia, coma, seizures (High serum cyanide level)	Antidote: kit includes amyl nitrite inhalant, parenteral sodium thiosulfate, and sodium nitrite
Digoxin	Example: Lanoxin Parenteral and oral	Nausea, vomiting, confusion, cardiac dysrhythmias	GI decontamination: activated charcoal Antidote: digoxin-specific Fab antibody (Digibind)
Iron	Examples: Sulfate, fumarate, gluconate	Nausea, diarrhea, GI bleeding, hypotension, metabolic acidosis, hepatic and renal failure (Serum iron level)	GI decontamination: whole-bowel irrigation Antidote: deferoxamine (Desferal)
Lithium	Example: Eskalith Liquid, capsules, and tablets	Blurred vision, polyuria, ataxia, myoclonic jerks, hyperthermia, seizures (Serum level of lithium)	GI decontamination: whole-bowel irrigation, hemodialysis, sodium polystyrene sulfonate

(continues)

Table 11.8 Clinical Features and Treatment of Specific Toxic Syndromes and Poisonings from Commonly Used Drugs and Industrial Solvents (*continued*)

Drug/Toxicant	Available Forms	Clinical Toxicity Features (Lab Findings)	Treatment
Opiates	Examples: morphine, heroin, methadone Oral and parenteral preparations	Respiratory and CNS depression, hypoxia, constipation, hypotension, bradycardia, seizures	Antidote: naloxone
Organophosphates	Pesticides and nerve gas agents	Lacrimation, salivation, diaphoresis, abdominal cramps, tachycardia, paralysis	GI decontamination Antidote: atropine, parlidoxim (2-PAM, Protopam)
Salicylates	Examples: acetyl salicylic acid (aspirin), methyl salicylate	Nausea, vomiting, tinnitus, lethargy, metabolic acidosis, GI bleeding	GI decontamination: multiple-dose activated charcoal, whole-bowel irrigation Urinary alkalization Hemodialysis
Theophylline	Example: Aerolate	Nausea, vomiting, seizures, cardiac dysrhythmias	GI decontamination: multiple-dose activated charcoal, whole-bowel irrigation Hemodialysis Antidote: β–blockers (e.g., esmolol)

Learning Bridge 11.3

ME is a 43-year-old female who presents to the emergency department with a history of ingesting more than 20 acetaminophen 500 mg tablets 5 hours ago. On presentation, her chief complaint is nausea. The patient reports consuming more than 10 cans of beer daily, but denies using any other medications.

A. What is the maximum daily dose of acetaminophen?
B. What is the mechanism of acetaminophen hepatotoxicity?
C. Would whole-bowel irrigation be of any benefit in treating ME? Why?
D. What is the most appropriate measure to treat ME?
E. Which other factors increase the acetaminophen hepatotoxicity risk in ME?

Learning Bridge 11.4

An 18-year-old teenager is brought to the emergency department by ambulance with chief complaints of nausea, vomiting, and ringing in her ears. Upon examination, she is found to have a BP of 120/60 mm Hg, HR 120 beats/min, and temperature of 39.5°C. Analysis of her blood gases and electrolytes shows pH 7.45, pCO_2 19, and bicarb 13.

A. What is the drug or class of drugs most likely responsible for this patient's symptoms?
B. Explain the observed values of her blood gases and electrolytes profile.
C. What are the most appropriate measures to treat this patient?

Target Organ Toxicity

Although most toxic substances target more than one organ, some are known to primarily affect a specific target organ. Such organ target toxicity may be attributed to the characteristics of the toxic substance (e.g., its physical nature, site of exposure, dose, and duration of exposure) or the unique anatomic and functional characteristics of the organ. Labeling a toxicant as "organ specific," however, does not preclude injury to other organs in the body. For example, designation of a drug as "hepatotoxic" means that the liver is the primary organ affected by the drug, but other organs may also incur less notable injury. Additionally, liver-induced injury by this "hepatotoxic" drug will undoubtedly have serious consequences for other organs depending on the exposure level and the patient's defense mechanisms.

Table 11.9 lists the drugs most frequently implicated in target organ toxicity. If a particular drug of concern is not included in this list, it should not be assumed that the drug is incapable of inducing such organ toxicity. Whenever possible, the exact or proposed mechanism of drug-induced organ toxicity is presented in Table 11.9 as well.

Table 11.9 Selected Examples of Target Organ Toxicity

Organ	Toxicity	Common Causative Agents	Comments
Blood	Aplastic anemia	Azidothymidine (Retrovir), carbamazepine, carbon tetrachloride (CCl_4), cimetidine (Tagamet), chloramphenicol, furosemide (Lasix), gold salts, sulfonamides, linezolid (Zyvox), NSAIDs,[1] phenytoin (Dilantin), ticlopidine	Aplastic anemia occurs when the bone marrow fails to produce red blood cells (RBCs), white blood cells (WBCs), and platelets (pancytopenia). Drug-induced aplastic anemia may represent either a predictable or an idiosyncratic reaction to an agent.
	Hemolytic anemia	Carbamazepine, CS,[2] ciprofloxacin (Cipro), cimetidine, isoniazide, methyldopa (Apo-Methyldopa, from Canada), NSAIDs,[1] pipracillin/tazobactam, probenecid (Benuryl, in Canada), quinidine	Hemolytic anemia occurs when RBCs are prematurely destroyed. Hemolytic anemia is often immune mediated.
	Megaloblastic anemia	*Vitamin B_{12} deficiency:* antimetabolites, carbamazepine, colchicine, ethanol, malabsorption syndrome *Folate deficiency:* neomycin, phenytoin, primidone (Mysoline), sulfasalazine, azidothymidine	Megaloblastic anemia is produced by disorders of DNA synthesis, most commonly as a result of folic acid and vitamin B_{12} deficiencies.
	Methemoglobinemia	Amyl nitrate, dapson, lidocaine (Xylocaine), methylene blue, nitroglycerin (Nitro-Dur), primaquine, sulfonamide	Methemoglobinemia occurs when the erythrocytes' metabolic mechanisms reduce heme iron back to the ferrous state. High levels of methemoglobin lead to tissue hypoxemia that is eventually fatal.

(continues)

Table 11.9 Selected Examples of Target Organ Toxicity (*continued*)

Organ	Toxicity	Common Causative Agents	Comments
Immune system	Immunosuppression	Aflatoxin, AIDS therapeutics, cocaine, ethanol, immunosuppressive drugs (azathioprine, cyclosporine A, glucocorticoids, leflunomide, rapamycin), ultraviolet radiation	Suppression of the immune system increases the host's susceptibility to infections.
	Hypersensitivity	Penicillins, metal salts, latex (surgical gloves), formaldehyde, procaine, sulfonamides, infectious agents (e.g., poison ivy)	Hypersensitivity reactions result from an exaggerated or inappropriate immune response following exposure to a xenobiotic.
	Autoimmunity	Hydralazine, halothane, isoniazid, methyldopa, procainamide	Autoimmunity occurs when the mechanisms of self-recognition break down. Immunoglobulins and T-cell receptors react with self-antigens, resulting in tissue damage.
Liver	Bile duct damage	Amoxicillin, methylene dianiline	The liver is particularly susceptible to drug-induced toxicity, mainly because of its unique anatomic location and physiological role in drug metabolism and excretion. The liver has specialized mechanisms for drug uptake and biliary secretion. Therefore, most drugs have high exposure levels in the liver compared to any other organ. Additionally, the abundant capacity of drug-metabolizing enzymes, especially cytochrome P450, in the liver affects the rate of exposure to proximate highly reactive metabolites. All of these factors make the liver a target site for many chemicals of diverse structure.
	Hepatic tumors	Aflatoxin, androgens, arsenic, vinyl chloride	
	Hepatic fibrosis and cirrhosis	CCl_4, ethanol, thioacetamide, vitamin A, vinyl chloride	
	Canalicular cholestasis	Chlorpromazine, cyclosporine A, estrogen	
	Hepatocyte death	Acetaminophen, ethanol, dimethylformamide	
	Fatty liver	Amiodarone (Cordarone), CCl_4, ethanol, tamoxifen (Nolvadex, in Canada), valproic acid	
	Immune-mediated	Diclophenac, ethanol, halothane	
Kidney	**Acute kidney injury** Hemodynamic-mediated	Diuretics (e.g., furosemide and hydrochlorthiazide), ACEI,[3] ARB,[4] NSAIDs,[1] cyclosporine (Neoral)	The kidney is a highly susceptible organ to drug-induced toxicity for the following reasons:
	Tubular necrosis	Aminoglycosides (e.g., gentamicin), amphotericin B (AmBisome), cisplatin, ifosfamide	• The kidneys receive 20–25% of the resting cardiac output. Therefore, they receive relatively large amounts of circulating drugs and chemicals.
	Interstitial nephritis	Allopurinol (Zyloprim), β-lactam antibiotics, ciprofloxacin, diuretics (e.g., furosemide and hydrochlorothiazide), NSAIDs[1]	• The process of forming concentrated urine also concentrates toxicants in the tubular fluid.

Kidney	Glomerulone-phritis	Allopurinol, gold, lithium, NSAIDs,[1] penicillamine (Cuprimine), propylthiouracil	• Metabolism of chemicals by kidney enzymes may also generate bioactive and nephrotoxic metabolites.
	Nephroli-thiasis	Acyclovir (Zovirax), allopurinol, furosemide, topiramate (Topamax), sulfonamides, indinavir (Crixivan)	
	Chronic kidney disease (CKD)	Carmustine (BiCNU), cidofovir (Vistide), cisplatin, cyclosporine, gold, lithium, mitomycin (Mutamycin, from Canada), penicillamine, tacrolimus (Prograf)	CKD is the progressive deterioration of renal function. It usually occurs with long-term exposure to nephrotoxic agents, but sometimes derives from acute renal failure that does not respond to treatment.
Respiratory system	Pulmonary fibrosis and interstitial lung disease	Amiodarone, bleomycin (Blenoxane, in Canada), bromocriptine (Parlodel), busulfan, carmustine, cyclophosphamide (Procytox, from Canada), dothiepin, gemcitabine, ifosfamide, infliximab (Remicade), methotrexate, mitomycin C, nitrofurantoin, nitrosoureas, penicillamine, rituximab (Rituxan), tamoxifen	Different drugs may cause lung injury via different mechanisms. Contributed mechanisms include cytokine imbalance (e.g., bleomycin), inhibition of lysosomal phospholipase and breakdown of phospholipid-laden macrophages (e.g., amiodarone), oxidant imbalance (e.g., cyclophosphamide and nitrofurantoin), and antioxidant imbalance (e.g., carmustin and cyclophosphamide).
	Asthma and bronchospasm	Acetaminophen, ACEI,[3] aspirin, β-blockers, colistin, cyclophosphamide, dipyridamol, heroin, hydrocortisone, interleukin-2, NSAIDs,[1] pentamidine, sulfites, tobramycin, verapamil	Mechanisms of drug-induced asthma and bronchospasm include imbalance of pro-inflammatory and anti-inflammatory eicosanoids (e.g., acetaminophen, aspirin, and NSAIDs), increased concentration of bradykinin (ACEI), increased plasma adenosine concentrations (dipyridamol), β-blockade (e.g., β-blockers, amiodarone, and propafenone), anaphylaxis (e.g., sulfites), and airway irritation (e.g., tobramycin).
Nervous system	Seizures	Bupropion (Wellbutrin SR), maprotiline, TCAs[8] Carbpenems, penicillins Isoniazid, theophylline Clozapine (Clozaril), phenothiazines Meperidine (Demerol) Cyclosporine	Proposed mechanisms are: • Increased noradrenergic activity • GABA[9] antagonists • Disturbance of pyridoxine metabolism • Dopamine antagonists • Metabolism to an excitatory metabolite • Direct neurotoxicity • Hypofunction of the dopaminergic mesocortical pathway, secondary to stimulation of the serotonin type 2 receptors. • Blockade of dopamine receptors in the mesocortical pathway • Blockade of striatal dopamine receptors • Depletion of neuronal dopamine • Decreased acetylcholine function • Increased dopamine function • GABA[9] antagonists • Decreased serotonin function
	Akathisia	SSRIs,[10] TCAs[8] Amoxapine, conventional neuroleptics[11]	
	Parkinsonism	Amoxapine, conventional neuroleptics[11] Methyldopa, reserpine	
	Delirium	TCAs,[8] clozapine, doxepin (Silenor), quetiapine (Seroquel)	

(continues)

Table 11.9 Selected Examples of Target Organ Toxicity (*continued*)

Organ	Toxicity	Common Causative Agents	Comments
Nervous system	Anxiety	Amantadine (Symmetrel, from Canada), levodopa (Sinemet), bromocriptine Benzodiazepines (e.g., diazepam) SSRIs[10] Amphetamine, methylphenidate (Ritalin), bupropion Caffeine, theophylline	• Inhibition of norepinephrine and dopamine reuptake • Inhibition of phosphodiesterase enzyme, resulting in excessive neurotransmitter activity • Antagonism at the α_2-adrenergic receptors resulting in increased outflow of norepinephrine from the CNS • Increased outflow of norepinephrine from the CNS and decreased GABA[9] activity • Increased dopamine concentrations • Antagonism of the NMDA[12] receptors • Increased dopamine and norepinephrine concentrations
	Psychosis	Yohimbine Benzodiazepines withdrawal Dopamine agonists (e.g., L-dopa) Ketamine, phencyclidine (PCP) Amphetamine, bupropion, cyclobenzaprine, pseudoephedrine	
Cardiovascular system	Myocardial ischemia and acute coronary syndrome	Cocaine, β-agonists, sympathomimetic agents, potent vasodilators Cocaine, triptans such as sumatriptan (Imitrex), ergot alkaloids (e.g., ergotamine), enalapril (Vasotec), nifedipine (Adalat), nitroprusside, dipyridamol (Persantine) Oral contraceptives, estrogens, NSAIDs[1]	Mechanisms include: • Increased myocardial oxygen demand due to increased heart rate, increased myocardial contractility, and increased left ventricular systolic wall tension • Decreased myocardial oxygen supply due to increased coronary vascular resistance, decreased oxygen-carrying capacity, and decreased coronary diastolic perfusion pressure • Coronary artery thrombosis.
	Heart failure	Cylcophosphamide Doxorubicin (Adriamycin) CCB[5], β-blockers, antiarrhythmic agents (e.g., propafenone, ecainide) NSAIDs,[1] pioglitazone (Actos), rosiglitazone, sodium-containing drugs	• Endothelial damage, formation of toxic metabolite • Generation of a toxic metabolite and oxygen radicals • Negative inotropic effect (i.e., decreased myocardial contractility) • Fluid retention and increased preload • Stimulation of sympathetic nervous system • Stimulation of mineralocorticoid receptors and fluid retention
	Hypertension	Amphetamines, cocaine, pseudoephedrine, MAOIs,[6] testosterone Corticosteroids, licorice NSAIDs[1] Calcineurin inhibitors (e.g., cyclosporine, tacrolimus), erythropoietin-alpha (Epogen)	• Inhibition of prostaglandins and increased fluid volume expansion • Increased fluid volume due to decreased sodium, water, and potassium excretion or stimulation of erythropoiesis • Inhibition of angiotensin II • Blockade of β-adrenergic receptors
	Hypotension	ACEI[3], ARB[4] β-blockers (e.g., atenolol, betaxolol, labetalol, propranolol, nadolol)	• Intravascular volume depletion • Blockade of calcium channels • Reduction of peripheral vascular resistance due to stimulation of central α-receptors

Cardio-vascular system		Diuretics (e.g., amiloride, furosemide, hydrochlorothiazide, mannitol) CCB[5] (e.g., amlodipine, nifedipine) Clonidine, methyldopa, guanabenz Antidepressant agents (e.g., amitriptyline, doxepin, trazodone) Amyl nitrate, nitroglycerin Dopaminergic drugs and dopamine agonists (e.g., levodopa, pergolide, pramipexole, ropinirole, selegiline)	• Reduction of systemic vascular resistance due to blockade of α-adrenoreceptors • Increase intracellular cyclic guanosine monophosphate concentrations • Dopamine leads to hypotension due to vasodilation, displacement of norepinephrine from nerve terminals, decreased and aldosterone renin secretion, and reduced sympathetic outflow • Inhibition of automaticity of sinus node • Reduced release of norepinephrine • Shortened atrial refractory period • Stimulation of sympathetic nervous system • Increased atrial automaticity
	Cardiac arrhythmias		• Inhibition of the Na^+/K^+-ATPase pump and increased intracellular Ca^{2+} concentration • Inhibition of Na^+ channel conductance • Inhibition of phosphodiesterase and increased intracellular Ca^{2+} concentration • Prolongation of ventricular repolarization and lengthening of action potential duration due to decreases in outward current or increases of inward current during plateau or repolarization phase of the action potential
	• Sinus bradycardia	Adrenergic β-blockers, neostigmine, physostigmine, pyridostigmine Clonidine	
	• Atrial fibrillation/flutter	Adenosine, dobutamine, flecainide Ethanol Theophylline	
	• Ventricular tachycardia	Digoxin Amiodarone, procainamide, propafenone (Rythmol) Theophylline	
	• Torsades de pointes	Amiodarone, cisapride, dofetilide, erythromycin, ibutilide, pentamidine (Pentam), sotalol (Betapace AF)	
Skin	SLE[7]-like syndrome	Chlorpromazine (Largactil, from Canada), disopyramide (Norpace), hydralazine, procainamide (Apo-Procainamide, in Canada), D-penicillamine, minoxidil (Loniten, in Canada), etanercept (Enbrel)	Exact mechanisms of drug-induced lupus are unknown. Proposed mechanisms are nucleic acid alterations, immunoregulatory alterations, interference in the complement pathway, generation of reactive metabolites, and genetic predisposition. Free-radical formation upon exposure to ultraviolet light, alteration in DNA synthesis, and increased melanin production.
	Photosensitivity	Amiodarone, fluoroquinolones (e.g., ciprofloxacin), NSAIDs,[1] furosemide, doxycycline, olanzapine, tetracycline, trimethoprim, sulfonamides	• Common mechanisms are androgenic stimulation of hair follicles and hyperinsulinemia. • Hypertrichosis usually becomes apparent after a few weeks/months of drug therapy.
	Hirsutism	Cyclosporine, nandrolone, progesterone, testosterone, testolactone, valproic acid	• The most common mechanism is the premature termination of the hair cycle resulting in an increased number of hair follicles shed. Another mechanism is through increasing androgen activity (androgenic alopecia)
	Hypertrichosis	Cyclosporine, minoxidil, phenytoin, prostaglandin analogs (e.g., travoprost, latanoprost), phenothiazines	

(continues)

Table 11.9 Selected Examples of Target Organ Toxicity (*continued*)

Organ	Toxicity	Common Causative Agents	Comments
Skin	Alopecia	Cancer chemotherapy agents (e.g., bleomycin, cyclophosphamide, doxorubicin, ifosfamide, paclitaxel, topotecan); other drugs including anabolic steroids, anticonvulsants, and dopamine agonists	
Endo-crine system	**Glucose and insulin dys-regulation** Hyperglyce-mia	Atypical antipsychotics, cyclosporine, didanosine, diuretics, glucocorticoids, growth hormone, niacin, oral contraceptives, pentamidine, phenytoin, protease inhibitors	Agents alter glucose regulation through different mechanisms, including alteration of insulin secretion or clearance, direct or indirect change in insulin sensitivity, alteration in glucose metabolism, and direct effect on pancreatic β cells. Major causes of drug-induced thyroid disorders include alteration in synthesis, transport, secretion, metabolism, or function of thyroid hormones; changes in synthesis or release of thyroid-stimulating hormone (TSH) from the pituitary gland; or disruption of thyroid-releasing hormone (TRH) from the hypothalamus.
	Hypoglyce-mia	ACEIs, ethanol, fluoroquinolones, insulin, quinidine, salicylates, sulfonamides, sulfonylureas	
	Thyroid disorders Hyperthy-roidism	Amiodarone, cyclosporine, interferon-α and -β, iodinated compounds, lithium	
	Hypothyroid-ism	Amiodarone, carbamazepine, imatinip, interferon-α and -β, iodinated compounds, lithium, paroxetine, phenytoin, rifampin, thalidomide, quetiapine	

Notes:

1. Nonsteroidal anti-inflammatory drugs (e.g., ibuprofen).
2. Cephalosporins (e.g., cafazolin).
3. Angiotensin-converting enzyme inhibitors (e.g., benzapril, captopril, ramipril).
4. Angiotensin receptor blockers (e.g., candesartan, losartan, valsartan).
5. Calcium-channel blockers (e.g., diltiazem, nifedipine, verapamil).
6. Monoamine oxidase inhibitors (e.g., phenelzine).
7. Systemic lupus erythematosus.
8. Tricyclic antidepressants (e.g., amitriptyline).
9. Gamma-aminobutyric acid.
10. Selective serotonin reuptake inhibitors (e.g., fluoxetine).
11. Examples: olanzapine, risperidone, chlorpromazine, haloperidol, thioridazine, perphenazine.
12. N-methyl-d-aspartic acid.

Learning Bridge 11.5

XYZ is a 40-year-old man who was rushed to the emergency department by his wife. Upon examination, he was revealed to have symptoms of dizziness, lightheadedness, and cyanosis. His wife reported that these symptoms appeared almost immediately after he ate lunch. The patient's oxygen saturation level by pulse oximetry is 72% (normal: > 92%). Blood drawn for routine testing is described as "black colored." Methemoglobin level is 35% (normal: 1–3%).

A. Which poison is most likely responsible for XYZ's symptoms?
B. What is the empiric therapy of choice to treat XYZ's condition?
C. If the antidote you mentioned in question B is provided as a 1% solution and the dose is 2 mg/kg infused intravenously over 5 minutes, how many milliliters is required for a 60-kg patient?

Golden Keys for Pharmacy Students

- Toxicology is concerned with studying the relationship between exposure level (dose) and its deleterious effects on the living organism, examining the nature of these effects, and predicting the probability of their occurrence.

- Dose–response curves can be used to derive dose estimates that may indicate safety, effectiveness, or toxicity of the substance under investigation.

- Generally, a drug with a higher therapeutic index (i.e., having a large difference between toxic and therapeutic doses) is preferred over a drug with a lower therapeutic index.

- Several factors appear to predispose an individual patient to drug toxicity. In most cases, these factors are associated with altering the pharmacokinetic or pharmacodynamic characteristics of the drug.

- General goals for treatment of poisoned patients should include clinical stabilization, prevention of further absorption of the poison, enhancement of poison elimination, administration of antidote, clinical follow-up, and prevention of reexposure.

- Although most toxic substances target more than one organ, some are known to primarily affect a specific target organ.

Learning Bridge Answers

11.1 The correct answer is B. As can be seen on the graph, 50% of the lethality response is approximately achieved at a dose of 17 mg/kg.

11.2

Exhibit 11.2 Interactions Between Drugs A and B

Patient Name	Drug A	Drug B	Result of Simultaneous Administration
MR	**Itraconazole** A potent inhibitor for CYP3A4	**Midazolam** It has a low bioavailability due to the substantial first-pass metabolism by CYP3A4 in the intestinal epithelium.	Itraconazole increases the area under the midazolam concentration–time curve 10–15 times and the mean peak concentrations 3–4 times. The end result is an increase in the hypnotic effect of midazolam.
PJ	**Nonsteroidal anti-inflammatory drugs** Competes with and displaces drugs from plasma protein-binding sites	**Warfarin** 98–99% plasma protein binding	Displacement of warfarin from its plasma protein-binding sites increases its free fraction and, therefore, increases the risk for gastrointestinal bleeding and the anticoagulant response of warfarin. Acetaminophen is the alternative of choice.
SK	**Probenecid** Acts as an active tubular secretion inhibitor	**Methotrexate** Excreted by active secretion by the kidneys	Reduction of methotrexate excretion by probenecid results in a 2- to 3-fold increase in methotrexate levels and may potentially cause toxicity. Symptoms of severe methotrexate toxicity include diarrhea, vomiting, diaphoresis, and renal failure, and this condition may result in death.
AR	**Ciprofloxacin** A potent inhibitor of CYP1A2	**Theophylline** Extensively metabolized by CYP1A2 and to a lesser extent by CYP3A4	Inhibition of the CYP-mediated elimination of theophylline results in increased theophylline levels and risk of toxicity. Signs of theophylline toxicity include headache, dizziness, hypotension, hallucinations, tachycardia, and seizures. (Levofloxacin or ofloxacin should be considered as an alternative to ciprofloxacin, as these medications have little effect on CYP1A2.)

11.3 A. The maximum daily dose of acetaminophen in an adult is 4,000 mg.

B. Toxicity of acetaminophen is due to production of its reactive metabolite, *N*-acetyl-*p*-benzoquinone imine (NAPQI) by the hepatic CYP2E1 enzyme. Excessive production of this electrophilic metabolite causes depletion of glutathione stores and binding of NAPQI to hepatocytes, leading to liver injury.

C. Whole-bowel irrigation would not have a high benefit-to-risk ratio 5 hours after acute acetaminophen toxicity, as a significant amount of the drug could be absorbed before the process clears unabsorbed material from the gastric lumen.

D. The most appropriate measure to treat ME is immediate initiation of antidotal therapy with *N*-acetylcysteine (NAC, Acetadote) to immediately restore glutathione stores.

E. Alcoholism increases the risk of hepatic injury from acetaminophen because alcohol is a potent inducer of CYP2E1.

11.4 A. The observed signs and symptoms, along with arterial blood gases, indicate acute poisoning from aspirin or salicylates. Patients with mild salicylate poisoning frequently have GI upset, nausea, vomiting, lethargy, ringing ears (tinnitus), and dizziness. Severe poisonings may result in more significant symptoms, such as hyperthermia, tachypnea, respiratory alkalosis, metabolic acidosis, hypokalemia, hypoglycemia, hallucinations, confusion, seizure, cerebral edema, and coma.

B. Blood gases and electrolyte results indicate respiratory alkalosis with a compensatory metabolic acidosis. Respiratory alkalosis develops from a direct stimulatory effect of aspirin (salicylate) on the medullary respiratory center. Metabolic acidosis can result from either compensatory mechanisms or accumulation of aspirin itself (an anion gap metabolic acidosis; these topics are explained in more detail in the *Introduction to Nutrients* chapter).

C. Management of salicylates poisoning include the following:

- *Supportive care*:
    - Fluid and electrolyte management to rehydrate the patient: Intravenous fluids containing dextrose such as D_5W are recommended to keep a urinary output in the range of 2–3 mL/kg/hr.
    - Hyperthermia: Sponge bath, fans, water submersion.

- *GI decontamination*: Repeated doses of charcoal have been proposed to be beneficial in case of aspirin overdose (induction of vomiting by using syrup of ipecac is not recommended).

- *Enhancement of elimination*: Urine alkalization through administration of sodium bicarbonate can enhance elimination of aspirin in the urine. Sodium bicarbonate is given until a urine pH between 7.5 and 8.0 is achieved.

11.5 A. These symptoms of methemoglobinemia may be due to overdose of sodium nitrite present in the meal as a food additive. Sodium nitrite may be added to certain foods to reduce microbial growth, reduce rancidity, and give taste and color to meat.

B. Methylene blue, by acting as a cofactor to increase the activity of NADPH-methemoglobin reductase, is an effective antidote for most patients with methemoglobinemia.

C. Methylene blue is provided as a 1% solution (i.e., 10 mg/mL). (The dose is 2 mg/kg, or 0.2 mL/kg of a 1% solution.) If the patient weighs 60 kg, the dose will be 12 mL infused intravenously over 5 minutes.

Problems and Solutions

Problem 11.1 Standard deviation is usually employed to indicate variability of response. In a dose–response relationship, one standard deviation represents _____ of the responses.

- **A.** 25%
- **B.** 45%
- **C.** 68%
- **D.** 95%

Solution 11.1 C is correct. Approximately 68% of the population lies within one SD of the mean; 95% of the population lies within two SD of the mean; 99.7% of the population lies within three SD of the mean.

Problem 11.2 Which of the following toxin antidote combinations is not correct?

   A. Morphine and naloxone

   B. Digoxin and calcium

   C. Propranolol and glucagon

   D. Iron and deferoxamine

Solution 11.2 B is correct. Digibind, the digoxin-specific Fab antibody fragment, is the specific antidote against digoxin overdose. Calcium chloride is frequently given to treat poisoning from calcium-channel blockers.

Problem 11.3 LD_{50} represents:

   A. The estimated dose that causes death in 50% of experimental animals.

   B. The estimated dose that causes toxicity in 50% of experimental animals.

   C. The estimated dose that causes a 50% reduction in liver functions.

   D. The effect resulting from administration of a 50-mg dose of a drug.

Solution 11.3 A is correct.

Problem 11.4 Which of the following is (are) component(s) of the "coma cocktail" that may be administered in an emergency to comatose individuals when the cause of the coma is not yet known?

   A. Dextrose

   B. Naloxone

   C. Thiamine

   D. All of the above

Solution 11.4 D is correct.

Problem 11.5 Which of the following might be used as an antidote for patients with Valium poisoning?

   A. Glucagon

   B. Flumazenil

   C. Digibind

   D. Deferoxamine

Solution 11.5 B is correct. Flumazenil is the specific antidote for benzodiazepine poisoning. Glucagon, Digibind, and deferoamine (Desferal) are specific antidotes for poisoning from β-blockers, digoxin (Lanoxin), and iron, respectively.

Problem 11.6 Which of the following medications can induce glomerulonephritis?

   A. Allopurinol

   B. Naproxen

   C. Penicillamine

   D. Gold salts

   E. All of the above

Solution 11.6 E is correct.

Problem 11.7 Which of the following statements is incorrect?

   A. Tetracycline increases the risk of toxicity from digoxin due to inactivation of gut flora.

   B. Ibuprofen increases the risk of toxicity from warfarin due to inhibition of CYP3A4, the major enzyme responsible for metabolism of warfarin.

   C. Hydrochlorothiazide increases the risk of toxicity from digoxin due to potassium depletion.

   D. Aspirin increases the risk of toxicity from methotrexate due to competition for the same transporter protein.

Solution 11.7 B is correct. Ibuprofen increases the risk of bleeding from warfarin because it displaces warfarin (approximately 99% plasma protein bound) from protein-binding sites and increases the unbound drug concentration. This is a common example of a drug–drug interaction that may influence the likelihood of drug toxicity.

Problem 11.8 True or false? A low serum poison level always indicates that toxicity is resolving.

Solution 11.8 False. Some drugs are formulated in such a way as to provide delayed or continuous absorption from the gastrointestinal tract. Therefore, lower serum levels do not always indicate resolving toxicity.

Problem 11.9 Which of the following statements is true regarding gastric decontamination of oral drug tablets taken as an overdose 2 hours prior to seeking assistance?

   A. Ipecac syrup should be administered at the scene regardless of the circumstances.

   B. Gastric lavage should be initiated immediately because studies have demonstrated that it leads to superior recovery of tablet material.

   C. Activated charcoal should be considered if contraindications are not present.

   D. Whole-bowel irrigation is all that should be utilized.

Solution 11.9 C is correct. Charcoal, through its binding to the poison in the gastrointestinal tract, prevents absorption and maintains a concentration gradient. The toxin passes continuously from the blood into the gut lumen, where it is adsorbed to charcoal.

Problem 11.10 Which of the following physiological facts make the kidney highly susceptible to drug-induced toxicity?

   A. The kidneys receive 20–25% of the resting cardiac output.

   B. The process of forming concentrated urine concentrates toxicants in the tubular fluid.

   C. Metabolism of chemicals by kidney enzymes may generate bioactive and nephrotoxic metabolites.

   D. All of the above.

Solution 11.10 D is correct.

Problem 11.11 The dose that causes toxic effects in 10% of the population is called:

   A. LD_{10}.

   B. LD_{90}.

   C. TD_{10}.

   D. TD_{90}.

Solution 11.11 C is correct. TD_{10} is the dose that causes toxic effects in 10% of the population.

References

1. Bauer LA, ed. *Applied clinical pharmacokinetics*, 2nd ed. New York, NY: McGraw-Hill; 2008.
2. Zastrow M. Drug receptors and pharmacodynamics. In: Katzung BG, Masters SB, Trevor AJ, eds. *Basic & clinical pharmacology*, 11th ed. New York, NY: McGraw-Hill; 2012. 15–36.
3. Chyka PA. Clinical toxicology. In: DiPiro JT, Talbert RL, Yee GT, et al., eds. *Pharmacotherapy: a pathophysiologic approach*, 8th ed. New York, NY: McGraw-Hill; 2011. 27–50.

4. Cohen MR. *Medication errors.* Washington, DC: American Pharmacist Association; 2010.

5. Eaton DL, Gilbert SG. Principles of toxicology. In: *Casarett & Doull's essentials of toxicology,* 2nd ed. New York, NY: McGraw-Hill; 2010. 5–20.

6. Gallo MA. History and scope of toxicology. In: *Casarett & Doull's essentials of toxicology,* 2nd ed. New York, NY: McGraw-Hill; 2010. 1–3.

7. Hajjar ER, Gray SL, Guay DR, et al. Geriatrics. In: DiPiro JT, Talbert RL, Yee GT, et al., eds. *Pharmacotherapy: a pathophysiologic approach,* 8th ed. New York, NY: McGraw-Hill; 2011. 173–189.

8. McCain KR, Foster HR. Clinical toxicology. In: McCain KR, Foster HR, eds. *McGraw-Hill's NAPLEX® Review Guide.* New York, NY: McGraw-Hill; 2011. 590–602.

9. Olson KR. Management of the poisoned patient. In: Katzung BG, Masters SB, Trevor AJ, eds. *Basic & clinical pharmacology,* 11th ed. New York, NY: McGraw-Hill; 2012. 1027–1038.

10. Osterhoudt KC, Penning TM. Drug toxicity and poisoning. In: Osterhoudt KC, Penning TM, eds. *Goodman & Gilman's the pharmacological basis of therapeutics,* 12th ed. New York, NY: McGraw-Hill; 2011. 73–88.

11. Shargel L, Wu-Pong S, Yu AB. Pharmacogenetics. In Shargel L, Wu-Pong S, Yu AB, eds. *Applied biopharmaceutics & pharmacokinetics,* 5th ed. New York, NY: McGraw-Hill; 2005. 301–320.

12. Teitelbaum DT. Introduction to toxicology: occupational and environmental. In: Katzung BG, Masters SB, Trevor AJ, eds. *Basic & clinical pharmacology,* 11th ed. New York, NY: McGraw-Hill; 2012. 1001–1012.

13. Tisdale JE, Miller DA. In: Tisdale JE, Miller DA, eds. *Drug-induced diseases: prevention, detection, and management,* 2nd ed. Bethesda, MD: ASHP; 2010.

14. UpToDate. Waltham, MA: 2012. Available at: http://www.uptodate.com/online with subscription.

Introduction to Pharmacogenomics

Sigrid C. Roberts

Sigrid C. Roberts

OBJECTIVES

1. Define *pharmacogenomics* and *pharmacogenetics*.

2. Describe polymorphism and genetic variation.

3. Define *genotype* and *phenotype*.

4. Explain the terms *heterozygous*, *homozygous*, *diploid*, and *alleles*.

5. Describe the common types of genetic variation: single-nucleotide polymorphism (SNP), indels, and copy number variations.

6. Comprehend how SNPs lead to restriction fragment length polymorphism (RFLP).

7. Define *haplotype*.

8. Recognize the nomenclature for genes.

9. Explain how genetic variation can influence the pharmacokinetic and pharmacodynamic properties of a drug.

10. Understand the concept of nonresponders and toxic response.

11. Summarize how enzymes affect drug metabolism; in this context, explain how variations in CYP enzymes lead to poor metabolism (PM), extensive metabolism (EM), intermediate metabolism (IM), and ultrarapid metabolism (UM).

12. Outline how variations in P-glycoprotein have an effect on drug import and export.

13. Comprehend how genetic variations influence the response to the following treatments: warfarin, clopidogrel, thiopurines, trastuzumab, cetuximab, and irinotecan.

14. Summarize the current and future impact of pharmacogenomics on drug treatment options.

15. Discuss the ethical considerations for pharmacogenomics.

16. Implement a series of Learning Bridge assignments at your experiential sites to bridge your didactic learning with your experiential experiences.

1. **Alleles:** the form or sequence of a gene. One particular gene can have several slightly different sequences (alleles).

2. **Copy number variations:** differences in the number of gene copies. This could be due to a gene deletion or a gene amplification (resulting in more than one gene copy).

3. **Cytochrome P450 monooxygenases (CYP):** a family of enzymes that catalyzes the metabolism (activation or inactivation) of approximately 80% of drugs.

4. **Diploid:** the presence of two sets of chromosomes—one of paternal origin and one of maternal origin.

5. **Drug metabolism:** activation or inactivation of a drug by enzymes of the body.

6. **Enhancer:** a regulatory DNA sequence that can be located near any of several thousand base pairs upstream or downstream of a gene. Transcription factors binding to enhancers usually increase transcription rates.

7. **Exon:** expressed region; a coding region that will remain in the mature mRNA after splicing.

8. **Genetic variations:** DNA sequence differences that occur normally within a species.

9. **Genome:** the entire genetic information of an organism.

10. **Genotype:** the genetic makeup of an organism or population.

11. **Haploid:** the presence of only one set of chromosomes.

12. **Heterozygous:** a diploid individual (two sets of chromosomes) is heterozygous for a gene if the two alleles have slightly different sequences.

13. **Homozygous:** a diploid individual (two sets of chromosomes) is homozygous for a gene if both alleles have the identical sequence.

14. **Indels**: insertion or deletion of one or more nucleotides.

15. **Intron:** intragenic region; a noncoding region that will be removed from the pre-mRNA by splicing.

16. **Mutation:** introduction of a change in the DNA sequence that is not part of the normal variations.

17. **Nonsense mutation:** a mutation that introduces a stop codon.

18. **Nonsynonymous or missense mutation:** a nucleotide substitution that changes the encoded amino acid.

19. **P-glycoprotein (P-gp):** transmembrane pump. This energy-dependent transporter is responsible for the majority of decreased drug uptake or increased drug efflux.

20. **Pharmacodynamics:** the study of how a drug affects the body, or the mechanism of action of a drug.

21. **Pharmacogenomics/pharmacogenetics:** the study of how genetic variations affect the drug response. Pharmacogenetics investigates how genetic variations in one or a few genes influence the response to a drug, whereas pharmacogenomics takes the entire genome into account. However, both terms are often used interchangeably.

22. **Pharmacokinetics:** the study of how the body affects a drug, or how a drug is absorbed, distributed, localized, and metabolized by the body.

23. **Phenotype:** the observable manifestation of the genotype (influencing physiology, metabolism, forms, and other characteristics).

24. **Polymorphism:** the occurrence of different forms and types in individuals (Greek origin: having multiple forms). Genetic polymorphism refers to genetic variations or differences in the DNA sequence.

25. **Promoter:** a regulatory DNA sequence located upstream of a gene where transcription factors and DNA polymerase bind and initiate transcription. Transcription factors binding to the promoter region can up- or down-regulate transcription levels.

(CONTINUED)

26. **Restriction enzyme endonucleases**: enzymes that recognize specific DNA sequences and endonucleolytically cleave the DNA at that site.

27. **Restriction fragment length polymorphism (RFLP)**: the generation of DNA fragments of different lengths when a restriction enzyme recognizes and cuts a specific sequence that is present in one DNA sample but not in another DNA sample. The sequence difference in these specific sites can be due to single-nucleotide polymorphisms.

28. **Single-nucleotide polymorphism (SNP)**: a difference in an individual nucleotide (or base pair).

29. **Synonymous mutation**: a nucleotide substitution that does *not* change the encoded amino acid (silent mutation).

30. **Wild type**: a DNA sequence that is shared by the majority of the population.

Introduction

It is well known that patients respond differently to drugs, and that sometimes these variations can be substantial and devastating. Some patients may experience toxicity from a drug or drug dose that is safe for others, while other patients may not respond to therapeutic treatment at all. These discrepancies can be due to gender, age, general health, or other medications used—but genetic variations in the population are also among the most important causes. Although the genome of humans is 99.9% identical across the population, the small percentage of differences represents approximately 1 million nucleotides (a considerable amount). Pharmacogenomics and pharmacogenetics investigate these variations, including how they correlate to the potential outcome of drug treatment. In other words, these fields study how the genetic inheritance of an individual affects the body's response to a drug. While pharmacogenetics investigates genetic variations in specific genes of interest, pharmacogenomics looks at the entire genome of a patient. However, the two terms are often used interchangeably. In this chapter, we review the genetic principles that underlie pharmacogenomics, discuss the impact of genetic variations on pharmacokinetic and pharmacodynamic properties of drugs, examine clinical examples, and provide a brief overview of ethical considerations and the impact of pharmacogenomics today and in the future.

Genetic Principles of Pharmacogenomics

Naturally occurring **variations** within our DNA result in polymorphism, whereby individuals within a population can have different physical or biochemical characteristics. By definition, these naturally occurring variations must be found in at least 1% of the population; otherwise, they would be considered "mutations." (The terms "mutation" and "variation" are often used interchangeably despite this distinction.) Changes in the DNA sequence determine the genotype. How this variation is displayed in observable changes in an organism is called the phenotype. Such differences can appear in metabolism or morphology, enzyme activity, growth phenotype, transporter activity, drug response, and so on. The differences in drug response that are due to genetic variations form the basis of pharmacogenomics.

DNA changes that affect the phenotype can occur in the coding region of a gene as well as other regulatory sequences. The efficacy of transcription is determined by regulatory DNA sequences such as promoters and enhancers. Changes in splice acceptor sites can alter the usage of exons and introns. Translational efficiency and mRNA stability can be influenced by changes in the sequence

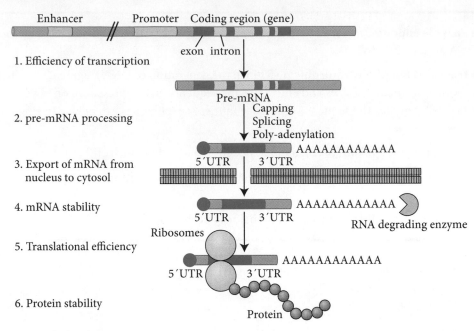

Figure 12.1 Regulation of gene expression.

of the 5′ and 3′ untranslated regions (flanking the coding region) of the mRNA. Fundamentally, genetic variations can influence gene expression if they modify processes such as transcriptional efficacy, mRNA maturation, export and degradation, translational efficiency, post-translational modifications, and protein stability (**Figure 12.1**).

Humans are diploid, which means that they have two sets of chromosomes. The paternal chromosomes are inherited from the father and the maternal chromosomes are inherited from the mother. Thus each individual has at least two copies of each gene. A gene can have several slightly different sequences, or alleles. If both gene copies have an identical sequence, the individual is homozygous for that particular gene; an individual is heterozygous if the two alleles have slightly different sequences (**Figure 12.2**). The sequence shared by the majority of individuals within a population is considered to be the wild type allele. Variants are alleles that contain slightly different sequences. These variants can be either very common among the population (just not as common as the wild type allele) or rare (but at least 1%).

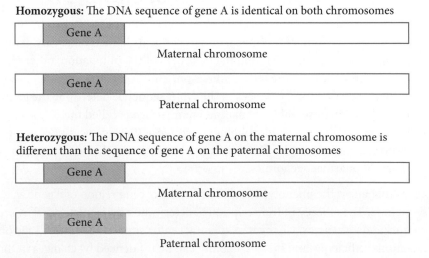

Figure 12.2 Homozygous and heterozygous alleles.

Wild type sequence

5'ATG CTT CAT CGT CGT TGC ACT AGT CAT GGT...
Met Leu His Arg Arg Cys Thr Ser His Gly...

Synonymous (silent) change
The amino acid sequence remains the same

5'ATG CTC CAT CGT CGT TGC ACT AGT CAT GGT...
Met Leu His Arg Arg Cys Thr Ser His Gly...

Nonsynonymous (missense) change
The amino acid sequence is different

5'ATG CTT CAA CGT CGT TGC ACT AGT CAT GGT...
Met Leu Gln Arg Arg Cys Thr Ser His Gly...

Nonsense change
The amino acid sequence is truncated

5'ATG CTT CAT CGT CGT TGA ACT AGT CAT GGT...
Met Leu His Arg Arg   STOP

Figure 12.3 Single-nucleotide polymorphisms.

There are three common types of genetic variations:

- Single-nucleotide polymorphisms (SNPs)
- Indels
- Gene copy number variations

Single-Nucleotide Polymorphism

A single-nucleotide polymorphism is just what the name indicates: a difference in a single nucleotide (**Figure 12.3**). These variations can occur in the coding region of a gene or in a regulatory sequence. If the single nucleotide difference occurs in the coding region, it may not necessarily translate into a different amino acid; this would be called a synonymous change (silent mutation). If the modification results in an amino acid exchange, it is called a nonsynonymous change or missense mutation. The consequence for protein function can be minimal if conservative substitutions occur or if the replacement is in a region of the protein that does not disturb its activity. Conversely, a single amino acid modification can be quite dramatic if the substrate binding or active site or the overall structure of a protein is altered. Sometimes, a variation in a single nucleotide can create a stop codon. Such a nonsense mutation will produce a truncated protein that may have little or no enzymatic activity.

Indels

An indel is defined as the insertion or deletion of one or more nucleotides (**Figure 12.4**). The addition or loss of three nucleotides will not change the reading frame because a codon consists of three nucleotides or bases. If one or two nucleotides are integrated or removed, however, the reading frame will shift. As a consequence, the remainder of the encoded protein will contain different amino acids. If such an insertion or deletion occurs early in the protein-coding sequence, the effect will be devastating and render the protein nonfunctional.

Wild type sequence

5'ATG CTT CAT CGT CGT TGC ACT
Met   Leu His Arg Arg Cys Thr

Indel: Insertion of a nucleotide

5'ATG CTT CCA TCG TCG TTG CAC T
Met   Leu Pro Ser Ser Leu His

Indel: Deletion of a nucleotide

5'ATG CTT ATC GTC GTT GCA CT
Met   Leu Ile Val Val Ala

Indel: Insertion of three nucleotides

5'ATG CTT CAT ACT CGT CGT TGC ACT
Met   Leu His Thr Arg Arg Cys Thr

Figure 12.4 Indels: Insertions or deletion of nucleotides.

A simple exercise to visualize this effect is to introduce a deletion or insertion into the following code:

Wild type: *THE CAT ATE THE RAT*

Insertion: *THE XCA TAT ETH ERA T…*

Deletion: *THE ATA TET HER AT…*

SNPs or indels can lead to differences in restriction enzyme recognition sites (**Figure 12.5**). Restriction enzymes, or restriction endonucleases, are enzymes that recognize very specific DNA sequences and endonucleolytically cut the DNA at this site. For example, the restriction

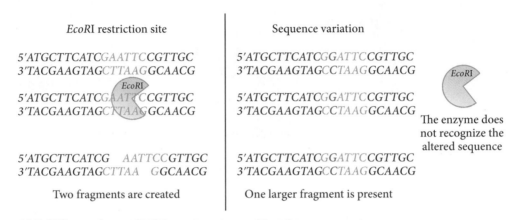

Figure 12.5 SNPs can change restriction enzyme recognition sites.

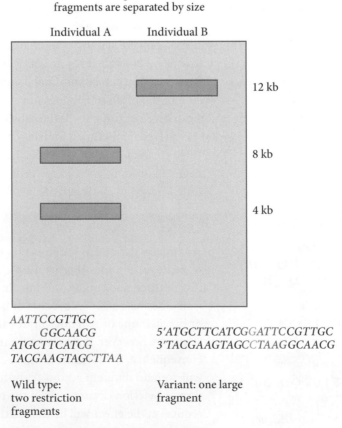

Figure 12.6 SNPs cause restriction fragment length polymorphism.

endonuclease *EcoRI* specifically cuts the DNA sequence GAATTC. If this sequence has been changed to GGATTC, the enzyme will not be able to recognize the sequence element and, therefore, cannot bind and cleave the DNA. Thus single nucleotide changes can lead to different lengths of restriction fragments generated by these enzymes, also called restriction fragment length polymorphism (RFLP) (**Figure 12.6**). DNA segments can be cut with a specific enzyme, and fragments of the same length will be generated if the restriction site is conserved. However, if a genetic variation occurred within the restriction site, the enzyme will no longer recognize the altered sequence element. As a consequence, larger DNA fragments will be generated. RFLPs are useful diagnostic tools that allow investigators to identify natural occurring variations in the population.

Diagnostic Technology

Several assays are available to determine genetic variations in patient samples in the clinical setting, and modern technologies related to genetic identification continue to change and improve. While classical methods relied on DNA sequencing, restriction enzyme digests, and gel electrophoresis, today automated systems are being applied. One high-throughput tool for the analysis of DNA and single nucleotide changes is mass spectrometry, such as MALDI-TOF (matrix-assisted laser desorption/ionization time-of-flight mass spectrometry). Other assays rely on polymerase chain reaction technologies, like the TaqMan SNP Genotyping Assays, which are easy to utilize and available for more than 4.5 million SNPs. Microarray technology, a microchip-based *in vitro* diagnostic tool, is also available. For example, the AmpliChip CYP450 test is used to analyze sequence variations in the *CYP2D6* and *CYP2C19* genes, which encode drug-metabolizing enzymes.

Gene Copy Number Variations

Gene duplication events can form multiple copies of a formerly single-copy gene (**Figure 12.7**). Conversely, genes can also be lost. The copy number of a gene often (though not always) directly affects the amount of protein being produced, where multiple genes generate more protein than one gene (gene copy number effect).

Haplotypes

Haplotypes are sets of DNA variations, or polymorphisms, that tend to be inherited together (**Figure 12.8**). Many groups of individuals share not just one SNP, but rather several SNPs within the same gene or several genes that are adjacent to each other. These variations are closely linked genetic markers and are passed on to the next generation together.

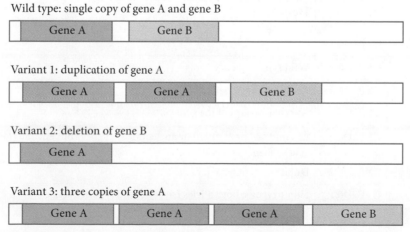

Figure 12.7 Examples of gene copy number variations.

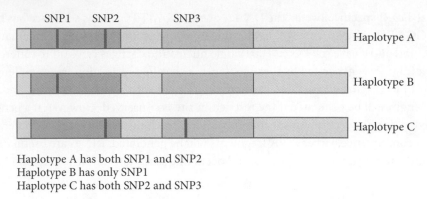

Haplotype A has both SNP1 and SNP2
Haplotype B has only SNP1
Haplotype C has both SNP2 and SNP3

Figure 12.8 Haplotypes.

Genetic Nomenclature

The abbreviation for a gene is usually written in italics (e.g., *CYP2D6*), whereas the protein is not italicized (e.g., CYP2D6). The gene may be followed by an asterisk and a number denoting a particular variant—for example, *CYP2D6*1*, where the number 1 designates the wild type. In contrast, *CYP2D6*2* and *CYP2D6*3* refer to two variations from the wild type sequence. If the *number is followed by a letter, it usually signifies a difference in nucleotide sequence that does not cause a variation in the amino acid sequence (a silent change). For example, *CYP2D6*2A* and *CYP2D6*2B* have genetic variations in their nucleotide sequence, but both encode proteins with identical amino acid sequences. If both gene copies in a diploid organism are being taken into consideration, the nomenclature is *CYP2D6*1/*1* for the homozygous wild type locus or *CYP2D6*1/*2* for a heterozygous locus. Gene amplification events can also be indicated in the terminology; for example, *CYP2D6*2X2* refers to a duplication event. **Table 12.1** provides more examples of genetic nomenclature.

The position and substitution in a SNP—as compared to the wild type sequence—can be specifically indicated in the nomenclature. For example, *3673 G>A* denotes the change of a guanosine to an adenosine at nucleotide position 3673. Similarly, the change of an amino acid in the protein can be indicated: Ala154Thr means that an alanine has been replaced by a threonine at amino acid position 154. **Table 12.2** provides more examples.

Table 12.1 Genetic Nomenclature

Gene	Protein	Denoting
CYP2D6	CYP2D6	
*CYP2D6*1*	CYP2D6.1	Wild type sequence
*CYP2D6*2*	CYP2D6.2	A variant of the gene
*CYP2D6*3*	CYP2D6.3	Another variant of the gene
*CYP2D6*2A* *CYP2D6*2B*	CYP2D6.2	*2A and *2B have different nucleotide sequences but encode the same amino acid sequence
*CYP2D6*2X2*	CYP2D6.2	Duplication of gene *CYP2D6*2*
*CYP2D6*1/*1*	CYP2D6.1	Homozygous; both alleles have the wild type sequence
*CYP2D6*1/*2*	CYP2D6.1 CYP2D6.2	Heterozygous; one wild type allele and one variant allele

Table 12.2 Examples of CYP2D6 Polymorphism

Gene	Nucleotide Change	Protein	Amino Acid Change	Enzyme Activity
CYP2D6*1	none	CYP2D6.1	None	Wild type activity
CYP2D6*1B	3828G>A	CYP2D6.1	None	Wild type activity
CYP2D6*2B	1039C>T 1661G>C 2850C>T 4180G>C	CYP2D6.2	R296C S486T	
CYP2D6*2X2	1661G>C 2850C>T 4180G>C	CYP2D6.2	R296C S486T	Increased
CYP2D6*4C	100C>T 1661G>C 1846G>A 3887T>C 4180G>C		L34S splicing defect L421P S486T	None
CYP2D6*3A	2549delA (deletion)		259 frameshift	None

The Human Genome Project

The Human Genome Project was a concerted effort to sequence the entire human genome and was completed in 2003. Several international institutions, led by the U.S. Department of Energy and the National Institutes of Health, collaborated over a span of 13 years to complete this enormous mission. The human genome sequencing project was simultaneously undertaken by a private company, Celera Genomics, which completed its task at the same time. The entire genome was sequenced, open reading frames or putative genes were identified, and the information was stored in publicly available databases.

The total number of genes in humans is estimated to be 30,000—a smaller number than previously estimated. Although the sequence of putative genes is available, we still do not know the function of approximately 50% of these genes. Thus, even though the sequencing project is finished, data analysis and identification of gene function are ongoing challenges. Another interesting finding from the Human Genome Project is that the vast majority of human DNA (approximately 98%) does not code for proteins. Some of these regions are regulatory sequences or influence the structure of the chromatin; others are "junk" sequences, often repetitive stretches of DNA, without any apparent function.

The Human Genome Project utilized DNA from several donors to generate a cumulative map of the human genome. However, several individual genomes have been sequenced, and such services are now available on a commercial basis. An estimated 1.4 million locations with SNPs have been identified. SNPs in individual genes are useful for pharmacogenetic analyses, whereas the sequencing of the entire genome of an individual will undoubtedly be used in the future for pharmacogenomic analyses.

Genetic Variations in Drug Response

Genetic variations often determine how an individual patient responds to certain medications. Specifically, polymorphism or genetic variation may affect the pharmacokinetic or pharmacodynamic properties of a drug. When polymorphism influences the absorption, distribution, metabolism, or excretion of a drug, it modifies the pharmacokinetic parameters and, therefore, will alter the available concentration of a drug in the body. Conversely, if genetic variations affect drug targets or other proteins involved in the physiological response, the pharmacodynamic properties of a medication may be altered. Simply stated, pharmacokinetics analyzes how the body acts on a drug, whereas pharmacodynamics examines how a drug acts on the body. Both pharmacokinetic and pharmacodynamic parameters determine the therapeutic outcome: A patient may respond to drug treatment as expected, may be a nonresponder, or may exhibit a toxic response.

Pharmacokinetics

The influence of genetic variations on drug metabolism has been studied extensively. Drug-metabolizing enzymes modify the chemical structure of compounds in biochemical reactions and can either detoxify or activate a drug. Thus they are critical in determining the concentration of active drug in the system, which in turn influences the body's response to the medication. Drug-metabolizing enzymes can be divided into Phase I and Phase II enzymes (see also the *Introduction to Medicinal Chemistry* chapter). Phase I enzymes catalyze a variety of reactions—such as oxidation, dealkylation, and hydroxylation reactions—that occur mainly in the liver. These enzymes typically belong to the cytochrome P450 monooxygenase (CYP) family, which is responsible for metabolizing approximately 80% of all drugs. The CYP family is undoubtedly the most important enzyme family for drug metabolism and is also the best-studied example for pharmacogenetics. Numerous genetic variations in these enzymes have been identified and associated with the therapeutic response to a multitude of drugs. Depending on the extent of drug metabolism by CYP enzymes, patients can be classified as poor metabolizers (PM), extensive metabolizers (EM), intermediate metabolizers (IM), or ultrarapid metabolizers (UM). Poor metabolism refers to slow drug metabolism, extensive metabolism means normal or wild type rates of drug conversion, intermediate metabolism denotes a response somewhere between slow and normal, and ultrarapid metabolism represents faster-than-normal reaction rates. Phase II enzymes catalyze conjugating reactions where a variety of enzymes add glutathione, sulfonate, or glucuronic acid to chemical compounds. The most prominent enzymes are glutathione-*S*-transferases, UDP-glucuronosyltransferases, and methyltransferases.

Another important contributor to pharmacokinetic outcomes is drug uptake. One of the best-studied examples is P-glycoprotein (P-gp), a transmembrane pump. This energy-dependent transporter belongs to the ATP-binding cassette (ABC) transporter superfamily and is responsible for decreased uptake or increased efflux of drugs. The protein transports a wide variety of compounds across membranes. Also known as multidrug resistance protein 1, it is responsible for resistance to a variety of drugs, ranging from antibiotics to chemotherapeutic agents. The *ABCB1* gene encodes this protein, and genetic variations in the *ABCB1* gene are responsible for differences in drug accumulation in individual patients. At least 50 SNPs have been identified in the promoter region and coding sequence of the *ABCB1* gene, which is responsible for overproduction of P-gp, modified activity, or altered substrate-binding specificity.

Pharmacodynamics

Genetic polymorphism that alters the physiological response to a drug will influence the pharmacodynamic properties of the medication. Examples include variations in genes encoding drug targets (such as enzymes or receptors) or proteins of signal transduction pathways (see also the *Introduction to Pharmacodynamics* chapter). If genetic variations alter the structure of a drug target, the compound may have increased or decreased affinity for this target. Genetic polymorphism, especially in DNA regulatory sequences such as promoters, can result in different amounts of the target protein being expressed and, therefore, can require dose adjustments to achieve the desired pharmaceutical outcome. Furthermore, genetic variations can occur in genes encoding proteins that do not directly interact with the drug, but still influence the body's response to the medication. Examples include proteins of the signal transduction pathways.

The best-studied examples involve polymorphism in receptors. Numerous drugs bind to receptors, which are usually present on the cell surface. Most compounds act as antagonists to inhibit the activation of signal transduction pathways. For instance, blood-pressure–lowering drugs act against a variety of receptors, and individuals have substantial variations in their response to these medications. Today, trial and error is often used to find a drug that an individual patient will respond to. Genetic variations in a variety of target genes and downstream modulators are often the basis for this unpredictability in drug treatment, so a better understanding and screening for these genetic variations would improve pharmacotherapeutic efficacy.

Clinical Examples

β-Blockers

One class of drugs that is used to treat high blood pressure (hypertension) comprises the β-blockers. These agents act as antagonists (inhibitors) of β-adrenergic receptors (see also the *Introduction to Pharmacology and Pathophysiology* chapter). Excessive activation of the adrenergic nervous system is the cause of hypertension and other cardiovascular disorders. Blocking the β-adrenergic receptors can effectively lower the heart rate, amount of blood pumped, and heartbeat, which in turn reduces blood pressure. However, a significant portion of patients—an estimated 30–60%—do not respond to treatment with β-blocker monotherapy. The cause of this variability in treatment outcome is genetic polymorphism in the β-adrenergic receptors and the drug-metabolizing enzymes.

CYP2D6 is responsible for the metabolism of β-blockers such as metoprolol (Lopressor; Toprol-XL), carvedilol (Coreg), and propranolol (Inderal LA, InnoPran XL). As a consequence, this enzyme affects the plasma concentration of the drug and determines the pharmacokinetic properties exerted by the β-blockers. The wild type or *CYP2D6*1/*1* genotype is an extensive metabolizer, whereas the *CYP2D6*2/*2* genotype causes ultrarapid metabolism. Conversely, the *CYP2D6*3*, *CYP2D6*4*, and *CYP2D6*5* alleles are associated with poor metabolism. Thus individuals homozygous for *CYP2D6*2/*2* have very low β-blocker plasma concentrations due to rapid turnover of the drug, whereas patients who are poor metabolizers have high concentrations of β-blockers in their system because they convert the drug poorly.

The *ADRB1* gene encodes the β-adrenergic receptor, and any individual variations in this target gene will affect the pharmacodynamic properties of the β-blockers (**Figure 12.9**). Clinical and *in vitro* studies have identified two SNPs that influence the drug response: codon 49 (Ser or Gly) and codon 389 (Arg or Gly). Patients with an Arg at position 389 have significantly higher diastolic blood pressure and heart rate and will experience the most benefit from β-blockers such as metoprolol. Indeed, one study suggested that patients with the Ser49 and Arg389 genotypes responded especially well to metoprolol therapy. Position 49 is on the extracellular domain of the receptor and presumably is important for ligand or drug binding, whereas position 389 is located in the intracellular domain of the transmembrane receptor and is postulated to interact with a G-protein that is involved in signal transduction. Interestingly, the Ser49 and Arg389 genotypes occur more frequently in African Americans than Caucasians.

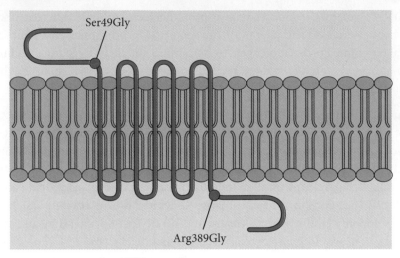

Figure 12.9 Common variations in the ADRB1 protein.

Genetic Testing

It may be possible to predict therapy outcome by genotyping the *CYP2D6* and *ADRB1* loci. Several clinical studies are seeking to correlate the benefits of genetic testing with clinical outcome of various β-blockers; however, as yet no such testing is required or recommended for patients.

Learning Bridge 12.1

An African American patient comes to your pharmacy to pick up his prescription for metoprolol. Although genetic testing is not required, his doctor wants him to have his *ADRB1* gene sequenced. The patient asks you for more information.

A. What does the gene code for, and why would it affect a prescription for metoprolol?

B. Does the fact that the patient is African American have any significance?

Warfarin

Warfarin (Coumadin, Jantoven) is an anticoagulant given to patients who have an increased risk of heart disease or stroke due to blood clotting. The drug, which is often called a "blood thinner," inhibits the formation of proteins that are part of the blood coagulation cascade. Warfarin was originally developed as a rat poison and is still sometimes used for this purpose.

Warfarin consists of a racemic mixture of two active enantiomers, the *R*- and *S*-forms, with the *S*-form being biologically more active (see also the *Introduction to Medicinal Chemistry* chapter). Both enantiomers are metabolized and inactivated by CYP enzymes. Warfarin acts by inhibiting the enzyme vitamin K epoxide reductase, an essential enzyme for the production of several blood clotting factors (see also the *Introduction to Nutrients* chapter) (**Figure 12.10**). Genetic variations in CYP enzymes will affect drug metabolism or the rate of warfarin inactivation, whereas genetic variations in the vitamin K epoxide reductase complex subunit 1 gene (VKORC1) will influence how potently warfarin inhibits the target enzyme. Thus both pharmacokinetic and pharmacodynamic aspects are important considerations for the dosing of warfarin.

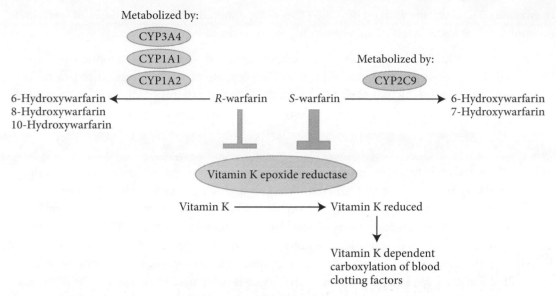

Figure 12.10 Warfarin inhibits vitamin K epoxide reductase and, therefore, the maturation of blood clotting factors.

Metabolism of Warfarin

CYP2C9 is responsible for metabolizing the more active *S*-enantiomer of warfarin to the inactive 7-hydroxywarfarin (as well as some 6-hydroxywarfarin), which will eventually be secreted. Thus warfarin clearance rates and dose requirements are influenced by genetic polymorphisms of the *CYP2C9* gene. Carriers of the *CYP2C9*2* and *CYP2C9*3* alleles have been found to have higher bleeding risks compared to patients who are homozygous for the wild type (*CYP2C9*1*) allele. The proteins encoded by *CYP2C9*2* and *CYP2C9*3* are less than 12% and 5% active, respectively, compared to normal (wild type) CYP2C9. As a consequence, warfarin is metabolized and inactivated at a slower rate in individuals with the *CYP2C9*2* and *CYP2C9*3* alleles, and these patients are at an increased risk of bleeding on a standard dose of warfarin. Such patients would benefit from lower doses of warfarin than are normally prescribed. Individuals carrying one wild type allele and either *CYP2C9*2* and *CYP2C9*3* (*CYP2C9*1/*2* or *CYP2C9*1/*3* heterozygotes) have an intermediate warfarin clearance, whereas *CYP2C9*2/*2* and *CYP2C9*3/*3* homozygotes have much lower clearance rates. Interestingly, the *CYP2C9*2* and *CYP2C9*3* variants are found in as many as 35% of Caucasians but far fewer Asians and African Americans. The interaction of warfarin with the different variants of the CYP2C9 enzyme is an example of how polymorphism can affect the pharmacokinetic properties of a drug, because the CYP2C9 enzyme influences drug inactivation and clearance.

Warfarin Targets the Vitamin K Epoxide Reductase Complex Subunit 1

The enzyme vitamin K epoxide reductase is responsible for reducing vitamin K to its active form, which in turn catalyzes the carboxylation of glutamic acid residues in some of the blood-clotting proteins. Warfarin inhibits vitamin K epoxide reductase, specifically interacting with subunit 1 (VKORC1). Several genetic variations have been identified in *VKORC1*, the gene encoding this subunit. Some of the polymorphism occurs in the promoter region; for example, *VKORC1*2* contains a single nucleotide exchange upstream of the coding region (-1639G>A). This variation does not affect the amino acid sequence of the enzyme but does lower its expression level. The sensitivity to warfarin is increased if fewer enzymes are produced (i.e., with a higher ratio of drug to enzyme). Thus patients with the *VKORC1*2* genotype should receive lower doses of warfarin to account for their lower levels of the vitamin K epoxide reductase enzyme.

Several other *VKORC1* polymorphisms have been identified—some leading to increased warfarin sensitivity (warfarin hypersensitivity), and others leading to warfarin resistance (warfarin hyposensitivity). The interaction of warfarin with the different variants of VKORC1 is an example of how polymorphism can alter the pharmacodynamic characteristics of a drug.

Genetic Testing

In 2007, the Food and Drug Administration (FDA) introduced additional information into the warfarin package insert stating that patients with certain genetic variations should potentially receive lower doses of warfarin. A paragraph on the insert announces that individuals carrying the *CYP2C9*2* or *CYP2C9*3* alleles have increased bleeding risks and that the *VKORC1*2* (-1639G>A) allele requires lower doses of warfarin. The impact of combined polymorphism in CYP2C9 and VKORC1 is also emphasized. Genetic testing is recommended before warfarin is administered. Although it is not yet routinely performed, such testing is being used more frequently. Fortunately, patients receiving warfarin are already monitored in anticoagulation clinics, where blood is drawn on a regular basis and bleeding time is established (INR: International Normalized Ratio). The INR values are used to adjust the warfarin dose to achieve the desired outcome.

Learning Bridge 12.2

A physician orders genetic testing for several patients before prescribing warfarin. What does the following information tell you about the two genes, and how would this information affect drug metabolism (pharmacokinetics) and drug–target interactions (pharmacodynamics)? Which general dose adjustments (increase or decrease of dose) would you recommend for these patients?

>   Patient A: *CYP2C9*1/*1, VKORC1*1/*1*
>   Patient B: *CYP2C9*3/*3, VKORC1*1/*1*
>   Patient C: *CYP2C9*1/*1, VKORC1*2/*2*
>   Patient D: *CYP2C9*3/*3, VKORC1*2/*2*

Clopidogrel

Clopidogrel (Plavix) is another medication prescribed as a blood thinner. In contrast to warfarin, which acts by inhibiting the proteins of the blood coagulation cascade, clopidogrel is an antiplatelet agent. Platelets are cell fragments in the bloodstream that, together with the proteins of the coagulation cascade, are responsible for blood clotting. Clopidogrel acts by binding irreversibly to a receptor ($P2Y_{12}$) on the platelet surface, thereby preventing binding of ADP, a physiological ligand and platelet activator. Thus this agent inhibits platelet activation and blood clotting. Not all patients respond to clopidogrel; that is, some patients may be nonresponders and, therefore, have an increased risk for stroke or heart attack despite receiving drug therapy.

Genetic variability influencing the response to clopidogrel has been found in a number of genes, including the gene encoding the $P2Y_{12}$ receptor on platelets, the gene encoding the P-glycoprotein responsible for drug efflux, and several of the CYP enzymes responsible for metabolism of clopidogrel. The receptor $P2Y_{12}$ is the actual drug target, while variations in the drug efflux system and metabolizing enzymes will affect the pharmacokinetic properties of the drug. Clopidogrel is a prodrug that requires activation via CYP2C19. In this example, drug metabolism is important for the activation of a prodrug, rather than for the inactivation or detoxification of a drug (as seen in the example of warfarin and CYP2C9 in the previous section).

Polymorphism in the *CYP2C19* gene has been extensively studied and is an important factor in drug unresponsiveness. Several genetic variations in *CYP2C19* have been identified. *CYP2C19*2* and *CYP2C19*3* are nonfunctional alleles and lead to poor metabolism and activation of clopidogrel. *CYP2C19*2* contains a SNP that causes aberrant splicing and results in a truncated, inactive protein. *CYP2C19*3* has a SNP that introduces a stop codon and also generates a truncated, inactive protein. These two SNPs or haplotypes account for the majority of poor metabolizers of clopidogrel. Other alleles that are associated with absent or reduced activity of CYP2C9 include *CYP2C19*4, *5, *6, *7,* and *8*.

Genetic Testing

Tests for *CYP1C19* genotyping are available and recommended. The FDA has included a statement about the importance of genetic variations in *CYP1C19* for drug metabolism in the package insert for clopidogrel.

Learning Bridge 12.3

The package insert for clopidogrel (Plavix) includes the following statement: "Poor metabolizers treated with Plavix at recommended doses exhibit higher cardiovascular event rates following acute coronary syndrome (ACS) or percutaneous coronary intervention (PCI) than patients with normal CYP2C19 function." How would you explain this statement to a patient?

Thiopurines

Thiopurines—mercaptopurine (Purinethol), thioguanine (Tabloid), and azathioprine (Azasan, Imuran)—are antimetabolites that are used as chemotherapeutic agents to treat acute lymphoblastic leukemia, autoimmune disorders, and organ transplant recipients. In the body, thiopurines are further metabolized and then falsely incorporated into DNA. Once these purine analogs are present in the DNA, replication is inhibited. As a consequence, thiopurines inhibit rapidly proliferating cells (e.g. cancer cells) and cells of the immune system that rely on extensive DNA synthesis for replication and proliferation. However, hematological toxicity will occur if the drug concentration is too high because blood cells are also affected. Indeed, it has been observed that approximately 10% of all patients experience life-threatening hematological side effects with thiopurine therapy.

A combination of clinical and molecular studies has revealed that genetic polymorphism in the gene encoding thiopurine-*S*-methyltransferase (TPMT) is responsible for different rates of thiopurine metabolism and toxic drug effects. If TPMT is less active, thiopurine metabolism and detoxification will be reduced; the increased amount of drug present in the body then causes toxicity. The genetics of TPMT has become one of the best-understood mechanisms of how genetic polymorphism can affect the drug response in patients by influencing pharmacokinetic parameters.

Thiopurine Metabolism

Azathioprine is a prodrug that is converted to 6-mercaptopurine, which is then further metabolized via several competing routes. Activation of 6-mercaptopurine is catalyzed by hypoxanthine guanine phosphoribosyltransferase (HPRT) and other enzymes that form 6-thioguanine-monophosphate or 6-thioinosine-monophosphate (**Figure 12.11** and **Figure 12.12**). Inactivation,

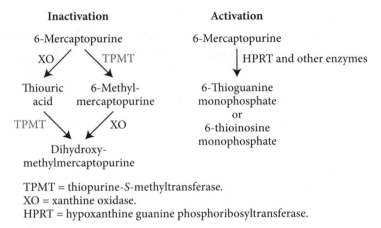

Figure 12.11 The structures of guanine and thiopurines.

Inactivation

6-Mercaptopurine

XO / \ TPMT

Thiouric acid   6-Methyl-mercaptopurine

TPMT \ / XO

Dihydroxy-methylmercaptopurine

Activation

6-Mercaptopurine

↓ HPRT and other enzymes

6-Thioguanine monophosphate

or

6-thioinosine monophosphate

TPMT = thiopurine-*S*-methyltransferase.
XO = xanthine oxidase.
HPRT = hypoxanthine guanine phosphoribosyltransferase.

Figure 12.12 Metabolism of 6-mercaptopurine.

in contrast, occurs by the action of TPMT and xanthine oxidase, which form 2,8-dihydroxy-6-methylmercaptopurine. TPMT catalyzes the *S*-methylation of 6-mercaptopurine and other aromatic and heterocyclic sulfhydryl compounds. Interestingly, the endogenous substrates for TPMT have not been identified and its normal biological role is unknown.

Genetic Polymorphism of TPMT

Approximately 28 variant alleles have been identified that lead to reduced activity of TPMT and, therefore, to increased thiopurine presence and toxicity. The most common haplotypes associated with reduced TPMT activity are *TPMT*3A*, **3B*, **3C*, and *TPMT*2* (see **Table 12.3**). The variations found in *TPMT*2* and *TPMT*3* enhance TPMT degradation at the protein level. Other sequence variations that have been recognized involve alterations in mRNA splice site consensus sequences, resulting in alternative TPMT mRNA splicing and decreased enzyme expression or truncated

Table 12.3 Common *TPMT* Haplotypes

Haplotype	Nucleotide Exchange	Amino Acid Substitution
TPMT*3A	G460A and A719G	Ala154Thr and Tyr240Cys
TPMT*3B	G460A	Ala154Thr
TPMT*3C	A719G	Tyr240Cys
TPMT*2	G238C	Ala80Pro

proteins (e.g., *TPMT*4* and *TPMT*15*). Patients who are heterozygous—one wild type copy (*TPMT*1*) and one variant allele—have reduced TPMT activity and experience moderate toxicity. This is an example of a gene dosage effect: one wild type allele in the heterozygous patient produces half as much protein as two wild type alleles in the homozygous individual. TPMT-deficient patients who have two variant alleles experience severe bone marrow suppression because the high levels of thiopurines inhibit the proliferation of red and white blood cells in the bone marrow.

Genetic Testing

The package inserts for mercaptopurine and thioguanine warn that patients with TPMT deficiency may be unusually sensitive to the myelosuppressive effect of the drugs. Pharmacogenetic testing for TPMT is available and recommended by the FDA. Testing can be performed either by genotyping (DNA sequence analysis) or by phenotyping (assay for enzyme activity).

Irinotecan

The drug irinotecan (Camptosar) is often given in combination with other chemotherapeutic drugs as a treatment for advanced colon cancer. However, some patients will suffer from severe side effects, such as neutropenia (reduced white blood cell count), and should be given a smaller dose. Irinotecan is a prodrug; it is metabolized to the active compound SN-38, which potently inhibits topoisomerase I. This enzyme is responsible for relieving the helical stress that occurs during replication, so it is especially important for rapidly proliferating cells, such as cancer cells. Inactivation of SN-38 occurs by glucuronidation (the addition of glucuronic acid), catalyzed by uridine diphosphate glucuronosyltransferase (UGT) 1A1. UGT is a typical example of a Phase II metabolizing enzyme, as it catalyzes a conjugation reaction. Genetic polymorphism in the *UGT1A1* gene has been found to be associated with decreased UGT activity, and the increased amount of SN-38 is responsible for the toxic side effects observed with irinotecan. Similar to the toxicity of thiopurine, hematological toxicity occurs because the proliferation of normal blood cells is inhibited.

The best-characterized variant is *UGT1A1*28*, which contains a TA repeat expansion in the promoter of *UGT1A1*. This increased number of TA dinucleotide repeats in the TATA promoter consensus sequence causes a reduced level of *UGT1A1* gene expression. The *UGT1A1*28* variant is present in approximately 10% of the U.S. population. Other, less frequently occurring polymorphisms have been identified that cause amino acid substitutions in the protein and reduced or absent enzyme activity.

Genetic Testing

The FDA now includes a warning in the package insert of irinotecan (Camptosar): "Individuals who are homozygous for the *UGT1A1*28* allele are at increased risk for neutropenia following initiation of Camptosar treatment." Neutropenia leads to reduced immune function. A DNA test is now recommended for patients considering irinotecan therapy.

Learning Bridge 12.4

A patient with advanced colon cancer has been treated with the chemotherapy drugs fluorouracil and leucovorin. After several weeks, the physician adds irinotecan to the treatment regimen. It soon becomes obvious that the patient is suffering from severe neutropenia. The physician contacts you as the pharmacist in charge and asks if you are aware of any potential problems with irinotecan. What is your advice?

Trastuzumab

Members of the epidermal growth factor receptor (EGFR) family are often found overexpressed in cancer. The epidermal growth factor receptor HER2 is overproduced in 25–30% of human breast cancers (HER2-positive breast cancer), and several drugs have been developed that target and inhibit the action of this receptor. Trastuzumab (Herceptin) is one such chemotherapy drug that is prescribed for HER2-positive breast cancer. This drug binds and inhibits HER2, and screening for HER2 overexpression is a prerequisite for treatment with this agent. This indication is an example where genetic screening is mandatory.

Mechanism of Action of Trastuzumab

Epidermal growth factor receptors are tyrosine kinase receptors that respond to ligand (epidermal growth factor) binding by dimerization. A conformational change is induced that activates the intracellular kinase domain of the receptor. The kinase, in turn, phosphorylates intracellular messengers, with the activated signal transduction cascade then causing increased cellular proliferation. Amplification of the gene encoding HER2 is usually the cause of the overexpression of this receptor. Because of the large number of receptors on the tumor cell surface, dimerization and activation occur spontaneously. The tumor cell is thus independent of extracellular proliferation signals, a feature typical of cancer cells.

Trastuzumab is a monoclonal antibody that binds specifically to the external domain of the HER2 receptor (**Figure 12.13**). Binding of the HER2 antibody acts via two modalities: (1) the prevention of dimerization and signal transduction and (2) the coating of tumor cells with antibodies. The coated tumor cell can then be recognized by the immune system and destroyed.

Genetic Testing

Patients are eligible for trastuzumab therapy only if the cancer cells overproduce HER2 at least twofold to threefold compared to normal protein expression. Commercially available test assays include HercepTest and PathVysion. HercepTest is based on immunohistochemistry and detects

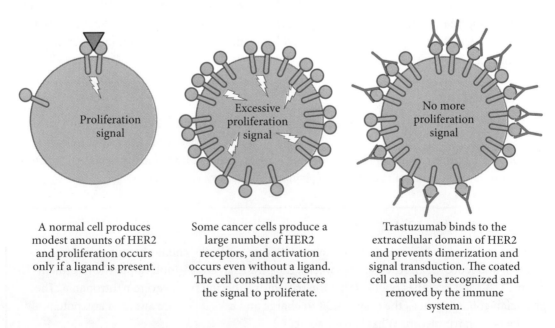

A normal cell produces modest amounts of HER2 and proliferation occurs only if a ligand is present.

Some cancer cells produce a large number of HER2 receptors, and activation occurs even without a ligand. The cell constantly receives the signal to proliferate.

Trastuzumab binds to the extracellular domain of HER2 and prevents dimerization and signal transduction. The coated cell can also be recognized and removed by the immune system.

Figure 12.13 Mechanism of action of trastuzumab.

the amount of protein expressed, whereas PathVysion uses fluorescence *in situ* hybridization (FISH) and detects gene amplification.

The drug lapatinib (Tykerb) also targets the HER2 receptor, although it interacts with HER2 in a different way than trastuzumab does. Lapatinib binds to the ATP binding pocket of the intracellular kinase domain of the receptor, thereby preventing kinase activity and signal transduction. Similar to the case for trastuzumab, testing for overexpression of HER2 is necessary before lapatinib therapy is initiated.

Cetuximab

Cetuximab (Erbitux) is an antibody that inhibits a different member of the epidermal growth factor receptor family, EGFR. This drug is being used for some patients with colorectal or head and neck cancer.

Clinical studies revealed that cetuximab is very effective in some patients but ineffective in others. Retroactive analysis found that the unresponsive patients had a mutation in *KRAS*, a protein that acts downstream of the signal transduction pathway. The *KRAS* mutation causes the signaling molecule to be constantly active and to induce a phosphorylation cascade that induces cellular proliferation (**Figure 12.14**). Thus patients with a *KRAS* mutation are invulnerable to any manipulation on the receptor level.

Cetuximab is an excellent example of how genetic polymorphism—or a mutation, in this case—can render an individual patient nonresponsive to a drug. Several other drugs target EGFR (see **Table 12.4**), and *KRAS* mutations also produce resistance phenotypes against these treatments.

Genetic Testing

Patients are required to undergo testing for overexpression of EGFR before cetuximab is prescribed. The National Cancer Institute now also recommends testing for the *KRAS* genotype. In Europe, treatment with cetuximab is restricted to patients with normal *KRAS* genes. **Table 12.5** identifies other genetic testing recommended or required by the FDA.

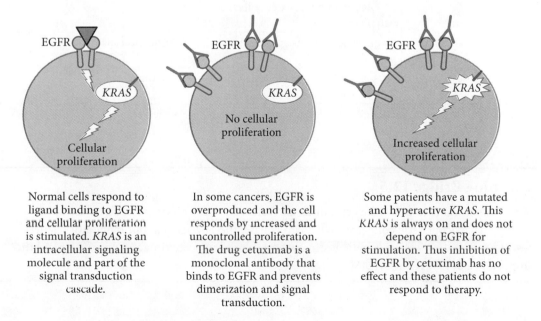

Normal cells respond to ligand binding to EGFR and cellular proliferation is stimulated. *KRAS* is an intracellular signaling molecule and part of the signal transduction cascade.

In some cancers, EGFR is overproduced and the cell responds by increased and uncontrolled proliferation. The drug cetuximab is a monoclonal antibody that binds to EGFR and prevents dimerization and signal transduction.

Some patients have a mutated and hyperactive *KRAS*. This *KRAS* is always on and does not depend on EGFR for stimulation. Thus inhibition of EGFR by cetuximab has no effect and these patients do not respond to therapy.

Figure 12.14 A mutation in *KRAS* renders cetuximab therapy ineffective.

Table 12.4 Drugs Targeting Members of the Epidermal Growth Factor Receptor Family

Receptor Type	Drug
EGFR (HER1, ErbB-1)	Cetuximab (Erbitux) Gefitinib (Iressa) Erlotinib (Tarceva) Panitumumab (Vectibix)
HER2 (Neu, ErbB-2)	Trastuzumab (Herceptin) Lapatinib (Tykerb)

Table 12.5 FDA Required or Recommended Genetic Testing

Clinical Presentation or Disease	Pharmacogenetic Marker	Drug
FDA-Required Genetic Testing		
Oncology	EGFR expression	Cetuximab, panitumumab, gefitinib
	HER2 overexpression	Trastuzumab, lapatinib
	Philadelphia chromosome presence	Dasatinib
AIDS	CCR5: chemokine C-C motif receptor	Maraviroc
FDA-Recommended Genetic Testing		
Oncology	TPMT (thiopurine methyltransferase) deficiency or lower activity	Azathioprine, thioguanine, mercaptopurine
	UGT1A1 (UDP-glucosyltransferase) variants	Irinotecan
Hematology	CYP2C9 variants Protein C deficiencies VKOR (vitamin K epoxide reductase) variants	Warfarin
	G6PD (glucose-6-phosphate dehydrogenase) deficiency	Rasburicase, dapsone
CNS/psychiatric disorders	*HLA-B*1502* allele (major histocompatibility complex, class I, B) presence	Carbamazepin
AIDS	*HLA-B*5701* allele presence	Abacavir

Learning Bridge 12.5

A physician wants to prescribe cetuximab and asks you as the pharmacist if you are aware of any pharmacogenetic concerns. What can you tell the physician about mandatory genetic testing and recommended genetic testing before prescribing cetuximab? Can you explain the importance of EGFR and *KRAS*?

Relevance of Pharmacogenomics Now and in the Future

Pharmacogenetics

The correlation of drug response with specific genotypes is increasingly useful in pharmacotherapy today. Approximately 10% of drug labels already contain pharmacogenetic information, and this proportion is steadily increasing. The usefulness of these recommendations in determining if a patient will be a responder or a nonresponder, or will have an increased risk of severe side effects, is clear. Adverse drug reactions are one of the leading causes of hospitalization and death in the United States, and pharmacogenetics has the potential to prevent these tragedies. Unfortunately, many healthcare professionals today are not trained adequately to recognize the importance of pharmacogenetics in treatment decisions. Pharmacists are in an ideal position to assume the role of educator and enabler in such cases because of their in-depth knowledge of drug metabolism, pharmacology, pharmacokinetics, and pharmacodynamics. Their training gives them a unique advantage in interpreting new pharmacogenetic findings and translating them into healthcare practice.

The usefulness of pharmacogenetics for scientific discovery should also not be underestimated. New genes and polymorphisms will undoubtedly be identified that affect drug response and disease pathology. Furthermore, pharmacotherapies that have not only additive but also synergistic effects may be discovered. Our increased understanding of how genetic variations influence drug efflux and metabolism as well as the interactions of compounds with their target proteins will allow for better comprehension of the complex interrelationship of drugs and the human body.

Pharmacogenomics

As noted earlier in this chapter, pharmacogenomics is most accurately defined as the knowledge of the entire genome of an individual and how it interacts with pharmacotherapy. While we do not currently understand everything there is to know about the genome–pharmacotherapy relationship, recent advances in biotechnology have made the sequencing of individual genomes possible, and such endeavors will become increasingly affordable and feasible in the future.

Personalized Medicine

Personalized medicine is a medical model based on detailed knowledge of all gene sequences affecting the health of an individual and the response to any given drug. Ideally, it would allow the prescription of the type and dosage of medicine that will most effectively treat a health condition and avoid adverse drug effects. In addition, cost-effectiveness would be increased, because more efficient pharmacotherapy will improve both the short- and long-term health of an individual. Not only pharmacogenomics, but other factors such as age, gender, weight, other medications, and even the environment need to be considered in any personalized treatment plan.

Of course, this is an idealized goal, and the reality is likely to be far less perfect. It will be difficult or nearly impossible to predict all drug responses, even with the complete genome information in hand. The examples discussed in this chapter identified only a few gene products that influence the pharmacokinetic and pharmacodynamic properties of a drug; many more gene products are likely to play roles in the physiological response to drug treatment. Furthermore, the cost and time required for genetic testing must be rationally evaluated.

Ethical Considerations in Pharmacogenomics

Ethics are the moral principles and values that our society holds in high esteem. In regard to health care, ethics consists of moral guidelines that are applied thoughtfully when considering and evaluating choices for patient treatment. Despite the undoubtedly large number of potential benefits that pharmacogenomics offers, ethical concerns will inevitably be associated with this field; indeed, some have already surfaced. Healthcare workers, politicians, and the public need to work together to raise awareness, increase education, and develop public health policies for use of pharmacogenomic data. Guidelines and regulations for such use are already being developed and implemented.

For example, should a patient keep genetic information private or should this knowledge be shared with family members who may have inherited the same genetic variant? Another challenge is to obtain genuine informed consent for testing for the presence of a genetic variation. Does the patient truly comprehend the complicated genetic issues? Some patients may merely scan the consent form before signing it, and healthcare providers may lack the time or patience to fully explain the issue. Furthermore, a healthcare professional needs to assess whether a genetic test should be performed. Currently, only a few drugs require genetic testing before they may be prescribed; other drug labels merely state recommendations. Some genetic tests may not be widely available, too expensive, or not covered by insurance. Testing for a certain gene may also provide more information than the patient bargained for. For example, the E4 variant in the *APOE* gene renders a patient nonresponsive to statin treatment but is also associated with an increased risk of developing Alzheimer's disease.

Several laws are in place to protect patients. The Health Insurance Portability and Accountability Act (HIPAA) of 1996 provides federal protection to keep personal health information private. The most important law in regard to pharmacogenomics, however, is the Genetic Information Nondiscrimination Act (GINA), which was passed into law in the United States in 2008. This law prevents people from being treated unfairly because of their DNA sequence and protects individuals against discrimination by both health insurance companies and employers.

Golden Keys for Pharmacy Students

- Pharmacogenetics and pharmacogenomics study the impact of genetic variations on drug response. Although both terms are often used interchangeably, pharmacogenetics evaluates just one or a few genes, whereas pharmacogenomics takes the entire genome into consideration.
- Pharmacists must be familiar with the genetic principles and terminology that form the foundation of pharmacogenomics.
- Single-nucleotide polymorphisms (SNPs) are the most common genetic variations.
- Genetic polymorphisms that affect drug uptake or efflux, distribution, and metabolism influence the pharmacokinetic properties of the drug.
- Genetic polymorphisms that modify the drug target, signal transduction pathways, or other disease-associated proteins influence the pharmacodynamic properties of a drug.
- The goal of pharmacogenomics is to optimize drug efficacy and to avoid drug toxicity.
- The pharmacist is in an ideal position to translate current and future pharmacogenomic discoveries into healthcare practice.
- Pharmacogenomics is still in its infancy but will have an increasingly profound impact on pharmacy practice in the future.

- Ethical concerns related to pharmacogenomics data need to be carefully discussed and evaluated.

Learning Bridge Answers

12.1 You explain to the patient that the *ADRB1* gene encodes the β-adrenergic receptor, which is the target for the drug metoprolol. Two SNPs have been identified that correlate with positive responsiveness to this drug: Ser49 and Arg389. This variation occurs more frequently in African Americans.

12.2 Patient A (*CYP2C9*1/*1, VKORC1*1/*1*) is homozygous for the wild type genes encoding the drug-metabolizing enzyme (CYP2C9) and the drug target (VKORC1). A normal standard dose of warfarin should be recommended.

Patient B (*CYP2C9*3/*3, VKORC1*1/*1*) is homozygous for a variant of CYP2C9 that is much less active than the wild type enzyme, which will reduce the metabolism of warfarin. The dose of warfarin should be lowered because this patient will have higher plasma levels of warfarin. The gene encoding the drug target VKORC1 is normal.

Patient C (*CYP2C9*1/*1, VKORC1*2/*2*) has wild type *CYP2C9* gene copies, but is homozygous for a genetic variation of *VKORC1* (*VKORC1*2/*2*) that will cause decreased expression of the target protein. Because there is less target protein present, a smaller amount of drug is required. Thus the dose of warfarin should be lowered.

Patient D (*CYP2C9*3/*3, VKORC1*2/*2*) expresses a variant of CYP2C9 that is much less active than the wild type. In addition, the patient has a variant of the *VKORC1* gene that will cause reduced expression of the target gene. The dose of warfarin should be lowered drastically, because higher plasma levels of warfarin will be present and less target protein will be available.

12.3 You would explain to your patient that Plavix is an antiplatelet agent that inhibits blood clotting, thereby preventing or reducing the risk of cardiovascular events, such as heart attacks. The effectiveness of Plavix depends on its activation to an active metabolite by the cytochrome P450 (CYP) system, principally CYP2C19. Some patients have sequence variations in the genes encoding CYP2C19 and may produce fewer enzymes or enzymes that are not as active. In that case, poor metabolism and activation of Plavix would occur and the drug will not be as effective. A higher dose or a different medication should be recommended.

12.4 You should counsel the physician on genetic variations in the uridine diphosphate glucuronosyltransferase (UGT) 1A1 gene. SN-38, the active metabolite of irinotecan, is inactivated by UGT via a glucuronidation reaction. However, some genetic variants cause decreased expression or activity of UGT. As a consequence, more active SN-38 will lead to severe side effects such as neutropenia. You should advise the physician that genetic testing is available for the *UGT1A1* locus.

12.5 You should explain to the physician that two genes are important to consider before prescribing treatment with cetuximab. One is the gene encoding EGFR, the receptor that is the target of the drug. Testing for EGFR is required, because only cancers that produce this type of receptor will respond to cetuximab therapy. Another gene to study is the *KRAS* gene. Patients with a mutation in *KRAS* will not respond to cetuximab therapy because the *KRAS* protein occurs downstream in the signal transduction cascade. Testing for *KRAS* mutations is not required but is recommended and may prevent unsuccessful treatment.

Problems and Solutions

Problem 12.1 Patients with the haplotype *CYP2D6*1/*17* are:

  A. Homozygous.
  B. Heterozygous.

Solution 12.1 B is correct. The patients have two different alleles, *1 and *17, so they are heterozygous for the *CYP2D6* gene.

Problem 12.2 You have sequenced the *VKORC1* gene (vitamin K epoxide reductase complex) in a patient and found that three nucleotides are deleted. This is an example of:

  A. An indel.
  B. A SNP.
  C. A copy number variation.

Solution 12.2 A is correct. This is an example of an indel, which is defined as the insertion or deletion of one or more nucleotides.

Problem 12.3 Which of the following statements about haplotypes is correct?

  A. A haplotype refers to the wild type gene sequence.
  B. A haplotype is defined by at least three SNPs.
  C. A haplotype is shared by a group of people and can contain one or several SNPs.
  D. A set of genetic mutations is called a haplotype if less than 1% of the population has them.

Solution 12.3 C is correct.

Problem 12.4 You are prescribing a standard dose of warfarin to a patient who is a slow metabolizer (*CYP2C9*3/*3*). What is the consequence?

  A. Warfarin will be active for a longer period of time.
  B. Warfarin will be inactivated more rapidly.

Solution 12.4 A is correct. CYP2C9 is the enzyme that converts warfarin to an inactive compound. Thus a slow metabolizer will have a reduced inactivation rate for the compound, and warfarin will remain active for a longer period of time.

Problem 12.5 Why is proof of HER2 overproduction required before trastuzumab is prescribed?

Solution 12.5 Trastuzumab is a monoclonal antibody that binds to the HER2 receptor and prevents its activation. Some cancers overproduce this receptor and, as a result, become independent of growth signals. The overproduced HER2 receptor will transmit the signal and cause increased cellular proliferation. If HER2 is not overexpressed in a particular cancer, trastuzumab, a very expensive medication, cannot be effective and should not be prescribed.

Problem 12.6 A patient with the genotype *CYP2D6*1/*1* exhibits extensive metabolism of the β-blocker metoprolol, and a patient with the genotype *CYP2D6*2/*2* displays ultrarapid metabolism of the same drug. Which type/speed of metabolism would you expect for a patient who has a *CYP2D6*1/*2* genotype?

Solution 12.6 The rate of metabolism of the β-blocker metoprolol would be somewhere in between extensive and ultrarapid metabolism.

Problem 12.7 How does a mutation in *KRAS* render cetuximab therapy ineffective?

Solution 12.7 *KRAS* is a signaling molecule that acts downstream of the EGFR receptor. A mutation in *KRAS*, which leads to an overactive *KRAS* protein, causes cells to proliferate independent of EGFR activation. Because *KRAS* is located downstream of EFGR in the signaling cascade, the drug cetuximab, which inhibits EGFR, will have no effect.

Problem 12.8 A single nucleotide polymorphism in the coding region of a gene:

  A. Will change the amino acid sequence.
  B. May change the amino acid sequence.

Solution 12.8 B is correct. The amino acid sequence will only change if the affected codon now encodes a different amino acid. Sometimes a nucleotide change will not alter the genetic code (the modified codon will still encode the same amino acid). Recall that the same amino acid can be encoded by 2–4 different codons.

Problem 12.9 The gene encoding Vitamin K Epoxide Reductase Complex (*VKORC1*) has slightly different sequences within the population. What determines which of these sequences is called the "wild type" sequence?

Solution 12.9 The sequence that is present in the majority of the population is called the wild type sequence.

Problem 12.10 Genetic variations in the gene encoding thiopurine-S-methyltransferase (TPMT) will influence the _____ properties of thiopurines.

  A. Pharmacokinetic
  B. Pharmacodynamic

Solution 12.10 A is correct. TMPT is responsible for metabolism of thiopurines. Thus, a mutation will affect how long the drugs will be present in the body and the pharmacokinetic properties of thiopurines.

References

1. Baudhuin LM, Miller WL, Train L, et al. Relation of ADRB1, CYP2D6, and UGT1A1 polymorphisms with dose of, and response to, carvedilol or metoprolol therapy in patients with chronic heart failure. *Am J Cardiol.* 2010;106(3):402–408.
2. Cavallari LM, Ellingrod VL, Kolesar JM. *Lexi-Comp's pharmacogenomics handbook*, 2nd ed. Hudson, OH: LexiComp; 2005.
3. Ford LT, Berg JD. Thiopurine *S*-methyltransferase (TPMT) assessment prior to starting thiopurine drug treatment: a pharmacogenomic test whose time has come. *J Clin Pathol.* 2010;63(4):288–295.
4. Ingelman-Sundberg M. Genetic polymorphisms of cytochrome P450 2D6 (CYP2D6): clinical consequences, evolutionary aspects and functional diversity. *Pharmacogenomics J.* 2005;5(1):6–13.
5. Limdi NA, Veenstra DL. Warfarin pharmacogenetics. *Pharmacotherapy.* 2008;28(9):1084–1097.
6. *Pharmacogenomics: applications to patient care.* Kansas City, MO: American College of Clinical Pharmacy; 2004.
7. Roden DM, Altman RB, Benowitz NL, et al. Pharmacogenomics: challenges and opportunities. *Ann Intern Med.* 2006;145(10):749–757.
8. Shin J, Kayser SR, Langaee TY. Pharmacogenetics: from discovery to patient care. *Am J Health Syst Pharm.* 2009;66(7):625–637.
9. Shin J, Johnson JA. Beta-blocker pharmacogenetics in heart failure. *Heart Fail Rev.* 2010;15(3):187–196.

10. UpToDate. Waltham, MA: 2012. Available at: http://www.uptodate.com/online with subscription.

11. Wang L, McLeod HL, Weinshilboum RM: Genomics and drug response. *N Engl J Med.* 2011, 364(12):1144-1153.

12. Weinshilboum R: Thiopurine pharmacogenetics. clinical and molecular studies of thiopurine methyltransferase. *Drug Metab Dispos.* 2001;29(4 Pt 2):601–605.

13. Zdanowicz MM. *Concepts in pharmacogenomics.* Bethesday, MD: American Society of Health-Systems Pharmacists; 2010.

14. Zhou S. Clinical pharmacogenomics of thiopurine *S*-methyltransferase. *Curr Clin Pharmacol.* 2006;1(1):119–128.

Introduction to Pharmacognosy

CHAPTER 13

Jennifer L. Rosselli
Miranda Wilhelm

OBJECTIVES

1. Describe the role of plants in the development and production of medications.
2. Identify and distinguish natural products that are available for common health conditions.
3. Understand the proposed mechanisms of action for various natural products.
4. Summarize the safety concerns related to various natural products.
5. Recognize and anticipate actual and potential drug–natural product interactions.
6. Implement a series of Learning Bridge assignments at your experiential sites to bridge your didactic learning with your experiential experiences.

KEY TERMS AND DEFINITIONS

1. **5-Alpha-reductase:** the enzyme responsible for converting testosterone to dihydrotestosterone.
2. **Alkaloids:** organic nitrogen-containing compounds that have significant pharmacologic activity.
3. **Antioxidant:** substances that protect cells from free-radical damage.
4. **Benign prostatic hypertrophy (BPH):** a hyperplastic process within the prostate due to an increase in epithelial and stromal cells that partially or completely obstruct the urethral canal, causing urinary tract symptoms.
5. **Chondroitin:** a hydrophilic glycosaminoglycan that promotes absorption of water in the articular cartilage.
6. **Complementary and alternative medicine (CAM):** health systems, therapies, and practices that are not a part of standard medical care.
7. **Congestive heart failure:** a chronic medical condition in which the heart is no longer able to maintain adequate blood circulation to tissues throughout the body.
8. **Cytochrome P450:** a family of enzymes that have an integral role in drug metabolism.
9. **Dementia:** a loss of cognitive function that interferes with normal functioning; may affect memory, perception, language, judgment, and behavior.
10. **Depression:** a psychiatric disorder characterized by a depressed mood or loss of interest in most activities, lasting at least 2 weeks.
11. **Diabetes mellitus:** a medical condition in which either the pancreas does not produce enough insulin or the cells in the body cannot adequately utilize insulin, resulting in elevated blood glucose levels.
12. **Dietary supplement:** a vitamin, mineral, herb or other botanical product, amino acid, or other dietary substance intended to supplement the diet and delivered as a concentrate, metabolite, constituent, extract, or combination of the ingredients described previously.
13. **Drug therapy problem:** a problem that is caused by a drug or that may be corrected or prevented by a drug.

(continues)

14. **Erectile dysfunction:** a medical condition in which a man has difficulty achieving or maintaining an erection for sexual performance.

15. **Flavonoid:** an organic compound found in plants that contains brightly colored pigments. Flavonoids have antioxidant properties and enhance the activities of other compounds in phytomedicinals.

16. **Gamma-aminobutyric acid (GABA):** a neurotransmitter that decreases central nervous system activity.

17. **Glucosamine:** a naturally occurring amino sugar present in many physiological fluids such as synovial fluid and articular cartilage.

18. **Good manufacturing practices (GMP):** regulations enforced by the Food and Drug Administration that require control of manufacturing processes such that the resulting drug products and dietary supplements meet quality standards.

19. **Hemoglobin A_{1c}:** a diagnostic and screening test used to determine the average glucose concentration within the blood during the previous 2- to 3-month time period.

20. **Hot flushes:** a common symptom of menopause, described as a sudden sensation of warmth that may be accompanied by sweating and a red, flushed face, neck, and chest; also known as hot flashes.

21. **Hyperemesis gravidarum:** a medical condition characterized by severe nausea and vomiting during pregnancy that results in weight loss, dehydration, and electrolyte disturbances.

22. **Hyperforin:** the active chemical in St. John's wort, which is believed to inhibit neuronal reuptake of neurotransmitters.

23. **Hypomanic symptoms:** atypical elevation in mood or irritable mood lasting for at least 4 days, but where psychosis is not present and hospitalization is not required. Hypomania consistent with bipolar disorder should be evaluated and treated by a health professional.

24. **International Normalized Ratio (INR):** a calculation used to standardize blood clotting time results as a measure of the extrinsic pathway of coagulation; it is used to monitor the effectiveness of anticoagulation medications.

25. **Irritable bowel syndrome (IBS):** a chronic medical condition of the intestine characterized by symptoms of constipation, diarrhea, or both, as well as abdominal pain that does not result in damage to the lining of the intestine.

26. **Manic symptoms:** atypical elevated mood that impairs normal daily functioning and may require hospitalization.

27. **Menopause:** loss of ovarian follicular activity causing permanent cessation of menses.

28. **Migraine:** a recurrent severe headache, often characterized by unilateral pain, lasting 4–72 hours, that interferes with daily activities.

29. **Neuropathy:** nerve damage resulting in pain; a common complication of diabetes.

30. **Nutraceutical:** a term encompassing vitamins, supplements, and herbal preparations.

31. **Osteoarthritis:** joint pain and tenderness caused by changes in the structure and function of the diarthrodial joint, largely involving the articular cartilage.

32. **P-glycoprotein:** a drug-transporting phosphoglycoprotein.

33. **Perimenopause:** a period of transition to menopause when the female experiences irregular menstruation during the previous 12 months.

34. **Pharmacognosy:** the study of medicinal products derived from nature.

35. **Phytoestrogens:** plants containing estrogenic chemicals.

(CONTINUED)

36. **Postmenopause:** the absence of menstruation during the previous 12 months.

37. **Proanthocyanidins:** nonhydrolyzable tannins.

38. **Rhabdomyolysis:** the breakdown of muscle tissue resulting in the cellular contents being released into the bloodstream, leading to damage to the kidney and subsequent renal failure.

39. **Rhizome:** a horizontal stem of a plant that is typically found underground and from which the roots of the plant extend.

40. **Saponins:** organic compounds found in plants that, when placed in water, result in a characteristic soapy lather.

41. **Sesquiterpene lactones:** the most abundant class of terpenoids; they contain functional groups that act as receptor sites and are involved in a wide variety of biological activities.

42. **Sterols:** solid chemical compounds, also known as phytosterols. Cholesterol is the most widely occurring sterol.

43. **Succulent:** a type of plant found in dessert climates that stores and retains water in the leaves and stems, giving them a thickened appearance.

44. **Tannins:** polyphenols that have astringent properties and precipitate proteins.

45. **Terpenoids:** natural products whose structures are divided into isoprene units (C_5H_8) and that are involved in a number of chemical reactions.

43. **Urinary tract infection:** the presence of microorganisms in the urinary tract that are capable of invading the immediate or adjacent tissues.

44. **Volatile oil:** a compound within oil that evaporates at room temperature and provides an aromatic aroma.

Introduction

Pharmacognosy is the study of drugs originating from natural sources. The word "pharmacognosy" is derived from the Greek *pharmakon*, meaning "drug or medicine," and *gnosis*, meaning "knowledge." The study of pharmacognosy encompasses many biologic and chemical sciences, such as botany, pharmaceutics, biochemistry, phytochemistry, and pharmacology.

This chapter introduces pharmacognosy and details how medicinal natural products have played an important role in the development of modern pharmacy. Regulatory and standardization practices related to natural products or dietary supplements in the United States are discussed. Evidence-based biomedical literature resources are identified that will assist the student pharmacist in researching and formulating responses to drug information inquiries related to natural products. Overviews of individual dietary supplements are provided that include therapeutic properties, pharmacology, summaries of clinical evidence, dosing, and safety concerns of each product.

The Role of Pharmacognosy in Pharmacy Practice

The practice of pharmacy began with the use of medicinal products derived from natural sources. The earliest documented use of medicinal plants dates back to the 4th century BC. In the 19th century, the molecules responsible for their pharmaceutical properties were isolated from plants and led to synthetic drug development. The term pharmacognosy was conceived to describe this scientific study of medicinal plants.

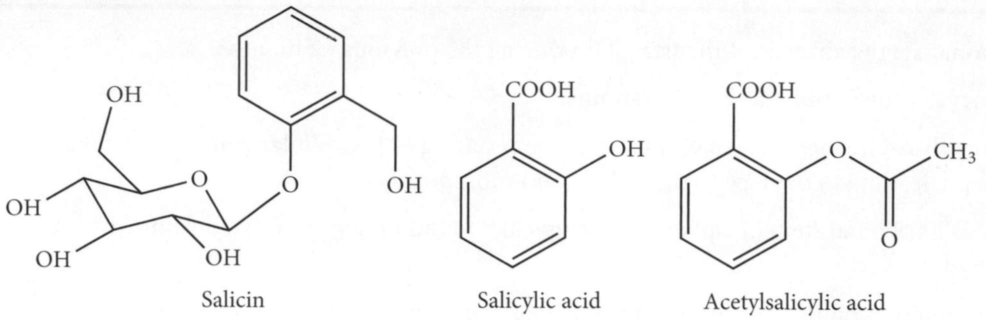

Figure 13.1 Structures of salicin, salicylic acid, and acetylsalicylic acid.

Aspirin is an example of a synthetic compound derived from modification of a natural chemical. It was discovered that salicin, a prodrug isolated from willow bark, converted to salicylic acid in the gastrointestinal tract. By replacing the acidic property with an acetyl group, the Bayer company was able to convert salicylic acid to acetylsalicylic acid, more commonly known as aspirin (**Figure 13.1**). Other examples of the first pure drug isolates from nature are included in **Table 13.1**.

Pharmacognosy is largely responsible for the evolution of pharmacy as a component of conventional medicine. Modern drug discovery techniques continue to utilize natural sources for the isolation of medicinal molecules to use as new drug prototypes. In addition, there is currently a substantial demand for natural remedies as part of complementary and alternative medicine (CAM) in Western medicine, while some cultures solely utilize natural products for the treatment and prevention of disease.

The 2007 United States National Health Interview Survey reported that 38% of adults and 12% of children used some form of CAM in the previous 12 months, with the highest rates found among the 50- to 59-year-old group. Pain and musculoskeletal problems have been identified as the most common reasons for CAM use. CAM encompasses mind–body medicine (i.e., meditation and acupuncture), manipulative and body-based practices (i.e., spinal manipulation and massage therapy), natural products, and other practices including Pilates, magnet therapy, and healing touch. Natural products and nutraceuticals are available without a prescription, are sold as dietary supplements, and are the most widely utilized type of CAM modalities. Fish oil/omega-3, glucosamine, Echinacea, and flaxseed have been cited as the most popular natural products. Many patients perceive CAM as being better than conventional care due to their belief that purely synthetic medications lack efficacy or due to their concerns about adverse drug events.

Table 13.1 Examples of Drugs Derived from Plants

Drug	Origin	Use
Atropine	Belladonna (*Atropa belladonna*)	Asthma, diarrhea, menopausal symptoms
Caffeine	Coffee shrub (*Coffea arabica*)	Stimulant
Digoxin	Foxglove (*Digitalis* spp.)	Heart failure or heart arrhythmias
Morphine	Opium poppy (*Papaver somniferum*)	Analgesic
Quinine	Cinchona bark (*Cinchona* spp.)	Malaria
Salicin	Willow bark (*Salix* spp.)	Analgesic, antipyretic, anti-inflammatory
Taxol	Pacific yew (*Taxus brevifolia*)	Anticancer treatment

Data from: Heinrich M, Barnes J, Gibbons S, Williamson EM. Phytotherapy and pharmacognosy. In: *Fundamentals of pharmacognosy and phytotherapy.* Edinburgh, UK: Churchill Livingstone; 2004:4–21.

Regulatory Information

The Dietary Supplement Health and Education Act (DSHEA) of 1994 provided regulation to establish standards with respect to dietary supplements. The DSHEA defined a dietary supplement as "a product (other than tobacco) intended to supplement the diet that bears or contains one or more of the following dietary ingredients:

- A vitamin;

- A mineral;

- An herb or other botanical;

- An amino acid;

- A dietary substance for use by man to supplement the diet by increasing the total dietary intake; or

- A concentrate, metabolite, constituent, extract or combination of an[y] ingredient described" previously.

The DSHEA classified dietary supplements as foods rather than drugs. Foods, including dietary supplements, are regulated by the U.S. Food and Drug Administration (FDA) under the Center for Food Safety and Applied Nutrition (CFSAN), whereas drugs are regulated by the FDA under the Center for Drug Evaluation Research (CDER). As a result, dietary supplements do not have to follow the strict standards of evidence for safety and efficacy that are required for nonprescription and prescription drugs. The manufacturers of nonprescription and prescription drugs are required to perform clinical trials to document the safety and efficacy of a drug prior to its approval for marketing by the FDA. Dietary supplements marketed before the DSHEA came into effect are not required to be approved by the FDA, as they are considered safe based on history and experience of use. However, a list of dietary supplements marketed before enactment of the DSHEA is not available, leaving the decision whether to claim this status up to the manufacturer. Manufacturers of new dietary supplements—that is, products marketed after the DSHEA became law—must provide the FDA with reasonable evidence that the product is safe for human use. Dietary supplements, in contrast to nonprescription and prescription drugs, are not approved by the FDA for safety and efficacy before the products are marketed. The DSHEA placed the burden of proof of safety on the FDA, thus requiring the FDA to prove a dietary supplement is harmful before the product can be removed from the market.

The DSHEA also provided guidance for ingredient and nutrition labeling of dietary supplements. All dietary supplements are required to carry a Supplement Facts label, which closely resembles the Nutrition Facts label found on food products, rather than the Drug Facts label found on nonprescription medications. Although manufacturers of dietary supplements do not have to provide evidence of efficacy of the product prior to marketing, certain restrictions apply to the claims that can be made on dietary supplement labels. Manufacturers of dietary supplements cannot claim that the product will diagnose, cure, mitigate, treat, or prevent a disease. Instead, three types of claims are allowed for dietary supplements: a health claim, a nutrient content claim, or a structure/function claim.

A health claim describes the connection between a food, food component, or dietary supplement and the resulting decreased risk of a disease or health-related condition. A statement that consuming a diet low in sodium may reduce the risk of high blood pressure is an example of a health claim. A nutrient content claim describes the amount of a nutrient or dietary substance in a product using comparative terminology (free, low, and reduced). An example of a nutrient content claim is stating that a product has "zero calories," which is defined as fewer than five calories per reference amount and per labeled serving. Both health and nutrient content claims require FDA approval for use on food and dietary supplement labels. A list of approved health and nutrient content claims can be found in Appendices C and A, respectively, of *A Food Labeling Guide*.

A structure/function claim describes how a nutrient or dietary supplement may affect organs or systems in the body, but cannot include statements about any specific disease. A statement that calcium maintains strong bones is an example of a structure/function claim. Structure/function claims are not approved by the FDA, and labeling on dietary supplement products must include the following disclaimer: "This statement has not been evaluated by the Food and Drug Administration. This product is not intended to diagnose, treat, cure, or prevent any disease." Dietary supplement manufacturers must provide the FDA with the wording of the structure/function claim that appears on the label within 30 days of marketing a product.

The DSHEA also allowed for the establishment of standards for good manufacturing practices (GMP) for the production of dietary supplements, which had been lacking. Prior to enactment of the DSHEA, determining the quality of a dietary supplement was difficult because manufacturers had to meet quality standards related to foods, not drugs. In 2007, the FDA released the final rule that describes the minimum requirements for GMP for dietary supplement manufacturers. Following GMP ensures that the dietary supplement contains the amount of ingredients listed on the label and does not include contaminants such as bacteria, heavy metals, or pesticides. Now dietary supplements are expected to be guaranteed by the manufacturer to meet standards related to the identity, purity, strength, and composition.

In an effort to improve reporting of safety information related to dietary supplements and nonprescription drugs, the Dietary Supplement and Nonprescription Drug Consumer Protection Act was passed in 2006. This law requires manufacturers of dietary supplements to report serious adverse events—defined as death, a life-threatening experience, inpatient hospitalization, a persistent or significant disability or incapacity, a congenital anomaly or birth defect, or an event that requires medical or surgical intervention—to the FDA. Improved reporting of adverse events allows the FDA to monitor and evaluate dietary supplements and take action to remove a product if it is deemed harmful.

Because dietary supplements are not required to be standardized or tested for safety and effectiveness before they are marketed, a number of organizations have implemented quality assurance programs. These programs test various dietary supplements to determine whether the product meets reference standards and then certify the product composition by providing a seal of approval. Such certification means that the product contains the ingredients in the quantity stated on the label but does not address safety or efficacy of the dietary supplement. Three reputable organizations that provide dietary supplement verification programs are the United States Pharmacopoeia (USP), ConsumerLab, and the National Sanitation Foundation International (NSFI).

Evidence-Based Resources

This chapter focuses on well-known natural products and is organized by common indications for their use. The intent is not to provide an extensive review of all nutraceuticals. There are hundreds of dietary supplements, and many references or databases are available as resources for this purpose (**Table 13.2**). Recommendations for the use of natural products should be provided with caution, as clinical trial data supporting the use of natural products are often lacking due to small sample sizes and flawed methodologies.

Drug information databases such as the Natural Standard and Natural Medicines Comprehensive Database contain monographs of natural products, and provide product efficacy and safety overviews. These drug compendia are updated periodically, but may not always include

Table 13.2 Reputable Natural Product Information Resources

Resource	Accessibility
National Center for Complementary and Alternative Medicine (NCCAM)	http://nccam.nih.gov
Natural Standard	Electronic database http//www.naturalstandard.com
Natural Medicines Comprehensive Database	Electronic database, print, personal digital assistant (PDA) http//www.naturaldatabase.com
Cochrane Library	http//www.cochrane.org

the most recently published information. MEDLINE (Medical Literature Analysis and Retrieval System) should be searched to find up-to-date biomedical information. Clinical trial data, meta-analyses, and review articles identified in MEDLINE and the Cochrane Database should be reviewed and interpreted to accurately answer drug information requests. The Cochrane Library provides systematic reviews and meta-analyses of biomedical research, and is a highly regarded resource for evidence-based information. The National Center for Complementary and Alternative Medicine (NCCAM) is part of the National Institutes of Health and is responsible for advancing research of nonconventional medicine. The NCCAM website provides information about CAM research opportunities and studies in progress, and contains concise natural product monographs.

Cardiovascular Health

Coenzyme Q10

Therapeutic Properties/Pharmacology

Coenzyme Q10 (CoQ10), also known as ubiquinone, is a natural substance found within the mitochondria of all cells. It is predominantly concentrated in the tissues of the heart, liver, pancreas, and kidney.

Clinical Evidence

Coenzyme Q10 has been studied for use in hypertension, congestive heart failure, myocardial infarction, Parkinson's disease, and migraine headaches, as well as some other disease states. Evidence supporting the use of coenzyme Q10 for these disease states is conflicting. Currently, the best evidence available supports the use of this product for its blood pressure lowering effects. Several small clinical trials have observed blood pressure reductions with supplementation of coenzyme Q10. A meta-analysis conducted by Rosenfeldt et al. showed clinically significant reductions in systolic blood pressure of as much as 17 mm Hg and diastolic blood pressure of as much as 10 mm Hg. A Cochrane review found coenzyme Q10 to produce reductions in systolic blood pressure of 11 mm Hg and diastolic blood pressure of 7 mm Hg when compared to placebo. However, the Cochrane review concluded that due to concerns about the reliability of the existing studies, it is unclear whether coenzyme Q10 is effective in reducing blood pressure on a long-term basis. Large, randomized, double-blind clinical trials assessing the impact of coenzyme Q10 on clinical end points such as stroke and death from cardiac causes, rather than surrogate markers, have not been completed. At this time coenzyme Q10 could be recommended as an adjunct to other antihypertensive therapies.

A theoretical use for coenzyme Q10 is in the treatment of statin-induced myopathy. One mechanism proposed for statin-induced muscle pain that does not stem from rhabdomyolysis is coenzyme Q10 deficiency. HMG-CoA reductase inhibitors (statins), by blocking cholesterol production, also block the endogenous synthesis of coenzyme Q10. Studies have shown that statins reduce blood levels of coenzyme Q10. It is unclear how statins might affect intramuscular levels of coenzyme Q10. If they take coenzyme Q10 supplements, patients with statin-induced myopathy might have decreased muscle pain and be able to continue with statin therapy. Review of the limited studies available shows inconsistent results, however. Until large clinical trials can definitively document the effectiveness of coenzyme Q10 supplementation, this product should not be recommended as a mainstay of therapy, but instead could be used on a trial basis for patients who develop muscle pain.

Dosage and Safety Considerations

Doses of coenzyme Q10 for the treatment of hypertension range from 120 200 mg taken by mouth daily in divided doses. The dose used for statin-induced myopathy ranges from 100 200 mg taken by mouth daily or 300 mg taken by mouth as 100 mg three times daily. Coenzyme Q10 is taken in divided doses to reduce the incidence of adverse effects. Overall, it is well tolerated, with gastrointestinal effects (abdominal pain, nausea, vomiting, diarrhea) being the most frequently reported adverse effects.

Coenzyme Q10 has a structure similar to vitamin K. Consequently, it is theorized that a drug interaction between coenzyme Q10 and warfarin could exist. One small randomized, double-blind, placebo-crossover study looking at the effects of coenzyme Q10 and warfarin found no interaction. Patients taking warfarin who initiate coenzyme Q10 supplementation should notify their physician and monitor the International Normalized Ratio (INR) more frequently.

Fish Oil

Therapeutic Properties/Pharmacology

Fish oil, obtained via food sources or supplementation, contains the omega-3 fatty acids docosahexaenoic acid (DHA) and eicosapentaenoic acid (EPA). It has been studied for use in lowering triglycerides, primary (those without coronary heart disease) and secondary (those with coronary heart disease) prevention of cardiovascular disease, and rheumatoid arthritis. Extensive research shows consistent benefits of omega-3 fatty acids in the reduction of triglycerides by 14% to 25%, with higher doses perhaps having a greater effect. These benefits are also supported by the FDA approval of the prescription product Lovaza (omega-3 acid ethyl esters). Lovaza is indicated as a primary therapy in addition to diet for adult patients with triglyceride levels greater than or equal to 500 mg/dL. Current treatment guidelines for cholesterol indications recommend supplementation of omega-3 fatty acids to lower triglycerides as an alternative to fibrates or nicotinic acid. The mechanism for reduction of triglycerides is a combination of a reduced synthesis in the liver and increased clearance.

Clinical Evidence

To date, clinical trials focusing on omega-3 fatty acid supplementation for primary prevention of coronary heart disease are lacking. The Japan EPA Lipid Intervention Study (JELIS), a large prospective study that included patients with hypercholesterolemia with and without coronary heart disease, found that the omega-3 fatty acid EPA was able to reduce risk of coronary events. However, more studies need to be completed to verify these effects in other populations. Data from secondary prevention trials are more impressive, with significant reductions in all-cause and cardiovascular mortality being reported, although many of these trials were completed prior to widespread use of statins. Again, more studies need to be completed to determine the benefits of omega-3 fatty acids in combination with modern lipid-lowering therapy.

Dosage and Safety Considerations

To treat elevated triglycerides, the American Heart Association (AHA) recommends a minimum of 2 grams of omega-3 fatty acids per day, but notes that higher doses of 4 grams per day may be needed. In patients without evidence of coronary heart disease, supplementation with omega-3 fatty acids is not routinely recommended. For these patients, the AHA recommends obtaining omega-3 fatty acids from food sources by including oily fish at a minimum of two meals per week. For patients with coronary heart disease, the AHA recommends 1 gram per day of omega-3 fatty acids. Clinical trials have used doses ranging from 1 to 6 grams per day.

A key component to dosing of omega-3 fatty acids is the content and ratio of DHA and EPA. The dosage recommendations described previously refer to the combined amount of DHA and EPA rather than the total dose listed for the fish oil capsule. For example, a bottle of fish oil might state that the capsules contain 1,200 mg of fish oil, but upon inspection of the Supplement Facts label it might become apparent that the DHA and EPA content is only 720 mg. It is also important to read the serving size to determine the number of capsules that will provide the amount of DHA and EPA. The best ratio of DHA and EPA has not been determined. Until clinical trials can appropriately evaluate and determine the concentrations, it is best to take a supplement that provides DHA and EPA in amounts similar to Lovaza (375 mg DHA and 465 mg EPA), as this product has the most data supporting its use.

Common adverse effects associated with omega-3 fatty acids include gastrointestinal upset and fish burps. These can be minimized by taking the supplements with meals, using enteric-coated products, and taking the products before bedtime. Observational studies have shown the potential for omega-3 fatty acids to prolong bleeding time, but clinical trials have not demonstrated alterations in bleeding time or warfarin dosing regimens.

Garlic

Therapeutic Properties/Pharmacology

Garlic is the common name of the culinary herb derived from the bulbs of *Allium sativum*. It has been studied for use in hyperlipidemia, in hypertension, as an anti-infective, and in the prevention of certain cancers. Most research conducted using garlic has been related to reduction in serum cholesterol levels. Two mechanisms have been proposed for the lipid-lowering effects of garlic: decreased absorption of cholesterol from the intestine and inhibition or deactivation of enzymes utilized for cholesterol synthesis.

Clinical Evidence

Previous evidence suggesting that garlic was an effective agent to lower cholesterol levels has now become controversial, as more recent meta-analyses have shown smaller reductions in cholesterol. Earlier studies focused on reductions in total cholesterol, whereas newer studies have incorporated measurement of the other lipid components, especially low-density lipoprotein (LDL) and high-density lipoprotein (HDL) cholesterol levels. A meta-analysis performed by Reinhart et al. found statistically significant reductions in total cholesterol and triglycerides of 4% and 22%, respectively. Although statistically significant, these modest reductions may have limited clinical relevance. The same study found very small changes in LDL and HDL, which did not achieve statistical or clinical significance. Another meta-analysis conducted by Khoo et al. failed to find any statistically significant changes on any lipid profile component. The various systematic reviews have yielded conflicting results, which does not provide convincing evidence of the effectiveness of garlic for use in hypercholesterolemia.

Dosage and Safety Considerations

Dosages of garlic studied to lower cholesterol have consisted of 3–5 mg or a product standardized to 1.3% allicin content daily. Garlic contains alliin, which when crushed is broken down by the enzyme alliinase and converted to allicin. Allicin is believed to be the active component and the part of garlic's volatile oil that gives it the characteristic aroma.

The most common adverse effects from garlic are bad breath and body odor. Although the adverse effects are mild, garlic can cause gastrointestinal discomfort such as nausea, vomiting, and heartburn. Enteric-coated products may reduce the unwanted gastrointestinal effects by delaying the release of allicin until the product reaches the intestine. While odorless garlic products may seem desirable, there is concern that these products may not contain the appropriate amount of allicin.

Garlic is also thought to inhibit platelet function. Consequently, it is theorized that a drug interaction between garlic and warfarin could exist. Patients taking warfarin who initiate garlic supplementation should notify their physician and receive more frequent monitoring of their INR.

Hawthorn

Therapeutic Properties/Pharmacology

Hawthorn is a popular herbal made from the leaves, flowers, and berries of the hawthorn bush. It is used for the treatment of angina, hypertension, and arrhythmias, with most research into its effects focusing on its use in congestive heart failure (CHF). Oligomeric procyanidins and flavonoids are considered the active components of hawthorn and are thought to be responsible for the pharmacologic effects. Oligomeric procyanidins have been proposed to increase coronary blood flow, have a positive inotropic effect, improve the force-frequency ratio, and act as free-radical scavengers. Flavonoids are thought to increase vasodilation, inhibit cholesterol synthesis, and inhibit platelet aggregation and adhesion.

Clinical Evidence

A Cochrane review published in 2009 assessed studies that compared hawthorn extract as an adjunct to conventional heart failure medications with placebo. The review found a 9% increase in the maximal workload in patients with CHF compared to placebo. Changes in such subjective measures are promising but do not always correlate to mortality. This study was not able to assess long-term outcomes such as cardiac death or nonfatal myocardial infarction.

The Hawthorn Extract Randomized Blinded Chronic Heart Failure Trial (HERB CHF) compared 450 mg twice daily of hawthorn to placebo for 6 months. The primary outcome was an increase in the 6-minute walking distance at 6 months. The study found no difference in the exercise capacity of patients who took hawthorn versus placebo when the supplement was added to standard medical therapy.

The first large-scale trial to assess morbidity and mortality outcomes related to hawthorn supplementation was the Efficacy and Safety of Crataegus Extract WS 1442 in Patients with Heart Failure: The SPICE Trial. This study compared 900 mg per day of a standardized hawthorn extract (WS 1442) to placebo in adult patients with New York Heart Association Class II or III heart failure who also had reduced left ventricular ejection fractions. The primary outcome was time to first cardiac event (cardiac death, nonfatal myocardial infarction, or hospitalization due to progressive heart failure). Although a small difference in average time to first cardiac event was found, the result did not reach statistical significance. A subgroup analysis of patients who had left ventricular ejection fractions in the range of 25% to 35% found sudden cardiac death was significantly reduced by 39.7%.

Proven conventional therapies are available for CHF, and hawthorn may be effective for symptom reduction when used as an adjunct. Widespread use of hawthorn should be limited until more data are available that support the safety and efficacy of this supplement for long-term use.

Dosage and Safety Considerations

Extracts of hawthorn are typically standardized to 18.75% oligomeric procyanidins and 2.2% flavonoids. Dosages used in clinical trials range 160 mg to 1,800 mg administered in two to three divided doses. Most studies to date have used WS 1442 and LI 132 standardized leaf and flower extracts of hawthorn.

Hawthorn is generally well tolerated and produces only minimal adverse effects, with vertigo and dizziness being the most common. Other mild, transient effects (gastrointestinal discomfort, headache, and palpitations) have been reported.

Drug interactions have not been well documented and are based on the various proposed mechanisms of action of hawthorn. These proposed interacting drugs include antihypertensives, vasodilators, antiarrhythmics, and (although somewhat controversial) digoxin. Patients taking digoxin who initiate hawthorn supplementation should notify their physician, and their digoxin levels should be monitored more frequently.

Policosanol

Therapeutic Properties/Pharmacology

Policosanol is a combination of eight long-chain alcohols extracted from the wax constituent of sugar cane. When derived from other sources (beeswax, rice, sunflower seed, and wheat germ), policosanol has not been shown to be effective medicinally. It has been studied for use in hyperlipidemia and intermittent claudication. The mechanism by which policosanol produces its lipid-lowering effects is not fully understood, but it is proposed to work by inhibiting cholesterol synthesis and potentially has a direct lipid-lowering effect in the intestine.

Clinical Evidence

Most of the original evidence supporting the use of policosanol for lowering cholesterol levels was published by one Cuban research group. More recently, studies published in other countries have failed to find an effect on lipid concentrations. This discrepancy has led to controversy over the true benefits of policosanol.

A meta-analysis of studies published from 1967 to 2003 was performed with a primary end point of reduction in LDL cholesterol levels. Using an average daily dose of 12 mg, the analysis found statistically significant reductions in total cholesterol (16.2%) and LDL (23.7%), along with a statistically significant increase in HDL (10.6%). Triglycerides were reduced by 12.4%, which was not statistically significant. The study concluded that policosanol lowered LDL levels similarly to prescription medications.

Two randomized, double-blind, placebo-controlled trials tested the effectiveness of policosanol 20 mg daily to determine its lipoprotein-lowering effects. Both studies found no statistically significant changes in any lipid profile component.

None of these studies addressed effects on mortality, but rather focused on surrogate markers of lipid profile data. Due to the recent uncertainty that has arisen regarding the effectiveness of policosanol, its use cannot be recommended at this time.

Dosage and Safety Considerations

Daily dosages of policosanol used in clinical trials have ranged from 5 mg to 40 mg, with typical starting doses of 5–10 mg and maintenance doses of 10–20 mg. The maximal clinical benefit seems to occur with doses of 20 mg per day. When daily dosages greater than 10 mg are taken, it is recommended that the supplement be given in divided doses. Policosanol should be taken in the evening, as that is when cholesterol synthesis in the liver occurs.

Policosanol is well tolerated with minimal adverse effects. The meta-analysis performed by Chen et al. found that adverse effects were more likely to be reported with use of placebo (4.81%) than with policosanol (0.86%). The most frequent adverse effects reported are central nervous system (somnolence, nervousness, dizziness, insomnia), gastrointestinal discomfort (polydipsia, polyphagia, diarrhea, nausea, heartburn), and hypotension. Drug interactions have not been well documented and are based on the various proposed mechanisms of action of policosanol.

Policosanol is also thought to inhibit platelet function. Therefore, it is theorized that a drug interaction between policosanol and warfarin could exist. Patients taking warfarin who initiate policosanol supplementation should notify their physician and undergo more frequent monitoring of their INR.

Learning Bridge 13.1

MW, a 45-year-old Caucasian male, presents to the community pharmacy with a new prescription for Lovaza and a bottle of 1,000-mg fish oil capsules containing a combination of 300 mg of DHA and EPA per capsule. He has a question and would like to talk to the pharmacist before the prescription is filled. "Is this Lovaza the same thing as fish oil? Can't I get that over the counter without a prescription?"

A. What is the mechanism of action of fish oil in lowering triglycerides?
B. What are adverse effects commonly associated with fish oil, and what are some ways to reduce them?
C. What is the difference between Lovaza and the over-the-counter fish oil dietary supplement that the patient selected?

Cold and Flu

AndrogrAPHIS

Therapeutic Properties/Pharmacology

Andrographis (*Andrographis paniculata*) is an annual herb whose leaves and rhizome are used for medicinal purposes. While not commonly used in the United States, andrographis has been used in Chinese and Thai herbal medicine for the treatment of various conditions. It is gaining popularity in Europe as a treatment for upper respiratory infections such as the common cold and influenza. Andrographolide and its derivatives are considered the active components of andrographis and are thought to be responsible for the pharmacologic effects. The mechanism by which andrographis works to treat cold symptoms is thought to be related to immune system stimulation, antipyretic, and anti-inflammatory properties.

Clinical Evidence

A systematic review of the literature performed by Kligler et al. identified two previously conducted systematic reviews and seven clinical trials of andrographis for the treatment of upper respiratory infections. The systematic reviews found statistically significant differences that favored andrographis over placebo in reducing upper respiratory infection symptom severity. Results from the seven clinical trials using andrographis were positive overall, but lacked consistency. The Kligler et al. systematic review also included one trial in which andrographis was used for prevention of upper respiratory infections. Patients were randomized to receive andrographis extract or placebo for 3 months. The study found a statistically significant reduction in diagnosis of upper respiratory infections in the andrographis treatment group compared to the placebo recipients.

It is important to point out some limitations of the studies conducted to date. Many of these studies were carried out in collaboration with the leading manufacturer of andrographis preparations. Another limitation is that the trials did not use a validated tool to assess upper respiratory infection symptoms and disease progression.

Overall, the evidence for use of andrographis in the treatment of symptoms related to upper respiratory infections is promising, but additional standardized studies are needed to clarify its effectiveness. Because only one trial has assessed the effectiveness of andrographis for prevention of upper respiratory infections, it cannot be recommended for this use at this time.

Dosage and Safety Considerations

Most of the clinical trials of andrographis have used a commercially available, standardized product known as Kan Jang. It is available both as a combination product that contains andrographis and eleutherococcus and as a single-herb product containing only andrographis. The combination product (andrographis 88.8 mg and eleutherococcus 10 mg per tablet) was dosed using two tablets three times daily. The single-herb product has been studied at a dose of 400 mg taken three times daily. Doses of 3–6 grams of dried leaves per day have been studied. It is recommended to use andrographis within 36–48 hours of symptom onset.

Short-term treatment with andrographis is associated with few adverse event reports. Allergic reactions and rash at typical doses and gastrointestinal upset (nausea, vomiting, abdominal discomfort) at high doses have been seen. No drug interactions have been documented with andrographis. Due to immune system stimulatory effects, it has been theorized that andrographis might potentially worsen autoimmune disorders or decrease the effectiveness of immunosuppressant medications, resulting in transplant rejection.

Echinacea

Therapeutic Properties/Pharmacology

Echinacea refers to the genus of plants frequently used for prevention and treatment of the common cold as well as other respiratory infections. The common cold is a viral infection of the upper respiratory tract; as there is no cure for this infection, treatment focuses on symptom management. Echinacea is thought to modulate the immune system by activating macrophages, increasing phagocytosis, enhancing cytokine production and natural killer cell activity, improving lymphocyte and monocyte cell counts, and improving antibody response. Activity of Echinacea against viruses, fungi, and inflammation has been observed.

Clinical Evidence

A Cochrane review evaluated two trials using Echinacea for 8 to 12 weeks for prevention of the common cold. The trials used the number of participants with one cold compared to the number of participants with more than one cold as outcomes. The results showed no statistically significant difference in the number of colds and reduction in cold symptom duration or severity.

The majority of clinical trials have studied the effectiveness of Echinacea for the treatment of the common cold, when the supplement was taken at the onset of cold symptoms to reduce the duration and severity of those symptoms. After reviewing the evidence, the Cochrane review concluded that supplementation with *Echinacea purpurea* might be effective to reduce symptom duration and severity when used for early cold treatment. The evidence relating to the effectiveness of other Echinacea preparations is lacking. Due to the differences in studied outcomes, cold symptom scoring systems, and types of Echinacea preparations, clarification is needed before Echinacea can be recommended for routine use.

Dosage and Safety Considerations

The dosages of Echinacea used in clinical trials have varied depending on the dosage form and the type of plant preparation. Echinacea extract of 2,000–3,000 mg, pressed juice of 6–9 mL, and 0.75–1.5 mL of tincture per day have all been studied. In addition, three different species of Echinacea have been studied (*E. angustifolia*, *E. pallida*, and *E. purpurea*). No standardization exists, such that commercial products could include various species of Echinacea as well as varying parts of the plant (roots, leaves, or flowers). There is no consensus as to which is most effective.

Echinacea is generally well tolerated, with infrequent adverse effects of gastrointestinal upset, headache, and rash being reported. Allergic reactions in patients with allergies to daisies, marigolds, ragweed, or other members of the Asteraceae family have been reported.

A review of the literature conducted by Freeman et al. concluded that Echinacea has a low potential to produce cytochrome P450 drug–herb interactions. Due to this product's immune system stimulatory effects, it has been theorized that Echinacea could worsen autoimmune disorders or decrease the effectiveness of immunosuppressant medications, resulting in transplant rejection.

Elderberry

Therapeutic Properties/Pharmacology

Elderberry or black elder is the common name for *Sambucus nigra*, whose berries have been used to treat influenza, the common cold, and herpes viral infections. Flavonoids found in elderberries are the component believed to exert an antiviral effect. Specifically related to influenza A and B, elderberry is thought to neutralize hemagglutinin, thereby preventing the virus from binding and entering cells, as well as inhibiting viral replication. Elderberry may exert immunomodulating effects by stimulating production of interleukins and tumor necrosis factor as well as cytokines. Elderberries contain vitamin A, various B vitamins, vitamin C, folic acid, and other components that may provide an antioxidant effect.

Clinical Evidence

Two clinical trials have evaluated the effectiveness of elderberry for treatment of influenza. Zakay-Rones et al. completed a randomized, placebo-controlled trial that included 60 patients who had confirmed cases of influenza. Patients received 15 mL of a standardized elderberry or placebo syrup with meals four times daily for 5 days; the first dose was administered within 48 hours of influenza-like symptoms onset. A clinically and statistically significant difference ($p < 0.001$) in "pronounced improvement" was found in patients in the treatment group 4 days sooner than in the placebo group. Mostly animal studies have been conducted on the use of elderberry, and additional studies are needed to verify this supplement's safety and effectiveness in humans.

Dosage and Safety Considerations

The Zakay-Rones et al. trial utilized a commercially available standardized elderberry extract called Sambucol (Raei Bar, Jerusalem, Israel). The dose was 15 mL of a 38% standardized extract of elderberry juice, taken four times daily for 3–5 days. Given that only one formulation of elderberry has been studied in clinical trials, it is not known if other elderberry products would offer the same benefit.

Elderberry is well tolerated, with no adverse effects being reported. Consuming fresh berries that have not been appropriately heated has caused nausea, vomiting, and diarrhea. No drug interactions have been reported. Due to its potential immune system stimulatory effects, elderberry could theoretically decrease the effectiveness of immunosuppressant medications, resulting in transplant rejection.

Diabetes

American Ginseng

Therapeutic Properties/Pharmacology

American ginseng is the common name for *Panax quinquefolius*, an herb whose root is used for the treatment of diabetes mellitus, immune modulation, and cognition. It is important not to confuse American ginseng and Asian ginseng (*Panax ginseng*), as the two species display different effects. Three proposed mechanisms by which American ginseng has effects on blood glucose are decreased carbohydrate absorption, increased cellular glucose uptake, and increased insulin production.

Clinical Evidence

Several small clinical trials have found statistically significant reductions in postprandial glucose levels with use of American ginseng. Vuksan et al. randomized patients, with ($n = 9$) and without ($n = 10$) diabetes, to receive 3 grams of American ginseng or placebo either 40 minutes prior to or with a 25-gram oral glucose challenge. The results showed statistically significant reductions in blood glucose concentrations for patients with and without diabetes when the American ginseng was administered 40 minutes before the glucose challenge.

Another trial randomized 10 patients (6 men, 4 women) with type 2 diabetes to receive placebo or 3, 6, or 9 grams of American ginseng at various time periods prior to a 25-gram oral glucose challenge. The results showed statistically significant reductions in blood glucose levels when using 3 grams of American ginseng regardless of the administration time. The study concluded that due to reductions in blood glucose levels 2 hours after the glucose challenge, American ginseng shows clinical significance for patients with diabetes.

The available data from clinical trials suggest a potential benefit may be realized with use of American ginseng for the treatment of diabetes. However, until long-term studies are able to verify the data collected in previous short-term trials, the limitations of the short treatment durations and small sample sizes in research conducted to date rule out recommending the widespread use of American ginseng.

Dosage and Safety Considerations

Dosages to lower postprandial blood glucose range from 1 to 9 grams of American ginseng administered up to 2 hours before a meal. The components in American ginseng believed to be active and to provide the medicinal benefit are ginsenosides. As more than 60 ginsenosides have been identified, different ginseng products or lots of the same product may contain inconsistent amounts of the active components. To date, ginseng extracts lack standardization. Due to the variability in type and quantity of ginsenosides found in commercial products, it is difficult to evaluate the safety and efficacy of American ginseng products.

American ginseng has been well tolerated in clinical trials, and adverse effects are rare. Monitoring for adverse effects should include blood pressure, heart rate, sleep patterns, and diarrhea.

There is potential for additive blood glucose lowering when this product is combined with other medications used to treat diabetes; this effect could result in severe hypoglycemia. American ginseng also reduces warfarin's anticoagulant effect. Patients taking warfarin who initiate American ginseng supplementation should notify their physician and receive more frequent INR monitoring.

Cinnamon

Therapeutic Properties/Pharmacology

Cinnamon is a spice obtained from the bark of *Cinnamonum* trees. There are two types of cinnamon: *Cinnamonum verum* (also known as *Cinnamomum zeylanicum*) and *Cinnamomum cassia*. *Cinnamonum cassia* is the type most commonly used medicinally and as a spice. Cinnamon is most notably known for lowering blood glucose to treat type 2 diabetes, insulin resistance, and metabolic syndrome. It is thought to work by increasing insulin sensitivity and cellular uptake of glucose.

Clinical Evidence

Conflicting evidence has been gathered related to the effectiveness of cinnamon when used to lower blood glucose. Several randomized, double-blind, placebo-controlled trials have shown reductions in fasting blood glucose and hemoglobin A_{1c} when patients took cinnamon for as long as 4 months. A study performed by Mang et al. randomized 79 patients with type 2 diabetes to either 3 grams of cinnamon daily or placebo for 4 months to determine the supplement's effects on fasting blood glucose and hemoglobin A_{1c}, as well as various lipid components. Cinnamon lowered fasting blood glucose by 10.3%, while placebo had a 3.4% reduction; this was a statistically significant difference ($p = 0.046$). No statistically significant differences in hemoglobin A_{1c} or any lipid component were observed.

In contrast, a Cochrane review found that the use of cinnamon did not improve hemoglobin A_{1c}, insulin levels, or postprandial blood glucose. Likewise, a meta-analysis of five prospective, randomized, controlled trials performed by Baker et al. found no statistically significant changes in hemoglobin A_{1c}, fasting blood glucose, or any lipid component when cinnamon was compared to placebo. Both the Cochrane review and the Baker et al. meta-analysis identified various limitations in the trials included. Poor-quality study design, short treatment duration, and inadequate sample size were limitations that led to an inability to detect statistically significant differences.

Long-term clinical trials with larger populations are needed to determine the efficacy of cinnamon. Proven conventional therapies for diabetes should be utilized initially, but cinnamon could be considered an adjunct to these therapies for interested patients.

Dosage and Safety Considerations

Studies with cinnamon have used divided daily dosages ranging from 1 to 6 grams, with the doses being taken with meals. The active component of cinnamon thought to be responsible for the increased insulin sensitivity is procyanidin type-A polymers. No standardization of supplements exists, however, so commercial products could use whole cinnamon or a water-soluble cinnamon extract.

Cinnamon is generally well tolerated, with no adverse effects reported in many clinical trials, although no clinical trials have lasted longer than 4 months. Adverse effects such as skin irritation, mucous membrane irritation, and stomatitis have been reported when using cinnamon as a flavoring spice but have not been reported when the product was used in clinical trials.

There is potential for additive blood glucose lowering when cinnamon is combined with other medications used to treat diabetes; this could result in severe hypoglycemia. Based on the coumarin component of cinnamon, there is a theoretical interaction with warfarin. Although no such interactions have been reported, patients taking warfarin who initiate cinnamon supplementation should notify their physician and receive more frequent INR monitoring.

Fenugreek

Therapeutic Properties/Pharmacology

Fenugreek is the common name for the plant *Trigonella foenum-graecum*, whose seeds are rich in fiber, protein, and saponins. Fenugreek is an herb commonly used in Indian cooking. It has been used for various indications including induction of labor, initiating lactation, and aiding digestion. The results of more recent trials suggest fenugreek may have hypoglycemic effects and would be useful for the treatment of type 2 diabetes. Among the proposed mechanisms for lowering blood glucose are delayed gastric emptying, slowed carbohydrate absorption from the intestine, and glucose-induced insulin release from pancreatic beta cells. A secondary mechanism relates to the fact that fenugreek seeds contain 50% fiber (30% soluble fiber and 20% insoluble fiber), which may help to lower postprandial glucose.

Clinical Evidence

Only a few clinical trials have evaluated the effectiveness of fenugreek as a means to lower blood glucose. A 2011 meta-analysis found two randomized placebo-controlled trials assessing the effectiveness of this herb in patients with type 2 diabetes for 8 weeks' duration that met the meta-analysis inclusion criteria. Pooled data from the clinical trials showed fenugreek significantly decreased hemoglobin A_{1c} ($p = 0.03$), whereas no effect on fasting blood glucose was observed. The evidence to date suggests fenugreek may be effective for lowering hemoglobin A_{1c} and potentially blood glucose, but further studies are needed to verify these effects.

Dosage and Safety Considerations

Dosages used in clinical trials range from 1 to 5 grams per day. Fifteen grams of ground fenugreek seeds taken with a meal has been shown to lower postprandial glucose in patients with type 2 diabetes. As much as 100 grams per day in divided doses has been used.

Fenugreek is generally well tolerated, with minimal adverse effects being reported. Due to its high fiber content, this herb can cause gastrointestinal upset such as nausea, diarrhea, and flatulence. The high fiber content could also interfere with the absorption of other oral medications from the intestine.

There is potential for additive blood glucose lowering when fenugreek is combined with other medications used to treat diabetes; this could result in severe hypoglycemia. Because fenugreek may contain coumarin, it might also potentially interact with warfarin. Although no such interactions have been reported, patients taking warfarin who initiate fenugreek supplementation should notify their physician and receive more frequent INR monitoring. Due to its potential to induce uterine contractions, fenugreek should not be used during pregnancy.

Learning Bridge 13.2

CS is a 63-year-old Caucasian female who presents to the community pharmacy with a question for the pharmacist and a recent laboratory result printout. The laboratory results show a hemoglobin A_{1c} of 6.4%, which the physician told CS was classified as prediabetes. The patient is interested in learning more about dietary supplements that could be used to lower blood glucose and to potentially slow the onset of type 2 diabetes.

A. Which of the dietary supplements discussed could potentially be used by this patient to lower blood glucose levels?

B. Which assessment questions should the pharmacist ask CS prior to recommending a potential therapy?

C. Which treatment option would you recommend for CS? Provide a rationale and justification for your answer.

Gastrointestinal Health

Ginger

Therapeutic Properties/Pharmacology

Ginger is the common name for the culinary spice from the *Zingiber officinale* plant. The rhizome is commonly used for the treatment of nausea and vomiting associated with pregnancy, motion sickness, chemotherapy, and surgery. Ginger has also been studied for use in arthritis due to its proposed anti-inflammatory effects. The potential mechanism of action whereby ginger acts as an antiemetic is attributed to serotonin antagonist effects locally in the gastrointestinal tract as well as potential central nervous system effects. Ginger is also thought to exert anticholinergic effects resulting in increased gastric tone and peristalsis. Ginger contains volatile oils and an oleoresin; the constituents of the oleoresin (gingerol, shogaol, galanolactone) are thought to be the active ingredients. Gingerol is believed to be the source of the antiemetic effects, while shogaol and galanolactone are associated with the antiserotonergic effects in the intestine.

Clinical Evidence

Evidence for the use of ginger in nausea and vomiting is conflicting. A Cochrane review published in 2010 searched the literature to determine the safety and effectiveness of various interventions for nausea and vomiting in early pregnancy; ginger was included in this meta-analysis. The review found nine randomized controlled trials with 1,077 patients that compared ginger to placebo, vitamin B_6, or dimenhydrinate and that met the meta-analysis inclusion criteria. While the results of many of the trials favored use of ginger, the effects were not statistically significant.

A 2012 systematic review was performed by Ding et al. to determine the effectiveness and safety of ginger for pregnancy-induced nausea and vomiting. The researchers concluded that ginger was more effective than placebo and as effective as vitamin B_6 in this indication. Limitations related to the inconsistent measurement of outcomes, however, mean the results are limited and difficult to generalize. Inadequate data are also available related to the use of ginger for the treatment of severe nausea and vomiting in pregnancy (hyperemesis gravidarum) and, therefore, ginger supplementation should not be recommended for this condition.

Dosage and Safety Considerations

Dosages of ginger used in clinical trials range from 250 mg to 1 gram of powdered root taken as a capsule one to four times daily. For nausea and vomiting related to pregnancy, the most common dose studied has been 250 mg taken by mouth four times per day.

Ginger is usually well tolerated, though with adverse effects of heartburn, diarrhea, and mouth irritation being reported. It is thought to inhibit thromboxane synthetase, thereby reducing platelet aggregation. Patients taking warfarin who initiate ginger supplementation, in larger quantities than found in food, should notify their physician and undergo more frequent INR monitoring. Ginger has been shown to lower blood glucose, so a potential synergistic effect could be seen in patients taking insulin or other medications for the treatment of diabetes.

Studies have not found any significant adverse effects of ginger on the developing fetus, and the United States recognizes this supplement as "Generally Regarded as Safe." In contrast, Finland and Denmark have issued warnings on products that contain high levels of ginger as being unsafe for use in pregnancy. In pregnant patients, given the concern for safety for the fetus, it is important to cautiously review the risk-versus-benefit profile of any agent used to treat nausea and vomiting.

Milk Thistle

Therapeutic Properties/Pharmacology

Milk thistle is the common name for the *Silybum marianum* plant, whose fruit and seeds have been used for medicinal purposes in the treatment of liver disease. Milk thistle is used as an adjunct to conventional therapies for the treatment of viral liver disease (hepatitis B and hepatitis C), cirrhosis, and fatty liver disease from alcohol or other toxins. The active ingredient in this plant is silymarin, which is a flavonoid complex made up of silybinin, isosilybin, silychristin, and silydianin. Silybinin is considered the most active compound. Milk thistle's proposed mechanism of action relates to the antioxidant effects of silymarin. Silymarin is thought to prevent liver damage by blocking the entrance of toxins into liver cells and by stimulating regeneration and formation of new hepatocytes.

Clinical Evidence

Due to the potential for protection and regrowth of liver cells, milk thistle has drawn increased interest in recent years. A Cochrane review evaluated 13 randomized clinical trials using milk thistle for the treatment of alcoholic or viral liver disease caused by hepatitis B or C, for any duration of time. In high-quality trials, when milk thistle was compared to placebo or no intervention, no statistically significant difference was found related to mortality, complications of liver disease, or liver histology. These results confirm the findings (no significant beneficial effects) of two meta-analyses of milk thistle for patients with liver disease. The review highlights the lack of high-quality clinical trials to support the use of this supplement. Due to the lack of supporting data for this treatment and the existence of proven conventional therapies for liver disease, milk thistle should not be recommended.

Dosage and Safety Considerations

Milk thistle products are standardized to contain 70–80% silymarin. Equivalent doses of silymarin range from 240 mg to 900 mg taken by mouth daily in two to three divided doses. For viral hepatitis, a dose of 420 mg of silymarin per day has been used.

Milk thistle is well tolerated, with no adverse effects being reported with various doses in multiple clinical trials. Pooled adverse effects were usually gastrointestinal and included bloating, nausea, heartburn, and diarrhea, which went away with continued use. Doses greater than 1,500 mg per day may produce a laxative effect. Patients allergic to ragweed should avoid use of milk thistle, as both of these plants are members of the Asteraceae family and allergic reactions to milk thistle have been reported. *In vitro* studies have shown a potential interaction with milk thistle and medications cleared by cytochrome P450 (CYP) 3A4 or CYP2C9, and caution should be used with concomitant administration.

Peppermint

Therapeutic Properties/Pharmacology

Peppermint is the common name of the *Menthe piperita* plant, which is commonly used for treatment of gastrointestinal complaints such as irritable bowel syndrome (IBS), nausea, and indigestion. Menthol is believed to be the active ingredient in peppermint. It is thought to work as an antispasmodic by antagonizing calcium channels, resulting in intestinal smooth muscle relaxation. An antiflatulent effect has also been seen and is produced by an unknown mechanism.

Clinical Evidence

A small number of studies have evaluated the effectiveness of peppermint for the treatment of IBS. A Cochrane review completed by Ruepert et al. evaluated the effectiveness of bulking agents, antispasmodics (including peppermint), and antidepressants for the treatment of IBS. The review identified 29 studies using antispasmodics, of which five utilized peppermint for the treatment of IBS and met the meta-analysis's inclusion criteria. Overall, antispasmodics produced statistically significant improvements in abdominal pain ($p < 0.001$), global assessment ($p < 0.001$), and symptom scores ($p < 0.01$) when compared to placebo. A subgroup analysis of peppermint revealed statistically significant improvements in global assessment and symptoms scores. While peppermint appears to be beneficial for the treatment of IBS symptoms, the methodologies used in the included studies were highly variable; the duration of treatment ranged from 1 week to 6 months, and other limitations need to be considered. When compared to conventional antispasmodic treatments, peppermint is not superior for reducing IBS symptoms but may be better tolerated.

Dosage and Safety Considerations

Clinical trials have used daily doses of three to six enteric-coated capsules containing 0.2–0.4 mL of peppermint oil. Adverse effects are not common with peppermint, but include nausea, heartburn, and perianal burning. Enteric-coated products release peppermint in the small intestine and can help to prevent nausea and heartburn due to lower esophageal sphincter relaxation.

Peppermint is contraindicated in patients with severe gastrointestinal disease such as biliary duct occlusion, gallbladder inflammation, and severe liver damage. Although evidence is lacking, drug interactions could potentially occur with medications metabolized by the CYP3A4 enzyme, owing to reduced activity of this enzyme. Due to smooth muscle relaxation and perianal irritation, the safety of peppermint during pregnancy is of concern.

Learning Bridge 13.3

TK is a 28-year-old African American female who presents to the community pharmacy. She is 6 weeks pregnant with her first child. Although very excited about the pregnancy, TK has been experiencing nausea throughout the day associated with rare vomiting. A parenting magazine recommended ginger supplements as a natural way to reduce pregnancy-induced nausea and vomiting.

A. What is the mechanism of action of ginger for reducing pregnancy-induced nausea and vomiting?

B. Which factors should the patient consider prior to initiating ginger therapy?

C. If approved by TK's OB/GYN, which dose of ginger is recommended for the treatment of pregnancy-induced nausea and vomiting?

Neurology and Mental Health

Ginkgo

Therapeutic Properties/Pharmacology

Ginkgo is most widely recognized as a treatment for cognitive impairment and dementia. Extracts from the leaves of the *Ginkgo biloba* maidenhair tree have been studied for age-related macular degeneration, memory disorder in multiple sclerosis, acute ischemic stroke, tinnitus, peripheral arterial disease, and migraines. The active constituents of ginkgo are flavonoids and unique terpenoids, known as ginkgolides and bilobalide. The flavonoids act as antioxidants and free radical scavengers, which are thought to prevent cell injury that might otherwise result in cerebrovascular disease. The ginkgolides have anti-inflammatory properties and prevent platelet aggregation through inhibition of platelet-activating factor; they are thought to improve cerebral blood flow. Bilobalide works synergistically with the ginkgolides to enhance cerebral circulation and cerebral tolerance to hypoxic states.

Clinical Evidence

A Cochrane review assessed ginkgo for the treatment of dementia or age-related cognitive impairment by analyzing 36 randomized, double-blind studies ($n = 4{,}423$) lasting 3 to 52 weeks. All trials except one used a standard extract, 24 mg of flavone glycosides and 6 mg of ginkgolides per 100 mg, in doses of 80–600 mg/day. Inconsistent and conflicting results were obtained in this review. Many trials showed no improvements with ginkgo compared to placebo, but a small number of trials found large treatment effects with ginkgo.

A more recent study ($n = 404$) found improvements in cognitive function, neuropsychiatric symptoms, and functional abilities in patients with Alzheimer's disease or vascular dementia who took *Ginkgo biloba* extract 240 mg/day for 24 weeks. A large, randomized, double-blind, placebo-controlled trial evaluated the effect of *Ginkgo biloba* extract for the prevention of Alzheimer's disease in patients aged 70 years or older with complaints of memory problems ($n = 2{,}820$). At 5 years, *Ginkgo biloba* extract 120 mg twice daily did not appear to reduce the progression to Alzheimer's disease compared to placebo (hazard ratio [HR] 0.84; 95% confidence interval [CI] 0.60–1.18; $p = 0.306$). Results of this trial are consistent with other studies of ginkgo for the prevention of dementia in elderly patients.

Overall, not enough consistent evidence exists to recommend *Ginkgo biloba* extract for the treatment or prevention of dementia or Alzheimer's disease.

Dosage and Safety Considerations

Recommended doses of ginkgo for cognitive effects in Alzheimer's disease range from 120 mg to 240 mg, divided two or three times daily, for at least 4–6 weeks. The ginkgo product should contain 24% flavone glycosides and 6% terpenoids.

There have been no reports of increased adverse effects with ginkgo compared to placebo. Ginkgo may increase bleeding risk through its inhibition of platelet aggregation, so this supplement should be avoided or used with caution in patients taking anticoagulants or antiplatelet agents. There is evidence that ginkgo may decrease concentrations of omeprazole and tolbutamide through induction of CYP2C9 and CYP2C19. Its use should be avoided in patients with a history of seizure, as there have been reports of seizure from consumption of the ginkgo seed.

Kava

Therapeutic Properties/Pharmacology

Kava, also known as kava-kava, is the dried root of *Piper methysticum* and has been used by Pacific Islanders for hundreds of years as a ceremonial beverage for relaxation. Kava has been used medicinally for anxiety, stress, and restlessness. Kavalactones are the active ingredients in this supplement that exert enhanced gamma-aminobutyric acid (GABA) effects without binding to the benzodiazepine receptor or to GABA directly. Other suggested mechanisms of action include inhibition of voltage-gated sodium channels, calcium channels, monoamine oxidase B, and neuronal uptake of norepinephrine and dopamine.

Clinical Evidence

A Cochrane review of the efficacy of kava in anxiety included 12 studies with 700 patients. Most trials used kava preparations containing 70% kavalactone and assessed efficacy using the Hamilton Anxiety (HAM-A) scale. A trend of improved anxiety on the HAM-A scale was observed in a pooled analysis of 380 patients taking kava versus placebo (weighted mean difference 3.9; 95% CI 0.1–7.7; $p = 0.05$). Other studies using various scoring assessments also reported improvements in anxiety with kava compared to placebo.

Kava has had a small effect in improving anxiety compared to placebo. It should not be widely recommended due to safety concerns and the need for long-term trials to further evaluate its efficacy and safety.

Dosage and Safety Considerations

Kava doses of 150–800 mg/day taken once daily or divided three times daily for 1–24 weeks were used in clinical trials.

In 2002, the FDA issued a warning that kava may increase the risk of severe liver damage. Several European countries and Canada have removed this supplement from the market due to numerous reports of liver toxicity. Some sources recommend the use of water-based extracts over acetone or ethanol-based extracts to prevent hepatotoxicity. A small trial ($n = 60$) evaluated aqueous kava extracts for 3 weeks and reported improvements in the HAM-A scale compared to placebo ($p < 0.0001$) with no hepatotoxicity. The mechanism underlying the hepatotoxicity is unknown, and this outcome seems to be a rare, but possibly serious event.

Cognitive impairment may occur with kava use and may impair driving abilities. Some reports indicate that long-term users of kava may develop dry, scaly skin called kava dermopathy. Gastrointestinal upset, restlessness, tremor, and headache have also been reported as adverse events.

Kava should not be taken with other centrally acting depressants such as alcohol, sedatives, and benzodiazepines to avoid excessive sedation. This supplement inhibits many cytochrome P450 enzymes and may theoretically interact with medications metabolized through this system.

St. John's Wort

Therapeutic Properties/Pharmacology

St. John's wort is a well-known herbal product used to treat depression. This supplement has also been studied for use in anxiety, sleep disorders, hot flushes (also known as hot flashes), premenstrual syndrome, and neuropathic pain. It is derived from the dried leaves and flowering tops of the plant *Hypericum perforatum* and was named St. John's wort because the flowers typically bloom around St. John's Day in June. The active component thought to provide the antidepressant activity is hyperforin. It is unknown whether other biologically active constituents of St. John's wort contribute to its pharmacological effects. The precise mechanism of action for St. John's wort is unknown. Studies suggest that it inhibits presynaptic neuronal reuptake of serotonin, norepinephrine, dopamine, and GABA.

Clinical Evidence

St. John's wort has been evaluated for mild to moderate depression in a Cochrane review including 29 studies with 5,489 patients. Included trials compared 4–12 weeks of St. John's wort therapy to placebo or synthetic antidepressant treatment (selective serotonin reuptake inhibitors and tricyclic antidepressants). Various formulations of the supplement were evaluated in the trials at doses ranging from 240 to 1,800 mg/day. St. John's wort was found to be superior to placebo and had similar efficacy compared to other antidepressants; however, the effect size was small. Publication bias was a concern in this review, and it was noted that German studies more often reported favorable effects of St. John's wort than trials conducted in other countries. Clinical trials since this review have provided mixed results regarding the product's efficacy.

Dosage and Safety Considerations

St. John's wort may be an effective antidepressant but has many potential drug–herb interactions, albeit fewer reported adverse events compared to synthetic antidepressants. Clinical trials have frequently used extracts of St. John's wort containing hypericin 0.3% at a dose of 300 mg three times daily. It is desirable that St. John's wort preparations contain 1–6% of the primary active constituent hyperforin. The herbal product should not be solely standardized based on the hypericin content. Patients with depression should not be treated with this supplement except under the supervision of a healthcare provider. If not treated adequately, depression can become serious and suicide risk may potentially increase with or without pharmacologic therapy.

The tolerability of St. John's wort in clinical trials was similar to that of placebo. The most commonly reported adverse events are skin rash, abdominal pain, and gastritis.

Numerous pharmacokinetic and pharmacodynamic drug–herb interactions have been documented with St. John's wort. This product is an inducer of P-glycoprotein as well as cytochrome P450 3A4, 1A2, 2E1, and 2C19 isoenzymes. Patients are at a higher risk of serotonin syndrome with concomitant use of St. John's wort and other medications that inhibit reuptake of serotonin.

Serotonin syndrome can result in nausea, vomiting, hypertension, myoclonus, hyperthermia, and mental status changes. Additionally, manic and hypomanic symptoms have been reported in patients taking St. John's wort and selective serotonin reuptake inhibitors.

Valerian

Therapeutic Properties/Pharmacology

Valerian is derived from the dried root of *Valeriana officinalis* and is popular as a sleep aid. Valerian has also been used for anxiety, depression, obsessive–compulsive disorder, and stress. Valerenic acid and derivatives from the volatile oil of valerian are the components thought to exert sedative effects through central nervous system depression. Studies have indicated that valerenic acid may also enhance GABA activity, although the exact mechanism by which this effect occurs is unknown.

Clinical Evidence

Well-designed clinical trials evaluating valerian are lacking. The efficacy of this supplement as a treatment for generalized anxiety disorder has been evaluated in a 4-week, double-blind, randomized study ($n = 36$). Patients were randomized to three times daily valerian 50 mg, placebo, or diazepam 2.5 mg. Improvements in anxiety based on the HAM-A scale were not significant between valerian and placebo (weighted mean difference –1.40; 95% CI –7.93 to 5.13) or between valerian and diazepam (weighted mean difference 0.40; 95% CI –6.22 to 7.02).

A large number of trials have evaluated valerian as a treatment for insomnia. A meta-analysis of 16 randomized controlled trials ($n = 1,093$) assessed the effects of valerian 225–1,215 mg/day on quality of sleep. Data were pooled from only 6 trials that reported sleep quality as an outcome; they showed valerian improved sleep quality versus placebo (relative risk [RR] of improved sleep 1.8; 95% CI 1.2–2.9).

Publication bias was identified as a major limitation in assessing studies of valerian. Methodologic issues have proved a significant barrier to combining and examining valerian trial data. In an attempt to overcome this problem, another systematic review provided a descriptive evaluation of 37 clinical trials, including controlled trials and open-label studies. According to this meta-analysis, ethanolic extracts of valerian 300–600 mg/day administered for 1–42 nights were not superior to placebo in improving sleep outcomes. Ethanolic valerian extracts were considered equivalent to benzodiazepines in improving subjective sleep quality, although these trials were not placebo controlled. Aqueous valerian extracts were studied using a variety of dosing regimens (400–900 mg at bedtime or 90–405 mg three times daily) administered for 1–30 days. Results were inconsistent, and many of the trials were of poor quality. Studies of valerian extracts containing valepotriate showed mild improvements in sleep quality after 9 nights of 120 mg. Sleep was improved with 100 mg valepotriate three times daily for 15 days in patients who were tapering and discontinuing long-term benzodiazepines. Results were also mixed when valerian was studied in combination with hops and lemon balm.

The utility of valerian for anxiety is unknown, and randomized studies are needed that include larger sample sizes, placebo or other standard treatments at therapeutic doses as comparator groups, and longer follow-up. For the treatment of insomnia, efficacy data supporting the use of valerian are conflicting and many studies have been hampered by poor trial designs.

Dosage and Safety Considerations

There is a lack of dosing consensus for the use of valerian. Valerian extract doses of 50 mg to 100 mg three times daily have been used for generalized anxiety disorder. For insomnia, doses ranging from 120 mg to 1,215 mg/day have been studied. Extracts containing valepotriate 120 mg at bedtime and 100 mg three times daily have shown to improve sleep in clinical trials.

The evidence is consistent in showing that valerian is a safe treatment. Minor adverse events reported include nausea, diarrhea, morning "hangover," drowsiness, and headache. Valerian should be avoided with other medications that increase sedation such as benzodiazepines, antihistamines, and alcohol.

Learning Bridge 13.4

A 22-year-old female college student would like to start taking St. John's wort. She states that she is too busy right now to drive the 5 hours back to her hometown where her primary care physician is located. She reports feeling sad since she and her boyfriend broke up. She has not had a desire to leave her apartment in the past 3 weeks, causing her to frequently miss class and work shifts. The only medications she takes are an oral contraceptive, ethinyl estradiol/drospirenone, and ibuprofen 200 mg 1–2 tablets three times daily once or twice per month for menstrual cramps.

A. Explain why St. John's wort is or is not an effective medication for depression.
B. Which possible drug interaction might this patient experience if she begins taking St. John's wort?
C. Would you recommend that this patient self-treat her depressed mood? Why or why not?

Pain

Alpha-Lipoic Acid

Therapeutic Properties/Pharmacology

Alpha-lipoic acid (ALA), also known as thioctic acid, is a natural antioxidant found in animal organ meats and plant food sources such as broccoli, spinach, and tomatoes. ALA has been used to treat many conditions, including dementia, kidney disease, multiple sclerosis, and diabetes. In diabetes studies, ALA has been shown to prevent oxidative stress and damage from hyperglycemia and to improve microvascular blood flow. There is also evidence that ALA may increase insulin sensitivity.

Clinical Evidence

A meta-analysis of four clinical trials ($n = 653$) assessed the effectiveness of ALA intravenous (IV) or oral 100–1,800 mg/day in patients with painful diabetic neuropathy. Duration of therapy for ALA IV was 3 weeks; oral ALA was given for 3 weeks to 6 months. Doses of 1,200 mg/day and

1,800 mg/day did not result in significantly improved symptoms over doses of 600 mg/day. All ALA regimens resulted in statistically significant total symptom score improvements compared to placebo ($p < 0.0001$). However, a daily infusion of 600 mg for 3 weeks was the only regimen considered to result in clinically meaningful symptom score improvements (30% change) compared to placebo.

A randomized placebo-controlled trial evaluated the long-term effects of oral ALA 600 mg/day in 460 patients with diabetic neuropathy. After 4 years of treatment, no significant differences in the primary outcome were found between treatment groups ($p = 0.105$).

A Cochrane review is currently in progress and should provide further evidence as to the role of ALA in neuropathy.

Dosage and Safety Considerations

ALA 600 mg daily is the recommended dose for diabetic peripheral neuropathy. Intravenously administered ALA for 2–3 weeks is a promising therapy.

ALA is generally well tolerated. Adverse effects more likely to be experienced with higher doses of 1,200–1,800 mg/day include nausea, vomiting, and diarrhea. Heart rate and rhythm abnormalities occurred more often in patients taking ALA, although discontinuation rates were extremely low.

Butterbur

Therapeutic Properties/Pharmacology

Extracts from the leaves and roots of the butterbur plant, *Petasites hybridus*, contain sesquiterpene lactones, petasin and isopetasin, that have antispasmodic and anti-inflammatory properties. Butterbur has been used in the treatment of urinary and gastrointestinal disorders, menstrual cramps, kidney stones, and migraine headaches; the rationale for its use in these indications is its induction of smooth muscle relaxation. The anti-inflammatory activity of butterbur is due to inhibition of leukotriene synthesis and may be useful in the management of allergic rhinitis and asthma.

Clinical Evidence

A randomized, controlled trial of 245 adult patients found *Petasites* extract 75 mg twice daily to be more effective than placebo in decreasing the number of monthly migraine attacks. Maximal effects were observed after 3 months of treatment, with the butterbur product resulting in a 58% migraine attack reduction compared to a 28% reduction seen with placebo. *Petasites* extract 50 mg twice daily was also studied and resulted in nonsignificant changes compared to placebo.

Butterbur has been studied in the pediatric population at doses (divided twice daily) of 50–75 mg/day in 6- to 9-year-old patients and doses of 100–150 mg/day in 10- to 17-year-old patients. The 4-month open-label, prospective study resulted in 77% of patients experiencing at least a 50% reduction in migraine attack frequency. Doses were increased in nonresponders after 2 months. Most patients experienced shortened attack duration, although a small percentage reported prolonged attack duration with therapy.

Butterbur appears to be a potential treatment for migraine prophylaxis in adults and children. Nevertheless, current data are limited, and larger randomized, placebo-controlled trials are needed.

Dosage and Safety Considerations

Petasites extract has been effective as a migraine preventive when administered for a minimum of 2 months at doses of 75 mg twice daily in adult patients, 25–37.5 mg twice daily in 6- to 9-year-old patients, and 50–75 mg twice daily in 10- to 17-year-old patients. The butterbur plant contains pyrrolizidine alkaloids (PA) that have the potential to be hepatotoxic and carcinogenic. The alkaloids are removed by an extraction process in commercially available butterbur products, and patients should be advised to consume only butterbur that is labeled as "PA free."

Butterbur is generally well tolerated. The most common adverse effects are belching and nausea. Allergic cross-sensitivity reactions may occur in patients with allergies to ragweed, marigolds, daisies, or chrysanthemums.

Capsaicin

Therapeutic Properties/Pharmacology

Capsaicin is a widely used topical product for relief of pain from conditions such as neuropathy, arthritis, and shingles. It consists of the cayenne pepper dried fruit and is available in over-the-counter formulations of creams, lotions, gels, liquids, and patches in strengths ranging from 0.025% to 0.15%. Additionally, a high-concentration capsaicin 8% patch has been approved as a prescription drug in the United States and Europe.

Capsaicin acts as an exogenous agonist of the transient receptor potential vanilloid 1 (TRPV1) receptor. Initial activation of TRPV1 causes sensory nerve depolarization and transmission of messages to the brain and spinal cord, with resultant sensations of warmth, burning, stinging, or itching. Repeated exposure or high concentrations of capsaicin cause defunctionalization of the sensory axons that express TRPV1, resulting in decreased neuronal excitability and responsiveness to pain. Capsaicin also stimulates the release and subsequent depletion of substance P from sensory neurons upon repeated exposure; however, the role of substance P in pain transmission appears to be much more limited than once thought.

Clinical Evidence

Treatment guidelines for diabetic peripheral neuropathy and hand osteoarthritis have recommended capsaicin as a drug therapy option, although robust clinical trial data on this therapy are lacking. Several small studies, many with flawed methodologies, have shown capsaicin 0.025% to 0.075%, applied three to four times daily, to be superior to placebo in reducing pain scores by 50% or more. In some instances, effects were not realized until 4 weeks of capsaicin use. The placebo response rates in these studies were high compared to capsaicin response rates (25–42% versus 38–60%, respectively). Further limitations of the capsaicin clinical trials were their small sample sizes and difficulties with double blinding due to the characteristic local burning sensation after capsaicin use. Capsaicin has limited clinical efficacy and should be reserved for use as an adjunctive treatment for pain disorders.

Dosage and Safety Considerations

Topical formulations of capsaicin 0.025% to 0.075% can be applied three to four times daily for arthritis and neuropathy, and the product is recommended to be applied three to five times daily for postherpetic neuralgia. Redness, burning, and stinging at the application site are the most common adverse drug reactions, largely due to the early response of the TRPV1 receptors to capsaicin. While this reaction is typically mild to moderate in intensity, it does lead many patients to discontinue therapy. Patients who are able to tolerate capsaicin notice the cutaneous adverse effects become less intense or dissipate after 1–2 weeks of use.

An FDA alert was issued to warn the public that over-the-counter topical analgesics, including capsaicin, have been reported to cause rare, but serious skin burns. Patients are advised to stop using the medication and seek medical attention if skin injury occurs.

Feverfew

Therapeutic Properties/Pharmacology

Feverfew is derived from the dried leaves of the weed plant *Tanacetum parthenium* and has been used as a treatment for migraines, fever, arthritis, and toothache. Similar to butterbur, feverfew plant leaves contain sesquiterpene lactones that provide the therapy's pharmacologic activity. Parthenolide is the active constituent responsible for the anti-inflammatory and antiplatelet effects through inhibition of prostaglandin synthesis and arachidonic acid. The antimigraine activity of feverfew is likely due to its inhibition of serotonin release from platelets and white blood cells. Serotonin is a vasoactive neurotransmitter involved in the vascular changes of the brain that result in migraine.

Clinical Evidence

In clinical trials, feverfew has demonstrated controversial efficacy. A 2004 Cochrane review of randomized, controlled trials of feverfew determined there was insufficient evidence of its superiority relative to placebo. The inconsistent results of these feverfew trials were thought to be due to use of poor-quality preparations or subtherapeutic concentrations. Consequently, a more stable extract of feverfew (MIG-99) was developed and evaluated in a randomized, double-blind, placebo-controlled study of 170 patients with 4–6 migraines per 28 days at baseline. MIG-99 6.25 mg three times daily was superior to placebo in reducing migraine frequency by 1.9 attacks per month compared to the reduction of 1.3 attacks per month seen with placebo ($p = 0.0456$). The onset of feverfew effectiveness is 1 month, with maximal effects seen at 2 months.

The inconsistent results from clinical trials preclude the recommendation of feverfew as migraine preventive treatment. Additional studies with stable feverfew products, such as MIG-99, are needed.

Dosage and Safety Considerations

The recommended dosage of feverfew for migraine prevention is 6.25 mg three times daily for at least 1 month. The MIG-99 formulation is the preferred extract.

Mouth ulcerations and dermatitis have been reported with feverfew. These adverse effects likely came from direct contact with the feverfew leaves or powder and are unlikely to occur if tablet or encapsulated preparations are used. Feverfew can induce uterine contractions and is contraindicated in pregnancy. Gastrointestinal disturbances and allergic reactions may occur; in particular, individuals with known hypersensitivity to plants in the daisy family should avoid feverfew. Feverfew should not be discontinued abruptly, as rebound headache, anxiety, insomnia, and muscle and joint stiffness may occur. Caution should be used in patients concurrently taking anticoagulants or antiplatelet agents due to a possible increased bleeding risk.

Glucosamine and Chondroitin

Therapeutic Properties/Pharmacology

Glucosamine is one of the most popular natural products used in the United States and is well recognized for its use in arthritis. A naturally occurring amino sugar, it is present in many physiological fluids such as synovial fluid and articular cartilage. Commercially available glucosamine is derived from extracts of shellfish exoskeletons or produced synthetically, and is readily available on an over-the-counter basis.

Glucosamine serves as a precursor for the biosynthesis of cartilage constituents: glycosaminoglycans, hyaluronic acid, and proteoglycans. Some evidence indicates that glucosamine stimulates production of hyaluronic acid within the synovial membrane, which surrounds the articular cartilage and protects the joints. Glucosamine also exerts anticatabolic activity through inhibition of proteoglycan breakdown and reverses damaging effects of interleukin-1β within the articular chondrocytes. When interleukin-1β is not expressed, anti-inflammatory activity results through inhibition of cyclooxygenase-2 and nitric oxide synthase.

Glucosamine is commonly combined with chondroitin as one formulation. Chondroitin is a hydrophilic glycosaminoglycan that promotes absorption of water in the articular cartilage to protect joints against compressive forces. Chondroitin is available commercially as a synthetic product, but may also be derived from bovine, shark, or avian sources.

Both glucosamine and chondroitin are slow acting. Indeed, it may take 2–3 weeks of regular use before benefits become apparent.

Clinical Evidence

Glucosamine and chondroitin have been studied in a variety of clinical trials, many with poor design quality. A 2005 Cochrane review of 25 trials including 4,963 patients found that only a specific preparation of glucosamine sulfate appeared to be superior to placebo for osteoarthritis pain and functional impairment. A large placebo-controlled study randomized 1,583 patients with osteoarthritis of the knee to receive either glucosamine hydrochloride 1,500 mg/day, chondroitin 1,200 mg/day, a combination of glucosamine and chondroitin, celecoxib 200 mg/day, or placebo. After 24 weeks, celecoxib was the only treatment found to decrease knee pain; a 20% reduction in pain was seen with this drug compared to placebo ($p = 0.0008$). A subanalysis of patients with moderate to severe osteoarthritis showed benefits from the combination therapy consisting of glucosamine and chondroitin ($p = 0.002$). An ancillary 2-year follow-up study with 662 patients from the aforementioned 24-week trial found no therapy to be superior to placebo in improving pain and function. The effect of the glucosamine/chondroitin combination in patients with moderate to severe baseline arthritis did not persist.

The lack of efficacy for these supplements in clinical studies may be a result of the limited glucosamine concentration available for joint uptake due to the competitive cellular uptake of glucosamine and glucose within the intestines, liver, and kidney. The American College of Rheumatology guidelines for knee and hip osteoarthritis provide specific recommendations that glucosamine and chondroitin not be used as treatment options for these conditions.

Dosage and Safety Considerations

The preferred dose of glucosamine is 1,500 mg/day, either taken as one dose or divided up to three times daily. Chondroitin can be used at doses of 600 mg to 1,200 mg/day, either taken as one dose or divided up to three times daily.

Glucosamine and chondroitin are considered to be safe products. Shellfish-allergic patients should use caution with glucosamine products extracted from crustacean exoskeletons, although a small study of 15 shrimp-allergic patients resulted in no adverse reactions during the 24 hours following glucosamine ingestion. Concerns have been raised that glucosamine might affect glucose metabolism and cause decreased insulin sensitivity; however, studies of this relationship have yielded inconclusive results. Chondroitin may have anticoagulant effects and should be used with caution in patients taking warfarin. Chondroitin is contraindicated in males with prostate cancer, as expression of chondroitin on cancer cells may contribute to metastatic and recurrent disease.

Willow Bark

Therapeutic Properties/Pharmacology

Willow bark (*Salix* spp.) has long been used for fever, headache, arthritis, and other acute and chronic pain disorders. Salicin is one of the active constituents in willow bark and is well known for being a precursor to acetylsalicylic acid (aspirin). The concentration of salicin in willow bark after ingestion and its metabolism to salicylic acid are likely not potent enough to produce analgesic effects. Other components of willow bark include phenolic acids, flavonoids, and tannins; those components—rather than salicin—are thought to be largely responsible for the anti-inflammatory and analgesic properties of willow bark.

Clinical Evidence

Salix alba has been evaluated as treatment for nonspecific low back pain. Compared to placebo ($n = 70$), salicin doses of 120 mg ($n = 70$) and 240 mg ($n = 70$) at week 4 resulted in more patients experiencing at least five pain-free days per week, fewer patients requiring tramadol as a rescue medication, and improved pain and impairment scores (Arhus Index, pain index, invalid index, physical impairment index). A dose-related trend of pain relief with *Salix alba* was noted in this study of acute episodes of chronic low back pain.

Another study of 228 patients with acute episodes of chronic nonspecific low back pain compared salicin 240 mg/day to rofecoxib 12.5 mg/day. At week 4, both the *Salix alba* and rofecoxib groups showed improved (by 44%) pain and impairment scores. Both treatments also resulted in fewer patients requiring rescue medication (10% *Salix alba*, 13% rofecoxib).

Willow bark has also been studied as a treatment for arthritis. In a 6-week study of treatments for hip or knee osteoarthritis, 127 patients were randomized to salicin 240 mg/day, diclofenac 100 mg/day, or placebo. The diclofenac group was the only one in which Western Ontario Macmaster University Osteoarthritis Index (WOMAC) pain scores significantly improved compared to placebo recipients ($p = 0.0002$). A study of 26 patients with rheumatoid arthritis did not find a difference between salicin 240 mg/day and placebo at 6 weeks ($p = 0.93$).

Willow bark has not been shown to be an effective treatment for arthritis, but it does seem to provide relief in cases involving acute low back pain.

Dosage and Safety Considerations

The recommended willow bark dose is 120 mg/day to 240 mg/day of the salicin component. Use beyond 4 weeks has not been studied. Larger, long-term clinical trials are needed to further evaluate the safety profile of this supplement. In contrast to aspirin, willow bark has not demonstrated gastrointestinal damage in animal studies and does not appear to impair platelet aggregation with salicin doses of 240 mg. Willow bark is contraindicated in patients with a history of allergic reactions to salicylates, as serious anaphylaxis may occur.

> ## Learning Bridge 13.5
>
> A 59-year-old male patient presents to the local pharmacy where you are working and asks which glucosamine and chondroitin product you recommend. He has osteoarthritis of the knee, has failed to respond to acetaminophen therapy, and was told not to take any anti-inflammatory medications because he had a heart attack a few years ago. His past medical history also includes hypertension and prostate cancer.
>
> **A.** If this patient is going to take a glucosamine formulation, which product and dose do you recommend?
>
> **B.** What do you tell the patient about the efficacy of glucosamine products?
>
> **C.** The patient notices that the product label states that individuals should consult a health-care professional if they are allergic to shellfish. He does experience a skin rash and nasal congestion after eating shellfish. Which advice will you give him about the shellfish warning and glucosamine?

Sexual Health

Dehydroepiandrosterone

Therapeutic Properties/Pharmacology

Dehydroepiandrosterone (DHEA) is a naturally occurring steroid hormone precursor to testosterone and estrogen that is produced in the adrenal gland, liver, testes, and ovaries. DHEA peak levels are reached between ages 15 and 45 years, but then steadily decline by approximately 5% per year. As a dietary supplement, DHEA has been studied for its antiaging properties and use in the following indications: systemic lupus erythematosus, assisted reproduction in females, mood disorders, cognitive function, postmenopausal females with impaired sexual function, and erectile dysfunction (ED).

Clinical Evidence

In a double-blind, placebo-controlled study, healthy men ages 41–69 years ($n = 40$) with ED of no organic etiology and low serum dehydroepiandrosterone sulfate (DHEAS) levels (less than 1.5 µmol/L) were randomized to DHEA 50 mg/day. After 24 weeks of treatment, the DHEA-treated group experienced increases in DHEAS levels and improvements in International Index of Erectile Function (IIEF) scores that assessed erectile function, orgasmic function, sexual desire, intercourse, and overall satisfaction. All IIEF scores in the placebo group decreased below the baseline at the end of the study, except in the sexual desire domain, and DHEAS levels did not change in these individuals. A follow-up 24-week study assessed the effects of DHEA 50 mg/day in erectile dysfunction. Men ages 35–69 years (mean = 62.7 years) were grouped according to ED etiology (hypertension, diabetes, neurological disorder, and no organic etiology). Improvements were observed in IIEF scores related to frequency of penetration and maintenance of erection in the group with hypertension and the group with ED of no organic etiology ($p < 0.005$).

In a study of men with sexual dysfunction and low androgen levels, patients were randomized to oral testosterone undecanoate 80 mg twice daily ($n = 29$), DHEA 50 mg twice daily ($n = 28$), or placebo ($n = 29$). Serum DHEA and testosterone levels did increase from DHEA supplementation; however, sexual dysfunction did not significantly improve from any intervention.

In a 12-month trial, 48 postmenopausal women were randomized to DHEA 10 mg/day, estradiol 1 mg plus dihydrogesterone 5 mg/day, or tibolone 2.5 mg/day. Vitamin D 4,000 IU/day was given to patients who refused hormonal therapy. Episodes of sexual intercourse increased compared to baseline with DHEA, estradiol plus dihydrogesterone, and tibolone ($p < 0.05$, all groups).

It appears that DHEA may potentially improve sexual function in men with erectile dysfunction from hypertension or no organic cause and in postmenopausal females. Large, long-term, placebo-controlled trials are needed before DHEA can be recommended for any indication.

Dosage and Safety Considerations

For the improvement of sexual function, DHEA is recommended at doses of 50 mg/day in men with ED and 10 mg/day in postmenopausal females. Possible risks of DHEA supplementation are related to its androgenic and estrogenic effects. Given the lack of long-term safety data, the same precautions and warnings for estrogen replacement therapy (breast and ovarian cancer) and testosterone (prostate cancer, acne, hirsutism) should be exercised with DHEA supplementation. Concerns about metabolic effects with DHEA use include increased insulin resistance and cardiovascular risk; however, a 52-week safety study of DHEA 50 mg/day in postmenopausal females did not show alterations in cholesterol or glucose compared to placebo. DHEA can significantly increase triazolam levels and is assumed to inhibit metabolism of other CYP3A4 substrates as well.

l-Arginine

Therapeutic Properties/Pharmacology

L-Arginine is an amino acid that is metabolized by nitric oxide synthase (NOS) through oxidation of the guanidium nitrogen group to nitric oxide (NO). Nitric oxide causes smooth muscle relaxation and increased blood flow. L-Arginine supplementation is thought to improve erection through relaxation of the corpus cavernosum, which results in increased blood retention and engorgement of the penis. L-Arginine has been studied in a variety of conditions, including cardiovascular disease, peripheral arterial disease, exercise enhancement, hypertension, and pre-eclampsia. Intravenous arginine has been FDA approved as a growth hormone reserve test.

Clinical Evidence

A randomized, placebo-controlled, crossover study assessed the efficacy of L-arginine 1,500 mg/day in 32 patients with ED. Patients took either L-arginine or placebo for 17 days, followed by a 7-day washout period, and then switched treatments for another 17 days. No statistically significant improvements in erectile function were found compared to placebo.

Larger doses of L-arginine were evaluated in a double-blind, placebo-controlled study. Men with ED ($n = 50$, age 55–75 years) were randomized to L-arginine 5 g/day or placebo divided three times daily for 6 weeks. More men reported subjective improvements in sexual function with L-arginine than with placebo (31% versus 12%, respectively); however, objective measures of sexual function did not significantly change in either group.

Some promising results have been obtained in studies of L-arginine given in combination with pycnogenol. Pycnogenol is an extract of French maritime pine bark that enhances NOS activity. The combination of pycnogenol 20 mg and L-arginine 700 mg was assessed in a randomized, double-blind, placebo-controlled, parallel study of 124 men with ED. After 6 months, the pycnogenol/L-arginine combination improved scores in all domains of the IIEF compared to placebo ($p < 0.05$).

More evidence is needed before recommendations for the general use of L-arginine can be made.

Dosage and Safety Considerations

L-Arginine appears to be more effective than placebo at improving subjective ED outcomes at doses of 5 g/day, and improved objective measures of erectile function at lower doses of 700 mg/day when combined with pycnogenol. This amino acid supplement is well tolerated with minimal adverse events. It may decrease blood pressure by approximately 10% and cause mild discomfort (e.g., headache, nausea, vomiting, diarrhea, flushing, numbness). L-Arginine should be avoided in patients with hypotension or a history of myocardial infarction. Use caution in patients taking antihypertensive agents, nitrates, or phosphodiesterase-5 inhibitors.

Yohimbe

Therapeutic Properties/Pharmacology

Yohimbe is derived from the bark of the West African tree, *Pausinystalia yohimbe*. Its active components are indole alkaloids, the primary one being yohimbine, an alpha$_2$-adrenergic blocker. Yohimbe has been used for ED and as an aphrodisiac—antagonism of the alpha$_2$-adrenergic receptor causes peripheral blood vessel dilation and increased blood flow. Yohimbine antagonizes norepinephrine effects and increases nitric oxide release at the smooth muscle, both of which decrease intracellular calcium and enhance vasodilation. This activity is thought to increase sensation to the genital tissue. Centrally, yohimbine increases sympathetic outflow. Yohimbine has been completely synthesized and is available by prescription as a 5.4-mg tablet.

Clinical Evidence

To date, there have been relatively few clinical trials evaluating yohimbe. Studies conducted with yohimbine have provided inconclusive evidence of its effectiveness for ED due to high placebo response rates, lack of validated symptom questionnaires, and poor trial designs. Yohimbe extracts contain approximately 6% active constituents, and it is unknown whether yohimbine and yohimbe extract exert similar effects. Neither yohimbe nor yohimbine should be recommended due to the lack of efficacy data and the potential for serious adverse events.

Dosage and Safety Considerations

Yohimbine has been used in clinical trials at doses of 5.4 mg three times daily, up to a maximum of 100 mg/day. This supplement increases catecholamine levels and can cause adverse effects such as hypertension, tachycardia, anxiety, and increased urinary frequency. Monoamine oxidase inhibitors should not be used with yohimbine to prevent additive effects. Yohimbe has been classified by the FDA as an unsafe herb that should be avoided in patients with hypertension, anxiety, psychiatric disorders, and benign prostatic hyperplasia.

Urogenital Heath

African Plum

Therapeutic Properties/Pharmacology

Pygeum africanum, also known as pygeum, is an extract of the African plum tree bark and has been used to treat mild to moderate benign prostatic hyperplasia (BPH). The active constituents of the African plum tree bark are sterols and pentacyclic triterpenes. The therapeutic activity of pygeum is not well understood, but is thought to target the etiologies of prostate hyperplasia.

The phytosterols are believed to competitively inhibit testosterone and exert anti-inflammatory properties in the prostate through inhibition of leukotriene and prostaglandin synthesis. Pentacyclic triterpenes decrease prostatic cholesterol, thereby reducing testosterone synthesis. Some evidence also indicates that pygeum may inhibit fibroblast proliferation in the bladder and the prostate, and improve bladder contraction. In addition to its administration for BPH, pygeum has been used to treat inflammation, kidney disease, malaria, upset stomach, and fever, and has been used as an aphrodisiac.

Clinical Evidence

A 1998 Cochrane review of 18 randomized controlled trials ($n = 1,562$) evaluated *Pygeum africanum* in the treatment of BPH for a mean duration of 64 ± 21.1 days. Only one study did not find a difference between pygeum and placebo. Assessment of the pooled data demonstrated that pygeum provided clinically significant improvements in global symptoms, nocturia, and urinary flow measures.

A more recent 1-year observational study of 1,456 patients newly diagnosed with lower urinary tract symptoms or BPH analyzed the effects of all therapies (medications and watchful waiting). Clinically significant changes, defined as an International Prostate Symptom Score (IPSS) reduction of 4 points, were reported by 43.3% of patients treated with pygeum ($n = 90$). Compared to watchful waiting, pygeum resulted in an IPSS mean change of –3.4 points ($p = 0.0002$). Alpha blockers and finasteride provided the largest reductions in IPSS (mean change = –6.3 points and –4.1 points, respectively).

Pygeum may be recommended for short-term treatment of BPH symptoms; however, non-phytotherapy medications (i.e., alpha blockers and 5-alpha-reductase inhibitors) may provide more symptomatic improvement. Large, long-term clinical trials are needed to further evaluate the efficacy and safety of pygeum.

Dosage and Safety Considerations

Pygeum africanum doses of 75 mg/day to 200 mg/day have been used to treat BPH in clinical studies. Tolerability of pygeum is similar to placebo in clinical trials. Bothersome adverse effects include nausea, diarrhea, constipation, and gastric pain. Some evidence suggests that pygeum activity may be enhanced when it is used in combination with other prostate-affecting products such as saw palmetto, stinging nettle, and 5-alpha-reductase inhibitors.

Cranberry

Therapeutic Properties/Pharmacology

Cranberry is a popular dietary supplement used to prevent and treat urinary tract infections (UTIs). It exerts antimicrobial effects by preventing adhesion of microorganisms to epithelial cells of the bladder wall. The constituents of *Vaccinium macrocarpon*, the American cranberry, responsible for its pharmacologic activity have not been fully described. Proanthocyanidins (PACs) containing A-type linkages are thought to be responsible for inhibiting the adhesion of uropathic P-fimbriated *Escherichia coli*. Cranberry is available as juice, concentrate, capsules, and tablets.

Clinical Evidence

The effectiveness of cranberry in UTI prevention was evaluated in a Cochrane review of 24 randomized controlled trials ($n = 4,473$). Patients with recurrent UTIs (defined as two or more UTIs in the past 12 months), elderly patients, patients with in-dwelling or intermittent catheterization, pregnant women, patients with urinary abnormalities, and children at risk of recurrent UTI (defined as having more than one recent UTI) were included. The 24 trials used multiple cranberry products (e.g., juice, concentrate, syrup, capsules, tablets). Overall, cranberry did not significantly reduce the occurrence of symptomatic UTIs when compared to placebo, water, or no treatment (RR 0.86; 95% CI 0.71–1.04). A small, nonsignificant reduction in repeat UTI risk was noted in women (RR 0.74; 95% CI 0.42–1.31). Three studies comparing cranberry capsules or syrup to antibiotic prophylaxis showed no difference between treatment groups (RR 1.31; 95% CI 0.85–2.02). Cranberry was similar to probiotics in two trials involving women and children (RR 0.42; 95% CI 0.24–0.74). Studies included in this Cochrane review had high dropout rates, largely due to adherence issues with consuming cranberry juice on a long-term basis, and did not use intention-to-treat protocols. Many studies did not describe the quantity of cranberry or the amount of PAC utilized.

Limited evidence suggests that cranberry juice is more effective than tablets or capsules. This difference may be related to better hydration of patients consuming the juice and the use of less than adequate concentrations of PACs in tablet or capsule formulations.

In another Cochrane review, not enough clinical trial data were available to determine the efficacy of cranberry in the treatment of UTIs. A double-blind, randomized, controlled trial evaluating the effects of cranberry juice three times daily in adult females with active UTI was recently completed; however, its results have not yet been published.

The use of cranberry products to prevent UTIs does not seem to provide benefits in most patient populations. Results from double-blind, randomized, controlled trials are needed before cranberry can be recommended as a UTI treatment.

Dosage and Safety Considerations

The recommended dose for prevention of UTI is 36–72 mg of proanthocyanidins daily, and can be consumed in 300 mL of cranberry juice cocktail or powder formulations. Only powder-containing capsules or tablets that have adequate amounts of active and correctly quantified PACs should be consumed to ensure potency. Cranberry should be administered two or three times daily. *In vitro* studies suggest that inhibition of bacterial adhesion lasts for approximately 8 hours after cranberry ingestion.

Cranberry does not appear to cause significant adverse events, although reporting of adverse outcomes in clinical trials has been inconsistent. When such events have been reported, gastrointestinal effects were not significantly different with cranberry than with placebo. The palatability of cranberry products and the need to ingest large amounts may be barriers to adherence, however. Consideration should be given to the caloric content of cranberry juice, and low-sugar formulations may be recommended to patients with diabetes.

Consuming large amounts of cranberry juice in conjunction with warfarin has been identified in case reports to increase the INR. Patients taking warfarin and cranberry should be closely monitored for INR alterations and bleeding events.

Saw Palmetto

Therapeutic Properties/Pharmacology

Saw palmetto (*Serenoa repens*), which is derived from the ripened fruit of the American dwarf palm tree, has been a widely used BPH treatment in the United States. Its active components include phytosterols, glycerides, fatty acids, and ethyl esters. Saw palmetto has many proposed mechanisms of action, including inhibition of 5-alpha-reductase, smooth muscle relaxation of the bladder detrusor and prostate, stimulation of apoptosis and inhibition of cell proliferation, and anti-inflammatory activity. In addition to treatment of BPH, saw palmetto has been used for urogenital infections, androgenic alopecia, diabetes, migraine headaches, and bronchitis.

Clinical Evidence

A Cochrane review evaluated the efficacy of saw palmetto in the treatment of BPH. The analysis included 5,666 men in 32 randomized controlled trials lasting 4–72 weeks. Limitations of the clinical trials included failure to use validated symptom rating scales and inadequate treatment allocation concealment. The majority of clinical trials used sabal extract 80–160 mg twice daily, which was not superior to placebo in improving urinary symptoms based on the American Urologic Association Symptom Index (AUA) or the IPSS (mean difference [MD] –0.77; 95% CI –2.88 to 1.34). Nocturia did not improve compared to placebo ($p = 0.19$), and there was no significant change in prostate size compared to placebo (MD 0.40 mL/s; 95% CI –3.91 to 1.47).

In a 72-week dose escalation trial, saw palmetto 320 mg/day, 640 mg/day, and 960 mg/day were not superior to placebo in improving AUA scores (MD 0.25; 95% CI –0.58 to 1.07).

Based on the results of these large trials that used sound methodologies, saw palmetto is not superior to placebo in reducing the urinary symptoms of BPH.

Dosage and Safety Considerations

The recommended dose of saw palmetto is 160 mg twice daily. Mild adverse effects associated with saw palmetto use have been reported, but were not statistically significant when compared to placebo. Commonly reported adverse effects include headache, decreased libido, nausea, diarrhea, and fatigue. Saw palmetto is contraindicated in pregnancy and should not be used with oral contraceptives or hormone therapy due to its antiandrogen and antiestrogen effects.

Learning Bridge 13.6

A 67-year-old female patient presents to the community pharmacy to pick up a new prescription of warfarin. The dose is different than that used in previous refills, and she is very concerned about the change. The physician's office called in a different dose after her recent INR. Upon questioning, she reports drinking cranberry juice over the past week because she thinks she has a bladder infection.

A. How does cranberry alter warfarin's effects?
B. Provide advice that should be given to the patient about using cranberry juice?

Weight Loss

Chitosan

Therapeutic Properties/Pharmacology

While not plant based, chitosan is a natural product obtained from the exoskeleton of shellfish, including crab, lobster, and shrimp. Treating shellfish exoskeleton with sodium hydroxide produces a polysaccharide molecule. Chitosan is commonly used for weight loss and is marketed as a "fat burner." The proposed mechanism of action for the weight loss effect is binding of the chitosan to cholesterol and bile acids within the intestine, which prevents their enterohepatic reabsorption. Considered a cellulose-like dietary fiber, chitosan exerts a local action in the gastrointestinal tract and is minimally absorbed from the intestine.

Clinical Evidence

A 2008 Cochrane review analyzed 15 trials that enrolled a total of 1,219 patients and that met the researchers' inclusion criteria. To be included in this meta-analysis, trials had to be randomized and controlled, with the duration of chitosan use ranging from a minimum of 4 weeks to 6 months in patients who were classified as overweight or obese. Although the results showed a mean weight-loss difference of 0.6 kg, this outcome did not reach statistical significance ($p = 0.09$). The researchers concluded that some evidence favors the use of chitosan when compared to placebo in short-term studies as an aid for weight loss in overweight and obese patients. Concerning limitations of the data included poor trial quality and lack of morbidity and mortality data. Until high-quality studies can evaluate the efficacy of chitosan, this supplement should be used with caution as a weight-loss aid.

Dosage and Safety Considerations

Dosages of chitosan used in clinical trials for weight loss have ranged from 1 gram to 5 grams per day in divided doses. Chitosan is generally well tolerated, but with gastrointestinal adverse effects such as nausea, diarrhea, constipation, bloating, and abdominal pain being reported. These adverse effects usually were not severe enough to cause discontinuation. No drug–natural product interactions have been reported. As a cholesterol binder, chitosan could theoretically bind to medications within the intestine, thereby preventing those drugs' absorption and reducing their effectiveness. There is also concern that chitosan might potentially block the absorption of fat-soluble vitamins, although this effect has not been seen clinically. Because this supplement is derived from shellfish exoskeletons, patients with shellfish allergy should use caution or avoid chitosan altogether.

Guarana

Therapeutic Properties/Pharmacology

Guarana is the common name of the *Paullinia cupana* plant, whose seeds are consumed for their caffeine content and stimulant effects. Guarana seeds have 2.5–7% caffeine content, compared to the 1–2% caffeine content in coffee. Guarana has been used for enhancement of cognition, mood, and athletic performance as well as for weight loss and to reduce fatigue. It is a common ingredient, used alone or in combination, in over-the-counter weight-loss aids and energy drinks.

Caffeine exerts its effects on numerous organ systems in the body. In the brain, it acts as an adenosine receptor antagonist, preventing adenosine from having its sleep-promoting or -inhibitory effects on neurons. To achieve its weight-loss effect, caffeine is thought to increase metabolic rate, energy expenditure, and fat metabolism, and potentially regulate body heat production due to its thermogenic activity.

Clinical Evidence

Relatively few clinical trials have been performed to document the safety and effectiveness of guarana. As it is believed that the active ingredient in guarana is caffeine, most clinical trials have used caffeine rather than the naturally derived guarana. Guarana and caffeine are often used in combination with other herbal ingredients for weight loss, making it difficult to determine which ingredient was actually effective. Moreover, the combination may have synergistic effects, resulting in enhanced weight loss.

Dosage and Safety Considerations

No specific dose of guarana has been identified in clinical trials as being safe and effective. This supplement is typically standardized based on its caffeine content. Doses range from 35 mg to 570 mg of caffeine per dose. In low doses, caffeine is generally well tolerated with limited adverse effects. Excessive doses of caffeine, however, can lead to headache, nausea, irritability, heart palpitations, anxiety, and other central nervous system adverse effects. Caffeine can increase blood pressure and heart rate, although tolerance to these adverse effects can develop over time. Patients who do not take or consume caffeine daily are at greater risk of unwanted adverse effects.

Patients with high blood pressure seem to be more sensitive to the cardiovascular effects of caffeine and have longer periods of elevated blood pressure after consuming this ingredient. Therefore, caffeine can decrease the effectiveness of antihypertensive medications. In addition, due to the stimulant effects of caffeine, it should be used with caution in patients taking antiarrhythmic and antianxiety medications.

Hoodia

Therapeutic Properties/Pharmacology

Hoodia gordonii is a flowering, slow-growing succulent plant found in South Africa. As a supplement, hoodia is used for weight loss and is marketed as an appetite suppressant. Indigenous Africans have used the plant for years to suppress appetite and quench thirst. Due to concerns about excessive harvesting of the plant that might potentially lead to endangered species status for *Hoodia gordonii*, hoodia cultivation and harvesting are regulated by the South African government. Owing to this regulation, many products claiming to contain hoodia actually have a lower concentration than that marked on the package.

The active ingredient in hoodia thought to exert the appetite suppressant effect is a glycoside identified as P57. The P57 glycoside has been proposed to exert its pharmacologic activity by increasing adenosine triphosphate content within the neurons of the hypothalamus and altering food intake in the body. The hypothalamus regulates hunger, appetite, and temperature control.

Clinical Evidence

No clinical trials to assess the safety or efficacy of hoodia in humans have been published in the medical literature. Animal models indicate that a 30–60% decrease in food intake may occur over the next 24 hours after injection of P57 into the brains of mice. Two different manufacturers of hoodia products have published preliminary human studies data on the Internet. Results were favorable, with reductions in daily caloric intake, body fat content, and body weight being reported. Limitations of the data are concerning, as the information was not published in a peer-reviewed journal and the authors did not provide study methods or demographic data with which to determine the generalizability of the results. Until high-quality studies can evaluate the safety and efficacy of hoodia, the risks associated with this supplement outweigh any potential benefits and, therefore, it should not be recommended as a weight-loss aid.

Dosage and Safety Considerations

As there are no reliable clinical trials demonstrating the safety and efficacy of hoodia, dosing is based on historical practices and anecdotal evidence. An unpublished trial conducted by Goldfarb used 500-mg hoodia capsules, where patients took two capsules by mouth daily for 28 days. Natural Standard lists dosages ranging from 400 mg to 800 mg per day for weight loss. No adverse effects have been reported, but insufficient reliable information is available to determine the true risks associated with taking hoodia. No drug interactions have been reported, but again insufficient reliable information is available to identify potential interactions.

Women's Health

Black Cohosh

Therapeutic Properties/Pharmacology

Black cohosh was traditionally used by Native Americans to treat a variety of women's health issues. This supplement has been studied for treatment of premenstrual syndrome and menopausal symptoms including hot flashes and sleep and mood disturbances. Black cohosh has also been used to treat snake bites, rheumatic symptoms, and chorea. The dried rhizomes and roots of the plant (*Actaea racemosa* or *Cimicifuga racemosa*) are used in the medicinal preparations.

The triterpene glycosides and flavonoids in black cohosh are considered to have pharmacologic activity, although their precise mechanism of action remains unknown. Initial reports indicated that black cohosh exerted estrogen-like activity, but this theory was refuted upon further testing. Reduction of luteinizing hormone secretion is another proposed mechanism of action that has not been validated by recent studies. More recent data indicate that black cohosh has central nervous system effects, possibly through serotonergic or dopaminergic activity. Dopaminergic-2 receptor stimulation has been demonstrated, which could increase libido and have positive effects on bone metabolism.

Clinical Evidence

In a recent Cochrane review, *Cimicifuga racemosa* (median dose = 40 mg/day, range 8–160 mg; mean duration = 23 weeks, range 4–52 weeks) was evaluated for efficacy and safety compared to placebo, hormone therapy, fluoxetine, or placebo. Sixteen randomized controlled trials that enrolled perimenopausal or postmenopausal females (*n* = 2,027) were analyzed. There were no statistically significant differences in frequency and intensity of hot flashes, frequency of night sweats, or menopausal symptom scores with black cohosh compared to placebo and red clover. Conversely, hormone therapy significantly reduced the frequency of hot flashes and night sweats and improved menopausal symptom scores compared to black cohosh. Statistically significant improvements in night sweat scores and menopausal symptoms scores were seen with black cohosh compared to fluoxetine (data from one trial).

Black cohosh is a promising treatment, but it cannot be confidently recommended for menopausal symptoms due to a lack of reliable data and large variations in trial designs. More studies with robust designs and improved reporting methods are needed to elucidate the value of this supplement. German health authorities have cited black cohosh as an effective treatment for PMS and painful menstruation, although only limited evidence supports this therapeutic benefit.

Dosage and Safety Considerations

The recommended dose of black cohosh is 20 mg twice daily for up to 6 months. Adverse events have not been adequately reported in clinical trials, but may include gastrointestinal upset and dizziness. Breast cancer was once a concern with black cohosh, but conclusions that the plant does not have estrogenic activity have helped alleviate this fear.

There have been case reports of hepatotoxicity with black cohosh use, although the *United States Pharmacopeia* review of the liver damage reports assigned possible causality to black cohosh versus probable or certain causality. Caution and monitoring for liver damage should be exercised before and during black cohosh use.

Phytoestrogens

Therapeutic Properties/Pharmacology

Phytoestrogens are plant compounds that exert estrogenic effects. Isoflavones (genistein and daidzein), lignans, and phytosterols are the pharmacologically active components that can be found in the red clover plant, soy products, chickpeas, beans, fruits, vegetables, and whole grains. Phytoestrogens attracted interest as a treatment for menopausal symptoms when it was observed that certain females who consumed large amounts of soy and other dietary sources of phytoestrogens had a lower incidence of such symptoms. Phytoestrogens also have the potential to act as antiestrogens through competitive binding of estrogen receptors.

Clinical Evidence

Phytoestrogen effects on hot flushes and night sweats in perimenopausal and postmenopausal women have been evaluated in a Cochrane review that included 30 randomized controlled trials ($n = 2,730$). Many different forms of phytoestrogen—such as dietary soy isoflavone, soy isoflavone extracts, and red clover extracts—were used as interventions in these trials, and most studies lasted 3 months. Studies of phytoestrogen used varying methodologies and inconsistent outcome assessments. As a consequence, only five studies of red clover extracts were included in a meta-analysis. These five studies of a standard extract of red clover (Promensil, 40 and 80 mg/day isoflavones) did not identify a significant reduction in frequency of hot flushes between groups or between dosages (weighted mean difference –0.57; 95% CI –1.76 to 0.62). Treatment with dietary soy did not prove more effective than the outcomes seen with the control group in 7 out of 9 trials. A 12-week study of soy powder containing 76 mg/day of isoflavones with casein did produce a reduction in daily hot flushes compared to placebo (weighted mean difference –1.6; 95% CI –1.95 to –1.2). Another study found that a diet high in phytoestrogens (more than 30 mg/day isoflavones) significantly reduced the severity of hot flushes more than diets that did not include phytoestrogens. Five studies using soy extract capsules or tablets (7–100 mg/day isoflavone or 50 mg/day genistin and daidzin, respectively) reported significant differences in the ability to reduce frequency of hot flushes, frequency of night sweats, or severity of flushes compared to placebo, while four other studies did not find a difference in symptoms. No difference in reduction of hot flushes was apparent when soy 120 mg/day was compared with estrogen; however, the soy-treated group experienced less genital bleeding as an adverse effect. Other phytoestrogen preparations (flaxseed, hops, lobata, genistein extract) did not improve vasomotor symptoms compared to placebo or hormone therapy.

Other systematic reviews suggest that phytoestrogens may have more of a beneficial impact on women who exhibit severe vasomotor symptoms at baseline. More data are needed to confirm this finding. To date, trials with inconsistent methodologies have yielded inconclusive evidence that phytoestrogens reduce menopausal vasomotor symptoms.

Dosage and Safety Considerations

Phytoestrogen sources containing 30 mg to 120 mg of isoflavones can be given daily for relief of postmenopausal symptoms. Higher rates of adverse events, including bloating, nausea, weight gain, and bowel function concerns, were reported in dietary phytoestrogen trials. The palatability of dietary phytoestrogens in the form of soy powder may limit many women's willingness to use this supplement. Phytoestrogens used for as long as 1 year do not appear to have estrogenic effects on the endometrium, as is frequently reported with hormone therapy. Until long-term safety data are available, phytoestrogens as a menopausal treatment should be used only with caution and perhaps avoided in patients with breast cancer. The inclusion of soy and other phytoestrogen-containing foods should not be restricted as part of a balanced diet.

Role of the Pharmacist

Nutraceuticals can be useful medicinal products, but should be subjected to the same efficacy and safety scrutiny as more conventional medicines. Pharmacists are responsible for encouraging appropriate use of medications to optimize therapeutic outcomes and improve patients' quality of life. This responsibility extends to nonprescription medications, herbal medicines, and dietary supplements, in just the same way that it applies to prescription drug use.

All healthcare providers should recognize that many patients today choose to use natural products, and they often do not seek guidance from healthcare providers when doing so or disclose their use of these treatments. When gathering a patient's medical history, data on present and past use of dietary supplements should be collected as part of this process. The healthcare team should routinely conduct a thorough evaluation of all current therapies for each patient. Pharmacists should contribute to this effort by identifying current and potential drug therapy problems such as duplication of therapy, adverse drug reactions, subtherapeutic doses, and drug interactions. Compatibility issues with natural products and other pharmaceuticals are frequently observed drug therapy problems. Common drug–herb interactions are summarized in **Table 13.3**.

In summary, pharmacists are in a unique position as medication experts to take a proactive role within the healthcare team by ensuring the appropriate use of all types of medicines, including prescription drugs, nonprescription products, and nutraceuticals.

Table 13.3 Summary of Drug–Dietary Supplement Interactions

Dietary Supplement	Drug	Possible Interaction
Blood Glucose Effects		
American ginseng Cinnamon Fenugreek Ginger	Antihyperglycemic agents	Enhanced blood-glucose–lowering effect
Coagulation Effects		
Chondroitin Feverfew Garlic Ginger Ginkgo Policosanol (theoretical) Yohimbine (theoretical)	Anticoagulants, antiplatelet agents	Increased bleeding risk through platelet inhibition, increased INR with garlic
Chitosan (theoretical) Coenzyme Q10 (theoretical)	Anticoagulants	Decreased anticoagulant effect
Cinnamon (theoretical) Fenugreek (theoretical)	Anticoagulants	Enhanced anticoagulation effects

(continues)

Table 13.3 Summary of Drug–Dietary Supplement Interactions (*continued*)

Dietary Supplement	Drug	Interaction
Cranberry	Warfarin	Increase in INR, increased bleeding risk
Ginseng		Decrease in INR, reduced anticoagulation effect
Fish oil	Anticoagulants	Prolonged bleeding time
Effects on Cytochrome P450 and P-Glycoprotein		
Dehydroepiandrosterone (DHEA) Peppermint (theoretical)	Drugs metabolized by CYP3A4	Increased concentrations of concomitant medications, DHEA significantly increases triazolam levels
Ginkgo	Omeprazole, tolbutamide	Induction of CYP2C9 and CYP2C19, decreased concentrations of concomitant medications
Kava (theoretical) Milk thistle (*in vitro*)	Drugs metabolized by CYP3A4, CYP2C9, and CYP2D6	Inhibition of CYP450 enzymes, increased concentrations of concomitant medications
St. John's wort	Substrates of P-glycoprotein, CYP1A2, CYP3A4, CYP2E1, and CYP2C19	Induction of P-glycoprotein and CYP450 enzymes, decreased concentrations of concomitant medications
	Serotonin-enhancing medications	Increased risk of serotonin syndrome
Miscellaneous Interactions		
Elderberry	Immunosuppressants	Immune system stimulation, possible transplant rejection
Kava Valerian	Central nervous system depressants	Increased sedation
Yohimbine	Clomipramine	Increased blood pressure
	Monoamine oxidase inhibitors	Enhanced monoamine oxidase inhibition, increased blood pressure
	Serotonin-enhancing medications (theoretical)	Increased risk of serotonin syndrome

CYP = cytochrome P450; INR = International Normalized Ratio.

Golden Keys for Pharmacy Students

- The study of plants for medicinal use led to drug discovery and synthetic drug production.

- Natural products are readily available without a prescription and are commonly used by the public.

- Natural products are regulated by the Food and Drug Administration according to the Dietary Supplement Health and Education Act (DSHEA).

- The DSHEA classifies dietary supplements as foods rather than as drugs.

- Three types of marketing claims are allowed for dietary supplements: a health claim, a nutrient content claim, or a structure/function claim. Manufacturers of dietary supplements cannot claim that the product will diagnose, cure, mitigate, treat, or prevent a disease.

- Patients should be encouraged to select a natural product from a reputable manufacturer and one whose label indicates that the product has been certified by a dietary supplement verification program.

- Limited and sometimes conflicting evidence is available to support or refute recommendations for dietary supplements.

- Because limited information is available about actual or potential drug interactions with natural products, caution should be exercised when selecting or recommending a dietary supplement.

- Drug information databases such as Natural Standard and Natural Medicines Comprehensive Database provide overviews of individual natural products.

- Cochrane reviews, clinical trial data, and other meta-analyses or systematic reviews should be utilized when responding to drug information requests.

- Coenzyme Q10 has been shown to reduce blood pressure and could be recommended as an adjunct to other antihypertensive therapies. A theoretical use for coenzyme Q10 is in the reduction of statin-induced muscle pain that is not due to rhabdomyolysis.

- Fish oil (i.e., omega-3 fatty acids) can be used to significantly lower triglycerides.

- Garlic and policosanol may have modest benefits in reducing cholesterol levels.

- Hawthorn has been studied for use in congestive heart failure. Until long-term data supporting its safety and efficacy are available, use of this supplement should be limited.

- American ginseng, cinnamon, and fenugreek have been studied as means to lower blood glucose for the treatment of diabetes.

- Andrographis, Echinacea, and elderberry are used for the treatment of the common cold and influenza.

- Ginger is commonly used for the treatment of nausea and vomiting associated with pregnancy, motion sickness, chemotherapy, and surgery.

- Milk thistle is used as an adjunct to conventional therapies for the treatment of liver diseases such as hepatitis B and hepatitis C, cirrhosis, and fatty liver disease from alcohol.

- *Ginkgo biloba* can be used for dementia or Alzheimer's disease, but does not have evidence supporting its ability to prevent these conditions.

- Kava may be an effective treatment of anxiety, but potentially increases the risk of severe liver injury.

- St. John's wort can be used as an antidepressant, but interacts with many medications through its cytochrome P450 activity.

- Valerian does not have adequate clinical data supporting it as a recommended treatment of insomnia or anxiety.

- Capsaicin exerts a characteristic burning, stinging, and tingling effect when applied topically, and it may cause severe skin burns.

- Butterbur and feverfew are used to prevent migraine headaches.

- Glucosamine and chondroitin, while generally safe, do not appear to be effective in improving osteoarthritis pain.

- Willow bark is used to relieve acute low back pain and is contraindicated in patients with an allergy to salicylates.

- DHEA is a precursor to testosterone and estrogen.

- L-Arginine is an amino acid that is metabolized to nitric oxide, which relaxes smooth muscles and increases blood flow.

- Yohimbe is an α_2-receptor blocker and is on the FDA's list of unsafe herbs due to its effects in stimulating central catecholamine release.

- Pygeum is used to improve urinary symptoms due to BPH.

- Cranberry inhibits bacterial adhesion to the bladder wall. This supplement has not been shown to be effective as a UTI preventive therapy and has not been studied extensively as a treatment of active UTI infections.

- Saw palmetto is no more effective than placebo for the treatment of BPH.

- Chitosan is obtained from the exoskeleton of shellfish. It is thought to work by binding to cholesterol and bile acids within the intestine, thereby preventing enterohepatic recycling.

- The active ingredient in guarana is caffeine.

- Hoodia is marketed as an appetite suppressant. Because no clinical trials on this supplement have been published in the medical literature, its safety and efficacy have not been established; consequently, hoodia should not be recommended.

- Peppermint is thought to work as an antispasmodic by antagonizing calcium channels, resulting in intestinal smooth muscle relaxation. It is commonly used for the treatment of irritable bowel syndrome.

- Black cohosh does not seem to have estrogenic activity, but rather is thought to have effects within the central nervous system.

- Phytoestrogens are found in red clover plant, soy products, chickpeas, beans, fruits, vegetables, and whole grains.

- Pharmacists need to be competent in educating patients and other members of the healthcare team on the appropriate use of dietary supplements.

- Information on dietary supplements use should be gathered as part of the patient's medical history.

Learning Bridge Answers

13.1 A. The mechanism of action for fish oil is a combination of reduced synthesis in the liver and increased clearance of triglycerides.

B. Common adverse effects associated with omega-3 fatty acids are gastrointestinal upset and fish burps. These effects can be minimized by taking the fish oil with meals, using enteric-coated products, and taking the supplements before bedtime. Fish oil also has the potential to prolong bleeding time, but clinical trials have not demonstrated alterations in bleeding time or warfarin dosing regimen.

C. Each 1-gram Lovaza capsule contains 375 mg of DHA and 465 mg of EPA (for a total of approximately 840 mg of omega-3 fatty acid ethyl esters). The 1,000-mg fish oil product that the patient presented to the pharmacist contained a combination of 300 mg of DHA and EPA. Thus one Lovaza capsule is approximately equal to three OTC fish oil capsules. The directions for Lovaza are to take 2 capsules by mouth twice a day. To equal the Lovaza dose, the patient would have to take 12 OTC fish oil capsules by mouth daily in divided doses.

13.2 A. American ginseng, cinnamon, and fenugreek have all been proposed to lower blood glucose.

B. A number of questions should be asked prior to recommending any treatment option. At a minimum, the pharmacist should inquire about current medications, current medical conditions, and allergies to medications and environmental factors. By asking these questions, the pharmacist can assess for potential drug–dietary supplement interactions or adverse effects.

C. Currently, limited evidence from randomized controlled clinical trials is available to support the use of American ginseng, cinnamon, and fenugreek. Proven conventional therapies, such as medical nutrition therapy (diet), physical activity, and medications, are available. Because the patient has a diagnosis of prediabetes, the best recommendation would be to avoid use of dietary supplements and to initiate lifestyle modifications.

13.3 A. Gingerol, shogaol, and galanolactone are thought to be the active ingredients in ginger. Ginger's mechanism of action as an antiemetic is attributed to its serotonin antagonist effects locally within the gastrointestinal tract as well as to its central nervous system effects. Ginger is also thought to exert anticholinergic effects, resulting in increased gastric tone and peristalsis.

B. Although ginger is "Generally Regarded as Safe" by the FDA in relation to the developing fetus, other countries have issued warnings that high doses of this product are unsafe for use in pregnancy. Prior to initiating ginger therapy, the patient should consult with her OB/GYN to weigh the risks versus the benefits of therapy. It is also important to consider adverse effects such as heartburn, increased risk of bleeding, and alterations of blood glucose levels.

C. For nausea and vomiting related to pregnancy, the most common dose studied is 250 mg of powdered root taken by mouth four times a day.

13.4 A. St. John's wort may be an effective antidepressant when taken for 4–12 weeks. Clinical trials have shown this supplement to be superior to placebo and to have similar efficacy compared to tricyclic antidepressants and selective serotonin reuptake inhibitors.

B. St. John's wort and the oral contraceptive will interact. St. John's wort induces the metabolism of the ethinyl estradiol component of this patient's oral contraceptive, which may result in contraceptive failure. St. John's wort should be avoided or the patient may use a nonhormonal contraceptive method.

C. Patients should use St. John's wort or any other antidepressant only under the supervision of a healthcare professional. Inadequate treatment can result in worsening of depression, and patients should be closely monitored when beginning drug treatment as anxiety and suicidal thoughts may increase initially.

13.5 A. Glucosamine sulfate 1,500 mg/day, given once or split three times daily, has been the most frequently studied regimen and has been found to be effective in a Cochrane review. The patient should not choose a product with chondroitin because he has a history of prostate cancer.

B. Glucosamine is not likely to be an effective treatment. A large clinical trial showed glucosamine and chondroitin to be effective for moderate to severe osteoarthritis during the first 6 months of treatment; however, this effect did not persist in a 2-year follow-up.

C. The risk of cross-reactivity with glucosamine is very small. Glucosamine is often derived from the exoskeletons of shellfish, although the extraction process likely removes the allergens. The patient should be cautious when first taking glucosamine. He should seek immediate medical attention if any swelling of the face, lips, tongue, or throat occurs. He could also look for a completely synthetic glucosamine product.

13.6 A. Consuming large amounts of cranberry juice while also taking warfarin has been reported to increase the INR. Patients taking warfarin and cranberry concomitantly should be closely monitored for INR alterations and bleeding events.

B. The patient should be advised that clinical trials evaluating cranberry as a UTI treatment are lacking, and that this supplement has not been shown to prevent UTIs in most populations. The patient should contact the healthcare providers who manage her warfarin to discuss stopping the cranberry. She also should follow up with her primary care provider for further evaluation of a possible UTI.

Problems and Solutions

Problem 13.1 Which of the following is the most widely used form of complementary and alternative medicine?

- **A.** Mind–body medicine
- **B.** Manipulative and body-based practices
- **C.** Dietary supplements
- **D.** Healing touch

Solution 13.1 C is correct.

Problem 13.2 A manufacturer is developing a marketing campaign for a new dietary supplement. Which of the following is an appropriate structure/function claim that can be used to market the product?

    A. "Promotes a healthy digestive system"
    B. "Prevents and treats symptoms of IBS"
    C. "Works with the body to naturally slow the progression of colon cancer"
    D. "Stimulates intestine enzyme production, curing ulcerative colitis"

Solution 13.2 A is correct. A structure/function claim describes how a nutrient or dietary supplement may affect organs or systems in the body, but cannot include statements about any specific disease. Structure/function claims are not approved by the FDA, and labeling on these products must include the following disclaimer: "This statement has not been evaluated by the Food and Drug Administration. This product is not intended to diagnose, treat, cure, or prevent any disease."

Problem 13.3 You are asked to answer the drug information question: "How safe and effective is St. John's wort?" Which resource should you use to find the most recently published St. John's wort clinical trials?

    A. Natural Standard
    B. Cochrane Library
    C. MEDLINE
    D. Internet search engine such as Google or Bing

Solution 13.3 C is correct. A MEDLINE search should be conducted to find the most recently published biomedical information. Cochrane reviews provide highly regarded systematic reviews and meta-analyses of clinical trial data; however, the most recent data may not be included due to the lengthy process involved in conducting such reviews. The Natural Standard is a good reference for natural product overviews and does contain evidence-based information, but is updated only periodically.

Problem 13.4 Dietary supplements that contain garlic are standardized to which active ingredient?

    A. Alliin
    B. Alliinase
    C. Allicin
    D. Allium

Solution 13.4 C is correct. Garlic contains alliin, which when crushed is broken down by the enzyme alliinase and converted to allicin. Allicin is believed to be the active component and is the part of garlic's volatile oil that gives it the characteristic aroma.

Problem 13.5 What is the proposed mechanism of action for cinnamon in relation to the treatment of diabetes?

    A. Increased insulin secretion by the pancreatic beta cells
    B. Increased uptake of glucose by cells in the liver, fat, and muscle
    C. Decreased hepatic glucose production
    D. Decreased breakdown of complex carbohydrates in the intestine

Solution 13.5 B is correct. Cinnamon is thought to work by increasing insulin sensitivity and cellular uptake of glucose.

Problem 13.6 What is the active ingredient in the commercially available product called Kan Jang?

    A. Andrographis
    B. Echinacea
    C. Elderberry
    D. Oscillococcinum

Solution 13.6 A is correct. Kan Jang (Swedish Herbal Institute) is available both as a combination product that contains andrographis and eleutherococcus and as a single-herb product containing only andrographis.

Problem 13.7 Echinacea is likely to have cross-hypersensitivity reactions (allergic reactions) with which of the following?

    A. Shellfish
    B. Pet dander
    C. Ragweed
    D. Pollen

Solution 13.7 C is correct. Echinacea, daisies, marigolds, and ragweed are all members of the Asteraceae family.

Problem 13.8 *Ginkgo biloba* may cause which of the following adverse effects?

    A. Hepatotoxicity
    B. Diarrhea
    C. Elevated blood sugars
    D. Increased bleeding risk

Solution 13.8 D is correct. *Ginkgo biloba* may increase bleeding risk through inhibition of platelet aggregation and may interact with antiplatelet medications or anticoagulants.

Problem 13.9 Which warning has the FDA issued concerning kava use?

    A. Increased risk of severe liver damage
    B. Increased risk of prostate cancer
    C. Increased risk of severe skin burns
    D. Increased risk of migraine headaches

Solution 13.9 A is correct. Numerous reports of liver toxicity related to kava resulted in an FDA warning in the United States and the removal of kava from markets in Canada and Europe.

Problem 13.10 Which constituent of butterbur has the potential to be hepatotoxic and carcinogenic?

    A. Sesquiterpene lactones
    B. Pyrrolizidine alkaloids
    C. Flavonoids
    D. Volatile oils

Solution 13.10 B is correct. The pyrrolizidine alkaloids found in butterbur can be hepatotoxic and carcinogenic. This component is removed from butterbur products through an extraction process, and patients should be educated to consume only butterbur labeled as "PA free."

Problem 13.11 What is the primary mechanism of action of capsaicin?

- **A.** Substance P depletion
- **B.** Anti-inflammatory effects
- **C.** Increased biosynthesis of cartilage constituents
- **D.** Prolonged activation of the TRPV1 receptor

Solution 13.11 D is correct. Prolonged and repeated activation of the TRPV1 receptor by capsaicin causes sensory nerve defunctionalization and decreased pain response. Capsaicin does cause depletion of substance P, but substance P has only a minor effect on the pain pathway.

Problem 13.12 A 52-year-old male patient would like a natural product to relieve his low back pain. He was instructed to stop using ibuprofen after he was diagnosed with a gastric ulcer 8 months ago. The patient has no known allergies to food or medications. Which of the following would be the best recommendation to treat this patient's low back pain?

- **A.** Willow bark
- **B.** Chondroitin
- **C.** Alpha lipoic acid
- **D.** Capsaicin

Solution 13.12 A is correct. Willow bark was observed in clinical trials to relieve acute low back pain and is not known to cause adverse gastrointestinal effects.

Problem 13.13 DHEA may improve sexual function in which patient population?

- **A.** Premenopausal females
- **B.** Men with erectile dysfunction from hypertension
- **C.** Men with erectile dysfunction from diabetes
- **D.** DHEA did not improve sexual function in any of these populations

Solution 13.13 B is correct. Small clinical trials have shown that sexual function may improve with DHEA 50 mg/day in men with ED from hypertension and of no organic etiology, and with DHEA 10 mg/day in postmenopausal women.

Problem 13.14 A 62-year-old male patient would like a recommendation for a natural product to treat BPH. He is not sleeping well because he must get up to urinate four to five times per night. He has been intolerant to the adverse effects of prescription alpha$_1$ blockers and cannot afford finasteride. Which of the following supplements would be the best recommendation based on efficacy?

- **A.** Saw palmetto
- **B.** Yohimbe
- **C.** Pygeum
- **D.** DHEA

Solution 13.14 C is correct. Pygeum has been shown to improve urinary symptoms in men with BPH, while saw palmetto is not more efficacious than placebo. Yohimbe can increase frequency of urination, and DHEA has not been studied as a BPH treatment.

Problem 13.15 A patient taking which of the following medications would be likely to experience an adverse effect when it is taken in combination with guarana (caffeine)?

   A. Lisinopril

   B. Amiodarone

   C. Alprazolam

   D. All of the above

Solution 13.15 D is correct. Due to the stimulant effects of caffeine, it can decrease the effectiveness of antihypertensive medications and should be used with caution in patients taking antiarrhythmic and antianxiety medications. Lisinopril is an angiotensin-converting enzyme (ACE) inhibitor used to lower blood pressure. Amiodarone is an antiarrhythmic. Alprazolam is a benzodiazepine used for anxiety.

Problem 13.16 Which portion of the *Zingiber officinale* plant is commonly used for the treatment of nausea and vomiting?

   A. Flowers

   B. Seeds

   C. Rhizome

   D. Leaves

Solution 13.16 C is correct.

Problem 13.17 Why have phytoestrogens been studied as a treatment for menopausal symptoms?

   A. Females consuming soy-rich foods had a lower incidence of menopausal symptoms.

   B. Isoflavones have high progestin activity.

   C. Phytoestrogens were commonly used by Native Americans for female complaints.

   D. Phytoestrogens were observed to reduce the risk of breast cancer.

Solution 13.17 A is correct. Females, particularly of Asian ethnicity, who regularly consumed soy and plant-based foods were observed to have a lower incidence of menopausal symptoms and less severe hot flushes.

References

1. Abenavoli L, Capasso R, Milic N, Capasso F. Milk thistle in liver diseases: past, present, future. *Phytotherapy Research.* 2010;24:1423–1432.

2. Altman RD, Barthel HR. Topical therapies for osteoarthritis. *Drugs.* 2011;71:1.

3. AltMedDex System [Internet database]. Greenwood Village, CO: Thomson Reuters (Healthcare); updated periodically.

4. Anand P, Bley K. Topical capsaicin for pain management: therapeutic potential and mechanisms of action of the new high-concentration capsaicin 8% patch. *Br J Anaesth.* 2011;107:490–502.

5. Anatomy of the new requirements for dietary supplement labels. Food and Drug Administration. Available at: http://www.preventivehealthtoday.com/fda/fdac/fdac_9811_fdsuppla.pdf. Accessed January 28, 2013.

6. Andreatini R, Sartori VA, Seabra ML, Leite JR. Effect of valepotriates (valerian extract) in generalized anxiety disorder: a randomized placebo-controlled pilot study. *Phytother Res.* 2002;16:650–654.

7. Appendix A: definitions of nutrient content claims. Guidance for industry: a food labeling guide. Food and Drug Administration; updated May 23, 2011. Available at: http://www.fda.gov/Food

/GuidanceComplianceRegulatoryInformation/GuidanceDocuments/FoodLabelingNutrition /FoodLabelingGuide/ucm064911.htm. Accessed January 28, 2013.

8. Appendix C: health claims. Guidance for industry: a food labeling guide. Food and Drug Administration; updated May 23, 2011. Available at: http://www.fda.gov/Food/Guidance ComplianceRegulatoryInformation/GuidanceDocuments/FoodLabelingNutrition/Food LabelingGuide/ucm064919.htm. Accessed January 28, 2013.

9. Aydin AA, Zerbes V, Parlar H, Letzel T. The medical plant butterbur (*Petasites*): analytical and physiological (re)view. *J Pharm Biomed Anal.* 2013;75:220–229.

10. Background information: dietary supplements. National Institute of Health Office of Dietary Supplements; reviewed June 24, 2011. Available at: http://ods.od.nih.gov/factsheets /DietarySupplements-HealthProfessional/. Accessed January 28, 2013.

11. Baker WL, Gutierrez-Williams G, White CM, et al. Effect of cinnamon on glucose control and lipid parameters. *Diab Care.* 2008;31:41–43.

12. Barbosa-Cesnik CT. Cranberry juice for treatment of urinary tract infections. In: ClinicalTrials. gov. Bethesda, MD: National Library of Medicine; 2004. Available at: http://clinicaltrials.gov/ct2 /show/NCT00093054. NLM Identifier: NCT00093054.

13. Barnes PM, Bloom B, Nahin R. CDC National Health Statistics Report #12. *Complementary and alternative medicine use among adults and children: United States, 2007.* December 10, 2008.

14. Basch E, Ulbricht C, Aukerman GF, et al., eds. *Natural standard.* Somerville, MA: The Natural Standard: The Authority on Integrative Medicine; 2013. Available at: www.naturalstandard.com.

15. Basch E, Ulbricht C, Kuo G, et al. Therapeutic applications of fenugreek. *Altern Med Rev.* 2003;8:20–27.

16. Bent S, Padula A, Moore D, et al. Valerian for sleep: a systematic review and meta-analysis. *Am J Med.* 2006;119:1005–1012.

17. Biegert C, Wagner I, Lüdtke R, et al. Efficacy and safety of willow bark extract in the treatment of osteoarthritis and rheumatoid arthritis: results of 2 randomized double-blind controlled trials [abstract]. *J Rheumatol.* 2004;31:2121–2130.

18. Birks J, Grimley EJ. *Ginkgo biloba* for cognitive impairment and dementia. *Cochrane Database System Rev.* 2009,1:CD003120.

19. Bonakdar RA, Guarneri E. Coenzyme Q10. *Am Fam Phys.* 2005;72:1065–1070.

20. Brattström A. Long-term effects of St. John's wort (*Hypericum perforatum*) treatment: a 1-year safety study in mild to moderate depression. *Phytomedicine.* 2009;16:277–283.

21. Bril V, England J, Franklin GM, et al. Evidence-based guideline: treatment of painful diabetic neuropathy: report of the American Academy of Neurology, the American Association of Neuromuscular and Electrodiagnostic Medicine, and the American Academy of Physical Medicine and Rehabilitation. *Neurology.* 2011:1758–1765.

22. Buvat J. Androgen therapy with dehydroepiandrosterone. *World J Urol.* 2003;21:346–355.

23. Capsaicin. In: *Lexi-Comp online.* Hudson, OH: Lexi-Comp, Inc.; February 15, 2013.

24. Chase CK, McQueen CE. Cinnamon in diabetes mellitus. *Am J Health-Syst Pharm.* 2007;64:1033–1035.

25. Chen J, Wollman Y, Chernichovsky T, et al. Effect of oral administration of high-dose nitric oxide donor L-arginine in men with organic erectile dysfunction: results of a double-blind, randomized, placebo controlled study. *BJU Int.* 1999;83:269–273.

26. Chen JT, Wesley R, Shamburek RD, et al. Meta-analysis of natural therapies for hyperlipidemia: plant sterols and stanols versus policosanol. *Pharmacotherapy.* 2005;25:171–183.

27. Chung EP. Cardiovascular disease. In: Shapiro K, ed. *Natural products: a case-based approach for health care professionals.* Washington, DC: American Pharmacists Association; 2006:147.

28. Claims that can be made for conventional foods and dietary supplements. Food and Drug Administration; September 2003. Available at: http://www.fda.gov/food/labelingnutrition /labelclaims/ucm111447.htm. Accessed January 28, 2013.

29. Clegg DO, Reda DJ, Harris CL, et al. Glucosamine, chondroitin sulfate, and the two in combination for painful knee arthritis. *N Engl J Med.* 2006;354:795–808.

30. *The Cochrane database of systematic reviews* [electronic resource]. Chichester, UK: Wiley; 2004.

31. Coon JT, Ernst E. *Andrographis paniculata* in the treatment of upper respiratory tract infections: a systematic review of safety and efficacy. *Planta Med.* 2004;70:293–298.

32. *Crataegus oxycantha* (hawthorn) monograph. *Altern Med Rev.* 2010;15:164–167.

33. Dahmer S, Scott E. Health effects of hawthorn. *Am Fam Physician.* 2010;81:465–469.

34. DeKosky ST, Williamson JD, Fitzpatrick AL, et al. *Ginkgo biloba* for prevention of dementia: a randomized controlled trial. *JAMA.* 2008;300:2253–2262.

35. Derry S, Moore RA. Topical capsaicin (low concentration) for chronic neuropathic pain in adults. *Cochrane Database System Rev.* 2012;9:CD010111.

36. Diener HC, Pfaffenrath V, Schnitker J, et al. Efficacy and safety of 6.25 mg t.i.d. feverfew CO_2-extract (MIG-99) in migraine prevention: a randomized, double-blind, multicentre, placebo-controlled study. *Cephalalgia.* 2005:15;1031–1041.

37. Dietary Supplement and Nonprescription Drug Consumer Protection Act. Food and Drug Administration; May 20, 2009. Available at: http://www.fda.gov/RegulatoryInformation /Legislation/FederalFoodDrugandCosmeticActFDCAct/SignificantAmendmentstotheFDCAct /ucm148035.htm. Accessed January 28, 2013.

38. Dietary Supplement Health and Education Act of 1994. Food and Drug Administration; updated May 20, 2009. Available at: http://www.fda.gov/RegulatoryInformation/Legislation /FederalFoodDrugandCosmeticActFDCAct/SignificantAmendmentstotheFDCAct/ucm148003 .htm. Accessed January 27, 2013.

39. Ding M, Leach M, Bradley H. The effectiveness and safety of ginger for pregnancy-induced nausea and vomiting: a systematic review. *Women Birth.* 2013;26:e26–e30.

40. Dulin MF, Hatcher LF, Sasser HC, Barringer TA. Policosanol is ineffective in the treatment of hypercholesterolemia: a randomized controlled trial. *Am J Clin Nutr.* 2006;84:1543–1548.

41. Dvorkin L, Song KY. Herbs for benign prostatic hyperplasia. *Ann Pharmacother.* 2002;36:1443–1452.

42. Edgar AD, Levin R, Constantinou CE, Denis L. A critical review of the pharmacology of the plant extract of *Pygeum africanum* in the treatment of LUTS. *Neurourol Urodyn.* 2007;26:458–463.

43. Eisenberg DM, Kessler RC, Van Rompay MI, et al. Perceptions about complementary therapies relative to conventional therapies among adults who use both: results from a survey. *Ann Intern Med.* 2001;135:344.

44. Eslick GD, Howe PR, Smith C, et al. Benefits of fish oil supplementation in hyperlipidemia: a systematic review and meta-analysis. *Int J Cardiol.* 2009;136:4–16.

45. Evans WC. Plants in medicine: the origins of pharmacognosy. In: *Trease and Evans pharmacognosy,* 16th ed. Edinburgh, UK: Elsevier; 2009:3–4.

46. FDA drug safety communication: rare cases of serious burns with the use of over-the-counter topical muscle and joint pain relievers. Food and Drug Administration; September 17, 2012. Available at: http://www.fda.gov/Drugs/DrugSafety/ucm318858.htm. Accessed February 25, 2013.

47. Francini-Pesenti F, Beltramolli D, Acqua SD, Brocadello F. Effect of sugar cane policosanol on lipid profile in primary hypercholesterolemia. *Phytother Res.* 2007;22:318–322.

48. Freeman C, Spelman K. A critical evaluation of drug interactions with *Echinacea* spp. *Mol Nutr Food Res.* 2008;52:789–798.

49. Gagnier JJ, van Tulder MW, Berman BM, Bombardier C. Herbal medicine for low back pain. *Cochrane Database System Rev.* 2006;2:CD004504.

50. Genazzani AR, Stomati M, Valentino V, et al. Effect of 1-year, low-dose DHEA therapy on climacteric symptoms and female sexuality. *Climacteric.* 2011;14:661–668.

51. Grigoleit HG, Grigoleit P. Peppermint oil in irritable bowel syndrome. *Phytomedicine.* 2005;12:601–606.

52. Guo R, Pittler MH, Ernst E. Hawthorn extract for treating chronic heart failure. *Cochrane Database System Rev.* 2008;1:CD005312.

53. Hartweg J, Farmer A, Perera R, et al. Meta-analysis of the effects of *n*-3 polyunsaturated fatty acids on lipoproteins and other emerging lipid cardiovascular risk markers in patients with type 2 diabetes. *Diabetologia.* 2007;50:1593–1602.

54. Heck AM, DeWitt BA, Lukes AL. Potential interactions between alternative therapies and warfarin. *Am J Health Syst Pharm.* 2000;57:1221–1227.

55. Heckman MA, Weil J, Gonzalez De Mejia E. Caffeine (1,3,7-trimethylxanthine) in foods: a comprehensive review of consumption, functionality, safety, and regulatory matters. *J Food Sci.* 2010;75:R77–R87.

56. Heinrich M, Barnes J, Gibbons S, Williamson EM. *Fundamentals of pharmacognosy and phytotherapy.* Edinburgh, UK: Churchill Livingstone; 2004.

57. Henroitin Y, Mobasheri A, Marty M. Is there any scientific evidence for the use of glucosamine in the management of human osteoarthritis? *Arthritis Res Ther.* 2012;14:201.

58. Hepler CD, Strand LM. Opportunities and responsibilities in pharmaceutical care. *Am J Hosp Pharm.* 1990;47:533–543.

59. Ho MJ, Bellusci A, Wright JM. Blood pressure lowering efficacy of coenzyme Q10 for primary hypertension. *Cochrane Database System Rev.* 2009;4:CD007435.

60. Hochberg MC, Altman RD, April KT, et al. American College of Rheumatology 2012 recommendations for the use of nonpharmacologic and pharmacologic therapies in osteoarthritis of the hand, hip, and knee. *Arthritis Care Res.* 2012;465:74.

61. Holubarsch CJ, Colucci WS, Meinertz T, et al. The efficacy and safety of *Crataegus* extract WS 1442 in patients with heart failure: the SPICE trial. *Eur J Heart Fail.* 2008;10:1255–1263.

62. Hutchison A, Farmer R, Verhamme K, et al. The efficacy of drugs for the treatment of LUTS/BPH: a study in 6 European Countries. *Eur Urol.* 2007;51:207–215.

63. Ihl R, Tribanek M, Bachinskaya N; GOTADAY Study Group. Efficacy and tolerability of a once daily formulation of *Ginkgo biloba* extract EGb 761® in Alzheimer's disease and vascular dementia: results from a randomised controlled trial [abstract]. *Pharmacopsychiatry.* 2012;45:41–46.

64. Jellin JM, Gregory PJ, Batz F, et al., eds. *Natural medicines comprehensive database.* Stockton, CA: Therapeutic Research Faculty. Available at: http//www.naturaldatabase.com. Accessed February 11, 2013.

65. Jepson RG, Mihaljevic L, Craig JC. Cranberries for treating urinary tract infections. *Cochrane Database System Rev.* 1998;4:CD001322.

66. Jepson RG, Williams G, Craig JC. Cranberries for preventing urinary tract infections. *Cochrane Database System Rev.* 2012;10:CD001321.

67. Jull AB, Ni Mhurchu C, Bennett DA, et al. Chitosan for overweight or obesity. *Cochrane Database System Rev.* 2008;3:CD003892.

68. Kar A. *Pharmacognosy and pharmacobiotechnology.* Tunbridge Wells, UK: Anshan; 2008.

69. Kasuli EG. Are alternative supplements effective treatment for diabetes mellitus? *Nutr Clin Pract.* 2011;26:352–355.

70. Kava linked to liver damage. National Center for Complementary and Alternative Medicine; December 13, 2012. Available at: http://nccam.nih.gov/news/alerts/kava?nav=gsa. Accessed February 25, 2013.

71. Khoo YS, Aziz Z. Garlic supplementation and serum cholesterol: a meta-analysis. *J Clin Pharm Ther.* 2009;34:133–145.

72. Kligler B, Ulbricht C, Basch E, et al. *Andrographis paniculata* for the treatment of upper respiratory infection: a systematic review by the natural standard research collaboration. *Explore.* 2006;2:25–29.

73. Klotz T, Mathers MJ, Braun M, et al. Effectiveness of oral L-arginine in first-line treatment of erectile dysfunction in a controlled crossover study [abstract]. *Urol Int.* 1999;63:220–223.

74. Leach MJ, Kumar S. Cinnamon for diabetes mellitus. *Cochrane Database System Rev.* 2012;9: CD007170.

75. Leach MJ, Moore V. Black cohosh (*Cimicifuga* spp.) for menopausal symptoms. *Cochrane Database System Rev.* 2012;9:CD007244.

76. Ledda A, Belcaro G, Cesarone MR, et al. Investigation of a complex plant extract for mild to moderate erectile dysfunction in a randomized, double-blind, placebo-controlled, parallel-arm study. *BJU Int.* 2010;106:1030–1033.

77. Lee RA, Balick MJ. Indigenous use of *Hoodia gordonii* and appetite suppression. *Explore.* 2007;3:404–406.

78. Lethaby A, Marjoribanks J, Kroneberg F, et al. Phytoestrogens for vasomotor menopausal symptoms. *Cochrane Database System Rev.* 2007;4:CD001395.

79. Linde K, Barrett B, Bauer R, et al. Echinacea for preventing and treating the common cold. *Cochrane Database of System Rev.* 2006;1:CD000530.

80. Linde K, Berner MM, Kriston L. St. John's wort for major depression. *Cochrane Database System Rev.* 2008;4:CD000448.

81. Lipton RB, Göbel H, Einhäupl KM, et al. *Petasites hybridus* root (butterbur) is an effective preventive treatment for migraine. *Neurology.* 2004;63:2240.

82. *Lovaza* [package insert]. Research Triangle Park, NC: GlaxoSmithKline; August 2102. Available at: https://www.gsksource.com/gskprm/htdocs/documents/LOVAZA-PI-PIL.PDF. Accessed February 2, 2013.

83. Luo JZ, Luo L. Ginseng on hyperglycemia: effects and mechanisms. *eCAM.* 2009;6423–6427.

84. Mahady GB, Low Dog T, Barrett ML, et al. *United States Pharmacopeia* review of the black cohosh case reports of hepatotoxicity. *Menopause.* 2008;15:628–638.

85. Mang B, Wolters M, Schmitt B, Kelb K. Effects of a cinnamon extract on plasma glucose, HbA$_{1c}$, and serum lipids in diabetes mellitus type 2. *Eur J Clin Invest.* 2006;26:340–344.

86. Marcoff L, Thompson P. The role of coenzyme Q10 in statin-associated myopathy: a systematic review. *J Am Coll Cardiol.* 2007;49:2231–2237.

87. Mason L, Moore RA, Derry S, et al. Systematic review of topical capsaicin for the treatment of chronic pain. *BMJ.* 2004;328:991.

88. Matthews A, Dowswell T, Haas DM, et al. Interventions for nausea and vomiting in early pregnancy. *Cochrane Database System Rev.* 2010;9:CD007575.

89. McQueen CE, Orr KK. Natural products. In: Krinsky DL, Berardi RR, Ferreri SP, et al., eds. *Handbook of nonprescription drugs: an interactive approach to self-care*, 17th ed. Washington, DC: American Pharmacists Association; 2012:967–1006.

90. Mijnhout GS, Kollen BJ, Alkhalaf A, et al. Alpha lipoic acid for symptomatic peripheral neuropathy in patients with diabetes: a meta-analysis of randomized controlled trials. *Int J Endocrinol.* 2012;2012:456279.

91. Miller KL, Clegg DO. Glucosamine and chondroitin sulfate. *Rheum Dis Clin North Am.* 2011;37:103–118.

92. Mirza N, Cornblath DR, Hasan S, Hussain U. Alpha-lipoic acid for diabetic peripheral neuropathy [intervention protocol]. *Cochrane Database System Rev.* 2005;4:CD005492.

93. Miyasaka LS, Atallah AN, Soares B. Valerian for anxiety disorders. *Cochrane Database System Rev.* 2006;4:CD004515.

94. Morales A, Black A, Emerson L, et al. Androgens and sexual function: a placebo-controlled, randomized, double-blind study of testosterone vs. dehydroepiandrosterone in men with sexual dysfunction and androgen deficiency. *Aging Male.* 2009;12:104–112.

95. Muriel P, Rivera-Espinoza Y. Beneficial drugs for liver diseases. *J Appl Toxicol.* 2008;28:93–103.

96. Nagels HE, Rishworth JR, Siristidis CS, Kroon B. Androgens (dehydroepiandrosterone or testosterone) in women undergoing assisted reproduction [protocol]. *Cochrane Database System Rev.* 2012;3:CD009749.

97. Nahas R, Balla A. Complementary and alternative medicine for prevention and treatment of the common cold. *Can Fam Physician.* 2011;57:31–36.

98. National Center for Complementary and Alternative Medicine. Available at: http://nccam.nih.gov. Accessed February 11, 2013.

99. National Cholesterol Education Program. *Third report of the Expert Panel on Detection, Evaluation, and Treatment of High Blood Cholesterol in Adults.* NIH Pub. No. 02-5215. Bethesda, MD: National Heart, Lung, and Blood Institute, 2002.

100. Panjari M, Bell RJ, Jane F, et al. The safety of 52 weeks of oral DHEA therapy for postmenopausal women. *Maturitas.* 2009;63:240–245.

101. Pepping J. Policosanol. *Am J Health Syst Pharm.* 2003;60:112–115.

102. Pirotta M. Irritable bowel syndrome: the role of complementary medicines in treatment. *Aust Fam Physician.* 2009;38:966–968.

103. Pittler MH, Ernst E. Feverfew for preventing migraine. *Cochrane Database System Rev.* 2004;1:CD002286.

104. Pittler MH, Ernst E. Kava extract versus placebo for treating anxiety. *Cochrane Database System Rev.* 2003;1:CD003383.

105. Pittler MH, Schmidt K, Ernst E. Adverse events of herbal food supplements for body weight reduction: systematic review. *Obes Rev.* 2005;6:93–111.

106. Poolsup N, Suthisisang C, Prathanturarug S, et al. *Andrographis paniculata* in the symptomatic treatment of uncomplicated upper respiratory tract infection: systematic review of randomized controlled trials. *J Clin Pharm Ther.* 2004;29:37–45.

107. Pothmann R, Danesch U. Migraine prevention in children and adolescents: results of an open study with a special butterbur root extract. *Headache.* 2005;45:196.

108. Rafehi H, Ververis K, Karagiannis TC. Controversies surrounding the clinical potential of cinnamon for the management of diabetes. *Diabetes Obes Metab.* 2012;14:493–499.

109. Rambaldi A, Jacobs BP, Gluud C. Milk thistle for alcoholic and/or hepatitis B or C virus liver diseases. *Cochrane Database System Rev.* 2007;4:CD003620.

110. Reinhart KM, Talati R, White CM, Coleman CI. The impact of garlic on lipid parameters: a systematic review and meta-analysis. *Nutr Res Rev*. 2009;22:39–48.

111. Reiter WJ, Pycha A, Schatzl G, et al. Dehydroepiandrosterone in the treatment of erectile dysfunction: a prospective, double-blind, randomized, placebo-controlled study. *Urology*. 1999;53:590–594.

112. Reiter WJ, Schatzl G, Märk I, et al. Dehydroepiandrosterone in the treatment of erectile dysfunction in patients with different organic etiologies. *Urol Res*. 2001;29:278–281.

113. Ricciardelli C, Sakko AJ, Stahl J, et al. Prostatic chondroitin sulfate is increased in patients with metastatic disease but does not predict survival outcome. *Prostate*. 2009;69:761–759.

114. Robbers JE, Speedie MK, Tyler VE. *Pharmacognosy and pharmacobiotechnology*. Baltimore, MD: Williams & Wilkins; 1996.

115. Robbers JE, Tyler VE. *Tyler's herbs of choice: the therapeutic use of phytomedicinals*. New York, NY: Haworth Herbal Press; 1999.

116. Rosenfeldt FL, Haas SJ, Krum H, et al. Coenzyme Q10 in the treatment of hypertension: a meta-analysis of the clinical trials. *J Hum Hypertens*. 2007;21:297–306.

117. Ross SM. Integrative therapeutic considerations in alcohol abuse. *Holist Nurs Pract*. 2009;23:69–72.

118. Roth EM, Harris WS. Fish oil for primary and secondary prevention of coronary heart disease. *Curr Atheroscler Rep*. 2010;12:66–72.

119. Roxas M, Jurenka J. Colds and influenza: a review of diagnosis and conventional, botanical, and nutritional considerations. *Altern Med Rev*. 2007;12:25–48.

120. Ruepert L, Quartero AO, de Wit NJ, et al. Bulking agents, antispasmodics and antidepressants for the treatment of irritable bowel syndrome. *Cochrane Database System Rev*. 2011;8:CD003460.

121. Saravanan P, Davidson N, Schmidt E, Calder P. Cardiovascular effects of marine omega-3 fatty acids. *Lancet*. 2010;375:540–550.

122. Sarris J, Kavanaugh DJ, Byrne G, et al. The Kava Anxiety Depression Spectrum Study (KADSS): a randomized, placebo-controlled crossover trial using an aqueous extract of *Piper methysticum*. *Psychopharmacology (Berl)*. 2009;205:399–407.

123. Sarris J, LaPorte E, Schweitzer I. Kava: a comprehensive review of efficacy, safety, and psychopharmacology. *Aust N Z J Psychiatry*. 2011;45:27–35.

124. Sawitzke AD, Shi H, Finco MF, et al. Clinical efficacy and safety of glucosamine, chondroitin sulphate, their combination, celecoxib or placebo taken to treat osteoarthritis of the knee: 2-year results from GAIT. *Ann Rheum Dis*. 2010;69:1459–1464.

125. Shapiro K. *Natural products: a case-based approach for health care professionals*. Washington, DC: American Pharmacists Association; 2006.

126. Shen YH, Nahas R. Complementary and alternative medicine for treatment of irritable bowel syndrome. *Can Fam Physician*. 2009;55:143–148.

127. Shi S, Klotz U. Drug interactions with herbal medicines. *Clin Pharmacokinet*. 2012;51:77–104.

128. Shields KM, Smock N, McQueen CE, Bryant PJ. Chitosan for weight loss and cholesterol management. *Am J Health Syst Pharm*. 2003;60:1310–1316.

129. Snitz BE, O'Meara ES, Carlson MC, et al. *Ginkgo biloba* for preventing cognitive decline in older adults: a randomized trial. *JAMA*. 2009;302;2663–2670.

130. Suksomboon N, Poolsup N, Boonkaew S, Suthisisang C. Meta-analysis of the effect of herbal supplement on glycemic control in type 2 diabetes. *J Ethnopharmacol*. 2011;137:1328–1333.

131. Sun-Edelstein C, Mauskop A. Alternative headache treatments: nutraceutical, behavioral and physical treatments. *Headache.* 2011:51;469–483.

132. Tacklind J, MacDonald R, Rutks I, et al. *Seronoa repens* for benign prostatic hyperplasia. *Cochrane Database System Rev.* 2012;12:CD001423.

133. Taibi DM, Landis CA, Petry H, Vitiello MV. A systematic review of valerian as a sleep aid: safe but not effective. *Sleep Med Rev.* 2007;11:209–230.

134. Taibi DM, Vitiello MV, Barsness S, et al. A randomized clinical trial of valerian fails to improve self-report, polysomnographic, and actigraphic sleep in older women with insomnia. *Sleep Med.* 2009;10:319–328.

135. Tam SW, Worcel M, Wyllie M. Yohimbine: a clinical review. *Pharmacol Ther.* 2001;91:215–243.

136. Tiran D. Ginger to reduce nausea and vomiting during pregnancy: evidence of effectiveness is not the same as proof of safety. *Complement Ther Clin Pract.* 2012;18:22–25.

137. Towheed TE, Maxwell L, Anastassiades TP, et al. Glucosamine therapy for treating osteoarthritis. *Cochrane Database System Rev.* 2005;2:CD002946.

138. Tsourounis C, Denneby, C. Introduction to dietary supplements. In: Krinsky DL, Berardi RR, Ferreri SP, et al, eds. *Handbook of nonprescription drugs: an interactive approach to self-care*, 17th ed. Washington, DC: American Pharmacists Association; 2012:956.

139. Uebelhart D. Clinical review of chondroitin sulfate in osteoarthritis. *Osteoarthritis Cartilage.* 2008;16:S19–S21.

140. Várkonyi T, Kempler P. Diabetic neuropathy: new strategies for treatment. *Diabetes Obes Metab.* 2008:10;99–108.

141. Vellas B, Coley N, Ousset PJ, et al. Long-term use of standardized *Ginkgo biloba* extract for the prevention of Alzheimer's disease (GuidAge): a randomized, placebo-controlled trial. *Lancet Neurol.* 2012;11:851–859.

142. Villacis J, Rice TR, Bucci LR, et al. Do shrimp-allergic individuals tolerate shrimp-derived glucosamine? *Clin Exp Allergy.* 2006;36:1457–1461.

143. Vlachojannis JE, Cameron M, Chrubasik S. A systematic review on the *Sambuci fructus* effect and efficacy profiles. *Phytother Res.* 2010;24:1–8.

144. Vlachojannis J, Magora F, Chrubasik S. Willow species and aspirin: different mechanisms of action. *Phytother Res.* 2011;25:1102–1104.

145. Vuksan V, Sievenpiper JL, Koo VY, et al. American ginseng (*Panax quinquefolius L*) reduces postprandial glycemia in nondiabetic subjects and subjects with type 2 diabetes mellitus. *Arch Intern Med.* 2000;160:1009–1013.

146. Vuksan V, Starvo MP, Sievenpiper JL, et al. Similar postprandial glycemic reductions with escalation of dose and administration time of American ginseng in type 2 diabetes. *Diab Care.* 2000;23:1221–1226.

147. Weitz D, Weintraub H, Fisher E, Schwartzbard A. Fish oil for the treatment of cardiovascular disease. *Cardiol Rev.* 2010;18:258–263.

148. Whelan AM, Jurgens TM, Szeto V. Efficacy of hoodia for weight loss: is there evidence to support the efficacy claims? *J Clin Pharm Ther.* 2010;35:609–612.

149. White B. Ginger: an overview. *Am Fam Physician.* 2007;75;1689–1691.

150. Wilt TJ, Ishani A. *Pygeum africanum* for benign prostatic hyperplasia. *Cochrane Database System Rev.* 1998;1:CD001044.

151. Wu J. Complementary and alternative medicine modalities for the treatment of irritable bowel syndrome: facts or myths? *Gastroenterol Hepatol (NY).* 2010;6:705–711.

152. Wu JW, Lin LC, Tsai TH. Drug–drug interactions of silymarin on the perspective of pharmacokinetics. *J Ethnopharmacol.* 2009;121:185–193.

153. Wyman M, Leonard M, Morledge T. Coenzyme Q10: a therapy for hypertension and statin-induced myalgia. *Cleve Clin J Med.* 2010;77:435–442.

154. Yeh GY, Eisenberg DM, Kaptchuk TJ, Phillips RS. Systematic review of herbs and dietary supplements for glycemic control in diabetes. *Diab Care.* 2003;26:1277–1294.

155. Yuan CS, Wei G, Dey L, et al. Brief communication: American ginseng reduces warfarin's effect in healthy patients: a randomized, controlled trial. *Ann Intern Med.* 2004;141:23–27.

156. Zakay-Rones Z, Thom E, Wollan T, Wadstein J. Randomized study of the efficacy and safety of oral elderberry extract in the treatment of influenza A and B virus infections. *J Int Med Res.* 2004;32:132–140.

157. Zick SM, Vautaw BM, Gillespie B, Aaronson KD. Hawthorn extract randomized blinded chronic heart failure (HERB CHF) trial. *Eur J Heart Fail.* 2009;11:990–999.

158. Ziegler D, Low PA, Litchy WJ, et al. Efficacy and safety of antioxidant treatment with alpha-lipoic acid over 4 years in diabetic polyneuropathy. *Diab Care.* 2011;34:2054–2060.

CHAPTER 14

Introduction to Nutrients

Reza Karimi

1. Understand the macronutrients (carbohydrates, fats, and proteins) that play important roles in daily calorie intake.

2. Understand the micronutrients (vitamins, minerals, and trace elements) that play important roles in physiologic, pharmacologic, and biochemical pathways.

3. Comprehend diseases associated with inadequate or excessive intake of macronutrients and micronutrients.

4. Understand the important role that bicarbonate plays in maintaining the physiological buffer system.

5. Learn about different acid–base disorders and the critical roles electrolytes play in patient care.

6. Understand obesity and the various factors, parameters, and hormones involved in obesity.

7. Implement a series of Learning Bridge assignments at your experiential sites to bridge your didactic learning with your experiential experiences.

1. **Anion gap:** to have neutral plasma, the number of Na^+ ions must equal the number of HCO_3^- and Cl^- ions. If the cations and anions are not equal, there is an existing gap, referred to as an anion gap.

2. **BMI:** body mass index; a measure of obesity.

3. **BMR:** basal metabolic rate; the energy expenditure by the body at nonsleeping rest, which is measured 12 hours after the last meal.

4. **Central obesity:** also referred to "metabolic syndrome"; fat that is concentrated on the abdomen and upper body in an individual, which is often used in the diagnosis of insulin resistance (diabetes type 2), hypertension, dyslipidemia, and cardiovascular disease.

5. **Chloride shift:** movement of chloride ions into cells from the plasma in an attempt to maintain electrochemical neutrality.

6. **Essential fatty acids:** fatty acids that are required for the synthesis of arachidonic acid.

7. **Gluconeogenesis:** synthesis of glucose by the liver.

8. **Glycemic index:** an indicator of how fast carbohydrates are hydrolyzed during digestion to release glucose into the bloodstream.

9. **Glycogen:** storage of glucose molecules in animals.

10. **Kwashiorkor:** a type of malnutrition caused by inadequate intake of protein.

11. **Macronutrients:** nutrients that include carbohydrates, fats, and protein.

12. **Marasmus:** a type of malnutrition caused by inadequate intake of protein and carbohydrates.

13. **Micronutrients:** nutrients that include electrolytes, trace elements, vitamins, and water.

(continues)

14. **Minerals:** inorganic elements that may serve as cofactors in an enzymatic reaction, as electrolytes to maintain cellular or physiologic function, or as structural building blocks in the body.

15. **Nitrogen balance:** the situation in which the amount of nitrogen consumed equals the nitrogen that is excreted in the urine and sweat, and by other means.

16. **Oncotic pressure:** a pressure generated by a capillary's proteins to prevent movement of water from the capillary's membrane into tissues.

17. **Oxidative phosphorylation:** generation of ATP molecules in the mitochondria.

18. **PLP:** pyridoxal phosphate that is derived from pyridoxine (vitamin B_6).

19. **RDA:** Recommended Dietary Allowance; an older nomenclature for RDI, which is used to formulate food guidelines.

20. **RDI:** Recommended Daily Intake; a dietary intake that is sufficient to meet the daily nutrient requirements of 97% of healthy individuals in a specific demographic population.

21. **REE:** resting energy expenditure; an estimate of the energy needs of an individual.

22. **TBW:** total body water.

23. **Trans fatty acids:** a type of fatty acid generated by hydrogenated polyunsaturated fatty acids in foods.

24. **Vitamins:** organic compounds that play a crucial role in many biochemical reactions; humans are unable to produce these compounds in an adequate quantity to meet the body's needs.

Introduction

Nutrients include both macronutrients and micronutrients. While macronutrients include carbohydrates, fats, and protein, micronutrients include electrolytes, trace elements, and vitamins. In addition, water has an important role in the overall use of nutrients. Macronutrients are broken down to their constituents to undergo different oxidation pathways to produce energy in the form of ATP molecules. By comparison, vitamins and minerals assist macromolecules in effectively and efficiently being oxidized to provide adequate amount of energy. Sufficient intake of macronutrients and micronutrients assists humans in maintaining the well-being of cellular, physiologic, and structural machineries of the body.

This chapter discusses the essential roles of both macronutrients and micronutrients in daily calorie intake. In addition, the principles underlying the actions of lipid- and water-soluble vitamins in different biochemical and physiological pathways are discussed. Physiologic consequences related to vitamin deficiency and toxicity in patient care are emphasized, and the significance of the most commonly used minerals in the diet is described. The critical roles that electrolytes play in acid–base homeostasis and the role of bicarbonate in the physiologic buffer system are addressed as well. Metabolic syndrome and obesity are covered, including the various factors, parameters, and hormones involved in obesity.

Digestion of Nutrients

All constituents of nutrients are essential for our daily well-being and survival. Humans receive daily requirements of these nutrients through daily food ingestion and digestion. The foods that we eat are broken into small nutrients within the digestive tract so that those nutrients can then be absorbed by the villi of the small intestine. We produce and release digestive enzymes from the salivary glands (for example, α-amylase), gastric glands (for example, pepsinogen), and intestinal glands (for example, lactase) to facilitate digestions of foods. For instance, the hydrolysis of starch is catalyzed by salivary and pancreatic amylases to produce a mixture of smaller carbohydrates such as dextrins, maltose, and glucose.

Three important organs play crucial roles in processing and absorbing nutrients by producing enzymes or hormones: the small intestine, liver, and pancreas.

Small Intestine

This absorptive organ, with its large surface area, is an important component of the gastrointestinal (GI) tract, which plays an essential role in the absorption of nutrients and drugs. The hormone known as gastrin is released from the gastric mucosa that lines the gastric glands of the stomach. Gastrin's role is to stimulate secretion of HCl and pepsinogen from gastric glands; these secretions then enter the stomach. Pepsinogen is a zymogen that becomes activated in the form of pepsin to degrade proteins in the stomach. The contents of stomach are acidic due to the presence of gastric acid. When the gastric contents travel from the stomach to the small intestine, the low pH of the small intestine triggers secretion of secretin from the duodenal and jejunal mucosa into the circulation and/or intestinal lumen. Secretin's role is to stimulate the pancreatic duct to release bicarbonate, which in turn increases the pH to about 7–8, an optimal pH for the activity of proteases that catalyze the digestion of proteins in the small intestine.

Cholecystokinin is a hormone produced by the small intestine. It stimulates the secretion of the pancreatic zymogens (i.e., chymotrypsinogen, trypsinogen, and procarboxypeptidases) into the small intestine. Enteropeptidase is a proteolytic enzyme, released from the duodenum, that activates trypsinogen by converting it into trypsin in the small intestine. Trypsin, in turn, activates chymotripsinogen, procarboxypeptidases, and proelastase. These proteases degrade proteins into their constituents that are polypeptides and/or amino acids.

Most nutrients that have been broken down into small enough molecules (e.g., amino acids, glucose, glycerol) are able to enter intestinal epithelial cells with a help of sodium ions and the brush border's carrier proteins (see Figure 6.2 in the *Introduction to Pharmacodynamics* chapter). For instance, a glucose molecule enters the epithelial cells together with two sodium ions. Because the sodium ions enter the cell down an electrochemical gradient, they provide enough energy to transport a glucose molecule against its concentration gradient into the cytoplasm. Through the help of glucose transporters that are embedded on the other side of the epithelial cells, glucose molecules enter the blood and are able to travel to other organs.

Liver

The liver is a large organ that produces bile acids to emulsify fats. Approximately 50% of body's cholesterol is used to synthesize bile acids in the hepatic peroxisomes. The storage site for bile acids is not the liver, however, but rather the gallbladder. Indeed, the synthesis of bile acids represents a major pathway to eliminate the water-insoluble cholesterol molecules from the body. The three bile acids most commonly found in the gallbladder are cholic acid, glycocholic acid, and taurocholic acid.

The structure of taurocholic acid is shown in **Figure 14.1** Taurocholic acid is released after ingestion of a lipid-rich meal. The hydrophobic component of taurocholic acid associates with lipids, and the hydrophilic functional groups (OH and SO_3 groups) associate with water molecules to emulsify lipids by making microscopic micelles. Therefore, lipids such as triacylglycerols must be converted to microscopic micelles before they can be digested by the hydrolytic enzyme, lipase, in the intestine.

Pancreas

The third important organ involved in the digestion of nutrients is the pancreas. The pancreas produces digestive enzymes, lipase, proteases, and amylase as part of the digestion of lipids, proteins,

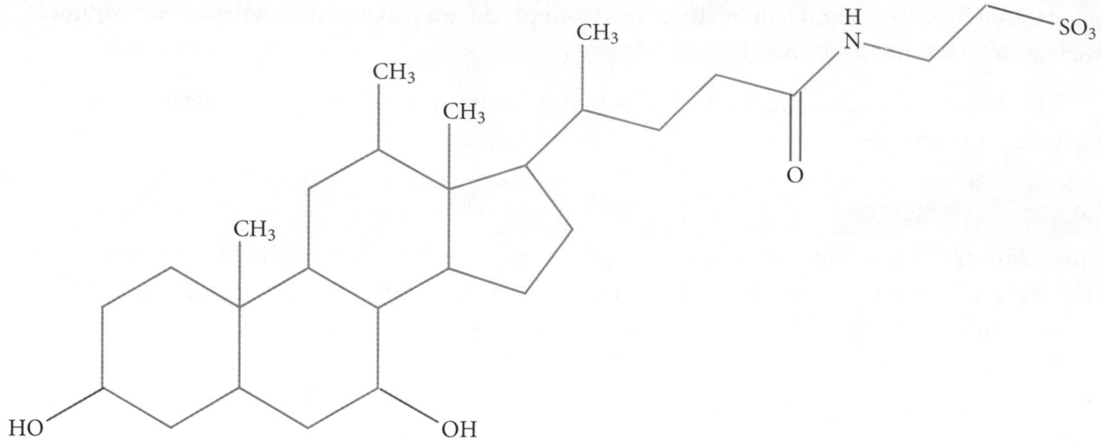

Taurocholic acid

Figure 14.1 Structure of taurocholic acid, an amphipathic molecule. The black functional groups indicate the hydrophilic components.

and carbohydrates, respectively (saliva also produces amylase, known as ptyalin, to facilitate digestion of carbohydrates in the mouth). As mentioned earlier, the pancreas also secretes bicarbonate to increase the pH of the small intestine. Some of the digestive enzymes are located in the brush border membrane of the small intestine. The formation of micelles by the bile acids significantly increases the accessibility of lipids to the pancreatic lipase. Lipase catalyzes the hydrolysis of triacylglycerols into glycerol (by removing all three fatty acids), monoacylglycerols (by removing two fatty acids), and diacylglycerols (by removing one fatty acid).

Human Nutritional Needs

While humans are able to synthesize glucose (gluconeogenesis), triacylglycerols (glyceroneogenesis), and proteins (gene expression and translation), none of these molecules is produced in quantities adequate to meet our daily nutrient needs. Similarly, humans do not produce adequate supplies of minerals or vitamins to assist our enzymes and other physiologic functions in maintaining homeostasis. In addition, humans need to balance our access to electrolytes. As a result, the human diet needs to include the required essential amino acids, essential fatty acids, glucose, fat-soluble and water-soluble vitamins, fiber, choline, and several minerals and electrolytes. The amounts of these ions or molecules that we require depend on our health, age, gender, pregnancy, and pathological conditions.

Recommended Dietary Allowances (RDA) for nutrients are established by the Food and Nutrition Board of the Institute of Medicine of the National Academy of Sciences. These RDAs define the amounts of nutrients adequate to meet our nutritional needs.

Under healthy and normal conditions, it is important to balance energy intake and energy output. Average energy intakes are about 1,900 and 2,600 kcal/day for women and men, respectively [1 kilocalorie (kcal) equals 4.18 kilojoules (kJ)]. The labels found on foods express the amount of energy in calories (1 calorie = 1 kcal). In biochemistry, one calorie (cal) is the amount of energy (in the form of heat) that raises the temperature of 1 gram of water by 1°C. Therefore, 1 kcal is equal to 1,000 cal. Thus, if a chocolate bar provides "100 Calories," it means the snack provides 100 kcal, which is equivalent to 100,000 cal. The misleading abbreviation of "C," which should be avoided, is sometimes used by some food manufacturers for calories.

The major nutrients in our foods (carbohydrates, fats, and protein) provide extensive amount of energy. While fats have the highest energy content (9 kcal/g), carbohydrate and protein both provide 4 kcal/g. For example, a banana provides 25 g carbohydrates and 1 g protein; thus this food provides 104 kcal of energy [(25 g × 4 kcal/g) + (1 g × 4 kcal/g)].

To estimate the energy needs of an individual, we can estimate the required resting energy expenditure (REE) by using the following equations: $900 + 10m$ (men) and $700 + 7m$ (women). The parameter m is mass in kilograms. These numbers can be adjusted based on the physical activities of individuals. For instance, the calculated REE is multiplied by 1.2 for sedentary (no exercise) individuals, 1.4 for moderately active individuals, and 1.8 for very active individuals. For instance, the REE for a moderately active man with a body weight of 70 kg is 2,240 kcal/day [(900 + 10 × 70) × 1.4].

The energy expenditure by the body at nonsleeping rest is called the basal metabolic rate (BMR) and is measured 12 hours after the last meal. BMR is affected by a series of factors, such as age, height, gender, lactation, pregnancy, emotional state, exercise, starvation, disease states, and weight. The highest BMR is reached during exercise. Greater age results in the replacement of muscle tissue by adipose tissue (which is metabolically less active); as a result, the older we get, the lower our BMR is. Also, because females have more fat than male, women have a lower BMR than men. BMR is often expressed as a percentage increase or decrease compared with the standard normal values. For instance, a value of +40 means that the BMR is 40% greater than the standard number.

The following equations can be used to calculate BMR for males (m) and females (f):

$$BMR(m) = 66 + [(13.7 \times kg) + (5 \times \text{Height in cm}) - (6.8 \times age)] \qquad (14.1)$$

$$BMR(f) = 655 + [(9.6 \times kg) + (1.8 \times \text{Height in cm}) - (4.7 \times age)] \qquad (14.2)$$

For instance, for an average 20-year-old man who weighs 70 kg and is 180 cm tall, the BMR per day is BMR(m) = 66 + [(13.7 × 70 kg) + (5 × 180 cm) − (6.8 × 20)] = 1,789 kcal/day.

A few disease states can result in hypermetabolism; that is, they can produce a higher BMR. For instance, patients with hyperthyroidism have a higher BMR. These patients produce too much of thyroid hormones because they overexpress the genes that control the citric acid cycle and oxidative phosphorylation pathways, which ultimately results in a higher metabolic rate. In addition, patients with advanced cancer, HIV infection, and AIDS often have a higher BMR.

Secretion of cytokines is stimulated in response to an infection or cancer. The release of cytokines results in stimulation of mitochondrial uncoupling proteins. These proteins cause thermogenesis in the oxidative phosphorylation pathway, which leads to increased oxidation of metabolic fuels and generation of heat (because the energy is released in the form of heat rather than ATP molecules). The latter mechanism, although independent of the cytokines' release, is also activated by the large amount of thyroid hormones in patients with hyperthyroidism—which explains why these patients are heat intolerant. In addition, many tumor cells oxidize glucose anaerobically and, as a result, they produce lactate. Lactate, via the Cori cycle (see the *Introduction to Biochemistry* chapter), is used by the liver to produce pyruvate and then glucose through the gluconeogenesis pathway. The use of gluconeogenesis, however, is an expensive pathway that requires six ATP molecules for the production of one glucose molecule. The overall effect is an increased catabolism to generate and supply ATP molecules.

Next, we explain each constituent of nutrients and explore their roles in our growth and endurance.

Carbohydrates

Carbohydrates should provide 45–55% of the daily energy in the diet, mostly in the form of complex carbohydrates (e.g., rice, wheat, corn) rather than simple carbohydrates (e.g., glucose, candy) (**Figure 14.2**). Complex carbohydrates are required because simple carbohydrates lack fiber.

Fiber

Fiber does not provide any energy, but it reduces cholesterol, the risk of colon cancer, and the risk of cardiovascular disease. Humans can achieve an adequate level of fiber by including fruits, vegetables, legumes, and whole-grain cereals in their diets. Dietary fiber has several effects. It adds bulk to water, drawing fluid into the lumen of the intestine and increasing bowl motility and, as a result, decreasing the risk of constipation. Fiber is also able to bind toxic compounds, including carcinogens, and reduce their absorption.

Too much fiber is not recommended (the optimal range is 20–35 g/day) because it can bind to trace elements (such as Zn^{2+}) and decreases the absorption of lipid-soluble vitamins. As will be discussed later in this chapter, zinc is an important element in gene expression and in the catalytic activities of many enzymes (e.g., alcohol dehydrogenase, methionine S-methyltransferase). The recommended daily intakes of fiber for men and women 50 years of age and younger are 38 g/day and 25 g/day, respectively. These numbers are reduced to 30 g/day and 21 g/day for men and women older than 50 years of age, respectively.

Worldwide, approximately 80% of consumed calories are based on carbohydrates (however, this number is reduced to 50% in the United States). Complex carbohydrates, in addition to fiber, provide B vitamins and minerals. Glucose is the most important energy-rich sugar of a complex

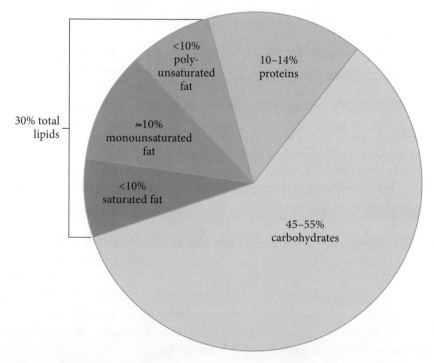

Figure 14.2 Recommended proportions of carbohydrates, lipids, and protein in daily food intake.

Adapted from: Dwyer J. Nutrient requirements and dietary assessment. In: Longo DL, Fauci AS, Kasper DL, et al., eds. *Harrison's principles of internal medicine*, 18th ed. New York: McGraw-Hill; 2012. Available at: http://www.accessmedicine.com/content.aspx?aID=9099636.

carbohydrate molecule. Humans have access to both endogenous glucose (from glycogen, the major form of stored carbohydrate) and exogenous complex carbohydrates (e.g., rice, wheat, corn). Glycogen is converted to monosaccharide (glucose) units by glycogen phosphorylase *a* enzyme to mobilize glucose for the glycolysis pathway or the pentose phosphate pathway (see also the *Introduction to Biochemistry* chapter) to supply energy or other important molecules such as amino acids and nucleic acids, respectively. Humans can also synthesize glucose by our own gluconeogenesis pathway. However, gluconeogenesis is not fast enough to meet a rapid demand for glucose, and, as mentioned earlier, it is an expensive pathway that requires many ATP molecules.

Glycemic Index

Exogenous carbohydrates are digested by being hydrolyzed first to produce oligosaccharides and then to produce monosaccharides and disaccharides. The glycemic index is a numerical index that ranges from 0 to 1 and defines how rapidly carbohydrates are hydrolyzed during digestion to release glucose into the bloodstream. It indicates an increase in the blood glucose level after ingestion of a carbohydrate dose and is normalized to ingestion of an equivalent amount of glucose that has a glycemic index of 1. For instance, starch has a glycemic index of 1 (or 100%) because it is readily hydrolyzed in the small intestine to produce glucose molecules. In contrast, the glycemic index for cellulose is 0 because it is not hydrolyzed at all (humans lack the necessary enzyme to hydrolyze cellulose). The glycemic index is 0.38 for apples and 0.52 for bananas. A comparison between these two fruits indicates that bananas can increase the blood glucose level faster than apples can.

Carbohydrates that have a low glycemic index are helpful for patients with type 2 diabetes because they cause less fluctuation in insulin secretion. A glycemic index of 0.55 or less is considered "low"; a glycemic index of 0.70 or greater is considered "high."

Lipids (Fats)

As was discussed in the *Introduction to Cell Biology* and *Introduction to Biochemistry* chapters, there are two types of lipids: simple lipids (fatty acids, triacylglycerols, cholesterol) and complex lipids (mainly membrane lipids). Lipids are not equally distributed in the body. For instance, adipose tissue is rich in triacylglycerols. By comparison, membrane lipids are rich in lipids that are attached to carbohydrates (glycolipids), phosphates (phosphatides or phospholipids), or proteins (some integral proteins), or are found in the plasma as soluble protein–lipid aggregates (lipoproteins).

The current guidelines for lipid intake state that fats should not exceed 30% of the daily calorie intake. Fatty acids found in lipids can be saturated or unsaturated. There is almost an equal (10%) requirement for saturated, polysaturated, and monosaturated fatty acids, although, whenever possible, saturated fats should be replaced by monounsaturated or polyunsaturated fats (Figure 14.2).

Humans consume fats in the form of triacylglycerols either from plants or from animals. Plant triacylglycerols contain more unsaturated fatty acids compared with those from animals (except fish). However, there are a few exceptions: coconut and palm oils, for example, are entirely saturated fatty acids. The major role of lipids are (1) to facilitate absorption and storage of lipid-soluble vitamins (A, D, E, and K); (2) serve as precursors for steroids and bile acids; (3) serve as precursors for arachidonic acids and eicosanoids (prostaglandins, leukotrienes, thromboxane); (4) supply energy (in the form of fatty acid β-oxidation); and (5) maintain the integrity of the plasma membrane of cells.

Whereas carbohydrates can be used to produce fatty acids (a process called lipogenesis), humans are unable to use fatty acids to produce glucose. Due to the unique structures of fatty

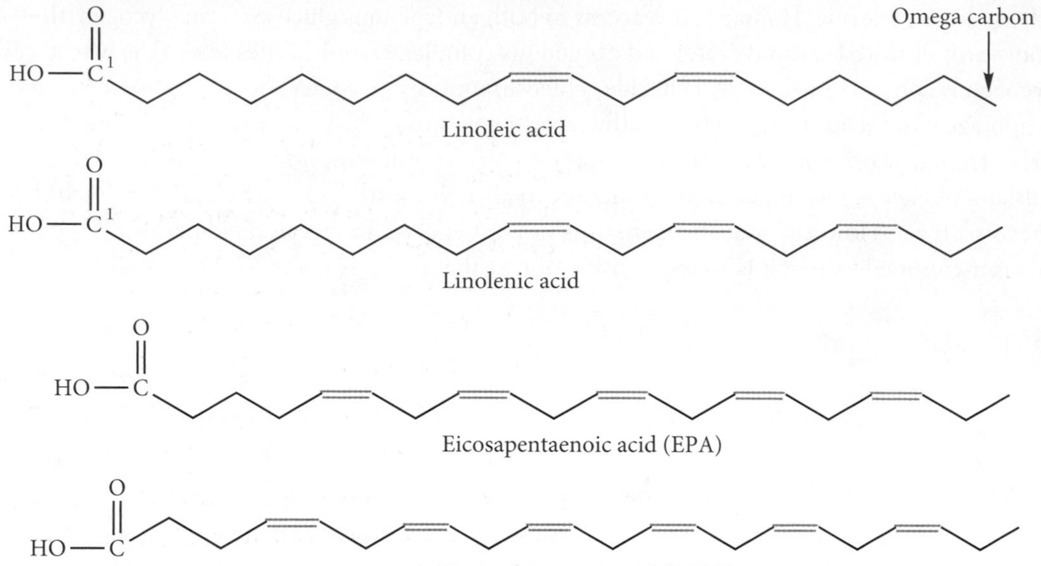

Figure 14.3 The structures of linolenic acid (an omega-3 fatty acid) and linoleic acid (an omega-6 fatty acid) and linoleic acid derivatives (EPA and EHA).

acids, they (1) provide the largest amount of energy compared with the other two sources, glucose and amino acid; (2) can be concentrated in small spaces; (3) enter the citric acid cycle as acetyl-CoA molecules; and (4) produce ketone bodies from acetyl-CoA.

There are two essential fatty acids that humans cannot synthesize endogenously: linolenic acid and linoleic acid (**Figure 14.3**). Because the essential fatty acids have important physiologic roles, it is important to emphasize their importance in our diet.

Essential Fatty Acids

Linolenic acid (also referred to as omega-3 fatty acid) and linoleic acid (also referred to as omega-6 fatty acid) are essential fatty acids that are crucial for the synthesis of arachidonic acid, which in turn is an important molecule for the synthesis of eicosanoids. While essential fatty acid deficiency is rare, it can occur due to a prolonged intake of lipid-free nutrition, administration of very-low-fat enteral feeding formulations, or severe malnutrition (i.e., when children or adults do not have access to fatty acid–containing foods). In addition, premature newborns, due to their limited fat stores, may develop essential fatty acid deficiency. Essential fatty acid deficiency can cause dermatitis, alopecia, impaired wound healing, growth failure, thrombocytopenia, and anemia.

Omega Oils

Both dietary linolenic acid and linoleic acid are absorbed from the GI tract. From the GI tract, they are transported to the liver as triacylglycerol in the plasma lipoproteins known as chylomicrons; triacylglycerol is then released into the blood in the form of other plasma lipoproteins. The final destination for these essential fatty acids is to be incorporated into cell membrane phospholipids or stored in adipose tissue as triacylglycerols.

All known eicosanoids are formed from the essential fatty acids. Linoleic acid can be found in vegetable, nut, and seed oils; it is called omega-6 because the first double bond occurs at carbon-6, counting from the opposite side from the carboxylic group of the fatty acid (see Figure 14.3). Oils from a fatty fish such as sardines, salmon, and mackerel consist of mostly linolenic acid; it is called omega-3 because the first double bond occurs at carbon-3, counting from the opposite side from carboxylic group of the fatty acid (see Figure 14.3). Linolenic acid tends to lower cardiovascular risk factors, although the exact mechanism is not fully understood. It has been suggested that linolenic acid increases hepatic β-oxidation of fatty acids, reduces hepatic synthesis of triacylglycerol, and increases plasma lipoprotein lipase activity. The roles of linolenic acid appear to involve reducing the amount of plasma triacylglycerols, producing antithrombotic effects, reducing the progression of atherosclerosis, reducing inflammation and oxidative stress, suppressing synthesis of pro-inflammatory cytokines, causing endothelial relaxation, and producing mild antihypertensive effects.

Omega-3 acid ethyl esters (fish oil) are available as Lovaza in the U.S. market; each 1 g of this medication contains 375 mg docosahexaenoic acid (DHA) and 465 mg eicosapentaenoic acid (EPA). DHA is a 22-carbon polyunsaturated fatty acid with six double bonds (see Figure 14.3). EPA is one carbon shorter than DHA and has five double bonds (see Figure 14.3). Both DHA and EPA are synthesized from linolenic acid and, as a result, they are omega-3 fatty acid derivatives. Based on clinical studies, it has been suggested that a daily dose of 3 g of omega-3 fatty acids may reduce morning stiffness and the number of tender joints in patients with rheumatoid arthritis. High doses of EPA (15–30 g/day) have been associated with thrombocytopenia and bleeding disorders.

Trans Fatty Acids

The hydrogenated polyunsaturated fatty acids found in foods may be manipulated to produce trans fatty acids. The hydrogenation process adds hydrogen atoms to unsaturated fatty acids, making them partially or completely saturated fatty acids. This hydrogenation process is convenient for the food industry because it solidifies vegetable oils, creating a form that is much easier to store and has a longer shelf-life. Consumption of trans fatty acids, however, has been linked to an increase risk of having a high level of low-density lipoprotein cholesterol (LDL-C) and a low level of high-density lipoprotein cholesterol (HDL-C). In addition, it has been suggested that trans fatty acids may compete with essential fatty acids, thereby limiting the positive effects of essential fatty acids in the body. As a result, the consumption of trans fatty acids should be as minimal as possible.

According to the U.S. Food and Drug Administration (FDA), the following foods typically include trans fatty acids: crackers, cookies, cakes, frozen pies, snack foods (such as microwave popcorn), frozen pizza, fast food, and stick margarines. Among these foods, stick margarine has the largest amount of trans fatty acids. In 2006, the FDA required that Nutrition Facts labels indicate trans fatty acids content.

Protein

Proteins are important molecules in our daily diets. They not only play a vital role by providing essential amino acids (the amino acids that humans cannot synthesize), but also support the protein synthesis process required to meet the needs created by rapid protein turnover. Proteins should account for 10–14% of the daily calorie intake (Figure 14.2). Generally, proteins from animal sources (such as meat, egg, and milk) are rich in essential amino acids, whereas proteins from plant sources (e.g., cereal, rice, wheat, corn) are low in essential amino acids. The body's demand for protein is higher during specific conditions such as growth, pregnancy, lactation, burning, and rehabilitation after injury or malnutrition.

In protein metabolism, the first step is to degrade the protein into its constituent polypeptide fragments and amino acids. Two classes of proteolytic enzymes, endopeptidases and exopeptidases, cleave proteins into smaller polypeptide fragments. Endopeptidases act first by catalyzing the cleavage of proteins into smaller fragments of polypeptides. As mentioned earlier, proteases such as pepsin, which is secreted in the stomach, and trypsin, chymotrypsin, and elastase, which are released from the pancreas into the small intestine, act on specific amino acids to degrade a polypeptide to smaller peptide fragments. For instance, trypsin catalyzes hydrolysis of lysine and arginine esters within polypeptides. In contrast, exopeptidases catalyze the cleavage of peptide bonds from the ends of peptides. Members of this enzyme class include carboxypeptidases, which cleave amino acids from the free carboxyl terminal, and aminopeptidases, which cleave amino acids from the amino terminal. In addition, other proteases such as dipeptidases and tripeptidases, located in the brush border of intestinal mucosal cells, serve as proteases to hydrolyze dipeptides and tripeptides, respectively.

The results of the actions of both endopeptidases and exopeptidases are production of oligopeptides, tripeptides, dipeptides, and free amino acids, which can then be absorbed across the GI tract. As mentioned earlier, membrane transporters exist on the epithelial cells that, in a sodium-dependent manner, assist amino acids in moving across the intestinal mucosa. These free amino acids are then transported into the hepatic portal vein to the liver before entering the circulation. Larger peptides are absorbed either by transcellular means (uptake into mucosal epithelial cells) or paracellular means (by going through epithelial cells; see also the *Introduction to Pharmacokinetics* chapter).

In the liver, an amino acid undergoes deamination to produce an amino group and a carbon skeleton. The amino group is converted into either other nitrogenous molecules (e.g., hormones, neurotransmitters, nucleic acid, heme) or a toxic molecule, ammonium. The urea cycle incorporates the harmful ammonium within a harmless molecule, urea. Urea is filtered through the kidneys and finally excreted into the urine. The carbon skeleton portion resulting from deamination of the amino acid takes different paths depending on the body's nutritional needs. For instance, it can be used for synthesis of other amino acids, undergo oxidization to generate ATP, serve as a precursor first to acetyl-CoA and then to ketone bodies (recall ketogenic amino acids from *Introduction to Biochemistry* chapter), and serve as a precursor to glucose by gluconeogenesis (recall glucogenic amino acids from *Introduction to Biochemistry* chapter) (**Figure 14.4**).

In addition to these molecules that are produced from proteins, proteins in the plasma play important roles in generating oncotic pressure and maintaining the blood's pH.

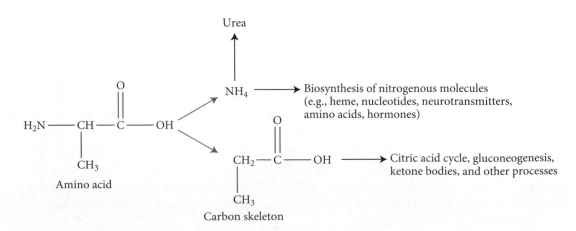

Figure 14.4 Different fates of an amino acid after a deamination process.

Oncotic Pressure

Proteins have a high molecular weight (an average of 70 kDa). Because of the relatively small amount of proteins in the plasma (70 g/L), the concentration of proteins in the plasma is usually approximately 1 mM. Oncotic pressure is a pressure generated by a capillary's proteins to prevent movement of water from the capillary into the interstitial fluid. The capillary is lined with endothelial cells (which separate the plasma from the interstitial fluid), which are impermeable to plasma proteins. The interstitial fluid contains fewer proteins than the plasma does. Oncotic pressure is important to prevent edema: because the concentration of proteins is higher in the capillary, water does not move from the capillary into the interstitial fluid (which otherwise would cause edema).

The three major proteins in the plasma are albumin, globulin, and fibrinogen. Albumin is the most abundant protein in plasma and is responsible for 80% of the oncotic pressure in plasma. There may be a correlation between peripheral edema and the oncotic pressure. In other words, peripheral edema may develop owing to a decrease in the oncotic pressure that could be explained by a low amount of plasma albumin.

Nitrogen Balance

In a healthy individual, a balance exists between the amount of nitrogen consumed and the nitrogen that is excreted in the urine. There is 1 g of nitrogen in 6.25 g of protein, and the RDA for protein is 0.66 g per 1 kg body weight. Nitrogen balance can be assessed by measuring urinary nitrogen excretion (as urea) and nitrogen intake (as protein). While nucleic acids also include nitrogen, they are not found to any significant level in the diet. As was mentioned in the *Introduction to Biochemistry* chapter, approximately 80% of the nitrogen atoms in our body are excreted as urea. Therefore, the amount of urea production (g/day) in a 24-hour urine urea collection is a reliable test to measure the nitrogen balance. However, one has to add 4 to the collected urine measurement to compensate for the loss of nitrogen that occurs through the skin, fecal, and respiratory systems.

There are three possible forms of nitrogen balance:

- *Equilibrium nitrogen balance.* This nitrogen balance occurs in healthy adults and is achieved when the intake of nitrogen equals the nitrogen excreted in the urine. There is no change in the total body content of protein in this nitrogen balance.
- *Positive nitrogen balance.* Positive nitrogen balance occurs when the nitrogen intake exceeds the nitrogen excretion. As a result, the excretion of nitrogen is less than the dietary intake of nitrogen, which ultimately causes retention of nitrogen in the body as proteins. This type of nitrogen balance is typically observed when tissues are growing—for instance, during the time a child is growing or during the pregnancy time frame.
- *Negative nitrogen balance.* This nitrogen balance occurs when the nitrogen loss exceeds the nitrogen intake. It is typically seen with inadequate protein intake, with a lack of the essential amino acids, and during stressful conditions such as trauma, burns, infection, or surgery.

High consumption of proteins does not result in a positive nitrogen balance. With such a protein-rich diet, the rates of both protein synthesis and degradation increase, with almost no net change in the amount of nitrogen present in the body.

Malnutrition

Malnutrition is often caused by starvation, impaired absorption of nutrients, or an increased demand on metabolism such as that exerted by neoplastic conditions. Malnutrition can result in both morbidity and mortality. While malnutrition can be associated with a lack of access to calories, vitamins, or trace elements, inadequate access to protein plays a major role in malnutrition.

Protein calorie malnutrition is often seen in hospitalized patients who have chronic illness, major trauma, or severe infection, or who have undergone major surgery. Malnutrition typically arises during these conditions because of enhanced oxygen consumption and metabolism. As a result, these highly catabolic patients may require intravenous administration of nutrients. In many cases, malnutrition leads to immune system suppression, which makes these patients prone to secondary infections and death.

Ideally, protein sources in the diet should include all nine essential amino acids: phenylalanine, valine, threonine, tryptophan, isoleucine, methionine, leucine, lysine, and histidine. These amino acids cannot be synthesized by eukaryotic organisms, including humans.

Extreme protein deficiency can lead to serious nutritional problems. A few of them are described in the following sections.

Kwashiorkor

Kwashiorkor is caused by inadequate intake of protein. This type of malnutrition has often been seen in children at about 1 year of age when their diet consists predominantly of carbohydrates. In addition, kwashiorkor is associated with an inadequate intake of antioxidants (such as zinc, copper, and vitamins C and E). Kwashiorkor is usually prevalent in areas experiencing famine and a limited food supply. While this condition is rarely seen in developed countries, it occurs when the feeding of children or elderly individuals is neglected. In contrast to marasmus (described in the following section), individuals with kwashiorkor appear well nourished due to relative adipose tissue preservation. However, edema is commonly seen in more advanced cases.

The concentration of hemoglobin is almost half the normal level (i.e., 8 g/dL as opposed to 12–16 g/dL) in patients with kwashiorkor. However, some children with kwashiorkor may show a normal hemoglobin concentration due to a reduced plasma volume. Typical symptoms of this malnutrition include anorexia, enlarged fatty liver, edema, and decreased plasma albumin concentration (hypoalbuminemia). A child with kwashiorkor shows a characteristic plump belly due to the developed edema.

Marasmus

Marasmus is another extreme form of malnutrition associated with protein deficiency. This malnutrition occurs because of inadequate intake of both calories and protein. Marasmus can affect both adults and children. Proteins from skeletal muscle (somatic proteins), particularly from the heart, liver, and kidneys (recall gluconeogenesis), and fat from the adipose tissue are degraded and oxidized. However, visceral proteins such as albumin and transferrin are preserved. Both cell-mediated immunity and muscle functions are impaired, and the former condition may increase the risk for infections.

Marasmus develops over a period of months and is characterized by loss of muscle tissue, loss of subcutaneous fat, wrinkled loose skin, and an inevitable weight loss. Patients with marasmus do not show the edema and changes in the plasma proteins that are readily apparent with kwashiorkor. As mentioned elsewhere in this chapter, patients with advanced cancer, HIV infection, and AIDS experience a high metabolic rate and, as a result, display physical signs of marasmus. However, there is a significant smaller protein loss in these patients compared with individuals having marasmus caused by starvation.

Table 14.1 Characteristics of Malnutrition Associated with Kwashiorkor, Marasmus, and Mixed Marasmus/Kwashiorkor

Features	Kwashiorkor	Marasmus	Mixed Marasmus/Kwashiorkor
Metabolic cause	Reduced protein intake and antioxidants, decreased concentration of plasma proteins	Reduced calorie intake	Reduced protein and calorie intake, reduced visceral protein synthesis
Onset	Fast (weeks)	Slow (months to years)	Fast (weeks)
Development	Associated with stress such as infections	In patients with advanced cancer, HIV infection, and AIDS	Associated with chronic illness, starvation, hypermetabolic, and stresses such as trauma, infection, and burns
Muscle wasting	Mild	Severe	Severe
Fat	Reduced	Absent	Reduced
Edema	Present	Absent	Present

Adapted from: Murray RK, Grossc PL. Biochemical case histories. In: Murray RK, Kennelly PJ, Rodwell VW, et al., eds. *Harper's illustrated biochemistry*, 29th ed. New York: McGraw-Hill; 2011. Available at: http://www.accesspharmacy.com/content.aspx?aID=55887347.

Mixed Marasmus/Kwashiorkor

Mixed marasmus/kwashiorkor is characterized by a severe protein-calorie malnutrition and often develops in chronically ill and starved patients. The visceral protein synthesis is reduced and wasting of somatic protein and energy (adipose tissue) stores is increased. Because of the reduction in cell-mediated immunity, the response to infection and wound healing are compromised in patients with mixed marasmus/kwashiorkor.

Table 14.1 highlights the differences between kwashiorkor, marasmus, and mixed marasmus/kwashiorkor.

Water

For each kilocalorie of energy produced in the body, we need 1–1.5 mL water. In total, then, a healthy individual adult man needs 1.7–2.5 L of water to meet his various physical activities and sweating. In turn, water is lost from the body through feces (50–100 mL/day), sweating and exhalation (500–1000 mL/day), and by urine (1,000 mL/day). The need for water is higher during pregnancy and lactation. In addition, in case of diarrhea, vomiting, or extensive sweating, the need for water is increased. The pediatric and geriatric populations have special needs related to water intake. For instance, infants require higher water intake due to their large surface area/volume ratio and their ongoing developing kidneys, whereas geriatric individuals have a higher body fat/water ratio (due to reduced total body water) and a reduced thirst sensation.

As mentioned in the *Introduction to Pharmacokinetics* chapter, the total body water (TBW) differs in men (60% of body weight) and women (50% of body weight, because women have more fat than men). While two-thirds of TBW is located in the intracellular compartment (intracellular fluid volume [ICFV]), one-third is located in the extracellular compartment (extracellular fluid volume [ECFV]). The interstitial fluid includes three-fourths of ECFV and the plasma accounts for one-fourth of ECFV.

Exposure to xenobiotics, including drug products, can change the water balance in all patients, including geriatric and pediatric populations. For instance, inotropic agents (such as dopamine and dobutamine) can change the glomerular filtration rate, and diuretics (such as thiazides and loop diuretics) can change the rate of Na^+ reabsorption. In addition, sympathomimetics, cholinergics, and uncoupling proteins of the oxidative phosphorylation pathway can increase fluid losses through excessive sweating.

Humans maintain plasma osmolality through water intake; actions of the hypothalamus, pituitary gland, and kidney; and the effects of hormones such as antidiuretic hormone (ADH; also called arginine vasopressin [AVP]) and adrenal mineralocorticoids. The urinary water loss is controlled by the hormone ADH. When the plasma osmolarity increases, the anterior hypothalamic osmoreceptors are stimulated, which in turn stimulates thirst. The posterior pituitary gland synthesizes and releases ADH. ADH, in turn, is transported to the kidney to stimulate the synthesis of cAMP molecules. An increase in cAMP molecules stimulates the insertion of aquaporin channels into the apical membrane of the distal convoluted tubule and collecting duct, which ultimately increases water reabsorption and reduces urinary water loss (see *Introduction to Cell Biology* chapter).

ADH also stimulates the insertion of the urea transporter protein, UT1, into apical membranes of collecting tubule cells to facilitate urea excretion. By the same token, if the plasma osmolality decreases, thirst and the release of ADH decrease as well. The latter effect results in decreased renal cAMP formation, which in turn reduces the water permeability of the distal convoluted tubule and collecting duct and increases the volume of the urine.

Aquaporins constitute a family of integral proteins that provide channels to facilitate rapid movement of water molecules across the plasma membrane in many tissues. More than 10 different mammalian aquaporins have been identified to date, and additional aquaporins may potentially emerge in the future. Diabetes insipidus is associated with inadequate release or action of ADH: Without ADH, aquaporin cannot reabsorb water from the collecting ducts, leading to reduced water retention. As a result, patients with nephrogenic diabetes insipidus, who have an inherited aquaporin-2 deficiency, develop polyuria (and polydipsia), which in turn results in hypernatremia. Consequently, these patients produce a large volume of daily urine (5–9 L). A number of pharmacologic agents such as ethanol, opioid antagonists, and β-adrenergic agonists, also suppress ADH release.

Ethanol (alcohol) can provide energy (calories) when consumed as part of the diet. However, its consumption has metabolic consequences that can affect a few important biochemical pathways. As discussed in the *Introduction to Biological Chemistry* and *Introduction to Pharmacology and Pathophysiology* chapters, the enzyme that catalyzes breakdown of alcohol is called alcohol dehydrogenase. This enzyme uses NAD^+ to metabolize (oxidize) alcohol to acetaldehyde by reducing NAD^+ to NADH. As a result, when alcohol is metabolized, the amount of NAD^+ decreases and the amount of NADH increases. Consequently, the normal NAD^+/NADH ratio will be changed and the cell will suffer from not having enough NAD^+. Many dehydrogenase enzymes need NAD^+ to perform cellular metabolism, particularly the ones that are involved in glycolysis and the citric acid cycle. As a result, ATP production will be reduced. In addition, alcohol can enhance the production of lactic acid, leading to acidosis, particularly in patients who are drinking alcohol and are at greater risk of developing this electrolyte imbalance.

Vitamins

Vitamins play a crucial role in many biochemical reactions in the body. These nutrients are organic compounds that the human body is unable to produce in an adequate quantity. In addition, some physiologic conditions such as pregnancy and lactation may require vitamin supplementation. Furthermore, medications can influence the absorption or elimination of vitamins.

A deficiency of a vitamin (or multiple vitamins) can lead to malfunction of a biochemical pathway, leading to severe physiologic consequences. Analytical tests often reveal vitamin deficiencies. For instance, measuring the plasma level of a vitamin or noting a decrease in the urinary excretion of a vitamin can alert the clinician to a particular vitamin deficiency. While the lipid-soluble vitamins are absorbed in the lipid micelles, the water-soluble vitamins are absorbed from the small intestine either by active transport or by carrier-mediated diffusion.

There are 13 vitamins that are divided into two major groups:

- Lipid-soluble vitamins such as A, D, E, and K
- Water-soluble vitamins such as B complex and C

These two groups are defined based on solubility and storage rather than function. The lipid-soluble vitamins are stored in association with body lipids and generally take an extended period of time to become depleted even in the presence of low-fat diets. In contrast, the water-soluble vitamins must be included in the daily diet because they are readily excreted by the kidneys and cannot be stored in the body. However, there is one exception to this rule: cobalamin (vitamin B_{12}). This vitamin is stored in the liver and, as a result, there is a risk of vitamin B_{12} toxicity if it is ingested in large amounts. B vitamins have a number of vital roles in the body, most notably serving as cofactors or coenzymes for enzymes involved in many of the metabolic and biochemical pathways that provide energy.

Vitamin deficiencies lead to diseases. A single-vitamin deficiency usually occurs as a result of a condition that interferes with vitamin uptake. Such a deficiency may be common in populations who eat a restricted diet (for instance, thiamin deficiency has been discovered in many vegans). Contrary to a general belief, vitamin deficiency exists in developed countries, including the United States. Indeed, multiple-vitamin deficiency is much more common in the United States than single-vitamin deficiency.

Four populations are especially prone to vitamin deficiencies: (1) children (because of their consumption of junk foods); (2) the elderly (because of their large consumption of tea and toast); (3) alcoholics (because of their poor diets); and (4) pregnant women (because of the continuous cell growth taking place in their bodies).

According to the American Medical Association, healthy individuals who eat a variety of foods do not need supplemental vitamins. However, pregnant women and individuals with poor diets should take supplemental vitamins. In 2006, it was reported that 73% of adults in the United States have used a dietary supplement within the past year. While there are misconceptions about the roles of vitamins (such as that they provide extra energy, promote muscle growth, or prevent or reverse chronic diseases), these nutrients are necessary molecules to maintain the normal level of biochemical reactions that are vital to our well-being.

Vitamin deficiency and vitamin toxicity both have severe biochemical consequences. Therefore, efforts have been made to provide standard recommendations regarding vitamin intakes. Given that some of the recommendations are still used in different nutrients' labeling, it is important to list the definitions for all of them.

- *Recommended Daily Intake (RDI):* a dietary intake that is sufficient to meet the daily nutrient requirements of 97% of healthy individuals in a specific demographic population.
- *Recommended Dietary Allowance (RDA):* an older nomenclature for RDI that is still used, particularly to formulate food guidelines.
- *Dietary Reference Intake (DRI):* a nutritional recommendation that is used in the United States and Canada. The DRI is the nutritional recommendation most recently established by

a joint effort from the National Academy of Sciences, the National Research Council, and the Institute of Medicine to replace the RDA (and it may replace the RDI in the future). Its goal was to expand the definition of RDI.

- *Adequate Intake (AI):* the nutrient intake necessary to maintain a healthy condition. AI is used for a given nutrient when there are not enough data to determine a RDI. For instance, AI is used for infants up to 1 year of age. In addition, for people of all ages, AI is used for calcium, chromium, vitamin D, fluoride, manganese, pantothenic acid (vitamin B_5), biotin (vitamin B_7), and choline.

- *Estimated Average Requirement (EAR):* a reference that indicates the amount of a nutrient estimated to be sufficient for 50% of healthy individuals of a specific age and sex. This reference is rarely used and is not helpful, as it refers to a median requirement for a group.

- *Tolerable Upper Level (UL):* the highest daily nutrient intake unlikely to cause adverse health effects for most of the population. Nutrient data are not available to estimate the UL for all vitamins. Thus a lack of UL does not mean the vitamin in question does not cause any toxicity.

Water-Soluble Vitamins

Water-soluble vitamins are divided into two groups: B vitamins and vitamin C.

Vitamin B_1 (Thiamine)

Thiamine plays a major role in the catalytic activity of a few enzymes involved in the synthesis of acetyl-CoA and nucleic acids. The pyruvate dehydrogenase complex (which catalyzes formation of pyruvate to acetyl-CoA; see also the *Introduction to Biochemistry* chapter) is affected by a thiamine deficiency. The availability of a smaller amount of acetyl-CoA results in a slower citric acid cycle, which in turn decreases ATP synthesis in the mitochondria—a factor that may explain the memory loss and confusion symptoms associated with thiamine deficiency. Similarly, the presence of thiamine is important for transketolase, an enzyme involved in the pentose phosphate pathway as part of the synthesis of nucleic acids from glucose-6-phosphate. In addition, the effects of thiamine deficiency on the pyruvate dehydrogenase complex result in an accumulation of pyruvate, which then can lead to lactic acidosis (i.e., pyruvate is catalyzed to lactic acid rather than being catalyzed to acetyl-CoA). Lactic acidosis is a severe metabolic consequence that, if untreated, is fatal.

Thiamine deficiency has a variable presentation, ranging from peripheral neuropathy to myocardial dysfunction. If a vitamin B_1 supplement is not adequately added to long-term total parenteral nutrition (TPN) in hospitals, the risk for patients to develop thiamine deficiency is high.

Sources of Thiamin

While pork, rice, and cereals contain large amounts of thiamine, milk, fruits, and vegetables are poor sources of thiamine. High temperature (cooking) and a high pH may inactivate thiamine. The RDIs for thiamine are 1.2 mg/day and 1.1 mg/day for men and women, respectively.

Thiamine is eliminated by renal clearance. A few drugs, such as furosemide (Lasix), acetazolamide (Diamox), chlorothiazide (Diuril), amiloride (Midamo, from Canada), and mannitol (Aridol), significantly increase the urinary elimination of thiamine. In addition, drugs such as furosemide and digoxin (Lanoxin) inhibit thiamine uptake into myocardial cells. Because the rate of excretion of thiamine depends on the ingested amount, with a small intake, the renal excretion decreases; conversely, with a high intake, the renal excretion increases. As a result, the risk of toxicity is fairly low. Keep in mind that while ethanol decreases thiamine absorption, consumption of foods rich in carbohydrates increases the thiamine requirement.

Thiamine Deficiency

Thiamine deficiency can cause "wet" beriberi (congestive heart failure) and "dry" beriberi (Wernicke encephalopathy and the Wernicke-Korsakoff syndrome). Patients who may develop thiamine deficiency include HIV patients who have a poor oral intake, patients who are receiving chemotherapy, and individuals who have impaired absorption (alcoholism). Beriberi symptoms may affect the gastrointestinal system (no appetite, indigestion), nervous system (fatigue, loss of memory and sensation), cardiovascular system (heart muscle weakness and edema), and musculoskeletal system (widespread muscle pain). Wernicke-Korsakoff syndrome is primarily seen in chronic alcoholism; its symptoms include loss of memory and vision, loss of muscle, and loss of coordination. In alcoholism, alcohol withdrawal and maintenance of a balanced diet help these individuals to recover and prevent future symptoms.

Treatment of Thiamine Deficiency

Patients with severe thiamine deficiency (Wernicke-Korsakoff syndrome) are given an initial dose of 100 mg of parenteral (intramuscularly or intravenously) thiamine hydrochloride (Betaxin); treatment then continues with 100 mg daily until the patient can consume a regular and balanced diet. In the case of beriberi, patients receive 5–30 mg/dose of parenteral (intramuscularly or intravenously) thiamine hydrochloride three times daily, and then 5–30 mg orally, daily for 1 month. However, patients with clinical deficiencies may require larger doses. For instance, a dose of as much as 1 g of thiamine hydrochloride can be given in the first 12 hours to a patient with persistent neurologic abnormalities.

Due to its low toxicity, thiamine is listed in pregnancy category A and is also safe for use in lactating mothers.

Vitamin B_2 (Riboflavin)

Riboflavin serves as a precursor for the coenzymes flavin mononucleotide (FMN) and flavin adenine dinucleotide (FAD). These coenzymes are essential for utilization of flavoproteins, which include enzymes in the mitochondrial oxidative phosphorylation, in fatty acid and amino acid oxidation, and in the citric acid cycle. While vitamin B_2 deficiency occurs in many countries, it does not lead to severe consequences because the body has an efficient conservation of tissue riboflavin and a recycling process; that is, when riboflavin is released from metabolic enzymes, it is rapidly incorporated into newly synthesized enzymes.

Riboflavin Sources

Vitamin B_2 can be found in milk, meat, fish, eggs, broccoli, legumes, and dark green vegetables. This nutrient is extremely sensitive to light, which causes photodegradation of riboflavin. Thus it is important to protect milk from photodegradation by storing it in light-proof containers.

Riboflavin Deficiency

Riboflavin deficiency is associated with malnutrition that leads to inflammation of the skin and tongue (cheilitis and glossitis, respectively) and seborrheic dermatitis. Due to a limited capacity of the GI tract to absorb riboflavin, vitamin B_2 toxicity is very rare.

Laboratory diagnosis of riboflavin deficiency can be made by the measurement of erythrocytes, urinary riboflavin concentrations, and erythrocyte glutathione reductase activity (FAD is important for the activity of glutathione reductase, so the enzyme activity of glutathione reductase is reduced in individuals with vitamin B_2 deficiency).

A number of medications can cause depletion of riboflavin. Examples include antibiotics, antimalarial agents, oral contraceptives, thiazide diuretics, thyroid hormones, and tricyclic antidepressants.

Treatment of Riboflavin Deficiency

Dietary supplements such as Ribo-100 are given as 100 mg once or twice daily to treat riboflavin deficiency. In addition, riboflavin is used in migraine prophylaxis (at higher doses, such as 400 mg/day).

Vitamin B₃ (Niacin)

Niacin is the precursor for the coenzymes nicotinamide adenine dinucleotide (NAD^+) and its phosphorylated derivative $NADP^+$. NAD^+ and $NADP^+$ function as coenzymes in many redox reactions. Niacin is absorbed well from the intestinal tract and can reach almost all tissues.

Niacin Sources

Meat, nuts, fish, and whole- and enriched-grain products are rich in niacin. In 1939, flour was supplemented with nicotinic acid, which assisted in eradicating pellagra in the United States.

Niacin supplements are also used (although not related to niacin's role as a vitamin) in the treatment of hyperlipidemia, because they increase the activity of lipoprotein lipase and decrease esterification of glycerols to form triacylglycerols in the liver.

Niacin Deficiency

Deficiency of niacin results in retarded growth and pellagra, a condition characterized by photosensitive dermatitis, diarrhea, and dementia. Originally, the niacin deficiency comes from tryptophan deficiency. Niacin is synthesized from the essential amino acid tryptophan (**Figure 14.5**). However, only 1 mg niacin is synthesized from 60 mg tryptophan. Tryptophan is

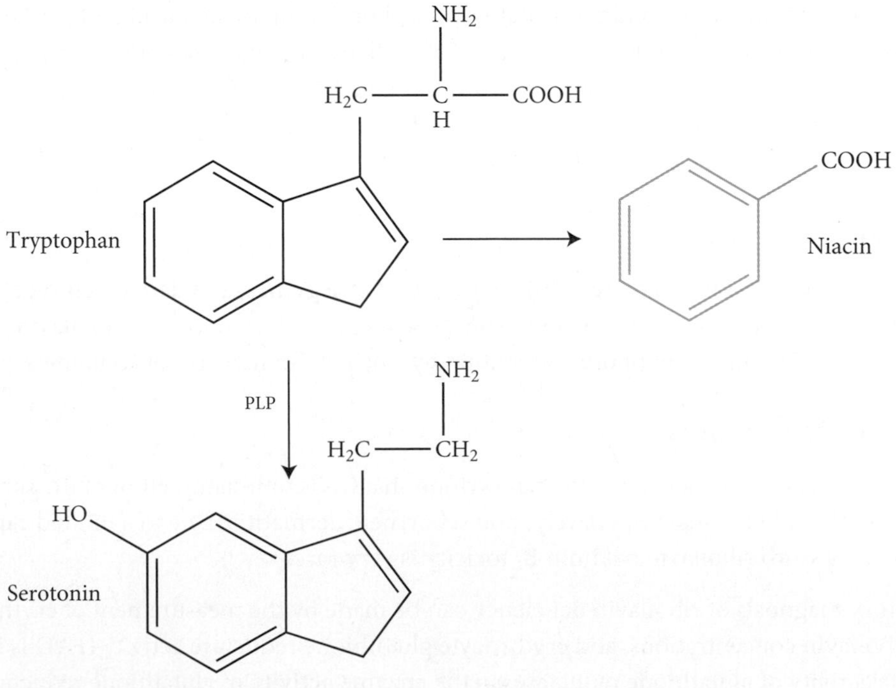

Figure 14.5 The essential amino acid tryptophan serves as a precursor in the synthesis of niacin.

also a precursor for the neurotransmitter serotonin (Figure 14.5). Thus a niacin deficiency may promote the endogenous synthesis of niacin and affect the synthesis of serotonin.

In most countries, niacin deficiency is rare. However, in many developed countries, because of the prevalence of alcoholism, pellagra remains a health issue.

In addition to tryptophan, other vitamins such as vitamins B_2 and B_6 are required for the synthesis of niacin from tryptophan. Women develop niacin deficiency twice as often as men, which may suggest a role for estrogen metabolites in inhibiting the synthesis of niacin from tryptophan. Niacin deficiency can also result from genetic factors such as a defect of the membrane transport mechanism for tryptophan, which results in the rare disease Hartnup.

Treatment of Niacin Deficiency

Oral supplementation of 100–200 mg of nicotinamide three times daily for 5 days is used to treat pellagra. As mentioned earlier, niacin is also used to reduce triacylglycerol synthesis and to lower the amount of LDL, albeit in much higher doses (1–6 g/day). This regimen is associated with side effects such as cutaneous flushing and pruritus. These side effects, which are caused by the production of prostaglandin D_2 and E_2, may be diminished by taking a dose of 325 mg aspirin 30 minutes before taking vitamin B_3.

Vitamin B_5 (Pantothenic Acid)

Pantothenic acid serves as a precursor for coenzyme A (CoA), which is a component of acetyl-CoA, and for the acyl carrier protein (ACP), which is a component of the fatty acid synthase complex. Therefore, a deficiency in vitamin B_5 affects many biochemical and physiologic pathways, including the citric acid cycle, β-oxidation of fatty acids, synthesis of cholesterol and steroid hormones, and synthesis of phospholipids, bile acids, porphyrin, and acetylcholine. It has also been suggested that pantothenic acid can reduce high levels of triacylglycerols and LDL-C and increase HDL-C levels.

Pantothenic Acid Sources

Pantothenic acid is found in liver, eggs, and yeast. While whole grains are rich in pantothenic acid (particularly the outer layers of the whole grains), milling reduces the amount of this vitamin present in grains. In addition, royal jelly is very rich in pantothenic acid.

Pantothenic Acid Deficiency

Deficiency of pantothenic acid is rare and has not been well characterized in humans. Similarly, there has not been any report of vitamin B_5 toxicity. However, some symptoms have been associated with vitamin B_5 deficiency, including GI upset, depression, muscle cramps, ataxia, and hypoglycemia. Because vitamin B_5 is excreted in the urine, the diagnosis of a vitamin B_5 deficiency is made through identification of a low urinary vitamin B_5 level.

Treatment of Pantothenic Acid Deficiency

The OTC drug Panto-250 is used to treat vitamin B_5 deficiency and does not cause any significant drug interaction.

Vitamin B_6 (Pyridoxine)

All of the aminotransferase enzymes that are involved in amino acid oxidation (to provide energy from proteins; see also the *Introduction to Biochemistry* chapter) require pyridoxal phosphate (PLP). PLP is derived from pyridoxine. PLP is also important for many decarboxylase enzymes that synthesize neurotransmitters such as dopamine, gamma amino-butyric acid (GABA), histamine, and serotonin (**Figure 14.6**).

Isoniazid (Isotamine, from Canada), a drug used in the treatment of tuberculosis, can bind to pyridoxal phosphate and induce a vitamin B_6 deficiency (**Figure 14.7**). Therefore, in the isoniazid treatment, vitamin B_6 supplement is required. In addition, levodopa, penicillamine, and cycloserine interact with PLP. For instance, PLP is required for the decarboxylase enzyme that converts levodopa to dopamine; carbidopa inhibits the decarboxylase enzyme. Therefore, vitamin B_6 counteracts the effect of carbidopa. When carbidopa and levodopa are combined, however, the carbidopa interaction with vitamin B_6 is minimal.

Pyridoxine Sources

Legumes, nuts, and meat are rich in vitamin B_6.

Pyridoxine Deficiency

Similar to the case with the other water-soluble vitamins, vitamin B_6 deficiency is rare. However, such a deficiency can cause abnormalities of tryptophan and methionine metabolism. A severe vitamin B_6 deficiency can lead to peripheral neuropathy, depression, and confusion. Some cases of photosensitivity and dermatitis have also been associated with vitamin B_6 deficiency. The most serious cause of vitamin B_6 deficiency is seizures due to a lack of GABA synthesis (Figure 14.6). In addition, vitamin B_6 is required to convert homocysteine to cystathionine, so a deficiency of this nutrient may result in accumulation of too much homocysteine, in turn increasing the risk of a cardiovascular disease (see also the discussion of folic acid deficiency in this chapter).

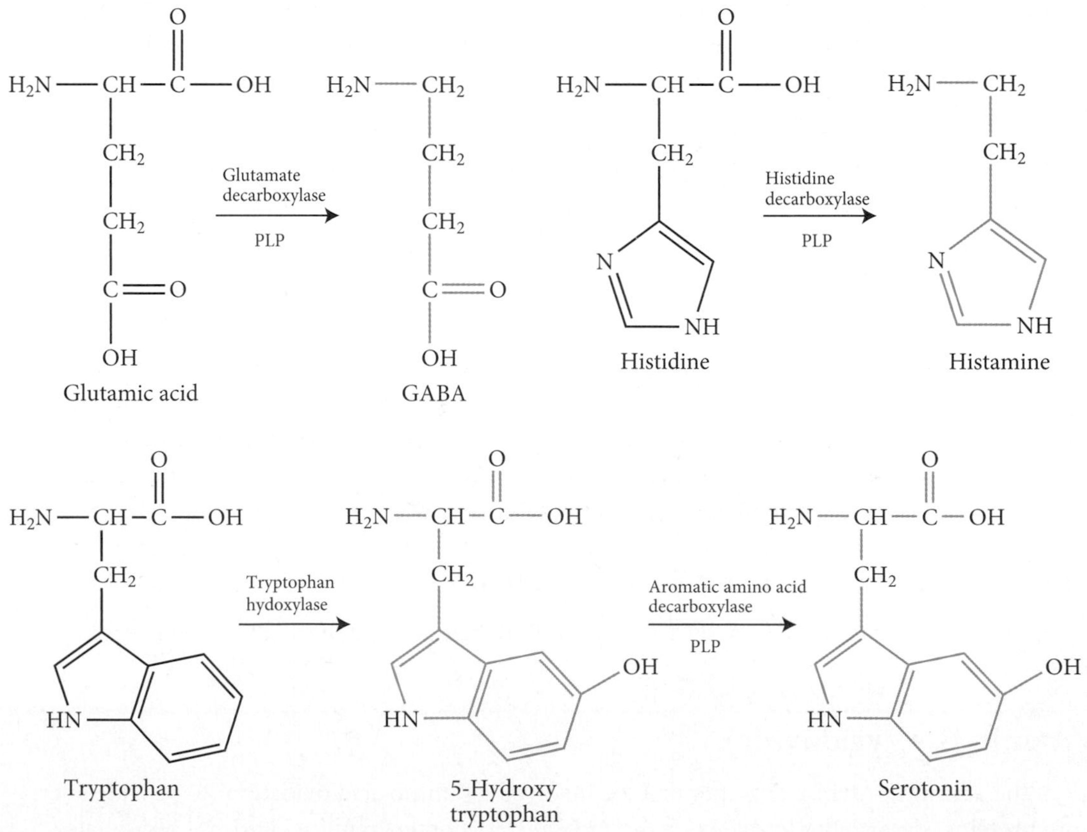

Figure 14.6 PLP is required for decarboxylase enzymes to catalyze the synthesis of a few neurotransmitters.

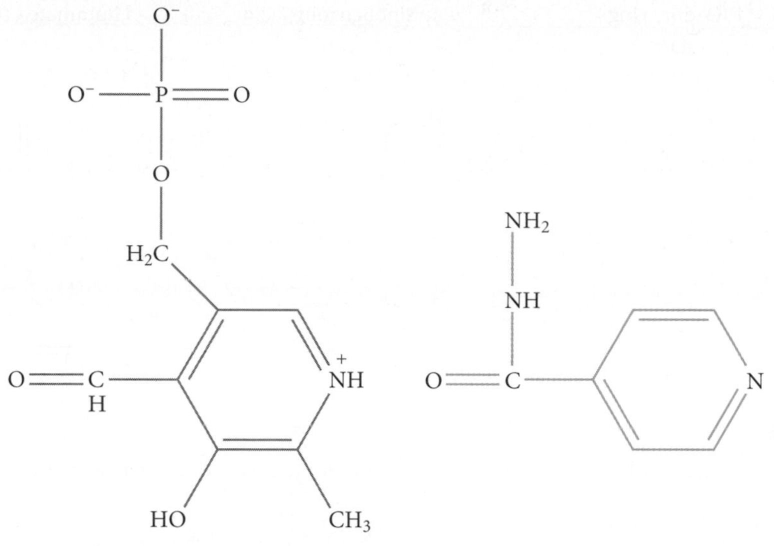

Figure 14.7 Isoniazid depletes PLP, which results in vitamin B_6 deficiency. Notice the similarity between PLP and isoniazid.

Treatment of Pyridoxine Deficiency

A vitamin B_6 deficiency is indicated by a low plasma PLP level (less than 20 nM) and is often resolved by administration of a vitamin B_6 supplement of 25-50 mg/daily. For isoniazid toxicity, patients are given a 100 mg IV dose of vitamin B_6 and then continue to take 25–100 mg/day as long as they use isoniazid. Toxicity of vitamin B_6 has been rarely seen, but when it happens, it results in a severe sensory neuropathy that leads to patients being unable to walk.

Although vitamin B_6 crosses the placenta, it is safe to be used during pregnancy. Indeed, it is used to treat nausea and vomiting during pregnancy.

Vitamin B_7 (Biotin)

Biotin is a coenzyme for a few important enzymes (there are nine known biotin-dependent enzymes), including playing a role in the catalysis of oxaloacetate formation (i.e., the transfer of a carboxyl group to pyruvate to form oxaloacetate). In addition, biotin is important for the acetyl-CoA carboxylase enzyme that converts acetyl-CoA to malonyl-CoA in the synthesis of fatty acids. Furthermore, this vitamin is required for the metabolism of odd-numbered fatty acids and a few essential amino acids (methionine, threonine, valine, and isoleucine) to synthesize succinyl-CoA. Succinyl-CoA is an intermediate molecule of the citric acid cycle. Consequently, biotin is important for gluconeogenesis, lipogenesis, fatty acid biosynthesis, the citric acid cycle, odd-numbered fatty acids metabolism, and the metabolism of methionine, threonine, valine, and isoleucine. Furthermore, it has been shown that this nutrient plays a role in the regulation of the cell cycle and gene expression by binding to a few nuclear proteins and also functions in the catabolism of another essential amino acid, leucine.

Biotin Sources

Good sources of vitamin B_7 include liver, nuts, and eggs. Biotin is also synthesized by intestinal bacteria.

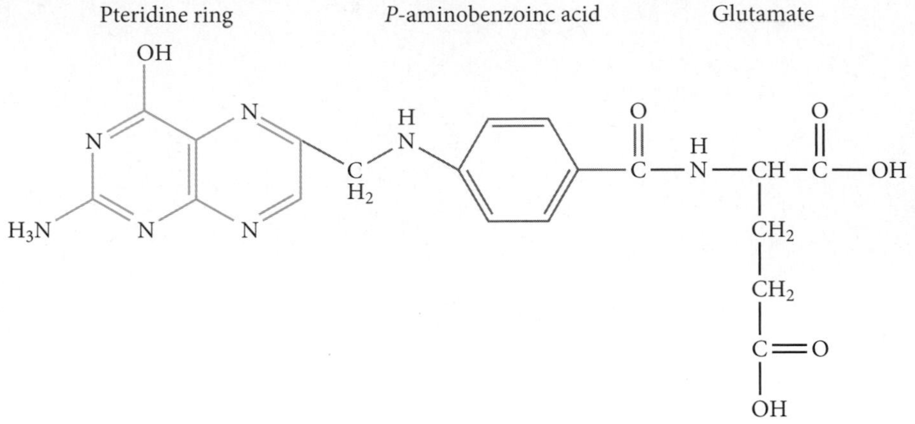

Pteridine ring   *P*-aminobenzoinc acid   Glutamate

Figure 14.8 The structure of folic acid, which consists of a pteridine ring, a *P*-aminobenzoic acid, and the amino acid glutamate.

Biotin Deficiency

A deficiency of biotin is uncommon. It can occur, however, in individuals who ingest large amounts of raw egg whites, in patients who receive biotin-free parenteral nutrition, and in patients who receive long-term antibiotic therapies that eliminate the intestinal bacteria that would otherwise synthesize biotin. The avidin glycoprotein in egg white has a high affinity to biotin; after binding to biotin, it can prevent biotin's absorption. Biotin deficiency causes alopecia, dermatitis, fatigue, depression, hallucinations, paresthesia, anorexia, and nausea.

Treatment of Biotin Deficiency

The treatment of vitamin B_7 deficiency requires biotin, using up to 10 mg/day. There is no report of vitamin B_7 toxicity.

Vitamin B_9 (Folic Acid)

The structure of folic acid consists of a pteridine ring, a *P*-aminobenzoic acid, and the amino acid glutamate (**Figure 14.8**). After absorption, folic acid is reduced by dihydrofolate reductase enzyme to dihydrofolate and then to tetrahydrofolate (THF) (the active form of folic acid; **Figure 14.9**). THF is important in the transfer of single carbon groups in the synthesis of glycine (amino acid) and nucleic acids (DNA).

Folic Acid Sources

Folic acid is found naturally in green leafy vegetables, mushrooms, oranges, and legumes. The synthetic form of vitamin B_9 is found in supplements and fortified grain products such as flour, cornmeal, rice, and pasta (since 1998, a requirement from the FDA in an attempt to reduce the risk of neural tube defects [NTDs]).

Folic Acid Deficiency

One of the most common vitamin deficiencies in the United States is folic acid deficiency. Two major causes of this deficiency are poor eating habits (as mentioned earlier, caused by tea-and-toast and junk food diets) and pregnancy (high cellular growth).

Neural tube defects are serious birth defects. The most severe variant, spina bifida, is caused by abnormalities in closing the fetal spinal cord, leading to a protruding spinal cord. Because folic

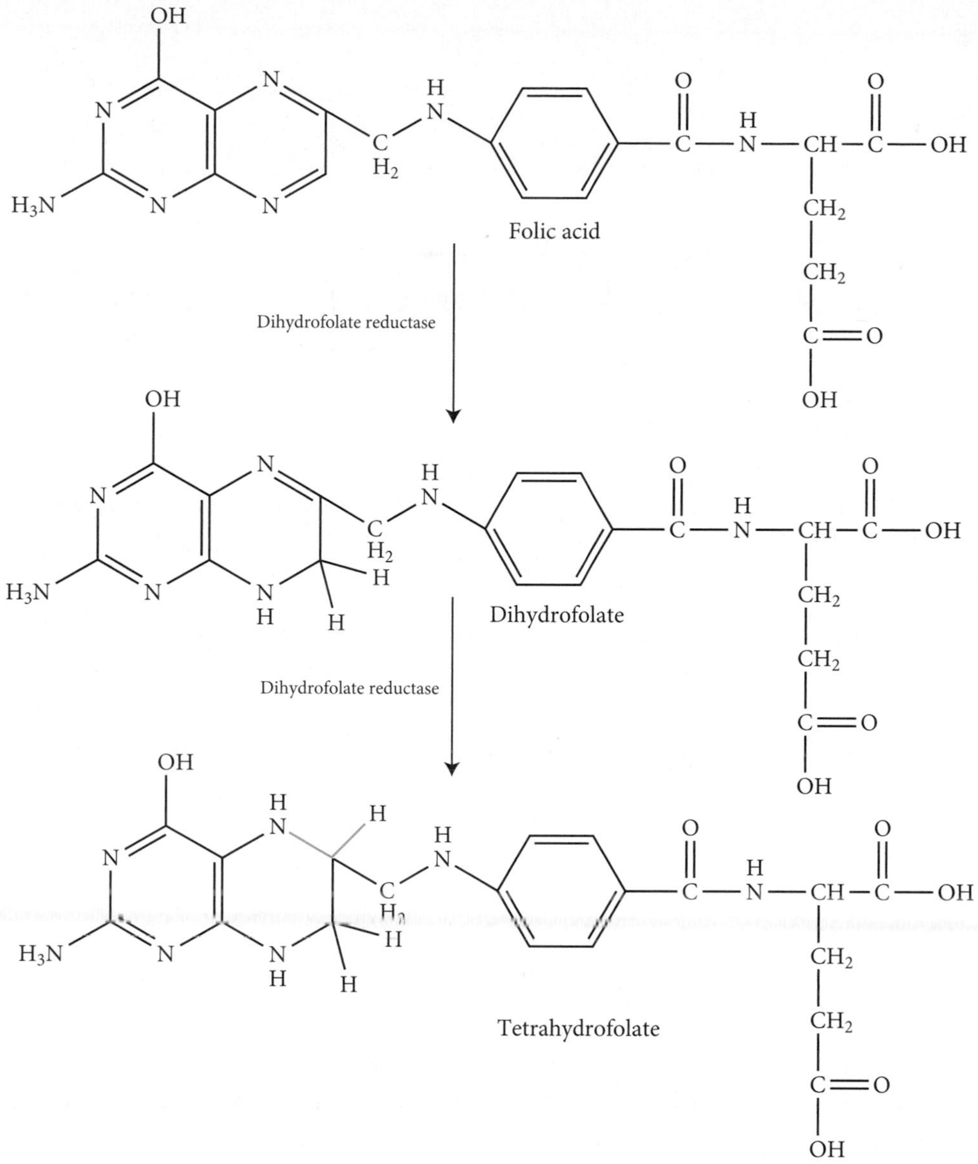

Figure 14.9 The dihydrofolate reductase enzyme plays a major role in the synthesis of tetrahydrofolate (THF), the active form of folic acid.

acid is required for the synthesis of nucleic acids (DNA), a folic acid deficiency may delay cell growth during the closure of the spinal cord. Folic acid deficiency can also result from therapy with drugs such as methotrexate (Rheumatrex) and trimethoprim (Primsol), which are known to inhibit dihydrofolate reductase and prevent the synthesis of THF. In addition, a high consumption of organic foods that lack folic acid fortification may lead to folic acid deficiency.

Treatment of Folic Acid Deficiency

Vitamin B_9 supplements before and during pregnancy can help to prevent most NTDs. To prevent NTDs in their children, females with childbearing potential require less than 1 mg (0.4–0.8 mg/day). However, this amount is increased to 4 mg/day for females at high risk of NTDs. During lactation, 0.5 mg is adequate to avoid any folic acid deficiency. Folic acid is also used for the treatment of megaloblastic and macrocytic anemias caused by folic acid deficiency.

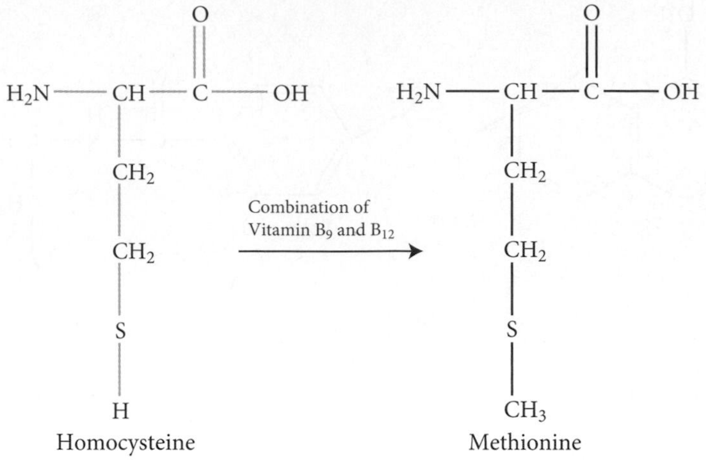

Figure 14.10 Conversion of the harmful homocysteine to the essential amino acid methionine requires both cobalamin and folic acid.

Drug interactions can occur between folic acid and other drugs. For instance, folic acid reduces serum levels of phenytoin (Dilantin), primidone (Mysoline), and raltitrexed (Tomudex, from Canada, which is used for the treatment of advanced colorectal cancer). Raltitrexed's effect is significantly reduced when taken with folic acid supplements; consequently, folic acid should not be taken immediately before or with raltitrexed.

Vitamin B_{12} (Cobalamin)

Cobalamin is a coenzyme with four pyrrole rings and a cobalt atom (Co) in the center. This vitamin is required as a coenzyme for at least three biochemical reactions: (1) methylation of homocysteine to produce methionine (**Figure 14.10**); (2) methyl rearrangement in methylmalonyl CoA to form succinyl-CoA; and (3) formation of the neurotransmitter acetylcholine.

Two mechanisms facilitate the absorption of cobalamin. One is an inefficient mechanism that occurs through buccal, duodenal, and ileal mucosa and contributes to less than 1% of the total absorption of cobalamin. The second mechanism is more active and is mediated by a glycoprotein called intrinsic factor (IF) that is secreted by the gastric parietal cells.

The absorption of cobalamin is a complex process that involves several proteins and enzymes. The GI enzymes dissociate dietary cobalamin from protein complexes to allow cobalamin to attach to a salivary glycoprotein known as haptocorrin. Haptocorrin is degraded by the pancreatic protease trypsin. When this degradation mechanism is activated, cobalamin is released and attaches to IF to form an IF–cobalamin complex. The IF–cobalamin complex is recognized by a specific receptor in the lining of the ileum, the IF is detached, and cobalamin enters the blood. In the blood, cobalamin attaches to another binding protein known as transcobalamin II (TC2). The role of transcobalamin II is to transport cobalamin to all body tissues.

Cobalamin and folic acid are both important vitamins for the synthesis of *S*-adenosylmethionine (SAMe) (Figure 14.10), which in turn is important in the synthesis of DNA (**Figure 14.11**) and myelination of nerve fibers. The SAMe molecule donates a methyl group to many other molecules in processes such as biosynthesis of epinephrine, phosphocreatine, and membrane phospholipids. It is available as an OTC product (oral 400–1,600 mg/day) for the treatment of depression and cardiovascular disease. Patients should be counseled to avoid SAMe if

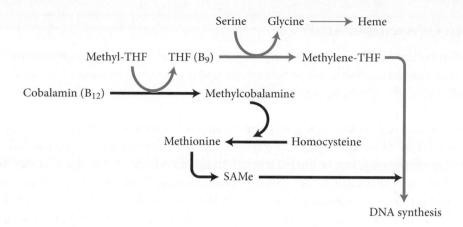

Figure 14.11 Cobalamin works closely with folic acid in the synthesis of nucleic acids, glycine, and heme, as well as the removal of homocysteine.

Adapted from: Bender DA. Micronutrients: vitamins and minerals. In: Murray RK, Kennelly PJ, Rodwell VW, et al., eds. *Harper's illustrated biochemistry*, 29th ed. New York: McGraw-Hill; 2011. Available at: http://www.accesspharmacy.com /content.aspx?aID=55885518.

they are using a monoamine oxidase (MAO) inhibitor or a tricyclic antidepressant, as the effects of these drugs may be enhanced by the concurrent use of SAMe (see also the *Introduction to Pharmacology and Pathophysiology* chapter).

Both cobalamin and folic acid are required for the biosynthesis of the amino acid glycine. Glycine, in turn, is important for the synthesis of heme. A lack of heme results in a low concentration of hemoglobin (Figure 14.11).

Cobalamin Sources

Cobalamin cannot be synthesized by plants or animals, but rather is produced only by microorganisms. Chicken, fish (salmon), yogurt, and milk are rich in cobalamin as well. Because vitamin B_{12} cannot be found in plants, strict vegetarians are prone to a type of vitamin B_{12} deficiency known as pernicious anemia. Humans have a 3- to 6-year supply of cobalamin stored in the liver; indeed, cobalamin is the only water-soluble vitamin that we can store in our body.

Cobalamin Deficiency

Pernicious anemia is caused by malabsorption of dietary cobalamin. This condition may arise from a variety of causes, such as an inherited defect, an autoimmune attack against the parietal cells (which decreases the synthesis of IF), a high intestinal pH, and a deficient pancreas. The last two conditions inhibit the release of vitamin B_{12} from haptocorrin. Incidence of pernicious anemia increases with age.

Treatment of Cobalamin Deficiency

Patients with pernicious anemia should receive vitamin B_{12} by injection or nasal spray. Intramuscular injection of 1 mg/day for 1 month or, alternatively, 1 mg/day for 5 days followed by 0.5–1 g/month has been recommended. A lower dose is recommended for the treatment of cobalamin deficiency caused by dietary deficiencies or malabsorption diseases (IM administration of 30 µg/day for 5–10 days). If patients do not have a malabsorption problem, they can use oral or intranasal cobalamin dosage forms (250 µg/day oral or 500 µg in one nostril once weekly).

Vitamin C (Ascorbic Acid)

Vitamin C is critical for the biosynthesis of collagen. It serves as a coenzyme for hydroxylase enzymes that hydroxylate lysine and proline amino acid residues in the collagen. As described in the *Introduction to Biochemistry* chapter, collagen is important in wound healing and bone formation (recall that collagen is part of tendons, connective tissues, bone structure, and skin). Vitamin C is also important in intestinal iron absorption because it can reduce Fe^{3+} to Fe^{2+} (Fe^{2+} is absorbed better than Fe^{3+}). In addition, vitamin C is important in the formation of carnitine and folic acid. A small fraction of vitamin C can be filtered through the glomeruli and is also able to undergo tubular resorption (see also the *Introduction to Pharmacokinetics* chapter). As a result of the latter process, vitamin C can compete with uric acid tubular resorption. Accordingly, vitamin C may reduce the plasma concentration of uric acid, an effect that may benefit patients with hyperuricemia and gout.

In addition, vitamin C is important for the action of the dopamine-β-hydroxylase enzyme in the synthesis of catecholamines (**Figure 14.12**). Dopamine-β-hydroxylase is a copper-containing enzyme; during the hydroxylation process, Cu^+ is oxidized to Cu^{2+}, with ascorbic acid then being required to reduce Cu^{2+} to back Cu^+ (in other words, to recycle Cu^+).

Furthermore, ascorbic acid is important in the blood coagulation process and the synthesis of the bile acids. Although ascorbic acid is synthesized from glucose, humans do not have the necessary enzyme to synthesize ascorbic acid; for this reason, we must take it in through our daily diet.

Ascorbic Acid Sources

Ascorbic acid is found in large amounts in vegetables and fruits such as tomatoes, spinach, blueberries, oranges, strawberries, watermelon, grapefruit, and cantaloupe. Organ juice is also rich in ascorbic acid. It is important to point out that ascorbic acid is heat sensitive and, consequently, cooking fruits diminishes ascorbic acid levels.

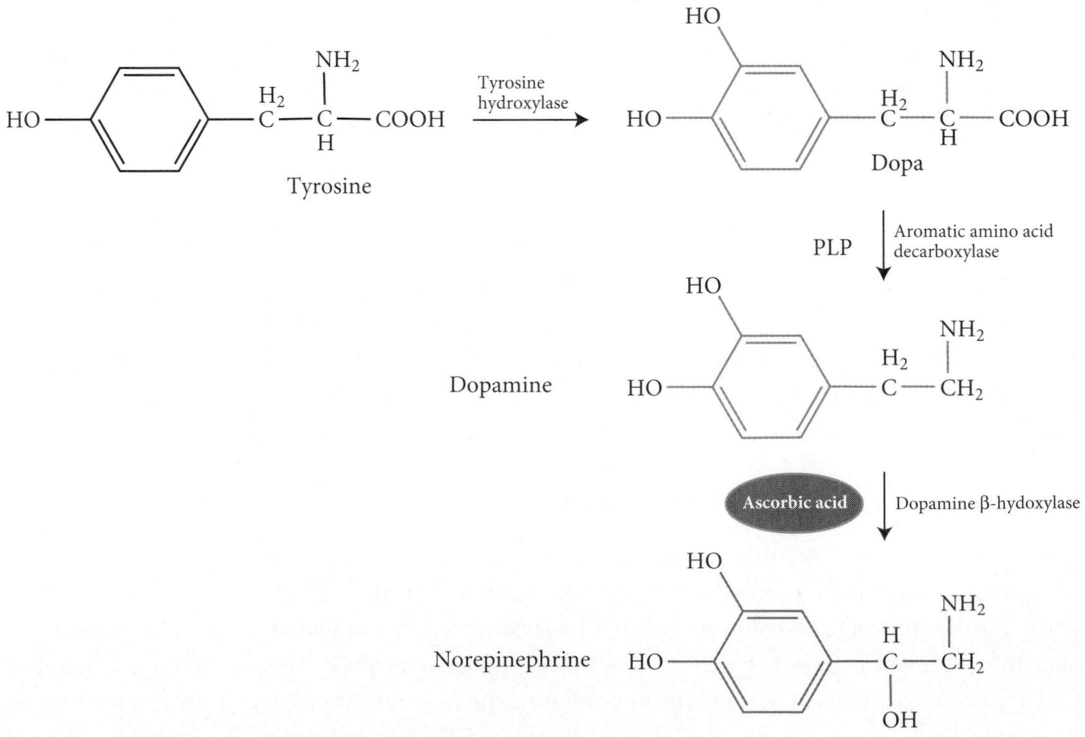

Figure 14.12 Ascorbic acid is important in the biosynthesis of norepinephrine.

Ascorbic Acid Deficiency

Deficiency in vitamin C is common among elderly persons and in alcoholics whose consumption of ascorbic acid is less than 10 mg/day. Deficiency of ascorbic acid results in scurvy, a defective collagen formation that causes sore, bleeding gums; fragile blood capillaries; loose teeth; and swollen joints.

Treatment of Ascorbic Acid Deficiency

Administration of ascorbic acid doses such as 100–250 mg/day twice daily for 2 weeks can improve the symptoms of scurvy. It has been suggested that higher doses such as 1–3 g/day may reduce the symptoms and duration of cold and upper respiratory tract infections. When counseling patients, it is imperative to avoid recommending multivitamins because the higher doses associated with multivitamin ingestion enhances the risk for other vitamin toxicity, particularly vitamin A toxicity (discussed later on in this chapter).

Table 14.2 summarizes the functions of water-soluble vitamins and the physiologic abnormalities that are associated with their deficiency.

Table 14.2 Characteristics of Water-Soluble Vitamins

Water-Soluble Vitamin	Function	Physiological Abnormalities Associated with Vitamin Deficiency
Thiamin (B_1)	Oxidative decarboxylation reactions, particularly for the synthesis of acetyl-CoA	Beriberi, Wernicke-Korsakoff syndrome
Riboflavin (B_2)	Synthesis of coenzymes FAD and FMN	Inflammation of skin and tongue, but does not lead to any severe consequences because of an efficient recycling process
Niacin (B_3)	Synthesis of coenzymes NAD^+ and $NADP^+$	Retarded growth, pellagra, Hartnup
Pantothenic acid (B_5)	Biosynthesis of acetyl-CoA	GI upset, depression, muscle cramps, ataxia, and hypoglycemia, but does not lead to any severe consequences
Pyridoxine (B_6)	Deamination of amino acids, decarboxylation involved in the biosynthesis of neurotransmitters	Rarely occurs by poor nutrition, rather it occurs by drug interactions; confusion and seizure, irritability
Biotin (B_7)	Important for the biosynthesis of oxaloacetate and fatty acids	Alopecia, fatigue, depression, and lethargy; rarely occurs
Folic acid (B_9)	Important for the synthesis of glycine amino acid and DNA	Megaloblastic anemia, neural tube defects
Cobalamin (B_{12})	Oxidation of odd-numbered fatty acids, conversion of homocysteine to methionine	Pernicious anemia, paresthesias, depression
Ascorbic acid (C)	Biosynthesis of collagen reduces oxidized vitamin E, synthesis of catecholamines, synthesis of bile acids from cholesterol	Scurvy, enhanced susceptibility to infections, hemorrhages under skin

Adapted from: Krebs NF, Primak LE, Haemer M. Normal childhood nutrition and its disorders. In: Hay WW, Levin MJ, Sondheimer JM, Deterding RR, eds. *Current diagnosis & treatment: pediatrics*, 20th ed. New York: McGraw-Hill; 2012. Available at: http://www.accessmedicine.com/content.aspx?aID=6578685.

Table 14.3 Recommended Daily Intakes for Water-Soluble Vitamins

Vitamin	Female	Male	Female (Pregnancy)
Thiamine (B$_1$)	1.1 mg/day	1.2 mg/day	1.4 mg/day
Riboflavin (B$_2$)	1.1 mg/day	1.3 mg/day	1.4 mg/day
Niacin (B$_3$)	14 mg/day	16 mg/day	18 mg/day
Pantothenic acid (B$_5$)	5 mg/day	6 mg/day	7 mg/day
Pyridoxine (B$_6$)	1.3 mg/day	1.3 mg/day	1.9 mg/day
Biotin (B$_7$)	30 µg/day	30 µg/day	30 µg/day
Folic acid (B$_9$)	0.4 mg/day	0.4 mg/day	0.8 mg/day
Cobalamin (B$_{12}$)	2.4 µg/day	2.4 µg/day	2.6 µg/day
Ascorbic acid (C)	75 mg/day	90 mg/day	85 mg/day

Table 14.3 indicates the RDIs for water-soluble vitamins for females, males, and pregnant females. Except for biotin and cobalamin, which are given in units of µg/day, the other vitamins are given in much higher amounts (mg/day).

Learning Bridge 14.1

During one of your introductory pharmacy practice experiences, your preceptor tells you about a tragic incident that occurred in 2003 in Israel. She explains that several infants who were fed with a brand of soy-based formula developed infantile beriberi. The infants showed symptoms of nystagmus, vomiting, and seizure. Your preceptor mentions that a blood test, if taken at that time, should have shown high levels of pyruvate and lactate in the blood. She further explains that a follow-up physical examination that occurred a few years after the incident indicated language and motor development impairment; in addition, many of the affected children developed chronic epilepsy.

Following her description of this tragic incident, your preceptor asks you the following questions to assess your understanding of nutrients:

A. What was the cause of the infantile beriberi?

B. What are the symptoms associated with infantile beriberi?

C. Why should a blood test reveal high levels of pyruvate and lactate?

D. Which nutrient should have been given to those young children to avoid the physical impairments described by your preceptor?

E. What is the Recommended Daily Intake (RDI) for the nutrient identified in question D for healthy males, healthy females, and pregnant females?

Fat-Soluble Vitamins

Fat-soluble vitamins include vitamins A, D, E, and K. Because toxicity is much more common with fat-soluble vitamins, their toxicity levels and the associated consequences are discussed here as well.

Vitamin A

Vitamin A plays an essential role in vision, bone growth, reproduction, cell division, cellular membrane stability, and cellular differentiation. Preformed vitamin A is found in animal foods such as whole eggs, whole milk, and liver. Provitamin A, also known as β-carotene, is abundant in darkly colored fruits and vegetables; it is metabolized to form retinol (known as vitamin A or vitamin A_1) and then is oxidized to form 11-*cis*-retinal, which is a visual pigment. The 11-*cis*-retinal compound is converted to the retinoic acid, a potent hormone that plays a major role in maintaining the normal growth and differentiation of epithelial cells in keratinizing tissue (**Figure 14.13**). In addition, 11-*cis*-retinal, in the presence of visible light, is converted to all-*trans*-retinal, which initiates a visual signal transduction by reducing cyclic GMP (cGMP) and closing gated ion channels so as to hyperpolarize the cell membrane. This chain of events ultimately triggers an electrical signal to the brain (see also the discussion of serpentine receptors in the *Introduction to Pharmacodynamics* chapter).

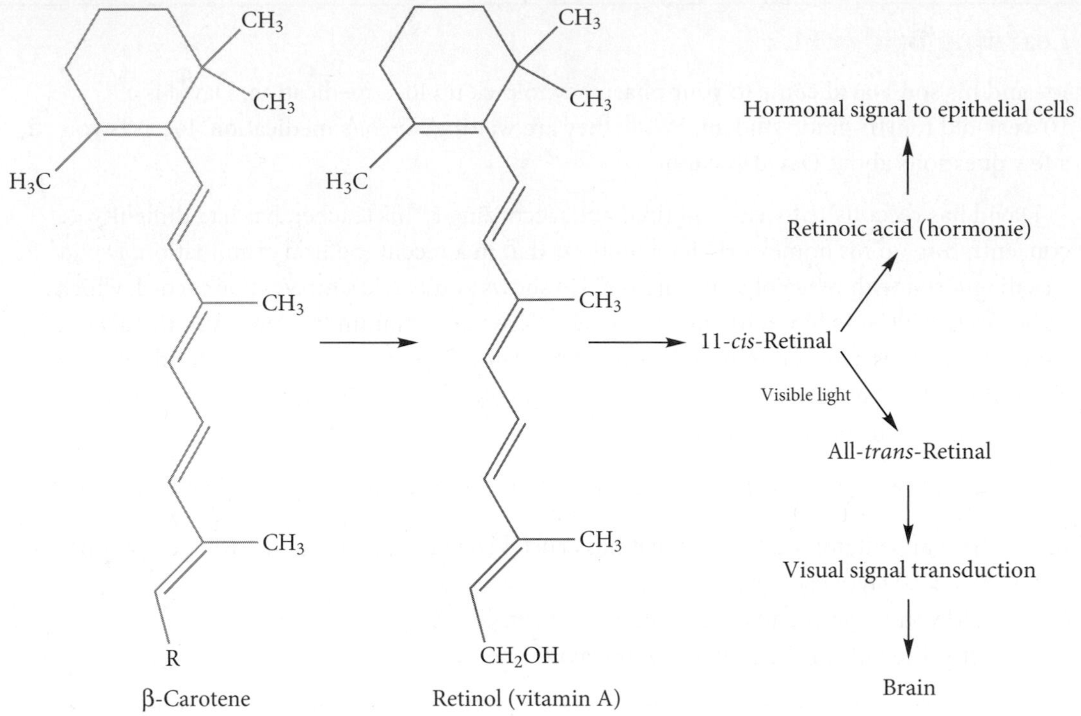

Figure 14.13 β-Carotene is an important precursor to retinol (vitamin A), 11-*cis*-retinal (visual pigment), and retinoic acid (hormone).

Adapted from: Nelson DL, Cox MM. *Lehninger principle of biochemistry*, 5th ed. New York: W. H. Freeman and Company; 2008: Chapter 10.

Vitamin A Sources

Dark green and yellow vegetables and fruits are rich in vitamin A, including spinach, turnips, carrots, broccoli, squash, and apricots. In addition, liver, milk, butter, cheese, and whole eggs are sources for vitamin A. In the United States, many cereal, grain, dairy, and other products, and infant formulas, are fortified with vitamin A.

Vitamin A Deficiency

Vitamin A deficiency causes the goblet mucus cells to be replaced by keratinized epithelium (i.e., when the outer layer of epidermis is keratinized). This replacement leads to dry skin and hair and broken fingernails. The worst effect occurs in the cornea, when hyperkeratization leads to blindness. In addition, the replacement of epithelial lining of other organ systems can lead to respiratory infections, diarrhea, and urinary calculi. Deficiency of 11-*cis*-retinal causes nyctalopia (night blindness).

Treatment of Vitamin A Deficiency

The RDA for healthy individuals has been recommended as 2,300–3,000 units/day (**Table 14.4**). However, higher intramuscular doses are often used to treat vitamin A deficiency, particularly in patients with oral absorption problems. Doses such as 100,000 units/day for 3 days followed by 50,000 units/day for 2 weeks are used in the treatment of vitamin A deficiency. In addition, it has been recommended that patients continue to receive oral doses, if feasible, of 10,000–20,000 units/day for an additional 2 months.

Vitamin A Toxicity

Vitamin A toxicity can cause pruritus, erythema (redness of skin), skin hyperfragility, and desquamation (skin peeling). Vitamin A toxicity can occur in individuals who eat large amounts of β-carotene–rich foods. For instance, vitamin A hepatotoxicity and neurotoxicity were reported in an 18-year-old woman who limited her diet for several years to β-carotene–rich foods (pumpkin, carrots, and liver). Hepatotoxicity is often indicated by a serum elevation of bilirubin, aminotransferases, and alkaline phosphatase.

To overcome vitamin toxicity, gastrointestinal decontamination is accomplished by administration of activated charcoal; alternatively, when large overdoses of vitamin A are taken, gastric lavage may be applied. In addition, bisphosphonates may be given. Because hypercalcemia also results from vitamin A toxicity, intravenous fluids, loop diuretics, and prednisone are given to patients. Keep in mind that thiazides cause hypercalcemia and should be avoided in patients with vitamin A toxicities.

In addition to foods, excessive ingestion of vitamin supplements results in vitamin A toxicity, particularly for those individuals who do not consult with healthcare providers before taking such supplements. It has been reported that hepatotoxicity can occur following ingestion of a high dose of vitamin A (more than 600,000 units). *In vitro* studies have shown that high doses of vitamin A stimulate bone resorption and inhibit bone formation, resulting in an increased fracture risk.

One important agent that includes vitamin A is isotretinoin (Amnesteem), a medication used to treat severe cystic acne. However, this drug has shown to have teratogenicity. This adverse effect is a serious concern, as approximately one-third of patients who use isotretinoin are females aged 13–19 years. Isotretinoin is known to interfere with cranial neural crest cells. These cells are important in the development of the ears and the conotruncal area of the heart. To avoid any potential teratogenicity risk in patients using isotretinoin, the FDA requires healthcare providers, patients, and pharmacists to review and comply with a risk management program called System to Manage Accutane-Related Teratogenicity (SMART). For instance, this program mandates that the female patient have two negative urine tests (or serum pregnancy tests) before using isotretinoin and have a negative pregnancy test before receiving each monthly prescription. Pharmacists can fill isotretinoin only if the healthcare provider and the patient have complied with the SMART program.

Retinyl ester is the storage form of vitamin A that is hydrolyzed to retinol (50–80% stored in the liver as retinyl esters). This enzymatic process is initiated by digestive enzymes in the intestinal lumen of the intestinal epithelial wall. In the intestinal epithelial cells, retinol is re-esterified to retinyl ester and is packed into chylomicrons, which are then released into the blood to be taken up by the Ito cells (fat-storing cells of the liver). Too much vitamin A leads to hypertrophy and hyperplasia of Ito cells. To maintain a constant level of retinol in tissue cells, the liver releases vitamin A into the bloodstream. The liver contains a supply of vitamin A that is sufficient to last approximately 2 years.

Vitamin D

Cholecalciferol (vitamin D_3) and ergocalciferol (vitamin D_2) are two related hydrophobic molecules that belong to the vitamin D family. While cholecalciferol is synthesized in the human's skin, ergocalciferol is synthesized only in plants and fungi. Vitamin D_2 is often found in commercial products. However, because both of these forms serve the same functions and have the same biological potency in humans, "vitamin D" is used as a collective term for both vitamins D_2 and D_3.

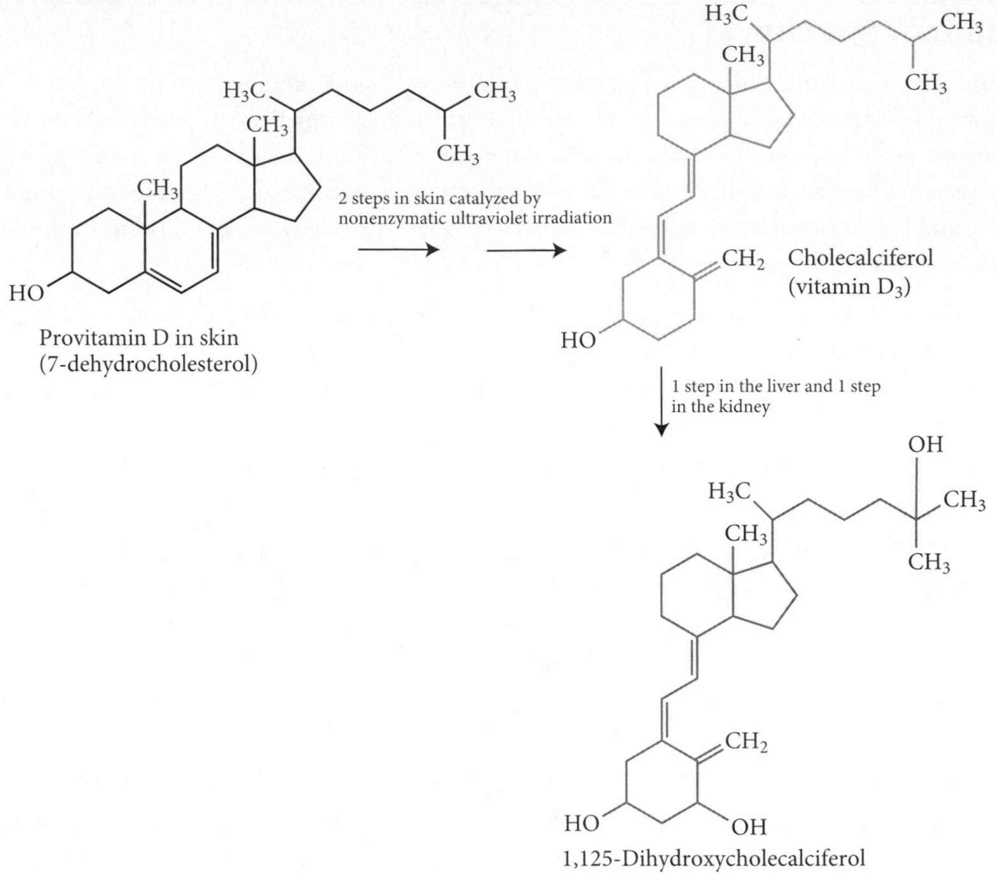

Figure 14.14 Synthesis and metabolism of cholecalciferol (vitamin D_3).
Adapted from: Nelson DL, Cox MM. *Lehninger principle of biochemistry*, 5th ed. New York: W. H. Freeman and Company; 2008: Chapter 10.

The most abundant form of vitamin D is vitamin D_3, which is synthesized in the skin from 7-dehydrocholesterol in a process catalyzed by a nonenzymatic photochemical reaction carried out by the UV component of sunlight (**Figure 14.14**). The newly synthesized vitamin D_3 is bound to a vitamin D–binding protein, which enables it to enter the circulation and then to reach the liver. In the liver's endoplasmic reticulum (ER), vitamin D_3 is metabolized to 25-hydroxyvitamin D by the vitamin D-25-hydroxylase enzyme. The 25-hydroxyvitamin D binds again to vitamin D–binding protein and is transported to the proximal convoluted tubule in the kidney, where it undergoes a hydroxylation process to become 1,25-dihydroxyvitamin D (calcitriol). This calcitriol is then secreted by kidneys into circulation to work as a hormone to regulate Ca^{2+} uptake in the intestine, bone, and kidney.

Because calcitriol is a hydrophobic hormone, it can enter cells and bind to a specific nuclear vitamin D receptor protein, thereby inducing gene expression of proteins that are important in the biological functions of vitamin D. In addition, in the intestines, calcitriol increases the production of calcium-binding proteins and calcium pump proteins in the cell membrane to enhance calcium absorption through the duodenum. Calcitriol also binds to vitamin D receptors in the parathyroid glands to decrease the synthesis and secretion of parathyroid hormone (PTH). Of note, a low serum phosphate level triggers the renal proximal tubular synthesis of calcitriol to enhance the absorption of phosphate.

Vitamin D is important for the reabsorption of calcium. When the body experiences hypocalcemia, the parathyroid gland releases PTH. PTH increases the release of Ca^{2+} from bones. Some of

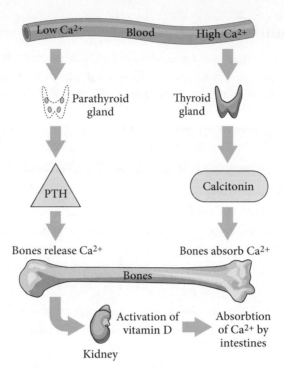

Figure 14.15 Vitamin D, parathyroid, and calcitonin hormones play important roles in the regulation of serum calcium levels.

the freed Ca^{2+} stimulates the kidneys to activate vitamin D, which in turn stimulates the intestines to absorb Ca^{2+}. The ultimate outcome of the PTH release is to increase the Ca^{2+} level in the blood. As a result, the major and primary role of vitamin D is to regulate calcium homeostasis. When the blood level of Ca^{2+} is high, the thyroid gland releases calcitonin hormone, which promotes the uptake of Ca^{2+} into bones so as to restore the normal blood levels of Ca^{2+} (**Figure 14.15**).

Vitamin D can be used for both prevention and treatment of rickets, osteomalacia, and osteoporosis. In addition, it is used to treat hypoparathyroidism and skin conditions including psoriasis. Calcitonin salmon (oral, nasal spray, and injection) is used by women for the treatment of osteoporosis. However, an increasing body of evidence suggests that long-term use of calcitonin may cause cancer.

Vitamin D Sources

Vitamin D is found in butter, milk, cheese, and cream; eggs; and fatty fish such as salmon and mackerel. In addition, fortified foods contain vitamin D, including cereals, bread, and milk. Indeed, rickets has been eliminated in many countries due to the fortification of milk with vitamin D. One microgram of vitamin D is equivalent to 40 IU of vitamin D.

Vitamin D Deficiency

Inadequate dietary intake of vitamin D or a defect in its biosynthesis leads to hypocalcemia and, in turn, increased secretion of PTH. Vitamin D deficiency results in rickets, in which bones are weak and malformed. If individuals have adequate access to sunlight and a well-balanced diet, they should not develop any vitamin D deficiency. In addition, normal exposure to sunlight during the summer should produce adequate vitamin D storage for the winter use. Because the vitamin D content of human milk is extremely low, infants who are breastfed and have limited access to sunlight require supplemental vitamin D.

Treatment of Vitamin D Deficiency

The daily adequate intake of vitamin D for people aged 1–70 years is 600 IU (many supplements contain this dose); this amount increases to 800 IU after age 71. These doses meet body's requirement to prevent rickets and osteomalacia. Larger doses of vitamin D, such as 800–1,000 units/day, are used for prevention of osteoporosis (for persons older than age 50) or for treatment of hyperparathyroidism. In the treatment of hypoparathyroidism and hyperparathyroidism, vitamin D supplement may be useful.

Vitamin D Toxicity

Vitamin D toxicity often occurs as a result of continued ingestion of vitamin D and calcium supplements due to treatment of hypoparathyroidism, osteoporosis, or osteomalacia. This toxicity is characterized by hypercalcemia. A high dose range, such as 50,000–150,000 IU, is associated with vitamin D toxicity. Excessive exposure to sunlight does not cause vitamin D toxicity because the human body has a limited ability to form 7-dehydrocholesterol.

Given that vitamin D toxicity results in hypercalcemia, signs and symptoms are characteristic of hypercalcemia, such as fatigue, somnolence, irritability, headache, dizziness, muscle and bone pain, nausea, abdominal pain, weight loss, and diarrhea or constipation. Severe hypercalcemia results in ataxia, confusion, psychosis, seizures, coma, and renal failure. Vitamin D toxicity should be suspected in all patients who have signs and symptoms of hypercalcemia. In addition, because vitamin D plays a role in the inhibition of erythropoietin production, its toxicity may result in anemia. Likewise, because vitamin D facilitates phosphate mobilization from bones and phosphate absorption in the small intestine, patients with vitamin D toxicity may show signs and symptoms of hyperphosphatemia.

To treat vitamin D toxicity, both vitamin D and calcium supplementation should be discontinued. In addition, patients need to be on a low-calcium diet, and adequate volumes of fluid should be given to increase renal calcium clearance. In addition, furosemide can be given to promote calcium excretion.

Vitamin E

The major role of vitamin E is to act as an antioxidant, particularly to protect polyunsaturated fatty acids embedded within cell membranes from the attacks of lipid peroxide radicals. In addition, it has been suggested that vitamin E inhibits phospholipase A_2, which in turn inhibits the synthesis of arachidonic acid. Vitamin E contains a phenol group (**Figure 14.16**) that prevents an oxidation reaction by donating its H atom to destroy the reactive forms of oxygen radicals and other free radicals, thereby protecting the cell membrane's unsaturated fatty acids (**Figure 14.17**). The oxidized vitamin E is regenerated in its reduced form by vitamin C and glutathione. The prevention of the oxidation process does not allow the free radical to make the cell membrane fragile—a particular concern with the most sensitive cell membranes, which are found in erythrocytes (oxidation of erythrocytes can lead to hemolytic anemia).

Similar to the fatty acids embedded in the cell membrane, unsaturated fatty acids in foods become rancid when oxygen from the air reacts with their double bonds. Both BHA (butylated hydroxyanisole) and BHT (butylated hydroxytoluene) are added as ingredients in many foods to prevent the oxidation of unsaturated fatty acids (**Figure 14.18**) and thereby prolong their shelf-life. The antioxidant mechanism described in Figure 14.17 is also employed by these two food ingredients.

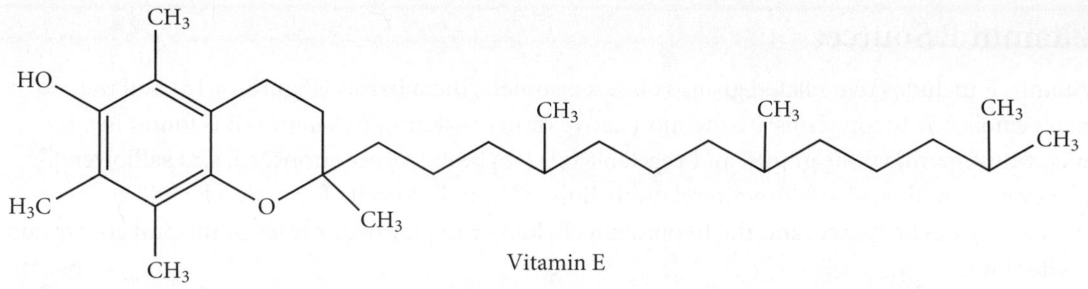

Figure 14.16 The structure of vitamin E. The hydroxyl group plays an important role in vitamin E's antioxidant effect.

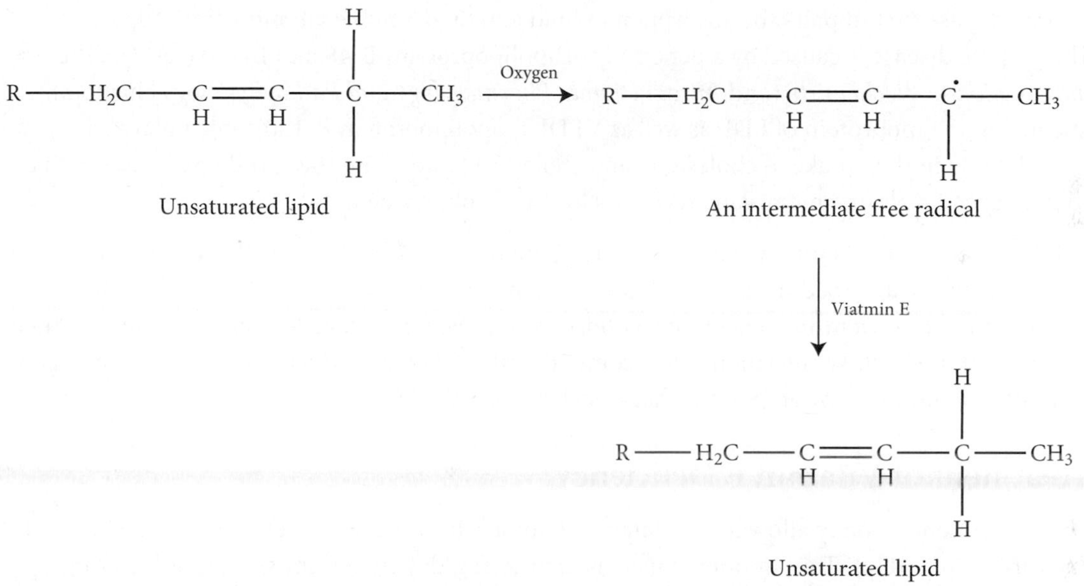

Figure 14.17 The free radicals built by oxidation of a cell membrane's unsaturated lipids makes the membrane fragile. Vitamin E counteracts this reaction.

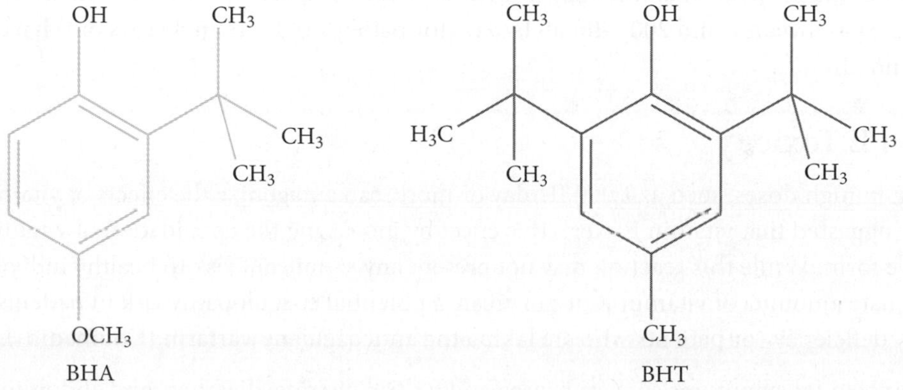

Figure 14.18 The hydroxyl groups from BHA (butylated hydroxyanisole) and BHT (butylated hydroxytoluene) play important roles in the protection of unsaturated fatty acids in foods.

Vitamin E Sources

Vitamin E includes two related groups of stereoisomers, tocopherols (Figure 14.16) and the tocotrienols; the tocopherols are the most active form of vitamin E. Vitamin E is found in nuts, wheat germ, whole grains, and vegetable oils (soybean, corn, cottonseed, and safflower). However, animal products contain relatively little vitamin E. Micelle formation by biliary secretions, erythrocyte uptake, and the lipoprotein chylomicron play major roles in the oral absorption of vitamin E.

Vitamin E Deficiency

Vitamin E deficiency is common in patients with malabsorption conditions. In addition, patients with abetalipoproteinemia are at risk for vitamin E deficiency. Abetalipoproteinemia is a rare genetic disease that impairs the absorption of lipid and lipid-soluble vitamins from foods. This genetic disease is caused by a deficiency of apolipoproteins B-48 and B-100 (see also the *Introduction to Biochemistry* and *Introduction to Pharmacology and Pathophysiology* chapters). The major apolipoprotein of LDL as well as VLDL is apolipoprotein B-100, which plays an essential role in the uptake of cholesterol and cholesteryl esters into the extrahepatic tissues that contain specific plasma membrane receptors for this apolipoprotein.

Bile acids are important for the absorption of vitamin E. Approximately 45% of a vitamin E dose is passively absorbed from the intestinal tract into the lymphatic circulation. From the lymphatic circulation, vitamin E enters the bloodstream in the form of chylomicrons, which are then taken up by the liver. While vitamin E becomes distributed to all of the body's tissues, the largest amounts are found in the adipocytes, hapatocytes, and myocytes.

Treatment of Vitamin E Deficiency

The recommended daily allowance of vitamin E for adults, including pregnant women, is 15 mg/day (or 25 units/day). This amount is increased to 19 mg/day (or 32 units/day) for lactating women. For the treatment of vitamin E deficiency, a higher dose is recommended (60–75 unit/day). It has been suggested that vitamin E may play an important role in protecting lung tissue from oxidative damage caused by free radicals. Patients with cystic fibrosis (CF) have an increased level of free radicals, as a result of the actions of their inflammatory cells. For patients with CF, doses such as 80–150 units/day (for patients aged 1–3 years), 100–200 units/day (for patients aged 4–8 years), and 200–400 units/day (for patients older than 8 years old) have been recommended.

Vitamin E Toxicity

Vitamin E in high doses, such as 1,000 IU/day or more, can antagonize the effects of vitamin K. It has been suggested that vitamin E exerts this effect by increasing the epoxidation of vitamin K to its inactive form. While this reaction may not present any significant risk to healthy individuals with adequate amounts of vitamin K, it can create a potential coagulopathy risk in patients with vitamin K deficiency (or patients who are taking the anticoagulant warfarin [Coumadin]).

Gastrointestinal symptoms such as nausea and gastric distress, diarrhea, and abdominal cramps have been reported when patients have ingested a high dose of vitamin E (such as 2,000 units/day or more). In addition, a high dose of vitamin E can displace other important antioxidants (e.g., *N*-acetylcysteine, vitamin C, glutathione) that protect the body from cellular oxidation reactions.

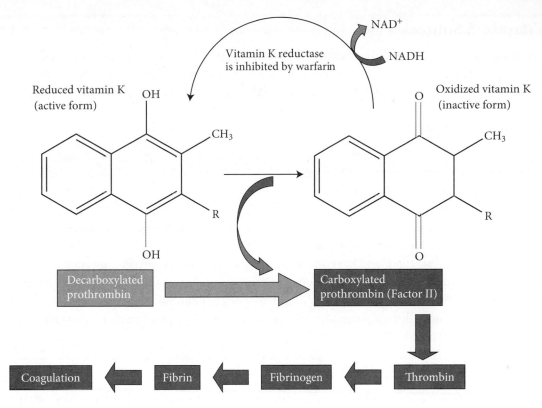

Figure 14.19 The vitamin K cycle is important for carboxylation of prothrombin to promote the blood coagulation cascade.

Adapted from: Weitz JI. Blood coagulation and anticoagulant, fibrinolytic, and antiplatelet drugs. In: Chabner BA, Brunton LL, Knollmann BC, eds. *Goodman & Gilman's the pharmacological basis of therapeutics,* 12th ed. New York, NY: McGraw Hill; 2011. Available at: http://www.accesspharmacy.com/content.aspx?aID=16668944.

Vitamin K

Vitamin K exists in three forms: vitamin K_1 (or phylloquinone), which is found in vegetables and animals; vitamin K_2 (or menaquinone), which is synthesized by vertebrate intestinal bacteria; and vitamin K_3 (menadione), which is produced synthetically. As newborn infants have a sterile intestinal tract, they are given a 1 mg vitamin K injection in the United States. Vitamin K, in its reduced form, serves as an essential cofactor and participates in post-translational carboxylation of glutamic acid residues in specific proteins, including prothrombin, to produce carboxyglutamate (factor II in the blood coagulation cascade) (**Figure 14.19**). The carboxylated prothrombin is converted to thrombin. Thrombin, in turn, cleaves fibrinogen to produce fibrin—the substance that builds the "net" within a blood clot. Because vitamin K counteracts the effect of warfarin, it is used to serve as an antidote to warfarin overdose.

Only the reduced form of vitamin K is biologically active. However, through the carboxylation mechanism of prothrombin, the reduced form is oxidized (to inactivated vitamin K). To participate in another cycle of carboxylation, vitamin K needs to be recycled into the reduced form, a mechanism catalyzed by vitamin K reductase enzyme. Warfarin is known to inhibit vitamin K reductase enzyme to block the regeneration (recycling) process of vitamin K (Figure 14.19).

Vitamin K is also important for the bone protein known as osteocalcin, which is an important protein for bone growth. This protein contains carboxyglutamate as well. Osteocalcin also contains hydroxyproline, so vitamin C is important for the formation of osteocalcin as well (see the discussion of vitamin C earlier in this chapter).

Vitamin K Sources

Green leafy vegetables such as spinach and lettuce, and margarine, olive, canola, soybean oils, and liver are rich in vitamin K. While the typical diet provides 50% of the vitamin K needed by humans, intestinal bacteria synthesize and provide the remaining 50% of vitamin K.

Vitamin K Deficiency

In vitamin K deficiency, the decarboxylated prothrombin is unable to adequately initiate the blood clotting cascade. Patients with chronic GI tract diseases such as celiac disease, Crohn's disease, or biliary cirrhosis may develop vitamin K deficiency. The symptoms of vitamin K deficiency consist of intracranial bleeding, bruisability, GI bleeding, and skin bleeding. Of particular concern is vitamin K deficiency in infants because they have a low fat/water ratio, which affects storage of vitamin K; are often fed by breast milk, which contains only low levels of vitamin K; have a sterile intestinal tract; and have an immature liver. As a result, severe consequences such as intracranial, GI, and skin bleeding can occur in vitamin K–deficient infants 1–7 days after birth, which can result in death. Administration of broad-spectrum antibiotics (e.g., amoxicillin, levofloxacin, tetracycline, chloramphenicol) can also reduce intestinal bacteria and, as a result, reduce the synthesis of vitamin K.

Treatment of Vitamin K Deficiency

Vitamin K deficiency is treated by administering a parenteral dose of 10 mg, which remedies the deficiency within 8–10 hours. In cases of chronic malabsorption, a parenteral dose of 10 mg/week is given.

Vitamin K Toxicity

Due to the important role that vitamin K plays in the blood clotting cascade, high doses of vitamin K can interfere with oral anticoagulants. For this reason, it is important to counsel patients who use warfarin to have a consistent amount of vegetables in their diet to avoid any fluctuation of warfarin's anticoagulation's effect.

Table 14.4 indicates the functions of fat-soluble vitamins and physiologic abnormalities that are associated with their deficiency.

Table 14.4 Characteristics of Lipid-Soluble Vitamins

Vitamin	Function	Physiological Abnormalities Associated with Vitamin Deficiency
A	Vision, bone growth, reproduction, cellular differentiation	Impaired night vision and keratinization of skin; growth retardation; increased susceptibility to infection
D	Calcium and phosphate metabolism	Osteomalacia (adults) or rickets (children)
E	Antioxidant	Fragile cell membrane; hemolytic anemia
K	Synthesis of blood coagulation enzymes; bone growth	Impaired blood coagulation; bruising or bleeding in GI tract

Adapted from: Krebs NF, Primak LE, Haemer M. Normal childhood nutrition and its disorders. In: Hay WW, Levin MJ, Sondheimer JM, Deterding RR, eds. *Current diagnosis & treatment: pediatrics*, 20th ed. New York, NY: McGraw-Hill; 2012. Available at: http://www.accessmedicine.com/content.aspx?aID=6578685.

Table 14.5 Daily Recommended Amounts of Fat-Soluble Vitamins

Vitamin	Female	Male	Female (Pregnancy)
A	2,330 units/day	3,000 units/day	2,560 units/day
D	600 units/day	600 units/day	600 units/day
E	25 units/day	25 units/day	25 units/day
K	55 µg/day	65 µg/day	55 µg/day

Table 14.5 summarizes the daily recommended amounts of fat-soluble vitamins.

Minerals

Minerals are inorganic elements that may serve as cofactors in an enzymatic reaction, as electrolytes to maintain cellular or physiologic function, or as structural building blocks in the body. The required daily intake of minerals varies from micrograms to grams depending on the nature of and need for the elements. Some of the most important mineral elements are calcium, phosphorus, zinc, iron, sodium, potassium, iron, magnesium, and chloride. Calcium and phosphorus are the most abundant mineral elements in the body.

Elemental electrolytes such as sodium, potassium, calcium, magnesium, phosphorus, and chloride are important to maintain many biological functions. Consequently, too high or too low amounts of these electrolytes lead to a series of clinical consequences that, if not corrected, can produce severe cellular or physiologic malfunctions. Electrolytes are available as single- or multiple-electrolyte solutions.

The concentrations of dissolved molecules in the blood (e.g., proteins, glucose, urea) are measured in units of mg/dL. In contrast, the concentrations of electrolytes in the body fluids and in intravenous solutions are often expressed in mEq/L (milliequivalents per liter; see also the *Introduction to Pharmaceutical Calculations* chapter). An exception is the concentration of phosphate, which will be explained later on in this chapter. The milliequivalents expression is more convenient to compare ions when different salt forms are used. For instance, 10 mEq of sodium acetate will contain the same amount of sodium as 10 mEq of sodium chloride. One equivalent of an ion is an amount equal to the molar mass of that ion (in grams) divided by the number of electrical charges. For instance, 1 Eq of Na^+ is equal to 23 g and 1 Eq of Cl^- is equal to 35.5 g because both of these two ions have only one electrical charge. In contrast, 1 Eq of Mg^{2+} is equal to 12.2 g because Mg^{2+} has two electrical charges (the molar mass for Mg^{2+} is 24.3, which is divided by 2).

Some drug products may affect patients' mineral and electrolytes' concentrations. For example, thiazide diuretics and loop diuretics increase Na^+, K^+, and Mg^{2+} depletion. While loop diuretics also increase Ca^{2+} depletion, thiazide diuretics decrease Ca^{2+} depletion.

Calcium (Ca^{2+})

Calcium exists in two forms with different functions. The first form is calcium phosphate complex, which gives the physical strength to the structure of bones and teeth. The second form is free calcium, which is important for muscle contraction and serves as a cofactor in the blood clotting cascade. The free form is also considered a potent second messenger in signaling processes (see the *Introduction to Pharmacodynamics* chapter). While 99% of calcium is stored in the bone and teeth, only 1% of the body's total calcium supply is involved in enzymatic reactions or other signaling processes. Calcium supplements, in combination with vitamin D supplements, reduce the risk of fracture in patients with osteoporosis. As was mentioned earlier, vitamin D is important for the intestinal absorption of calcium. In patients with impaired fat absorption, the presence of a large amount of fatty acids in the intestinal lumen can lead to formation of insoluble calcium salts, which reduce calcium absorption.

Foods that are rich in calcium include milk, yogurt, salmon, broccoli, and calcium-fortified orange juice. Deficiency of calcium can occur as a result of dietary intake that is low in calcium, decreased calcium absorption, or increased calcium excretion. Indeed, patients with osteoporosis (or at risk to develop osteoporosis) require supplemental calcium intake. Some clinical data indicate that calcium supplements can also reduce blood pressure, cholesterol, and colorectal cancer risk.

Several types of calcium supplements are available, such as calcium carbonate, calcium citrate, calcium acetate, and tricalcium phosphate. The elemental calcium is the actual amount of calcium in each formulation. For instance, if a woman needs 500 mg calcium and each calcium carbonate tablet is identified as "600 mg," she should ensure that her elemental calcium intake reaches 500 mg. Calcium carbonate contains 40% elemental calcium, which means that each tablet has 240 mg elemental calcium. To reach the 500 mg calcium level, the patient would need to take two 600 mg calcium carbonate tablets. Most multivitamin supplements have 200 mg calcium carbonate (80 mg elemental calcium) in each tablet.

The RDA for adult males, females, and females during pregnancy and lactation is 1,000 mg/day. Most men and women in the United States obtain 650 mg/day and 850 mg/day, respectively, from foods.

Because calcium carbonate is a basic supplement, it needs the stomach's acidity for its optimal absorption. As a result, this mineral needs to be taken with foods. In addition, due to its basicity, calcium carbonate is used in antacid products such as Tums and Rolaids. In contrast, calcium citrate is acidic and does not need to be taken with foods, but it is more expensive compared with other calcium supplements. Calcium citrate contains 21% elemental calcium. In addition, calcium citrate has fewer GI side effects compared with the calcium carbonate; the latter formulation builds gas and causes stomach upset. Tricalcium phosphate contains 38% elemental calcium, but formation of calcium–phosphate complexes could reduce calcium absorption when it is used. This supplement is useful for patients who have also a low serum phosphate level (hypophosphatemia). Keep in mind that an adult can absorb only 500 mg elemental calcium or less at a time.

Calcium supplements that are labeled "USP Verified" or "United States Pharmacopeia," should be used or recommended, as these products have reliable identity, strength, purity, and quality (see also the *Introduction to Pharmacognosy* chapter). If a patient has a swallowing problem, alternative dosage forms, such as chewable or dissolvable tablets or liquid, can be recommended. Intravenous calcium is reserved for acute situations such as acute hypoparathyroidism following head and neck cancer treatments or acute decreases in serum calcium (i.e., to less than 7.5 mg/dL; the normal range is 8.8–10.3 mg/dL).

Zinc (Zn^{2+})

Zinc is a cofactor for the lactate dehydrogenase enzyme (recall its role in anaerobic glycolysis) and for many metalloproteases, including the collagenases (which play important roles in wound remodeling). Spermatogenesis (formation of sperm) is a zinc-dependent process as well, because of zinc's role in testosterone metabolism. In addition, zinc is an important mineral for the synthesis and stabilization of proteins, DNA, and RNA. This element is essential for the binding of steroid hormone receptors, and a few other transcription factors, to different genes, which affects gene expression. Zinc also binds to the phosphate backbone of ribosomes and plays an important role in the structures of ribosomes.

Zinc deficiency affects growth in infants. In animal models, it has been shown to be required for embryonic development. Some evidence suggests that zinc plays a role in immunology. Zinc is involved in the regulation of T lymphocytes and natural killer cells (see also the *Introduction to Immunology* chapter). In a meta-analysis conducted in 2012 that included 17 randomized controlled trials with more than 2,000 participants, researchers found that those individuals who received zinc had a shorter duration of cold symptoms, although it did not help children with the cold symptoms. A few factors were mentioned that contributed to the lack of an effect from zinc to the pediatric population—namely, differences in the host inflammatory responses, different infectious agents, and the use of lower doses of zinc in the pediatric groups.

Zinc is found in meat, shellfish, nuts, and legumes, but several dietary minerals and drugs can inhibit its absorption. For instance, minerals such as copper, calcium, and iron compete with zinc for absorption sites. Drugs such as penicillamine (Cuprimine), valproic acid (Depacon), and ethambutol (Myambutol) can inhibit the absorption of zinc. In addition, a few disease states can cause zinc deficiency. Most notably, mild zinc deficiency can occur in conjunction with diabetes, HIV/AIDS, cirrhosis, alcoholism, inflammatory bowel disease (IBD), malabsorption syndromes, and sickle cell anemia.

Symptoms of zinc deficiency include white spots on the fingernails, loss of sense of smell or taste, joint pain, menstrual irregularities, slow wound healing, acne, and recurrent infections. Severe chronic zinc deficiency has been associated with hypogonadism and dwarfism in several Middle Eastern countries. A rare genetic disease, acrodermatitis enteropathica, is characterized by abnormalities in zinc absorption. Symptoms such as diarrhea, alopecia, muscle wasting, depression, irritability, and rashes are associated with acrodermatitis enteropathica.

The RDAs for zinc for men and women in the United States are 11 mg/day and 8 mg/day, respectively. However, during pregnancy and lactation, a higher dose is recommended (12 mg/day). Zinc supplements are available in the form of oral tablets, lozenges, and topical cream. Zinc deficiency may be treated with elemental zinc 25–50 mg in three divided doses per day (many multivitamin supplements contain 20–25 mg zinc). In 1997, zinc acetate was approved by the FDA for maintenance therapy of Wilson's disease. Patients with Wilson's disease develop copper overload, and zinc induces the formation of metallothionein, which has a high affinity for copper; thus zinc treatment assists patients in the elimination of copper from their blood and body tissues.

Zinc is the least toxic of all the trace metals. Nevertheless, increased oral doses of zinc may result in a deficiency of copper. Zinc toxicities include GI distress and diarrhea, fever, chest pain, chills, cough, dyspnea, nausea, muscle soreness, and fatigue. In addition, chronic use of large doses of zinc may impair the immune system. The nasal mucosa are sensitive to zinc and can be irreversibly damaged. Consequently, intranasal zinc preparations should be avoided.

Iron (Fe^{2+})

Iron is an essential component of oxygen-storing proteins, hemoglobin and myoglobin, heme-containing enzymes (cytochromes; recall their role in the mitochondrial inner membrane from the *Introduction to Biochemistry* chapter and the discussion of CYP450 in the *Introduction to Medicinal Chemistry* chapter), catalase, peroxidase, and a few other enzymes. In addition, iron plays an important role in the metabolism of catecholamines.

Iron deficiency is a common nutritional disorder and is the most common underlying cause of anemia. Indeed, 75% of all anemia cases are caused by iron deficiency, anemia of chronic disease, and acute bleeding. The remaining 25% of anemia cases are caused by bone marrow damage, decreased erythropoiesis, and hemolysis. Iron deficiency can cause muscle fatigue and a reduced heat production by affecting metabolism in muscles—specifically, by reducing the activity of iron-dependent mitochondrial proteins.

Anemia

Three types of anemia are distinguished based on the shape and structure of erythrocytes:

- Macrocytic anemia (large cells) is caused by vitamin B_{12} deficiency or folic acid deficiency, or both. As noted earlier, vitamins B_9 and B_{12} are both important for the synthesis of nucleic acids. Macrocytic anemia is characterized by nondividing cells, which explains the enlarged erythroid precursor cells characteristic of this condition. Pernicious anemia is a typical type of macrocytic anemia.

- Normochromic anemia (normal cells) is caused by acute blood loss or the bone marrow's failure to produce three blood cell types—erythrocytes, leukocytes (neutropenia is indicated by a decreased number of white blood cells), and platelets (thrombocytopenia is indicated by a decreased number of platelets). In addition, normochromic anemia may be caused by hemolysis and G6PD deficiency (recall the role of this enzyme in the pentose phosphate pathway, as discussed in the *Introduction to Biochemistry* chapter). Furthermore, autoimmune diseases, such as anemia of chronic disease, renal failure, and endocrine disorders, cause normochromic anemia.

- Hypochromic anemia (low hemoglobin content, small cells) is caused by iron deficiency, sickle cell anemia, and thalassemia.

Iron Sources

Iron-rich foods (containing more than 5 mg/100 g) include liver and heart, egg yolks, and oysters. Foods that have a low amount of iron (less than 1 mg/100 g) include milk (and milk products) and most nongreen vegetables.

Iron Deficiency

Iron-deficiency anemia is caused by depletion of the body's iron stores. The lack of iron store may be attributable to inadequate oral intake of iron, increased iron demand (caused by pregnancy, lactation, rapid growth, or elderly age), blood loss (caused during menstruation, trauma, or GI ulcers), and inadequate absorption (caused by reduced gastric acid secretion, medications such as tetracyclines, gastrectomy, enteritis, persistent diarrhea, or carcinoma). In addition, blood donations and the use of NSAIDs (which may cause bleeding in some individuals) contribute to iron deficiency. Iron fortification of flour and formulas for infants and the widespread availability of iron supplements have contributed to reducing the incidence of iron deficiency in the United States. The risk of developing iron deficiency is high in premature infants, especially when they are not fed by breast milk or iron-fortified formula.

The first sign of iron-deficiency anemia is a decreased level of ferritin. Free iron is a toxic mineral; consequently, in the blood iron is bound to the iron transport protein transferritin and in the tissues iron is bound to ferritin. There are two forms of irons: ferric (Fe^{3+}) and ferrous (F^{2+}). Whereas ferric iron is the oxidized form, ferrous iron is the reduced form. Iron, in the ferrous form, is absorbed in mammals. The ferric state has very limited biological availability unless it is solubilized by an acidic environment (such as in the stomach). The iron-storing protein known as ferritin is found in two sites, the reticuloendothelial system and hapatocytes. To a lesser extent, it is also found in muscle. Because the serum ferritin level correlates well with the total amount of stored iron, a plasma level of ferritin lower than 12 mg/L is an indication of depletion of iron stores.

A significant amount of the serum's iron (80%) goes to the erythroid marrow, where it is packaged into new erythrocytes. The life span of erythrocytes is 3 months. These cells are then catabolized by the reticuloendothelial system (which encompasses a series of phagocytic cells, including macrophages, that are capable of ingesting bacteria, colloidal particles, and dead erythrocytes). A portion of the iron is recycled and returns to the serum in the form of transferrin, while another portion stored in the ferritin of reticuloendothelial cells. The latter cells gradually release iron to the circulation.

Treatment of Iron Deficiency

Different conditions result in different losses of iron. On average, we lose 0.5–1 mg iron every day through biliary or urinary secretions, sweating, exfoliation of dermatologic cells, and gastrointestinal blood loss. It is important to treat iron deficiency. Nevertheless, therapy for this condition is affected by a few factors, including the severity of anemia, the rate of iron absorption and tolerance, and the presence of other diseases (e.g., inflammatory illnesses reduce the rate of erythrocyte production). The effectiveness of iron therapy is assessed based on the increase in the rate of erythrocyte production. If oral iron therapy has not produced the desired result within 3–4 weeks, the medication should be discontinued and a new diagnosis must be considered. By the same token, once a response to an oral iron therapy is achieved for a patient, the therapy should be continued until his or her hemoglobin returns to normal level (normal ranges are 14–18 g/dL for men and 12–16 g/dL for women).

For the treatment of iron-deficiency anemia, 200 mg of elemental iron per day (2–3 mg/kg) is given in three equal doses of 65 mg; for children weighing 15–30 kg, half the average adult dose is given. Iron deficiency may be treated with any of the several ferrous (Fe^{2+}) salts (e.g., ferrous sulfate, ferrous gluconate). A maximum of 300 mg of elemental iron per day can be administered. However, because humans do not fully absorb iron, a dose of 300 mg of elemental iron per day results in the absorption of approximately 50 mg of elemental iron per day (i.e., approximately 15% absorption). This normally low absorption rate is exacerbated in patients with iron deficiency.

The RDAs of elemental iron for healthy individuals aged 19–50 years are 8 mg/day (male) and 18 mg/day (female). For pregnant women, the RDA is 27 mg/day. Interestingly, the RDA for children aged 1–3 years is 7 mg/day due to their rapid growth. The RDA for males and females 50 years or older is 8 mg/day. Because of their increased need for iron owing to expansion of blood volume, increased hemoglobin concentration, and increased muscle mass in adolescence, boys and girls require higher daily iron intake during their pubertal growth periods.

The most widely administered iron supplements in the United States are ferrous sulfate (Feosol 325 mg; least expensive), which contains 20% elemental iron; ferrous gluconate (Fergon, 300 g), which contains 12% elemental iron; and ferrous fumarate (Femniron, 300 mg), which contains 33% elemental iron. All three of the agents have almost the same absorption profile; the major difference between them is the presence of elemental iron. Keep in mind that it is the amount of elemental iron that is important, rather than the mass of the total salt in the iron tablets. To achieve the maximum absorption of iron, the coating of the tablet should dissolve rapidly in the stomach. Iron should be administered intravenously only if the patient is noncompliant, has iron malabsorption, has oral iron intolerance, is receiving erythropoietin, or refuses blood transfusion therapy. The IV dosage forms include iron dextran, sodium ferric gluconate, and iron sucrose.

When counseling patients who use iron supplements, it is important to advise them to take the medication with orange juice and to take it 1 hour before or 3 hours after antacids; patients should also be warned that iron may darken stools or cause constipation. Drugs such as tetracyclines and quinolone bind iron and reduce its absorption. In addition, to reduce GI side effects, particularly upper gastric discomfort, it is preferable to administer iron 1–2 hours before consuming food.

Iron should be kept out of the reach of children, particularly given that children between the ages of 12 and 24 months are highly vulnerable to iron toxicity. As little as 1–2 g of iron may cause death in members of this age group. Therefore, it is critical to advise patients to make iron supplements not available in the household, particularly given that many formulations are colored sugar-coated tablets that look like candy. Because iron toxicity has a lethal effect, it is important to recognize the signs and symptoms when this toxicity occurs. Iron toxicity may occur rapidly (as early as 30 minutes after ingestion), and its signs and symptoms include abdominal pain, diarrhea, vomiting of brown or bloody stomach contents containing iron supplement tablets, blue or purple coloration of the skin (cyanosis), lethargy, drowsiness, hyperventilation due to acidosis, and cardiovascular collapse.

Learning Bridge 14.3

Today is your first day at the pharmacy, and you feel ready to help a patient manage his disease state. It is around 2 PM when David comes to your pharmacy for his medication. David is a 71-year-old retired electrician who was first diagnosed with a neurodegenerative disease when he was 65 years old. While he is giving his prescription to you, you notice that he has extensive tremor in his hands and a slowness of movement. You immediately identify these symptoms as characteristic of Parkinson's disease (PD). You ask David to have a seat, and you mention it will take 20 minutes to fill the prescription.

The prescription reads as follows:

> Sinemet 50/200, immediate release
> Sig: two tablet daily
> Quantity: 90 tablets

After 5 minutes of waiting, David comes to the counter and asks you a few questions.

A. Why does this drug have two doses (50/200)?

B. David also wants to buy vitamin B_6 capsules and an iron supplement. What advice do you have for him in regard to these supplements?

C. Should David take this medication with food or without food? Why?

Copper (Cu²⁺)

Similar to iron, copper is an important cofactor for many enzymes, such as ferroxidase (catalyzes oxidation of Fe^{2+} to Fe^{3+}), cytochrome *c* oxidase (oxidative phosphorylation), melanin synthesis (skin and hair color), and dopamine hydroxylase (dopamine synthesis). In addition, copper is important for a few antioxidant enzymes. Furthermore, this mineral affects iron absorption because copper is a component of ferroprotein, which is involved in the transfer of iron during absorption from enterocytes (almost all iron is absorbed through the duodenum's enterocytes, which line the lumen, into the blood).

Copper Sources

Free cellular copper does not exist; rather, copper is stored by metallothioneins and distributed by specific chaperones to different sites and tissues. Foods such as shellfish, liver, nuts, legumes, bran, and organ meats are rich in copper.

Copper Deficiency

Copper deficiency has rarely been seen because the amount present in foods is more than adequate. However, it can occur for infants with malabsorption. Copper deficiency can also cause anemia in patients who use high doses of zinc for the treatment of Wilson's disease. A low serum level of copper (less than 65 µg/dL) is an indication of copper deficiency. Copper deficiency causes symptoms such as lower limb paresthesias, weakness, spasticity, and gait difficulties (difficulty in walking), discoloration of hair and skin, anemia, and inflammation.

Copper toxicity is often accidental. In severe cases, it can lead to kidney failure, liver failure, and coma.

Treatment of Copper Deficiency

The daily RDA for copper is 0.9 mg for adults, 1 mg for pregnant women, 1.3 mg for nursing women, and 0.2–0.5 mg for adolescents. Most multivitamin dietary supplements include 1–2 mg of copper. As much as 3–5 mg/day copper can be ingested with no toxicity consequences. In addition, vegan diets provide adequate amounts of copper. Copper gluconate, copper amino acid chelates, and copper glycinate are a few of the copper supplements available in the U.S. market.

Learning Bridge 14.4

Joe is a student at the University of Northeast Lake in Pennsylvania. Joe plays football for his university's football team every weekend. He has large muscles and a naturally athletic physique. He comes to your pharmacy to receive some advice. Joe exercises in the university's gym for 1 hour every evening. Recently, he has experienced abdominal pain, diarrhea, and muscle pain. In addition, he feels out of energy when he gets home and has difficulty concentrating with his homework from his daily classes. You ask Joe to tell you more about his medications, diet, and alcohol consumption. He denies drinking any alcohol or taking any medications. However, every morning he eats 7 raw eggs to be "in good fit."

A. Does Joe's diet reveal anything about his symptoms? Justify your answer.
B. Why does Joe have a lack of energy and difficulty concentrating?
C. Which OTC product will you suggest to Joe to remedy his symptoms? What is the appropriate dose for Joe?
D. What are other suggestions and advice do you have for Joe?

Magnesium (Mg^{2+})

Magnesium is an abundant intracellular cation and can tightly bind to ATP molecules. It is involved in many cellular functions (more than 300 biochemical reactions), which range from ensuring accuracy of protein synthesis, replication, and secretion of parathyroid hormone, to the functions of cell membrane and mitochondria. Magnesium is highly distributed in bones and muscle. Indeed, 50% (25 g) of the body's total store of magnesium (50 g) is distributed in the bones; the remainder is bound to intracellular proteins and enzymes or is loosely bound to phosphate and other anions. Only 1% of the body's total magnesium is found in the ECF. As a result, measurement of the serum magnesium does not accurately represent the body's magnesium level.

The serum concentration of magnesium is closely regulated and is within the range of 1.5–2 mEq/L. A concentration outside this range can significantly change neuromuscular and cardiovascular activities, which in turn can cause cardiac arrhythmias and paralysis. Because cellular influx and outflow of magnesium are not hormonally regulated, there is a risk of magnesium abnormalities. For instance, it has been estimated that two-thirds of patients in intensive care units develop hypomagnesemia. In contrast, toxicity—that is, hypermagnesemia (serum level >2 mEq/L)—is rarely seen.

Magnesium Sources

Chlorophyll-containing vegetables (dark green vegetables such as spinach) are rich in magnesium. In addition, baked potatoes with skin, rice, legumes, nuts, whole unrefined grains, and tap water contain magnesium and, if consumed on a daily basis, will adequately meet the daily requirement for magnesium.

Magnesium Deficiency

The RDAs for magnesium are 400 mg/day and 310 mg/day for men and women, respectively. While during lactation the amount of magnesium remains the same (310 mg/day), during pregnancy it is increased to 350 mg/day. Approximately 30–40% of the magnesium in the human diet is absorbed in the small intestine. This mineral is predominantly reabsorbed in the loop of Henle, although approximately 20% is reabsorbed in the proximal tubule. Accordingly, a hypomagnesemia condition (serum level <1.4 mEq/L) can be caused by either decreased absorption of magnesium (owing to a small bowel disease) or increased renal elimination (owing to diuretic therapy).

Signs and symptoms of hypomagnesemia include involuntary muscle contraction and relaxation (muscular fasciculation), convulsions, palpitations, ECG changes, arrhythmias, and hypertension. In addition, hypokalemia and hypocalcemia are often associated with hypomagnesemia.

Treatment of Magnesium Deficiency

Oral or IV administration of supplemental magnesium is provided to treat hypomagnesemia. IM injection, however, is a painful way of giving magnesium and is reserved as the last-resort route of administration. Magnesium therapy occurs over several weeks due to the fact that 50% of the administered dose is eliminated in the urine.

Available oral magnesium supplements in the United States include magnesium oxide, magnesium sulfate, and magnesium carbonate, taken as 400–800 mg daily. The oral supplement is often given to patients with magnesium levels less than 1 mEq/L who are asymptomatic. In contrast, patients with signs and symptoms of hypomagnesemia receive IV magnesium with hourly monitoring of the serum level until the signs and symptoms disappear and the serum level is at least 1.5 mEq/L. Products containing large amounts of magnesium often cause diarrhea, and a few drug interactions occur with magnesium supplements. For instance, while magnesium reduces the serum levels of bisphosphonate derivatives, it enhances the hypotensive effect of calcium-channel blockers.

For the treatment of hypermagnesemia (a rare condition), patients should be advised to reduce the intake or increase the elimination of magnesium. In such a case, educating patients to reduce their consumption of magnesium-rich foods and magnesium-containing OTC supplements is often helpful. Diuretics (particularly loop diuretics such as furosemide) can also be given to increase the elimination of magnesium and thereby achieve a normal level of serum magnesium concentration.

Potassium (K⁺)

Potassium (K^+) is the major intracellular cation that is essential for excitability of nerve cells and for muscle functions. The intracellular concentration of K^+ is 130–140 mEq/L, whereas the extra-cellular concentration is 3.5–5.0 mEq/L. As a result, the total body potassium is distributed 98% intracellularly and 2% extracellularly. Even a small change in the distribution of potassium can lead to hypokalemia or hyperkalemia.

Potassium Sources

Many fruits are good sources of potassium, including apricots, dried avocados, bananas, canta-loupes, dried dates, melons, nectarines, oranges, and pears. In addition, orange juice, peanut butter, hummus, milk, baked potatoes, tomatoes, lima beans, spinach, and potassium-containing salt are rich in potassium.

Potassium Deficiency (Hypokalemia)

When output of potassium exceeds input, potassium depletion occurs. A low amount of K^+ leads to hypokalemia. Hypokalemia produces hyperpolarization of excitable membranes, which in turn results in decreasing excitability. This causes disturbances of neuromuscular functions and conse-quently muscle weakness, hyperreflexia, and constipation.

While some potassium is lost in sweat under intensive physical exertion and through vomit-ing, hypokalemia is often a result of drug therapy. Corticosteroids, diuretics, aldosterone, and amphotericin B (Fungizone) are all medications that can cause potassium depletion. To increase the level of serum K^+, one has to either increase potassium intake or decrease potassium output—for instance, by using K^+-sparing diuretics. Different diuretics have different effects on the serum level of potassium. For instance, thiazides' effect on the serum level is greater than the effect of loop diuretics. In addition to diuretics, high doses of penicillin-related antibiotics (e.g., nafcillin, dicloxacillin, carbenicillin) are able to increase K^+ excretion. Aldosterone is also known to increase the driving force for K^+ excretion. As a result, hyperaldosteronism—that is, an unusually high level of circulating aldosterone—can lead to hypokalemia. Hyperaldosteronism can be caused by Cushing's syndrome (a syndrome associated with an excessive level of cortisol production).

Because many disorders of the distal nephrons result in excretion of both potassium and magnesium, it is common for patients to have both hypokalemia and hypomagnesemia. Furthermore, magnesium depletion increases K^+ secretion by the distal nephrons due to the reduced magnesium-dependent blockage of K^+ efflux from principal cells (principal cells in the collecting ducts are the major site for regulation of K^+ excretion). In addition, the muscles' Na^+/K^+-ATPase pump requires magnesium ions to function effectively; consequently, magnesium depletion has inhibitory effects on these active pumps as well.

Potassium is an important cation for cardiac, skeletal, and intestinal muscle cells, so hypokalemia can affect the function of these cells. In particular, it can lead to both ventricular and atrial arrhyth-mias. Potassium also competes with digoxin (Lanoxin) for shared binding sites on the cardiac $Na^+/$

K^+-ATPase pump, so hypokalemia can cause digoxin toxicity. Hypokalemia impairs the muscle contraction process, which can lead to weakness and even paralysis. Paralysis of the intestinal smooth muscle causes intestinal ileus (blockage of the small or large intestine).

Insulin can stimulate the activity of the Na^+/K^+-ATPase pumps on myocytes and hepatocytes, thereby increasing the influx of potassium into these cells. Therefore, the IV administration of insulin to treat diabetic ketoacidosis may cause hypokalemia.

Treatment of Potassium Deficiency

Treatment goals for potassium deficiency should focus on preventing and identifying the underlying cause of the hypokalemia. Because hypokalemia is often caused by laxatives, diuretics, antibiotics, and diet, the provider must explore the patient's habits and lifestyle, including signs of periodic weakness, hypertension, hyperthyroidism, hyperinsulinemia, and Cushing's syndrome. A 24-hour urine collection of less than 15 mM is indicative of hypokalemia. As mentioned earlier, the kidney partly regulates potassium excretion. For instance, with the normal potassium intake of 40–120 mEq/day, a large amount of potassium is excreted into the urine by the kidney; when there is a risk of hypokalemia, however, the kidney can significantly reduce the amount of potassium excretion.

The severity of the hypokalemia greatly influences the treatment administered. As hypokalemia often is associated with the depletion of other electrolytes, the provider may give potassium phosphate to patients with combined hypokalemia and hypophosphatemia, potassium bicarbonate or potassium citrate to patients with metabolic acidosis, or a combination of magnesium and potassium to patients with both hypokalemia and hypomagnesemia.

Excess Potassium (Hyperkalemia)

An excess intake or redistribution of potassium from the intracellular compartment to the extracellular compartment or a transfusion of outdated blood (due to K^+ release from old erythrocytes) will lead to hyperkalemia. As healthy kidneys have a large excretory capacity for potassium (90% of daily potassium intake is excreted by the kidneys), hyperkalemia does not develop in healthy individuals.

Although hyperkalemia is less common than hypokalemia, it has severe effects on the heart and can cause a deadly electrolyte imbalance that arises without warning. As a result, hyperkalemia is considered a medical emergency. The excess of K^+ increases the excitability of the nerve and muscle cells. In the hyperkalemia condition, the patient has more K^+ in the ECF than normal. Because the difference in K^+ concentrations between the ICF and the ECF is small, K^+ tends to stay inside of the cells, which results in depolarization (the inside of the cell becomes positively charged). The accumulation of K^+ inside cells results in the production of more action potentials and, in turn, causes a cardiac arrest.

Administration of intravenous calcium can protect the heart while lab data are being analyzed to confirm the diagnosis of hyperkalemia. Calcium increases the action potential threshold and reduces excitability to maintain a resting membrane potential.

Hyperkalemia is indicated when the plasma concentration of potassium is 5.5 mM or greater. This condition occurs in approximately 10% of all hospitalized patients. Severe hyperkalemia (plasma concentration > 6.0 mM) occurs in only 1% of hospitalized patients.

The most common cause of hyperkalemia is a decrease in renal K^+ excretion rather than an excessive intake of K^+. As mentioned earlier, the latter condition is rare because the kidney has a remarkable adaptive capacity to increase renal secretion. Chronic kidney disease and end-stage kidney disease, therefore, may cause hyperkalemia. Potassium-sparing diuretics, such as spirono-lactone (Aldactone), triamterene (Dyrenium), and amiloride (Midamor, from Canada), and drugs that affect the renin–angiotensin–aldosterone system, such as ACE inhibitors, ARBs, and renin inhibitors (see also the *Introduction to Pharmacology and Pathophysiology* chapter), can result in hyperkalemia as well.

As noted earlier, insulin causes hypokalemia and, therefore, is used to treat hyperkalemia. Insulin is administered intravenously to provide a rapid reduction in plasma K^+ concentration. The recommended dose of insulin is 10 units followed immediately by 50 mL of dextrose ($D_{50}W$ or 50%). If the patient has a high blood glucose level (200–250 mg/dL), it is important that insulin be given without glucose and that close monitoring of the patient's blood glucose level be performed.

In acidosis conditions, hydrogen ions move into the cell; in an exchange mechanism, potassium ions move out of the cell. Consequently, patients with an acidosis condition will develop hyperkalemia as well.

Sodium (Na^+)

Sodium is largely confined in the ECF and plays an important role in maintaining the size of the ECF volume (ECFV). Consequently, the amount of sodium in the ECF is approximately equivalent to the total body sodium. The extracellular concentration of sodium is 135–1,405 mEq/L, whereas the intracellular concentration is 12 mEq/L. The kidneys play a vital role in maintaining the amount of sodium in the ECF by adjusting the excretion of sodium. If ECFV increases, the kidneys increase their excretion of sodium. In contrast, if ECFV decreases, the kidneys decrease their excretion of sodium.

Sodium Sources

The recommended amount of daily intake of sodium is 0.5 g. However, the average daily intake in the United States is approximately 10 times higher than this level. Sodium plays an important role in maintaining the blood pressure. Indeed, the prevalence of essential hypertension in many countries, including the United States, is associated with an average sodium intake of 2.3 g or more. Imbalances of sodium lead to either hypernatremia or hyponatremia.

Hyponatremia

Hyponatremia is the condition in which there is an abnormally small amount of sodium in the blood (less than 135 mEq/L). This imbalance is often a result of too much water excretion (through extensive sweat or urine). As mentioned elsewhere in this chapter, the antidiuretic hormone (ADH), which is released from the posterior pituitary, increases water absorption in the collecting ducts of the nephron. This function is carried out by placing aquaporin-2 water channels in the collecting ducts of the kidney. Therefore, an increase in circulating ADH may indicate hyponatremia. The two most important factors to maintain the serum osmolality are water intake and circulating ADH. In the case of heart failure and cirrhosis, the circulating ADH level is increased, which results in water retention and hyponatremia.

Hyponatremia is a very common electrolyte disorder in hospitalized patients (occurring in approximately 22% of such patients). However, vomiting, diarrhea, sweating, and burns may also cause hyponatremia. In addition, reduced circulation of aldosterone can lead to hyponatremia, which is often a cause of adrenal insufficiency or hypoaldosteronism.

A few drug products and disorders can cause hyponatremia. For instance, while thiazides cause polydipsia and diuretic-induced volume depletion, loop diuretics inhibit Na^+/Cl^- and K^+

absorption, thereby reducing the ability of the kidneys to concentrate urine. Glycosuria (in patients experiencing starvation or untreated diabetes) or ketonuria (in alcoholic ketoacidosis) can also lead to volume depletion and hyponatremia.

Hyponatremia is also caused by a very low salt intake. For instance, alcoholics whose sole nutrient is beer can develop hyponatremia, as beer has a very low salt content. In addition, individuals with nutrient-restricted diets (e.g., extreme vegetarian diets) can develop hyponatremia.

Symptoms of acute hyponatremia include headache, poor skin turgor, tachycardia, hypotension, nausea and vomiting, seizures, and confusion. In contrast, patients with chronic hyponatremia (which often lasts more than 48 hours) often do not develop these symptoms.

Hypernatremia

Hypernatremia develops when the concentration of sodium is high in the blood (more than 145 mEq/L). Because of high intake or impaired excretion of Na^+, water may rapidly move out of the intracellular compartment, which can in turn lead to cerebral dehydration. Hypertension, water retention, and edema are other consequences. Hypernatremia is often caused by a combination of water and electrolyte deficits. In addition, it can result from increased water loss caused by fever, exercise, diarrhea, heat, severe burns, and diuresis secondary to hyperglycemia. The prevalence of hypernatremia is high among geriatric patients, many of whom have a reduced thirst or reduced access to fluids.

Genetic factors such as mutations in the ADH-responsive aquaporin-2 water channel can cause nephrogenic diabetes insipidus. In addition, hypokalemia inhibits the renal response to ADH and down-regulates aquaporin-2 expression. A few drugs may cause acquired nephrogenic diabetes insipidus, including lithium (Lithobid) and ifosfamide (Ifex). Lithium causes acquired nephrogenic diabetes by directly inhibiting renal glycogen synthase kinase-3 (GSK3). GSK3 is an important enzyme that enables principal cells to respond to ADH.

When there is a high concentration of Na^+ in the ECF, the osmolality of the ECF is increased, which causes an efflux of intracellular water and cellular shrinkage. Similar to the symptoms of hyponatremia, the signs and symptoms of hypernatremia are neurologic in nature, ranging from mild confusion and lethargy to deep coma. However, in severe hypernatremia (particularly in neonatal and pediatric patients), a sudden shrinkage of brain cells may cause parenchymal or subarachnoid hemorrhages and/or subdural hematomas. Hypernatremic rhabdomyolysis is another consequence of a high plasma level of sodium; it is caused by an osmotic damage to muscle membranes. In 2006 in Ohio, a pharmacy technician accidentally compounded and prepared a chemotherapy solution as a hypertonic saline solution (23.4%) instead of a 0.9% NaCl solution, and the pharmacist did not detect the error. The solution was injected into a 2-year-old cancer patient who, due to the ensuring severe hypernatremia, was in coma for a few days and eventually died. A 0.9% NaCl solution, often referred to as "normal saline," is isotonic to our blood cells (see the *Introduction to Pharmaceutics* and *Introduction to Pharmaceutical Calculations* chapters).

Treatment of Hyponatremia and Hypernatremia

Treatment of hyponatremia begins with slow correction by fluid restriction (less than 800 mL/day fluid intake) or a vasopressin receptor antagonist such as tolvaptan (Samsca). Overly rapid correction of severe hyponatremia can result in osmotic demyelination, which leads to irreversible neurologic damage. If volume depletion is present, administration of an isotonic saline can be helpful to slowly enhance the serum sodium level by approximately 1 mEq/L for each infused 1 L of the isotonic saline solution. In January 2013, the FDA warned healthcare providers that tolvaptan may cause liver damage and its use should be discontinued if any signs of liver damage occur, such as dark urine or jaundice, fatigue, or elevated serum alanine aminotransferase (ALT) or bilirubin.

In the treatment of hypernatremia, the focus should be on identifying risk factors, including the presence or absence of thirst, polyuria, drugs, hyperglycemia, and diarrhea. In addition, a detailed neurologic examination and an assessment of the ECFV are considered, and knowledge of daily fluid intake and daily urine output is important. Laboratory analysis often includes a measurement of serum and urine osmolality, urine electrolytes, and daily urine volume. To avoid cerebral edema, similar to the correction of hyponatremia, it is important to correct hypernatremia slowly and to replace the calculated free-water deficit over 48 hours. The plasma Na^+ level correction should not exceed 10 mEq/L per day. However, in the case of acute hypernatremia, the healthcare provider can safely and rapidly correct the Na^+ level at a rate of 1 mEq/L per hour.

Phosphate (PO_4^{2-})

Phosphorus exists in both the ICF and the ECF in several anion forms, which collectively are referred to as phosphate. These anion forms are mainly $H_2PO_4^-$ and $NaHPO_4^-$ and, to a lesser extent, $HPO4_2^-$. There is approximately 600 g of phosphorus present in the body, with a significant amount (85%) being found in the bone. Phosphorus is one of the major intracellular electrolytes that exists as free anions; as a negative ion, it can be found in complexes formed with structural proteins (particularly collagen), enzymes, transcription factors, carbohydrate and lipid intermediates, ATP molecules, creatine phosphate, and nucleic acids. Interestingly, and in contrast to calcium, potassium, and sodium, there are not dramatic differences between intracellular and extracellular concentrations of phosphorus.

Approximately 12% of the body's store of phosphorus is bound to proteins in the serum. Because the volume of the ICF is greater than the volume of the ECF, a measurement of phosphate in the ECF does not accurately represent phosphate availability in the ICF. Recall that most of the electrolytes are expressed in units of mEq/L—the exception is phosphate. The phosphate injection is a mixture of phosphate salts (a mixture of monobasic potassium phosphate, KH_2PO_4, and dipotassium phosphate, K_2HPO_4), and the body phosphate is measured in units mmol/kg/day; thus it is more convenient to express the concentration of phosphate in mM or mmol/L units. The normal range of elemental phosphorus in the blood and ECF is 2.5–4.5 mg/dL, which corresponds to 0.75–1.45 mmol/L.

Phosphate is absorbed in the proximal tubules, and its absorption is regulated by changes in the apical expression and activity of Na^+/PO_4^{2-} co-transporters proteins in the proximal tubules of the kidney. The parathyroid hormone (PTH) has a dual effect on the plasma level of phosphate. While PTH increases intestinal absorption of phosphate, through the activation of vitamin D it reduces the expression of Na^+/PO_4^{2-} co-transporters proteins in the proximal tubules of the kidney. Accordingly, PTH enhances urinary excretion of phosphate. The inhibitory effect of PTH on renal phosphate absorption indicates that hypocalcemia increases urinary excretion of phosphate (**Figure 14.20**). PTH's renal effect in lowering the plasma phosphate concentration predominates in patients with normal renal function.

FGF23 is a hormone that is synthesized by osteocytes. Consumption of foods that are high in phosphate increase FGF23 levels. It is known that FGF23 regulates phosphate metabolism because it decreases phosphate absorption in the proximal tubules and suppresses the expression of the 1-hydroxylase enzyme, which is responsible for synthesis of calcitonin.

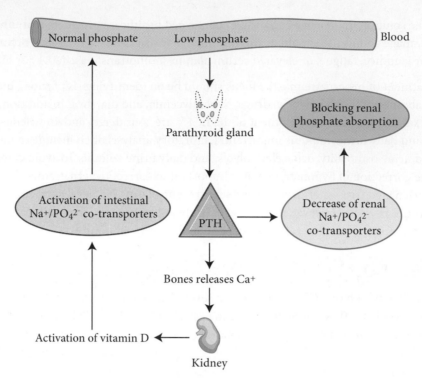

Figure 14.20 Parathyroid hormone (PTH) plays an essential role in the regulation of serum phosphate levels.

Phosphate Sources

Most foods are rich in phosphate, and the small intestine effectively (65% absorption) facilitates the absorption of phosphate even in the absence of vitamin D. However, calcitriol can enhance (up to 90%) the intestinal absorption of phosphate by activating intestinal Na^+/PO_4^{2-} co-transporters (Figure 14.20). Depending on the nature of food ingestion, the daily intestinal phosphate absorption ranges from 500 mg to 1,000 mg. These numbers can be reduced by large doses of calcium salts, ingestion of aluminum hydroxide antacids, or drugs such as sevelamer (Renagel). Foods rich in phosphate include whole-wheat bread, cottage cheese and cheddar cheese, peanut butter, corn, broccoli, and garlic.

Phosphate Deficiency (Hypophosphatemia)

Hypophosphatemia can induce bone resorption and in chronic cases, particularly in children, may result in osteomalacia, rickets, and short stature. The underlying mechanisms of hypophosphatemia include the following:

- Reduced intestinal phosphate absorption, which is often caused by fasting or starvation or occurs in the presence of aluminum hydroxide antacids.
- Increased renal phosphate excretion.
- Reduced renal phosphate absorption (caused by diuretics or a few toxins).
- Rapid influx of phosphate from the ECF into bone or soft tissue. This often occurs in hospitalized patients when insulin therapy is required (such as in the treatment of DKA), with administration of IV glucose without other nutrients, with high release of catecholamines (endogenous or exogenous), and in respiratory alkalosis.

Because foods are rich in phosphate, inadequate intestinal absorption is rarely seen. Other factors that can cause hypophosphatemia include low levels of serum calcitonin and calcium (Figure 14.20).

Phosphate is an important component of ATP molecules, and hypophosphatemia (less than 0.75 mmol/L or less than 2.5 mg/dL) results in reduced cellular energy metabolism and greater utilization of cellular glycolysis, rather than the activation of the oxidative phosphorylation pathway that occurs in mitochondria (to compensate for the low ATP synthesis). Acute and severe hypophosphatemia mainly occur in hospitalized patients due to medical illness and preexisting phosphate depletion due to high urinary losses or severe malabsorption and malnutrition. Chronic hypophosphatemia is less severe and often is indicated by bone pain, osteomalacia, pseudofractures, and proximal muscle weakness. A progressive hypophosphatemia can cause rhabdomyolysis.

Mild and severe hypophosphatemia are indicated by low serum phosphate concentrations (less than 0.75 mmol/L and less than 0.32 mmol/L, respectively). While mild hypophosphatemia rarely causes recognizable signs and symptoms, severe hypophosphatemia is symptomatic and is indicated by life-threatening symptoms such as seizures, coma, and rhabdomyolysis. A severe imbalance should be corrected immediately. Hypophosphatemia has been seen in 18–28% of hospitalized critically ill patients.

Hyperphosphatemia

Hyperphosphatemia is indicated by a fasting serum level of more than 1.8 mmol/L. It is often caused by impaired glomerular filtration, an abnormally low amount of PTH, high delivery of phosphate from the bones and gut into the ECF, administration of large amounts of phosphate-containing laxatives, extensive soft-tissue injury or necrosis (e.g., with crush injuries, rhabdomyolysis, or cytotoxic chemotherapy), or recent parenteral phosphate therapy. Of particular concern is a massive soft-tissue injury that can cause severe hyperphosphatemia (concentrations as high as 7 mmol/L). The clinical manifestations of severe hyperphosphatemia include formation of calcium–phosphate precipitations that reduce calcium levels and cause hypocalcemia.

Treatment of Hypophosphatemia and Hyperphosphatemia

In severe hypophosphatemia, patients often receive IV phosphate therapy. In adults, this therapy can be administered as neutral mixtures of sodium and potassium phosphate salts at initial doses of 0.2–0.8 mmol/kg of elemental phosphorus over a 6-hour time frame. If hypocalcemia is also present, it should be corrected before IV phosphate therapy is initiated. For this reason, it is important to closely monitor serum levels of phosphate and calcium every 6–12 hours throughout the treatment. To avoid precipitation, phosphorus must be added separately into multiple-electrolyte solutions.

It is important to differentiate between hyperphosphatemia caused by impaired renal phosphate excretion and a high delivery of phosphate into the ECF. For instance, a reduced GFR in chronic renal deficiency results in phosphate retention, which in turn leads to hyperphosphatemia. This type of hyperphosphatemia leads to reduced renal synthesis of calcitonin and stimulates secretion of PTH. Consequently, hyperphosphatemia causes secondary hyperparathyroidism of renal failure.

In contrast to the case with hypophosphatemia, treatments of hyperphosphatemia are limited. A few drugs are able to bind phosphate in the GI tract and reduce phosphorus absorption by forming insoluble complex compounds (i.e., chelating effect), which are then excreted in feces. These drugs include phosphate-binding agents such as calcium-, aluminum-, and magnesium-containing compounds and sevelamer carbonate. It is important to counsel patients to take these agents with meals to increase the binding of phosphorus in the GI tract. Another effective treatment is hemodialysis, which lowers serum phosphorus and calcium, particularly in cases of a renal failure.

Chloride (Cl⁻)

Chloride is the major extracellular anion (compare it with potassium, which is the major intracellular cation). The normal serum chloride concentration is 90–110 mEq/L. Chloride is an important electrolyte to maintain normal acid–base balance and osmolality. For instance, when chloride is lost, patients can develop alkalosis. The reabsorption of chloride is dependent on the reabsorption of sodium.

Chloride Sources

Table salt, cheese, tomatoes, bacon, butter, and olives are rich in chloride. In addition, foods such as raisins, dates, cherries, coconut, grapes, and grapefruit are rich in potassium chloride.

Chloride Deficiency (Hypochloremia)

A low serum concentration of chloride (less than 90 mEq/L) is an indication of hypochloremia, but there are no symptoms associated with this imbalance. Hypochloremia is caused either by metabolic alkalosis (when the urinary chloride concentration is 10 mE/L) or by expansion of extracellular fluid volume (when the urinary chloride concentration is 40 mE/L). This condition is often associated with prolonged vomiting, gastric suctioning, metabolic alkalosis, congestive heart failure (CHF), Addison's disease, or use of H_2 blockers or proton pump inhibitors. In addition, chronic use of diuretics, chronic respiratory acidosis, DKA, excessive sweating, acute intermittent porphyria, adrenal insufficiency, hyperaldosteronism, and metabolic alkalosis result in hypochloremia. Keep in mind that hyperaldosteronism causes retention of HCO_3^- and Na^+ and promotes excretion of H^+, K^+, and Cl^-.

Hyperchloremia

In contrast to hypochloremia, if too much chloride is gained or retained, acidosis can develop. Hyperchloremia is often associated with metabolic acidosis, respiratory alkalosis, dehydration, diabetes insipidus, convulsions, renal failure, overtreatment with saline, hyperparathyroidism, diabetes insipidus, and hyperadrenocorticism.

Treatment of Hypochloremia and Hyperchloremia

In the case of hypochloremia, an IV normal saline infusion is administered. In the case of hyperchloremia, the underlying cause first needs to be identified and corrected.

Learning Bridge 14.5

During one of your introductory pharmacy practice experiences, Eva comes to the counter and asks you a question. Eva is a history teacher. Her father has recently (2 months ago) been diagnosed with Alzheimer's disease. Eva's father has lived alone since 6 months ago, and Eva has been worried about his well-being and diet. She explains that her father's doctor has prescribed an OTC product, Key-E Kaps (150 units/day), to help him with his memory loss. Eva read an article about Key-E Kaps, which seems to contain vitamin E. The article described how vitamin E could prevent neuronal damage that was caused by oxidative stress and free radicals. However, Eva admits that she does not understand how vitamin E works as an antioxidant.

Use your knowledge and assist Eva in understanding how vitamin E works to prevent oxidative stress and the accumulation of free radicals. Could her father's Alzheimer's disease be associated with having a vitamin E–deficient diet during the last 6 months? Which kind of vitamin E–rich foods do you suggest her father to eat?

Acid–Base Disorders

The role of a buffer in a buffered solution is to resist a pH change in the solution. Because blood contains buffers, there is a resistance to pH changes in the blood. The body can tolerate only a minimal change in the blood pH (7.4 ± 0.3). Above or below this range, many essential proteins lose their structural and functional integrity, which ultimately leads to many physiological dysfunctions (**Figure 14.21**).

Before explaining acid–base disorders, it is important to discuss bicarbonate formation, as it has a major role in metabolic acid–base disorders and in the physiologic buffering systems.

Bicarbonate (HCO_3^-)

Bicarbonate plays an important role in maintaining the buffer systems of the blood and all body fluids and tissues, including the interstitial fluid and lymph. Actions of the lungs, hydrogen ions, and carbon dioxide also assist bicarbonate in maintaining the pH of the blood (**Figure 14.22**).

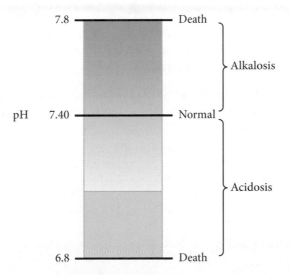

Figure 14.21 The buffer system in the blood plays a crucial role in maintaining the pH of the blood.

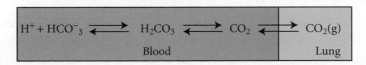

Figure 14.22 The reversible formation of carbonic acid, bicarbonate, and carbon dioxide in the blood and lungs.

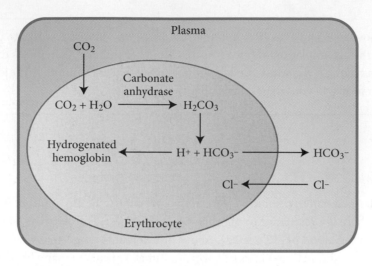

Figure 14.23 Formation of carbonic acid, bicarbonate, and carbon dioxide in the erythrocytes, catalyzed by carbonate anhydrase.
Adapted from: Marshall WJ, Bangert SK. *Clinical chemistry*, 5th ed. Edinburgh: Mosby; 2004: Chapter 3.

Bicarbonate Formation in Erythrocytes

Carbon dioxide (CO_2) is produced as a waste molecule in the tissue cells during metabolism (recall the citric acid cycle) and diffuses into the ECF. In the ECF, CO_2 reacts with water to form carbonic acid, which then is dissociated to hydrogen and bicarbonate ions. The hydrogen ions formed in this way are responsible for reducing the pH of the ECF.

Erythrocytes do not have mitochondria, so no citric acid cycle occurs there. As a result, carbon dioxide moves into erythrocytes down the concentration gradient. In the erythrocytes, carbon dioxide mixes with water to form carbonic acid (H_2CO_3), a mechanism catalyzed by the erythrocyte enzyme, carbonic anhydrase. Degradation of carbonic acid produces bicarbonate and hydrogen ions inside the erythrocytes (**Figure 14.23**).

The bicarbonate buffer system (HCO_3^-/H_2CO_3) plays an important role in controlling the blood's pH. One can calculate the normal ratio of HCO_3^- to H_2CO_3 in the blood. The pK_a for carbonic acid is 6.1 and the pH of the blood is 7.4. The Henderson-Hasselbalch equation (Equation 14.3) can help us to calculate the ratio between bicarbonate and carbonic acid (see also the *Introduction to Biological Chemistry*):

$$pH = pK_a + \log \frac{[HCO_3^-]}{[H_2CO_3]} \tag{14.3}$$

$$\text{Antilog } (7.4 - 6.1) = \frac{[HCO_3^-]}{[H_2CO_3]} = 20 \tag{14.4}$$

Equation 14.4 indicates that the ratio of HCO_3^- to H_2CO_3 is about 20:1 in the blood. An increase in the concentration of HCO_3^- results in a higher ratio, which in turn results in alkalosis. The normal range of bicarbonate in the plasma is 22–26 mEq/L.

This bicarbonate buffering system assists the body in maintaining acid–base homeostasis. Interestingly, we are able to manipulate the bicarbonate buffering system to avoid prolonged alkalosis or acidosis. For instance, during a 100-meter dash running competition, athletes produce a large amount of lactic acid (recall the discussion of anaerobic glycolysis in the *Introduction to Biochemistry* chapter), which in turn reduces their blood pH during their run. However, many

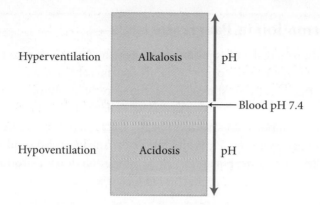

Figure 14.24 Hyperventilation and hypoventilation result in alkalosis and acidosis, respectively.

of these athletes hyperventilate (breathe rapidly and deeply) for about 30 seconds before they run. The short hyperventilation causes a large amount of CO_2 to be expelled from the lungs. This condition results in the body taking up more H^+ ions to make more carbonic acid and CO_2 (**Figure 14.24**). Decreasing the amount of H^+ ions increases the pH of the blood and tissues, which compensates for the acidosis that would arise during the athletes' short run. Figure 14.24 describes the alkalosis and acidosis caused by hyperventilation and hypoventilation, respectively.

Bicarbonate diffuses out of the erythrocytes down the concentration gradient into the plasma. To maintain the electrochemical balance of erythrocytes, chloride ions move into these cells, a mechanism called chloride shift (Figure 14.23). The hydrogen ions inside of erythrocytes are attached to hemoglobin to maintain the pH of erythrocytes. Because bicarbonate is synthesized from carbon dioxide, approximately 90% of the body's total store of carbon dioxide exists as bicarbonate in the blood. The remaining 10% of carbon dioxide is found either as carbon dioxide or carbonic acid.

Bicarbonate Formation in Parietal Cells

Bicarbonate is also produced in the gastric parietal cells (**Figure 14.25**). Carbonate dehydrogenase enzyme combines water with carbon dioxide to make carbonic acid, which then dissociates into bicarbonate and hydrogen ions. The hydrogen ions are released into the stomach to reduce the pH of the gastric acid, and the bicarbonate is released into the blood. Here, the chloride shift occurs as well (i.e., chloride moves into the parietal cells and bicarbonate moves into the blood). The chloride ions are then secreted from parietal cells into the stomach.

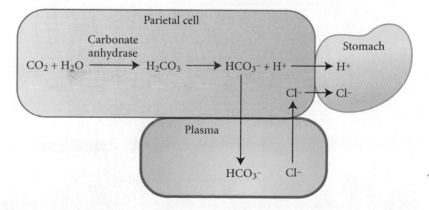

Figure 14.25 Formation of carbonic acid, bicarbonate, and hydrogen ion in a parietal cell, catalyzed by carbonate anhydrase.

Adapted from: Marshall WJ, Bangert SK. *Clinical chemistry*, 5th ed. Edinburgh: Mosby; 2004: Chapter 3.

Bicarbonate Formation in Pancreatic Cells

Similar to parietal cells, pancreatic cells produce bicarbonate that moves into the pancreatic duct (**Figure 14.26**). The cells that line the pancreatic duct (ductal cells) secrete bicarbonate into the small intestine. These ductal cells are stimulated by the secretin hormone (secretin is released from the duodenum). The neurotransmitter acetylcholine stimulates the ductal cells to secrete bicarbonate as well. Bicarbonate is important to neutralize gastric acid in the small intestine and thereby promote the activity of pancreatic enzymes and bile acids. The liver also produces bicarbonate from the metabolic carbon dioxide, but almost all of the carbon dioxide produced in the liver is used in the synthesis of urea (see the *Introduction to Biochemistry* chapter).

Bicarbonate Formation in Renal Tubular Cells

Every day we produce hydrogen ion in our bodies through the metabolism of proteins (i.e., from protein-rich food). For instance, oxidation of the amino acid cysteine results in the release of hydrogen ions in amounts as high as 60 mmol per day (**Figure 14.27**). To determine how much this amount increases the concentration of H^+ in the ECF, we need to divide it by the volume of the ECF in the body.

An adult body contains approximately 40 liters of water: two-thirds as ICF (26 L), and one-third as ECF (14 L). Thus, every day, the concentration of H^+ in the ECF increases by 60 mmol/14L (or 4 mM—100,000 times higher than the normal value in the blood, which is 40 nM). This significant increase in the number of protons in the ECF is a deadly condition. However, the same extracellular fluid (about 14 liters) that has 100,000 times more H^+ ions than the blood also has a concentration of 24 mM HCO_3^-. This indicates that as the number of H^+ ions increases, more H_2CO_3 (carbonic acid) is formed by using HCO_3^-. In other words, we reduce the concentration of HCO_3^-.

The body's buffering system does not remove the excess of H^+ ions, but rather takes care of it for a short period of time. Indeed, it is the renal excretion system that manages the excess of H^+ ions (**Figure 14.28**). In the peritubular capillary, H^+ joins HCO_3^- to form carbonic acid. The carbonic anhydrase enzyme, found at the brush border of the tubular cells, catalyzes the breakdown of carbonic acid to water and CO_2, which both diffuse freely to the tubule cells. The CO_2 is hydrated in the tubular cells back to carbonic acid, which again is broken down by the intracellular carbonic anhydrase enzyme. Basically, what a person needs is a good source of bicarbonate (HCO_3^-, 24 mM) in the extracellular fluid to take care of the excess H^+ ions (see step 1 in Figure 14.28) and

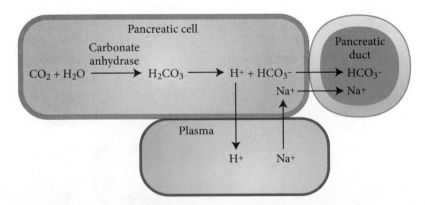

Figure 14.26 Formation of carbonic acid, bicarbonate, and hydrogen ion in a pancreatic cell, catalyzed by carbonate anhydrase.
Adapted from: Marshall WJ, Bangert SK. *Clinical chemistry*, 5th ed. Edinburgh: Mosby; 2004: Chapter 3.

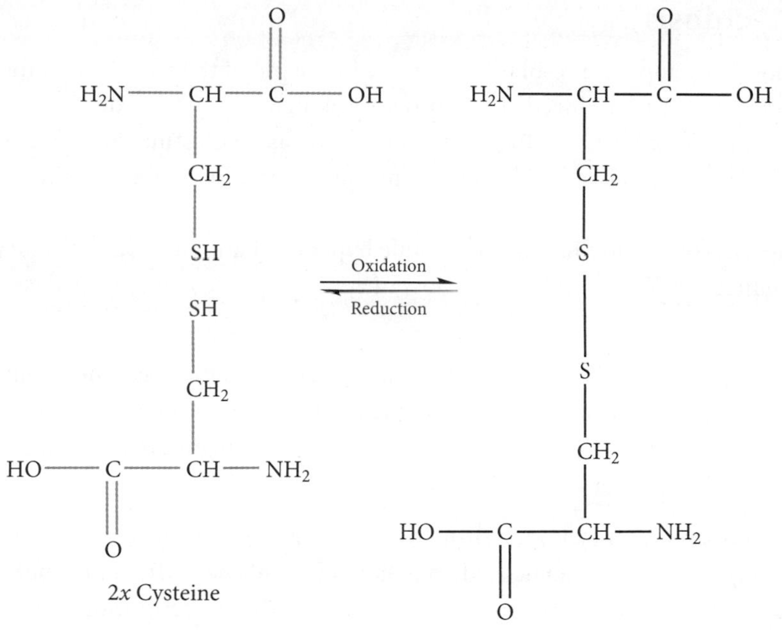

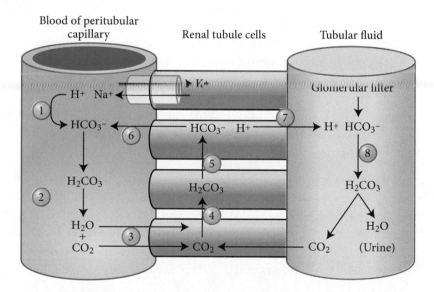

Figure 14.27 Oxidation of cysteine amino acids results in the release of protons (hydrogen ions).

Figure 14.28 Kidney, bicarbonate, and carbonic anhydrase play important roles in removing the excess of protons produced by protein degradation so as to prevent an increase in the blood's pH.
Adapted from: Lee M. *Basic skills in interpreting laboratory data*, 4th ed. Bethesda: ASHP, Inc.; 2009; Chapter 8.

functional kidneys to regenerate bicarbonate to maintain the plasma concentration of HCO_3^- within normal limits (steps 5 and 6). A carbonic anhydrase inhibitor agent diuretic such as acetazolamide (Diamox), however, can disrupt this buffering system, which in turn may result in a metabolic acidosis condition.

There are three forms of acid–base disorders: metabolic acid–base disorders, respiratory acid–base disorders, and mixed acid–base disorders.

Metabolic Acidosis

Metabolic acidosis develops as a result of a decrease in the pH of the blood when the serum bicarbonate concentration is reduced. Two causes are associated with the development of metabolic acidosis: (1) a loss of HCO_3^-, which can result from gastrointestinal loss (diarrhea and small bowel drainage), and (2) a gain of acid, which can result from endogenous H^+ production (e.g., from ketoacidosis, drug intoxication, or hypokalemia) or ingestion of methanol or ethylenglycol solutions. Symptoms of metabolic acidosis include hyperventilation (a compensatory mechanism that is often the first sign of this imbalance), loss of appetite, nausea, vomiting, dyspnea, and lactic acidosis.

Two forms of metabolic acidosis are distinguished: increased anion gap metabolic acidosis and normal anion gap metabolic acidosis. Upon diagnosis of metabolic acidosis, therefore, it is important to analyze and determine the serum anion gap. These two forms are explained further when the anion gap is described later in this chapter.

Metabolic acidosis may, for example, ensue from an overdose of acidic drugs or ingestion of some alcohols. Aspirin (acetylsalicylic acid) is metabolized into salicylic acid, whereas methanol is metabolized into formic acid. These metabolites increase the concentration of H^+ ions, which in turn leads to use of more HCO_3^- to take care of the excess H^+. Consequently, the concentration of HCO_3^- drops in the blood—an indication of metabolic acidosis.

Metabolic acidosis usually occurs in patients with impaired circulation from cardiac arrest. One way to eliminate the acidosis condition is to use mechanical hyperventilation. Mechanical hyperventilation removes CO_2 form the lungs (Figure 14.22), which increases the pH and thereby brings the patient's pH back to the normal level. Another treatment is to give a sodium bicarbonate ($NaHCO_3$) solution to remedy the acidosis condition. A mild to moderate degree of metabolic acidosis is indicated by a lower than normal concentration of serum bicarbonate (12–20 mEq/L versus the normal 22–26 mEq/L). Administration of $NaHCO_3$ over a period of 1–2 weeks can increase the concentration of serum bicarbonate to the normal level. Recall that $NaHCO_3$ is a salt that, upon dissociation, produces Na^+ and HCO_3^- in which HCO_3^- serves as a base to pick up the excess H^+ by forming first carbonic acid and then CO_2.

Because a large amount of CO_2 is produced with either mechanical hyperventilation or administration of $NaHCO_3$ and if the patient experiences cardiac arrest, he or she often has an acute lung injury that makes it very challenging to exhale the large amount of the produced CO_2. It has been suggested that administration of hydroxylmethylaminomethane (tris; **Figure 14.29**) may help patients with acidosis and cardiac arrest. Tris is a base that removes the excess of H^+ without forming any CO_2; the protonated tris is then excreted into the urine.

Metabolic Alkalosis

Metabolic alkalosis commonly occurs in hospitalized patients and is indicated by an elevated serum bicarbonate concentration. Two mechanisms are associated with development of metabolic alkalosis: (1) a loss of H^+ or (2) a gain of HCO_3^-. For instance, excessive use of $NaHCO_3$ (baking soda, which is a common remedy for upset stomach), loss of H^+ ions either through vomiting, or a potassium deficiency condition all increase the serum concentration of HCO_3^-. In otherwise healthy individuals, however, the kidney has a remarkable ability to excrete the excess of endogenous or exogenous bicarbonate.

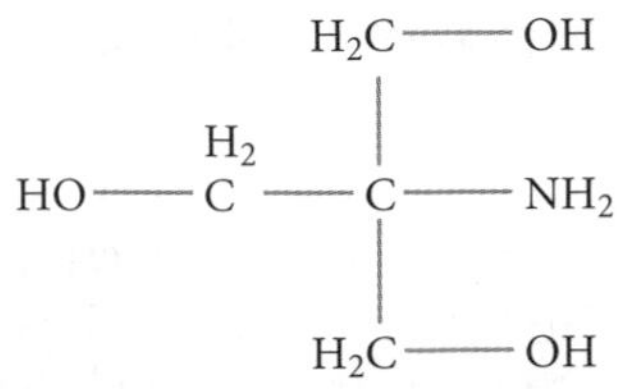

Figure 14.29 Structure of hydroxylmethylaminomethane (tris).

The potassium deficiency that leads to metabolic alkalosis has to do with the sodium–potassium exchange mechanism in the renal tubule cells (Figure 14.28). Upon potassium depletion, H^+ (rather than K) is exchanged for Na^+ in the renal tubules. Thus, despite an alkalosis condition, the urine has an acidic pH. This mechanism is commonly observed among patients who take diuretic therapies, particularly loop diuretics and thiazides, because of over-excretion of potassium in the urine (i.e., because of potassium depletion).

Metabolic alkalosis is not associated with any specific symptoms. However, if potassium depletion is one of the underlying mechanisms, patients may complain of muscle weaknesses. Because metabolic alkalosis is less tolerable than metabolic acidosis, a treatment plan is necessary to treat affected patients. It is important to eliminate the underlying cause. For instance, if vomiting is the cause, an antiemetic agent needs to be administered; if potassium depletion is the cause, either a potassium supplement or a potassium-sparing diuretic can be used. If feasible, the original diuretic therapy should be discontinued.

Respiratory Acidosis

Respiratory acidosis occurs when lungs cannot adequately expel carbon dioxide, which results in an increase in hydrogen ions that consequently reduces the pH of the blood (Figure 14.22). For instance, choking and chronic obstructive airway diseases such as bronchitis and emphysema can lead to respiratory acidosis. Respiratory acidosis can be a life-threatening condition if it leads to hypoxemia (characterized by a low oxygen concentration within the arterial blood: $PaO_2 < 40$ mm Hg) and hypercarbia (characterized by a high concentration of CO_2 within the arterial blood: $PaCO_2 > 80$ mm Hg). Symptoms of respiratory acidosis are neurological in nature, and include confusion, headache, seizures, stupor, and coma. Adequate oxygenation and mechanical ventilation are necessary to reduce these symptoms.

Respiratory Alkalosis

Respiratory alkalosis is characterized by decreased arterial $PaCO_2$, a condition that arises when more CO_2 is expelled than is created through metabolic production. Respiratory alkalosis is relatively common and often occurs during pregnancy, in people living at high altitudes, or with hysterical over-breathing (hyperventilation). If the decreased $PaCO_2$ is not treated, it can lead to a decrease in cerebral blood flow, which in turn can cause muscle cramps, confusion, syncope, and seizures. In severe cases, cardiac arrhythmias can occur as well. In mild cases, using a paper bag to allow for rebreathing is useful to control the hyperventilation. However, oxygen therapy and mechanical ventilation are required for severe cases.

Table 14.6 summarizes the characteristics of acid–base disorders.

Mixed Acid–Base Disorder

While a mixed metabolic acidosis and alkalosis or a mixed respiratory acidosis and alkalosis cannot coexist, a cross-combination of metabolic and respiratory disorders can coexist. Metabolic acidosis and respiratory alkalosis commonly occur together. For instance, salicylic acid poisoning (aspiring overdose, 200–300 mg/kg) results in a metabolic acidosis/respiratory alkalosis. Salicylic acid stimulates the respiratory center in the brain stem, reducing CO_2 and causing hyperventilation, and consequently causes respiratory alkalosis. However, salicylic acid is also a weak acid that, in toxic concentrations, can titrate 2–3 mEq/L of plasma bicarbonate (decreases HCO_3^-), which results in a metabolic acidosis.

Table 14.6 Characteristics of Acid–Base Disorders

Condition	Laboratory Data	Symptoms
Metabolic acidosis	Low concentration of HCO_3^- (<12–20 mEq/L); increased H^+ production	Hyperventilation, loss of appetite, nausea and vomiting, dyspnea, lactic acidosis
Metabolic alkalosis	Loss of H^+ or retention of HCO_3^-	Lacks specific symptoms but muscle weakness as a result of potassium depletion can occur
Respiratory acidosis	Low oxygen and high carbon dioxide concentrations within the arterial blood	Confusion, headache, seizures, stupor, coma
Respiratory alkalosis	Low carbon dioxide concentration within the arterial blood	Muscle cramps, confusion, syncope, seizures

Anion Gap

It is ideal to have neutral plasma by having an equal number of sodium cations (the predominant plasma cations) and anions such as HCO_3^- and Cl^-. However, it is known that the sum of the latter anions does not equal the number of sodium cations. As a result, there must be other anions that can make the plasma neutral. These extra anions are usually albumin, phosphate, sulfate, lactic acid, and the conjugate bases of ketoacids.

These extra anions are not routinely measured and, as a result, they are called unmeasured anions (UA). Cations that similarly are not measured include Ca^{2+}, K^+, and Mg^{2+} (however, as mentioned earlier, K^+ is largely confined in the cells and consequently does not contribute to any significant extent to the number of plasma cations). These cations are referred to as unmeasured cations (UC). To have neutral plasma, the number of Na^+ cations and the number of HCO_3^- and Cl^- anions must be equal. If the cations and anions are not equal, there is an imbalance referred to as an anion gap, with a normal value of 7 ± 4 mEq/L. Simply put, the anion gap is a useful metric for evaluating underlying causes of metabolic acidosis.

We can write an equation to express the balance between plasma cations and anions:

$$([Na^+]+[UC]=([HCO_3^-]+[Cl^-]+[UA])$$ (14.5)

Therefore, the anion gap is equal to

Anion gap $=[UA]-[UC]$ (14.6)

This is also equal to

Anion gap $=[Na^+]-([HCO_3^-]+[Cl^-])$ (14.7)

As Equation 14.6 indicates, an elevated anion gap may be caused by a decrease in UC, an increase in UA, or an error in the laboratory measurement of Na^+, Cl^-, or HCO_3^-. While a decreased UC is rare, it can occur due to severe calcium or magnesium depletion. Overall, the existence of an anion gap indicates that there are more unmeasured anions than cations.

When metabolic acidosis occurs in conjunction with an increased anion gap, toxic alcohol poisoning should be suspected. A toxic ingestion of ethylene glycol or methanol increases the amount of lactic acid, which in turn increases the UA and, consequently, the anion gap. Drugs that increase the amount of UA (e.g., amiloride, metformin, niacin, propofol, NSAIDs, valproic acid, verapamil) can increase the anion gap as well. After diagnosis of metabolic acidosis, it is important to analyze the serum anion gap. There are two forms of metabolic acidosis:

- *Caused by an increased amount of UA.* In this form, one or more agents (such as toxic organic acids) contribute to the increased UA. This form is referred to as "increased anion gap metabolic acidosis." Some clinicians use the mnemonic "AT MUD PILES" to remember the names of the toxic agents that cause an increased anion gap: Alcohol, Toluene, Methanol, Uremia, DKA, Paraldehyde, Iron and Isoniazid, Lactic acid, Ethylene glycol, and Salicylic acid. In one study in which 57 hospitalized patients were evaluated to identify the cause of their increased anion gap, patients who had an anion gap greater than 30 mEq/L were identified as having lactic acidosis or ketoacidosis.
- *Caused by a normal anion gap.* In this form, the metabolic acidosis is not caused by an increase in an anion, but rather by a low bicarbonate concentration and a normal anion gap in plasma (i.e., the anion gap is approximately 7 ± 4 mEq/L).

Occasionally, the term "hyperchloremic" metabolic acidosis is used to describe normal anion gap metabolic acidosis. The reasoning is that many patients develop metabolic acidosis due to a high concentration of chloride. However, the descriptor "hyperchloremic" metabolic acidosis is accurate only if the concentration of plasma Na^+ is normal. If the Na^+ plasma concentration is low (i.e., hyponatremia), the chloride concentration may be normal or even low. Therefore, the most accurate term to use is normal anion gap metabolic acidosis. To correct for a low plasma albumin concentration, it is necessary to reduce the anion gap by 2.5 mEq/L for each 1 g/dL decrease in the plasma albumin concentration.

Learning Bridge 14.6

As an intern pharmacist working at your first introductory pharmacy practice experience site in a health system, you receive a phone call from a physician. The physician orders potassium phosphate for an IV injection, 20 mEq/L. Potassium phosphate is available as concentrates. You immediately notice that there is something wrong with the order.

A. What is wrong with the order? Justify your answer to the physician.
B. Name at least three underlying mechanisms of hypophosphatemia.
C. What is the water that you will use to dilute the potassium phosphate concentrate for the IV administration?

Obesity

Obesity occurs as the result of an imbalance between energy intake and energy expenditure, marked by an increased energy storage. Many factors play important roles in the development of obesity, including genetics, environmental factors, medical conditions, and adverse effects of some medications.

Obesity is a growing nutritional problem in the United States. It is estimated that 60–65% of U.S. adults are overweight or obese. By 2020, obesity is predicted to affect 80% of adults in the United States, and the prevalence of overweight in children is expected to double by 2030. Obesity and overweight can progressively increase the risk for and exacerbate the development of many diseases and, as a result, can significantly impair patients' quality of life and increase the costs of their health care.

Guidelines have been established to distinguish between overweight and obesity. For example, body mass index (BMI), which is an acceptable measure of obesity, is used to for this purpose. BMI is calculated as weight in kilograms divided by height in meters squared (kg/m^2). For instance, individuals with a BMI of 18.5–24.9 kg/m^2 have normal weight; those with a BMI of 25–29.9 kg/m^2 are overweight; those with a BMI of 30–39.9 kg/m^2 are obese; and those with a BMI of 40 kg/m^2 or greater are referred to as severely obese. A reduction in life expectancy and increased mortality have been associated with BMI values greater than 35, mainly as a result of the increased risk of cardiovascular disease. Not all fat threatens health in the same way, however. For instance, superficial subcutaneous fat has a weak association with insulin production or resistance, whereas deep subcutaneous fat has shown a correlation with the insulin resistance phenomenon.

As mentioned earlier, environmental and genetic factors play important roles in obesity. Indeed, in some individuals, genetic factors are the sole cause of obesity. It has been estimated that BMI and body fat distribution are 50–80% attributable to genetic factors. While the role of genetic factors is currently under intense research investigation, the exact genes that are involved in obesity remain to be determined. By comparison, we know more about the environmental impacts on the development of obesity. For instance, reduced physical activity, sedentary lifestyle, consumption of high-fat foods, culture, and socioeconomic status may influence eating habits and body weights.

Some patients develop obesity secondary to a medical condition. For instance, Cushing's disease, growth hormone deficiency, insulinoma, leptin deficiency, and some psychiatric disorders can cause obesity. In addition, medications can contribute to obesity. For instance, anticonvulsants such as carbamazepine (Carbatrol), gabapentin (Neurontin), pregabalin (Lyrica), and valproic acid (Depacon) have been shown to increase likelihood of a weight gain. Other medications that have similar effect on obesity include tricyclic antidepressants, atypical antipsychotics, conventional antipsychotics such as haloperidol (Haldol), and hormones such as corticosteroids and insulin. However, the exact role of these agents in weight gain is not fully understood.

Appetite is another factor that contributes to the development of obesity. Appetite is a complex process that involves the hypothalamus, limbic system, brain stem, hippocampus, and elements of the cortex. In addition, many neurotransmitters and neuropeptides have been shown to either stimulate or depress the appetite network. For instance, neurotransmitters such as neuropeptide Y (NPY) and dopamine and the hormones ghrelin (produced in the distal stomach and duodenum right before a meal) and orexin (produced in the lateral and posterior hypothalamus) have been suggested to increase eating. Indeed, the lateral hypothalamus has been referred to as the "hunger" center within the brain. Conversely, glucagon-like peptide-1 (GLP-1), which increases insulin secretion and slows gastric emptying, appears to reduce the risk of obesity. Bariatric surgery, a surgical weight-loss procedure, has been shown to increase the serum concentration of GPL-1. The National Institutes of Health has recommended this surgical procedure for obese patients with a BMI of 40 kg/m^2 or greater.

Leptin is a small polypeptide hormone that is expressed by the OB gene produced in adiopocytes and is transported by the blood to the brain. This hormone is produced when there are adequate stores of lipids in the adiopocytes, and it interacts with its receptor in the hypothalamus. The interaction of leptin with the hypothalamus produces a cascade of effects that suppress appetite and increase energy expenditure. For example, leptin stimulates the oxidation of fatty acids and inhibits the accumulation of fats in nonadipose tissue. It reduces food intake by up-regulating anorexigenic (appetite-reducing) neuropeptides, such as corticotropin-releasing hormone (CRH), cocaine- and amphetamine-regulated transcript (CART), and proopiomelanocortin (POMC). The role of these neuropeptides is to down-regulate orexigenic (appetite-stimulating) factors (e.g., NPY). Genetic defects in anorexigenic signaling, such as mutations in the leptin receptors, may cause obesity. Interestingly, research studies have shown that in leptin-deficient mice, exogenous leptin administration can produce significant weight loss. Leptin has several other biochemical roles, such as increasing insulin and glucocorticoid secretion and glucose transport within the small intestine.

Orlistat (Xenical, 120 mg) is a synthetic derivative of lipstatin; lipstatin is a natural hormone that inhibits gastric and pancreatic lipases. These lipases are known to facilitate absorption of long-chain triacylglycerols. Because high fat intake contributes to the development of obesity, orlistat may be helpful in reducing the absorption of triacylglycerols. Orlistat, 120 mg three times daily with meals, has been shown to reduce fat absorption by as much as 30%. An OTC version of this drug (Alli, 60 mg) has been approved by the FDA. To be effective, orlistat must be taken within 1 hour of ingestion of fat-containing foods.

Phentermine (Adipex-P) has also been used to treat obesity. Its structure is similar to amphetamine, but it has less severe CNS effects and, as a result, carries a lower risk for drug abuse. Its role is to stimulate the hypothalamus to release norepinephrine. In 2012, the FDA approved a new diet drug called phentermine/topiramate (Qsymia). Qsymia is believed to be a potent drug to treat obesity, however, concerns about heart and birth defect risks have been raised in conjunction with this medication. Both phentermine (an appetite suppressant) and topiramate (an anticonvulsant) are separately available on the market.

Diethylpropion (Tenuate) is another drug that stimulates the release of norepinephrine, which in turn activates hypothalamic centers to decrease appetite and food intake. This drug is recommended only for obese patients with a BMI of 30 or greater and for patients with a BMI of 27 or greater who also have other risk factors such as hypertension, diabetes, or dyslipidemia. Fluoxetine (Prozac), a selective serotonin-reuptake inhibitor (SSRI), has also been prescribed as an appetite-suppressing agent (60 mg, as opposed to 20 mg that is used to treat depression).

Drug therapy should be implemented along with diet, exercise, and lifestyle modifications in patients with obesity. However, the roles of drugs in reducing weight have been questioned due to the efficacy and safety concerns associated with these agents. For this reason, clinicians should always carefully evaluate the risks and benefits when considering drug therapy for their patients with obesity.

As mentioned in the *Introduction to Biochemistry* chapter, there are two major types of adipose tissue: white and brown adipose tissue. While the major roles of the white adipose tissue are to synthesize, store, and release lipids, the major role of the brown adipose tissue is to dissipate energy through an uncoupled mitochondrial respiration process to generate heat. Initially, it was believed that the brown adipose tissue was exclusively found in infants, but this tissue is now known to exist in adults as well.

Central obesity is often considered as a factor in the diagnosis of insulin resistance (diabetes type 2), hypertension, dyslipidemia, and cardiovascular disease. Central obesity, or "metabolic syndrome," refers to the fat that is concentrated on the abdomen and upper body in an individual. While the amount of intra-abdominal fat is best estimated by computed tomography (CT) and magnetic resonance imaging (MRI), it can also be estimated by measuring the waist circumference (WC). A high-risk WC is defined as greater than 102 cm in men and greater than 89 cm in women.

Hypertension and heart failure are associated with obesity. The cause of hypertension in obese patients has been associated with thickening of the ventricular wall, ischemia, and increased heart volume. Sleep apnea has also been associated with obesity. While the exact mechanism is not known, weight loss has been shown to significantly improve sleep apnea. There are indications that insulin resistance is associated with obesity. A growing body of evidence suggests that bariatric surgery may assist patients with type 2 diabetes to manage their diabetic complications.

The amount of adiponectin (an anti-inflammatory cytokine) appears to be low and the amount of resistin hormone high in individuals with obesity. While adiponectin inhibits gluconeogenesis in hapatocytes and increases glucose transport and fatty acid oxidation in myocytes, resistin hormone blocks the action of insulin.

Perhaps the best method to treat obesity is to encourage patients to lose weight and implement a weight management process by a balanced dietary intervention, exercise, changing eating practices, reduced caloric intake, and/or surgical intervention. An initial 5–10% weight loss is an ideal goal for most obese patients. The national guidelines recommend a weight-loss goal for adults to be 10% of the initial weight over 6 months.

Learning Bridge 14.7

While you are in a hospital to complete your summer experiential program, Eva, a 71-year-old retired bank clerk, is admitted to the hospital with severe muscular weakness. Her record indicates that she is currently using a large amount of a bulk laxative agent on a daily basis and takes a thiazide agent for mild hypertension. Her serum sample reveals low T_3 and T_4 hormones, a potassium concentration of 2.30 mEq/L, and an HCO_3^- concentration of 19 mEq/L. The pH of her blood is 7.37 and the pH of her urine is 4.7.

A. Why does Eva have constipation, and for how long she should use the laxative agent?
B. Why is the pH high in her blood and low in her urine?
C. Has Eva developed an acid–base disorder? Why?
D. What would you suggest to Eva and her physician to help Eva with her medical conditions?

Learning Bridge 14.8

Amy is a 23-year-old cashier who works for the Portlander Theater in Portland, Oregon. She comes to your pharmacy to receive her refill of Qsymia (phentermine 7.5 mg/topiramate 46 mg), which she has been using during the last 2 months to lose weight. Amy tells you that she feels good about her medication and that she has lost 5% of her total body weight since she began using Qsymia. However, she mentions that each time she eats fast food, she has pain in the upper-right portion of her abdomen and feels bloating.

Her symptoms remind you of gallstones. After a short discussion with Amy, you perform a drug utilization review (DUR) and notice that Amy is also using an OTC product, Pepcid Complete, for treatment of her heartburn. In addition, her medical record indicates that Amy has a BMI of 35 kg/m².

A. Identify the cause for gallstones in this patient.
B. Do you have any suggestion in regard to Amy's medications?
C. If laboratory data confirm that Amy has gallstones, which drug(s) would you suggest to her provider to prescribe to treat her gallstones? Why?

Golden Keys for Pharmacy Students

1. Three important organs play crucial roles in processing and absorbing nutrients by producing enzymes or hormones: the small intestine, the liver, and the pancreas.

2. Approximately 50% of the body's cholesterol is used to synthesize bile acids in the hepatic peroxisomes. The storage site for bile acids is not the liver, but rather the gallbladder.

3. The average energy intake is about 1,900 and 2,600 kcal/day for women and men, respectively.

4. While fats have the highest energy content (9 kcal/g), carbohydrates and proteins both provide 4 kcal/g.

5. Fiber does not provide any energy, but it reduces cholesterol levels, the risk of colon cancer, and the risk of cardiovascular disease.

6. Linolenic acid (omega-3 fatty acid) and linoleic acid (omega-6 fatty acid) are crucial for the synthesis of arachidonic acid, which in turn is important for the synthesis of eicosanoids.

7. Trans fatty acids may compete with essential fatty acids and cause essential fatty acid deficiency.

8. Generally, proteins from animal sources (such as meat, eggs, and milk) are rich in essential amino acids, whereas proteins from plant sources (such as cereal, rice, wheat, and corn) are low in essential amino acids.

9. Single-vitamin deficiency is usually common in populations that eat a restricted diet.

10. Isoniazid is used in the treatment of tuberculosis. It can bind to pyridoxal phosphate and induce a vitamin B_6 deficiency.

11. One of the most common vitamin deficiencies in the United States is folic acid deficiency.

12. To prevent neural tube defects (NTDs) in their offspring, females of childbearing potential require less than 1 mg of folic acid on a daily basis (0.4–0.8 mg/day). This amount is increased to 4 mg/day for females at high risk of NTDs.

13. Cobalamin (vitamin B_{12}), together with folic acid, is important for the synthesis of S-adenosylmethionine (SAMe), which in turn is important in the synthesis of DNA and promotes myelination of nerve fibers.

14. Cobalamin cannot be synthesized by plants or animals, but rather is produced only by microorganisms.

15. Vitamin C is critical for biosynthesis of collagen; it serves as a coenzyme for the hydroxylase enzymes that hydroxylate lysine and proline residues in the collagen, and is important in wound healing and bone formation.

16. Calcitriol is secreted by the kidneys into the circulation and works as a hormone to regulate Ca^{2+} uptake in the intestines, bones, and kidneys.

17. Vitamin D is important for the reabsorption of calcium. When the body experiences hypocalcemia, the parathyroid gland releases PTH. PTH increases release of Ca^{2+} from the bones. Some of the freed Ca^{2+} stimulates the kidneys to activate vitamin D, which in turn stimulates the intestines to absorb Ca^{2+}.

18. The concentrations of dissolved molecules in body fluids (e.g., proteins, glucose, urea) are measured in units of mg/dL. The concentrations of electrolytes in the body fluids and in intravenous solutions are often expressed in units of mEq/L.

19. Because calcium carbonate is a basic supplement, it needs the stomach's acidity to ensure its optimal absorption. As a result, it needs to be taken with foods.

20. There are two forms of irons: ferric (Fe^{3+}) and ferrous (F^{2+}). While ferric iron is the oxidized form, ferrous iron is the reduced form. Iron, in the ferrous form, is absorbed in mammals.

21. The most widely administered iron supplements in the United States are ferrous sulfate (Feosol, 325 mg) with 20% elemental iron, ferrous gluconate (Fergon, 300 g) with 12% elemental iron, and ferrous fumarate (Femniron, 300 mg) with 33% elemental iron.

22. Potassium (K^+) is the major intracellular cation; it is essential for excitability of nerve cells and for muscle functions.

23. Although hyperkalemia is less common than hypokalemia, it has a severe effect on the heart and can be a deadly electrolyte disorder that arises without warning.

24. Because insulin causes hypokalemia, insulin is used to treat hyperkalemia.

25. Because the volume of the ICF is greater than the volume of the ECF, measurement of phosphate in the ECF does not accurately represent phosphate availability in the ICF.

26. Bicarbonate plays an important role in maintaining the physiologic buffer systems.

27. Hyperventilation and hypoventilation result in alkalosis and acidosis, respectively.

28. Metabolic acidosis is caused by a loss of HCO_3^- or a gain of acid.

29. Metabolic alkalosis is caused by a loss of H^+ or a gain of HCO_3^-.

30. Respiratory acidosis occurs when lungs cannot adequately expel carbon dioxide, which results in an accumulation of hydrogen ions that consequently reduces the pH of the blood.

31. If the cations and anions are not equal in the plasma, the imbalance is referred to as an anion gap; its normal value is 7 ± 4 mEq/L.

32. Obesity occurs as a result of an imbalance between energy intake and energy expenditure, marked by increased energy storage.

33. When metabolic acidosis occurs with an increased anion gap, toxic alcohol poisoning should be suspected.

34. Body mass index (BMI) is used to differentiate between overweight and obesity.

Learning Bridge Answers

14.1 **A.** Thiamin (vitamin B_1) deficiency is known to cause infantile beriberi.

B. Thiamine is essential to produce acetyl-CoA. A lack of thiamine results in the following effects:

- A slow citric acid cycle (low ATP/energy), which affects the brain
- A high pyruvate concentration (lactic acidosis)
- A slow pentose phosphate pathway, which affects nucleic acid synthesis

C. A high level of pyruvate in the blood suggests a deficiency in the mitochondrial pyruvate dehydrogenase complex, which catalyzes the conversion of pyruvate to acetyl-CoA. If pyruvate accumulates, the level of lactate becomes high as well, because lactate is synthesized from pyruvate by the enzyme known as lactate dehydrogenase.

D. Thiamine should initially have been included in the formula. A lack of thiamine causes irreversible brain damage, so providing thiamine to children a few years after the incident would not have helped remedy their symptoms.

E. The RDIs are 1.1 mg/day, 1.2 mg/day, and 1.4 mg/day for females, males, and pregnant females, respectively.

14.2 A. David's vitamin B_{12} level is normal, so he is suffering from folic acid deficiency. Folic acid is required for the biosynthesis of the amino acid glycine. Glycine, in turn, is important for the synthesis of heme. A lack of heme results in a low amount of hemoglobin—a finding confirmed by the measurement of the amount of hemoglobin in David's erythrocytes.

B. Folic acid is important in the synthesis of DNA as well. Cells that are inefficient in synthesizing DNA are nondividing cells, which explains the enlarged erythroid precursor cells (macrocytosis).

C. Do not recommend a high level of multivitamin ingestion because of the risk for vitamin A toxicity. Instead, the best treatment for David is 0.8–1 mg/day of single folic acid (vitamin B_9) for 4 months (to clear all vitamin B_9–deficient erythrocytes from the circulation). High doses of folic acid, such as 0.8–1 mg, require a prescription.

D. The DRIs are 0.4 mg/day for females and males and 0.8 mg/day for pregnant women. Children older than 4 years receive the same doses as adults.

14.3 A. There are two doses because Sinemet includes two agents: levodopa (50 mg) and carbidopa (200 mg). Levodopa is converted to dopamine in the peripheral tissue. However, this synthesized dopamine (a polar molecule) cannot cross the blood–brain barrier, but rather is metabolized in the peripheral tissue. Carbidopa inhibits the peripheral aromatic amino acid decarboxylase enzyme that is responsible for peripheral conversion of levodopa to dopamine. This inhibition reduces the synthesis of dopamine in the peripheral tissue and allows more of the levodopa to reach the brain. In the brain, levodopa is converted to dopamine.

B. Vitamin B_6 is a precursor to PLP (pyridoxal phosphate). PLP is required by the decarboxylase enzyme, which converts levodopa to dopamine; in other words, vitamin B_6 counteracts the effects of carbidopa. When carbidopa and levodopa are combined, however, the counter-effect of vitamin B_6 is minimal. In contrast, an iron supplement reduces the absorption of levodopa because iron chelates levodopa, thereby reducing levodopa's absorption by 50%. Vitamin B_6 should be an acceptable choice, but suggest that the patient avoid the iron supplement unless it is truly necessary to use iron (in which case it may be necessary to increase the doses).

C. Food, particularly protein-rich food, delays absorption of levodopa. System L (a specific transport system in the CNS) is saturated with high plasma concentrations of amino acids generated from a protein-rich meal. Therefore, the patient should take his medication at least 1 hour before a meal.

14.4 A. Raw eggs contain a significant amount of the protein called avidin. Avidin has a very high affinity for biotin (vitamin B_7). As a result, Joe has developed biotin deficiency—a condition that his symptoms match well.

B. The avidin from the raw eggs sequesters biotin. Biotin is necessary for a few enzymes that are involved in biochemical reactions that provide energy. For instance, it is important for the enzyme pyruvate carboxylase to be active. A lower activity of the pyruvate carboxylase results in lower rates of gluconeogenesis and glyceroneogenesis. Consequently, it is likely that the patient is experiencing a buildup of pyruvate, which in turn can be converted to lactic acid—an outcome that could explain his muscle pain during exercise. In addition, biotin is important in the metabolism of odd-numbered fatty acids and essential amino acids such as methionine, threonine, valine, and isoleucine to synthesize succinyl-CoA. The last molecule is important in the citric acid cycle to generate NADH and $FADH_2$. These two electron carrier coenzymes provide ATP molecules during oxidative phosphorylation. A low rate of ATP production leads to difficulty concentrating and a lack of energy. Furthermore, biotin is important for the acetyl-CoA carboxylase enzyme, which converts acetyl-CoA to malonyl-CoA to synthesize fatty acids.

C. Suggest biotin (vitamin H) supplement to Joe, 5 mg/day for 2 weeks. In addition, advise him to stop eating raw eggs.

D. Ask Joe to see a physician to check his serum lactic acid as well.

14.5 As an intern pharmacist, just by looking at the structure of vitamin E, you should be able to tell how it works as an antioxidant (see Figure 14.16). Vitamin E has a hydroxyl group that prevents oxidation by donating a hydrogen atom to the free radicals. Humans have the capacity to store 3–8 g vitamin E in their adipose tissue—an amount sufficient to meet the body's requirements for at least 4 years during a vitamin E–deficient diet. Thus the patient's Alzheimer's disease cannot be attributed to a vitamin E deficiency. Vitamin E is a fat-soluble vitamin and is found in vegetable oils, cereal grains, animal fats, meat, eggs, and fruits.

14.6 A. Recall that most electrolyte solutions are ordered in concentrations of mEq/L. The exception is potassium phosphate. Because the phosphate injection contains a mixture of phosphate salts (monobasic potassium phosphate, KH_2PO_4, and dipotassium phosphate, K_2HPO_4), it is more convenient to express the concentration of phosphate in mM or mmol/L units. Tell the physician that to avoid a medication error, the physician should give the phosphate concentration in mM than in mEq/L. Alternatively, convert 20 mEq/L to mM.

B. The underlying mechanisms of hypophosphatemia are as follows:

- Reduced intestinal phosphate absorption, often caused by fasting or starvation or in the presence of aluminum hydroxide antacids.
- Increased renal phosphate excretion.
- Reduced renal phosphate absorption (by diuretics or a few toxins).
- Rapid influx of phosphate from the ECF into bone or soft tissue. This type of hypophosphatemia often occurs in hospitalized patients when insulin therapy is required (such as in the treatment of DKA), with administration of IV glucose without other nutrients, with high release of catecholamines (endogenous or exogenous), and during respiratory alkalosis.
- Low levels of serum calcitonin and calcium.

C. Water for injection USP is a purified water that is pyrogen free and has been prepared by distillation or reverse osmosis (the reverse osmosis effectively removes viruses and bacteria). This ready-made water needs to be added under aseptic techniques in an appropriate laminar flow hood.

14.7 A. Eva's constipation is most likely caused by hypothyroidism. Suggest that her physician prescribe levothyroxine (T_4), which may alleviate her need for a laxative agent.

B. Eva's serum potassium is low and she has hypokalemia. Thiazide diuretics cause potassium depletion. The sodium–potassium exchange mechanism in the renal tubule cells exchanges H^+ (rather than K^+) for Na^+. This phenomenon explains why the patient's urine is acidic. This mechanism is common among patients who take diuretic therapies, particularly loop and thiazide diuretics, because of over-excretion of potassium in the urine. In addition, a loss of H^+ in a potassium-deficient patient increases the serum concentration of HCO_3^-, which explains why her blood is alkalotic.

C. To determine the patient's acid–base disorder, one needs to look at the serum analysis of her cation and anion electrolytes. Her bicarbonate concentration is lower than normal, which is an indication of metabolic alkalosis. Her anion gap analysis is normal, which means there is no anion toxicity.

D. The laxative and thiazide agents most likely are the key factors contributing to her metabolic alkalosis and hypokalemia. A potassium supplement is a good choice to prescribe when diuretics (e.g., thiazides) are prescribed. Keep in mind that hypokalemia can lead to end-stage renal disease in patients with chronic hypokalemia because of eating disorders or laxative abuse. Consequently, it is critical (particularly in elderly patients) to treat hypokalemia immediately. Alternatively, Eva's physician can switch her thiazide diuretic to a potassium-sparing diuretic agent or another appropriate hypertensive agent. In addition, lifestyle and dietary modifications, such as regular daily fiber intake of 20–25 g/day, can help with her constipation problem.

14.8 A. Amy's BMI indicates that she is obese; obese individuals who are experiencing rapid weight loss may develop gallstones. Both Amy's symptoms and her rapid loss of 5% of her body weight are indicative of gallstones. Gallstones block the gallbladder and inhibit the flow of bile acids.

B. Qsymia includes both phentermine and topiramate; phentermine's role is to release norepinephrine, similar to the action of amphetamine. Antacids are known to decrease the excretion of amphetamines and amphetamine-like molecules (such as phentermine). This may also explain the rapid weight-loss effect of Qsymia. Ask Amy to stop taking antacids to avoid any drug interaction with phentermine.

C. Ursodiol (Actigall) is effective in the treatment of gallstones. Ursodiol is a bile acid that will help Amy replace the lack of her endogenous bile acids and thereby improve her lipid metabolism until she produces her own bile acids.

Problems and Solutions

Problem 14.1 Which of the following digestive enzymes is used to facilitate digestions of foods?

A. α-Amylase, hydroxylase, reductase, and lactase
B. α-Amylase, pepsinogen, lipase, and lactase
C. Reductase, pepsinogen, enteropeptidase, and lactase
D. Enteropeptidase, lactase, carboxylase, and lipase

Solution 14.1 B is correct. Humans produce digestive enzymes from the salivary glands (α-amylase), gastric glands (pepsinogen), pancreas (lipase), and intestinal glands (lactase) to facilitate digestion of foods.

Problem 14.2 Calculate REE for a moderately active man with a body weight of 80 kg.

Solution 14.2 REE: $900 + 10 \times$ weight (kg). The calculated REE is multiplied by 1.2 for a sedentary individual (no exercise), by 1.4 for a moderately active individual, and by 1.8 for a very active individual.

$$[(900 + 10 \times 80) \times 1.4] = 2{,}380 \text{ kcal/day}$$

Problem 14.3 Why does a patient with hyperthyroidism have a high BMR?

Solution 14.3 The patient produces too much of thyroid hormones that over-express the genes that control the citric acid cycle and oxidative phosphorylation pathways, which ultimately results in a higher metabolic rate.

Problem 14.4 Which of the following roles do lipids *not* play in the body?

A. Facilitate absorption and storage of lipid-soluble vitamins (A, D, E, and K)
B. Provide precursors for steroids and bile salts
C. Provide precursors for arachidonic acids and eicosanoids
D. Provide glucose upon β-oxidation of fatty acids

Solution 14.4 D is correct. Humans are unable to convert fatty acids to glucose, but we can produce fatty acids from glucose.

Problem 14.5 Which of the following statements about the OTC product Lovaza is correct?

A. Each 1-g capsule contains docosahexaenoic acid (DHA) and eicosapentaenoic acid (EPA), which are linolenic acid derivatives.
B. Each 1-g capsule contains both linoleic acid and linolenic acid.
C. Each 1-g capsule contains essential fatty acids and phospholipids.
D. Each 1-g capsule contains essential fatty acids and at least one cholesterol-reducing agent.

Solution 14.5 A is correct. Omega-3 acid ethyl esters (fish oil) in the form of Lovaza are available in the U.S. market. Each 1 g capsule contains 375 mg DHA and 465 mg EPA.

Problem 14.6 Which of the following statements about water is incorrect?

A. While TBW accounts for 60% of total body weight in men, it accounts for 50% of total body weight in women.
B. Two-thirds of TBW is located in the intracellular compartment, also called the intracellular fluid volume (ICFV).
C. Interstitial fluid makes up approximately half of the ECFV.
D. The plasma makes up approximately one-fourth of the ECFV.

Solution 14.6 C is correct. TBW accounts for 60% of men's body weight and 50% of women's body weight (because women have more fat than men). Interstitial fluid makes up approximately three-fourths of the ECFV.

Problem 14.7 Which vitamin is important for the synthesis of the glycine amino acid and DNA?

Solution 14.7 Folic acid (vitamin B_9).

Problem 14.8 Which of the following water-soluble vitamins is inactivated by high temperature (cooking) and high pH?

A. Thiamine (B_1)
B. Riboflavin (B_2)

C. Niacin (B$_3$)

D. Pantothenic acid (B$_5$)

E. Biotin (B$_7$)

Solution 14.8 A is correct.

Problem 14.9 Which of the following vitamin deficiencies results in retarded growth and pellagra?

A. Thiamine (B$_1$)

B. Riboflavin (B$_2$)

C. Niacin (B$_3$)

D. Pantothenic acid (B$_5$)

E. Biotin (B$_7$)

Solution 14.9 C is correct. Pellagra is characterized by a photosensitive dermatitis, diarrhea, and dementia.

Problem 14.10 Which of the following vitamins provides PLP, which is a required prosthetic group for all of the aminotransferase enzymes that are involved in the amino acid oxidation?

A. Thiamine (B$_1$)

B. Riboflavin (B$_2$)

C. Niacin (B$_3$)

D. Pantothenic acid (B$_5$)

E. Pyridoxine (B$_6$)

Solution 14.10 E is correct.

Problem 14.11 Which of the following fat-soluble vitamins is important for carboxylation of pro-thrombin to promote the blood coagulation cascade?

A. Vitamin A

B. Vitamin D

C. Vitamin E

D. Vitamin K

Solution 14.11 D is correct.

Problem 14.12 Which of the following hormones is secreted by the kidneys into the circulation to regulate Ca^{2+} uptake in the intestines, bones, and kidneys?

A. Vitamin A

B. Vitamin D

C. Vitamin E

D. Vitamin K

Solution 14.12 B is correct. 1,25-Dihydroxyvitamin D (calcitriol) is secreted by the kidneys into the circulation to serve as a hormone to regulate Ca^{2+} uptake in the intestines, bones, and kidneys.

Problem 14.13 Which of the following conditions leads to metabolic acidosis?

A. When the serum bicarbonate concentration is increased and the pH of the blood is reduced

B. When the serum bicarbonate concentration and the pH of the blood are reduced

   C. When the serum CO_2 concentration and the pH of the blood are reduced
   D. When the serum bicarbonate and serum CO_2 concentrations are increased

Solution 14.13 B is correct. Metabolic acidosis has two origins: (1) a loss of HCO_3^-, which can result from gastrointestinal loss (diarrhea and small bowel drainage), and (2) a gain of acid, which can result from endogenous H^+ production.

Problem 14.14 Which of the following conditions leads to metabolic alkalosis?

   A. When the serum bicarbonate concentration and the pH of the blood are increased
   B. When the serum bicarbonate concentration and the pH of the blood are reduced
   C. When the serum CO_2 concentration and the pH of the blood are reduced
   D. When the serum bicarbonate and CO_2 concentrations are increased

Solution 14.14 A is correct. Metabolic alkalosis has two origins: (1) a loss of H^+ or a gain of HCO_3^-, such as from excessive use of $NaHCO_3$ (baking soda, a common remedy for upset stomach), a loss of H^+ in vomiting, or a loss of H^+ in a potassium-deficient patient, and (2) an abnormal retention of HCO_3^-.

Problem 14.15 Joe Smith is a bank clerk in Washington County, Oregon. In his recent medical examination (2 weeks ago), he reacted positively to a tuberculosis skin test. He was immediately placed on prophylactic isoniazid, 300 mg/day. During the last 4 days, Joe has developed two seizures. Which vitamin deficiency has caused his seizures and a loss of memory?

Solution 14.15 Vitamin B_6; isoniazid is known to sequester PLP.

Problem 14.16 Why does a hepatocyte have a large number of mitochondria?

Solution 14.16 The liver plays a central role in the biosynthesis and metabolism of many molecules. As a result, the liver needs many ATP molecules to perform its functions.

Problem 14.17 Prepare a 1 liter intravenous dextrose solution that includes 1 mg/mL elemental calcium. You have access to calcium carbonate.

Solution 14.17 Calcium carbonate contains 40% elemental calcium. We need 1,000 mg calcium to make the 1 mg/mL solution; thus we need 2.5 g calcium carbonate ($2,500 \text{ mg} \times 0.4 = 1,000 \text{ mg}$).

Problem 14.18 Calculate the amount of sodium (Na^+) in ECF for a woman who weighs 60 kg. The normal sodium concentration is approximately 140 mEq/L.

Solution 14.18 First calculate the TBW which is $60 \text{ kg} \times 0.5 = 30$ L. Out of this volume, one-third is the ECFV—that is, 10 L. The normal sodium concentration is approximately 140 mEq/L. Thus the amount of sodium, for this woman, in her ECF is 1,400 mEq or 1.4 Eq.

Problem 14.19 Which of the following statements related to the daily food intake is false?

   A. Individuals should decrease their consumption of saturated fats.
   B. Individuals should increase their consumption of polyunsaturated fats.
   C. Individuals should increase their fiber consumption to 20–35 g/day.
   D. Individuals should have no more than 40% of their total intake in the form of fat consumption.

Solution 14.19 D is false; fat consumption should be no more than 30% of the total dietary intake.

Problem 14.20 A patient comes to your pharmacy with a prescription for methotrexate (Rheumatrex), 7.5 mg once a week. Which of the following vitamins is the patient recommended to take as well?

A. Thiamine (B_1)
B. Folic acid (B_9)
C. Niacin (B_3)
D. Pantothenic acid (B_5)
E. Biotin (B_7)

Solution 14.20 B is correct. Methotrexate irreversibly inhibits dihydrofolate reductase enzyme and can cause folic acid deficiency. Dihydrofolate reductase plays a major role in the synthesis of tetrahydrofolate (THF), which is the active form of folic acid.

References

1. Ahearn GA. Absorption (biology). In: *AccessScience*. New York, NY: McGraw-Hill; 2012. Available at: http://www.accessscience.com.

2. Amanzadeh J, Reilly RF. Hypophosphatemia: an evidence-based approach to its clinical consequences and management. *Nat Clin Pract Nephrol*. 2006:2:136–148.

3. Bender DA, Mayes PA. Micronutrients: vitamins and minerals. In: Murray RK, Kennelly PJ, Rodwell VW, et al., eds. *Harper's illustrated biochemistry*, 28th ed. New York, NY: McGraw-Hill; 2009. Available at: http://www.accesspharmacy.com/content.aspx?aID=5229785, 2009.

4. Bender DA, Mayes PA. Nutrition, digestion, and absorption. In: Murray RK, Kennelly PJ, Rodwell VW, et al., eds. *Harper's illustrated biochemistry*, 28th ed. New York, NY: McGraw-Hill; 2009. Available at: http://www.accesspharmacy.com/content.aspx?aID=5229716.

5. Borja-Hart N, Whalen KL. Interpretation of clinical laboratory data. In: Kier KL, Nemire RE, eds. *Pharmacy student survival guide*, 2nd ed. New York, NY: McGraw-Hill; 2009. Available at: http://www.accesspharmacy.com/content.aspx?aID=5257616.

6. Braen GR, Joshi P. Vitamins and herbals. In: Tintinalli JE, Stapczynski JS, Cline DM, et al., eds. *Tintinalli's emergency medicine: a comprehensive study guide*, 7th ed. New York, NY: McGraw-Hill 2011. Available at: http://www.accessmedicine.com/content.aspx?aID=6378672.

7. Bringhurst FR, Demay MB, Krane SM, Kronenberg HM. Bone and mineral metabolism in health and disease. In: Longo DL, Kasper DL, Jameson JL, et al., eds. *Harrison's principles of internal medicine*, 18th ed. New York, NY: McGraw-Hill; 2012. Available at: http://www.accesspharmacy.com/content.aspx?aID=9142739.

8. Cantilena LR Jr. Clinical toxicology. In: Cantilena LR Jr., ed. *Casarett & Doull's essentials of toxicology*, 2nd ed. New York, NY: McGraw-Hill; 2012. Available at: http://www.accesspharmacy.com/content.aspx?aID=6487627.

9. Chen JT, Sheehan AH, Yanovski JA, Calis KA. Obesity. In: DiPiro JT, Talbert RL, Yee GC, et al., eds. *Pharmacotherapy: a pathophysiologic approach*, 8th ed. New York, NY: McGraw-Hill; 2011. Available at: http://www.accesspharmacy.com/content.aspx?aID=8013538.

10. Chessman KH, Kumpf VJ. Assessment of nutrition status and nutrition requirements. In: DiPiro JT, Talbert RL, Yee GC, et al., eds. *Pharmacotherapy: a pathophysiologic approach*, 8th ed. New York, NY: McGraw-Hill; 2011. Available at: http://www.accesspharmacy.com/content.aspx?aID=8011919.

11. Dominguez C, Gartner S, Linan S, et al. Enhanced oxidative damage in cystic fibrosis patients. *Biofactors*. 1998;8:149–153.

12. Dwyer J. Nutrient requirements and dietary assessment. In: Longo DL, Kasper DL, Jameson JL, et al., eds. *Harrison's principles of internal medicine*, 18th ed. New York, NY: McGraw-Hill; 2012. Available at: http://www.accesspharmacy.com/content.aspx?aID=9099636.

13. Ellison DH. Core curriculum in nephrology: disorders of sodium and water. *Am J Kidney Dis*. 2005;46:356–361.

14. Findling RL, Maxwell K, Scotese-Wojtila L, et al. High-dose pyridoxine and magnesium administration in children with autistic disorder: an absence of salutary effects in a double-blind, placebo-controlled study. *J Autism Dev Disord*. 1997;27:467–478.

15. Flomenbaum NE. Salicylates. In: Flomenbaum NE, ed. *Goldfrank's toxicologic emergencies*, 9th ed. New York, NY: McGraw-Hill; 2011. Available at: http://www.accesspharmacy.com/content.aspx?aID=6510436.

16. Friedman PA. Agents affecting mineral ion homeostasis and bone turnover. In: Friedman PA, ed. *Goodman & Gilman's the pharmacological basis of therapeutics*, 12th ed. New York, NY: McGraw-Hill; 2011. Available at: http://www.accesspharmacy.com/content.aspx?aID=16674741.

17. Gabow PA, Kaehny WD, Fennessey PV, et al. Diagnostic importance of an increased serum anion gap. *N Engl J Med*. 1980;303:854–858.

18. Ginsburg BY. Vitamins. In: Ginsburg BY, ed. *Goldfrank's toxicologic emergencies*, 9th ed. New York, NY: McGraw-Hill; 2011. Available at: http://www.accesspharmacy.com/content.aspx?aID=6511992.

19. Gourley DR, Eoff JC. *The APhA complete review for pharmacy*, 9th ed. Washington, DC: APhA. 2012.

20. Hall GD and Reiss BS. *Appleton & Lange's review of pharmacy*, 2nd ed. New York, NY: McGraw-Hill; 2001.

21. Haluzik M, Parizkova J, Haluzik MM. Adiponectin and its role in the obesity-induced insulin resistance and related complications. *Physiol. Res.* 2004;53:123–129.

22. Henness S, Perry CM. Orlistat: a review of its use in the management of obesity. *Drugs*. 2006;66(12):1625–1656.

23. Hoffman RS. Antidotes in depth (A25): thiamine hydrochloride. In: Hoffman RS, ed. *Goldfrank's toxicologic emergencies*, 9th ed. New York, NY: McGraw-Hill; 2011. Available at: http://www.accesspharmacy.com/content.aspx?aID=6537739.

24. Hoffman RS, Charney AN. Fluid, electrolyte, and acid–base principles. In: Hoffman RS, Charney AN, eds. *Goldfrank's toxicologic emergencies*, 9th ed. New York, NY: McGraw-Hill; 2011. Available at: http://www.accesspharmacy.com/content.aspx?aID=6505554.

25. Hudson JQ. Chronic kidney disease: management of complications. In: DiPiro JT, Talbert RL, Yee GC, et al., eds. *Pharmacotherapy: a pathophysiologic approach*, 8th ed. New York, NY: McGraw-Hill; 2011. Available at: http://www.accesspharmacy.com/content.aspx?aID=7981679.

26. Jones KM, Neill KK, Warmack TS. Electrolyte disorders. In: Jones KM, Neill KK, Warmack TS, eds. *McGraw-Hill's NAPLEX® review guide*. New York, NY: McGraw-Hill; 2011. Available at: http://www.accesspharmacy.com/content.aspx?aID=7252925.

27. Kallet RH, Jasmer RM, Luce JM, et al. The treatment of acidosis in acute lung injury with trishydroxymethyl aminomethane (THAM). *Am J Respir Crit Care Med*. 2000;161(4 Pt 1):1149–1153.

28. Karimi R, Brumfield T, Brumfield F, et al. Zellweger syndrome: a genetic disorder that alters lipid biosynthesis and metabolism. *Internet J Pharmacol*. 2007;5:1.

29. Kaushansky K, Kipps TJ. Hematopoietic agents: growth factors, minerals, and vitamins. In: Kaushansky K, Kipps TJ, eds. *Goodman & Gilman's the pharmacological basis of therapeutics*, 12th ed. New York, NY: McGraw-Hill; 2011. Available at: http://www.accesspharmacy.com/content.aspx?aID=16672174.

30. Klein BP. Food. In: *AccessScience*. New York, NY: McGraw-Hill; 2008. Available at: http://www.accessscience.com, 2008.

31. Kolasinski SL. Complementary and alternative therapies. In: Imboden JB, Hellmann DB, Stone JH, eds. *Current rheumatology diagnosis & treatment*, 2nd ed. New York, NY: McGraw-Hill; 2007. Available at: http://www.accessmedicine.com/content.aspx?aID=2730173.

32. Kowalski TE, Falestiny M, Furth E, Malet PF. Vitamin A hepatotoxicity: a cautionary note regarding 25,000 IU supplements. *Am J Med*. 1994;97:523–528.

33. Krebs NF, Primak LE, Haemer M. Normal childhood nutrition and its disorders. In: Hay WW, Levin MJ, Sondheimer JM, Deterding RR, eds. *Current diagnosis & treatment: pediatrics*, 20th ed. New York, NY: McGraw-Hill; 2012. Available at: http://www.accessmedicine.com/content.aspx?aID=6578685.

34. Kris-Etherton PM, Harris WS, Appel LJ. Fish consumption, fish oil, omega-3 fatty acids, and cardiovascular disease. *Circulation*. 2002;106:2747–2757.

35. Lee M. *Basic skills in interpreting laboratory data*, 4th ed. Bethesda, MD: ASHP; 2009.

36. Lee S, Lee G, Turner M. *BrainChip for biochemistry*. Williston, VT: Blackwell; 2002.

37. Lee YS. The role of genes in the current obesity epidemic. *Ann Acad Med Singapore*. 2009;38(1):45–43.

38. Lerner V, Miodownik C, Kaptsan A, et al. Vitamin B_6 as add-on treatment in chronic schizophrenic and schizoaffective patients: a double-blind, placebo-controlled study. *J Clin Psychiatry*. 2002;63:54–58.

39. Majlesi N. Zinc. In: Majlesi N, ed. *Goldfrank's toxicologic emergencies*, 9th ed. New York, NY: McGraw-Hill; 2011. Available at: http://www.accesspharmacy.com/content.aspx?aID=6526245.

40. Marshall WJ, Bangert SK. Hydrogen ion homoeostasis and blood gases. In: *Clinical chemistry*, 5th ed. Edinburgh, UK: Elsevier Health Sciences; 2004.

41. Matzke GR. Acid–base disorders. In: DiPiro JT, Talbert RL, Yee GC, et al., eds. *Pharmacotherapy: a pathophysiologic approach*, 8th ed. New York, NY: McGraw-Hill; 2011. Available at: http://www.accesspharmacy.com/content.aspx?aID=7984321.

42. Meacham S, Grayscott D, Chen JJ, et al. Review of the dietary reference intake for calcium: where do we go from here? *Crit Rev Food Sci Nutr*. 2008;48:378–384.

43. Mount DB. Fluid and electrolyte disturbances. In: Longo DL, Kasper DL, Jameson JL, et al., eds. *Harrison's principles of internal medicine*, 18th ed. New York, NY: McGraw-Hill; 2012. Available at: http://www.accesspharmacy.com/content.aspx?aID=9097635.

44. Murray RK, Grossc PL. Biochemical case histories. In: Murray RK, Kennelly PJ, Rodwell VW, et al., eds. *Harper's illustrated biochemistry*, 29th ed. New York, NY: McGraw-Hill; 2011. Available at: http://www.accesspharmacy.com/content.aspx?aID=55887347.

45. Nagai K, Hosaka H, Kubo S, et al. Vitamin A toxity secondary to excessive intake of yellow-green vegetables, liver and laver. *J Hepatol*. 1999;31:142–148.

46. Nelson DL, Cox MM. *Lehninger principle of biochemistry*, 5th ed. New York, NY: W. H. Freeman; 2008.

47. Nicolaou DD, Kelen GD. Acid–base disorders. In: Tintinalli JE, Stapczynski JS, Cline DM, et al., eds. *Tintinalli's emergency medicine: a comprehensive study guide*, 7th ed. New York, NY: McGraw-Hill; 2011. Available at: http://www.accessmedicine.com/content.aspx?aID=6353829.

48. Obesity gene map database. Human Genomics Laboratory. Available at: http://obesitygene .pbrc.edu/.

49. O'Connell MB, Vondracek SF. Osteoporosis and other metabolic bone diseases. In: DiPiro JT, Talbert RL, Yee GC, et al., eds. *Pharmacotherapy: a pathophysiologic approach*, 8th ed. New York, NY: McGraw-Hill; 2011. Available at: http://www.accesspharmacy.com/content .aspx?aID=7996689.

50. Office of Dietary Supplements, National Institutes in Health. Available at: http://ods.od.nih.gov .proxy.lib.pacificu.edu:2048/. Accessed November 2012.

51. Ouellette RJ. *Introduction to general, organic and biological chemistry*. 4th ed. Upper Saddle River, NJ: Prentice Hall; 1997.

52. Pai AB. Disorders of calcium and phosphorus homeostasis. In: DiPiro JT, Talbert RL, Yee GC, et al., eds. *Pharmacotherapy: a pathophysiologic approach*, 8th ed. New York, NY: McGraw-Hill; 2011. Available at: http://www.accesspharmacy.com/content.aspx?aID=7983818.

53. Perreault MM, Ostrop NJ, Tierney MG. Efficacy and safety of intravenous phosphate replacement in critically ill patients. *Ann Pharmacother.* 1997;31:683–688.

54. Peters SA, Kelly FJ. Vitamin E supplementation in cystic fibrosis. *J Pediatr Gastroenterol Nutr.* 1996;22(4):341–345.

55. Poirier P, Giles TD, Bray GA, et al. Obesity and cardiovascular disease: pathophysiology, evaluation, and effect of weight loss: an update of the 1997 American Heart Association scientific statement on obesity and heart disease from the Obesity Committee of the Council on Nutrition, Physical Activity, and Metabolism. *Circulation.* 2006;113(6):898–918.

56. Poon BB, Witmer C, Pruemer J. Coagulation disorders. In: DiPiro JT, Talbert RL, Yee GC, et al., eds. *Pharmacotherapy: a pathophysiologic approach*, 8th ed. New York, NY: McGraw-Hill; 2011. Available at: http://www.accesspharmacy.com/content.aspx?aID=8000061.

57. Pratt CW, Cornely K. *Essential biochemistry*, 2nd ed. Hoboken, NJ: John Wiley & Sons; 2011.

58. Pray WS. *Nonprescription product therapeutics*, 2nd ed. Baltimore, MD: Lippincott Williams & Wilkins; 2006.

59. Russell RM, Suter PM. Vitamin and trace mineral deficiency and excess. In: Longo DL, Kasper DL, Jameson JL, et al., eds. *Harrison's principles of internal medicine*, 18th ed. New York, NY: McGraw-Hill; 2012. Available at: http://www.accesspharmacy.com/content.aspx?aID=9099706.

60. Sardesai VM. Requirements for energy, carbohydrates, fat, and proteins. In: *Introduction to clinical nutrition*, 3rd ed. New York, NY: CRC Press; 2003.

61. Science M, Johnstone J, Roth DE, et al. Zinc for the treatment of the common cold: a systematic review and meta-analysis of randomized controlled trials. *CMAJ.* 2012;184(10):E551–E561.

62. Shargel L, Mutnick AH, Souney PF, Swanson LN. *Comprehensive pharmacy review*, 7th ed. Philadelphia, PA: Lippincott Williams and Wilkins; 2010.

63. Timberlake KC. *Organic and biological chemistry: structures of life*. San Francisco, CA: Benjamin Cummings; 2001.

64. Tong GM, Rude RK. Magnesium deficiency in critical illness. *J Intensive Care Med.* 2005;20:3–17.

65. UpToDate. Waltham, MA: 2012. Available at: http://www.uptodate.com/online with subscription.

66. U.S. Food and Drug Administration. Talking about trans fat: what you need to know. Available at: http://www.fda.gov/food/resourcesforyou/consumers/ucm079609.htm?&lang=en_us&output =json. Accessed November 2012.

67. van Haaften RI, Haenen GR, van Bladeren PJ, et al. Inhibition of various glutathione *S*-transferase isoenzymes by RRR-alpha-tocopherol. *Toxicol In Vitro.* 2003;17:245–251.

68. Wang Y, Beydoun MA, Liang L, et al. Will all Americans become overweight or obese? Estimating the progression and cost of the US obesity epidemic. *Obesity.* 2008;16(10):2323–2330.

69. Weitz JI. Blood coagulation and anticoagulant, fibrinolytic, and antiplatelet drugs. In: Chabner BA, Brunton LL, Knollmann BC, eds. *Goodman & Gilman's the pharmacological basis of therapeutics*, 12th ed. New York, NY: McGraw-Hill; 2011. Available at: http://www.accesspharmacy.com /content.aspx?aID=16668944.

70. Wu BU. Acute and chronic pancreatitis. In: Longo DL, Kasper DL, Jameson JL, et al., eds. *Harrison's principles of internal medicine*, 18th ed. New York, NY: McGraw-Hill; 2012. Available at: http://www.accessmedicine.com/content.aspx?aID=9135863.

Introduction to Pharmaceutical Calculations

CHAPTER
15

Pauline A. Low
Jeffery Fortner

OBJECTIVES

1. Review the basic systems of measurements used in pharmacy.

2. Review core calculation principles, including fractions, algebra, and dimensional analysis, required to accurately perform pharmaceutical calculations.

3. Define commonly used methods to describe the concentrations of mixtures of liquids and solids, including percent strength and ratio strength.

4. Describe a systematic method to convert between the units used for electrolytes: milligrams, millimoles, milliosmoles, and milliequivalents.

5. Apply commonly used patient-specific calculations used to describe body surface area, ideal body weight, body mass index, kidney function, and weight-based dosing.

6. Demonstrate commonly used calculations used to both make intravenous medications and safely administer them.

7. Calculate the nutrition provided by nutrition formulas that are administered into the gastrointestinal tract, as well as those administered intravenously.

8. Implement a series of Learning Bridge assignments at your experiential sites to bridge your didactic learning with your experiential experiences.

KEY TERMS AND DEFINITIONS

1. **Actual body weight:** a patient's actual body weight.

2. **Adjusted body weight:** a dosing weight that is higher than the ideal body weight, but less than the actual body weight; its use allows for a higher dose in obese patients for drugs that may be partially distributed into fat tissue.

3. **Alligation alternate:** a visual method of calculating proportional parts in a mixture of two or more components.

4. **Body mass index:** an indicator of a patient's actual weight versus a "normal" weight, which is calculated based on the individual's height and weight.

5. **Body surface area:** an estimate of the surface area of a patient's body, which is calculated based on the individual's height and weight.

6. **Concentration:** a description of how much of a substance is contained within a total weight or volume of a mixture.

(continues)

7. **Creatinine clearance:** creatinine is a physiological by-product of muscle breakdown and is excreted from the kidneys. By measuring or estimating the clearance, or removal, of creatinine through the kidneys, a patient's kidney function can be quantified.

8. **Dimensional analysis:** a calculation method that uses the concept of proportions to solve a problem by using ratios, such as conversion factors, to cancel out all unwanted units, leaving only the correct answer and its desired units.

9. **Electrolyte:** an ion such as sodium, potassium, magnesium, phosphate, and calcium, which is necessary for physiologic functions such as nerve impulse conduction and muscular contraction.

10. **Enteral:** a route of drug administration to the patient via the throat and stomach, either by swallowing or by using a gastric tube.

11. **Fraction:** an expression of a quantity in which two whole numbers are written one above the other, most commonly for a quantity less than 1. The number above the fraction line is called the numerator; the number below the fraction line is the denominator.

12. **Ideal body weight:** a calculated "normal" weight based on the height of a person; also known as lean body weight.

13. **Intramuscular:** a route of drug administration to the patient by injection into a muscle.

14. **Intravenous:** a route of drug administration to the patient by injection into a vein.

15. **Isotonicity:** a term describing the osmotic pressure, or tonicity, of fluid mixtures (e.g., drug solutions, IV fluids) in relation to human blood. When compared to the osmotic pressure of human blood, fluids may be hypertonic, isotonic, or hypotonic when they have more, the same, or less osmotic pressure respectively.

16. **Macronutrients:** the major nutrient types necessary for healthy nutrition, which include protein, carbohydrates, and fat.

17. **Micronutrients:** the minor nutrient types necessary for healthy nutrition, which include vitamins, trace elements, and electrolytes.

18. **Molarity:** an expression of concentration in which the number of moles of a substance is given per liter (mol/L). A mole is the molecular weight (MW) of a substance expressed in grams.

19. **Molecular weight:** an expression of the atomic weight of a molecule based on its component elements.

20. **Parenteral:** a route of drug administration to the patient by injection into the fat layer under the skin (subcutaneous), muscle (intramuscular), artery (intra-arterial), or vein (intravenous).

21. **Percent strength:** an expression of the concentration of a drug mixture that is standardized to $X\% = \frac{x \text{ g or mL}}{100 \text{ g or mL}}$ with the units depending on whether the solute and solvent are solids or liquids.

22. **Percentage:** a quantity, denoted by the percent sign (%), which represents a given number "in a hundred" and is basically a fraction with a set denominator of 100.

23. **Proportion:** when two ratios are equal to each other, they can be expressed as a proportion such as $10:1 = 20:2$, which may also be expressed as $\frac{10}{1} = \frac{20}{2}$.

24. **Ratio:** an expression of the relative amounts of two values that is similar to a fraction. While a fraction may be expressed as $\frac{2}{3}$ and is read as "two thirds," a ratio is expressed as 2:3 and is read as "two to three."

25. **Ratio strength:** describes the quantity relationship of two substances using a ratio of parts, commonly the number of parts of solute to solvent.

(continues)

(CONTINUED)

26. **SI units:** units of measurement from the International System of Units (abbreviated as SI from the French name *Système international d'unités*, also known as the metric system). Examples include the gram, liter, and meter.

27. **Solute:** a solid or liquid substance that is dissolved into another substance (solvent) to form a mixture.

28. **Solvent:** a solid or liquid substance into which other substances (solutes) are dissolved to form a mixture.

29. **Species:** an expression of how many pieces or parts an electrolyte molecule may split into when in a solution.

30. **Stock solution:** a mixture of a drug in a solution that is the highest concentration possible under normal storage conditions before the drug precipitates out of the solution.

31. **Valency:** an expression of the relative molecular charge of an electrolyte molecule.

Introduction

Pharmaceutical calculations are at the cornerstone of providing medications to a patient. It is essential that pharmacists are proficient in accurately performing an extensive variety of calculations when preparing, dispensing, or recommending/prescribing medications. In addition to being fully proficient with the various measurement systems used, and knowledgeable in the various specialized equations and formulas used in pharmacy, pharmacists must be able to apply all of the basic mathematical concepts such as fractions and algebra with high precision and accuracy.

Basic Units and Measures

Any word or abbreviation that describes the type or kind of a numerical value in an equation could be called a "unit." For instance, in the equation $3 \text{ boxes} \times \frac{20 \text{ apples}}{1 \text{ box}} = 60 \text{ apples}$, both "boxes" and "apples" are units that describe what the numbers represent. Units are necessary to help keep track of numbers and to ensure accuracy when performing calculations, which is critically important in any healthcare field. It is critical that you use units to label all your calculations to help ensure accuracy and to allow others to understand and check your work. In the pharmacy, the most common use of units are the formal "units of measurement" that represent an exactly defined measurement of weight, volume, distance, and so on.

> Example 15.1: A medication may be dosed as a 500-*milligram* tablet, or an injectable drug made available in a 100-*milliliter* bag, or a patient dosed using an equation based on his height of 74 *inches*.

Both milligram and milliliter are units from the International System of Units (abbreviated as SI, from the French name *Système international d'unités*, also known as the *metric system*), while inches are a unit of the system of United States Customary Units (USCU, also known as the *Household system*). The United States is one of only three nations worldwide that do not primarily use the SI system, so despite the SI system's extensive use in the practice of pharmacy, an understanding of both measurement systems is needed to effectively communicate with patients who tend to be more comfortable with the U.S. Customary Units system. The SI system has achieved widespread adoption due to its benefits, which include an understandable base-10 decimal system, specific base units and prefixes, and ease of international communication regarding measurements. The SI units most commonly used in pharmacy are shown in Table 15.1.

Table 15.1 SI Units Commonly Encountered in Pharmacy

Quantity	Name	Symbol	SI Value	USCU Conversion*
Length	Meter	m	Base unit for length and volume	1 m = 3.28 ft
Length	Centimeter	cm	1 cm = 0.01 m	1 cm = 0.394 in.
Volume	Liter	L	1 L = 1,000 cm³ = 1 dm³ = 0.001 m³	1 L = 0.264 gal
Volume	Milliliter	mL	1 mL = 1 cm³ = 0.001 L = 0.000001 m³	1 mL = 0.0338 fl oz
Mass	Kilogram	kg	Basc unit for mass	*1 kg = 2.2 lb*
Mass	Gram	g	1 g = 0.001 kg	1 g = 0.0353 oz
Mass	Milligram	mg	1 mg = 0.000001 kg	1 mg = 0.0000353 oz
Mass	Microgram	mcg	1 mcg = 0.000000001 kg	1 mg = 0.0000000353 oz

* See the next section for a discussion of the U.S. Customary Units (USCU) system.
The conversion in italics is commonly used in pharmacy—definitely memorize it.

The SI system is organized around seven official base units (meter, kilogram, second, ampere, kelvin, mole, and candela), of which all but the kilogram are based on measurable natural events. Three of the SI base units are commonly used in pharmacy: the meter, kilogram, and second. The meter (m) is the official base unit of distance; its definition is "the length of the path traveled by light in a vacuum during a time interval of 1/299,792,458 of a second." The centimeter (cm) may be used to describe length and patient height, and the meter squared (m^2) is used to describe body surface area. The official definition of a liter (L) is the volume of a cube with sides 10 centimeters long (see **Figure 15.1**). The most common units of volume in pharmacy are the liter and the milliliter (mL); the milliliter is equivalent to, and may sometimes be referred to as, a cubic centimeter (cc).

The kilogram is the official base unit of mass; its definition is "the mass of the international prototype of the kilogram." The international prototype is a human-made cylinder of a platinum–iridium alloy that is kept under specific controlled conditions in France. The kilogram is routinely used to describe patient weights in dosing calculations for many medications. The gram, milligram, and microgram are used to describe amounts or doses of various medications or products. Because seconds, minutes, and hours are currently in universal use as values, they are not discussed in detail here.

As mentioned earlier, the SI system uses a set of prefixes to describe different orders of magnitude of numbers (see **Table 15.2**). These prefixes make it easy to describe varying amounts quickly and to easily convert between them.

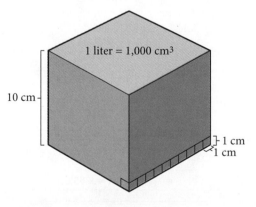

Figure 15.1 Common units of volume.

Table 15.2 Commonly Encountered SI Prefixes

Prefix	Abbreviation (Example)	Value Relative to the Base Unit
micro-	mc- (mcg)	One millionth of (0.000001)
milli-	m- (mL)	One thousandth of (0.001)
centi-	c- (cm)	One hundredth of (0.01)
deci-	d- (dL)	One tenth of (0.1)
kilo-	k- (kg)	One thousand times (1,000)

> Example 15.2: One milligram equals one thousandth of a gram, 1 mg = 0.001 g.

In pharmacy, the most common SI conversions are 1,000-fold differences between similar base units, which simply need a three-decimal-point shift to convert the values. For instance, a conversion from 1 gram (g) to *X* milligrams (mg) can be accomplished by shifting the decimal point three spaces to the right: 1 g = 1,000 mg. This decimal shifting technique works only if you know which direction to shift the decimal—which requires remembering what the SI prefixes represent. It is critical to *double-check* your calculations when shifting decimals because a misplaced decimal can cause at a minimum a 10-fold error either greater or less than the intended value.

Another cause of 10-fold errors is a misread decimal point—meaning someone does not see a decimal point, which causes the number to be interpreted as 10 times too great. For this reason, in pharmacy, and in health care in general, it is critical to *use leading zeroes,* which precede a decimal point, and to *avoid trailing zeroes*, which follow a decimal point.

Good	Leading zeroes: <u>0.</u>1 mg → Less likely to be misread as 1 mg
Bad	Trailing zeroes: 1<u>.0</u> mg → May be misread as 10 mg, so use 1 mg

As mentioned earlier, most patients in the United States do not regularly use the SI system of measurement, but instead use the USCU system, which is based on the British Imperial system and incorporates elements of the older Avoirdupois and Apothecary systems. **Table 15.3** lists the most common measures in the USCU system, along with conversions to their SI equivalents.

Table 15.3 U.S. Customary Units Commonly Encountered in Pharmacy

Quantity	Name	Symbol	USCU Conversion	SI Conversion
Length	Inch	in. or "	12 in = 1 ft	*1 in. = 2.54 cm*
Length	Foot	ft or '	1 ft = 12 in	1 ft = 0.305 m
Volume	Teaspoon	tsp or t	N/A	*1 tsp ≈ 5 mL**
Volume	Tablespoon	Tbsp or T	1 Tbsp = 3 tsp	*1 Tbsp ≈ 15 mL**
Volume	Fluid ounce	fl oz or oz	1 fl oz = 2 Tbsp	*1 fl oz ≈ 30 mL**
Volume	Cup	cp	1 cp = 8 fl oz	1 cp ≈ 240 mL*
Volume	Pint	pt	1 pt = 2 cp = 16 fl oz	*1 pt ≈ 480 mL+*
Volume	Quart	qt	1 qt = 2 pt	1 qt = 946 mL
Volume	Gallon	gal	1 gal = 4 qt	1 gal = 3785 mL
Mass	Ounce	oz	N/A	1 oz = 28.35 g
Mass	Pound	lb	1 lb = 16 oz	1 lb = 453.6 g

* The FDA uses these values for simplicity but precise conversions to mL are 1 tsp = 4.93 mL, 1 Tbsp = 14.79 mL, 1 oz = 29.57 mL, and 1 cp = 236.59 mL.

+ The FDA does not specify a simplification for the pint, but 480 mL is commonly used, despite 473mL being the precise number.

Conversions in italics are commonly used in pharmacy—definitely memorize them.

Learning Bridge 15.1

You are working at your pharmacy when a concerned-looking woman approaches to ask a question about an over-the-counter (OTC) pain medicine. She says a doctor told her to buy acetaminophen solution for her child and give 1½ teaspoonfuls every 4 hours. She is concerned because she is visiting from Europe and is familiar with the SI system but not the USCU system, so she asks you how many milliliters to give her child for each dose. What is your answer to her?

Basic Calculation Principles

Many of the calculations used in the practice of pharmacy may be completed using some of the seemingly mundane concepts of standard arithmetic and basic algebra. Despite their apparent simplicity, a solid understanding of these concepts is essential to prevent harm to patients. The following is a brief review of concepts such as fractions, percentages, units of measurement, basic algebra, ratio and proportion, and dimensional analysis.

Fractions

Some calculations in pharmacy involve fractions or conversion between fractions and decimals. A fraction uses two whole numbers, written one above the other, to represent a quantity, most commonly a quantity less than 1. The number above the fraction line is called the numerator, while the number below the fraction line is the denominator. One way to remember this arrangement is to think of the letter "d" in "denominator" as standing for $\overline{\text{Down under}}$ the fraction line.

Example 15.3:

In the fraction $\frac{1}{3} \rightarrow \frac{\text{1 is the numerator}}{\text{3 is the denominator}}$.

If multiple fractions have the same number as a denominator, the fractions are said to have a common denominator.

Example 15.4:

$\frac{1}{6}, \frac{3}{6}$ and $\frac{5}{6}$ all have a common denominator of 6.

There are three main types of fractions: proper, improper, and mixed number fractions.

Proper fractions represent values less than 1 by having a numerator that is smaller than the denominator.

Example 15.5:

$\frac{3}{4}$ is a proper fraction: the numerator (3) is smaller than the denominator (4).

Improper fractions represent values greater than 1 by having a numerator that is larger than the denominator.

Example 15.6:

$\frac{4}{3}$ is an improper fraction: the numerator (4) is larger than the denominator (3).

Mixed number fractions represent values greater than 1 by having a whole number followed by a fraction.

Example 15.7:

$1\frac{1}{4}$ is a mixed number fraction.

Another concept that may be used when dividing fractions is the reciprocal, which is a fraction in which the numbers of the numerator and denominator have been switched.

Example 15.8:

The fraction $\frac{2}{3}$ has a reciprocal of $\frac{3}{2}$.

The following are a set of commonly used rules when calculating with fractions:

1. To add or subtract fractions, they must have a common denominator, then add or subtract the numerators.

Example 15.9:

$$\frac{1}{3}+\frac{3}{8}-\frac{5}{12}=\frac{4}{24}+\frac{9}{24}-\frac{10}{24}=\frac{3}{24}=\frac{1}{8}$$

2. To multiply fractions, multiply all the numerators to determine the answer's numerator, then repeat for the denominators.

Example 15.10:

$$\frac{1}{3}\times\frac{2}{5}\times\frac{5}{12}=\frac{6}{60}=\frac{1}{10}$$

3. To divide one fraction into another, multiply by the reciprocal of the divisor fraction.

Example 15.11:

$$\frac{1}{4}\div\frac{2}{5}\rightarrow\frac{1}{4}\times\frac{5}{2}$$

Percentages

Percentages are commonly used in the practice of pharmacy to represent relative amounts of substances such as active drug in medications (i.e., 5% cream). The percent sign (%) represents a given number "in a hundred" and is simply a fraction with a set denominator of 100. For instance, 75% is equal to $\frac{75}{100}$, or 75 in 100. A percentage, or any fraction, may be converted to a decimal by dividing the number by 100 or moving the decimal point two spots to the left.

Example 15.12:

$$50\% = \frac{50}{100} = 0.5$$

$$22\% = \frac{22}{100} = 0.22$$

Basic Algebra

Many pharmacy calculations involve using known values to solve an equation for an unknown quantity, such as using a patient's height, weight, or age to help determine an appropriate dose of a medication. Basic algebra is used to analyze relationships between numbers using equations. Its most common use is to calculate the value of an unknown variable when other factors are known. The unknown variable is usually represented by the letter X.

Example 15.13: Three times an unknown number plus four is equal to 16, or $3X + 4 = 16$.

If both sides of the equation are equal and the same mathematical functions (e.g., multiplication, division) are applied to both sides, then both sides remain equal. To solve most basic algebraic equations, you must isolate the variable X onto one side of the equal sign by adding/subtracting or multiplying/dividing by the known values on the same side as X to cancel them out.

Example 15.14: First subtract 4 from both sides of the equation, and next divide both sides of the equation by 3:

$$3X + 4 = 16 \rightarrow 3X + 4 - 4 = 16 - 4 \rightarrow \frac{3X}{3} = \frac{12}{3} \rightarrow X = 4.$$

Ratio and Proportion

A ratio is basically a different way to express a fraction or describe the relative amounts of two values. While a fraction may be expressed as $\frac{2}{3}$ and is read as "two thirds," a ratio is expressed as 2:3 and is read as "two to three." Rather than separating terms above and below a dividing line, a ratio uses a colon to separate the numerator on the left and denominator on the right. Note that all of the rules of fractions apply to calculations with ratios.

Example 15.15: A school has a student-to-teacher ratio of 10:1, which is read as "ten to one" and can also be expressed as $\frac{10 \text{ students}}{1 \text{ teacher}}$, meaning for every 10 students there is 1 teacher.

When two ratios are equivalent, or equal to each other, they can be expressed as a proportion such as 10:1 = 20:2, which may also be expressed as $\frac{10}{1} = \frac{20}{2}$. A benefit of expressing proportions as fractions is that it makes certain calculations more straightforward. For instance, one helpful characteristic of proportions set up as equal fractions is that their cross-products are always equal.

Example 15.16:

$$\frac{10}{1} = \frac{20}{2} \rightarrow \frac{10}{1} \times \frac{20}{2} \rightarrow 10 \times 2 = 1 \times 20 \rightarrow 20 = 20$$

Given the relationships between the four numbers in a proportion, if you have known quantities for three of the numbers, you can calculate the fourth unknown number.

Example 15.17:

$$\frac{10}{2} = \frac{40}{X} \rightarrow 10X = 80 \rightarrow \frac{10X}{10} = \frac{80}{10} \rightarrow X = 8$$

Applying this process of using the known quantities to solve for a fourth unknown, proportions can be routinely used to help answer many pharmacy calculation problems. However, if set up incorrectly, a proportional calculation may yield an incorrect answer. Therefore, when calculating proportions in pharmacy, you must *always include units of measurement and check your answer carefully.*

Example 15.18: A drug is available as a solution in a concentration of 100 mg of drug per 5 mL of solution, or 100 mg/5 mL. A doctor orders a prescription that calls for a dose of 60 mg of the drug. How many milliliters is needed?

Answer

$$\frac{100 \text{ mg}}{5 \text{ mL}} = \frac{60 \text{ mg}}{X \text{ mL}} \rightarrow 100 \text{ mg} \times X \text{ mL} = 60 \text{ mg} \times 5 \text{ mL} \rightarrow X \text{ mL} = \frac{60 \, \cancel{\text{mg}} \times 5 \text{ mL}}{100 \, \cancel{\text{mg}}} \rightarrow X = 3 \text{ mL}$$

You must check your calculation by using your answer to compare the values of each side of the original proportion. If they are equal, your answer is correct.

$$\frac{100 \text{ mg}}{5 \text{ mL}} = \frac{60 \text{ mg}}{3 \text{ mL}} \rightarrow \frac{20 \text{ mg}}{\text{mL}} = \frac{20 \text{ mg}}{\text{mL}}$$

Dimensional Analysis

Dimensional analysis is an expansion of the concept of proportions, wherein you may solve a problem by using ratios, such as conversion factors, to cancel out all unwanted units, leaving only the correct answer and its desired units. "Dimensions" is another term for "units," meaning the descriptors that appear after numbers (as discussed earlier). By analyzing the dimensions, or units, of the ratios in an equation and inverting (or making the reciprocal) of certain ratios, the unwanted units will cancel out, leaving only the units of the desired answer. Example 15.19 demonstrates the steps necessary to complete a dimensional analysis problem.

Example 15.19: You are processing a prescription for a child's liquid antibiotic. The prescription calls for a dose of 15 mg/kg given twice a day for 7 days. The drug is available in a concentration of 200 mg/5 mL of liquid drug, and you know the patient weighs 33 lb. How many milliliters of the drug is needed for each dose?

Answer

1. *Identify the desired units.* Begin by placing the units you desire on the right side of the equal sign.

$$= \frac{mL}{dose}$$

2. *Enter known data.* Add all known and necessary data values and conversion factors.

$$\frac{15\ mg}{kg/dose} \times \frac{200\ mg}{5\ mL} \times 33\ lb \times \frac{1\ kg}{2.2\ lb} = \frac{mL}{dose}$$

3. *Invert units as needed.* Set up the equation and invert ratios by replacing them with their reciprocal (as with the **bolded** ratio below) to cancel out all unwanted units, leaving only the desired answer's units on the left side of the equation.

$$\frac{15\ \cancel{mg}}{\cancel{kg}/dose} \times \frac{\mathbf{5\ mL}}{\mathbf{200\ mg}} \times 33\ \cancel{lb} \times \frac{1\ \cancel{kg}}{2.2\ \cancel{lb}} = \frac{mL}{dose}$$

   If you have extra units after canceling out what you can, you have likely included values that you do not need to solve the equation (such as if the "7 days" value mentioned in the problem statement were included). If you cancel units and do not obtain your desired units, then you are likely forgetting to include a conversion or other ratio (such as if the "15 mg/kg/dose" value in our example was left out).

4. *Finish calculations.* Complete the equation's calculations by multiplying all the numerators together and then dividing by all of the denominators to determine a final answer.

$$\frac{15\ \cancel{mg}}{\cancel{kg}/dose} \times \frac{5\ mL}{200\ \cancel{mg}} \times 33\ \cancel{lb} \times \frac{1\ \cancel{kg}}{2.2\ \cancel{lb}} = \frac{5.6\ mL}{dose}$$

Learning Bridge 15.2

Albuterol sulfate (ProAir) is a medication used to treat bronchospasm, or asthma. It is available in a metered-dose inhaler (MDI) that consists of a pressurized canister of drug mixture and a plastic mouthpiece to direct the spray into the patient. An MDI delivers a specific amount of drug to the patient with each use. For every 200 doses, ProAir delivers 21.6 mg of albuterol sulfate. How many milligrams of drug are delivered with each dose?

Concentration Units and Expressions

Pharmaceutical products usually consist of an active medication combined with other nonactive substances that act as diluents or excipients. A diluent ("solvent") is a nondrug liquid that is present to help get a drug ("solute") into a solution, or to provide a certain total volume of fluid (see the *Introduction to Pharmaceutics* chapter). An excipient is also a nondrug substance; it is added to a drug to enhance the product in some way, such as to act as a sweetener, binder, or preservative. The dose of the active component in a medication liquid or solid is, therefore, often described as a unit of concentration. For example, a solution may contain 10% active drug, with the other 90% being water used as a diluent. The following expressions of concentration are described with associated examples.

Concentration

Concentration is the most basic description of how much of a substance is contained within a total weight or volume. A basic concentration is expressed as a specific weight or volume of active drug in a specific weight or volume of the total mixture, which includes the drug and any diluents or excipients.

Example 15.20: Suppose 4.5 g NaCl (sodium chloride) is dissolved in a sufficient quantity of water to total 500 mL. This can also be converted to a "per mL" concentration:

$$\frac{4.5\,\text{g NaCl}}{500\,\text{mL}} = \frac{0.009\,\text{g NaCl}}{\text{mL}} \text{ or } \frac{0.009\,\text{g}}{\text{mL}} \times \frac{1{,}000\,\text{mg}}{1\,\text{g}} = \frac{9\,\text{mg}}{\text{mL}}$$

Percent Strength

The units of concentration most commonly used in pharmacy involve percent strength. These concentration units have been standardized for consistency of calculations, which enhances medication safety. A liquid or solid, for example, can be described in terms of percent strength. In the case of a solid drug (solute) that is present in a liquid (solvent, or diluent), the percent strength is described as a weight of active drug per volume (w/v) concentration. Similarly, for a liquid drug that is present in a liquid diluent, the percent strength is described as a volume of active drug per volume of diluent (v/v) concentration. In the case of a solid drug (solute) that is present in a solid (diluent), the percent strength is described as a weight of active drug per weight (w/w) concentration.

- The w/v ("weight per volume") percent strength is standardized so that the active drug is described as grams per 100 mL of the total volume.

- The v/v ("volume per volume") percent strength is described as the volume in milliliters of active drug per 100 mL of the total volume.

- The w/w ("weight per weight") percent strength is standardized so that the active drug is described as grams per 100 grams of the total substance.

Example 15.21: (w/v Percent Strength)

An intravenous fluid that is often administered to patients in the hospital is called D_5W. The "D" is short for dextrose, and the "W" stands for water. D_5W refers to a w/v solution of dextrose 5% in water. Applying the standardized definition for w/v of grams per 100 mL, this means 5 grams of dextrose per 100 mL. Other dextrose solution concentrations are also commercially available, such as $D_{10}W$. This is a dextrose-in-water solution containing 10 grams of dextrose per 100 mL.

Example 15.22: (w/v Percent Strength)

A commonly used antibiotic is amoxicillin (Moxatag). It comes in many different forms, including a liquid suspension that is designed for administration to children. **Figure 15.2** diagrams one of the commercially available preparations and demonstrates the difference between basic concentration and ratio strength.

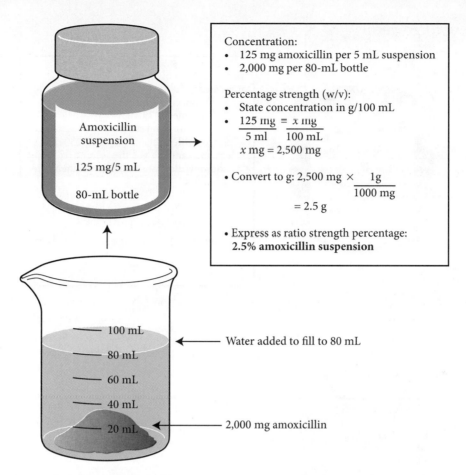

Figure 15.2   Amoxicillin suspension concentration.

Example 15.23: (v/v Percent Strength)

Isopropyl alcohol (also known as "rubbing alcohol") is an example of a liquid commonly used in pharmacy as both a solvent and a disinfectant. A 75% v/v solution is used in some hand sanitizers. This means that out of 100 mL total hand sanitizer solution, 75 mL is isopropyl alcohol (such a high concentration is needed to effectively kill bacteria; **Figure 15.3**).

Example 15.24: (w/w Percent Strength)

Hydrocortisone cream 1% is available as an OTC anti-itch cream. It is made commercially by combining hydrocortisone powder with a cream base. A 1% cream concentration means this formulation is made with 1 g hydrocortisone powder per 100 g of cream (**Figure 15.4**).

Ratio Strength

Ratio strength describes the quantity relationship of two substances using a ratio of parts, commonly the number of parts of solute to solvent. By convention, the number of parts of solute is always expressed as a constant (1), and the number of parts of solvent for each 1 part of solute appears after the colon. The units for both solute and solvent are either grams or milliliters depending on whether they are a solid or liquid.

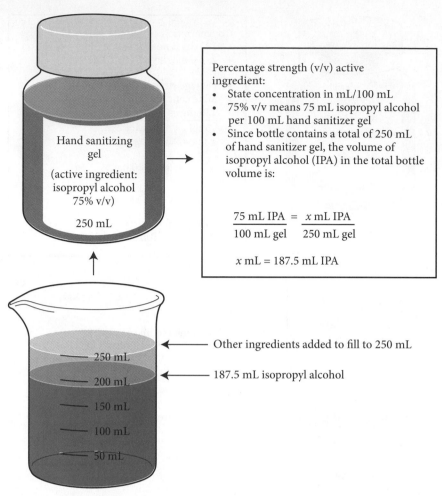

Hand sanitizing gel

(active ingredient: isopropyl alcohol 75% v/v)

250 mL

Percentage strength (v/v) active ingredient:
- State concentration in mL/100 mL
- 75% v/v means 75 mL isopropyl alcohol per 100 mL hand sanitizer gel
- Since bottle contains a total of 250 mL of hand sanitizer gel, the volume of isopropyl alcohol (IPA) in the total bottle volume is:

$$\frac{75 \text{ mL IPA}}{100 \text{ mL gel}} = \frac{x \text{ mL IPA}}{250 \text{ mL gel}}$$

x mL = 187.5 mL IPA

Other ingredients added to fill to 250 mL

187.5 mL isopropyl alcohol

250 mL

200 mL

150 mL

100 mL

50 mL

Figure 15.3 Isopropyl alcohol concentration.

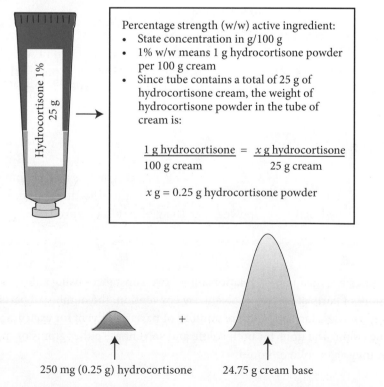

Hydrocortisone 1%
25 g

Percentage strength (w/w) active ingredient:
- State concentration in g/100 g
- 1% w/w means 1 g hydrocortisone powder per 100 g cream
- Since tube contains a total of 25 g of hydrocortisone cream, the weight of hydrocortisone powder in the tube of cream is:

$$\frac{1 \text{ g hydrocortisone}}{100 \text{ g cream}} = \frac{x \text{ g hydrocortisone}}{25 \text{ g cream}}$$

x g = 0.25 g hydrocortisone powder

+

250 mg (0.25 g) hydrocortisone   24.75 g cream base

Figure 15.4 Hydrocortisone cream concentration.

Example 15.25: "1:1" indicates 1 part of solute for every 1 part of solvent (this is read as "1 to 1"). Similarly, "1:100" indicates a "1 to 100 ratio" or 1 part solute per 100 parts solvent.

For a drug such as an epinephrine injection, USP 1:1000 the ratio strength may be read as 1 g epinephrine in 1000 mL of solution.

Ratio strength can easily be converted to percent strength by using the following equation:

Ratio strength (w/v) 1:200

$$\text{Percent strength} = \frac{1}{200} \times 100\% = 0.5\% \text{ or } 0.5\,\text{g per } 100 \text{ mL}$$

Percent strength can be converted to ratio strength by using the method shown in Example 15.26.

Example 15.26: NaCl 3% (w/v) contains 3 g NaCl per 100 mL.

Step 1: Express percent strength as a fraction, then as a ratio.

$$3\% = 3/100 = 3:100$$

Step 2: To make the first number in the ratio equal to 1, divide the entire ratio by the first number.

$$= \frac{3:100}{3}$$

Step 3: Perform the calculation to find the final 1:x ratio.

$$\frac{3:100}{3} = 1:33.33$$

Therefore, 3% = 1:33.33 ratio strength.

Figure 15.5 provides an example of ratio strength and percent strength interconversion using the drug epinephrine as an example.

Alligation Alternate

Alligation alternate is a visual method of calculating proportional parts in a mixture of two or more components. This method may be used if you need to mix a high-strength product and a low-strength product to create a mixture with a strength in between the two. For instance, if a prescription calls for a 0.2% cream of a certain drug, but you have only 0.5% and 0.1% creams available, you may use the alligation alternate method to calculate the amounts of each cream to mix together.

To set up this method, first write the concentration of the high-strength product on top, and below that write the low-strength concentration. Then in the middle and off to the right, put the desired concentration (see the example below). The concentration units used may be in a variety of forms, such as percent, mg/mL, or g/5 mL, as long as all three concentrations are in the same form and have the same units.

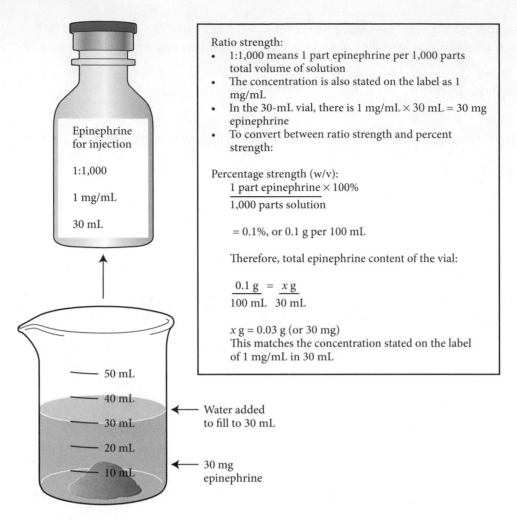

Ratio strength:
- 1:1,000 means 1 part epinephrine per 1,000 parts total volume of solution
- The concentration is also stated on the label as 1 mg/mL
- In the 30-mL vial, there is 1 mg/mL × 30 mL = 30 mg epinephrine
- To convert between ratio strength and percent strength:

Percentage strength (w/v):

$$\frac{1 \text{ part epinephrine} \times 100\%}{1{,}000 \text{ parts solution}}$$

$$= 0.1\%, \text{ or } 0.1 \text{ g per } 100 \text{ mL}$$

Therefore, total epinephrine content of the vial:

$$\frac{0.1 \text{ g}}{100 \text{ mL}} = \frac{x \text{ g}}{30 \text{ mL}}$$

x g = 0.03 g (or 30 mg)
This matches the concentration stated on the label of 1 mg/mL in 30 mL

Water added
to fill to 30 mL

30 mg
epinephrine

Figure 15.5 Epinephrine concentration.

0.5%

0.2%

0.1%

Now that the concentrations are set up, the next step is to cross diagonally from the high strength and the low strength through the medium concentration and find the difference between the two. Whether that difference is positive or negative is unimportant.

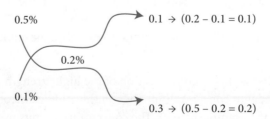

The difference between the high and medium strengths is placed across from the low strength, and the difference between the low and medium strengths is placed across from the high strength. These differences represent the parts of the high- and low-strength products that need to be mixed to achieve the medium-strength mixture.

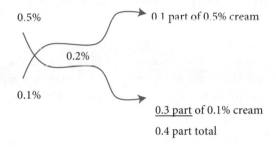

0.5% → 0.1 part of 0.5% cream

0.2%

0.1% → 0.3 part of 0.1% cream

0.4 part total

Once you know the parts of each product, a proportion calculation may be used to determine the volumes or quantities of the high- and low-strength products to combine into a medium-strength mixture. The proportion calculation may be arranged depending on the known and unknown amounts of products. For instance, in the preceding example, if you want a final amount of 30 g of 0.2% cream, then the parts of the 0.5% and 0.1% creams can be calculated with the following two proportions:

$$\frac{0.1 \text{ part } 0.5\% \text{ Cr}}{0.4 \text{ part}} = \frac{X \text{ g } 0.5\% \text{ Cr}}{30 \text{ g total Cr}} \rightarrow \frac{0.1 \times 30}{0.4} = X = 7.5 \text{ g of } 0.5\% \text{ Cr}$$

$$\frac{0.3 \text{ part } 0.1\% \text{ Cr}}{0.4 \text{ part}} = \frac{Y \text{ g } 0.1\% \text{ Cr}}{30 \text{ g total Cr}} \rightarrow \frac{0.3 \times 30}{0.4} = Y = 22.5 \text{ g of } 0.1\% \text{ Cr}$$

Or skip the second proportion: 30 g total Cr − 7.5 g 0.5% Cr = 22.5 g 0.1% Cr.

Alternatively, if you did not need a specific final amount but you wanted to use up 30 g of the 0.1% cream, then the following proportions would work, although solving for X is a bit more difficult:

$$\frac{0.3 \text{ part } 0.1\% \text{ Cr}}{0.4 \text{ part}} = \frac{30 \text{ g } 0.1\% \text{ Cr}}{30 + X \text{ g total Cr}} \rightarrow$$

$$30 \text{ g } 0.1\% \text{ Cr} \times \left(\frac{0.4 \text{ total part}}{0.3 \text{ part } 0.1\% \text{ Cr}} \right) - 30 \text{ g } 0.1\% \text{ Cr} = X$$

$X = 10$ g of 0.5% Cr to add to 30 g of 0.1% Cr to make 0.2% Cr

Molarity

In chemistry, it is common to express concentration in molar form, which is the number of moles of a substance per liter (mol/L). A mole is the molecular weight (MW) of a substance expressed in grams. For example, calcium has a MW of 40, so 1 mole of calcium weighs 40 g (40 g/mol). This can also be expressed as 1 mol/L of calcium = 40 g/L.

In pharmacy, the unit millimoles per liter (mmol/L) is more commonly used because the amounts and concentrations used are typically much smaller. A very useful concept to know for calculations is that while the concentration of calcium is 40 *g/mol*, it is also equal to 40 *mg/mmol*. If the conversion of one thousandth is applied to both the numerator (g → mg) and the denominator (mol → mmol), then the number value (in this case, 40) remains unchanged.

Example 15.27: Some laboratories report the concentration of calcium in the blood in units of mmol/L, while others report it in units of mg/dL. If a blood calcium level is reported as 2.5 mmol/L, this can be converted to mg/dL by knowing that calcium has a molecular weight of 40 and, therefore, can be expressed as 40 mg/mmol:

$$\frac{2.5 \text{ mmol}}{1 \text{ L}} \times \frac{40 \text{ mg}}{\text{mmol}} \times \frac{1 \text{ L}}{10 \text{ dL}} = \frac{10 \text{ mg}}{\text{dL}}$$

Isotonicity

Another concentration expression that is commonly used in pharmacy is tonicity. This term is often used in conjunction with "osmosis." Osmosis refers to the process that occurs when a semipermeable membrane separates two solutions of different concentration, and allows only the solvent to move freely across the membrane, leaving the solutes to stay in place (see also the *Introduction to Pharmaceutics* chapter). This concentration difference creates an osmotic pressure difference, with a higher osmotic pressure on the side of the membrane that has more concentrated solute. The osmotic pressure causes the solvent to move down the concentration gradient from the side of higher concentration and osmotic pressure to the side of lower concentration and osmotic pressure, until an equal concentration is present on each side. At this equal concentration point, "iso-osmosis" is reached. A common example of a biological semipermeable membrane is the membrane surrounding blood cells, but most other tissue cells in the body are also semipermeable.

The term "isotonicity" refers specifically to fluid mixtures (i.e., drug solutions, IV fluids) with the same osmotic pressure or tonicity as blood. One example of a fluid considered to be isotonic to blood is a 0.9% NaCl solution. This saline (sodium salt) solution of 0.9% NaCl is also called "normal saline" or "NS." Based on percent strength, 0.9% NaCl means 0.9 gram NaCl per 100 mL of fluid. Each liter of normal saline has 308 milliosmoles of NaCl/L, which is approximately the same osmotic pressure as human blood. Solutions that have a lower osmotic pressure than normal saline are called "hypotonic"; they cause a net movement of water through a semipermeable membrane from outside to inside a cell, leading to swelling of the cell. Solutions that have a higher osmotic pressure than normal saline are called "hypertonic"; they cause a net movement of water through a semipermeable membrane from inside to outside a cell, leading to intracellular dehydration and shriveling of the cell. In pharmacy, the infusion of solutions into a vein that are hypotonic or hypertonic can lead to tissue damage and pain. It is therefore important for pharmacists to understand the concept of tonicity and to know how to calculate an isotonic solution (see also the *Introduction to Pharmaceutics* chapter).

Example 15.28: An intravenous fluid contains 45 g NaCl/L. Is this fluid isotonic, hypotonic, or hypertonic?

Answer

Step 1: Express as a w/v percent strength. A shortcut to solving this problem is to express the 45 g/L as 45 g/1,000 mL:

$$\frac{45 \text{ g}}{1,000 \text{ mL}} = \frac{X \text{ g}}{100 \text{ mL}} = 4.5 \text{ g or } 4.5\%$$

Step 2: Compare to w/v percent strength of NS. NS contains 0.9% NaCl, which means 0.9 g per 100 mL. This solution contains 4.5 g per 100 mL. Since this solution is far more concentrated than NS, it is described as being *hypertonic*.

Example 15.29: An intravenous fluid contains 120 mOsm/L. Would this fluid be categorized as isotonic, hypotonic, or hypertonic?

Answer

Since human blood is normally 280–310 mOsm/L, this fluid with far fewer mOsm/L is described as *hypotonic*.

Learning Bridge 15.3

The medication epinephrine may be used in emergency situations to treat severe allergic reactions such as anaphylactic shock. It is administered intramuscularly (IM) and is commonly supplied in an automatic injection device called an EpiPen. You are working at a pharmacy that is supplying flu vaccine. To be prepared for any severe allergic reactions to the vaccine, the pharmacy usually stocks EpiPen devices. Because EpiPens are out of stock and unavailable to order at this time, the pharmacist has asked you to order an equivalent form of the medication. From looking at an expired EpiPen, you learn the strength is epinephrine 1:1,000. When you look for an equivalent form, you see that all the strengths are listed in units of mg/mL. What is EpiPen's strength in mg/mL?

Concepts and Units for Electrolytes

The human body needs certain electrolytes such as sodium, potassium, magnesium, phosphate, and calcium for key physiologic functions, including nerve impulse conduction and muscular contraction. Electrolytes are found in many of the foods we eat, but additional supplementation may be required in certain circumstances (see also the *Introduction to Nutrients* chapter). Electrolytes are supplied as salts, such as calcium carbonate, magnesium sulfate, and potassium chloride. The units used for dosing each type of electrolyte can be mg (milligrams), mmol (millimoles), or mEq (milliequivalents). Therefore, it is important for a pharmacist to be able to accurately interchange between any of these dosing units. Additionally, the mOsm (milliosmoles) provided by an intravenous preparation of electrolytes may need to be calculated to ensure the correct type of vein is used for infusion to prevent tissue damage and pain; for example, a hypertonic solution should

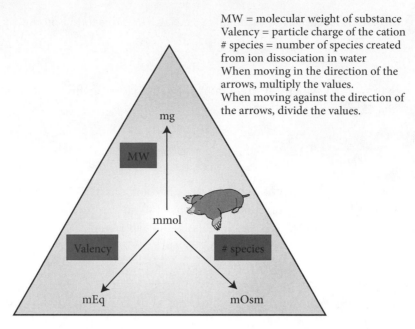

MW = molecular weight of substance
Valency = particle charge of the cation
# species = number of species created
from ion dissociation in water
When moving in the direction of the
arrows, multiply the values.
When moving against the direction of
the arrows, divide the values.

Figure 15.6 Unit interconversions.
Courtesy of Eric J. Mack, PhD.

be injected into a large vein to dilute it quickly. The diagram in **Figure 15.6**, which we like to call the Magic Triangle, defines the interchange of units between mg, mmol, mEq, and mOsm. To use the Magic Triangle one must know at least one of the three outer units (mg, mEq, or mOsm) for a given molecule, as well as that molecule's three conversion factors: molecular weight (MW) expressed as mg/mmol; valency which is also known as the charge of the molecule and is usually expressed as 1, 2, or 3 mEq/mmol; and lastly species, which is also known as parts or pieces of that molecule in solution expressed as mOsm/mmol. To convert between the three outer units of the Magic Triangle, move from the known to the unknown unit while *dividing* by the conversion factor (MW, valency, or species) when *moving against* an arrow's direction and *multiplying* by the conversion factor when *moving with* the arrow's direction (see examples below). Note that the unit mmol is in the center of the triangle because it is necessary for each conversion factor, but it is also cancelled out during each conversion between mg, mEq, or mOsm.

Table 15.4 lists some of the commonly encountered salts in pharmacy together with the accompanying data for unit conversions.

Example 15.30: Calculate the number of mEq of sodium (Na^+) contained within 9,000 mg of sodium chloride (NaCl).

Answer

Following the Magic Triangle diagram:

Step 1: Convert from mg to mmol.

- 9,000 mg divided by the MW of NaCl (58.5 g/mol or mg/mmol) converts the mg into mmol

- 9,000 mg/58.5 mg/mmol = 153.85 mmol

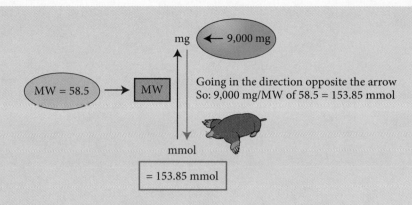

Step 2: Convert from mmol to mEq.

- 153.85 mmol multiplied by the valence of the cation in NaCl (1+) converts the mmol into mEq
- 153.85 mmol × 1 mEq/mmol = 153.85 mEq
- Therefore, 9,000 mg NaCl = 153.85 mEq Na^+

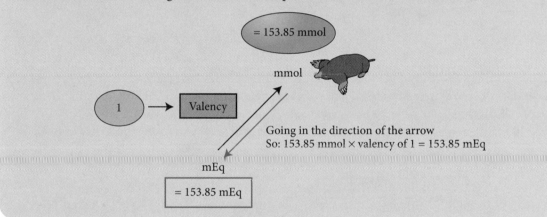

Table 15.4 Common Electrolyte Salts

Components of Unit Conversions		Examples		
MW	Molecular weight of product	*Salt*	*MW*	
		NaCl	58.5	
		$MgSO_4$	120	
		$CaCl_2$	111	
		$Al(OH)_3$	78	
Valency	Particle charge of cation	*Salt*	*Cation*	*Valency*
		NaCl	Na^+	1
		$MgSO_4$	Mg^{2+}	2
		$CaCl_2$	$Ca2^+$	2
		$Al(OH)_3$	Al^{3+}	3
# species	Ion dissociation in water	*Salt*	*Species*	*# species*
		NaCl	Na^+, Cl^-	2
		$MgSO_4$	$Mg2^+$, SO_4^{2-}	2
		$CaCl_2$	$Ca2^+$, Cl^-, Cl^-	3
		$Al(OH)_3$	$Al3^+$, OH^-, OH^-, OH^-	4

Example 15.31: Calculate the mOsm provided by 77 mEq NaCl.

Answer

Step 1: Convert from mEq to mmol.

- 77 mEq Na^+ provided by NaCl is divided by the valence of Na^+
- 77 mEq/1 = 77 mmol

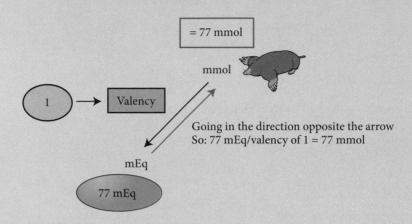

Step 2: Convert from mmol to mOsm.

- 77 mmol multiplied by the number of species generated by NaCl in water (which is 2 – Na^+ and Cl^-) converts the mmol into mOsm
- 77 mmol × 2 mOsm/mmol = 154 mOsm

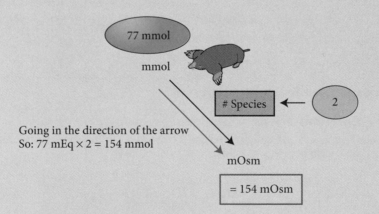

Learning Bridge 15.4

A patient takes two 500-mg chewable calcium carbonate tablets three times a day for heartburn. His doctor advised him to limit his calcium intake to less than 100 mEq per day. How many milliequivalents of calcium carbonate are ingested each day?

Patient-Specific Calculations

Dosing Based on Weight or Body Size

Certain drugs are dosed based on the actual body weight (ABW) of a patient. Dosing for such drugs is described as a certain amount of dosing units per unit of weight.

Example 15.32: One dose for an adult receiving gentamicin is 6 mg/kg/day in divided doses every 8 hours. How many milligrams per dose should be given to a patient who weighs 150 lb?

Answer

$$\text{Dimensional Analysis: } 150\ \text{lb} \times \frac{1\ \text{kg}}{2.2\ \text{lb}} \times \frac{6\ \text{mg}}{\text{kg}/\text{day}} \times \frac{1\ \text{day}}{3\ \text{doses}} = \frac{136\ \text{mg}}{\text{dose}}$$

$$\text{Ratio: } 1\ \text{kg} = 2.2\ \text{lb} \qquad \frac{2.2\ \text{lb}}{150\ \text{lb}} = \frac{6\ \text{mg}/\text{day}}{x\ \text{mg}/\text{day}} \qquad x = \frac{409\ \text{mg}}{\text{day}} \qquad \frac{409\ \text{mg}/\text{day}}{3\ \text{doses}/\text{day}} = \frac{136\ \text{mg}}{\text{dose}}$$

Ideal Body Weight

Besides actual body weight, there are accepted "normal" ranges for weight based on the height of a person. People who weigh either more or less than these ranges may need special considerations for drug dosing. Probably the most common equation to assess weight is that used to calculate ideal body weight (IBW, also sometimes referred to as "lean body weight"). For a given height, there is an ideal weight for males and females. The ideal body weight for a male is higher than that for a female of the same height, based on the assumption that a male body has a higher percentage of lean muscle, which weighs more.

The chemical structure of a drug will affect how it becomes distributed in the body once it enters the bloodstream. Drugs that become distributed well into fat are termed lipophilic ("fat-loving"), whereas those that do not distribute well into fat tissue are termed hydrophilic ("water loving"). Hydrophilic drugs are often dosed based on IBW—if they were dosed based on total body weight in an overweight individual, that calculation might lead to an overdose. There are two versions of the IBW equation, depending upon whether weight is reported in kilograms or pounds:

Males: IBW = **50 kg** + (2.3 kg × each inch > 60 in.)
Females: IBW = **45.5 kg** + (2.3 kg × each inch > 60 in.)
Round the answer to nearest tenth of a kilogram

Males: IBW = **110 lb** + (5 lb × each inch > 60 in.)
Females: IBW = **100 lb** + (5 lb × each inch > 60 in.)
Round to nearest tenth of a pound

Example 15.33: What are the ABW and IBW of a female who is 5'9" tall and weighs 165 lb?

Answer

$$\text{ABW (kg)} = 165 \text{ lb} \times \frac{1 \text{ kg}}{2.2 \text{ lb}} = 75 \text{ kg} \quad \text{IBW (kg)} = 45.5 \text{ kg} + (2.3 \text{ kg} \times 9) = 66.2 \text{ kg}$$

Adjusted Body Weight

An adjusted body weight is sometimes calculated for obese patients. The adjusted body weight calculates a dosing weight that is higher than the IBW but less than the ABW, allowing for a higher dose in obese patients for drugs that may become partly distributed into fat tissue. Guidelines for when to use an adjusted body weight for dosing are provided in the drug package insert from the drug manufacturer. Additionally, the degree to which the IBW is adjusted may be found in the drug package insert. The following equation shows how to calculate the adjusted body weight (IBW_{ADJ}) and includes the variable conversion factor, which depends on the particular drug or situation:

$$\text{IBW}_{\text{ADJ}} = \text{IBW} + X(\text{ABW} - \text{IBW})$$

where X = conversion factor specific to the drug or situation (X typically ranges from 0.1 to 0.4, or 10–40% of the difference between ABW and IBW).

Example 15.34: A patient with an ABW of 75 kg and an IBW of 63 kg is being dosed with a drug based on an adjusted IBW using a conversion factor of 0.3. What is the patient's IBW_{ADJ}?

Answer

$$\text{IBW}_{\text{ADJ}} = 63 \text{ kg} + 0.3(75 \text{ kg} - 63 \text{ kg}) = 63 \text{ kg} + 3.6 \text{ kg} = 66.6 \text{ kg}$$

Body Surface Area

Another method of calculating drug dosing that accounts for the size of a patient is to use body surface area (BSA). It is common to use BSA when calculating drug dosing for pediatric patients and when dosing chemotherapy agents. Various equations are available for use with pediatric patients, but they require specific knowledge of which equation to use for which specific circumstance. For adult patients, there are two commonly used equations, depending upon whether SI units are used:

$$\text{BSA in m}^2 = \sqrt{\frac{\text{Ht} \times \text{Wt}}{3,131}} \qquad \text{Ht} = \text{height in } \textit{inches} \qquad\qquad \text{Wt} = \text{weight in } \textit{pounds}$$

The alternative formula substitutes SI units:

$$\text{BSA in m}^2 = \sqrt{\frac{\text{Ht} \times \text{Wt}}{3,600}} \qquad \text{Ht} = \text{height in } \textit{centimeters} \qquad \text{Wt} = \text{weight in } \textit{kilograms}$$

BSA values are traditionally rounded to the nearest tenth for adults and nearest hundredth for pediatric patients.

Example 15.35: What is the BSA of a patient who is 6'2" tall and weighs 185 lb?

Answer

6'2" = 74 inches

$$BSA = \sqrt{\frac{74 \times 185}{3,131}} = 2.1 \text{ m}^2$$

Body Mass Index

The National Institutes of Health (NIH) uses body mass index (BMI) as an indicator of a patient's actual weight versus a "normal" weight (**Table 15.5**). There are two versions of the BMI equation. The standard equation uses SI units:

$$BMI = \frac{\text{Weight (kg)}}{\text{Height (m)}^2}$$

The alternative equation uses U.S. units:

$$BMI = \frac{\text{Weight (lb)}}{\text{Height (in.)}^2} \times 704.5$$

Example 15.36: Calculate the BMI of a patient who is 5'6" and weighs 145 lb.

Answer

$$66 \text{ in.} \times \frac{1 \text{ m}}{39.37 \text{ in.}} = 1.68 \text{ m} \qquad 145 \text{ lb} \times \frac{1 \text{ kg}}{2.2 \text{ lb}} = 65.9 \text{ kg}$$

$$BMI = \frac{65.9 \text{ kg}}{1.68 \text{ m}^2} = 23.4 \qquad BMI = \frac{145 \text{ lb}}{66 \text{ in.}^2} \times 704.5 = 23.5$$

Dosing Based on Kidney Function

Many drugs are eliminated in the urine and, therefore, are dosed according to the degree of the patient's kidney function. Several equations can be used to *estimate* kidney function. The most commonly used equation used for drug dosing purposes, called the Cockcroft-Gault equation, estimates

Table 15.5 NIH Weight Definitions

BMI	Definition
<18.5	Underweight
18.5–24.9	Normal
25–29.9	Overweight
>30–39.9	Obese
>40	Extreme obesity

creatinine clearance (CrCl). It is based on measuring a muscle by-product called creatinine in the blood that is cleared by the kidneys (see also the *Introduction to Nutrients* chapter). If the serum creatinine (SCr) value in the blood is high, it is usually indicative of poor kidney clearance, and hence poor overall kidney function. The equation is adjusted downward for females because they typically have less muscle mass and, therefore, produce less creatinine. Note that the units of CrCl are mL/min, but the equation is odd because the units of the variables do not cancel out to mL/min.

$$\text{Males}: \text{CrCl} = \frac{(140 - \text{Age}) \times \text{Body Weight}}{72 \times \text{Scr}}$$

$$\text{Females}: \text{CrCl} = \frac{(140 - \text{Age}) \times \text{Body Weight}}{72 \times \text{Scr}} \times 0.85$$

$$\text{Units: Age in years} \quad \text{SCr in} \frac{\text{mg}}{\text{dL}} \quad \text{BW in kg}$$

The Cockcroft-Gault equation is usually calculated using a patient's IBW, unless the person is either underweight or overweight. In that case, the person's ABW or IBW_{ADJ} is used as follows:

- Underweight (ABW < IBW): use ABW

- Overweight (ABW > 130% of IBW): use IBW_{ADJ} with a conversion factor of 0.4 (see the section on adjusted body weight for details)

Once CrCl has been calculated, the value is compared to the normal range:

- Males: ~100 to ~140 mL/min

- Females: ~90 to ~130 mL/min

Patients with low CrCl values who require medications that have significant kidney elimination may, therefore, need to take a lower dose. The package insert for drugs includes information on how to adjust the dose of drugs based on diminished kidney function.

Example 15.37: What is the estimated creatinine clearance (CrCl) of a male patient who is 57 years old, is 5'9" tall, and weighs 165 lb with a SCr of 1.6 mg/dL? Is this within the normal range or above/below normal?

Answer

1. Calculate ABW: $\text{ABW} = 165\,\text{lb} \times \dfrac{1\,\text{kg}}{2.2\,\text{lb}} = 75\,\text{kg}$

2. Calculate IBW: $\text{IBW} = 50\,\text{kg} + (2.3 \times 9) = 70.7\,\text{kg}$

3. Compare ABW and IBW: $\dfrac{\text{ABW}}{\text{IBW}} \times 100\% = \dfrac{75\,\text{kg}}{70.7\,\text{kg}} \times 100\% = 106.1\%$

    Because the ABW is less than 130% of IBW, use IBW.

4. Calculate CrCl: $\text{CrCl} = \dfrac{(140 - 57) \times 70.7}{72 \times 1.6} = 50.9\,\text{mL / min}$

This CrCl is below the normal range.

Example 15.38: What is the estimated CrCl of a female patient who is 41 years old, is 5'5" tall, and weighs 121 lb with a SCr of 0.7 mg/dL? Is this within the normal range or above/below normal?

Answer

1. Calculate ABW: $ABW = 121\,lb \times \dfrac{1\,kg}{2.2\,lb} = 55\,kg$

2. Calculate IBW: $IBW - 45.5\,kg + (2.3 \times 5) = 57\,kg$

3. Compare ABW and IBW: $\dfrac{ABW}{IBW} \times 100\% = \dfrac{55\,kg}{57\,kg} \times 100\% = 96.5\%$

   Because the ABW is less than IBW, use ABW.

4. Calculate CrCl: $CrCl = \dfrac{(140-41) \times 55}{72 \times 0.7} \times 0.85 = 91.8\,mL\,/\,min$

This CrCl is within the normal range.

Learning Bridge 15.5

A 78-year-old female is admitted into the hospital to be treated with intravenous antibiotics for a severe infection. She is 5'4" tall and weighs 225 lb. When her blood work was done today, her creatinine was 2.6 mg/dL. Ampicillin sodium, an IV antibiotic, was ordered at a dose of 2 g IV every 6 hours.

   You assess the order for appropriateness of dosing and find the following dosing guidelines:

Ampicillin sodium dosing

- Normal kidney function: 2 g IV every 4 to 6 hours

- CrCl between 10 and 50 mL/min: change the dosing interval to every 6 to 12 hours

- CrCl less than 10 mL/min: change interval to every 12 to 16 hours

Reference: Bennett WM, Aronoff GR, Golper TA, et al. *Drug prescribing in renal failure*, 3rd ed. Philadelphia, PA: American College of Physicians; 1987.

A. Calculate the patient's IBW.
B. Calculate the patient's $IBW_{ADJ.}$
C. Calculate the patient's kidney function using the Cockcroft-Gault equation.
D. Based on this patient's kidney function, how should the ampicillin dosing be adjusted?

Parenteral Preparation and Administration

Medications that are swallowed or placed down a tube that goes into the stomach or small intestine are called "enteral" medications, whereas those supplied to the patient by injection into the fat layer under the skin (subcutaneous), muscle (intramuscular), artery (intra-arterial), or vein (intravenous), are called "parenteral" medications. Pharmacists and technicians must be able to accurately calculate medications that are prepared for parenteral administration. Because the medication is being directly injected into the body and begins to affect the patient almost immediately, there is no room for calculation error. Calculations are performed both when making preparations for intravenous administration and when ensuring that the correct dose, or rate of drug delivery, is being administered.

Parenteral Medication Preparation

When preparing a parenteral medication, the drug may be provided as a sterile liquid or a powder that must be reconstituted with a liquid (usually Sterile Water for Injection [SWI]) to get the drug into solution. Parenteral medications are prepared in a special sterile cabinet to avoid bacterial contamination.

Preparing a Liquid Medication for Administration by Syringe

The required dose of a medication is drawn up into a syringe. The concentration of the drug in solution will dictate the volume of the drug needed to provide the dose.

> Example 15.39: Diphenhydramine (Benadryl) is an antihistamine that is administered in certain cases of allergic reactions. It is commercially supplied for parenteral use in a 1-mL vial with a concentration of 50 mg/mL. If a 25 mg dose is to be given intravenously, then the correct volume needed to supply the dose is drawn up into a syringe. This volume is calculated as follows (**Figure 15.7**):
>
> $$\frac{50\ \text{mg}}{1\ \text{mL}} = \frac{25\ \text{mg}}{X\ \text{mL}} = 0.5\ \text{mL diphenhydramine to supply a 25 mg dose}$$

Preparing a Powder Medication for Administration by Syringe

If the medication is supplied as a powder, it must first be reconstituted before drawing up the correct volume needed to supply the dose into a syringe.

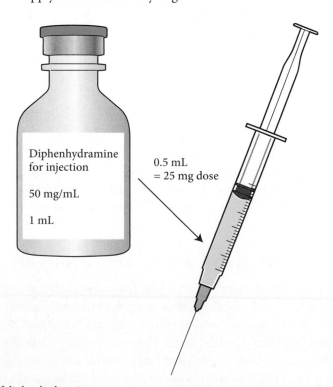

Diphenhydramine for injection

50 mg/mL

1 mL

0.5 mL = 25 mg dose

Figure 15.7 Volume of diphenhydramine.

Example 15.40: Ceftriaxone is an antibiotic that is supplied commercially as a powder for reconstitution. It is usually administered into a vein, but for certain infections it is administered via intramuscular injection. The volume of liquid that can be injected into a muscle is limited to approximately 4–5 mL in order to avoid patient discomfort.

Drug manufacturers usually provide specific recommendations for how to prepare the injection safely. In the case of ceftriaxone, the product instructions indicate that a final drug concentration of 250 mg/mL be used. If a dose of 1 g is to be administered intramuscularly, then the manufacturer has already calculated the volume of SWI to add to ensure the correct final concentration. In this case, the product instructions state that a 1-g vial of powder should have 3.6 mL of SWI added, and the final concentration will be 250 mg/mL (**Figure 15.8**).

If the dose was 750 mg instead of 1 g, the same procedure would be used to reconstitute the drug, but the volume of final drug solution drawn up into the syringe would be adjusted to achieve the desired dose. In this case, because the concentration is 250 mg/mL, the volume needed to supply 750 mg would be

$$\frac{250 \text{ mg}}{1 \text{ mL}} = \frac{750 \text{ mg}}{X \text{ mL}} = 3 \text{ mL reconstituted drug solution to supply 750 mg dose}$$

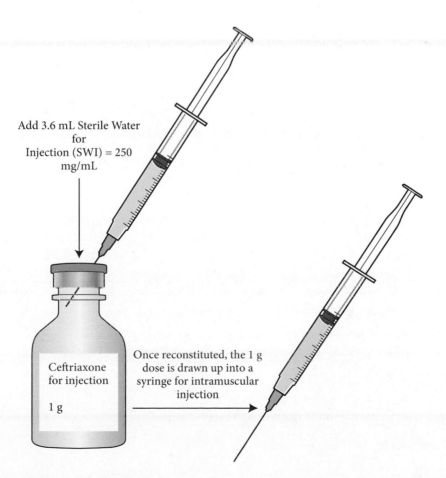

Add 3.6 mL Sterile Water for Injection (SWI) = 250 mg/mL

Ceftriaxone for injection

1 g

Once reconstituted, the 1 g dose is drawn up into a syringe for intramuscular injection

Figure 15.8 Reconstitution of ceftriaxone.

Preparing a Small-Volume Bag of Intravenous Medication

Drugs that are administered intravenously are often prepared in IV bags of volume ranging from 50 mL to 500 mL. These bags contain solutions such as dextrose 5% (D_5W), 0.9% NaCl (NS), or 0.45% NaCl (½ NS), and a particular diluent is selected based on drug compatibility as well as patient-specific factors. Traditionally, these preparations are termed "small-volume" IV bags.

The volume of fluid chosen for a particular medication is based on several factors, including the volume that a patient can tolerate, the compatibility of the drug in solution, the stability of the solution over time, and the time period over which the medication needs to be administered. The majority of small-volume IV bags are used to deliver medications such as intravenous antibiotics over a period of 0.5–2 hours. Sometimes, a small-volume bag is used for a continuous infusion if the dose is low and the bag volume does not need to be large to provide 24 hours' worth of medication. In most cases, medications are discarded if they have been infusing at room temperature for 24 hours due to concerns about potential bacterial contamination, although medications may need to be discarded after a much shorter duration due to drug stability concerns.

Example 15.41: Insulin is often administered as a continuous drip to patients in the intensive care unit. The dose used is typically quite small, so a small-volume bag is mixed and supplied. Although hospitals may have different protocols for insulin concentration and volume supplied, a very commonly used concentration is 1 unit of insulin per mL fluid, supplied in a 100-mL bag. Patients are then started on a certain rate of X units per hour, and this dose is adjusted based on regular monitoring of the blood glucose level. If a patient is to be initially started on 5 units of insulin per hour, then the volume per hour would be

$$\frac{1 \text{ unit}}{\text{mL}} = \frac{5 \text{ units per hour}}{X \text{ mL}} = 5 \text{ mL per hour}$$

Based on this rate, a 100-mL bag of insulin, infused at a concentration of 1 unit/hr, would be expected to last $\frac{5 \text{ units}}{1 \text{ hour}} = \frac{100 \text{ units}}{X \text{ hours}} \rightarrow X = 20$ hours, if the dose does not change.

Example 15.42: Gentamicin is an intravenous antibiotic that is used for severe infections. It is supplied in a 20-mL vial for injection at a concentration of 40 mg/mL. The dosing recommendations are typically based on the weight of the patient. One dose recommendation is for 5 mg/kg/day. If a patient weighs 70 kg, then the dose required is calculated as follows and supplied in a small-volume IV bag for administration over 30 minutes.

Step 1: Calculate the required daily dose.

$$5 \frac{\text{mg}}{\text{kg}} \times 70 \text{ kg} = 350 \text{ mg}$$

Step 2: Calculate the volume of drug needed to supply the daily dose.

$$\frac{40 \text{ mg gentamicin}}{1 \text{ mL}} = \frac{350 \text{ mg gentamicin}}{X \text{ mL}} = 8.75 \text{ mL}$$

Step 3: Draw up the needed volume of drug and add to the small-volume IV bag. The volume of diluent used is based on recommendations from manufacturers, or other reliable sources of drug information. In the case of gentamicin, the manufacturer recommends dilution in 50–200 mL of either D_5W or NS.

Each hospital typically has a protocol that standardizes how this medication is mixed. Let's assume the standard bag is 100 mL of NS. In this case, 8.75 mL of gentamicin would be drawn out of the stock vial and added to a 100-mL bag of NS. The total volume inside the bag would therefore be 100 mL + 8.75 mL = 108.75 mL. Sometimes it is critical that a particular volume or concentration of final product is reached, in which case the volume of diluent is adjusted before adding the drug, but for this drug it is fine to end up with a total volume greater than 100 mL.

The drug is then thoroughly mixed with the diluent and then administered over 30 minutes to the patient, which is the equivalent rate of 200 mL per hour (100 mL in 0.5 hour) (**Figure 15.9**).

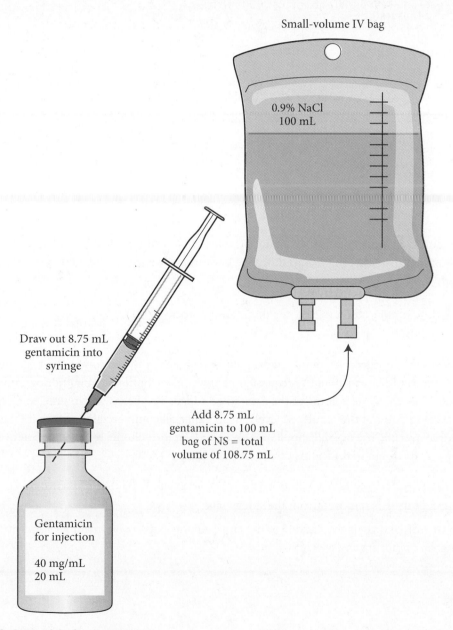

Small-volume IV bag

0.9% NaCl
100 mL

Draw out 8.75 mL
gentamicin into
syringe

Add 8.75 mL
gentamicin to 100 mL
bag of NS = total
volume of 108.75 mL

Gentamicin
for injection

40 mg/mL
20 mL

Figure 15.9 Gentamicin dose preparation.

Preparing a Large-Volume Bag of Intravenous Medication

A large-volume intravenous bag usually refers to volumes greater than 500 mL. The most common volume used is 1,000 mL, although 2,000 mL and 3,000 mL volumes are also seen.

Large volumes are typically used for administering general intravenous fluid to a patient or for delivering medications in doses that require larger volumes of fluid due to the recommended concentration.

Example 15.43: A patient is to receive D_5W with 0.45% NaCl (also known as "D_5W with ½ NS") at a rate of 125 mL/hr continuously. This mixture of fluid is available commercially in 1,000-mL bags. While there are no calculations needed to mix the actual fluid, pharmacists will calculate the number of bags needed to supply the prescribed fluid for a 24-hour period.

$$\frac{125 \text{ mL}}{\text{hour}} = \frac{X \text{ mL}}{24 \text{ hours}} = 3,000 \text{ mL, or } 3 \times 1,000 \text{ mL bags}$$

Example 15.44: Dobutamine is used in patients in the intensive care unit if their hearts are not pumping well. It is supplied in 40-mL vials at a concentration of 12.5 mg/mL. The physician has asked for a 1,000-mL bag to be prepared at a concentration of 2 mg/mL.

Step 1: Calculate the amount of dobutamine that must be added to a 1,000-mL bag of D_5W to achieve the desired concentration:

$$\frac{2 \text{ mg dobutamine}}{1 \text{ mL}} = \frac{X \text{ mg dobutamine}}{1,000 \text{ mL}} = 2,000 \text{ mg dobutamine}$$

Step 2: Calculate how many milliliters of dobutamine stock solution must be added to the 1,000-mL bag to obtain the desired concentration. We know that we need to add 2,000 mg, and each vial is 12.5 mg/mL:

$$\frac{12.5 \text{ mg dobutamine stock}}{1 \text{ mL}} = \frac{2000 \text{ mg dobutamine stock}}{X \text{ mL}} = 160 \text{ mL dobutamine stock}$$

Step 3: Because a considerable volume of drug must be added to the large-volume bag, the concentration would be less than the requested 2 mg/mL. One option is to withdraw from the large-volume bag the same volume as the drug to be added. This keeps the volume equal and the concentration remains at the requested level. (In actuality, all commercially provided IV bags contain some overfill. The overfill should not exceed 5% of the volume, but as this exact volume is unknown, it is often ignored.) In this case, following **Figure 15.10**:

1. 160 mL of D_5W is removed from the large-volume bag, leaving 840 mL.

2. 160 mL of drug is removed from the stock vials.

3. The 160 mL of drug is then added to the large-volume bag to obtain a final concentration of 2 mg/mL, ignoring any overfill.

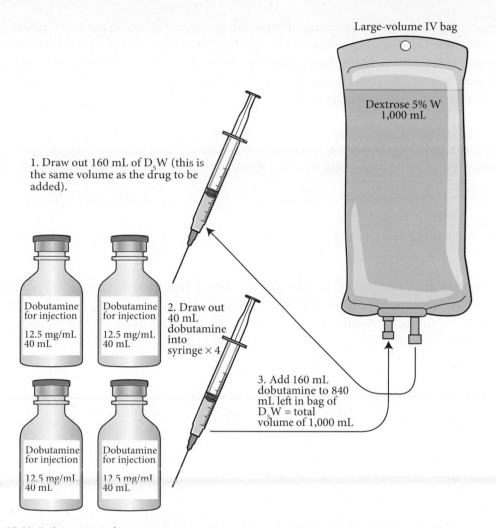

Large-volume IV bag

Dextrose 5% W
1,000 mL

1. Draw out 160 mL of D$_5$W (this is the same volume as the drug to be added).

Dobutamine for injection

12.5 mg/mL
40 mL

Dobutamine for injection

12.5 mg/mL
40 mL

2. Draw out 40 mL dobutamine into syringe × 4

3. Add 160 mL dobutamine to 840 mL left in bag of D$_5$W = total volume of 1,000 mL

Dobutamine for injection

12.5 mg/mL
40 mL

Dobutamine for injection

12.5 mg/mL
40 mL

Figure 15.10 Dobutamine infusion preparation.

Parenteral Medication Delivery

Medications that are administered directly into the blood usually must be injected over a specific duration of time to safely provide the drug to the patient.

Example 15.45: Vancomycin is an intravenous antibiotic that can cause adverse effects such as low blood pressure and skin flushing if administered to a patient too quickly. It is recommended that the rate of delivery should not exceed 1 gram per hour. A dose of 1,250 mg must therefore be administered over 75 minutes:

Infusion time: $\dfrac{1,000 \text{ mg}}{60 \text{ min}} = \dfrac{1,250 \text{ mg}}{X \text{ min}}$

$X \text{ min} = \dfrac{1,250 \text{ mg} \times 60 \text{ min}}{1,000 \text{ mg}} = 75 \text{ min}$

Sometimes the medication infusion rate is expressed as a certain dose per unit time, such as X mcg/min. These types of medications are usually administered to a patient using a programmable electronic infusion pump. Some pumps allow programming in units such as mcg/min, whereas others must be programmed as a dose per hour. It is important to be able to interconvert the rate of drug delivery between the different units.

Example 15.46: Norepinephrine is a drug that is used to treat severe low blood pressure. The initial dosing recommendation is to start the dose between 8 and 12 mcg/min. To convert the starting dose of 8 mcg/min to an hourly rate:

$$\frac{8 \text{ mcg}}{1 \text{ min}} \times \frac{60 \text{ min}}{1 \text{ hr}} = 480 \text{ mcg/hr}$$

Pharmacists may also calculate how long an intravenous bag of medication will last so they can anticipate when to mix and supply a new one. They will calculate the rate of medication delivery and use the volume of the bag to determine how long that individual bag will last, assuming the dose does not change.

Example 15.47: A patient is receiving norepinephrine continuous infusion at 12 mcg/min, and the volume of the bag supplied is 4 mcg/mL in 500 mL. To calculate how long the bag is anticipated to last:

Step 1: Calculate the amount of drug provided in the 500-mL bag.

$$4\,\frac{\text{mcg}}{\text{mL}} \times 500 \text{ mL} = 2{,}000 \text{ mcg}$$

Step 2: Calculate the amount of drug provided in 1 hour.

$$\frac{12 \text{ mcg}}{\text{min}} = \frac{60 \text{ min}}{1 \text{ hr}} = 720 \text{ mcg/hr}$$

Step 3: Calculate how long the bag will last based on the 2,000 mcg of drug supplied in the bag.

$$\frac{720 \text{ mcg}}{1 \text{ hr}} = \frac{2{,}000 \text{ mcg}}{X \text{ hr}} \rightarrow X = 2.78 \text{ hr}$$

Thus, the bag will need to be replaced after a little more than 2½ hours.

Nutrition Provision

In addition to providing medications, pharmacists provide specialist types of nutrition to certain patients who are unable to eat normally. There are two ways to administer specialized nutrition: send nutrition down a tube into the stomach or small intestine, or infuse it directly into the blood. Specialized nutrition therapy employs many of the calculation skills described thus far. Nevertheless, to clarify the types of calculations that a pharmacist will perform in this area, a little explanation and terminology must first be provided.

Parenteral Nutrition Versus Enteral Nutrition

Enteral nutrition describes food that enters the gut, where it is digested and processed into smaller units. This could be food we put into our mouths or liquid food that enters the gut through a feeding tube. Parenteral nutrition describes the provision of nutrients in "predigested" liquid form straight into the bloodstream (intravenous; i.e., as a sterile liquid straight into the venous circulation). **Figure 15.11** shows the difference between parenteral and enteral nutrition.

Components of Parenteral Nutrition

Two major categories of components make up parenteral nutrition: macronutrients and micronutrients (see also the *Introduction to Nutrients* chapter). When designing what goes into parenteral nutrition, both the macronutrients and micronutrients can be adjusted to meet the needs of a specific patient (**Figure 15.12**).

Macronutrients

There are four macronutrients: protein, fat, carbohydrates, and water.

- Protein is available as a sterile solution of *amino acids*.

- Fat is available as a sterile solution of *lipids*.

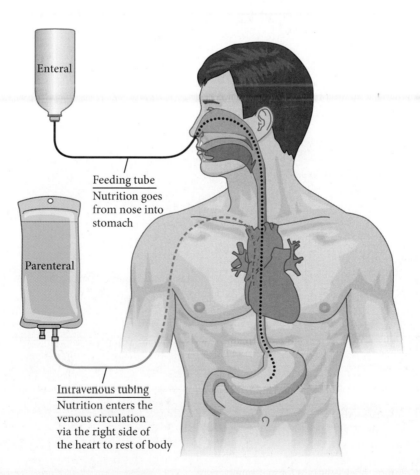

Figure 15.11 Routes of nutrition administration.

- Carbohydrate is available as a sterile solution of *dextrose*.
- Water is available as *Sterile Water for Injection*.

Amino acids, lipids, and dextrose are all available commercially in different percentage strength solutions that can be used as stock solutions when compounding a parenteral nutrition bag (**Figure 15.13**).

Each macronutrient supplies a certain amount of kcal per gram. **Table 15.6** shows the kilocalories of energy provided by 1 gram of each macronutrient.

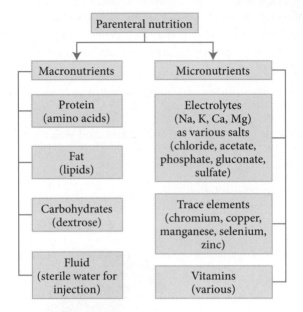

Figure 15.12 Major components of parenteral nutrition.

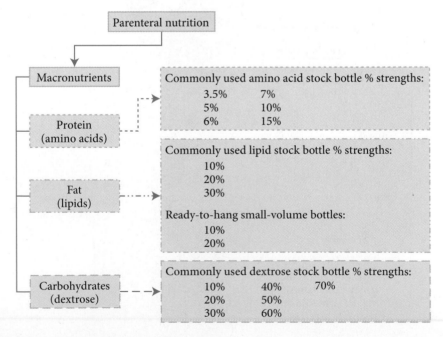

Figure 15.13 Common stock solutions for macronutrients.

Table 15.6 Energy Content of Macronutrients

Macronutrient	Energy (kcal/g)
Amino acids	4
Dextrose	3.4
Lipids	9

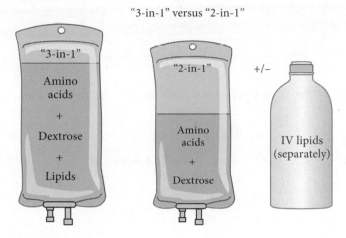

Figure 15.14 Types of parenteral nutrition.

A parenteral nutrition bag containing all the macronutrients together in one bag is called a "3-in-1" (referring to the inclusion of protein, fat, and carbohydrates). Alternatively, commercially available products containing preset volumes of amino acids and dextrose, in varying concentrations, are available. These products, called "2-in-1" nutrition bags, are provided in special packaging that allows the amino acid and dextrose solutions to be mixed together without having to compromise their sterility. If a patient receiving a "2-in-1" nutrition bag is to receive lipids as well, these are supplied separately using a different intravenous line (**Figure 15.14**).

A typical parenteral nutrition prescription provides the desired protein kilocalories, and then makes up the remaining kilocalories with as much as 30% of the daily kilocalories as fat, and the remainder as dextrose. **Figure 15.15** shows the typical kilocalorie percentage breakdown of the macronutrients.

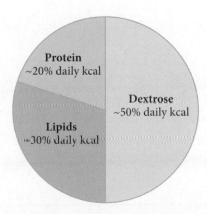

Figure 15.15 Parenteral nutrition typical calorie percentage from each macronutrient.

Example 15.48: A parenteral nutrition solution contains 900 mL of dextrose 70%, 800 mL of amino acid 8%, and 150 mL lipid 30%.

A. How many grams of dextrose are in the solution?

Dextrose 70% means 70 g per 100 mL, so 900 mL contains

$$\frac{70 \text{ g dextrose}}{100 \text{ mL}} = \frac{X \text{ g dextrose}}{900 \text{ mL}} = 630 \text{ g dextrose}$$

B. How many kilocalories of dextrose are in the solution?

From Table 15.6, each 1 g of dextrose provides 3.4 kcal, so 630 g dextrose provides

$$630 \text{ g dextrose} \times \frac{3.4 \text{ kcal}}{\text{g dextrose}} = 2,142 \text{ kcal}$$

C. How many grams of protein are in the solution?

The protein in the solution comes from amino acids. Amino acid 8% means 8 g per 100 mL, so 800 mL contains

$$\frac{8 \text{ g amino acids}}{100 \text{ mL}} = \frac{X \text{ g amino acids}}{800 \text{ mL}} = 64 \text{ g amino acids}$$

D. How many protein kilocalories are in the solution?

From Table 15.6, each 1 g of amino acids provides 4 kcal, so 64 g amino acids provides

$$64 \text{ g amino acids} \times \frac{4 \text{ kcal}}{\text{g amino acids}} = 256 \text{ kcal}$$

E. How many grams of fat are in the solution?

The fat in the solution comes from lipids. Lipids 30% means 30 g lipids per 100 mL, so 150 mL contains

$$\frac{30 \text{ g lipids}}{100 \text{ mL}} = \frac{X \text{ g lipids}}{150 \text{ mL}} = 45 \text{ g lipids}$$

F. How many fat kilocalories are in the solution?

From Table 15.6, each 1 g of fat provides 9 kcal, so 45 g lipids provides

$$45 \text{ g lipids} \times \frac{9 \text{ kcal}}{\text{g lipids}} = 405 \text{ kcal}$$

G. How many total kilocalories of energy does this parenteral nutrition solution provide?

Dextrose kcal = 2,142 kcal

Protein kcal = 256 kcal

Fat kcal = 405 kcal

Total kcal = 2,803 kcal

Fluid Requirements

The final macronutrient in a parenteral nutrition formula is water. The fluid requirements of a given patient can vary tremendously depending on factors such as the individual's medical conditions, degree of fluid loss from wounds, or sweating. As a general guide, typical daily fluid needs for a standard patient, without special fluid needs or restriction, are 30–40 mL/kg/day. When supplying a patient with parenteral nutrition, the volume provided by the other macronutrients and micronutrients is first calculated, and any deficit between what is supplied and what the patient needs is added in the form of Sterile Water for Injection.

Example 15.49: What are the estimated daily fluid needs for an adult patient weighing 72 kg?

Answer

The daily fluid needs, assuming no special fluid restrictions or need for additional fluid, are estimated at 30–40 mL/kg/day. Therefore, for a 72-kg patient:

$$72 \text{ kg} \times \frac{30 \text{ mL}}{\text{kg}} = 2{,}160 \text{ mL} / \text{day}$$

$$72 \text{ kg} \times \frac{40 \text{ mL}}{\text{kg}} = 2{,}880 \text{ mL} / \text{day}$$

Therefore, the estimated daily fluid needs would be 2,160–2,880 mL/day.

Calories

The macronutrients protein, carbohydrates, and fat all contain calories (kcal). When designing a nutrition regimen for a specific patient, there is a goal number of kilocalories to provide. In addition to calculating the needed daily kilocalories, the grams of protein needed per day are calculated. The American Society for Parenteral and Enteral Nutrition (ASPEN) provides guidelines for how many kilocalories and grams of protein per day are recommended for specific types of patients. These guidelines are summarized in **Table 15.7**. Note that the table refers to actual body weight (ABW) and ideal body weight (IBW); these were described in the "Patient-Specific Calculations" section.

Table 15.7 Guidelines for Nutrient Provision

Type of Patient	Kilocalories	Protein
Hospitalized, not critically ill	20–25 kcal/kg ABW/day	0.8–1 g/kg ABW/day
Critically ill, BMI < 30	25–30 kcal/kg ABW/day	1.2–2 g/kg ABW/day
Critically ill, BMI 30–39	11–14 kcal/kg ABW	≥ 2 g/kg IBW/day
Critically ill, BMI ≥ 40	11–14 kcal/kg ABW	≥ 2.5 g/kg IBW/day

Adapted from: McClave SA, Martindale RG, Vanek VW, et al. Guidelines for the provision and assessment of nutrition support therapy in the adult critically ill patient: Society of Critical Care Medicine (SCCM) and American Society for Parenteral and Enteral Nutrition (A.S.P.E.N.). *J Parenter Enteral Nutr.* 2009;33(3): 277–316.

Example 15.50: What are the goal daily kilocalories for a critically ill patient who is 5'6" tall and weighs 78 kg?

Answer

Step 1: To find the correct category of goal kilocalories, the BMI must be calculated:

$$BMI = \frac{Weight\ (kg)}{Height\ (m)^2}$$

Because the height is reported in inches, this must first be converted to meters:

$$66\ in. \times \frac{1\ m}{39.37\ in.} = 1.68\ m$$

Now the BMI can be calculated:

$$BMI = \frac{70\ kg}{1.68\ m^2} = 27.6$$

As the patient's BMI is less than 30, the goal daily kilocalories is 25–30 kcal/kg ABW/day.

Step 2: Calculate the goal kilocalories range. The goal range daily kilocalories is 25–30 kcal/kg ABW/day.

$$25\ kcal/kg \times 78\ kg = 1,950\ kcal$$

$$30\ kcal/kg \times 78\ kg = 2,340\ kcal$$

Therefore, goal daily kilocalories range is 1,950–2,340 kcal.

Micronutrients

In addition to the macronutrients that provide energy, other vital nutrients are provided in the parenteral nutrition formula. These so-called micronutrients consist of vitamins, trace elements, and electrolytes—all of which are normally provided by the food we eat, and all of which are vital for normal physiologic functions (see also the *Introduction to Nutrients* chapter).

The electrolytes are salts such as sodium chloride, potassium chloride, sodium phosphate, potassium phosphate, calcium gluconate, and magnesium sulfate. ASPEN also provides guidelines for typically required daily quantities of these salts; the exact amounts in any patient-specific parenteral nutrition prescription will vary depending on the patient's organ function (such as kidney and liver function) as well as the patient's medical conditions and medications provided. Pharmacists monitor electrolyte blood levels for patients receiving parenteral nutrition and make adjustments accordingly. The calculations already covered in the section "Concepts and Units for Electrolytes" are further applied here.

Example 15.51: Potassium chloride 60 mEq is ordered to be added to the parenteral nutrition solution. The stock vial comes in a concentration of 2 mEq per mL fluid. How many milliliters of stock KCl should be added to the formula?

Answer

$$\frac{2 \text{ mEq KCl}}{\text{mL}} = \frac{60 \text{ mEq KCl}}{X \text{ mL}} = 30 \text{ mL KCl to be added}$$

Calculating a Parenteral Nutrition Order

The calculations required for compounding a parenteral nutrition order utilize many of the calculations already covered in this chapter, so they offer an excellent opportunity to review all the major concepts. To ascertain the goal daily kilocalories and grams of protein, the patient's weight must be assessed for correct dosing weight, based on BMI. The daily fluid requirements must be known, and the percentage breakdowns between the macronutrients must be calculated.

Once the amino acid, dextrose, and lipid calculations have been performed, the volumes of electrolyte solutions to be added must be calculated. Then, the volume of water to be added is determined, and the hourly rate for delivery can finally be calculated (**Figure 15.16**).

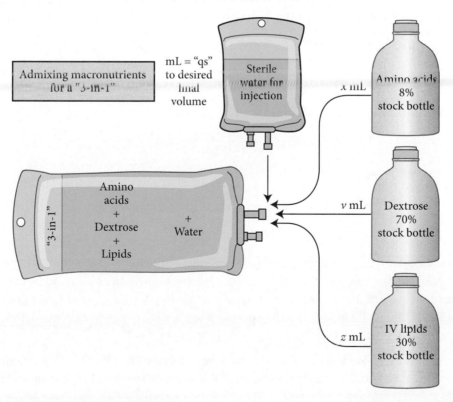

Figure 15.16 Parenteral nutrition preparation.

Example 15.52: A 5'8", 70-kg, critically ill male is to be started on parenteral nutrition. The stock solutions of macronutrients available for this preparation are amino acids 7%, dextrose 70%, and lipids 20%.

Step 1: Select the goal nutrition ranges. To select the correct goal range, the BMI must first be calculated:

$$BMI = \frac{Weight\ (kg)}{Height\ (m)^2}$$

As the height is reported in inches, it must first be converted to meters:

$$68\ in. \times \frac{1\ m}{39.37\ in.} = 1.73\ m$$

Now the BMI can be calculated:

$$BMI = \frac{70\ kg}{1.73\ m^2} = 23.4$$

Because the patient's BMI is less than 30, the goal daily kilocalories is 25–30 kcal/kg ABW/day, and the goal daily protein grams is 1.2–2 g protein/kg ABW/day.

Step 2: Calculate the goal daily kilocalories and grams of protein.

A. The goal range daily kilocalories is 25–30 kcal/kg ABW/day

$$25\ kcal/kg \times 70\ kg = 1,750\ kcal$$

$$30\ kcal/kg \times 70\ kg = 2,100\ kcal$$

Therefore, the goal daily kilocalories range is 1,750–2,100 kcal.

B. The goal range daily protein grams is 1.2–2 g protein/kg ABW/day.

$$1.2\ g/kg \times 70\ kg = 84\ g\ protein$$

$$2\ g/kg \times 70\ kg = 140\ g\ protein$$

Therefore, goal daily protein g range is 84–140 g protein.

Step 3: Calculate the volume of amino acid stock solution required to deliver the goal protein grams. To calculate the volume of amino acid stock solution to use, an absolute amount of protein to provide to the patient must be selected. Typically, a value somewhere around the middle of the range is selected, unless there is a clinical reason to select a value closer to either end of the range. In this case, we will pick a goal of delivering 110 g protein per day.

Using an amino acid stock solution of 7%, the volume required to provide 110 g protein can be calculated using the ratio and proportion method. Recall that a 7% amino acid solution means 7 g per 100 mL.

$$\frac{7\ g\ amino\ acids}{100\ mL} = \frac{110\ g\ amino\ acids}{X\ mL} = 1571\ mL\ stock\ solution$$

Step 4: Calculate how many kilocalories are provided by the amino acids. Using Table 15.6, we see that each 1 g of amino acids supplies 4 kcal/g.

110 g protein × 4 kcal/g = 440 kcal

Since the goal range of kcal was between 1,750 and 2,100 kcal, if the kilocalories supplied by the amino acids is subtracted, the remaining number of kilocalories to provide with the other macro-nutrients can be calculated:

1,750 kcal − 440 kcal = 1,310 kcal

2,100 kcal − 440 kcal = 1,660 kcal

Therefore, the remaining kilocalories to be provided with dextrose and lipids is in the range of 1,310–1,660 kcal.

Step 5: Calculate how many grams of lipids to provide. As the maximum kilocalories provided by lipids is approximately 30%:

1,750 kcal × 30% = 525 kcal

2,100 kcal × 30% = 700 kcal

We will select 600 kcal to be supplied as lipids.

Step 6: Calculate the number of grams of lipids delivered by the selected 600 lipid kcal.

$$\frac{1 \text{ g lipids}}{9 \text{ kcal}} = \frac{X \text{ g lipids}}{600 \text{ kcal}} = 66.7 \text{ g lipids}: \text{ round to 67 g}$$

Step 7: Calculate the volume of lipid stock solution required to deliver the selected lipid kilocalories. The lipid stock solution is 30%.

$$\frac{30 \text{ g lipids}}{100 \text{ mL}} = \frac{67 \text{ g lipids}}{X \text{ mL}} = 223 \text{ mL}$$

Step 8: Calculate the remaining kilocalories to be supplied as dextrose. The remaining kilocalories to be provided by dextrose and lipids was 1,310–1,660 kcal. With 600 kcal supplied as lipids, the remaining kilocalories to provide as dextrose can now be calculated:

1,310−600 kcal = 710 kcal

1,660−600 kcal = 1,060 kcal

Therefore, the kilocalories range remaining to supply as dextrose is 710–1,060 kcal.

Step 9: Calculate the number of grams of dextrose to provide the remaining kilocalories. We will provide 900 kcal as dextrose (the remaining range is 710–1,060 kcal). The grams of dextrose provided by 900 kcal is calculated as follows:

$$\frac{1 \text{ g dextrose}}{3.4 \text{ kcal}} = \frac{X \text{ g dextrose}}{900 \text{ kcal}} = 264.7 \text{ g; rounded to 265 g}$$

Step 10: Calculate the volume of dextrose 70% stock solution needed to provide 265 g dextrose.

$$\frac{70 \text{ g dextrose}}{100 \text{ mL}} = \frac{265 \text{ g dextrose}}{X \text{ mL}} = 379 \text{ mL}$$

Step 11: Review the final macronutrient formula (**Table 15.8**).

Table 15.8 Macronutrient Formula for Example 15.52

Macronutrient	Stock Solution	Grams	Volume (mL)	Energy (kcal)
Amino acids	7%	110 (see step 3)	1,571 (see step 3)	440
Lipids	30%	67 (see step 6)	223 (see step 7)	603
Dextrose	70%	265 g (see step 9)	379 (see step 10)	901
Total			2,173	**1,944** (compare to goal range of 1,750–2,100 kcal)

Step 12: Calculate the fluid requirements. The usual recommended daily fluid needs are 30–40 mL/kg/day.

$$30 \text{ mL/kg} \times 70 \text{ kg} = 2,100 \text{ mL}$$

$$40 \text{ mL/kg} \times 70 \text{ kg} = 2,800 \text{ mL}$$

The formula without any additional fluid provides 2,173 mL. The micronutrient additives typically provide an additional 100–150 mL. This would bring the total volume to 2,183–2,323 mL. Thus no additional fluid needs to be added to this formula to meet the daily goal fluid delivery. If the patient for any reason needs additional fluid, a separate IV bag of fluid can be provided.

Step 13: Calculate the volume of each of the micronutrients ordered. In this example, the following daily micronutrients are ordered:

Sodium chloride	40 mEq
Sodium phosphate	30 mmol
Potassium chloride	40 mEq
Potassium acetate	20 mEq
Calcium gluconate	10 mEq
Magnesium sulfate	10 mEq
Trace elements	5 mL
Multivitamins	10 mL

To calculate the volume of each of the electrolytes ordered, the concentration of each commercially available vial needs to be known. Once this is known, the volume for each micronutrient can be calculated by using the ratio and proportion method (**Table 15.9**).

Step 14: Calculate the total volume of the parenteral nutrition formula.

Macronutrients: 1,944 mL

Micronutrients: 89 mL

Total: 2,033 mL

Table 15.9 Micronutrient Formula for Example 15.52

Micronutrient	Amount Ordered	Concentration of Vial Used	Volume to Add to Parenteral Nutrition Formula
Sodium chloride	40 mEq	23.4% (4 mEq/mL)	$\dfrac{4\ \text{mEq}}{1\ \text{mL}} = \dfrac{40\ \text{mEq}}{X\ \text{mL}} = 10\ \text{mL}$
Sodium phosphate	30 mmol	3 mmol phosphate/mL	$\dfrac{3\ \text{mmol}}{1\ \text{mL}} = \dfrac{30\ \text{mmol}}{X\ \text{mL}} = 10\ \text{mL}$
Potassium chloride	40 mEq	2 mEq/mL	$\dfrac{2\ \text{mEq}}{1\ \text{mL}} = \dfrac{40\ \text{mEq}}{X\ \text{mL}} = 20\ \text{mL}$
Potassium acetate	20 mEq	2 mEq/mL	$\dfrac{2\ \text{mEq}}{1\ \text{mL}} = \dfrac{20\ \text{mEq}}{X\ \text{mL}} = 10\ \text{mL}$
Calcium gluconate	10 mEq	10% (0.465 mEq/mL)	$\dfrac{0.465\ \text{mEq}}{1\ \text{mL}} = \dfrac{10\ \text{mEq}}{X\ \text{mL}} = 21.5\ \text{mL}$
Magnesium sulfate	10 mEq	50% (4 mEq/mL)	$\dfrac{4\ \text{mEq}}{1\ \text{mL}} = \dfrac{10\ \text{mEq}}{X\ \text{mL}} = 2.5\ \text{mL}$
Trace elements	5 mL		5 mL
Multivitamins	10 mL		10 mL
Total volume			89 mL

Enteral Nutrition

Calculations relating to enteral nutrition ascertain the goal hourly rate needed to meet the desired daily kilocalories and protein grams goals. The goal daily kilocalories and protein grams are the same for enteral nutrition as for parenteral nutrition (see Table 15.7).

Enteral nutrition formulas come in pre-prepared containers that are ready to hang by the patient and be connected to the feeding tube that is inserted into the patient's gastrointestinal tract. Different formulations are designed to provide different amounts of protein and kilocalories per milliliter of solution. When calculating the goal rate for enteral nutrition delivery, the two key pieces of information needed are the kcal/mL and the grams of protein/L (the latter is more typically reported on the product label than grams of protein/mL).

Example 15.53: A patient has a goal daily kilocalorie range of 1,300–1,625 kcal, and a goal daily protein of 52–65 g. The nutrition formula ordered contains 1.8 kcal/mL and 85 g protein/L (1,000 mL). The goal rate in mL/hr of this enteral formula can be calculated as follows:

Step 1: Select a goal for the protein grams. We will select 55 g protein per day, as a value in the middle of the goal range.

Step 2: Calculate the daily volume of formula needed to deliver 55 g protein.

$$\frac{85\ \text{g protein}}{1,000\ \text{mL}} = \frac{55\ \text{g protein}}{X\ \text{mL}} = 647\ \text{mL}$$

Step 3: Calculate the kilocalories provided by the volume selected.

$$\frac{1.8 \text{ kcal}}{1 \text{ mL}} = \frac{X \text{ kcal}}{647 \text{ mL}} = 1,165 \text{ kcal}$$

Step 4: Compare the kilocalories delivered by the selected protein goal to the goal for daily kilocalories. The kilocalorie goal range is 1,300–1,625 kcal. If 55 g protein is selected, only 1,165 kcal is provided every day, which is below the goal range. We therefore select a higher goal for protein—65 g per day—and reassess the number of kilocalories per day this amount provides.

$$\frac{85 \text{ g protein}}{1,000 \text{ mL}} = \frac{65 \text{ g protein}}{X \text{ mL}} = 765 \text{ mL}$$

$$\frac{1.8 \text{ kcal}}{1 \text{ mL}} = \frac{X \text{ kcal}}{765 \text{ mL}} = 1,377 \text{ kcal}$$

Changing the protein grams to 65 g per day, which is at the higher end of the goal range, will provide a number of kilocalories within the daily goal range. Sometimes a different type of nutrition formula that is higher in protein per liter must be selected to meet the patient goals.

Step 5: Calculate the hourly rate required to deliver the required volume. The total daily volume of nutrition formula required is 765 mL. We can calculate the hourly rate required to deliver this volume in 24 hours:

$$\frac{765 \text{ mL}}{\text{day}} \times \frac{1 \text{ day}}{24 \text{ hr}} = 32 \frac{\text{mL}}{\text{hr}}$$

Learning Bridge 15.6

Milrinone is an intravenous medication that is used in critically ill patients to help the heart pump more efficiently. This drug is commercially available as 40 mg/200 mL. It is dosed at 0.375mcg/kg/min for a patient who weighs 69 kg. If the dose is maintained at this level, for how many hours would this bag last?

Learning Bridge 15.7

A critically ill patient who weighs 68 kg (non-obese) is receiving parenteral nutrition daily with the following formula:

Dextrose 242 g

Amino acids 136 g

Lipids 60 g

A. How many kilocalories (kcal) per day are provided by this formula?
B. How many kcal/kg are provided by this formula?
C. How many g protein/kg are provided by this formula?

Medication Errors Related to Calculations

The Institute for Safe Medication Practices (ISMP) provides guidelines for reducing the possibility of medication errors. Unfortunately, pharmaceutical calculation errors can result in severe patient harm, even death.[1] For this reason, it is essential to follow the recommendations for best practices related to calculations. ISMP recommends that calculations be double-checked. However, it is known that the likelihood of noticing a calculation error is much higher if the double-check is performed *independently*—that is, if two people perform the calculation separately. Performing a calculation together with another person tends to lead to both persons making the same mistake, whereas independent calculation checking tends to avoid this possibility. When asked to double-check a calculation, it is important to treat this task as if you were doing the entire calculation alone from scratch, rather than taking any assumptions made by the other person.

ISMP also encourages that medication doses based on patient-specific information, such as weight, be written in such a way that an independent check can be performed. For example, if a medication is dosed as 5 mg/kg once daily and the patient weighs 10 kg, then it is recommended that the medication order include the final dose calculated in addition to providing the patient weight and dosing information. This allows the pharmacist to check the actual dose that was calculated as well as the basis for the dose.

Golden Keys for Pharmacy Students

1. Memorize common conversion factors used in pharmacy to convert between the SI and USCU systems of measurement.

2. In pharmacy and health care in general, it is critical to *use leading zeroes*, which precede a decimal point (0.5), and to *avoid trailing zeroes*, which follow a decimal point (0.50).

3. The percent sign (%) represents a given number "in a hundred" and is simply a fraction with a set denominator of 100.

4. To solve most basic algebraic equations, you must isolate the variable X onto one side of the equal sign by adding/subtracting or multiplying/dividing by the known values on the same side as X to cancel them out.

5. If set up incorrectly, a proportional calculation may yield an incorrect answer. To avoid this problem, when calculating proportions, you must *always include units of measurement and check your answer carefully*.

6. To use dimensional analysis to solve a problem, (1) identify the desired units, (2) enter the known data, (3) invert units as needed, and (4) finish the calculation.

7. When using dimensional analysis, if you have extra units after canceling out what you can, you have likely included values or conversions you do not need to solve the equation. If you cancel out what you can and do not have the desired units, you have likely forgotten to include a conversion or other ratio.

8. In a fraction or ratio, if both the numerator and the denominator are multiplied or divided by the same amount, then the number value of the fraction or ratio remains unchanged.

9. Percent strength concentration is standardized according to the type of mixture. An x% w/v solution means x g/100 mL, an x% v/v solution means x mL/100 mL, and an x% w/w mixture means x g/100g.

10. The "Magic Triangle" (Figure 15.6) provides a systematic method to interconvert between mg, mEq, mmol, and mOsm.

11. The safe administration of parenteral nutrition requires pharmacists to accurately apply many calculation concepts such as percent strength and unit interconversion.

12. The nutritional kilocalories value provided by each of the three major macronutrients must be known to ensure correct nutrition provision: carbohydrate = 3.4 kcal/g, protein = 4 kcal/g, and fat = 9 kcal/g.

13. Inaccuracies in pharmaceutical calculations have resulted in severe patient harm, including death. Extreme care must always be taken when performing calculations, and a second check is always warranted. Do not be afraid to ask for assistance when checking your calculations. Ensure all calculation double-checks are performed independently.

Learning Bridge Answers

15.1

$$1.5 \text{ tsp} \times \frac{5 \text{ mL}}{1 \text{ tsp}} = 7.5 \text{ mL}$$

15.2

$$\frac{21.6 \text{ mg}}{200 \text{ doses}} = \frac{X \text{ mg}}{1 \text{ dose}} \rightarrow 21.6 \text{ mg} \times 1 \text{ dose} = X \text{ mg} \times 200 \text{ dose} \rightarrow X \text{ mL} = \frac{21.6 \text{ mg} \times 1 \text{ dose}}{200 \text{ doses}} \rightarrow X$$
$$= 0.108 \text{ mg}$$

15.3

$$1:1,000 = \frac{1}{1,000} \times 100\% = 0.1\% = \frac{0.1 \text{ g}}{100 \text{ mL}} \times \frac{1,000 \text{ mg}}{\text{g}} = \frac{1 \text{ mg}}{\text{mL}}$$

15.4

Total dose of calcium carbonate ingested each day = 6 × 500 mg tablets = 3,000 mg

Using the Magic Triangle:

Step 1: Convert 3,000 mg into mmol (**Exhibit 15.1**).

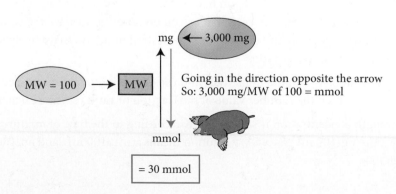

Exhibit 15.1 Calcium carbonate conversion mg to mmol.

Step 2: Convert 30 mmol into mEq (**Exhibit 15.2**).

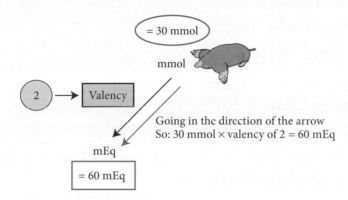

Exhibit 15.2 Calcium carbonate conversion mmol to mEq.

15.5

A. $\text{ABW} = 185 \text{ lb} \times \dfrac{1 \text{ kg}}{2.2 \text{ lb}} = 84.1 \text{ kg}$

$\text{IBW} = 45.5 \text{ kg} + (2.3 \times 4) = 54.7 \text{ kg}$

B. $\dfrac{\text{ABW}}{\text{IBW}} \times 100\% = \dfrac{84.1 \text{ kg}}{54.7 \text{ kg}} \times 100\% = 153.7\%$; ABW > 130% of IBW, so use IBW_{ADJ}.

$\text{IBW}_{\text{ADJ}} = 54.7 \text{ kg} + 0.4(84.1 \text{ kg} - 54.7 \text{ kg}) = 66.5 \text{ kg}$

C. $\text{CrCl} = \dfrac{(140 - 78) \times 66.5}{72 \times 2.6} = 22 \text{ mL / min}$

D. Ampicillin 2 g IV every 12 hours or ampicillin 2 g IV every 16 hours, depending on how aggressive the prescriber wishes to be

15.6

Step 1: Calculate concentration in mg/mL.

$\dfrac{40 \text{ mg milrinone}}{200 \text{ mL}} = 0.2 \text{ mg / mL}$

Step 2: Calculate the dose in mcg/min.

$69 \text{ kg} \times \dfrac{0.375 \text{ mcg}}{\dfrac{\text{kg}}{\text{min}}} = 25.875 \text{ mcg / min}$

Step 3: Calculate the dose in mg/hr.

$\dfrac{25.875 \text{ mcg}}{\text{min}} \times \dfrac{60 \text{ min}}{1 \text{ hr}} \times \dfrac{1 \text{ mg}}{1,000 \text{ mcg}} = 1.5525 \text{ mg/hr}$; round to 1.55 mg/hr

Step 4: Calculate the number of hours that 40 mg/200 mL of drug will last.

$\dfrac{1.55 \text{ mg}}{1 \text{ hr}} = \dfrac{40 \text{ mg}}{X \text{ hr}} = 25.81 \text{ hr}$

As most hospitals have a policy of discarding intravenous bags once they have been hanging for 24 hours to avoid infectious complications, this bag would be replaced at 24 hours.

15.7

A. Dextrose 242 g × 3.4 kcal/g = 822.8 kcal

Amino acids 136 g × 4 kcal/g = 544 kcal

Lipids 60 g × 9 kcal/g = 540 kcal

Total kcal = 1,906.8; round to 1,907 kcal

B. 1,907 kcal/68 kg = 28 kcal/kg

C. Amino acids 136 g/68 kg = 2 g protein/kg

Problems and Solutions

Problem 15.1 Convert the following values and round to one digit after the decimal point:

A. 25 mg = _____ g
B. 1.25 g = _____ mg
C. 500 g = _____ kg
D. 70 mg = _____ mcg
E. 55 mcg = _____ mg
F. 250 mL = _____ L
G. 1.75 L = _____ mL
H. 45 cm = _____ m
I. 2.15 m = _____ cm

Solution 15.1

A. $25 \text{ mg} \times \dfrac{1 \text{ g}}{1,000 \text{ mg}} = 0.025 \text{ g}$

B. $1.25 \text{ g} \times \dfrac{1,000 \text{ mg}}{1 \text{ g}} = 1,250 \text{ mg}$

C. $500 \text{ g} \times \dfrac{1 \text{ kg}}{1,000 \text{ g}} = 0.5 \text{ kg}$

D. $70 \text{ mg} \times \dfrac{1,000 \text{ mcg}}{1 \text{ mg}} = 70,000 \text{ mcg}$

E. $55 \text{ mcg} \times \dfrac{1 \text{ mg}}{1,000 \text{ mcg}} = 0.055 \text{ mg}$

F. $250 \text{ mL} \times \dfrac{1 \text{ L}}{1,000 \text{ mL}} = 0.25 \text{ L}$

G. $1.75 \text{ L} \times \dfrac{1,000 \text{ mL}}{1 \text{ L}} = 1,750 \text{ mL}$

H. $45 \text{ cm} \times \dfrac{1 \text{ m}}{100 \text{ cm}} = 0.45 \text{ m}$

I. $2.15 \text{ m} \times \dfrac{100 \text{ cm}}{1 \text{ m}} = 215 \text{ cm}$

Problem 15.2 Convert the following values and round to one digit after the decimal point:

   A. 66 in. = _____ ft
   B. 2 Tbsp = _____ tsp
   C. 1.5 pt = _____ fl oz
   D. 1.5 tsp = _____ mL
   E. 240 mL = _____ pt
   F. 12 oz = _____ mL
   G. 30 mL = _____ Tbsp
   H. 73 cm = _____ in
   I. 2.3 lb = _____ g

Solution 15.2

A. $66 \text{ in.} \times \dfrac{1 \text{ ft}}{12 \text{ in}} = 5.5 \text{ ft}$

B. $2 \text{ Tbsp} \times \dfrac{3 \text{ tsp}}{1 \text{ Tbsp}} = 6 \text{ tsp}$

C. $1.5 \text{ pt} \times \dfrac{16 \text{ fl oz}}{1 \text{ pt}} = 0.5 \text{ kg}$

D. $1.5 \text{ tsp} \times \dfrac{5 \text{ mL}}{1 \text{ tsp}} = 7.5 \text{ mL}$

E. $240 \text{ mL} \times \dfrac{1 \text{ pt}}{480 \text{ mL}} = 0.5 \text{ pt}$

F. $12 \text{ oz} \times \dfrac{30 \text{ mL}}{1 \text{ oz}} = 360 \text{ mL}$

G. $30 \text{ mL} \times \dfrac{1 \text{ Tbsp}}{15 \text{ mL}} = 2 \text{ Tbsp}$

H. $73 \text{ cm} \times \dfrac{1 \text{ in}}{2.54 \text{ cm}} = 28.7 \text{ in}$

I. $2.3 \text{ lb} \times \dfrac{453.6 \text{ g}}{1 \text{ lb}} = 1043.3 \text{ g}$

Problem 15.3 A patient is starting a new prescription mouth rinse with directions to swish and spit 30 mL by mouth four times a day. The patient asks you, "How many tablespoons do I take each time?" What is your answer?

Solution 15.3 $30 \text{ mL} \times \dfrac{1 \text{ Tbsp}}{15 \text{ mL}} = 2 \text{ Tbsp}$

Problem 15.4 You are entering a patient's information into a computer database and you note her height as 5 ft 9 in. The database asks for the height in centimeters. What do you enter?

Solution 15.4 $5 \text{ ft} \times \dfrac{12 \text{ in.}}{1 \text{ ft}} = 60 \text{ in.} + 9 \text{ in.} = 69 \text{ in.} \times \dfrac{2.54 \text{ cm}}{1 \text{ in.}} = 175.3 \text{ cm}$

Problem 15.5 Add, subtract, multiply, or divide the following fractions:

A. $\dfrac{3}{4}+\dfrac{5}{8}-\dfrac{3}{16}$

B. $\dfrac{1}{2}\times\dfrac{3}{5}\times\dfrac{4}{9}\times\dfrac{6}{25}$

C. $\dfrac{9}{10}\div\dfrac{4}{15}$

D. $\dfrac{2}{7}+\dfrac{53}{32}-\dfrac{22}{28}+\dfrac{17}{4}$

E. $\dfrac{12}{25}\times\dfrac{5}{11}\times\dfrac{8}{18}\times\dfrac{10}{21}\times\dfrac{24}{3}\times\dfrac{15}{4}$

F. $\dfrac{5}{22}\div\dfrac{7}{32}\div\dfrac{1}{11}$

Solution 15.5

A. $\dfrac{3}{4}+\dfrac{5}{8}-\dfrac{3}{16}=\dfrac{12+10-3}{16}=\dfrac{12}{16}-\dfrac{10}{16}-\dfrac{3}{16}=\dfrac{19}{16}$

B. $\dfrac{1}{2}\times\dfrac{3}{5}\times\dfrac{4}{9}\times\dfrac{6}{25}=\dfrac{1\times3\times4\times6}{2\times5\times9\times25}=\dfrac{72}{2,250}=\dfrac{36}{1,125}$

C. $\dfrac{9}{10}\div\dfrac{4}{15}\rightarrow\dfrac{9}{10}\times\dfrac{15}{4}=\dfrac{135}{40}=\dfrac{27}{8}$

D. $\dfrac{2}{7}+\dfrac{53}{32}-\dfrac{22}{28}+\dfrac{17}{4}=\dfrac{64+371-176+952}{224}=\dfrac{1,211}{224}=\dfrac{173}{32}$

E. $\dfrac{12}{25}\times\dfrac{5}{11}\times\dfrac{8}{18}\times\dfrac{10}{21}\times\dfrac{24}{3}\times\dfrac{15}{4}=\dfrac{12\times5\times8\times10\times24\times15}{25\times11\times18\times21\times3\times4}=\dfrac{1,728,000}{1,247,400}=\dfrac{320}{231}$

F. $\dfrac{5}{22}\div\dfrac{7}{32}\div\dfrac{1}{11}\rightarrow\dfrac{5}{22}\times\dfrac{32}{7}\times\dfrac{11}{1}=\dfrac{1,760}{154}=\dfrac{80}{7}$

Problem 15.6 Convert the following percentages to decimals:

A. 12.5%
B. 40%
C. 88%

Solution 15.6

A. $12.5\%=\dfrac{12.5}{100}=0.125$

B. $40\%=\dfrac{40}{100}=0.4$

C. $88\%=\dfrac{88}{100}=0.88$

Problem 15.7 Convert the following decimals to percentages:

    A. 0.45

    B. 0.257

    C. 0.095

Solution 15.7

    A. $0.45 \times 100\% = 45\%$

    B. $0.257 \times 100\% = 25.7\%$

    C. $0.095 \times 100\% = 9.5\%$

Problem 15.8 In the following equations, solve for X:

    A. $45.5 + 2.3X = 66.2$

    B. $110 + \left(5 \times (X - 60)\right) = 170$

    C. $15X \times \dfrac{5}{150} \times \dfrac{1}{15} = 2$

    D. $154 \times \dfrac{1}{X} \times 30 = 2{,}100$

    E. $\dfrac{625}{1{,}000} \times 14X = 35$

Solution 15.8

    A. $45.5 + 2.3X = 66.2 \rightarrow 2.3X = 66.2 - 45.5 \rightarrow X = \dfrac{20.7}{2.3} = 9$

    B. $110 + \left(5 \times (X - 60)\right) = 170 \rightarrow \left(5 \times (X - 60)\right) = 170 - 110 \rightarrow X - 60 = \dfrac{60}{5} \rightarrow X = 12 + 60 = 72$

    C. $15X \times \dfrac{5}{150} \times \dfrac{1}{15} = 2 \rightarrow 15X \times \dfrac{5}{150} = \dfrac{2}{\frac{1}{15}} \rightarrow 15X = \dfrac{30}{\frac{5}{150}} \rightarrow X = \dfrac{900}{15} = 60$

    D. $154 \times \dfrac{1}{X} \times 30 = 2{,}100 \rightarrow \dfrac{1}{X} = \dfrac{\frac{2{,}100}{154}}{30} \rightarrow \dfrac{1}{X} = 0.45454 \rightarrow X = \dfrac{1}{0.45454} = 2.2$

    E. $\dfrac{625}{1{,}000} \rightarrow 14X = 35 \rightarrow 14X = \dfrac{35}{0.625} \rightarrow X = \dfrac{56}{14} = 4$

Problem 15.9 If one tablet contains 250 mg of active drug, how many milligrams are in a bottle of 30 tablets?

Solution 15.9

$$\frac{250 \text{ mg}}{1 \text{ tab}} = \frac{X \text{ mg}}{30 \text{ tab}} \rightarrow 250 \text{ mg} \times 30 \text{ tab} = X \text{ mg} \times 1 \text{ tab} \rightarrow X \text{ mL} = \frac{250 \text{ mg} \times 30 \text{ tab}}{1 \text{ tab}} \rightarrow X = 7,500 \text{ mg}$$

Problem 15.10 If a drug costs \$83.50 for a bottle of 50 tablets, how much do 12 tablets cost?

Solution 15.10

$$\frac{\$83.50}{50 \text{ tab}} = \frac{\$X}{12 \text{ tab}} \rightarrow \$\,83.50 \times 12 \text{ tab} = \$X \times 50 \text{ tab} \rightarrow \$X = \frac{\$83.50 \times 12 \text{ tab}}{50 \text{ tab}} \rightarrow X = \$20.04$$

Problem 15.11 Ibuprofen (Advil) is available as a suspension that contains 50 mg of drug per 1.25 mL. How many milligrams are in 1.875 mL?

Solution 15.11

$$\frac{50 \text{ mg}}{1.25 \text{ mL}} = \frac{X \text{ mg}}{1.875 \text{ mL}} \rightarrow 50 \text{ mg} \times 1.875 \text{ mL} = X \text{ mg} \times 1.25 \text{ mL} \rightarrow X \text{ mg}$$

$$= \frac{50 \text{ mg} \times 1.875 \text{ mL}}{1.25 \text{ mL}} \rightarrow X = 75 \text{ mg}$$

Problem 15.12 Insulin is commonly available at a strength of 100 units per milliliter, or 100 U/mL. How many milliliters are needed for a dose of 85 units?

Solution 15.12

$$\frac{100 \text{ units}}{1 \text{ mL}} = \frac{85 \text{ units}}{X \text{ mL}} \rightarrow 100 \text{ units} \times X \text{ mL} = 85 \text{ units} \times 1 \text{ mL} \rightarrow X \text{ mL}$$

$$= \frac{85 \text{ units} \times 1 \text{ mL}}{100 \text{ units}} \rightarrow X = 0.85 \text{ mL}$$

Problem 15.13 Drug E is dosed at 25 mg/kg/day and is available as an injection with 100 mg of drug in every milliliter of solution, or 100 mg/mL. How many milliliters will a patient receive each day if he weighs 67 lb?

Solution 15.13

$$\frac{25 \text{ mg}}{\text{kg}\Big/\text{day}} \times \frac{1 \text{ mL}}{100 \text{ mg}} \times 67 \text{ lb} \times \frac{1 \text{ kg}}{2.2 \text{ lb}} = \frac{7.6 \text{ mL}}{\text{day}}$$

Problem 15.14 Drug Q is dosed at 40 mg/kg/day divided twice daily, meaning the daily dose is divided into two doses given 12 hours apart, and the drug comes as a 500 mg/mL solution. How many milliliters will a patient receive with each dose if she weighs 175 lb?

Solution 15.14

$$\frac{40\ \cancel{mg}}{\cancel{kg}\Big/day} \times \frac{1\ \cancel{day}}{2\ doses} \times \frac{1\ mL}{500\ \cancel{mg}} \times 175\ \cancel{lb} \times \frac{1\ \cancel{kg}}{2.2\ \cancel{lb}} = \frac{3.2\ mL}{dose}$$

Problem 15.15 Drug U is dosed at 7.5 mg/kg/day divided four times daily for a total of 7 days, and the drug comes as a 200 mg/5 mL solution. How many milliliters will a patient receive over the entire 7-day regimen if he weighs 88 lb?

Solution 15.15

$$\frac{7.5\ \cancel{mg}}{\cancel{kg}\Big/day} \times 7\ \cancel{days} \times \frac{5\ mL}{200\ \cancel{mg}} \times 88\ \cancel{lb} \times \frac{1\ \cancel{kg}}{2.2\ \cancel{lb}} = 52.5\ mL$$

Problem 15.16 A solution contains 10 mg of Drug A per 0.8 mL of solution, and the dosing is 1.5 mg/kg/dose. How many milliliters will a patient receive with each dose if she weighs 39 lb?

Solution 15.16

$$\frac{0.8\ mL}{10\ \cancel{mg}} \times \frac{1.5\ \cancel{mg}}{\cancel{kg}\Big/dose} \times 39\ \cancel{lb} \times \frac{1\ \cancel{kg}}{2.2\ \cancel{lb}} = \frac{2.1\ mL}{dose}$$

Problem 15.17 A powdered medication in a bottle containing 500 g of Drug T is dosed at 100 mg/kg/day.

A. How many grams per day are needed for a patient who weighs 110 lb?

B. How many days will a single bottle last this patient?

Solution 15.17

A. $$\frac{100\ \cancel{mg}}{\cancel{kg}\,/\,day} \times 110\ \cancel{lb} \times \frac{1\ \cancel{kg}}{2.2\ \cancel{lb}} = \frac{g}{1000\ \cancel{mg}} = \frac{5\ g}{day}$$

B. $$500\ \cancel{g} \times \frac{1\ day}{5\ \cancel{g}} = 100\ days$$

Problem 15.18 A nasal spray bottle measures out 0.15 mL of solution, which contains 30 mcg of Drug E in each spray, and the bottle contains enough solution for 150 sprays.

A. How many milligrams of Drug E are in the entire bottle?
B. How many milliliters of solution are in the entire bottle?

Solution 15.18

A. $$\frac{30\ mcg}{spray} \times 150\ sprays \times \frac{1\ mg}{1,000\ mcg} = 4.5\ mg$$

B. $$\frac{0.15\ mL}{spray} \times 150\ sprays = 22.5\ mL$$

Problem 15.19 Express the following as mg/mL concentrations:

    A. 3 g potassium chloride in 250 mL water

    B. 2 g magnesium sulfate in 50 mL water

    C. 3.375 g piperacillin/tazobactam (an antibiotic) in 150 mL water

Solution 15.19

    A. Step 1: Express the 3 g as milligrams.

$$3\ g \times \frac{1,000\ mg}{1\ g} = 3,000\ mg$$

Step 2: Calculate the concentration in mg/mL.

$$\frac{3,000\ mg}{250\ mL} = 12\ \frac{mg}{mL}$$

    B. Step 1: Express the 2 g as milligrams.

$$2\ g \times \frac{1,000\ mg}{1\ g} = 2,000\ mg$$

Step 2: Calculate the concentration in mg/mL.

$$\frac{2,000\ mg}{50\ mL} = 40\ mg\,/\,mL$$

    C. Step 1: Express the 3.375 g as milligrams.

$$3.375\ g \times \frac{1,000\ mg}{1\ g} = 3,375\ mg$$

Step 2: Calculate the concentration in mg/mL.

$$\frac{3,375\ mg}{150\ mL} = 22.5\ mg\,/\,mL$$

Problem 15.20 What percentage w/v is a solution of 6,500 mg of magnesium sulfate in 250 mL water?

Solution 15.20

Step 1: Convert milligrams to grams.

$$6,500\ mg \times \frac{1\ g}{1,000\ mg} = 6.5\ g$$

Step 2: Calculate the number of grams per 100 mL.

$$\frac{6.5\ g\ magnesium\ sulfate}{250\ mL} = \frac{X\ g}{100\ mL} = 2.6\ g$$

Step 3: Express as a w/v concentration.

2.6 g per 100 mL = 2.6 % w/v concentration

Problem 15.21 What percentage w/v is a solution of 4g NaCl in 1,000 mL?

Solution 15.21

Step 1: Calculate the number of grams per 100 mL.

$$\frac{4 \text{ g NaCl}}{1,000 \text{ mL}} = \frac{X \text{ g}}{100 \text{ mL}} = 0.4 \text{ g}$$

Step 2: Express as a w/v concentration.

0.4 g per 100 mL = 0.4 % w/v concentration

Problem 15.22 What percentage w/w is a cream made with 25 g hydrocortisone cream in 50 g of cream base?

Solution 15.22

Step 1: Calculate the number of grams per 100 g.

$$\frac{25 \text{ g hydrocortisone}}{50 \text{ g cream}} = \frac{X \text{ g}}{100 \text{ mL}} = 50 \text{ g}$$

Step 2: Express as a w/v concentration.

50 g per 100 g = 50% w/w concentration

Problem 15.23 What percentage v/v is 250 mL isopropyl alcohol mixed with 150 mL liquid?

Solution 15.23

Step 1: Calculate the number of milliliters per 100 mL.

$$\frac{250 \text{ mL isopropyl alcohol}}{150 \text{ mL liquid}} = \frac{X \text{ mL}}{100 \text{ mL}} = 167 \text{ mL}$$

Step 2: Express as a v/v concentration.

250 mL per 100 mL = 167% v/v concentration

Problem 15.24 Convert a 1:250,000 solution into percentage w/v.

Solution 15.24

Step 1: Express as a fraction and convert to a percentage.

$$\frac{1}{250,000} \times 100\% = 0.0004\%$$

Step 2: Express as a w/v percent strength.

0.0004% or 0.0004 g/100 mL

Problem 15.25 Express a 16% w/v solution as a ratio strength.

Solution 15.25

Step 1: Express the percent strength first as a fraction, then as a ratio.

16% = 16/100 = 16:100

Step 2: To make the first number in the ratio equal to 1, divide the entire ratio by the first number.

$$\frac{16:100}{16}$$

Step 3: Perform the calculation to find the final 1:x ratio.

$$\frac{16:100}{16} = 1:6.25$$

Therefore, 16% = 1:6.25 ratio strength.

Problem 15.26 How many milligrams are contained in 50 mL of a 1:250 solution?

Solution 15.26

Step 1: Express as a fraction and then convert to a percentage.

$$\frac{1}{250} \times 100\% = 0.4\ \%$$

Step 2: Express as a w/v percent strength.

$$0.4\ \% = 0.4\ g/100\ mL$$

Step 3: Calculate grams per 50 mL.

$$\frac{0.4\ g}{100\ mL} = \frac{X\ g}{50\ mL} = 0.2\ g$$

Step 4: Convert to milligrams per 50 mL.

$$0.2\ g \times \frac{1,000\ mg}{1\ g} = 200\ mg$$

Problem 15.27 You are mixing a custom dosed nasal spray and need 5 mL of a 1.5% solution, which you will mix from two standard strengths, 1% and 3%.

    A. How many milliliters of the 1% solution will you need?
    B. How many milliliters of the 3% solution will you need?

Solution 15.27

A.

    3%   0.5 part of 3% solution

           1.5%

    1%

                 1.5 parts of 0.1% solution

                 2 parts total

$$\frac{0.5\ part\ 3\%\ soln}{2\ parts} = \frac{X\ mL\ 3\%\ soln}{5\ mL\ total\ soln} \rightarrow X = 1.25\ mL\ of\ 3\%\ soln$$

B. $$\frac{1.5\ parts\ 1\%\ soln}{2\ parts} = \frac{X\ mL\ 1\%\ soln}{5\ mL\ total\ soln} \rightarrow Y = 3.75\ mL\ of\ 1\%\ soln$$

Problem 15.28 You are mixing an injectable drug for veterinary use and need 20 mL of 10 mg/mL solution. You have a concentrated solution of drug that is 75 mg/mL and normal saline, which has no active drug (0 mg/mL), to use as a diluent.

A. How many milliliters of the 75 mg/mL solution will you need?

B. How many milliliters of the normal saline will you need?

Solution 15.28

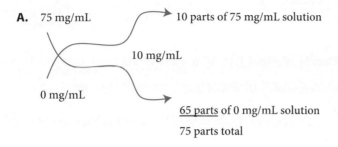

A. 75 mg/mL → 10 parts of 75 mg/mL solution

10 mg/mL

0 mg/mL → 65 parts of 0 mg/mL solution

75 parts total

$$\frac{10 \text{ parts } 75 \text{ mg}/\text{mL soln}}{75 \text{ parts}} = \frac{X \text{ mL } 75 \text{ mg}/\text{mL soln}}{20 \text{ mL total soln}} \rightarrow X = 2.67 \text{ mL of } \frac{75 \text{ mg}}{\text{mL}} \text{ soln}$$

B. $$\frac{65 \text{ parts } 0 \text{ mg}/\text{mL soln}}{75 \text{ parts}} = \frac{X \text{ mL } 0 \text{ mg}/\text{mL soln}}{20 \text{ mL total soln}} \rightarrow Y = 17.33 \text{ mL of } \frac{0 \text{ mg}}{\text{mL}} \text{ soln}$$

Problem 15.29 You are asked to mix 2.5 mL of a 0.5% eye drop solution using a low-strength 0.2% solution and a high-strength 50 mg/mL solution.

A. How many milliliters of the 0.2% solution will you need?

B. How many milliliters of the 50 mg/mL solution will you need?

Solution 15.29

A. 50 mg/mL → 8 parts of 50 mg/mL solution

5 mg/mL

2 mg/mL → 45 parts of 2 mg/mL solution

53 parts total

$$\frac{8 \text{ parts } 50 \text{ mg}/\text{mL soln}}{53 \text{ parts}} = \frac{X \text{ mL } 50 \text{ mg}/\text{mL soln}}{2.5 \text{ mL total soln}} \rightarrow X = 0.38 \text{ mL of } \frac{50 \text{ mg}}{\text{mL}} \text{ soln}$$

B. $$\frac{45 \text{ parts } 2 \text{ mg}/\text{mL soln}}{53 \text{ parts}} - \frac{X \text{ mL } 2 \text{ mg}/\text{mL soln}}{2.5 \text{ mL total soln}} \rightarrow Y = 2.12 \text{ mL of } \frac{2 \text{ mg}}{\text{mL}} \text{ soln}$$

Problem 15.30 Express 4 mmol/L potassium as mg/dL (MW of K is 39).

Solution 15.30

$$\frac{4 \text{ mmol}}{1 \text{ L}} \times \frac{39 \text{ mg}}{\text{mmol}} \times \frac{1 \text{ L}}{10 \text{ dL}} = \frac{15.6 \text{ mg}}{\text{dL}}$$

Problem 15.31 Express 12.4 mg/dL calcium as mmol/L (MW of Ca is 40).

Solution 15.31

$$\frac{12.4 \text{ mg}}{1 \text{ dL}} \times \frac{1 \text{ mmol}}{40 \text{ mg}} \times \frac{10 \text{ dL}}{L} = \frac{3.1 \text{ mmol}}{L}$$

Problem 15.32 Express 102 mEq/L chloride as mmol/L (MW of Cl is 35.5).

Solution 15.32 102 mEq/L divided by valency of = 02 mmol/L.

Problem 15.33 For each of the following intravenous fluids, determine whether they are isotonic, hypotonic, or hypertonic.

  A. NaCl 22.5%
  B. Dextrose 5% (253 mOsm/L)
  C. NaCl 45g/250 mL

Solution 15.33

  A. This IV solution would be described as hypertonic because it is far more concentrated than NS:

   NaCl 22.5% = 22.5 g NaCl/100 mL

   NaCl 0.9% normal saline [NS]) = 0.9 g NaCl/100 mL

  B. The normal mOsm/L value for human blood is 280–310. Because this IV solution has only 253 mOsm/L, it would be described as hypotonic.

  C. To assess this IV fluid, we need to ascertain the grams of NaCl per 100 mL:

   $$\frac{2.25 \text{ g}}{250 \text{ mL}} = \frac{X \text{ g}}{100 \text{ mL}} = 0.9 \text{ g per 100 mL, or } 0.9\% \text{ NaCl}$$

   This IV fluid is normal saline and is therefore isotonic.

Problem 15.34 How many milligrams of calcium chloride are provided by 27 mOsm?

Solution 15.34

Step 1: Convert from mOsm to mmol.

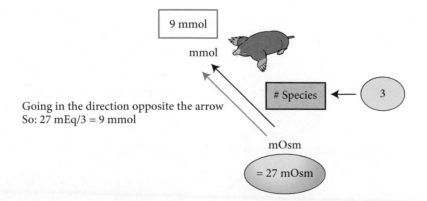

Going in the direction opposite the arrow
So: 27 mEq/3 = 9 mmol

Step 2: Convert from mmol to mg.

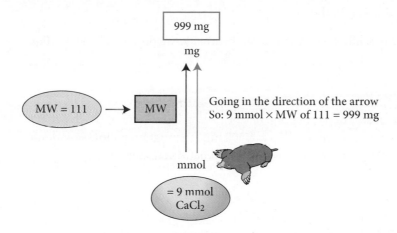

Therefore, 27 mOsm calcium chloride is provided by 999 mg (rounded to 1 g).

Problem 15.35 How many milligrams of magnesium sulfate are needed to supply 10 mEq?

Solution 15.35

Step 1: Convert from mEq to mmol.

10 mEq / valency of 2 = 5 mmol

Step 2: Convert mmol to mg.

5 mmol × MW of 120 = 600 mg

Problem 15.36 How many milliequivalents of sodium chloride are contained with 3 L of normal saline?

Solution 15.36

Step 1: Use the definition of "normal saline" together with fluid volume to calculate how many milligrams of salt are present.

- Normal saline, as described earlier, is by definition 0.9% NaCl.

- Because 0.9 % NaCl means 0.9 g NaCl per 100 mL, and we have 3 L of solution, the number of milligrams of NaCl can be calculated:

$$\frac{0.9 \text{ g NaCl}}{100 \text{ ml}} = \frac{X \text{ g}}{3,000 \text{ mL}} = 27 \text{ g NaCl}$$

- Express as milligrams: $27 \text{ g NaCl} \times \frac{1,000 \text{ mg}}{1 \text{ g}} = 27,000 \text{ mg}$

Step 2: Convert mg to mmol.

27,000 mg/MW of 58.5 = 462 mmol

Step 3: Convert mmol to mEq.

$$462 \text{ mmol} \times \text{valency of } 1 = 462 \text{ mEq}$$

Problem 15.37 How many millimoles of aluminum hydroxide are provided by 900 mEq?

Solution 15.37 Convert mEq to mmol.

$$900 \text{ mEq} / \text{valency of } 3 = 300 \text{ mmol}$$

Problem 15.38 A doctor orders dopamine at a rate of 15 mcg/kg/min for a 210-lb patient. The drug is available at a concentration of 400 mg/500 mL. To program an infusion pump, a nurse asks you for an infusion rate in units of mL/hr. What is your answer?

Solution 15.38

$$210 \text{ lb} \times \frac{1 \text{ kg}}{2.2 \text{ lb}} \times \frac{15 \text{ mcg}}{\text{kg}\big/\text{min}} \times \frac{500 \text{ mL}}{400 \text{ mg}} \times \frac{60 \text{ min}}{\text{hr}} \times \frac{1 \text{ mg}}{1,000 \text{ mcg}} = \frac{15.3 \text{ mL}}{\text{hr}}$$

Problem 15.39 A doctor orders the following drug for a 133-lb patient who is 5'6"tall: vancomycin 15 mg/kg/dose IV every 8 hr. You have the drug in a premixed solution of 500 mg/100 mL. How many milliliters per dose will the patient need?

Solution 15.39

$$133 \text{ lb} \times \frac{1 \text{ kg}}{2.2 \text{ lb}} \times \frac{15 \text{ mg}}{\text{kg}\big/\text{dose}} \times \frac{100 \text{ mL}}{500 \text{ mg}} = \frac{181 \text{ mL}}{\text{dose}}$$

Problem 15.40 Calculate the ABW and IBW of the following patients:

   A.   5'4", 180-lb male
   B.   5'1", 95-lb female
   C.   180-cm, 77-kg male
   D.   195-cm, 89-kg female

Solution 15.40

   A. $\text{ABW} = 180 \text{ lb} \times \dfrac{1 \text{ kg}}{2.2 \text{ lb}} = 81.8 \text{ kg} \quad \text{IBW} = 50 \text{ kg} + \left(2.3 \text{ kg} \times 4\right) = 59.2 \text{ kg}$

   B. $\text{ABW} = 95 \text{ lb} \times \dfrac{1 \text{ kg}}{2.2 \text{ lb}} = 43.2 \text{ kg} \quad \text{IBW} = 45.5 \text{ kg} + \left(2.3 \text{ kg} \times 1\right) = 47.8 \text{ kg}$

   C. $\text{ABW} = 77 \text{ kg} \times \dfrac{2.2 \text{ lb}}{1 \text{ kg}} = 169.4 \text{ lb}$

$$\text{IBW} = 50 \text{ kg} + \left(2.3 \text{ kg} \times \left(\frac{180 \text{ cm} - 152.4 \text{ cm}}{2.54}\right)\right) = 75 \text{ kg}$$

   D. $\text{ABW} = 89 \text{ kg} \times \dfrac{2.2 \text{ lb}}{1 \text{ kg}} = 195.8 \text{ lb}$

$$\text{IBW} = 45.5 \text{ kg} + \left(2.3 \text{ kg} \times \left(\frac{195 \text{ cm} - 152.4 \text{ cm}}{2.54}\right)\right) = 84 \text{ kg}$$

Problem 15.41 A patient with an ABW of 83.2 kg and an IBW of 68.4 kg is being dosed with a drug based on an adjusted IBW using a conversion factor of 0.35. What is the patient's IBW$_{ADJ}$?

Solution 15.41

$$IBW_{ADJ} = 68.4 \text{ kg} + 0.35(83.2 \text{ kg} - 68.4 \text{ kg}) = 73.6 \text{ kg}$$

Problem 15.42 A male patient who is 5'10" tall and weighs 164 lb is being dosed with a drug based on his IBW$_{ADJ}$ using a conversion factor of 0.25. What is the patient's IBW$_{ADJ}$?

Solution 15.42

$$ABW = 164 \text{ lb} \times \frac{1 \text{ kg}}{2.2 \text{ lb}} = 74.5 \text{ kg} \quad IBW = 50 \text{ kg} + (2.3 \text{ kg} \times 10) = 73 \text{ kg}$$

$$IBW_{ADJ} = 73 \text{ kg} + 0.25(74.5 \text{ kg} - 73 \text{ kg}) = 73.4 \text{ kg}$$

Problem 15.43 A female patient who is 6'1" tall and weighs 181 lb is being dosed with a drug based on her IBW$_{ADJ}$ using a conversion factor of 0.4. What is the patient's IBW$_{ADJ}$?

Solution 15.43

$$ABW = 181 \text{ lb} \times \frac{1 \text{ kg}}{2.2 \text{ lb}} = 82.3 \text{ kg} \quad IBW = 45.5 \text{ kg} + (2.3 \text{ kg} \times 13) = 75.4 \text{ kg}$$

$$IBW_{ADJ} = 75.4 \text{ kg} + 0.4(82.3 \text{ kg} - 75.4 \text{ kg}) = 78.2 \text{ kg}$$

Problem 15.44 Calculate the BSAs of the following patients:

A. 5'4" and 180 lb
B. 5'1" and 95 lb
C. 180 cm and 77 kg
D. 195 cm and 89 kg

Solution 15.44

A. $BSA = \sqrt{\dfrac{64 \times 180}{3131}} = 1.9 \text{ m}^2$

B. $BSA = \sqrt{\dfrac{61 \times 95}{3131}} = 2.1 \text{ m}^2$

C. $BSA = \sqrt{\dfrac{180 \times 77}{3600}} = 2 \text{ m}^2$

D. $BSA = \sqrt{\dfrac{195 \times 89}{3600}} = 2.2 \text{ m}^2$

Problem 15.45 Calculate the BMIs of the following patients:

A. 5'11" and 183 lb
B. 6'4" and 235 lb

C. 5'4" and 135 lb

D. 6'7" and 292 lb

Solution 15.45

A. $71 \text{ in.} \times \dfrac{1 \text{ m}}{39.37 \text{ in.}} = 1.8 \text{ m}$ $183 \text{ lb} \times \dfrac{1 \text{ kg}}{2.2 \text{ lb}} = 83.2 \text{ kg}$

$\text{BMI} = \dfrac{83.2 \text{ kg}}{1.8 \text{ m}^2} = 25.7$ $\text{BMI} = \dfrac{183 \text{ lb}}{71 \text{ in}^2} \times 704.5 = 25.6$

B. $76 \text{ in.} \times \dfrac{1 \text{ m}}{39.37 \text{ in.}} = 1.93 \text{ m}$ $235 \text{ lb} \times \dfrac{1 \text{ kg}}{2.2 \text{ lb}} = 106.8 \text{ kg}$

$\text{BMI} = \dfrac{106.8 \text{ kg}}{1.93 \text{ m}^2} = 28.7$ $\text{BMI} = \dfrac{235 \text{ lb}}{76 \text{ in}^2} \times 704.5 = 28.7$

C. $64 \text{ in.} \times \dfrac{1 \text{ m}}{39.37 \text{ in.}} = 1.63 \text{ m}$ $135 \text{ lb} \times \dfrac{1 \text{ kg}}{2.2 \text{ lb}} = 61.4 \text{ kg}$

$\text{BMI} = \dfrac{61.4 \text{ kg}}{1.63 \text{ m}^2} = 23.1$ $\text{BMI} = \dfrac{135 \text{ lb}}{64 \text{ in}^2} \times 704.5 = 23.2$

D. $79 \text{ in.} \times \dfrac{1 \text{ m}}{39.37 \text{ in.}} = 2 \text{ m}$ $292 \text{ lb} \times \dfrac{1 \text{ kg}}{2.2 \text{ lb}} = 132.7 \text{ kg}$

$\text{BMI} = \dfrac{132.7 \text{ kg}}{2 \text{ m}^2} = 33.2$ $\text{BMI} = \dfrac{292 \text{ lb}}{79 \text{ in}^2} \times 704.5 = 33$

Problem 15.46 What is the estimated creatinine clearance (CrCl) of a male patient who is 69 years old, is 6'2" tall, and weighs 245 lb, with a SCr of 1.9 mg/dL? Is this within the normal range or above/below normal?

Solution 15.46

A. $\text{ABW} = 245 \text{ lb} \times \dfrac{1 \text{ kg}}{2.2 \text{ lb}} = 111.4 \text{ kg}$

B. $\text{IBW} = 50 \text{ kg} + (2.3 \times 14) = 82.2 \text{ kg}$

C. $\dfrac{\text{ABW}}{\text{IBW}} \times 100\% = \dfrac{111.4 \text{ kg}}{82.2 \text{ kg}} \times 100\% = 135.5\%; \text{ ABW} > 130\% \text{ of IBW, so use IBW}_{\text{ADJ}}.$

D. $\text{IBW}_{\text{ADJ}} = 82.2 \text{ kg} + 0.4(111.4 \text{ kg} - 82.2 \text{ kg}) = 93.9 \text{ kg}$

E. $\text{CrCl} = \dfrac{(140 - 69) \times 93.9}{72 \times 1.9} = 48.7 \dfrac{\text{mL}}{\text{min}}; \text{ this CrCl is below the normal range.}$

Problem 15.47 What is the estimated CrCl of a female patient who is 56 years old, is 5'10" tall, and weighs 184 lb, with a SCr of 1.3 mg/dL? Is this within the normal range or above/below normal?

Solution 15.47

A. $\text{ABW} = 184 \text{ lb} \times \dfrac{1 \text{ kg}}{2.2 \text{ lb}} = 83.6 \text{ kg}$

B. $\text{IBW} = 45.5 \text{ kg} + (2.3 \times 10) = 68.5 \text{ kg}$

C. $\dfrac{\text{ABW}}{\text{IBW}} \times 100\% = \dfrac{83.6 \text{ kg}}{68.5 \text{ kg}} \times 100\% = 122\%$; ABW < 130% of IBW, so use IBW.

D. $\text{CrCl} = \dfrac{(140 - 56) \times 68.5}{72 \times 1.3} \times 0.85 = 52.3 \dfrac{\text{mL}}{\text{min}}$; CrCl is within the normal range.

Problem 15.48 Piperacillin/tazobactam is an antibiotic that is excreted from the body primarily through the kidneys. In patients with poor kidney function, the dose may need to be adjusted downward to avoid an excessive dose. The following table shows doses given to patients with decreased kidney function.

Piperacillin/Tazobactam Renal Dosing

Patient's CrCl	Recommended Dose
> 40 mL/min	3.375 g IV every 6 hr
20–40 mL/min	2.25 g IV every 6 hr
< 20 mL/min	2.25 g IV every 8 hr

What dose would you recommend for a male patient who is 72 years old, is 5'7" tall, and weighs 144 lb, with a SCr of 1.8 mg/dL?

Solution 15.48

A. $\text{ABW} = 144 \text{ lb} \times \dfrac{1 \text{ kg}}{2.2 \text{ lb}} = 65.5 \text{ kg}$

B. $\text{IBW} = 50 \text{ kg} + (2.3 \times 7) = 66.1 \text{ kg}$

C. $\dfrac{\text{ABW}}{\text{IBW}} \times 100\% = \dfrac{65.5 \text{ kg}}{66.1 \text{ kg}} \times 100\% = 99.1\%$; ABW < IBW, so use ABW.

D. $\text{CrCl} = \dfrac{(140 - 72) \times 65.5}{72 \times 1.8} = 34.4 \dfrac{\text{mL}}{\text{min}}$; recommend 2.25g IV every 6 hr.

Problem 15.49 How many milliliters of morphine, a potent pain medication, should be drawn up into a syringe to provide a 6 mg dose, if the stock vial contains 15 mg/mL?

Solution 15.49

$$\dfrac{15 \text{ mg morphine}}{\text{mL}} = \dfrac{6 \text{ mg morphine}}{X \text{ mL}} = 0.4 \text{ mL}$$

Problem 15.50 How many milliliters of prochlorperazine, an injectable antinausea drug, should be drawn up into a syringe to provide a 10 mg dose, if the stock vial contains 5 mg/mL?

Solution 15.50

$$\frac{5 \text{ mg prochlorperazine}}{\text{mL}} = \frac{10 \text{ mg prochlorperazine}}{X \text{ mL}} = 2 \text{ mL}$$

Problem 15.51 How many milliliters of tobramycin, an antibiotic, should be added to a small-volume IV bag (50 mL) to provide a dose of 280 mg to a patient?

Solution 15.51

$$\frac{40 \text{ mg tobramycin}}{\text{mL}} = \frac{280 \text{ mg tobramycin}}{X \text{ mL}} = 7 \text{ mL}$$

Problem 15.52 How many milliliters of NaCl 23.5% must be added to a large-volume IV bag (1,000 mL) to make 1 L of normal saline?

Solution 15.52

Step 1: Define normal saline.

Normal saline = 0.9% NaCl

This means 0.9 g NaCl/100 mL, and therefore for 1,000 mL (1 L):

$$\frac{0.9 \text{ g NaCl}}{100 \text{ mL}} = \frac{X \text{ g NaCl}}{1,000 \text{ mL}} = 9 \text{ g}$$

Step 2: Calculate the volume of NaCl 23.5% needed to supply the desired amount of NaCl.

$$\frac{23.5 \text{ g NaCl stock}}{100 \text{ mL}} = \frac{9 \text{ g NaCl}}{X \text{ mL}} = 38.3 \text{ mL}$$

Step 3: To make the large-volume solution, remove 38.3 mL from a 1,000-mL bag of SWI, and replace it with 38.3 mL of NaCl 23.5% solution, to make 1 L of NS.

Problem 15.53 Phenytoin is an antiseizure medication that should not be administered to a patient at a rate greater than 50 mg/min. A 900 mg dose is prepared in a small-volume IV bag (100 mL). What is the maximum rate, in mL/hr, at which this dose can be administered?

Solution 15.53

Step 1: Determine over how many minutes the dose can be administered.

$$\frac{900 \text{ mg phenytoin}}{\dfrac{50 \text{ mg}}{\text{min}}} = 18 \text{ min}$$

Step 2: Determine the rate in mL/hr needed to deliver 900 mg in 18 minutes.

$$\frac{100 \text{ mL}}{18 \text{ min}} = \frac{X \text{ mL}}{60 \text{ min}} = 333 \text{ mL} / \text{hr}$$

Problem 15.54 Dopamine is an agent to increase blood pressure. It is available as a premixed drug in a 500-mL bag at a concentration of 0.8 mg/mL. This solution is to be administered as a continuous infusion to a patient weighing 75 kg. The dose ordered is 2 mcg/kg/minute. At what rate, in mg/hr, should this drug be administered?

Solution 15.54

Step 1: Calculate the dose in mcg/min.

$$\frac{2 \text{ mcg}}{\frac{\text{kg}}{\text{min}}} \times 75 \text{ kg} = 150 \frac{\text{mcg}}{\text{min}}$$

Step 2: Convert mcg/min to mg/hr.

$$\frac{150 \text{ mcg}}{\text{min}} \times \frac{60 \text{ mins}}{1 \text{ hr}} \times \frac{1 \text{ mg}}{1,000 \text{ mcg}} = 9 \frac{\text{mg}}{\text{hr}}$$

Problem 15.55 At what rate, in mL/h4, must magnesium sulfate be administered to provide a 2 g dose if it is supplied in a small-volume IV bag (50 mL) over 4 hours?

Solution 15.55

$$\frac{50 \text{ mL magnesium sulfate}}{4 \text{ hr}} = \frac{X \text{ mL}}{1 \text{ hr}} = 12.5 \text{ mL/hr}$$

Problem 15.56 A premature infant is to receive a continuous drip of fentanyl, a drug to treat pain. The dose of 0.75 mcg/kg/hr is to be administered using a fentanyl IV bag that has a concentration of 10 mcg/mL. What rate of administration, in mL/hr, is needed to deliver this dose?

Solution 15.56

Step 1: Calculate the dose in mcg/hr.

$$\frac{0.75 \text{ mcg fentanyl}}{\frac{\text{kg}}{\text{hr}}} \times 1.6 \text{ kg} = 1.2 \frac{\text{mcg}}{\text{hr}}$$

Step 2: Convert mcg/hr to mL/hr.

$$\frac{1.2 \text{ mcg}}{\text{hr}} \times \frac{1 \text{ mL}}{10 \text{ mcg}} = \frac{0.12 \text{ mL}}{\text{hr}}$$

As you can see, the administration rate for an infant is extremely low. In situations such as these, a special IV pump that controls the rate of drug delivery from a syringe is used. This allows for a higher degree of precision for such low delivery rates.

Problem 15.57 A patient with a spinal cord injury is to receive methylprednisolone, a steroid used to reduce swelling, at a dose of 30 mg/kg over 15 minutes. What rate of infusion, in mL/hr, must be administered to provide this dose?

Solution 15.57

Step 1: Calculate the mg dose to be provided.

$$\frac{30 \text{ mg methylprednisolone}}{\text{kg}} \times 82 \text{ kg} = 2,460 \text{ mg}$$

Step 2: Calculate the rate in mL/hr.

$$\frac{250 \text{ mL}}{20 \text{ min}} = \frac{X \text{ mL}}{60 \text{ min}} = 750 \frac{\text{mL}}{\text{hr}}$$

Putting this together: 2,460 mg methylprednisolone would be prepared in a 250-mL IV bag and administered over 20 minutes at a rate of 750 mL/hr.

Problem 15.58 How many grams of lipids provide 800 kcal of energy?

Solution 15.58

$$\frac{1 \text{ g lipid}}{9 \text{ kcal}} = \frac{X \text{ g lipids}}{800 \text{ kcal}} = 89 \text{ g lipids}$$

Problem 15.59 How many kilocalories of energy is provided by 400 mL of an 8% amino acid solution?

Solution 15.59

Step 1: Calculate how many grams of amino acids are provided by 400 mL of an 8% solution.

$$\frac{8 \text{ g amino acids}}{100 \text{ mL}} = \frac{X \text{ g amino acids}}{400 \text{ mL}} = 32 \text{ g amino acids}$$

Step 2: Calculate how many kilocalories are provided by 32 g amino acids:

$$32 \text{ g amino acids} \times \frac{4 \text{ kcal}}{\text{g amino acids}} = 128 \text{ kcal}$$

Problem 15.60 How many milliliters of dextrose 70% is required to provide 500 dextrose kcal?

Solution 15.60

Step 1: Calculate the number of grams of dextrose that provides 500 kcal.

$$\frac{1 \text{ g dextrose}}{3.4 \text{ kcal}} = \frac{X \text{ g dextrose}}{500 \text{ kcal}} = 147 \text{ g dextrose}$$

Step 2: Calculate the number of milliliters of dextrose 70% that will provide 147 g.

$$\frac{70 \text{ g dextrose}}{100 \text{ mL}} = \frac{147 \text{ g dextrose}}{X \text{ mL}} = 210 \text{ mL dextrose}$$

Problem 15.61 How many kilocalories of energy is provided by the following parenteral macronutrient solution: amino acids 7%, 1,250 mL; dextrose 70%, 550 mL; lipids 20%, 300 mL?

Solution 15.61

Step 1a—Amino acids: Calculate the number of grams of amino acids in 1,250 mL of a 7% solution.

$$\frac{7 \text{ g amino acids}}{100 \text{ mL}} = \frac{X \text{ g amino acids}}{1250 \text{ mL}} = 87.5 \text{ g amino acids}$$

Step 1b—Amino acids: Calculate the kilocalories provided by 87.5 g amino acids.

$$87.5 \text{ g amino acids} \times \frac{4 \text{ kcal}}{\text{g}} = 350 \text{ kcal}$$

Step 2a—Dextrose: Calculate the grams of dextrose in 550 mL of a 70% solution.

$$\frac{70 \text{ g dextrose}}{100 \text{ mL}} = \frac{X \text{ g dextrose}}{550 \text{ mL}} = 385 \text{ g dextrose}$$

Step 2b—Dextrose: Calculate the kilocalories provided by 385 g dextrose.

$$385 \text{ g dextrose} \times \frac{3.4 \text{ kcal}}{\text{g}} = 1,309 \text{ kcal}$$

Step 3a—Lipids: Calculate the number of grams of lipids in 300 mL of a 20% solution.

$$\frac{20 \text{ g lipids}}{100 \text{ mL}} = \frac{X \text{ g lipids}}{300 \text{ mL}} = 60 \text{ g lipids}$$

Step 3b—Lipids: Calculate the kilocalories provided by 60 g lipids.

$$60 \text{ g lipids} \times \frac{9 \text{ kcal}}{\text{g}} = 540 \text{ kcal}$$

Step 4: Calculate the total kcal.

Amino acids: 350 kcal

Dextrose: 1,309 kcal

Lipids: 540 kcal

Total: 2,199 kcal

Problem 15.62 If a patient's daily kilocalories goal is 1,680 kcal, and 30% of this goal is to be provided by lipids, how many grams of lipid solution should be added to the parenteral nutrition solution?

Solution 15.62

$$1,680 \text{ kcal} \times \frac{30}{100} = 504 \text{ kcal to be provided by lipids}$$

$$504 \text{ kcal} \times \frac{1 \text{ g}}{9 \text{ kcal}} = 56 \text{ g lipids}$$

Problem 15.63 What are the estimated daily fluid requirements for a patient weighing:

A. 85 kg
B. 68 kg
C. 91 kg

Solution 15.63

A. $85 \text{ kg} \times \dfrac{30 \text{ mL}}{\text{kg}} = 2,550 \text{ mL per day}$

$85 \text{ kg} \times \dfrac{40 \text{ mL}}{\text{kg}} = 3,400 \text{ mL per day}$

Estimated daily fluid needed: 2,550–3400 mL/day

B. $68 \text{ kg} \times \dfrac{30 \text{ mL}}{\text{kg}} = 2,040 \text{ mL per day}$

$68 \text{ kg} \times \dfrac{40 \text{ mL}}{\text{kg}} = 2,720 \text{ mL per day}$

Estimated daily fluid needed: 2,040–2,720 mL/day

C. $91 \text{ kg} \times \dfrac{30 \text{ mL}}{\text{kg}} = 2,730 \text{ mL per day}$

$91 \text{ kg} \times \dfrac{40 \text{ mL}}{\text{kg}} = 3,640 \text{ mL per day}$

Estimated daily fluid needed: 2,730–3,640 mL/day

Problem 15.64 Calculate the volumes of each of the following micronutrients to be added to a parenteral nutrition formula:

A. Sodium chloride 40 mEq (vial concentration is 2 mEq/mL)
B. Potassium acetate 60 mEq (vial concentration is 2 mEq/mL)
C. Magnesium sulfate 18 mEq (vial concentration is 4 mEq/mL)
D. Calcium gluconate 12 mEq (vial concentration is 0.465 mEq/mL)

Solution 15.64

A. $\dfrac{2 \text{ m Eq NaCl}}{\text{mL}} = \dfrac{40 \text{ mEq}}{X \text{ mL}} = 20 \text{ mL}$

B. $\dfrac{2 \text{ mEq K acetate}}{\text{mL}} = \dfrac{60 \text{ mEq}}{X \text{ mL}} = 30 \text{ mL}$

C. $\dfrac{4 \text{ mEq magnesium sulfate}}{\text{mL}} = \dfrac{18 \text{ mEq}}{X \text{ mL}} = 4.5 \text{ mL}$

D. $\dfrac{0.465 \text{ mEq calcium gluconate}}{\text{mL}} = \dfrac{12 \text{ mEq}}{X \text{ mL}} = 25.8 \text{ mL}$

Problem 15.65 A patient is to receive the following parenteral nutrition formula:

Dextrose 70%	337
Amino acids 10%	1280
Lipids 20%	640
Total	**2,257 mL**

A. Calculate the number of kilocalories provided by this parenteral nutrition formula.
B. Calculate the grams protein/kg provided by this parenteral nutrition formula for a patient weighing 70 kg.
C. Calculate the rate, in mL/hr, needed to administer this volume of parenteral nutrition over 24 hours.
D. Calculate the percentage of total kilocalories provided as fat kilocalories.

Solution 15.65

A.

Macronutrient	mL	g	kcal
Dextrose 70%	337	$\dfrac{70\ g}{100\ mL}=\dfrac{X\ g}{337\ mL}=236\ g$	$236\ g\times\dfrac{3.4\ kcal}{g}=802\ kcal$
Amino acids 10%	1,280	$\dfrac{10\ g}{100\ mL}=\dfrac{X\ g}{1,280\ mL}=128\ g$	$128\ g\times\dfrac{4\ kcal}{g}=512\ kcal$
Lipids 20%	640	$\dfrac{20\ g}{100\ mL}=\dfrac{X\ g}{640\ mL}=48\ g$	$48\ g\times\dfrac{9\ kcal}{g}=432\ kcal$
Total	**2,257 mL**		**1,746 kcal**

B. Total grams protein = 128 g/70 kg = 1.83 g/kg protein
C. Total volume of formula = 2,257 mL/24 hr = 94 mL/hr
D. Total kcal = 1,746
Fat kcal = 432

Percentage of fat kcal $=\dfrac{432}{1,746}\times100\%=24.7\%$

Problem 15.66 Calculate the goal daily kilocalories for the following patients:

A. Hospitalized patient, not critically ill, who is 5'4" tall and weighs 62 kg
B. Critically ill patient who is 5'4" tall and weighs 62 kg
C. Critically ill patient who is 5'4" tall and weighs 114 kg

Solution 15.66

A. Goal daily kcal: 20–25 kcal/kg ABW/day
20 kcal/kg × 62 kg = 1,240 kcal
25 kcal/kg × 62 kg = 1,550 kcal
Goal daily kcal range: 1,240–1,550 kcal

B. Step 1: To find the correct category of goal kcal, the BMI must be calculated:

$$BMI=\dfrac{Weight\ (kg)}{Height\ (m)^2}$$

Since the height is reported in feet and inches, it must first be converted to meters:

64 in. × 1 m/39.37 in. = 1.63 m

Now the BMI can be calculated:

$$BMI=\dfrac{62\ kg}{1.63\ m^2}=23.3$$

Since the patient's BMI < 30, goal daily kcal = 25–30 kcal/kg ABW/day.

Step 2: Calculate the goal kcal range.

Goal range daily kcal: 25–30 kcal/kg ABW/day

25 kcal/kg × 62 kg = 1,550 kcal

30 kcal/kg × 62 kg = 1,860 kcal

Goal daily kcal range: 1,550–1,860 kcal

C. Step 1: To find the correct category of goal kcal, the BMI must be calculated:

$$BMI = \frac{Weight\ (kg)}{Height\ (m)^2}$$

Since the height is reported in feet and inches, it must first be converted to meters:

64 in. × 1 m/39.37 in. = 1.63 m

Now the BMI can be calculated:

$$BMI = \frac{114\ kg}{1.63\ m^2} = 42.9$$

Since the patient's BMI ≥ 40, goal daily kcal = 11– 4 kcal/kg ABW/day.

Step 2: Calculate the goal kcal range.

Goal range daily kcal: 11–14 kcal/kg ABW/day

11 kcal/kg × 114 kg = 1,254 kcal

14 kcal/kg × 114 kg = 1,596 kcal

Goal daily kcal range: 1,254–1,596 kcal

Problem 15.67 A patient is to be started on enteral nutrition with a goal daily kilocalories range of 2,200–2,640 kcal. The goal daily grams of protein is 106–176. The enteral formula ordered contains 1.4 kcal/mL and 74 g protein/L. What is the goal rate for this nutrition to administered, in mL/hr, that will meet the kilocalories goal range and supply 130 g protein per day?

Solution 15.67

Step 1: Calculate the daily volume of formula needed to deliver 130 protein grams.

$$\frac{74\ g\ protein}{1,000\ mL} = \frac{130\ g\ protein}{X\ mL} = 1,756\ mL$$

Step 2: Calculate the kilocalories provided by the volume selected.

$$\frac{1.4\ kcal}{1\ mL} = \frac{X\ kcal}{1,756\ mL} = 2,458\ kcal$$

Step 3: Compare the kilocalories delivered by the selected protein goal to the goal for daily kilocalories. The kcal goal range is 2,200–2,640 kcal/day, so using this formula and providing 130 g protein per day will meet the daily kcal goal.

Step 4: Calculate the hourly rate required to deliver the required volume. The total daily volume of nutrition formula required is 1,756 mL. To calculate the hourly rate required to deliver this volume in 24 hours:

$$\frac{1,756\ mL}{day} \times \frac{1\ day}{24\ hr} = 73\ mL/hr$$

References

1. http://www.ismp.org/newsletters/acutecare/articles/20070920.asp. Accessed May 17, 2012.

2. http://www.ismp.org/newsletters/acutecare/articles/20030306.asp. Accessed May 17, 2012.

3. http://www.ismp.org/newsletters/acutecare/articles/19990421.asp. Accessed May 17, 2012.

4. http://www.bipm.org/en/. Accessed April 15, 2012.

Introduction to Drug Information, Literature Evaluation, and Biostatistics

CHAPTER 16

Kristine Marcus

OBJECTIVES

1. Explain the need for the pharmacist to be a drug information master throughout his or her career.
2. Locate references that are most likely to yield answers efficiently for the following drug information question types commonly encountered by students of pharmacy during their early curriculum:
    a. Chemical structure and properties
    b. Drug names, manufacturers, and pronunciations
    c. Product presentations, formulations, and manufacturers
    d. Mechanism of action
    e. Pharmacokinetic parameters
    f. Dosing
    g. Side effects
    h. Drug interactions
    i. Indications for use
3. Describe the importance of critically appraising an article from the biomedical literature.
4. List the factors that are considered in choosing the correct statistical test.
5. Apply foundational principles in biostatistics when interpreting descriptive and analytic data.
6. Implement a series of Learning Bridge assignments at your experiential sites to bridge your didactic learning with your experiential experiences.

KEY TERMS AND DEFINITIONS

1. **Abstracting service:** a database that indexes and provides titles, abstracts, and citations for biomedical journal articles. *See also Secondary literature.*
2. **Alpha:** the probability of concluding that there is a difference between groups when there really is no difference between them (making a Type I error). Alpha is traditionally set at 0.05.
3. **Alternate hypothesis:** the hypothesis that there is a difference between treatment groups in a study; may be referred to as the research hypothesis by the investigators.
4. **Article abstract:** a digest of the key aspects of a biomedical journal article. Abstracts appear at the beginning of the article, are usually limited to 250 words, and are indexed by abstracting services.
5. **Beta:** the probability of concluding that there is no difference between treatment groups when there really is a difference (making a Type II error). Beta is traditionally set at 0.20.
6. **Boolean search terms:** logical operators (i.e., AND, OR, NOT) used to expand or contract sets of retrieved articles from searchable databases when searching the primary literature.

(continues)

(CONTINUED)

7. **Clinical significance:** study results that an individual clinician feels are important enough to change his or her practice. The clinician's decision to apply the findings may be made irrespective of whether the study results were statistically significant.

8. **Clinical trial:** an experimental study that is designed to compare the therapeutic benefits of two or more treatments. *See also Phase 3 studies and Phase 4 studies.*

9. **Confidence interval (CI):** the interval computed from sample data associated with a given probability that the studied parameter is contained within that interval. The confidence level is traditionally set at 95%, but could be as narrow as 90% or as wide as 99%. This interval may be stated as the estimate of the range of values within which the investigators are 95% certain that the true value lies. If the confidence interval for the difference between study samples includes the point of no effect, then the possibility that there is no difference between the groups cannot be excluded.

10. **Confounder:** a variable in a study that affects the statistical relationship between the independent variable and the dependent variable. A confounding factor can make it appear that there is a direct relationship between the two variables of interest when, in reality, the confounder is responsible for the relationship.

11. **Control:** a treatment (placebo, active, historical) used for comparison in a study to measure a difference in effect against an investigational agent.

12. **Cross-over study design:** a study design in which each patient receives both treatments, serving as his or her own control. The two phases of the study are usually separated by a washout period.

13. **Drug compendium (pl: compendia):** a print or electronic tertiary reference containing a concise summary of the body of knowledge about marketed drugs that is generally presented as a collection of individual drug monographs. It may also contain drug class summaries or product comparisons.

14. **Drug monograph:** a structured compilation of the major features of a drug product.

15. **Evidence-based medicine (EBM):** the practice of integrating clinical experience and judgment with the most current and relevant evidence when making decisions about the care of patients.

16. **Journal club:** a group of individuals who meet regularly to critically evaluate recent journal articles in the biomedical literature. Journal clubs are usually organized around a defined subject or learning purpose.

17. **Medication list:** a record of all the patient's medications, including prescription drugs and any over-the-counter drugs or supplements purchased at a pharmacy or grocery store.

18. **Nonparametric data:** discrete or non-normally distributed data. Analyzing these data requires a statistical test that does not make assumptions regarding the distribution of the observations. Nonparametric statistical tests are commonly used to analyze dichotomous and categorical data, but can also be used for continuous data that have an abnormal dispersion.

19. **Null hypothesis:** the hypothesis being tested about a population. This hypothesis concludes that there is no difference between treatment groups in a study.

20. **p-value:** the level of statistical significance. A value of $p < 0.05$ means that the probability that the result is due to chance is less than 1 in 20; the smaller the p-value, the greater the statistical significance. The p-value does not provide any information about the size of an effect, but rather simply describes the strength of the result.

21. **Package insert:** printed prescription drug labeling information subject to detailed regulatory specifications by the U.S. Food and Drug Administration, which accompanies each package of medication sold to pharmacies.

22. **Parallel study design:** a study in which two or more groups receive different treatments and the outcomes are compared.

(continues)

23. **Parameter:** a measurement that describes part of the population.

24. **Parametric data:** normally or near-normally distributed data. Analyzing these data requires a statistical test that assumes a normal bell-shaped distribution. Parametric statistical tests are commonly used to analyze continuous data. If the continuous data are skewed, however, a nonparametric test is more appropriate.

25. **Patient medication profile:** records and notes kept in the pharmacy detailing the patient's demographic information, medication list, and pattern of medication use.

26. **Pharmacy care plan:** pharmacy documentation organized according to medical condition or indication for drug therapy that outlines the pharmacist's plan to achieve the patient's goals of therapy, resolve and prevent any drug therapy problems, and follow up.

27. **Phase 1 studies:** clinical trials testing a new biomedical intervention in a small group of people for the first time to evaluate safety. These studies often seek to identify the optimal dosage route and dosage range, and to characterize possible side effects.

28. **Phase 2 studies:** clinical trials testing a biomedical or behavioral intervention in a larger group of people (several hundred) to determine efficacy and to further evaluate safety.

29. **Phase 3 studies:** clinical trials investigating the efficacy of a biomedical or behavioral intervention in a large group of human subjects (several hundred to several thousand) by comparing the intervention to other standard or experimental interventions. Monitoring for adverse effects and collection of information to allow the intervention to be used safely are often carried out during such clinical trials. These studies provide the clinical practice experience for FDA drug approval.

30. **Phase 4 studies:** investigations conducted after the intervention is available on the market. These studies are designed to monitor effectiveness of the approved intervention in the general population and to collect information about any adverse effects associated with widespread use. They are often referred to as postmarketing surveillance studies.

31. **Population:** the entire collection of observations or subjects that have something in common and to which conclusions are inferred.

32. **Prescription brown bag review:** an event in which patients are encouraged to bring all of their medications and supplements to an appointment or health fair, so that the pharmacist can review and discuss the patient's medications.

33. **Primary literature:** original studies or reports published in biomedical journals.

34. **Sample:** a subset of the population.

35. **Secondary literature:** resources that index and/or abstract literature from primary biomedical journals.

36. **Statistical significance:** a result is usually considered statistically significant if the probability of a Type I error is less than 5% ($p < 0.05$). Statistical significance does not automatically mean that a clinical difference in the effect between the intervention and control groups exists (*see also Clinical significance*).

37. **Tertiary literature:** textbooks and drug compendia (including print and electronic formats) that collect established knowledge.

38. **Top 200 prescription drug:** annually published list of the most prescribed pharmaceuticals in the United States by retail sales and volume.

39. **Translational research:** research that fosters the multidirectional integration of basic research, patient-oriented research, and population-based research, with the long-term aim of improving the health of the public.

(*continues*)

(CONTINUED)

40. **Type I error:** the conclusion that there is a difference between treatments when there is really no difference between them; rejection of the null hypothesis when it is actually true.

41. **Type II error:** the conclusion that there is no difference between treatments when there really is a difference between them; accepting the null hypothesis when it is actually false.

42. **Variable:** a characteristic of the study sample that is being measured or observed. The independent variable (e.g., the intervention) causes a change in the dependent variable (e.g., the outcome of interest).

Introduction

Pharmacists today are viewed by the public and other care providers as drug experts. The number of hours dedicated in pharmacy curricula to the study of balancing the benefits and harms of medications far supersedes the time devoted to this topic in any other healthcare discipline. Accessibility and recognition of their unique contributions in guiding therapy and improving the health and well-being of patients have increased the demands on pharmacists to find, decode, and communicate complex information about medications and disease states to a wide variety of audiences.

As health care continues to emphasize the importance of evidence-based medicine (EBM) as the foundation for clinical decision making, pharmacists are being trained in these methods as well. Practicing EBM requires a number of skills that are the focus of this chapter: efficiently searching for quality information about medications, critically appraising the biomedical literature relevant to the drug information need, and interpreting and applying the found information. EBM principles can be used when making decisions about an individual patient or in anticipation of the needs of many patients. They are also an essential component of the lifelong learning process undertaken by pharmacists, who are duty bound to stay abreast of new medical developments so that they can continue to solve drug-related problems and optimize therapies for patients based on the latest published articles and practice guidelines.

Building Drug Information Skills

The Ultimate Question

Upon initially receiving a request for drug information, the query is reformulated into what drug information pharmacists refer to as "the ultimate question." A structured, organized approach to information gathering renders a final question that accurately defines the genuine information need of the requestor. Sometimes requestors do not provide enough patient context or particulars about the issue they are seeking consultation for. Pharmacists have to use their knowledge, practice experience, and questioning skills to elicit missing details so that they do not provide an incorrect or inadequate response. When pharmacists can explain how the requestor plans to use the information, they have sufficiently characterized the ultimate question and can begin searching for relevant information pertaining to the request.

Types of Drug Information Questions

During their training, students of pharmacy will encounter a variety of types of drug information questions (**Table 16.1**). The complexity of questions they are given to research will deepen in relationship to their acquisition of a stronger drug knowledge base and more practical experience.

Table 16.1 Examples of Common Drug Information Question Types by Phase of Pharmacy Training

Drug Information Types	Early Coursework	Later Coursework
Adverse effects	Frequency of side effects occurrence	Severity assessment, clinical management of adverse effects and medication errors, drug-induced diseases
Compatibility/stability	Nonsterile compounding	Sterile compounding, intravenous and nutritional administration, and extemporaneously compounded liquids
Dosing and administration	Usual doses and routes of administration	Dose escalation, optimal dose, maximal dose limits, method and rate of administration, alternative routes of administration
Drug identification	Product dispensing verification	Clinical management of poisoning
Drug interactions	Mechanisms of drug–drug interactions	Clinical management of drug–drug, drug–disease, drug–lab test, and drug–food interactions
Herbal products and dietary supplements	Availability and quality of natural products and supplements	Effectiveness and safety of natural products and supplements
Pharmaceutics/physical chemistry	Dosage form design, medicinal chemistry structure–activity relationships	Impact of altered drug delivery, formulating recipes for compounding
Pharmacokinetics	Absorption, distribution, metabolism, and excretion (ADME); pharmacogenomics	Extracorporeal clearance, therapeutic drug monitoring, pharmacodynamics
Pharmacology	Mechanism of action	Predicting adverse effects, impact of concurrent therapies, toxicology
Pregnancy and lactation	FDA safety rating categories	Assessment of medication risk and benefit during pregnancy or breastfeeding
Product availability	Drug names and manufacturers, marketed dosage forms, cost	Foreign and investigational drugs
Therapeutic use	FDA-approved uses	Unlabeled uses, regimen recommendations

Searching for Answers

Once the question has been categorized, an organized approach can ensure that sufficient references and documentation will be acquired to answer the question. For many years, pharmacy students have been taught a modified systematic approach to responding to drug information questions that begins with searching the tertiary literature, then proceeds to secondary sources that index the primary literature. Final steps involve reviewing the primary literature found through the secondary search and, if necessary, speaking with experts when literature-derived guidance does not exist. This preferred order for looking for information was established prior to the wide availability of the Internet, user-friendly search engines, and electronic books and clinical knowledge databases. It remains a practical method for searching for answers to many questions likely to be posed to students of pharmacy in their early coursework and to front-line entry-level pharmacists. The broad scope and easy navigation of a tertiary resource remains the most efficient route for responding to a question that can be answered using digested data. Because the tertiary literature often aims for broad coverage, some topics may not be addressed in sufficient depth to meet the requestor's needs. When this occurs, pharmacists need to consult the primary literature.

The multitude of steps needed to effectively use the primary literature require skill and practice to complete:

1. Identify the most appropriate secondary literature abstracting service to run the search.

2. Compose a search strategy using high-yield subject headings, text words, Boolean operators, and limits.

3. Execute the search strategy.

4. Review and refine the search results.

5. Review abstracts and select articles for full-text review.

6. Access full text if available or request via interlibrary loan.

7. Critically analyze the identified primary literature for relevance and applicability to the question.

8. Re-execute the strategy in other secondary literature services that index other journal titles.

In reviewing the source articles, the reader is allowed to interpret all the available data and decide whether they are useful and valid instead of accepting what is presented in a book verbatim without knowing the choices the author made in presenting the data. Because it can take multiple years to produce a book, there is also a risk that the information will be outdated compared to what can be retrieved from the primary literature. Electronic drug compendia and clinical knowledge systems are updated more frequently, but not every monograph or disease consult is updated annually. The publisher generally has a rotating review plan for the content but will add alerts or other safety-driven information as soon as they become available.

Useful Tertiary Resources

This next section is not exhaustive but contains lists of tertiary resources that are included in the American Association of Colleges of Pharmacy's Basic Resources for Pharmacy Education "recommended for first purchase" list or that are widely used by drug information pharmacists. Many of these titles may also be available to pharmacy students through electronic book collections or reference databases available through their library. Some are also downloadable onto mobile devices. Students are encouraged to check with their drug information faculty or reference librarian about on-campus and off-campus access to these titles.

Core Pharmaceutical Science Textbooks

Many student questions can be answered by a textbook, but these resources are often overlooked as reference material.

Biochemistry

-   Devlin TM. *Textbook of biochemistry: with clinical correlations*, 7th ed. Hoboken, NJ: John Wiley & Sons; 2011. ISBN: 9780470281734. $219.35.

-   *Lehninger principles of biochemistry*, 5th ed. New York, NY: W. H. Freeman and Company; 2008. ISBN: 9780716771081. $178.50.

-   Voet D, Voet JG. *Biochemistry*, 4th ed. Hoboken, NJ: John Wiley & Sons; 2010. ISBN: 9780470570951. $182.55.

Medicinal Chemistry

-   *Foye's principles of medicinal chemistry*, 6th ed. Philadelphia, PA: Lippincott Williams & Wilkins; 2007. ISBN: 9780781768795. $92.95.

- Lemke TL. *Review of organic functional groups: introduction to medicinal organic chemistry*, 4th ed. Baltimore, MD: Lippincott Williams & Wilkins; 2002. ISBN: 9780781743815. $49.95.

- *Wilson and Gisvold's textbook of organic medicinal and pharmaceutical chemistry*, 12th ed. Baltimore, MD: Lippincott Williams & Wilkins 2011. ISBN: 9780781779296. $92.50.

Pharmaceutics

- *Ansel's pharmaceutical dosage forms and drug delivery systems*, 9th ed. Philadelphia, PA: Lippincott Williams & Wilkins; 2011. ISBN: 9780781779340. $64.95.

- *Martin's physical pharmacy and pharmaceutical sciences: physical chemical and biopharmaceutical principles in the pharmaceutical sciences*, 6th ed. Philadelphia, PA: Lippincott Williams & Wilkins; 2011. ISBN: 9780781797665. $82.95.

- Shrewsbury RP. *Applied pharmaceutics in contemporary compounding*, 2nd ed. Englewood, CO: Morton; 2008. ISBN: 9780895827449. $69.95.

Pharmacology

- *Goodman & Gilman's the pharmacological basis of therapeutics*, 12th ed. New York, NY: McGraw-Hill; 2011. ISBN: 9780071624428. $179.00.

- Katzung BG, Masters SB, Trevor AJ, eds. *Basic and clinical pharmacology*, 11th ed. London, UK: McGraw-Hill; 2009. ISBN: 9780071604055. $64.95.

Pharmacokinetics

- Hedaya MA. *Basic pharmacokinetics*. Boca Raton, FL: CRC Press; 2007. ISBN: 9781420046717. $98.25.

- Shargel L, Wu-Pong S, Yu A. *Applied biopharmaceutics and pharmacokinetics*, 5th ed. New York, NY. McGraw-Hill; 2004. ISBN: 9780071375504. $71.95.

- Winter ME. *Basic clinical pharmacokinetics*, 5th ed. Philadelphia, PA: Lippincott Williams & Wilkins; 2009. ISBN: 9780781779036. $67.95.

Pharmacy Calculations

- Ansel HC. *Pharmaceutical calculations*, 13th ed. Philadelphia, PA: Lippincott Williams & Wilkins; 2010. ISBN: 9781582558370. $77.95.

- O'Sullivan TA. *Understanding pharmacy calculations*. Washington, DC: American Pharmaceutical Association; 2002. ISBN: 9781582120331. $48.00.

- Zatz JL, Teixeira MG. *Pharmaceutical calculations*, 4th ed. New York, NY: Wiley-Interscience; 2005. ISBN: 9780471433538. $76.50.

Package Inserts: FDA- and Manufacturer-Provided Drug Information

The National Library of Medicine provides DailyMed, an open access website that provides high-quality information about marketed drugs (dailymed.nlm.nih.gov/). This information includes the official FDA drug labels (package inserts). Drugs@FDA allows you to search for information about FDA-approved innovator and generic drugs and therapeutic biological products (accessdata.fda.gov/scripts/cder/drugsatfda/). Manufacturer websites are another useful source of prescribing and patient information. Many companies buy the trade name of their drug as a website (e.g., www.Lovenox.com) to host their product materials. New drugs in the pipeline to market are indexed in the clinicaltrials.gov database of publicly and privately supported clinical studies of human participants conducted around the world.

Drug Compendia

Drug compendia will be one of the pharmacy student's most frequently consulted references (**Table 16.2**). If students have access to more than one compendium, they are encouraged to learn how to use all of them, although they will likely develop a favorite "go-to" resource. Once in practice, most pharmacies purchase only a single compendium resource. Thus getting experience using different ones while in school will allow students to quickly adapt to whichever is the preferred resource of their work site. While these compendia have fair depth in niche areas such as over-the-counter drug products and natural products, specialty compendia on these topics may need to be consulted for some requests.

Table 16.2 Strengths and Limitations of Commonly Available Electronic Drug Compendia

Compendium Resource	Strengths	Limitations
Facts & Comparisons eAnswers	• Drug identifier • Comparison tables • Don't crush/don't chew list • Pregnancy and lactation (Brigg's) • Chemotherapy resources • Product/manufacturer information • Use of natural products • Formulary monograph service • Medication safety programs/REMS/black box warnings • Orphan drugs • Normal lab values (including drug levels)	• More limited information outside of the package insert
Lexi-Comp Online	• Drug interactions • Natural products • Patient education (many languages) • Calculators • Allergy • Pregnancy and lactation • Don't crush/don't chew list • IV compatibility (King Guide)	• More limited information outside of the package insert • Toxicology • Off-label use
Micromedex 2.0	• Off-label use • Adverse drug reactions • Toxicology • Trissel's IV compatibility	• Drug identifier • Calculators • Manufacturer information • Product availability • Natural products only by extra subscription

Acknowledgment: Table co-created with Kristen Malabanan, PharmD, Academic Fellow.

Learning Bridge 16.1

As part of an orientation activity during your first pharmacology class, each student is given the name of a Top 200 prescription drug (http://www.pharmacytimes.com/publications/issue/2012/July2012/Top-200-Drugs-of-2011) and is asked to complete the following tasks:

A. Write the pronunciation of the generic name of the drug.
B. State whether the drug is available only as a brand-name product or if a generic equivalent is marketed.
C. Find a picture of the drug.
D. File their completed research in the correct folder at the front of the classroom. The folders are labeled with the names of each of the pharmacology courses that are arranged by body system (e.g., Pharmaceutical Sciences—Pulmonary).

You are assigned the drug carvedilol (Coreg) tablets for the activity. Where will you look to complete assignment parts A–C? In which body system folder will you file your completed assignment?

Learning Bridge 16.2

As a member of a pre-pharmacy club, you have been invited to shadow the club advisor at a prescription brown bag review event at the local senior day-care center. Your advisor introduces you to a second-year pharmacy intern on IPPE with him and asks the two of you to work together to gather information from the patients before the pharmacist meets with them to review their medications. Your primary duty is to accurately record each patient's medication list on a provided form.

Your IPPE colleague reviews Ms. White's prescription labels and asks the patient to describe her current medication regimen. The intern records the information and highlights in yellow the areas that she wants you to double check. Using a standard drug compendium, research the following yellow-highlighted items before handing off the list to the pharmacist:

A. What does the abbreviation ASA stand for?
B. What would be the medically appropriate terms for the ASA indication for use?
C. What is the brand name of metoprolol succinate?
D. Can a metoprolol succinate extended-release tablet be cut in half?
E. What is the brand name of atorvastatin?
F. What would be the medically appropriate term for the atorvastatin indication for use?
G. What does the abbreviation SL stand for?
H. What does the abbreviation prn stand for? Is prn a sufficient direction for use?

(continues)

(*continued*)

Exhibit 16.1

Ms. White, 70 yo F; no known drug allergies

123 Notting Hill Lane, Anytown, USA

Drug	Dosage Form	Dose	Directions for Use	Qty Supply	Refills	Pre-scriber	Indication for Use
ASA	EC tablet	325 mg	1 tablet once daily	60	5	Dr. Heart	**"Heart and brain protection"**
Metoprolol succinate **(generic of brand name)**	Extended-release tablet	100 mg	½ tablet orally daily	30	5	Dr. Heart	Angina
Atorvastatin **(generic of brand name)**	Tablet	40 mg	1 tablet once daily	30	11	Dr. Heart	**"High cholesterol"**
Nitroglyc-erin	**SL** tablet	0.4 mg	**prn**	Bottle of 25	11	Dr. Heart	Chest pain

The Drug–Disease Interface

Certain textbooks and clinical knowledge systems provide information on both disease states and the medications used to treat them. Many pharmacists rely on these drug–disease interface sources because of their currency and focus on drugs of choice. The electronic versions also have the great utility offered by an integrated index that provides within-monograph mapping to other related source material that may be of interest.

Pharmacotherapy Textbooks

- Chisholm-Burns MA, Wells BG, Schwinghammer TL, et al., eds. *Pharmacotherapy: principles and practice*, 3rd ed. New York, NY: McGraw-Hill Medical; 2013. ISBN: 9780071804233. $160.00.

- Dipiro, J, Talbert RL, Yee GC, et al., eds. *Pharmacotherapy: a pathophysiologic approach*, 8th ed. New York, NY: McGraw-Hill; 2011. ISBN: 9780071703543. $203.00.

- Helms RA, Quan DJ, eds. *Textbook of therapeutics: drug and disease management*, 8th ed. Philadelphia, PA: Lippincott Williams & Wilkins; 2006. ISBN: 9780781757348. $191.99.

- *Koda-Kimble and Young's applied therapeutics: the clinical use of drugs*, 10th ed. Philadelphia, PA: Lippincott Williams & Wilkins; 2012. ISBN: 9781609137137. $193.95.

Clinical Knowledge System

- *MD Consult*. Maryland Heights, MD: Elsevier; 2012. Available at www.mdconsult.com with subscription.

- *UpToDate*. Waltham, MA: Wolters Kluwer Health; 2012. Available at www.uptodate.com/online with subscription.

Table 16.3 Pathfinder for Common Drug Information Needs Encountered During Early Pharmacy Coursework

Recommended Resource	Chemical Structure, Drug Properties	Drug Names, Pronunciations	Product Presentations, Formulations, Manufacturers	Mechanism of Action, Pharmacology	Pharmacokinetic Parameters (ADME), Drug Levels	Dosing	Side Effects	Drug Interactions	Indication, Therapeutic Use
Textbook—MedChem	XXX							X	
Textbook—pharmacology				XXX	X		X		
Drug compendia	X	XXX	XX	XX	XX	XXX	XXX	XXX	XXX
Package insert	XX	XX	X	XX	XX	X	XX	XX	X
Drug–disease interface resource						XX	XXX		XX

Drug Information Resource Pathfinder for Early Pharmacy Coursework

The most common questions that pharmacy students are likely to pose to themselves during their education and the questions they may be asked during early experiential rotations have been plotted against recommended resources to assist students in quickly identifying a high-yield reference (**Table 16.3**). Relative usefulness is indicated by an increased number of X's.

Learning Bridge 16.3

You are working as a first-year pharmacy intern at the intake window of your IPPE community pharmacy site. As you are processing a middle-aged woman's request for a refill of her lisinopril (Zestril) 10 mg, she asks you if this medication can cause a cough. You call your pharmacist preceptor over, and she reviews the patient's medication profile. Your preceptor also asks the patient to describe the nature and timing of her cough and confirms that she is taking the lisinopril for her blood pressure. Your preceptor tells the patient that it is possible that the lisinopril is causing the cough and that she will speak with the doctor about changing to another medication. After the patient has left, your preceptor turns to you and asks you to research the following questions:

A. To which pharmacologic class does lisinopril belong?
B. Is this side effect consistent with lisinopril's mechanism of action?
C. Could the patient be switched to fosinopril (Monopril) or losartan (Cozaar) without risk of the same side effect?

Getting to the Source: The Secondary Literature

Much as they should become familiar with tertiary resources so that search efficiency and effectiveness can be enhanced with future use, students should build a base of expertise with one indexing/abstracting service but also be able to recognize when searching another archive is needed. PubMed Medline and Google Scholar are open-access resources used widely by pharmacists. Other useful secondary literature sources are available by subscription:

- EMBASE
- Inpharma
- International Pharmaceutical Abstracts (IPA)
- Iowa Drug Information Service (IDIS)
- OVID
- Reactions
- Web of Science

Receiving and Responding to Requests for Drug Information

The provision of drug information is a skill that is common to all areas of pharmacy practice. First and foremost, pharmacists receive and respond to their own needs for drug information when going about their daily work of reviewing patient medication profiles, developing and revising pharmacy care plans, and overseeing the acquisition and dispensing of medications.

Whether they work in a compounding pharmacy or in an intensive care unit pharmacy satellite at a hospital, as the drug experts, pharmacists are frequently asked by their healthcare colleagues and patients for their advice and counsel about available products and the best ways to use them safely and effectively. These requests can span the continuum of requiring only a quick verbal response to needing hours of research and a formal written response. It is common for the requestor to ask for a written email or chart note follow-up as documentation to a provided verbal response. Pharmacy students who are requested to provide written drug information consultations should ask their preceptor for examples of acceptable responses from prior students and any institutional standards or templates that must be followed. Elements frequently encountered in a written drug information response include the following:

- Month date, year
- Salutation
- Restatement of question being answered
- Summary of the information resources/data sources used in the search strategy
- Literature review
- Applicability of the literature to the patient/scenario
- Summary/recommendations
- Closing
- References

If students are not provided with specific guidance from their work site, then the "friendly letter" format can be followed. This written response format works well in many practice settings.

Example Drug Information Response in Friendly Letter Format Prepared by a First-Year Intern

Month Date, Year

Dear Doctor,

This letter is in response to the information you requested about which statins have to be dose adjusted for patients with renal impairment who have a creatinine clearance of less than 30 mL/min. This question was in regard to a patient with severe renal impairment and hyperlipidemia whom you would like to start on a formulary statin.

My primary sources of information on this subject were two drug compendia, *Facts and Comparisons* and *Lexi-Comp*. I searched all formulary statins (atorvastatin, lovastatin, rosuvastatin, and simvastatin) and evaluated their dosing in renally compromised patients.

Table 16.4 shows which statins require dose adjustments. I have also included the suggested starting dose and the maximum dose for each statin in patients with severe renal impairment. The percentage of the oral dose excreted in the urine is included as well, as an indicator of how much the drug is dependent on renal clearance.

Table 16.4 Statins Require Dose Adjustments

Statin	Patients with CrCl < 30 mL/min or "Severe Renal Impairment"		% of Oral Dose Excreted in Urine
	Starting Dose Suggested	Maximum Dose Suggested	
Atorvastatin	No adjustment	No adjustment	< 2%
Lovastatin	No adjustment	20 mg/day	10%
Rosuvastatin	5 mg	10 mg	90% excreted in feces
Simvastatin	5 mg	No adjustment	13%

Summary: All available statins, except atorvastatin, have suggested dosing recommendations for use in patients with CrCl < 30 mL/min or "severe renal impairment." Atorvastatin would be the best choice for your patient with severe renal impairment because no dose adjustment would be required. The dose on which you start your patient will depend on your patient's LDL goal. Generally a starting dose of atorvastatin 10–20 mg per day is acceptable. If, however, your patient requires a drop in LDL that is greater than 45%, you may want to consider a dose as high as 40 mg per day. Doses greater than 80 mg daily are not recommended.

I hope this information is useful to you. Please let me know if you have additional questions or need any clarification.

Sincerely,

Student Name, PharmD candidate, Your School of Pharmacy

P1student@yourschool.edu

References

Drug Facts and Comparisons 4.0. St. Louis, MO: Wolters Kluwer; 2012 [cited 2012 Month Date]. Available at: http://online.factsandcomparisons.com with subscription.

Lexi-Comp Online. Hudson, OH: Lexi-Comp; 1978–2012 [cited 2012 Month Date]. Available at: http://online.lexi.com with subscription.

Providing drug information is viewed as the dispensing of medication knowledge and is covered under state pharmacy practice acts. Early pharmacy students should be aware of the laws and regulations in their state and their school's policies concerning their ability to provide this service. As with other pharmacy practice skills, preceptors will need to review student research and responses before their conclusions are shared with patients or other healthcare providers.

Building Literature Evaluation Skills

Pharmacists are expected not only to retain and apply what they learned in pharmacy school, but also to enhance and expand that knowledge as new information becomes available so that they can provide the best care for their patients. It is impossible for any pharmacist to comprehensively keep up with all new drug developments and shifts in medical practices that are detailed in the biomedical literature. In addition to following a continuous professional development plan to keep abreast of the most relevant EBM findings and trends in practice that affect their pharmacy setting and patient mix, pharmacists must rely on their ability to find and interpret data as needed. A key skill in accomplishing this goal is critically reading and appraising the primary literature.

A good place to begin when reading a journal article is to consider the "three preliminary questions to get your bearings" suggested by Greenhalgh:

Question 1: Why was the study done and which hypothesis were the authors testing?

Question 2: Which type of study was done?

- Primary studies are original research and include true experiments, clinical trials, and surveys.
- Secondary studies attempt to summarize and draw conclusions from primary studies and include reviews, systematic reviews, meta-analyses, guidelines and pharmacoeconomic analyses.

Question 3: Does the design seem appropriate to the field of research addressed?

The first consideration begins to address whether the study is asking the right question and what the likelihood is that it will contribute findings beyond what is already known about the subject. The second and third questions are key to allowing the reader to determine whether the methods (and subsequently the results) are subject to bias and whether they are reproducible, generalizable, and of importance to their practice.

Early students of pharmacy will most likely be reviewing true experiments as part of their coursework. Speaking with pharmaceutical science faculty about usual methods and accepted research practices can help when students are still building their skills in thinking critically about the quality of the chosen study design. Examples of critical points to consider are shown in **Table 16.5**. Analyzing the results section requires an understanding of introductory biostatistical principles and interpretation of presented data.

Table 16.5 Examples of Key Considerations When Evaluating Pharmacy Literature Encountered in Early Coursework

Primary Literature Study Example	Key Considerations When Critically Evaluating the Study
Stability study	• Complete description of study methods and test conditions? • Validated assays used? • Sample collection scheme includes a baseline at time zero, intermediate time points, and a relevant practice-based end point?
Bioequivalence study	• Are the subjects included defined by the protocol? • Were confounding factors identified and controlled through either exclusion criteria or statistical analysis? • Was a cross over design used? • Was a washout period needed? • Was the study randomized and blinded?
Natural product efficacy and safety study	• Was a standard botanical extract or formulation utilized? • Was product quality assessed? • Was the study dose appropriate? • Was the trial length appropriate to perceive treatment effects or differences? • Was safety monitoring conducted? • Were enough patients compared to detect a difference?

Assessing the methodological quality and results of a clinical trial requires iterative practice. This ability is often enhanced in the later years of pharmacy school, when students can apply their newly gained foundational knowledge of drugs and diseases by using structured critical appraisal checklists found in drug information textbooks when preparing for journal club or when providing drug information responses.

Types of Study Results

Students of pharmacy are likely to encounter two different types of findings and their associated biostatistics when interpreting biomedical and pharmaceutical sciences articles: descriptive and analytic results. Descriptive results involve only one variable and are used to describe and summarize data collected from an experiment. Analytic results compare multiple variables, members within groups, or multiple groups. For any comparisons, statistical testing will be performed to see if the groups are mathematically similar or different.

For example, in a study of a potential metabolic drug interaction between an inhibitor and a substrate, descriptive results might portray the types of patients included in the experiment as depicted in a study subjects' demographics table showing which percentage of the participants were male or female, and which mean age (± standard deviation) was observed. In the analytic section of the same study, the reader is likely to find statistical comparisons of observed drug levels in those study subjects when only the substrate drug is present and after its combination with the interacting inhibitor drug.

Relationships between variables can be described through the methods of correlation and regression. Correlation measures the strength of association between two variables but does not assume causation. Regression analysis can predict one variable based on another variable and assumes a cause-and-effect relationship.

Choice of Biostatistical Test

The random variables studied in the experiment generate data that are evaluated using the appropriate statistical test. The choice of the appropriate statistical test is based on the following factors:

- The study design, including the number of samples being studied and the relationship between the samples
- The type of data being analyzed
- Whether the data distribution is parametric or nonparametric
- Whether any confounding variables are present

Study Design

In early pharmacy coursework, students are more likely to encounter foundational science studies in drug discovery, translational research, preclinical trials (phase 1 and 2), and experiments unique to each pharmaceutical science discipline, such as structural biochemistry, the biochemistry of disease, drug exposure–response, pharmacokinetics, drug interactions, pharmacogenomics, dosage form design, drug stability and quality assurance, and bioequivalence assessment. In later pharmacy curricula, students will be exposed to study designs that explore the clinical efficacy and safety of drugs, such as phase 3 and 4 clinical studies, epidemiological studies, observational studies, and meta-analyses. These later study designs are not the focus of this chapter. Nevertheless, for all study types, it is important to be able to determine whether the samples drawn from the population were independent or related (dependent) and how many samples were compared to determine which statistical test is most appropriate to the research question. Independent samples are not related, paired, or matched to each other. Samples are dependent or related if members of one sample can be used to determine the members from the other sample. The following terminology used in studies would indicate the samples are related: before and after, cross-over, dependent, matched, paired, repeated, related, "subjects served as their own control," or within-subject comparison. Other terms would indicate the samples are not related: independent, parallel, and unrelated.

Types of Data

Variables and their observed data can be described as either discrete or continuous (**Table 16.6**). The discrete category includes both dichotomous and categorical variables. Dichotomous variables are binary and can be only one thing or another. Categorical variables can be sorted into mutually exclusive groupings. These categorical groupings can be further subdivided into nominal or ordinal. As implied by its name, ordinal data have a logical order, whereas nominal data do not. In contrast, continuous variables can take on any number of values along a specified continuum. Two types of continuous data exist that are differentiated by the presence or absence of an absolute zero; however, interval and ordinal data are handled similarly in statistical testing.

When reading the methods and results section of the biomedical literature, pharmacy students should practice classifying the type of data being analyzed. It is important to be aware that many variables can be treated either as discrete or continuous depending on how the investigators collect and report the data (**Table 16.7**).

Data Distribution

Descriptive statistics are used to summarize and describe data that are generated in research studies. Such description can be done both visually and numerically. Visual methods include frequency distribution, histograms, and scatter plots. The numeral representations focus on measures of central tendency and dispersion.

Table 16.6 Discrete and Continuous Variables and Example Observed Data

Variable Type		Description	Example Data	Often-Observed Forms of Data
Discrete	Dichotomous	Binary, one or the other but not both	Mortality status: dead or alive	Counts, percentages
	Categorical—nominal	Nonordered mutually exclusive groupings	Race: white, Hispanic, black, Asian, other	
	Categorical—ordinal	Ordered groupings may indicate increase in severity but no consistent magnitude of difference between ranks	Functional category: New York Heart Association Stage of Heart Failure—Class I (mild), Class II (mild), Class III (moderate), Class IV (severe)	
Continuous	Continuous—interval	Ordered data with a consistent change in magnitude between units; zero point is arbitrary	Physical measurement: body temperature in degrees Fahrenheit	Measure of central tendency and distribution of data
	Continuous—ratio	Same as interval but zero point is absolute	Physical measurement: blood pressure in mm Hg	

Table 16.7 Example of Age as Both a Discrete Variable and a Continuous Variable

Variable Type		Example Data Collected
Discrete	Dichotomous	Nonelderly ($n = 95$)
		Elderly ($n = 5$)
	Categorical—ordinal	Newborn ($n = 0$)
		Infant ($n = 2$)
		Child ($n = 5$)
		Adolescent ($n = 13$)
		Adult ($n = 75$)
		Elderly ($n = 5$)
Continuous	Continuous—ratio	Age in years (mean = 35.6 years, range 3 months–67 years)

Table 16.8 Examples of Calculated Measures of Central Tendency

Example Data Set: 5, 5, 5, 5, 10, 15, 15, 20, 25, 25, 25, 100, 100, 100, 100	Definition	Measure of Central Tendency
5, 5, 5, 5 10 15, 15 20 25, 25, 25 75 100, 100, 100, 100	Most common value in a distribution	Bimodal = 5, 100
5, 5, 5, 5, 10, 15, 15, 20, 25, 25, 25, 100, 100, 100, 100	Midpoint of the values when placed in order from highest to lowest; half of the observations are above and half are below	Median = 20
$5 + 5 + 5 + 5 + 10 + 15 + 15 + 20 + 25 + 25 + 25 + 100 + 100 + 100 + 100 =$ 555/15	Sum of all values divided by the total number of values	Mean = 37

The central tendency value that is reported should depend on the scale of measurement of the data being evaluated (**Table 16.8**). The mode is used as the measure of central tendency for dichotomous or nominal data, as such data have no specific order or rank. Sometimes there can be more than one mode. The median is appropriately used with ordinal data but can also be reported for continuous data because it is helpful in highlighting whether the data are skewed from the mean. The mean can be very sensitive to outliers; the median is not. The mean is used with continuous data on the interval or ratio scale.

Studies that present only measures of central tendency can be misleading. Ideally, they should provide some idea of the data spread or variability around that central measure as well.

In evaluating dichotomous or nominal data, there is no measure of dispersion to report; instead, a description of the number of categories is helpful. The range is the difference between the smallest and largest values in a data set and is very sensitive to outliers. The same data types that can

Table 16.9 Commonly Encountered Descriptive Data Presentations by Data Type

Type of Data Reported		Mode	Median	Mean	Range	Interquartile Range (IQR)	Standard Deviation (SD)
Discrete	Dichotomous or categorical—nominal	X					
	Categorical—ordinal	X	X		X	X	
Continuous	Continuous—interval or ratio	X	X	X	X	X	X

be described by a range can also be described by the interquartile range (IQR). The IQR does not assume the population has a certain distribution pattern, so it can be used for parametric or non-parametric data. This value is commonly used to describe distribution around the median; because it takes into account data between the 25th and 75th percentiles, it is less likely to be affected by extreme values in the data set compared to the range.

The standard deviation (SD) is a measure of the variability about the mean and is appropriately applied only to continuous data that are normally or near-normally distributed or that can be transformed to be parametric. By the empirical rule, 68% of the sample values are found within ±1 SD, 95% are found within ±2 SD, and 99% are found within ±3 SD.

Commonly encountered descriptive data presentations are summarized in **Table 16.9**.

Presence of Confounding Variables

Variables that can affect the outcome of the study results even though they were not the main intervention being studied are commonly encountered and are dealt with in two general ways. Proper selection of study patients can prevent some confounding by excluding patients with those known influential factors. Often, however, it is not possible to exclude all covariates. Instead these covariates can be controlled through statistical analysis techniques such as analysis of variance (ANOVA) or analysis of covariance (ANCOVA) (**Table 16.10**).

Covariate analysis is performed for the following reasons:

- The covariate naturally occurs in close association with the other variable of interest.
- The covariate precedes the other variable and cannot be avoided.
- The investigator wants to explore a number of potential covariates to see if they will be influential factors.

Biostatistical Significance

Once researchers have gathered their observations, they will perform a mathematical assessment of the data based on their stated hypotheses. Statistical testing is used to determine whether the null hypothesis, H_0 (no effect), can be rejected in favor of the alternate hypothesis, H_A (there is a difference). Instead of trying to prove that a difference exists, statistical testing estimates the probability that what is observed is due to chance. This probability is reported as a p-value. The lower the probability that chance is responsible for the observed differences, the more likely the investigator is to believe that any differences observed are due only to the research intervention.

Table 16.10 Selected Representative Statistical Tests

Type of Variable	Two Samples (Independent; e.g., Parallel Design)	Two Samples (Related; e.g., Cross-over Design)	More Than Two Samples (Independent, Parallel Design)	More Than Two Samples (Related; e.g., Cross-over Design)
Dichotomous or nominal	Chi squared or Fischer Exact test	McNemar test	Chi squared (Bonferroni)	Cochran Q (Bonferroni)
Ordinal	Wilcoxan rank sum Mann-Whitney U-test	Wilcoxan signed rank	Kruskal-Wallis ANOVA (MCP or Bonferroni)	Friedman ANOVA
Continuous: no confounders	Student *t*-test	Paired Student *t*-test	One-way ANOVA (MCP)	Repeated-measures ANOVA (MCP)
Continuous: one confounder	ANCOVA	Two-way repeated measures ANOVA	Two-way ANOVA (MCP)	Two-way repeated measures ANOVA

ANCOVA = analysis of covariance; ANOVA = analysis of variance; MCP = multiple comparison procedures.

Adapted from: DiCenzo R, ed. *Clinical pharmacist's guide to biostatistics and literature evaluation*. Lenexa, KS: American College of Clinical Pharmacy; 2011.

By convention, most investigators utilize a cut-off point of $p < 0.05$ in determining that the null hypothesis can be rejected. This is often referred to as a "statistically significant difference" between the observed values. Values of $p = 0.05$ or $p > 0.05$ indicate a degree of chance the researchers are unwilling to accept (i.e., $p = 0.10$ means there is a 10% chance that any observed difference may not be real but is instead due to chance). However, readers are cautioned that the decision to use $p < 0.05$ as the cut-off point is not law. There is nothing magical about the value of 0.05; it is just a number that most researchers agree with as an acceptable level of probability of committing a Type I error. When investigators plan their research, they determine beforehand which levels of false positive (alpha) and false negative (beta) error they are willing to accept (**Figure 16.1**). Unfortunately, it is not possible to reduce both risks to zero. Most researchers adopt standard levels of alpha (5%) and beta (20%); the chosen levels should be disclosed in the statistical methods section.

Healthcare providers may be convinced of the need to alter therapy when a *p*-value is nonsignificant or to refuse to alter therapy when a *p*-value is significant. Clinicians use confidence intervals to get an idea of the magnitude of the difference between groups as well as the statistical significance. The point estimate and its associated 95% confidence interval can help pharmacists decide whether a study has clinical significance. The point estimate is a single value that estimates the true effect of the intervention in the population. The confidence interval is interpreted as the range of values that are statistically plausible. As long as the confidence interval does not include the point of no effect, then the results are statistically significant.

Differences between statistical significance and clinical significance are hotly debated topics at pharmacy journal clubs. Adding this layer of clinical knowledge and judgment to the interpretation of study results will be discussed in the therapeutics curriculum during the last years of pharmacy school.

Interpreting Study Results and Their Biostatistics

Once readers are convinced that the study methods fit the research question and that the biostatistical test chosen was appropriate, they should closely inspect the observed data, including the data's dispersion and the statistical significance of the reported results. Many pharmacists rely on

		"Underlying truth in the universe"	
		In reality: H_0 is TRUE (no difference exists)	In reality: H_0 is FALSE (difference does exist)
"Investigator decision"	*Accept null hypothesis, H_0 (no difference)*	No error (correct decision)	Type II error (beta error) "false negative"
	Reject null hypothesis, H_0 *By rejecting the null = Accepting the alternate hypothesis, H_A (difference)*	Type I error (alpha error) "false positive"	No error (correct decision)

Figure 16.1 Hypothesis testing: decision errors.

their core drug information texts, an excellent six-part introductory biostatistics series by Gaddis in *Annals of Emergency Medicine*, and a quick guide designed for clinical pharmacists by ACCP to become more comfortable with interpreting the medical literature including biostatistical results. The *JAMA Users' Guides to the Medical Literature: A Manual for Evidence-Based Clinical Practice* in another popular resource used by clinicians practicing evidence-based medicine.

Learning Bridge 16.4

During an Introduction to Drug Information and Literature Evaluation course, the class is asked to perform the following tasks:

A. Search the primary literature for pharmacokinetic studies on a topic assigned by the professor.

B. Review the titles and abstracts of all recent literature on the topic to find the most relevant articles.

C. Choose and read the most relevant article, focusing on the study design/methods and results sections.

D. Come prepared the next day to share impressions of the study results related to application of key concepts that were discussed during the Pharmaceutics and Pharmacokinetic blocks—in particular, dosage design of the new formulation versus the control formulation, pharmacokinetic blood sampling and observed drug concentrations, and the pharmacokinetic parameters of AUC, C_{max}, and C_{min}.

You are assigned the following topic: pharmacokinetics of a combination tablet of zidovudine (ZDV)/lamivudine (3TC)/nevirapine (NVP) in HIV-infected children. How will you search and use the primary literature to complete assignment parts A–C? In which section of the article are you likely to find discussion of the items in part D?

Golden Keys for Pharmacy Students

1. Pharmacists practice evidence-based medicine every day by ensuring that drug information is appropriately interpreted and correctly applied.

2. Needs for drug information may be for a specific patient, for a group of patients, or to increase the pharmacist's medication knowledge base.

3. Providing responses and consulting without knowledge of pertinent patient information, the context of the request, or the way in which the information will be applied, or without the preceptor's approval, is unacceptable and can potentially harm patients.

4. Tertiary sources provide valuable information that has been filtered and synthesized to provide a quick summary of a topic.

5. Comprehensive searches for drug information will require the use of multiple databases and resources.

6. Using a structured, organized approach when searching for, interpreting, and formulating a response to drug information involves critical thinking and clear communication skills.

7. There are five scales of measurement: dichotomous, nominal, ordinal, interval, and ratio.

8. The appropriateness of a statistical test used to analyze experimental data is based on several factors: the data scale of measurement, the number of groups compared, the study design, and the degree of confounding.

9. The mean is the most appropriate measure of central tendency for normally distributed continuous data, while the median is the most appropriate measure for ordinal data or skewed distributions.

10. While statistical significance is important, pharmacists are more likely to debate the clinical significance of a study's findings.

Learning Bridge Answers

16.1 Choosing any of the core drug compendia would be the most efficient way to research the elements requested in the assignment. Once you have accessed the correct drug monograph, you will have to navigate to the appropriate section of the monograph to find the relevant details.

Where to Find It	A. Pronunciation	B. Brand or Generic?	C. Picture	D. Which Body System?
Lexi-Comp Online	Monograph > Pronunciation; includes sound file of pronunciation	Monograph > Preparations > Generic Available	Images tab	Monograph > Uses
Facts & Comparisons eAnswers	Monograph > Patient Handouts Monograph > Sound file of pronunciation next to drug name in banner	Monograph > Product List > Product Name, including generic equivalency (Orange Book) rating	Monograph > Product List > Product Name > Product Image/Description	Monograph > Indications

Clinical Pharmacology	Monograph > Patient Education	Monograph > Product	Monograph top of page	Monograph > Classification
Micromedex 2.0	360° View Dashboard > Other Information	360° View Dashboard > Product Lookup—Redbook Online, including generic equivalency (Orange Book) rating	360° View Dashboard > Drug Images	360° View Dashboard > Micromedex Drug Summary Information > FDA Labeled Indications
Answers: carvedilol (Coreg) tablets	KAR ve dil ole	Generic and brand are both available		Cardiovascular

Photo: **Courtesy of National Library of Medicine, National Institutes of Health, U.S. Dept. of Health & Human Services.**

16.2 The missing details could be obtained from any drug compendium, including Lexi-Comp, Facts & Comparisons, Micromedex, or Clinical Pharmacology. Many of these databases are now available for mobile devices or as printed pocket guides for times when the pharmacist is away from the pharmacy but still needs access to detailed drug information.

Ms. White, 70 yo F; no known drug allergies 123 Notting Hill Lane, Anytown, USA							
Drug	**Dosage Form**	**Dose**	**Directions for Use**	**Qty Supply**	**Refills**	**Prescriber**	**Indication for Use**
Aspirin	EC tablet	325 mg	1 tablet once daily	60	5	Dr. Heart	Prevention of myocardial infarction or stroke
Metoprolol succinate (generic of Toprol-XL)	Extended-release tablet	100 mg	½ tablet orally daily (confirmed this XL tablet is scored and can be split in half without disrupting its drug delivery system)	30	5	Dr. Heart	Angina
Atorvastatin (generic of Lipitor)	Tablet	40 mg	1 tablet once daily	30	11	Dr. Heart	Hypercholesterolemia
Nitroglycerin	Sublingual tablet	0.4 mg	1 tablet under tongue every 5 minutes as needed for chest pain; maximum of 3 doses in 15 minutes, then seek emergency care	Bottle of 25	11	Dr. Heart	Chest pain

16.3 This Learning Bridge illustrates a common type of clinical problem encountered by pharmacists that requires them to recall, look up, and synthesize foundational knowledge from the disciplines of pathophysiology, pharmacology, medicinal chemistry, and pharmacokinetics. It also necessitates their accessing the right resources to efficiently look up information to address the drug information need.

A. Your pharmacology textbook or a drug compendium would reveal that lisinopril is an angiotensin-converting enzyme inhibitor (ACE-I). Lisinopril's action is directed at the renin–angiotensin system (RAS), which contributes to hypertension. Inhibiting the production of angiotensin II leads to a lowered systemic vascular resistance and blood pressure.

B. Drug compendia or the package insert would indicate that this is a known side effect of lisinopril and would cite a frequency of its occurrence somewhere between 5% and 20%. Finding out why side effects occur generally requires looking more deeply in the adverse reactions section, considering the pharmacology/mechanism of action section, and reviewing pathophysiologic connections. A resource such as your pharmacology textbook or a drug–disease interface reference (e.g., UpToDate) may be helpful for understanding the reasons why the adverse reaction is associated with the drug and describing its usual clinical presentation. Because ACE has many substrates, it is possible that lisinopril might also induce effects unrelated to its RAS targeted use for blood pressure control. ACE-I agents also increase bradykinin, substance P, and prostaglandins, which accumulate in the lungs and stimulate the cough reflex. Current research is looking into whether this side effect is associated with certain genetic polymorphisms. This side effect is characterized as a bothersome, nonproductive, hacking cough that usually begins within 1–2 weeks of instituting therapy, but can be delayed up to 6 months. On stopping the ACE-I, the cough typically resolves in 1–4 days but can be prolonged for a month.

C. Your medicinal chemistry or pharmacology textbook would show that ACE-I chemical structures belong to one of three general groups. The main differences conferred by these structural groups are related to drugs' potency, pharmacokinetic profiles, and prodrug status. A pharmacy therapeutics textbook or EBM point-of-care knowledge base (e.g., MDConsult) that discusses the clinical use of drugs would likely discuss management of the side effect and therapeutic alternatives. Although some patients respond to a dose reduction of the ACE-I, more than two-thirds of patients rechallenged with the same or a different ACE-I from any structural class will experience a return of the cough. Patients who responded well to the antihypertensive effects of the ACE-I can be switched to an angiotensin II receptor blocker (ARB), as these drugs are associated with a much lower rate of cough, even in patients with a prior history of ACE-I–induced cough.

16.4 To search the primary literature, you have your choice of PubMed Medline, which is open access, or available subscription-only primary literature indexing systems, such as Ovid Medline, EMBASE, and Web of Science.

A. Searching the primary articles indexed in these systems requires you to combine terms that are relevant to your inquiry and then sort through the results or further refine your search. Typing each term in succession in the main search bar of PubMed automatically combines the terms behind the scenes using the Boolean search term "AND," which will return only those articles that have all of those concepts indexed. Returned results can be further reduced by applying limits such as age, article type, and full-text availability. Another approach using the PubMed Advanced Search Builder allows you to see the impact of each new subject as you add it to your search string (**Exhibit 16.2**).

Search	Add to builder	Query	Items found	Time
#5	Add	Search (#1 AND #2 AND #3 AND #4)	6	13:03:49
#4	Add	Search pediatric	429521	13:03:36
#3	Add	Search HIV	253450	13:03:30
#2	Add	Search pharmacokinetics	332800	13:03:26
#1	Add	Search (((zidovudine) AND lamivudine) AND nevirapine)	473	13:03:14

History   Download history Clear history

Exhibit 16.2 PubMed advanced search builder screenshot showing how to do a stacked search.

Limits can also be later applied to these search results.

B. A search with the appropriately applied aged-based limits should result in a list of fewer than 10 articles to review. A quick scan of the article titles reveals that 2 of them look promising and should be selected for further review of the article abstracts.

C. On closer reading, only the first article (1) is relevant to pediatric patients and is the more recent publication. The full text of the article is available for free through PubMed Central as an NIH Public Access Author Manuscript.

D. The "Methods" section (especially the subsections "Study Design" and "Antiretroviral Drug Level Measurement and Analysis") addresses the dosage forms that are being compared and explains how the blood samples will be drawn and the pharmacokinetic parameters calculated—information that ensures other investigators could replicate the study. The "Results section" and associated figures and tables describe the authors' findings and should be read critically, with readers forming their own impressions of the data before reviewing the authors' "Discussion" section.

Reference: Chokephaibulkit K, Cressey TR, Capparelli E, et al. Pharmacokinetics and safety of a new paediatric fixed-dose combination of zidovudine/lamivudine/nevirapine in HIV-infected children. *Antivir Ther.* 2011;16(8):1287–1295.

Problems and Solutions

Problem 16.1 Why do the public and the pharmacist's healthcare colleagues consider the pharmacist to be the medication expert?

Solution 16.1 Pharmacists receive the most intensive education in medication management and continue to maintain their knowledge base and skills in this area. Because it is impossible to stay abreast of every medication development, it is important to be a master of drug information so that information can be quickly accessed and interpreted on demand to meet patient care needs.

Problem 16.2 Why is it necessary for pharmacists to gather further information about the background of the question from the requestor when asked to provide a drug information response?

Solution 16.2 Pharmacists need to inquire and obtain additional details so that they can be sure the question they are going to research and respond to is the "ultimate question." This ensures that the requestor gets the answer he or she needs even if the requestor was not able to articulate it plainly.

Problem 16.3 Which reference is likely to be the most useful in efficiently addressing the following information request: "Compare the chemical structures of diphenhydramine and loratadine and comment on differences in their structure–activity relationships."

Solution 16.3 A medicinal chemistry textbook, pharmacology textbook, or the package inserts of the two drugs. Certain drug compendia also show chemical structures. Of these resources, the medicinal chemistry text is likely to be the most useful because in addition to providing a drawing of the chemical structures, it is more likely to discuss their similarities and differences related to their functional groups.

Problem 16.4 Which reference is likely to be the most useful in efficiently addressing the following information request: "How long is amoxicillin–clavulanate oral suspension good for after it has been reconstituted?"

Solution 16.4 All major drug compendia and the package insert would provide this information. It is generally found under a section titled "Storage" or "Stability," or at the end of the "Dosage and Administration" section. The stability of a dosage form depends on a number of factors, including the drug concentration, diluting solution, and storage temperature. The *United States Pharmacopeia* (USP) designates beyond-use-dates for both sterile and nonsterile dosage forms. For sterile products such as intravenous solutions, sterility concerns can result in shorter beyond-use-dating than the stability of the drug would indicate.

Problem 16.5 Which reference is likely to be the most useful in efficiently addressing the following information request: "How long will it take for amiodarone to be cleared from the body?"

Solution 16.5 Any drug compendium or the package insert will provide the pharmacokinetic parameters studied for the drug, including the drug's half-life and its routes of clearance. The compendium may prove the best reference because the logical next question may be related to an adverse event the patient is experiencing. Compared to the package insert, the compendium will be more useful in identifying and managing any reactions, including possibly needing to identify another drug to which the patient could be switched. Additionally the compendium may have abstracted more data from multiple patient populations—not just the ones studied for drug approval, as noted in the package insert.

Problem 16.6 Which reference is likely to be the most useful in efficiently addressing the following information request: "Can midazolam be used for status epilepticus?"

Solution 16.6 Searching drug compendia will be more likely to return a confirmative answer that the drug is or is not used for that purpose, as these resources list both FDA-approved and unlabeled but medically acceptable uses. The package insert lists only FDA-approved uses that could mislead the pharmacist into thinking there is no role for that drug in the disease, when that is not really the case. A drug–disease reference may also be helpful, especially if the drug search does not turn up a matching indication, as the next logical step would be to search by disease or indication to see which drugs are available to treat that condition.

Problem 16.7 Why must pharmacists have the skill of reading and critically appraising the biomedical literature?

Solution 16.7 To keep up with new evidence concerning the benefits and risks of medicines, pharmacists have to actively seek new knowledge, which includes reading the biomedical literature and assessing the quality and importance of published studies.

Problem 16.8 Describe the difference between a parallel study design and a cross-over study design.

Solution 16.8 In a parallel study, the samples never overlap. In a cross-over study, the samples receive both interventions. For example, in a study of a new antihypertensive agent using a parallel design, one group of patients would get the new drug and the other group would get the comparator antihypertensive agent. In the cross-over design, half of the patients would first get the new drug while the others got the standard drug, then they would switch treatments for the last part of the study so that every patient will have data on their blood pressure control on the two different medications.

Problem 16.9 Explain the impact of confounding on a study and how it can be controlled.

Solution 16.9 Confounding can lead to erroneous conclusions if not controlled for, as these factors influence the results but are not the intervention under study. Such confounding factors can be controlled through study design (e.g., exclusion criteria) or through biostatistical methods (e.g., ANOVA or ANCOVA).

Problem 16.10 Describe what is meant by statistical significance, and identify the value at which the significance level is traditionally set.

Solution 16.10 The value $p < 0.05$ is the traditional cut-off point at which statistical significance is set. This means that the chance of the observed results being different due to chance alone is less than 5%, which is a generally acceptable level of risk of Type I error.

Problem 16.12 Explain why pharmacists may disagree about the clinical significance of study findings.

Solution 16.12 Because clinical significance is in the eye of the beholder, individual pharmacists may disagree about whether they find the observed results to be clinically relevant regardless of their statistical significance. For example, a pharmacist who specializes in the management of patients with diabetes may find a smaller difference in blood glucose lowering from a new, high-cost antidiabetic agent to be beneficial in patients who have failed to respond to other therapies, while a health insurance pharmacist who decides which diabetic drugs should be added to the Medicaid formulary for coverage of all diabetic patients may feel the additional cost is not worth the level of blood glucose lowering for most patients.

References

1. Bryant PJ, Norris KP, McQueen CE, Poole EA. Appendix 5-1: beyond the basics: questions to consider for critique of primary literature. In: Malone PM, Kier KL, Stanovich JE, eds. *Drug information: a guide for pharmacists*. 4th ed. New York, NY: McGraw-Hill; 2012. Available at: http://www.accesspharmacy.com with subscription.
2. DiCenzo R, ed. *Clinical pharmacist's guide to biostatistics and literature evaluation*. Lenexa, KS: American College of Clinical Pharmacy; 2011.
3. Gaddis ML, Gaddis GM. Introduction to biostatistics. Part 1, basic concepts. *Ann Emerg Med*. 1990;19:86–89.
4. Gaddis ML, Gaddis GM. Introduction to biostatistics. Part 2, descriptive statistics. *Ann Emerg Med*. 1990;19:309–315.
5. Gaddis ML, Gaddis GM. Introduction to biostatistics. Part 3, sensitivity, specificity, predictive value, and hypothesis testing. *Ann Emerg Med*. 1990;19:591–597.
6. Gaddis ML, Gaddis GM. Introduction to biostatistics. Part 4, statistical inference techniques in hypothesis testing. *Ann Emerg Med*. 1990;19:820–825.
7. Gaddis ML, Gaddis GM. Introduction to biostatistics. Part 5, statistical inference techniques for hypothesis testing with nonparametric data. *Ann Emerg Med*. 1990;19:1054–1059.
8. Gaddis ML, Gaddis GM. Introduction to biostatistics. Part 6, correlation and regression. *Ann Emerg Med*. 1990;19:1462–1468
9. Gaebelein CJ, Gleason BL. *Contemporary drug information: an evidence-based approach*. Philadelphia, PA: Lippincott Williams & Wilkins; 2008.

10. Giovenale S, Nanstiel B, eds. *AACP basic resources for pharmacy education*. Alexandria, VA: American Association of Colleges of Pharmacy; 2012. Available at: http://www.aacp.org/governance /SECTIONS/libraryeducationalresources/Pages/LibraryEducationalResourcesSpecialProjectsand Information.aspx.

11. Greenhalgh T. *How to read a paper: the basics of evidence based medicine*, 2nd ed. London, UK: BMJ Books; 2001.

12. Guyatt G, Rennie D, Meade MO, Cook DJ. *Users' guides to the medical literature: a manual for evidence-based clinical practice*, 2nd ed. New York, NY: American Medical Association; 2008.

13. Kendrach M, Freeman MK, Wensel TM, Hughes PJ. Appendix 4-1: questions for assessing clinical trials. In: Malone PM, Kier KL, Stanovich JE, eds. *Drug information: a guide for pharmacists*, 4th ed. New York, NY: McGraw-Hill; 2012. Available at: http://www.accesspharmacy.com with subscription.

14. Malone PM, Kier KL, Stanovich JE, eds. *Drug information: a guide for pharmacists*, 4th ed. New York, NY: McGraw-Hill; 2012.

INDEX